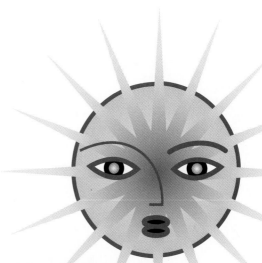

COMMUNITY HEALTH NURSING
Promoting and Protecting the Public's Health

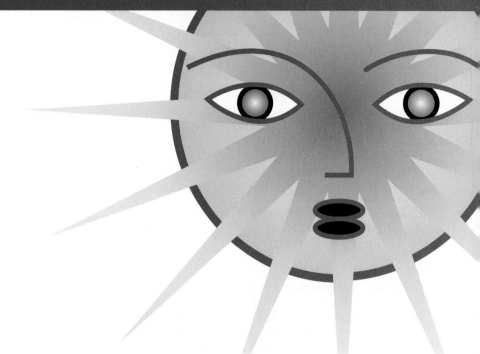

COMMUNITY HEALTH NURSING
Promoting and Protecting the Public's Health

● **Judith Ann Allender**, EdD, MSN, MEd, RN,C
Professor
Department of Nursing, College of Health and
**   Human Services**
California State University
Fresno, California

● **Barbara Walton Spradley**, MN, RN
Associate Professor, Emerita
School of Public Health
University of Minnesota
Minneapolis, Minnesota

sixth edition

6

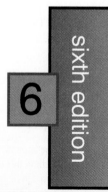

LIPPINCOTT WILLIAMS & WILKINS
A Wolters Kluwer Company

Philadelphia • Baltimore • New York • London
Buenos Aires • Hong Kong • Sydney • Tokyo

Acquisitions Editor: Margaret Zuccarini
Managing Editor: Joe Morita
Editorial Assistant: Carol DeVault
Senior Production Editor: Tom Gibbons
Director of Nursing Production: Helen Ewan
Managing Editor / Production: Erika Kors
Art Director: Brett MacNaughton
Cover Designer: Melissa Walter
Interior Designer: BJ Crim
Senior Manufacturing Manager: William Alberti
Indexer: Ann Cassar
Compositor: Peirce Graphic Services
Printer: Courier-Westford

6th Edition

9 8 7 6 5 4 3 2 1

Library of Congress Cataloging-in-Publication Data

Allender, Judith Ann.
  Community health nursing : promoting and protecting the public's health / Judith Ann Allender, Barbara Walton Spradley.—6th ed.
       p. ; cm.
    Includes bibliographical references and index.
    ISBN 0-7817-4449-0 (hardcover : alk. paper)
  1. Community health nursing.   2. Public health nursing.   I. Spradley, Barbara Walton.
    II. Title.
    [DNLM: 1. Community Health Nursing.   2. Health Promotion.   WY 106 A425c 2005]
  RT98.S68 2005
  610.73'43—dc22

                                          2004007777

LWW.com

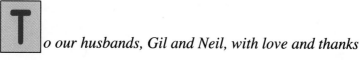

o our husbands, Gil and Neil, with love and thanks

Contributors

Tina Bayne, MS, APRN, BC
Associate Professor
Assistant Dean, Undergraduate Intercollegiate Center for
    Nursing Education
Washington State University
Spokane, Washington

Nancy Clark, RN, MSN, MPA, EdD (c)
Chair & Professor, Department of Nursing
California State University, Stanislaus
Turlock, California

Donald C. Johnson, DrPH
Adjunct Professor
Department of Nursing
California State University, Stanislaus
Turlock, California
Chief of Health Education (Retired)
World Health Organization
Geneva, Switzerland

Cherie Rector, PhD, RN,C
Professor, Department of Nursing
California State University, Bakersfield
Bakersfield, California

Kristine D. Warner, PhD, MPH, RN
Assistant Professor
California State University, Sacramento
Sacramento, California

Lynette Zimmerman, BSN, RN, PHN
Child Care Coordinator
Children's Hospital
Madera, California

Reviewers

Joan T. Bickes, MSN, APRN, BC
Assistant Professor (Clinical)
Wayne State University
Detroit, Michigan

Margaret M. Craig, RN, MS
Associate Dean, Nursing
Napa Valley College
Napa, California

Sharon A. Denham, DSN, RN
Professor, School of Nursing
Ohio University
Athens, Ohio

Nancy L. Dillard, DNS, RN, CS, ANP
Associate Director, Baccalaureate Nursing Program
School of Nursing
Ball State University
Muncie, Indiana

Gail Gerding, RN, MS, PhD
Lecturer
University of Michigan
Ann Arbor, Michigan

Leigh Hart, RN, PhD, CCRN
Assistant Professor
Jacksonville University
St. Augustine, Florida

Bonnie Kellogg, RN, MS, DrPH
Professor
California State University, Long Beach
Long Beach, California

Jeanne Leffers, PhD, RN
Assistant Professor
University of Massachusetts Dartmouth
North Dartmouth, Massachusetts

Sandra Kundrik Leh, RN, MSN, CNS
Assistant Professor
Cedar Crest College
Allentown, Pennsylvania

Carrie A. McCoy, PhD, MSPH, RN, CEN
Associate Professor of Nursing
Northern Kentucky University
Highland Heights, Kentucky

Nancy J. Michela, DA (c), MS, RN
Associate Professor
The Sage Colleges
Troy, New York

Anne K. Oboyski, MS, RN, CS
Associate Professor
School of Nursing
SUNY Institute of Technology at Utica/Rome
Utica, New York

Judith Pratt, MSN, RN
Associate Professor
Weber State University
Ogden, Utah

Mattie Tolley, RN, BSN, MSN, & British SRM (State Registered Midwife)
Faculty, Coordinator of Community Health Nursing
Southwestern Oklahoma State University
Weatherford, Oklahoma

Euphemia G. Williams, RN, PhD
Professor, Department of Nursing
University of Southern Colorado
Pueblo, Colorado

Preface

The sixth edition of *Community Health Nursing: Promoting and Protecting the Public's Health* represents a continuing effort to capture the essence and clarify the practice of community health nursing. It is written to share the authors' enthusiasm for a field whose dynamic nature calls for nursing creativity, leadership, and innovation with you, the student community health nurse. The potential for community health nurses to protect and enhance the health of at-risk populations and to influence the quality of health services poses exciting challenges and opportunities.

As a basic text, the sixth edition, like the other five, is designed to give you, the undergraduate nursing student, a comprehensive introduction to the field of community health nursing. It is also designed to be a professional resource in order to enlarge the vision and enhance the impact of practicing community health nurses.

With a continuing and escalating demand for nurses to practice in the community, it is important that the meaning of community health nursing as a specialized field of nursing practice be clearly understood. The challenge for the nurse who wishes to practice community health nursing lies in incorporating public health principles with nursing knowledge and skills to offer preventive, health-promoting, and protective services that benefit aggregates and populations. As a beginning practitioner in this field, you may have limited impact on aggregates, but an aggregate or population-based orientation must be germane to your practice. With experience and advanced preparation in public health, you can become a specialist in public or community health.

The sixth edition of this text continues to use the term *community health nurse* to describe a practitioner in the community whose work incorporates public health philosophy, theory, and skills with an emphasis on aggregates and populations.

ABOUT THE SIXTH EDITION

This edition of *Community Health Nursing: Promoting and Protecting the Public's Health* continues to be written with you, the undergraduate nursing student, in mind. It is "user friendly" with many mini-case studies woven throughout the text in order for you to more easily apply the information with your clients. The text is comprehensive and incorporates the impact of the global health status. We are a small planet with big health problems that impact each person's health and the role of the community health nurse now and in the future. As a nation, we have a new and continuing health agenda through *Healthy People 2010* that gives direction to our work. These new goals and objectives are incor-

porated throughout the text. Finally, the text format is designed to provide you with the comprehensive, globally sensitive information and skills you need to be an effective practitioner with aggregates, groups, and individuals in the community.

Organization of the Text

In this edition the text remains 37 chapters in length and is organized into seven units. Unit sequence has been changed, two chapters have been combined, and a new chapter on populations with disabilities has been added. Some unit titles as well as some chapter titles have been reworded to include more descriptive language, provide greater continuity for the reader, and expand the work with specific populations.

Unit I, Foundations of Community Health Nursing, introduces you to the conceptual and historical bases for practice in this field. Seven chapters compose this unit, describing first the basic concepts of community and health that provide the opportunities and challenges in the field of community health nursing (Chapter 1); the history and nature of community health nursing (Chapter 2); its traditional and innovative roles and settings for practice (Chapter 3); the impact of culture on health and community health nursing practice (Chapter 4); and the values and ethical decision-making that influence community health nursing (Chapter 5). The unit concludes with two broad chapters providing the structure and function of community health services (Chapter 6) and the economic considerations that influence community health practice (Chapter 7).

Unit II, Public Health Principles in Community Health Nursing, contains three very important chapters embracing essential elements of public health practice germane to community health nursing and has been moved forward in the text, now coming before the unit on tools of community health nursing. It begins with the principles of epidemiology as the foundation for prevention and control of negative health consequences (Chapter 8). Next is an expanded and comprehensive chapter on communicable disease control (Chapter 9). The unit concludes with environmental health and safety concerns (Chapter 10). Throughout the unit the role of the community health nurse is emphasized.

Unit III, Tools of Community Health Nursing, provides you with an understanding of the tools needed for practice in this field and how to develop and use them. The unit has six chapters that encompass the specific tools the community health nurse must develop to be effective with community aggregates. The unit focuses on communication and collaboration, two essential skills of the community health nurse (Chapter 11); health promotion through education (Chapter

12); leadership and management responsibilities (Chapter 13); examples of nursing research and discussion of practicing nurses' involvement in and use of research (Chapter 14); and promoting quality in health care services through quality measurement and improvement (Chapter 15). Finally, Chapter 16 describes the ways in which community health nurses can influence the health care system through leadership, power, effecting change, policy-making, and advocacy for the health of the community.

Unit IV, Community as Client, is the first of two units that follow a similar nursing process organizational format. This five-chapter unit begins with the theoretical basis for the practice of community health nursing (Chapter 17). Next, the assessment of communities (Chapter 18) and the planning, intervention, and evaluation of health care in communities (Chapter 19) are discussed. Treatment of communities in crisis (Chapter 20) is expanded in this edition to include post-9/11/01 concepts of communities suffering from disasters, group violence, and terrorism. The final chapter in this unit focuses on the global community, exploring international health concerns (Chapter 21).

Unit V, The Family as Client, is a four-chapter unit. It begins with the theoretical basis for promoting family health (Chapter 22), followed by the assessment of families (Chapter 23). The planning, intervention, and evaluation of health care to families follow (Chapter 24). The unit concludes with examination of families in crisis and those experiencing domestic violence and abuse (Chapter 25). These chapters were organized under different units in previous editions. Although nurses work with individual families in the community, this text also supports the need to view clusters of families as aggregates for community health nursing intervention.

Unit VI, Promoting and Protecting the Heath of Aggregates With Developmental Needs, examines client populations based on age-appropriate needs. In this unit you are helped to understand their needs and how to intervene with each population group. The five chapters in this unit emphasize promoting and protecting the health of populations in each major life cycle stage. First is maternal, perinatal, and newborn populations (Chapter 26), and then infants, toddlers, and preschool populations (Chapter 27). The next chapter, on school-age children and the adolescent population (Chapter 28), emphasizes the role of the school nurse and school-based health care services. Adult men and women and the working population (Chapter 29) is expanded in this edition to include separate sections on men's and women's health issues, while the role of the occupational health nurse is presented in detail. Finally, Chapter 30 describes the older adult population and the need to compress the years of morbidity and extend the years of wellness. *Healthy People 2010* goals are included throughout the chapters.

Unit VII, Promoting and Protecting the Health of Vulnerable Aggregates, has seven chapters; one is new to this sixth edition. Because community health nurses are expected to work more frequently with vulnerable populations, this unit focuses on specific groups you may encounter in the community. First, the rural populations at-risk for health care accessibility are discussed (Chapter 31). Next we examine the needs of clients living in urban areas, poverty, and the homeless (Chapter 32), in addition to the complex and often unmet needs of migrant populations (Chapter 33). New to this edition, we have included a chapter on clients with disabilities and chronic illnesses (Chapter 34). Many clients in the community have unmet mental health needs or various addictions, such as substance abuse, eating disorders, or gambling, and are discussed together as they often cannot be separated (Chapter 35). Many of the clients we serve in the community live high-risk lifestyles often bringing them in contact with law enforcement and the corrections/incarceration systems in the country. Clients in correctional facilities and the needs of their families are explored (Chapter 36). Finally, we examine the role of the community health nurse working with clients and their families through home care services and hospices (Chapter 37).

New and Changed Chapters

To keep abreast of changes in society and among populations community health nurses serve, many new topics have been introduced or expanded on in this edition. Chapter 4 expands our view of the cultural influence on a person's or group's health status and the need for community health nurses to become more familiar with diversity in our nation. Chapter 8 provides a more thorough view of the changing world of epidemiology and provides enhanced examples of "webs of causation," the more complex causes of disease or ill health that we face today. Chapter 14, on research and the community health nurse's role, provides richer applications of the research process when used in the community. Chapter 20, Communities in Crisis, provides you with current information about our vulnerablity as a nation and how the community health nurse can assist groups using the three levels of prevention when disasters threaten or have struck a community. Chapter 29 is newly organized, with separate sections on the promotion and protection of women's and men's health while continuing to discuss the role of the occupational health nurse. Chapter 32, which focused only on clients in poverty in the fifth edition, has an added focus on urban health. A new chapter on clients with disabilities and chronic illnesses (Chapter 34) has been created for this edition. Chapter 35 was previously presented in two chapters. In this edition we have combined the topics of clients with mental health issues and addictions. These difficult health issues are often found in combination in clients, and to discuss them together in one chapter provides a more seamlesss approach. Finally, in the last chapter (Chapter 37) we have strengthened the approach to home care and those involved with hospices. The role of the nurse in end-of-life care also has been broadened. All chapters have been updated to include the latest research and information on populations' needs and delivery of services using the most recent references possible.

Key Features

The sixth edition of *Community Health Nursing: Promoting and Protecting the Public's health* includes key features from previous editions as well as new features.

Features continued from previous editions include:

- An emphasis on aggregate-level nursing and the community health nurse's opportunity and responsibility not only to serve individuals and families but also to promote and protect the health of communities and populations.
- An emphasis on health promotion, health protection, and illness prevention. This, in addition to the aggregate emphasis, reflects the view set forth in this text that community health nursing is the amalgamation of nursing science with public health science. Public health philosophy, values, knowledge, and skills are an essential part of community health nursing practice.
- A balance of theory with application to nursing practice. The sixth edition continues the presentation of theoretical and conceptual knowledge to provide you with an understanding of human needs and a rationale for nursing actions. At the same time the text presents practical information on how you can use theory to undergird practice.
- A summary of highlights at the end of each chapter provides you with an overview of material covered and serves as a review for study.
- References and Selected Readings at the end of each chapter provide you with classic sources, current research, and a broad base of authoritative information for furthering knowledge on each chapter's subject matter.
- A student-friendly writing style has been a hallmark of this text since the first edition. Topics are expressed and concepts explained to enhance your understanding and capture your interest. Writing style remains consistent throughout the text (including contributed chapters) to promote an uninterrupted flow of ideas for your learning.
- Internet Resources have been enhanced and are included in nearly every chapter for quick and easy student reference.
- Learning Objectives and Key Terms sharpen your focus and provide a guide for learning the chapter content.
- Activities to Promote Critical Thinking at the close of each chapter are designed to challenge you, promote critical-thinking skills, and encourage your active involvement in solving community health problems. They include activities using the Internet.
- Recurring displays throughout the text highlight important content and create points of interest for student learning.
- Levels of Prevention boxes are redesigned in this edition. Each follows a similar matrix to enhance your understanding of the levels of prevention concept, basic to community health nursing. Each box addresses a chapter topic, describes nursing actions at each of the three levels of prevention, and is unique to this text.
- Research: Bridge to Practice boxes describe a current public health or nursing research study related to the chapter subject matter.
- The Global Community boxes emphasize an international perspective on chapter topics.
- In Voices From the Community displays, clients, practicing nurses, and students share their feelings about the topic presented in the chapter in which they appear. This personalizes the material and lets you feel what the person is expressing.
- Sixteen Clinical Corner case studies have been incorporated in key chapters throughout the text. Each Clinical Corner includes a case study and concludes with questions for critical thinking. These cases do not always get easily solved, just as in the real world of community health nursing, and give you a "real" picture of the community.
- Bridging Financial Gaps displays explore examples from practice and the nursing literature when services are more easily and clearly delivered to clients. They demonstrate innovative approaches to "cutting red tape" that often impedes clients from getting services.
- Additional assessment tools can be found throughout the chapters. They are added to enhance your assessment skills of aggregates, families, or individuals in unique situations.
- New art has been added throughout the text to clarify important concepts and enhance your interest in and understanding of material.
- A Glossary provides definitions of all key terms highlighted throughout the text.

Features New to This Edition

Additional recurring displays new to this edition include:

- Using the Nursing Process When…. This new feature was created to assist you in thinking through a situation in the community using the steps of the nursing process as a framework to your approach with clients. Ofen the nursing process is associated with inpatient nursing care and is not emphasized as nursing education experiences expand outside hospital walls. Through these displays you can see how the steps of the nursing process apply in the community.
- What Do You Think? is a feature that occurs at least once in most chapters. It gives a challenging, innovative, or controversial tidbit of information related to the chapter content. It is designed to give you "food for thought" or a new way of looking at a subject. Some topics lend themselves to more thought, and you will find two or three of them in some chapters.

ANCILLARY TEACHING-LEARNING SERVICES

A complete supplemental teaching-learning service is available to students and faculty on the Internet. This innovative feature is provided through Lippincott Williams & Wilkins' website, called *Connection,* and includes both student and faculty features.

STUDENT FEATURES

The student-focused *Connection* website includes several features found in the text that are updated regularly and are designed to be companion learning tools for the student:

- Clinical Corner—regularly updated interactive case studies designed to enhance your application of the pedagogic material in the text.
- Research: Bridge to Practice—regularly updated summaries of public health and public health nursing research that has an impact on practice.
- Bridging Financial Gaps—regularly updated information about the latest ways that government, local communities, or neighborhood programs are bridging financial gaps for clients.
- Voices From the Community—input from professionals, peers, and clients in the community regarding their feelings about current public health issues.

The following features are also included:

Interactive Exercises. The website includes interactive exercises based on key concepts recurring throughout the text. For example, an interactive exercise may focus on your role as a community health nurse in eliminating a communicable disease in a particular community. In order to accomplish this you may need to access resources to conduct a community assessment, explore issues related to school-age children, use principles of epidemiology, and update yourself on communicable disease control. The exercise takes you to four chapters in the text and may necessitate your accessing other Internet resources, which encourages you to integrate information from a variety of sources in order to solve the problem, just as community health nurses must do.

Chapter Outlines. These outlines are designed to assist you with organizing your thoughts about each chapter. They can be used as highlights for studying material to prepare you for testing.

Sample Test Questions. Sample test questions are included. An analysis is given for each distractor chosen and why it is the best answer or why it is not a good answer choice. This will help you understand community health nursing content and should prepare you better for the NCLEX.

FACULTY FEATURES

The ancillary Internet teaching package for faculty includes the following:

Chapter Outlines. These outlines will assist you in your classroom planning and weighing numbers and types of test items you will use.

PowerPoint Slides. Over 400 PowerPoint slides are provided as a companion to the text. They are available for faculty use to enhance classroom discussion and promote student learning.

Suggested Classroom Activities. Approximately 100 suggested classroom activities are provided to enhance discussion and student learning. They will assist you in creating a more active learning environment.

Testbank. Test questions for each chapter are included. There are approximately 145 NCLEX-style multiple-choice questions, and a key is provided for all questions with rationale for the correct answers and distractors.

Judith Ann Allender, EdD, MSN, MEd, RN,C
Barbara Walton Spradley, MN, RN

Acknowledgments

We are grateful to many individuals for their assistance in completing this sixth edition. To acknowledge them all would be impossible, given the limitations of space and memory. Many have unwittingly enriched the writing by sharing their experiences and expertise. Others have directly provided ideas, criticism, encouragement, and support. To all we offer our sincere gratitude.

Many individuals have made important new contributions to this sixth edition. Ten chapters were written in whole or in part by contributing authors. These experts in the field were sought out specifically for their expertise and currency in the area explored in their chapters. Many are faculty members in universities and colleges around the country. Some are in practice and teach part-time. All have contributed excellent information to enhance this edition of *Community Health Nursing: Promoting and Protecting the Public's Health*. We wish to thank the contributors to past editions whose work, in many cases, is still entwined in the chapters of this edition. We are grateful to each of them.

We wish to thank our faculty colleagues for their ideas and encouragement. Others have made a variety of contributions to this sixth edition. First, we want to thank two new graduates for assistance with research, stimulation, and support: Biana Grogg, BSN, RN, PHN, and Lynette Zimmerman, BSN, RN, PHN. We are also grateful to the many community colleagues in both nursing and other fields who have supported and contributed to our efforts.

We would like to thank the many people who provided their suggestions and assistance as reviewers throughout the revision process.

Many people at Lippincott Williams & Wilkins have provided invaluable assistance. We are grateful to Margaret Zuccarini, our editor for most of this revision, for her direction, support, and patience, and to Joe Morita, our managing editor who "burned the midnight oil" to help us edit and meet printer deadlines. Several editorial assistants took part in making this edition happen; Hilarie Surrena and Helen Kogut worked early on the project and Carol DeVault helped us see it through to publication. We are grateful to all the other helpful people at Lippincott Williams & Wilkins.

Finally, we are grateful to the many friends and family members who provided essential encouragement and assistance. Most importantly, we are grateful to our husbands, Gil Allender and Neil Kittlesen, for their unflagging support, interest, and encouragement. Their lives in our lives make the effort worthwhile.

Contents

U N I T

Public Health Principles in Community Health Nursing

UNIT

Tools of Community Health Nursing

U N I T

Community as Client

U N I T

5

The Family as Client

UNIT

6

Promoting and Protecting the Health of Aggregates With Developmental Needs

UNIT 7
Promoting and Protecting the Health of Vulnerable Aggregates

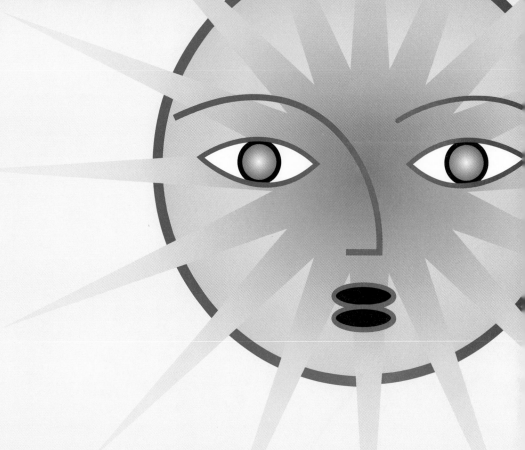

Foundations of Community Health Nursing

1

Opportunities and Challenges of Community Health Nursing

Learning Objectives

Upon mastery of this chapter, you should be able to:

- Define community health and distinguish it from public health.
- Explain the concept of community.
- Describe three types of communities.
- Diagram the health continuum.
- Differentiate among the three levels of prevention.
- Analyze the six components of community health practice.
- Describe the eight characteristics of community health nursing.

s we enter the new millennium, the opportunities and challenges in nursing are boundless and ever-changing. New biotechnologies offer opportunities not experienced before: women can give birth to eight living babies in one delivery; multiple defective organs can be replaced; and through genomic typing we soon will be able to anticipate the anomalies that lead to illness. However, challenges abound: millions of people die each year from conflicts resulting in wars and terrorism, drought, and starvation; from preventable ancient, new, and reemerging infectious diseases; and from unhealthy lifestyle choices. In addition, opportunities and challenges confront the nurse personally and professionally. The complexity of career decisions for the individual with a professional degree in nursing is compounded by the expanding arenas in which nurses practice.

As a specialty in nursing practice, community health nursing offers unique challenges and opportunities. For the nurse entering this field, there is the challenge of understanding and the opportunity to enrich the heritage of early public health nursing efforts while realizing that the world is much changed since the 1900s. There is the challenge of expanding nursing's focus from the individual and family to encompass communities and the opportunity to affect the health status of populations. There also is the challenge of determining the needs of populations at risk and the opportunity to design interventions to address their needs. There is the challenge of learning the complexities of a constantly changing health care system and the opportunity to shape its service delivery. Community health nursing is community based and, most importantly, it is population focused. Operating within an environment of rapid change and increasingly complex challenges, this field of nursing holds the potential for positively shaping the quality of community health services and improving the health of the general public.

You have provided nursing care in familiar acute care settings with the very ill, both young and old, with other professionals at your side. You worked as part of a team, in close proximity, to welcome a new life, to reestablish a client's health, or to comfort someone toward a peaceful death. Now, you are being asked to leave the familiarity of the acute care setting and go out into the community—into homes, schools, recreational facilities, the work setting, parishes, and even street corners that are familiar to clients and unfamiliar to you. Here, there are minimal or no monitoring devices, charts full of laboratory data, or professional and allied health workers at your side to assist you. You will be asked to use the nontangible skills of listening, assessing, planning, teaching, coordinating, evaluating, and referring. Often, your practice will be solo and you will need to combine creativity, ingenuity, and resourcefulness along with the above-mentioned skills. You will be providing care not only to individuals but also to families and other groups in a variety of settings within the community. Talk about boundless opportunities and challenges!

But perhaps, just perhaps, you might find this a rewarding kind of nursing—one that constantly challenges you, interests you, and allows you to use your skills holistically with clients of all ages, at all stages of illness and wellness; one that absolutely demands the use of your critical-thinking skills. And you may decide, when you finish your community health nursing course, that you have found your career choice. Finding out begins with understanding the concepts of community and health.

This chapter provides an overview of the basic concepts of community and health, the components of community health practice, and the salient characteristics of contemporary community health nursing practice, so that you can enter this field of nursing in concert with its intentions. The opportunities and challenges of community health nursing will become even more apparent as the chapter progresses. The discussion of the concepts and theories that make community health nursing an important specialty within nursing begins with the broader field of community health, which provides the context and essential content for community health nursing practice.

COMMUNITY HEALTH

Human beings are social creatures. All of us, with rare exception, live out our lives in the company of other people. An Eskimo lives in a small, tightly knit community of close relatives; a rural Mexican lives in a small village with hardly more than 200 members. In contrast, someone from New York City might be a member of many overlapping communities, such as professional societies, a political party, a religious group, a neighborhood, and the city itself. Even those who try to escape community membership always begin their lives in some type of group, and usually they continue to depend on groups for material and emotional support. Communities are an essential and permanent feature of the human experience.

The communities in which we live and work have a profound influence on our collective health and well-being. Here are three examples:

- Research has established that both smoking and passive exposure to tobacco smoke are directly associated with serious negative health effects and premature mortality among more than 1 billlion smokers worldwide (Institute of Medicine, 2001). Many states, communities, and organizations (including hospitals, schools, restaurants, and airlines) have developed regulatory approaches to smoking. They have removed cigarette vending machines, conducted antismoking advertising campaigns, prohibited televised commercials, increased cigarette taxes, and restricted smoking in public places. Such community rules and educational efforts protect nonsmokers, promote quitting smoking, and generally decrease the potential for heart and lung disease on a community-wide basis. These efforts have contributed to the downward trend in cigarette smoking, especially in high-income countries such as the United States, Australia, Italy, and the United

Kingdom in the last three decades (Jha et al., 2002). Community-wide efforts to identify causative lifestyle factors followed by appropriate interventions to reduce chronic diseases related to tobacco use are ongoing areas of research (Nordstrom et al., 2000; McGrady & Pederson, 2002; Pollack, 2001).

- State laws that require the use of a seat belt, child restraints, and placing young children in the back seat and that severely penalize the combination of drinking and driving protect motorists and reduce the risk of vehicular crashes, injuries, and death. Research has shown that if young children sit in the back seat with seat belts on, their risk of injury and death is significantly reduced. Based on many studies conducted in the 1990s, the state of Rhode Island passed a law in 1998 requiring children younger than 6 years old to sit in the rear seat of motor vehicles. A later study found that children in Rhode Island were more likely to be sitting in the back seat, whereas no significant changes in child passenger seating behavior occurred in Massachusetts, a state without such a law, during the same period (Segui-Gomez et al., 2001).
- On a larger scale, "Theory and research suggest that behavioral interventions to prevent HIV/AIDS may be most effective when they are personalized and affectively compelling, when they provide models of desired behaviors, and when they are linked to social and cultural narratives" (Galavotti, Pappas-Delucca, & Lansky, 2001, p. 1602). Using "entertainment-education" and interpersonal reinforcement at the community level creates the foundation of the MARCH (Modeling and Reinforcement to Combat HIV) initiative being implemented in 14 sub-Saharan African countries. The countries are in various phases of this major initiative, and thorough, continuous follow-up will provide much information about this long-term behavioral change approach to combating human immunodeficiency virus (HIV) and the acquired immunodeficiency syndrome (AIDS).

Just as a whole is greater than the sum of its parts, the health of a community is more than the sum of the health of its individual citizens. A community that achieves a high level of wellness is composed of healthy citizens, functioning in an environment that protects and promotes health. Community health, as a field of practice, seeks to provide organizational structure, a broad set of resources, and the collaborative activities needed to accomplish the goal of an optimally healthy community.

In acute care, the health of an individual is the primary focus. Community health broadens that focus to concentrate on families, populations, and the community at large. The community becomes the recipient of service, and health becomes the product. Viewed from another perspective, community health is concerned with the interchange between population groups and their total environment, and with the impact of that interchange on collective health.

Although many believe that health and illness are individual issues, evidence indicates that they also are community issues. The spread of the HIV pandemic, nationally and internationally, is a dramatic and tragic case in point (Berkman, 2001). Other community and national concerns include the rising incidence and prevalence of sexually transmitted diseases, substance abuse, tuberculosis, teen pregnancy, family and teen violence, terrorism, and pollution-driven environmental hazards. Communities can influence the spread of disease, provide barriers to protect members from health hazards, organize ways to combat outbreaks of infectious disease, and promote practices that contribute to individual and collective health (American Nurses Association [ANA], 2000; Clark, 2002; Wurzbach, 2002).

Many different professionals work in community health to form a complex team. The city planner designing an urban renewal project necessarily becomes involved in community health. The social worker providing counseling about child abuse or the use of chemical substances among adolescents is involved in community health. A physician treating clients affected by a sudden outbreak of hepatitis and seeking to find the source is engaged in community health practice. Prenatal clinics, meals for the elderly, genetic counseling centers, and educational programs for the early detection of cancer all are part of the community health effort.

The professional nurse is an integral member of this team, a linchpin and a liaison between physicians, social workers, government officials, and law enforcement officers. Community health nurses work in every conceivable kind of community agency, from a state public health department to a community-based advocacy group. Their duties range from examining infants in a well-baby clinic, or teaching elderly stroke victims in their homes, to carrying out epidemiologic research or engaging in health policy analysis and decision-making. Despite its breadth, however, community health nursing is a specialized practice. It combines all of the basic elements of professional clinical nursing with public health and community practice. This text examines the unique contribution made by community health nursing to our health care system.

Community health and public health share many features. Both are organized community efforts aimed at the promotion, protection, and preservation of the public's health. Historically, as a field of practice, public health has been associated primarily with the efforts of official or government entities—for example, federal, state, or local tax-supported health agencies that target the whole range of health issues. In contrast, private health efforts, such as those of the American Lung Association or the American Cancer Society, work toward solving selected health problems. The latter augments the former. Currently, public health practice encompasses both approaches and works collaboratively with all health agencies and efforts, public or private, that are concerned with the public's health. In this text, community health practice refers to a focus on specific, designated communities. It is a part of the larger public health effort and recognizes the fundamental concepts and principles of public health as its birthright and foundation for practice.

Winslow's classic 1920 definition of **public health** still holds true and forms the basis for our understanding of community health in this text:

> *Public health is the science and art of preventing disease, prolonging life, and promoting health and efficiency through organized community efforts for the sanitation of the environment, the control of communicable infections, the education of the individual in personal hygiene, the organization of medical and nursing services for the early diagnosis and preventive treatment of disease, and the development of the social machinery to insure everyone a standard of living adequate for the maintenance of health, so organizing these benefits as to enable every citizen to realize his birthright of health and longevity (Pickett & Hanlon, 1990, p. 5).*

Turnock (1997, p. 375) offered a more concise definition of public health and stated that it includes "activities that society undertakes to assure the conditions in which people can be healthy. This includes organized community efforts to prevent, identify, and counter threats to the health of the public."

Given this understanding of public health, the concept of community health can be defined. **Community health** is the identification of needs and the protection and improvement of collective health within a geographically defined area.

One of the challenges community health practice faces is to remain responsive to the community's health needs. As a result, its structure is complex; numerous health services and programs are currently available or will be developed. Examples include health education, family planning, accident prevention, environmental protection, immunization, nutrition, early periodic screening and developmental testing, school programs, mental health services, occupational health programs, and the care of vulnerable populations. A community health and safety service developed in the aftermath of the terrorist attack on New York City and Washington, DC, on September 11, 2001, is the Department of Homeland Security.

Community health practice, a part of public health, sometimes is misunderstood. Even many health professionals think of community health practice in limiting terms such as sanitation programs, clinics in poverty areas, or massive campaigns to prevent communicable disease. Although these are a part of its ever-broadening focus, community health practice is much more. To understand the nature and significance of this field, it is necessary to more closely examine the concept of community and the concept of health.

THE CONCEPT OF COMMUNITY

The concepts of community and health together provide the foundation for understanding community health. Broadly defined, a community is a collection of people who share some important feature of their lives. In this text, the term **community** refers to a collection of people who interact with one another and whose common interests or characteristics form the basis for a sense of unity or belonging. It can be a society of people holding common rights and privileges (eg, citizens of a town), sharing common interests (eg, a community of farmers), or living under the same laws and regulations (eg, a prison community). The function of any community includes its members' collective sense of belonging and their shared identity, values, norms, communication, and common interests and concerns (Bruce & McKane, 2000; Clark, 2002). Some communities—for example, a tiny village in Appalachia—are composed of people who share almost everything. They live in the same location, work at a limited number of jobs, attend the same churches, and make use of the single health clinic with its visiting physician and nurse. Other communities, such as members of Mothers Against Drunk Driving (MADD) or the community of professional nurses, are large, scattered, and composed of individuals who share only a common interest and involvement in a certain goal. Although most communities of people share many aspects of their experience, it is useful to identify three types of communities that have relevance to community health practice: geographic, common interest, and health problem.

Geographic Community

A community often is defined by its geographic boundaries and thus is called a **geographic community**. A city, town, or neighborhood is a geographic community. Consider the community of Hayward, Wisconsin. Located in northwestern Wisconsin, it is set in the north woods environment, far removed from any urban center and in a climatic zone characterized by extremely harsh winters. With a population of approximately 2200, it is considered a rural community. The population has certain identifiable characteristics, such as age and sex ratios, and its size fluctuates with the seasons: summers bring hundreds of tourists and seasonal residents. Hayward is a social system as well as a geographic location. The families, schools, hospital, churches, stores, and government institutions are linked in a complex network. This community, like others, has an informal power structure. It has a communication system that includes gossip, the newspaper, the "co-op" store bulletin board, and the radio station. In one sense, then, a community consists of a collection of people located in a specific place and is made up of institutions organized into a social system.

Local communities such as Hayward vary in size. A few miles south of Hayward lie several other communities, including Northwoods Beach and Round Lake; these three, along with other towns and isolated farms, form a larger community called Sawyer County. If a nurse worked for a health agency serving only Hayward, that community would be of primary concern; however, if the nurse worked for the Sawyer County Health Department, this larger community would be the focus. A community health nurse employed by the State Health Department in Madison, Wisconsin, would have an interest in Sawyer County and Hayward, but only as part of the larger community of Wisconsin.

Frequently, a single part of a city can be treated as a community. In Seattle, for example, the district near the waterfront forms a community of many transient and homeless people. In New York City, the neighborhood called Harlem is a community, as is the Haight-Ashbury district of San Francisco.

In community health, it is useful to identify a geographic area as a community. A community demarcated by geographic boundaries, such as a city or county, becomes a clear target for analysis of health needs. Available data, such as morbidity and mortality figures, can augment assessment studies to form the basis for planning health programs. Media campaigns and other health education efforts can readily reach intended audiences. Examples include distributing educational information on safe sex, self-protection, the dangers of substance abuse, or where to seek shelter from abuse and violence. A geographic community is easily mobilized for action. Groups can be formed to carry out intervention and prevention efforts that address needs specific to that community. Such efforts might include more stringent policies on day care, shelters for battered women, work site safety programs in local hazardous industries, or improved sex education in the schools. Furthermore, health actions can be enhanced through the support of politically powerful individuals and resources present in a geographic community.

On a larger scale, the world can be considered as a global community. Indeed, it is overwhelmingly important to view the world this way. Borders of countries change with political revolution. Communicable diseases are not aware of arbitrary political boundaries. A person can travel around the world in less than 24 hours, and so can diseases. Children starving in Africa affect persons living in the United States. Political uprisings in the Middle East have an impact on people in Western countries. Floods in southeast Asia have meaning for other national economies. The world is one large community that needs to work together to ensure a healthy today and a healthier and safer tomorrow. *Global health* has become a dominant phrase in international public health circles. It frames World Health Assembly discussions and presidential addresses. Global health raises an expectation of health for all, for if good health is possible in one part of the world, the forces of globalization should allow it elsewhere (Bunyavanich & Walkup, 2001). Governments need to work together to develop a broader base for international relations and collaborative strategies that will place greater emphasis on global health security.

Common-Interest Community

A community also can be identified by a common interest or goal. A collection of people, even if they are widely scattered geographically, can have an interest or goal that binds the members together. This is called a **common-interest com-**munity. The members of a church in a large metropolitan area, the members of a national professional organization, and women who have had mastectomies are all common-interest communities. Sometimes, within a certain geographic area, a group of people become a community by promoting their common interest. Disabled individuals scattered throughout a large city may emerge as a community through a common interest in promoting adherence to federal guidelines for wheelchair access, parking spaces, toilet facilities, elevators, or other services for the disabled. The residents of an industrial community may develop a common interest in air or water pollution issues, whereas others who work but do not live in the area may not share that interest. Communities form to protect the rights of children, stop violence against women, clean up the environment, promote the arts, preserve historical sites, protect endangered species, develop a smoke-free environment, or provide support after a crisis. The kinds of shared interests that lead to the formation of communities are widely varied.

Common-interest communities whose focus is a health-related issue can become useful to agencies to promote. A group's single-minded commitment is a mobilizing force for action. Many successful prevention and health promotion efforts, including improved services and increased community awareness of specific problems, have resulted from the work of common-interest communities.

Community of Solution

A type of community encountered frequently in community health practice is a group of people who come together to solve a problem that affects all of them. The shape of this community varies with the nature of the problem, the size of the geographic area affected, and the number of resources needed to address the problem. Such a community has been called a **community of solution**. For example, a water pollution problem may involve several counties whose agencies and personnel must work together to control upstream water supply, industrial waste disposal, and city water treatment. This group of counties forms a community of solution focusing on a health problem. In another instance, several schools may collaborate with law enforcement and health agencies, as well as legislators and policy makers, to study patterns of substance abuse among students and design possible preventive approaches. The boundaries of this community of solution form around the schools, agencies, and political figures involved. Figure 1–1 depicts some communities of solution related to a single city.

In recent years, communities of solution have formed in many cities to attack the spread of HIV infection. More recently, communities of solution have worked with community members to assess public safety and security and create plans to make the community a safer place in which to live. Public health agencies, social service groups, schools, and media personnel have banded together to create public awareness of dangers that are present and to promote preventive

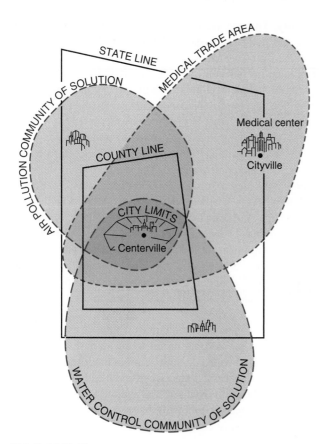

FIGURE 1–1. A city's communities of solution. State, county, and city boundaries (*solid lines*) may have little or no bearing on health solution boundaries (*dashed lines*).

behaviors. A community of solution is an important medium for change in community health.

Populations and Aggregates

The three types of communities just discussed underscore the meaning of the concept of community: in each instance, a collection of people choose to interact with one another because of common interests, characteristics, or goals. The concept of population has a different meaning. In this text, the term **population** refers to all of the people occupying an area, or to all of those who share one or more characteristics. In contrast to a community, a population is made up of people who do not necessarily interact with one another and do not necessarily share a sense of belonging to that group. A population may be defined geographically, such as the population of the United States or a city's population. This designation of a population is useful in community health for epidemiologic study and for collecting demographic data for purposes such as health planning. A population also may be defined by common qualities or characteristics, such as the elderly population or the homeless population. In community health, this meaning becomes useful when a specific group of people (eg, homeless individuals) is targeted for intervention: the population's common characteristics (eg, the

health-related problems of homelessness) become a major focus of the intervention.

In this text, the term **aggregate** refers to a mass or grouping of distinct individuals who are considered as a whole and who are loosely associated with one another. It is a broader term that encompasses many different-sized groups. Both communities and populations are types of aggregates. The aggregate focus, or a concern for groupings of people in contrast to individual health care, becomes a distinguishing feature of community health practice.

The continuing shift away from acute care settings and toward community-based services as the focus of the health care system, along with a rising emphasis on managed care of populations, underscores the importance of community health nursing's aggregate focus. In fact, some say it validates the focus of community health nursing as practiced over many decades (Porter-O'Grady, 2001). With the community as central to the health care model, it becomes essential for nurses to understand the meaning of community health and to assume leadership in aggregate-level health care (see What Do You Think?).

Community health workers, including community health nurses, need to define the community targeted for study and intervention: Who are the people who compose the community? Where are they located, and what are their characteristics? A clear delineation of the community or population must be established before the nurse can assess needs and design interventions. The complex nature of communities also must be understood. What are the characteristics of the people in terms of age, sex, race, socioeconomic level, and health status? How does the community interact with other communities? What is its history? What are its resources? Is the community undergoing rapid change, and, if so, what are the changes? These questions, as well as the tools needed to assess a community for health purposes, are discussed in detail in Chapter 18.

THE CONCEPT OF HEALTH

Health in the abstract refers to a person's physical, mental, and spiritual state; it can be positive (as being in good health) or negative (as being in poor health). The World Health

Organization defines health positively as "a state of complete physical, mental, and social well-being and not merely the absence of disease or infirmity" (Venes, 2001, p. 930). Our understanding of the concept of health builds on this classic definition. **Health**, in this text, refers to a holistic state of well-being, which includes soundness of mind, body, and spirit. Community health practitioners place a strong emphasis on **wellness**, which includes the definition of health just mentioned but incorporates the capacity to develop a person's potential to lead a fulfilling and productive life, one that can be measured in terms of quality of life.

There is increasing awareness of the strong relationship of health to environment. This is not a new concept. Almost 150 years ago, Florence Nightingale explored the health and illness connection with the environment. She believed that a person's health was greatly influenced by ventilation, noise, light, cleanliness, diet, and a restful bed. She laid down simple rules about maintaining and obtaining "health," which were written for lay women caring for family members to "put the constitution in such a state as that it will have no disease" (Nightingale, 1859, preface).

In some cultures, health is viewed differently. Some see it as the freedom from and absence of evil. Illness, to some, is seen as punishment for being bad or doing evil (Spector, 2000). Many nurses come from or know families in which health and illness beliefs are heavily influenced by religion, superstition, folk beliefs, or "old wives' tales." This is not unusual, and encountering such beliefs when working with various groups in the community is common. Chapter 4 explores these beliefs more thoroughly for a better understanding of how health beliefs influence every aspect of a person's life.

Although health is widely accepted as desirable, the nature of health often is ambiguous. Consumers and providers often define health and wellness in different ways. To clarify the concept for nurses who are considering community health practice, the distinguishing features of health are briefly characterized here; the implications of this concept for professionals in the field can then be examined more fully.

The Health Continuum: Wellness–Illness

Society suggests a polarized or "either/or" way of thinking about health: people either are well or they are ill. Yet wellness is a relative concept, not an absolute, and **illness** is a state of being *relatively* unhealthy. There are many levels and degrees of wellness and illness, from a robust 70-year-old woman who is fully active and functioning at an optimal level of wellness, to a 70-year-old man with end-stage renal disease. Someone recovering from pneumonia may be mildly ill, whereas a teenaged boy with limitations in functioning because of episodic depression may be described as mildly well.

The Human Genome Project, completed in 2001, and the coming of a genomics foundation for health care may skew the health continuum toward the more healthy end. **Genomics**, the identification and plotting of human genes for future disease occurrence, will alter how we view disease. Primary and secondary preventive services will be individually designed based on gene findings, and client lifestyle modifications will be recommended from birth. The capacity for this kind of health care will be a reality in the early decades of the 21st century.

Because health involves a range of degrees from optimal health at one end to total disability or death at the other (Fig. 1–2), it often is described as a continuum. This **health continuum** applies not only to individuals but also to families and communities. A nurse might speak of a dysfunctional family, meaning one that is experiencing a relative degree of illness; or a healthy family might be described as one that exhibits many wellness characteristics, such as effective communication and conflict resolution, as well as the ability to work together and use resources appropriately. Likewise, a community, as a collection of people, may be described in terms of degrees of wellness or illness. The health of an individual, family, group, or community moves back and forth along this continuum throughout life.

A healthy community, first described by Cottrell (1976) as a competent community, is one in which the various organizations, groups, and aggregates of people making up the community do at least four things:
1. They collaborate effectively in identifying the problems and needs of the community.
2. They achieve a working consensus on goals and priorities.
3. They agree on ways and means to implement the agreed-on goals.
4. They collaborate effectively in the required actions.

By thinking of health relatively, as a matter of degree, the scope of nursing practice can be broadened to focus on preventing illness or disability and promoting wellness. Traditionally, most health care has focused on treatment of acute and chronic conditions at the illness end of the continuum. Gradually, the emphasis is shifting to focus on the wellness end of the continuum, as outlined in the government document, *Healthy People 2010* (U. S. Department of Health and Human Services [UDHHS], 2000). Community health practice ranges over the entire continuum; it always works to improve the degree of health in individuals, families, groups, and communities. In particular, community health practice emphasizes the promotion and preservation of wellness and the prevention of illness or disability.

Health as a State of Being

Health refers to a state of being, including many different qualities and characteristics. An individual might be described in terms such as energetic, outgoing, enthusiastic, beautiful, caring, loving, and intense. Together, these qualities become the essence of a person's existence; they describe a state of being. Similarly, a specific geographic community, such as a neighborhood, has many characteristics. It might be characterized by the terms congested, deteriorating, unattractive, dirty, and disorganized. These characteristics

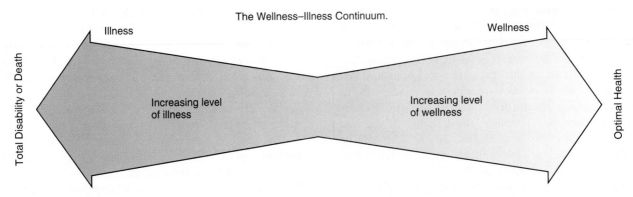

The Wellness–Illness Continuum.

The level (degree) of illness increases as one moves toward total disability or death; the level of wellness increases as one moves toward optimal health. This continuum shows the relative nature of health. At any given time a person can be placed at some point along the continuum.

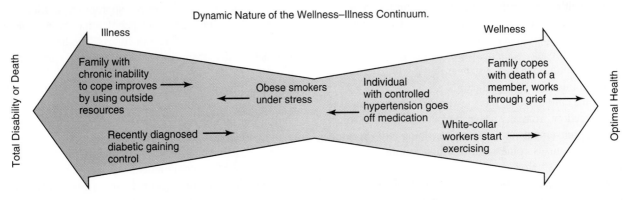

Dynamic Nature of the Wellness–Illness Continuum.

A person's relative health is usually in a state of flux, either improving or deteriorating. This diagram of the wellness–illness continuum shows several examples of people in changing states of health.

FIGURE 1–2.   The health continuum.

suggest diminishing degrees of vitality. A third example might be a population, such as workers involved in a massive layoff who band together to provide support and share resources to effectively seek new employment. This community shows signs of healthy and positive coping.

Health involves the total person or community. All of the dimensions of life affecting everyday functioning determine an individual's or a community's health, including physical, psychological, spiritual, economic, and sociocultural experiences. All of these factors must be considered when dealing with the health of an individual or community. The approach should be holistic. A client's placement on the health continuum can be known only if the nurse considers all facets of the client's life, including not only physical status but also the status of home, family, and work.

When considering an aggregate or group of people in terms of health, it becomes useful for intervention purposes to speak of the "health of a community." With aggregates as well as individuals, health as a state of being does not merely involve that group's physical state but also includes psychological, spiritual, and socioeconomic factors. The health of south central Los Angeles after the riots in the early 1990s is an example. Extensive damage from interracial fighting,

burning, and looting left the community totally devastated. Littleton, Colorado, in the late 1990s was a damaged and vulnerable community after the shootings and multiple deaths at Columbine High School. And in 2001, thousands of lives were lost in New York City and Washington, DC, while an airline and its passengers were sacrificed over Somerset County, Pennsylvania, to prevent further deaths. The trauma of these events left our nation shaken. The health of many communities was dangerously low. Communities needed to be restored, and the entire country needed to heal.

Subjective and Objective Dimensions of Health

Health involves both subjective and objective dimensions; that is, it involves both how people feel (subjective) and how well they can function in their environment (objective). Subjectively, a healthy person is one who feels well, who experiences the sensation of a vital, positive state. Healthy people are full of life and vigor, capable of physical and mental productivity. They feel minimal discomfort and displeasure with the world around them. Again, people experience varying degrees of vitality and well-being. The state of feeling well

VOICES FROM THE COMMUNITY

"I never thought much about being healthy or not, now that you ask. I keep busy, I cook like I'm expecting company, I have a good appetite. I really think all these so-called healthy things people suggest are fads, just so someone can get rich—like tofu and low fat this and that. Don't give me margarine, only butter, . . . and skim milk, it's like drinking water! I work in my garden, I read, and I eat fresh foods, and don't talk to me about my smoking, it's the one pleasure I have left."

—Bettie, age 81

fluctuates. Some mornings we wake up feeling more energetic and enthusiastic than we do on other mornings. How people feel varies day by day, even hour by hour; nonetheless, how they feel overall is a strong indicator of their state of health.

Health also involves the objective dimension of ability to function. A healthy individual or community carries out necessary activities and achieves enriching goals. Unhealthy people not only feel ill but are limited, to some degree, in their ability to carry out daily activities. Indeed, levels of illness or wellness are measured largely in terms of ability to function (Roach, 2000). A person confined to bed is labeled sicker than an ill person managing self-care. A family that meets its members' needs is healthier than one that has poor communication patterns and is unable to provide adequate physical and emotional resources. A community actively engaged in crime prevention or policing of industrial wastes shows signs of healthy functioning. The degree of functioning is directly related to the state of health (see Voices from the Community).

The ability to function can be observed. A man dresses and feeds himself and goes to work. Despite financial exigencies, a family nourishes its members through a supportive emotional climate. A community provides adequate resources and services for its members. These performances, to some degree, can be regarded as indicators of health status. Some community health agencies assess clients' ability to function as a measure of client progress and nursing care effectiveness (Beckerman & Tappen, 2000).

The actions of an individual, family, or community are motivated by their values. Some activities, such as walking and taking care of personal needs, are functions valued by most people. Other actions, such as bird watching, volunteering to help a charity, or running, have more limited appeal. In assessing the health of individuals and communities, the community health nurse can observe people's ability to function but also must know their values, which may contrast sharply with those of the professional. The influence of values on health is examined more closely in Chapter 5.

The subjective dimension (feeling well or ill) and the objective dimension (functioning) together provide a clearer picture of people's health. When they feel well and demonstrate functional ability, they are close to the wellness end of the health continuum. Even those with a disease such as arthritis or diabetes may feel well and perform well within their capacity. These people can be considered healthy or closer to the wellness end of the continuum. Figure 1–3 depicts the relationships between the subjective and objective views of health.

Continuous and Episodic Health Care Needs

Community health practice encompasses populations in all age groups with birth-to-death developmental health care needs. These **continuous needs** may include, for example, assistance with providing a toddler-proof home or establishing positive toilet-training techniques, help in effectively dealing with the progressive emancipation of preteens and teenagers, anticipatory guidance for reducing and managing the stress associated with retirement, or help coping with the death of an aged parent. These are developmental events experienced by most people and represent typical life occurrences. The community health nurse has the skills to work at the individual, family, and group level to meet these needs. On an individual and family level, a home visit may be the appropriate place for intervention. If the nurse sees that the community has many young and growing families and sev-

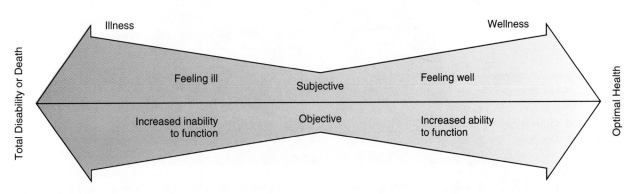

FIGURE 1–3.   Subjective and objective views of the wellness–illness continuum.

eral families have similar developmental issues, a class for mothers and babies, parents and teenagers, or preretirement adults may be formed to meet weekly at the library or health clinic waiting room. In these instances, the nurse works with groups ranging from small to large.

In addition, populations may have one-time, specific, negative health events, such as an illness or injury, that are not an expected part of life. These **episodic needs** might derive from the birth of an infant with Down syndrome, a head injury incurred from an automobile crash, or a diagnosis of HIV/AIDS.

In a given day, the community health nurse may interact with clients having either continuous or episodic health care needs, or both. For example, when can parents expect a child with Down syndrome to begin toilet training? How do middle-aged adults, planning their retirement and preparing for the death of an aged parent, deal with their adult child's AIDS diagnosis? Complex situations such as these may be positively influenced by the interaction with and services of the community health nurse.

COMPONENTS OF COMMUNITY HEALTH PRACTICE

Community health practice can best be understood by examining six basic components, which, when combined, encompass its services and programs. These components are (1) promotion of health, (2) prevention of health problems, (3) treatment of disorders, (4) rehabilitation, (5) evaluation, and (6) research.

Promotion of Health

Promotion of health is recognized as one of the most important components of public health and community health practice (UDHHS, 2000). **Health promotion** includes all efforts that seek to move people closer to optimal well-being or higher levels of wellness. Nursing, in particular, has a social mandate for engaging in health promotion (Pender, 2001). Health promotion programs and activities include many forms of health education—for example, teaching the dangers of drug use, demonstrating healthful practices such as regular exercise, and providing more health-promoting options such as heart-healthy menu selections. Community health promotion, then, encompasses the development and management of preventive health care services that are responsive to community health needs. Wellness programs in schools and industry are examples; they are useful when they are accompanied by desire, opportunity, and resources that encourage more healthful practices (Brownson, Baker, & Novick, 1999; Rockhill et al., 2001). Demonstration of such healthful practices as eating nutritious foods, either vegetarian (Fig. 1–4) or nonvegetarian (Fig. 1–5), and exercising

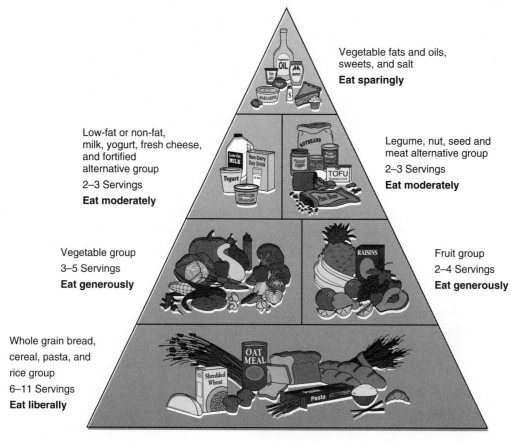

FIGURE 1-4.   The Vegetarian Food Pyramid. (Adapted from the Vegetarian Resource Group of the American Dietetic Association, The Health Connection.)

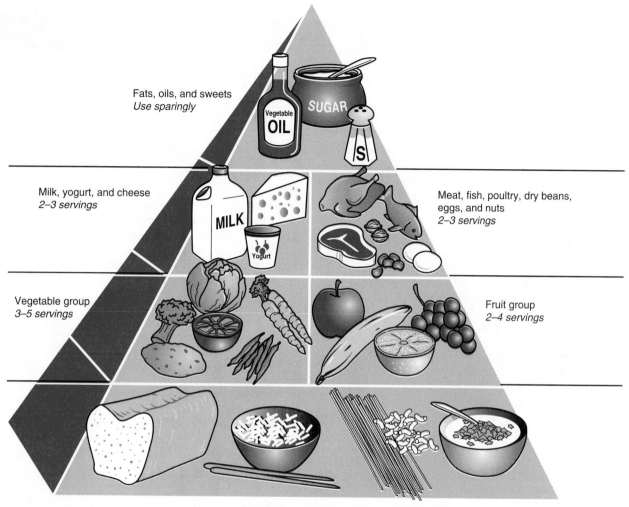

FIGURE 1–5.   The Food Guide Pyramid. In 1992, the U.S. Department of Agriculture replaced the old four food groups, in use since 1946, with the food guide pyramid. It emphasizes grains, fruits, and vegetables as the basis of a healthy diet. Recommended daily servings in each group are noted. In 2004 plans were revealed to redesign this pyramid, offering 12 diet plans for all ages and activity levels.

more regularly often is performed and promoted by individual health workers. In addition, groups and health agencies that support a smoke-free environment, encourage physical fitness programs for all ages, or demand that food products be properly labeled underscore the importance of these practices and create public awareness.

The goal of health promotion is to raise levels of wellness for individuals, families, populations, and communities. Community health efforts accomplish this goal through a three-pronged effort to:
1. Increase the span of healthy life for all citizens
2. Reduce health disparities among population groups
3. Achieve access to preventive services for everyone

Specifically, in the 1980s, the U.S. Public Health Service published the Surgeon General's report, *Healthy People,* and continued with *Promoting Health, Preventing Disease: 1990 Health Objectives for the Nation* and *Healthy*

People 2000. The third set of health objectives for the nation, *Healthy People 2010* (USDHHS, 2000), built on the previous two decades of success in Healthy People initiatives.

The Surgeon General's report provided vision and an agenda for significantly reducing preventable death and disability nationwide, enhancing quality of life, and greatly reducing disparities in the health status of populations. It emphasized the need for individuals to assume personal responsibility for controlling and improving their own health destiny. It challenged society to find ways to make good health available to vulnerable populations whose disadvantaged state placed them at greater risk for health problems. Finally, it called for an intensified shift in focus from treating preventable illness and functional impairment to concentrating resources and targeting efforts that promote health and prevent disease and disability (Allison, Kiefe, & Weissman, 1999).

In 2000, the U.S. Public Health Service (USDHHS) out-

DISPLAY 1.1

Issues in Community Health Nursing

Priority Areas for National Health Promotion and Disease Prevention

The context in which *Healthy People 2010* was developed differs from that in which Healthy People 2000 was framed—and will continue to evolve through the decade. Advances in preventive therapies, vaccines and pharmaceuticals, assistive technologies, and computerized systems will all change the face of medicine and how it is practiced. New relationships will be defined between public health departments and health care delivery organizations. Meanwhile, demographic changes in the United States—reflecting an older and more radically diverse population—will create new demands on public health and the overall health care system. Global forces—including food supplies, emerging infectious diseases, and environmental interdependence—will present new public health challenges (U.S. Department of Health and Human Services, 2000).

Its report, *Healthy People 2010*, states two broad goals: to (1) increase the quality and years of healthy life, and (2) eliminate health disparities. To accomplish these goals, measurable objectives were established under each of the following 28 priority areas:

Healthy People 2010 Focus Areas
1. Access to Quality Health Services
2. Arthritis, Osteoporosis, and Chronic Back Conditions
3. Cancer
4. Chronic Kidney Disease
5. Diabetes
6. Disability and Secondary Conditions
7. Educational and Community-Based Programs
8. Environmental Health
9. Family Planning
10. Food Safety
11. Health Communication
12. Heart Disease and Stroke
13. HIV
14. Immunization and Infectious Diseases
15. Injury and Violence Prevention
16. Maternal, Infant, and Child Health
17. Medical Product Safety
18. Mental Health and Mental Disorders
19. Nutrition and Overweight
20. Occupational Safety and Health
21. Oral Health
22. Physical Activity and Fitness
23. Public Health Infrastructure
24. Respiratory Diseases
25. Sexually Transmitted Diseases
26. Substance Abuse
27. Tobacco Use
28. Vision and Hearing

This national listing is a guide to policy makers and health planners at all levels. It provides a framework for prioritizing and addressing specific health needs in designated communities.

---

lined 28 priority areas for intervention in its publication, *Healthy People 2010* (Display 1–1). Under each of the 28 areas, *Healthy People 2010* outlined several objectives, stated in measurable terms, that specified targeted incidence and prevalence changes and that addressed age, gender, and culturally vulnerable groups along with improvement in public health systems. Healthy people make healthy communities and a healthy society.

The implications of this national agenda for health have far-reaching consequences for persons engaged in health care. For centuries, health care has focused on the illness end of the health continuum, but health professionals can no longer justify concentrating most of their efforts exclusively on treating the sick and injured. We now live in an age when it is not only possible to promote health and prevent disease and disability but our mandate and responsibility to do so (UDHHS, 2000).

Prevention of Health Problems

Prevention of health problems constitutes a major part of community health practice. Prevention means anticipating and averting problems or discovering them as early as possible to minimize potential disability and impairment. It is practiced on three levels in community health: (1) primary pre-

vention, (2) secondary prevention, and (3) tertiary prevention (Neuman, 2001). These concepts recur throughout the chapters of this text, in narrative format and in the Levels of Prevention Matrix Boxes, because they are basic to community health nursing. Once the differences among the levels of prevention are recognized, a sound foundation on which to build additional community health principles can be developed.

Primary prevention obviates the occurrence of a health problem; it includes measures taken to keep illness or injuries from occurring. It is applied to a generally healthy population and precedes disease or dysfunction. Examples of primary prevention activities by a community health nurse include encouraging elderly people to install and use safety devices (eg, grab bars by bathtubs, hand rails on steps), to prevent injuries from falls; teaching young adults healthy lifestyle behaviors so that they can adopt changes for a lifetime, for themselves and their children; or working through a local health department to help control and prevent communicable diseases such as rubeola, poliomyelitis, or varicella by providing regular immunization programs.

Primary prevention involves anticipatory planning and action on the part of community health professionals, who must project themselves into the future, envision potential needs and problems, and then design programs to counteract

LEVELS OF PREVENTION MATRIX

SITUATION: Promotion of community nutritional status through healthy dietary practices.

GOAL: Using the three levels of prevention, negative health conditions are avoided, or promptly diagnosed and treated, and the fullest possible potential is restored.

PRIMARY PREVENTION		SECONDARY PREVENTION		TERTIARY PREVENTION		
Health Promotion and Education	*Health Protection*	*Early Diagnosis*	*Prompt Treatment*	*Rehabilitation*	*Primary Prevention*	
					Health Promotion and Education	*Health Protection*
Provide nutrition educational programs to promote awareness at schools, work sites, food stores, etc. Encourage restaurants to offer healthy menu items Complete a kitchen cupboard survey in collaboration with client Recommend nutrition classes offered at neighborhood centers or health care facilities Use educationally significant tools (literature, posters, food guide pyramid) to enhance educational programs	Supplement diet with vitamins and minerals that offer health protection (eg, vitamins A, B, C, E)	Provide dietary screening programs for high-risk groups: infants, adolescents, young female adults, elderly individuals Refer clients with eating disorders (underweight/ overweight, anorexia, bulimia, compulsive eating) to nutritionist or primary care provider	Initiate educational and incentive programs to improve dietary practices Teach clients (individuals or families) on a one-to-one basis to modify dietary practices	Encourage long-term follow-up for diagnosed eating disorders Reassess client dietary practices as necessary	Encourage healthy meal preparation and consumption	Use vitamin and mineral supplements as needed

them so that they never occur. A community health nurse who instructs a group of overweight individuals on how to follow a well-balanced diet while losing weight is preventing the possibility of nutritional deficiency (see Levels of Prevention Matrix). Educational programs that teach safe-sex practices or the dangers of smoking and substance abuse are other examples of primary prevention. In addition, when the community health nurse serves on a fact-finding committee exploring the effects of a proposed toxic waste dump on the outskirts of town, the nurse is concerned about primary prevention. The concepts of primary prevention and planning for the future are foreign to many social groups, who may resist on the basis of conflicting values. The Parable of the Dangerous Cliff (Display 1–2) illustrates such a value conflict.

Secondary prevention involves efforts to detect and treat existing health problems at the earliest possible stage when dis-ease or impairment already exist. Hypertension and cholesterol screening programs in many communities help to identify high-risk individuals and encourage early treatment to prevent heart attacks or stroke. Other examples are teaching breast and testicular self-examination, encouraging regular mammograms and Pap smears for early detection of possible cancer, and providing skin testing for tuberculosis (in infants at 1 year of age and periodically throughout life, with increasing frequency for high-risk groups). Secondary prevention attempts to discover a health problem at a point when intervention may lead to its control or eradication. This is the goal behind testing of water and soil samples for contaminants and hazardous chemicals in the field of community environmental health. It also prompts community health nurses to watch for early signs of child abuse in a family, emotional disturbances in a group of widows, or alcohol and drug abuse among adolescents.

DISPLAY 1.2

Parable of the Dangerous Cliff

Twas a dangerous cliff, as they freely confessed,
　　Though to walk near its crest was so pleasant;
But over its terrible edge there has slipped
　　A duke, and full many a peasant.
The people said something would have to be done
　　But their projects did not at all tally.
Some said, "Put a fence around the edge of the cliff";
　　Some, "an ambulance down in the valley."
The lament of the crowd was profound and was loud,
　　As their hearts overflowed with their pity;
But the cry of the ambulance carried the day
　　As it spread through the neighboring city.
A collection was made to accumulate aid
　　And the dwellers in highway and alley
Gave dollars or cents
Not to furnish a fence
But "an ambulance down in the valley."
"For the cliff is all right if you're careful," they said.
"And if folks ever slip and are dropping,
　　It isn't the slipping that hurts them so much
As the shock down below when they're stopping."
So for years (we have heard), as these mishaps occurred,
　　Quick forth the rescuers sally,
To pick up the victims who fell from the cliff,
　　With the ambulance down in the valley.
Said one in his plea, "It's a marvel to me

That you'd give so much greater attention
To repairing results than to curing the cause;
You had much better aim at prevention.
　　For the mischief, of course, should be stopped at its
　　　source,
Come neighbors and friends, let us rally.
　　It is far better sense to rely on a fence
Than an ambulance down in the valley."
"He is wrong in his head," the majority said;
　　"He would end all our earnest endeavor.
He's a man who would shirk this responsible work,
　　But we will support it forever.
Aren't we picking up all, just as fast as they fall,
　　and giving them care liberally?
A superfluous fence is of no consequence,
If the ambulance works in the valley."
The story looks queer as we've written it here,
　　But things oft occur that are stranger.
More humane, we assert, than to care for the hurt,
　　Is a plan for removing the danger.
The very best plan is to safeguard the man,
　　And attend to the thing rationally;
To build up the fence and try to dispense
　　With the ambulance down in the valley.
Better still! Cut down the hill!
—Author Unknown

Tertiary prevention attempts to reduce the extent and severity of a health problem to its lowest possible level, so as to minimize disability and restore or preserve function. Examples include treatment and rehabilitation of persons after a stroke to reduce impairment, postmastectomy exercise programs to restore functioning, and early treatment and management of diabetes to reduce problems or slow their progress. The individuals involved have an existing illness or disability whose impact on their lives is lessened through tertiary prevention. In broader community health practice, tertiary prevention is used to minimize the effects of an existing unhealthy community condition. Examples of such prevention are insisting that businesses provide wheelchair access, warning urban residents about the dangers of a chemical spill, and recalling a contaminated food or drug product. When a community experiences a disaster such as an earthquake, a fire, or even a terrorist attack, preventing injuries among the survivors and volunteers during rescue is another example of tertiary prevention—eliminating additional injury to those already experiencing a tragedy.

Health assessment of individuals, families, and communities is an important part of all three levels of preventive practice. Health status must be determined to anticipate problems and select appropriate preventive measures. Community health nurses working with young parents who themselves have been victims of child abuse can institute early

treatment for the parents to prevent abuse and foster adequate parenting of their children. If the assessment of a community reveals inadequate facilities and activities to meet the future needs of its growing senior population, agencies and groups can collaborate to develop the needed resources.

Health problems are most effectively prevented by maintaining healthy lifestyles and healthy environments. To these ends, community health practice directs many of its efforts to providing safe and satisfying living and working conditions, nutritious food, and clean air and water. This area of practice includes the field of preventive medicine, which is a population-focused, or community-oriented, branch of medical practice that incorporates public health sciences and principles (Barton, 1999; Kriebel & Tickner, 2001).

Treatment of Disorders

The third component of community health practice is treatment of disorders. It focuses on the illness end of the continuum and is the remedial aspect of community health practice. This occurs by three methods: (1) direct service to people with health problems, (2) indirect service that helps people to obtain treatment, and (3) development of programs to correct unhealthy conditions. Examples of direct service include the following scenarios: a nursing center serving a homeless population provides health screening, education, and referral services; elderly persons confined to home with disabling chronic illness obtain home visits from a nursing agency for assistance with treatment regimens, supervision of medications, and personal care; and a neighborhood health center provides an educational program and support group for people wanting to stop smoking or lose weight. Many kinds of community agencies provide direct health care or health-related services.

The second method of treating disorders is indirect service, which consists of assisting people with health problems to obtain treatment. In many instances, a community agency is not able to provide needed care and refers the individuals or groups concerned to a more appropriate resource. A young woman with postpartum bleeding, assisted by the community health nurse, can obtain an immediate appointment with a physician at the local clinic. A social worker can help a family that is plagued by personal and economic problems to enter a family therapy and counseling program. Several community agencies provide information and referral services. An effective community health nurse works diligently to develop partnerships with health care workers in agencies that provide services to potential clients. The quality of this partnership is paramount in ensuring that clients' needs are met. It builds a bridge between the client who has a health care need and the individual or group who provides a service to meet that need. A strong relationship may make the difference between resolution of a problem and frustration with the health care system.

The third method of treatment of disorders is the development of programs to correct unhealthy conditions. One community with a high incidence of alcoholism and drug abuse initiated a chemical dependency counseling and treatment center. In another community, the health department developed new regulations for industrial waste disposal as a result of increased pollution of the water supply. Individual community members and health workers also take corrective action to remedy situations such as a case of apparent child abuse, poor nutrition in a school lunch program, or inhumane conditions and treatment in a nursing home.

Rehabilitation

Rehabilitation, the fourth component of community health practice, involves efforts to reduce disability and, as much as possible, restore function. People whose handicaps are congenital or are acquired through illness or accident (eg, stroke, heart condition, amputation, mental illness) can be helped to regain some measure of lost function or to develop new compensating skills. For example, a factory worker who lost his leg in an industrial accident received good medical and nursing care, prosthetic fittings, and physical and occupational therapy; he then retrained to assume an office job.

In community health, the need to reduce disability and restore function applies equally to families, groups, communities, and individuals. Many groups form for rehabilitation and offer support and guidance for those recuperating from some physical or mental disability. Examples include Alco-

holics Anonymous, halfway houses for psychiatric patients discharged from acute care settings, ostomy clubs, and drug rehabilitation programs. Rehabilitation services often are needed and sought by whole communities, such as when an inner city area desires to provide decent, safe playgrounds for its children.

As an element of community health practice, rehabilitation becomes increasingly significant when disease trends and changes in life expectancy are considered. Chronic diseases, such as cancer, heart disease, diabetes, and mental illness, are major cripplers. So, too, are accidents and injuries from many causes, including violence. Abuse of drugs, alcohol, and tobacco further adds to the list of disabling conditions. As a result, the need for rehabilitation services and long-term care has increased, stimulated further by the rising number of elderly persons with chronic health problems (Stone, 2000).

Evaluation

Evaluation, the fifth component of community health practice, is the process by which that practice is analyzed, judged, and improved according to established goals and standards. Evaluation of health and health care should be an integral part of every kind of health service, from individual practice to national and international programs. Whether done on a single-case basis or at the program level, evaluation helps to solve problems and provides direction for future health care efforts. Its goals are to determine the needs and success of activities and to develop improved services. In one study, evaluation of mental health services revealed a drastic need for adequate comprehensive psychiatric care, especially for serious mental illness in young adults and African-Americans living in the South. Researchers saw the gaps in service as an enormous public health problem for which public policies and cost-effective interventions were needed to improve both access to treatment and quality of treatment (Wang, Demler, & Kessler, 2002). In another instance, the CHIPS Study evaluated the effects of pricing and promotion efforts on purchases of low-fat snacks from vending machines. It revealed that reducing relative prices of low-fat snacks was effective in promoting their purchase from vending machines in both adult and adolescent populations (French et al., 2001). Evaluation studies of many types of community health interventions exist in the literature and provide insights and direction for further community health planning.

A comprehensive discussion of evaluation is provided in Chapters 19 and 24.

Research

Research, the sixth component of community health practice, is systematic investigation to discover facts affecting community health and community health practice, solve problems, and explore improved methods of health service. Community health practitioners conduct and use scientific investigations at all levels, from federal agencies such as the

U. S. Public Health Service to state and local groups conducting research. **Epidemiology** (the study of health and disease determinants and distribution in populations) and **biostatistics** (the science of statistically measuring population health conditions) are the primary public health measurement and analytic sciences underlying community health practice. Chapter 14 addresses these sciences more extensively.

Researchers in community health investigate the characteristics and patterns of illness and health. Conditions such as food poisoning, trauma, alcoholism, lung cancer, child abuse, drug dependency, and suicide are studied for possible causes and means of prevention. Health and healthful behavior are analyzed, for example, in nutrition projects and in studies of normal human growth and behavior for a better understanding of ways to promote healthful living.

Community health researchers also explore ways to improve health care. For example, an experimental intervention program among 22 work sites was aimed at increasing consumption of fruits and vegetables. It was found that interventions that included work site plus family involvement were more successful in increasing fruit and vegetable consumption than was work site intervention alone (Sorensen et al., 1999). A review of community-based nursing research provided evidence that "community-based nursing practice includes quality services that can control costs; a focus on disease prevention and health promotion; the organization of services where people live, work, and learn; partnerships and coalitions; service to people across the life span; services to culturally diverse populations; access to services for at-risk populations; development of the community's capacity for health; work with policy makers for policy change; and efforts to make the environment healthier" (Flynn, 1998, p. 165). Other research projects focus on the effectiveness of drug treatment programs, long-term stroke rehabilitation, improved treatment approaches to obesity, or empowerment of the disenfranchised and underserved.

Chapter 14 expands on the community health nurse's role in research interpretation, use, and conduct.

Community health researchers also examine the impact of social and environmental factors on health and health services provision. For example, one study sought to identify factors associated with recovery in a sample of urban residential fire survivors. A set of predictor variables was identified to help clinicians target survivors who are at high risk for psychological distress and plan needed interventions (Keane et al., 2002). More studies have centered on the needs and care of age-specific groups such as the maternal-infant population regarding the effects of smoke and smoking (Gantt, 2001; Gaffney, 2001) or the health and safety of elders in their homes (Berg, Hines, & Allen, 2002). Researchers have looked at study participant compliance, eliminating dropouts, and enhancing retention—important factors that affect the outcome of research (Moser, Dracup, & Doering, 2000; Davis, Broome, & Cox, 2002). Others have investigated ways to improve health services planning and policy development through efforts such as studying the community's needs and program utilization.

CHARACTERISTICS OF COMMUNITY HEALTH NURSING

Eight characteristics of community health nursing are particularly salient to the practice of this specialty: (1) it is a field of nursing; (2) it combines public health with nursing; (3) it is population focused; (4) it emphasizes prevention, health promotion, and wellness; (5) it promotes client responsibility and self-care; (6) it uses aggregate measurement and analysis; (7) it uses principles of organizational theory; and (8) it involves interprofessional collaboration.

Field of Nursing

The two characteristics of any specialized nursing practice are (1) specialized knowledge and skills, and (2) focus on a particular set of people receiving the service. These two characteristics are true for community health nursing. As a specialty field of nursing, community health nursing adds public health knowledge and skills that address the needs and problems of communities and aggregates and focuses care on communities and vulnerable populations.

Confusion over the meaning of "community health nursing" arises when it is defined only in terms of where it is practiced. Because health care services have shifted from the hospital to the community, many nurses in other specialties now practice in the community. Examples of these practices include home care, mental health, geriatric nursing, long-term care, and occupational health. Although community health nurses today practice in the same or similar settings, the difference lies in applying the public health principles to large groups and communities of people (Fig. 1–6). For nurses moving into this field of nursing, it requires a shift in focus — from individuals to aggregates. Nursing and other theories undergird its practice (see Chapter 17), and the nursing process (incorporated in Chapters 18 and 19) is one of its basic tools (see levels of prevention discussed earlier).

Community health nursing, then, as a field of nursing, combines nursing science with public health science to formulate a community-based and population-focused practice (Williams, 2000). It "synthesizes the knowledge from the public health sciences and professional nursing theories" (ANA, 1999, 2000) to improve the health of communities and vulnerable populations. For instance, community health nurses are nursing when their concern for homeless individuals sleeping in a park leads to development of a program providing food and shelter for this population. Community health nurses are nursing when they collaborate to institute an AIDS education curriculum in the local school system. When they assess the needs of elderly people in retirement homes to ensure necessary services and provide health instruction and support, they are, again, nursing.

During the first 70 years of the 20th century, community health nursing was known as **public health nursing.** The later title of community health nursing was adopted to better describe where the nurse practices. As used in this text, the terms are interchangeable.

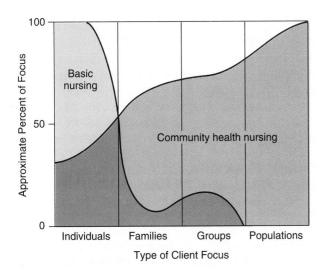

FIGURE 1–6. Difference in client focus between basic nursing and community health nursing.

Combines Public Health with Nursing

Community health nursing is grounded in both public health science and nursing science, which makes its philosophical orientation and the nature of its practice unique. It has been recognized as a subspecialty of both fields. Recognition of this specialty field continues with a greater awareness of the important contributions made by community health nursing to improve the health of the public.

Knowledge of the following elements of public health is essential to community health nursing (ANA, 1999; Williams, 1977, 2000):

1. History and philosophy of public health, including emphasis on the greatest good for the greatest number
2. Concept of aggregates—assessing needs, planning and providing services, and evaluating services' impact on population groups—including aggregate-level decision-making
3. Priority of preventive, protective, and health-promoting strategies over curative strategies
4. Means for measurement and analysis of community health problems, including epidemiologic concepts and biostatistics
5. Influence of environmental factors on aggregate health
6. Principles underlying management and organization for community health, because the goal of public health is accomplished through organized community efforts
7. Public policy analysis and development
8. Health advocacy and the political process

There are many ways in which community health nursing incorporates public health knowledge into its research and practice. For example, it is general knowledge that physical activity may contribute to important health and well-being outcomes among people of all ages. A group of nurse-researchers examined exemplars of physical activity research in nursing that illustrated the importance of physical activity research across the lifespan, and recommended directions for theory development and research. They looked at studies of physical activity and exercise currently being conducted by nurse investigators and those conducted during the past decade, searching multiple databases. What they found is that investigators have emphasized the need to evaluate the effects of theory-based physical activity interventions designed to alter key correlates of physical activity identified through descriptive research. They concluded that regular physical activity is necessary for health promotion and disease prevention for all populations and that continued research in this area of health behavior is critical to identify the most effective interventions to increase physical activity among diverse populations (Robbins et al., 2001). This gives the community health nurse valuable information about the outcomes of exercise from many well-done studies among people of various ages, races, and socioeconomic situations.

In another study, a researcher was concerned with the limited emphasis nurse educators place on the assessment and treatment of people living in violence. The Parenting Profile Assessment (PPA) tool was assessed for efficacy in assisting nurses to assess violent families. This 20-item screening tool was developed by nurses in 1985 and has since gone through additional reliability testing. Sensitivity and specificity were considered together as a measure of validity. Sensitivity is the probability that a case will be correctly identified, and specificity is the probability that a noncase will be correctly identified. In a follow-up study, estimates from 71 abusive and 71 nonabusive mothers indicated that sensitivity and specificity were 95.8% and 98.6% respectively, indicating a validity estimate of 97.18% (Anderson, 2000). This information contributed to showing that the PPA is a valid and reliable screening tool for identifying abusive behaviors. The tool can alert nurses to potential abuse when it is used along with nursing judgment and additional assessment parameters. Nurse educators can recommend this tool when students complete assessments of families they serve during a community health nursing clinical experience in homes, clinics, homeless shelters, and other settings.

Population Focused

The central mission of public health practice is to improve the health of population groups. Community health nursing shares this essential feature: it is **population focused**, meaning that it is concerned for the health status of population groups and their environment. A population may consist of the elderly living throughout the community or of southeast Asian refugees clustered in one section of a city. It may be a scattered group with common characteristics, such as people at high risk of developing coronary heart disease or battered women living throughout a county. It may include all people living in a neighborhood, district, city, state, or province. Community health nursing's specialty practice serves populations and aggregates of people.

Working with individuals and families as parts of aggregates has been common for community health nursing; however, such work must expand to incorporate a population-oriented focus, a feature that distinguishes it from other nursing specialties. Basic nursing focuses on individuals, and community health nursing focuses on aggregates, but the many variations in community needs and nursing roles inevitably cause some overlap (Display 1–3).

A population-oriented focus requires the assessment of relationships. When working with groups and communities, the nurse does not consider them separately but rather in context—that is, in relationship to the rest of the community. When an outbreak of hepatitis occurs, for example, the community health nurse does more than work with others to treat it. The nurse tries to stop the spread of the infection, locate possible sources, and prevent its recurrence in the community. As a result of their population-oriented focus, community health nurses seek to discover possible groups with a common health need, such as expectant mothers or groups at high risk for development of a common health problem (eg, potential diabetics, victims of child abuse). Community health nurses continually look for problems in the environment that influence community health and seek ways to increase environmental quality. They work to prevent health problems, such as promoting school-based education about safe sex or exercise programs for groups of seniors.

DISPLAY 1.3

Parable of the Trees: Population-Focused Practice

There were once two sisters who inherited a large tract of heavily forested land from their grandmother. In her will, the grandmother stipulated that they must preserve the health of the trees. One sister studied tree surgery and became an expert in recognizing and treating diseased trees. She also was able to spot conditions that might lead to problems and prevent them. Her work was invaluable in keeping single or small clusters of trees healthy. The other sister became a forest ranger. In addition to learning how to care for individual trees, she studied the environmental conditions that affected the well-being of the forest. She learned the importance of proper ecologic balance between flora and fauna and the impact of climate, geography, soil conditions, and weather. Her work was to oversee the health and growth of the whole forest. Although she spent time walking through the forest assessing conditions, her aerial view from their small plane was equally important for spotting fires, signs of disease, or other potential problems. Together, the sisters preserved a healthy forest.

Nursing also has tree surgeons and forest rangers. Various nursing specialties, like the tree surgeons, serve the health needs of individuals and families. Community health nurses, like the forest rangers, study and address the needs of populations. Both are needed and must work together to ensure healthy communities.

A population-oriented focus involves a new outlook and set of attitudes. Individualized care is important, but prevention of aggregate problems in community health nursing practice reflects more accurately its philosophy and benefits more people. The community or population at risk is the client. Furthermore, because community health nurses are concerned about several aggregates at the same time, service will, of necessity, be provided to multiple and overlapping groups.

Emphasizes Prevention, Health Promotion, and Wellness

In community health nursing, the promotion of health and prevention of illness are of first-order priority. There is less emphasis on curative care. Some corrective actions always are needed, such as cleanup of a toxic waste dump site, stricter enforcement of day care standards, or home care of the disabled; however, community health best serves its constituents through preventive and health-promoting actions (UDHHS, 2000). These include services to mothers and infants, prevention of environmental pollution, school health programs, senior citizens' fitness classes, and "workers' right-to-know" legislation that warns against hazards in the workplace.

Another distinguishing characteristic of community health nursing is its emphasis on positive health, or wellness (Porter-O'Grady, 2001; Clark, 2002). Medicine and acute care nursing have dealt primarily with the illness end of the health continuum. With the potential of genomics just around the corner, the wellness end of the continuum may be the focus in the near future. In contrast, community health nursing always has had a primary charge to prevent health problems from occurring and to promote a higher level of health. For example, although a community health nurse may assist a population of new mothers in the community with postpartum fatigue and depression, the nurse also works to prevent such problems among women of child-bearing age by developing health education programs, establishing prenatal classes, and encouraging proper rest and nutrition, adequate help, and stress reduction.

Community health nurses concentrate on the wellness end of the health continuum in a variety of ways. They teach proper nutrition or family planning, promote immunizations among preschool children, encourage regular physical and dental checkups, assist with starting exercise classes or physical fitness programs, and promote healthy interpersonal relationships. Their goal is to help the community reach its optimal level of wellness.

This emphasis on wellness changes the community health nursing role from a reactive to a proactive stance. It places a greater responsibility on community health nurses to find opportunities for intervention. In clinical nursing and medicine, the patients seek out professional assistance because they have health problems. As Williams put it decades ago, "patients select themselves into the care system, and the providers' role is to deal with what the patients bring to them" (1977, p. 251). Community health nurses, in contrast, seek out potential health problems. They identify high-risk groups and institute preventive programs. They watch for early signs of child neglect or abuse and intervene when any occur, often long before a request for help is made. They look for possible environmental hazards in the community, such as smoking in public places, and work with appropriate authorities to correct them. A wellness emphasis requires taking initiative and making sound judgments, which are characteristics of effective community health nursing.

Promotes Client Responsibility and Self-Care

The goal of public health, "to increase quality and years of healthy life and eliminate health disparities" (UDHHS, 2000), requires a partnership effort. Just as learning cannot take place in schools without student participation, the goals of public health cannot be realized without consumer participation. Community health nursing's efforts toward health improvement go only so far. Clients' health status and health behavior will not change unless people accept and apply the proposals (developed in collaboration with clients) presented by the community health nurse.

Community health nurses can encourage individuals' participation by promoting their autonomy rather than permitting a dependency. For example, elderly persons attending a series of nutrition or fitness classes can be encouraged to take the initiative and develop health or social programs on their own. Independence and feelings of self-worth are closely related. By treating people as independent adults, with trust and respect, community health nurses help promote self-reliance and the ability to function independently.

Consumers frequently are intimidated by health professionals and are uninformed about health and health care. They do not know what information to seek and are hesitant to act assertively. For example, a migrant worker brought her 2-year-old son, who had symptoms resembling those of scurvy, to a clinic. Recognizing a vitamin C deficiency, the physician told her to feed the boy large quantities of orange juice but gave no explanation. Several weeks later, she returned; the child was much worse. After questioning her, the nurse discovered that the mother had been feeding the child large amounts of an orange soft drink, not knowing the difference between that and orange juice. Obviously, the quality of care is affected when the consumer does not understand and cannot participate in the health care process.

When people believe that their health, and that of the community, is their own responsibility, not just that of health professionals, they will take a more active interest in promoting it. The process of taking responsibility for developing one's own health potential is called **self-care**, a concept discussed in Chapter 19. As people maintain their own lives, health, and well-being, they are engaging in self-care. Some examples of self-care activities at the aggregate level include building safe playgrounds, developing teen employment opportunities, and providing senior exercise programs.

When people's ability to continue self-care activities drops below their need, they experience a **self-care deficit**. At this point, nursing may appropriately intervene. However,

nursing's goal is to assist clients to return to or reach a level of functioning at which they can attain optimal health and assume responsibility for maintaining it (Orem, 2001). To this end, community health nurses foster their clients' sense of responsibility by treating them as adults capable of managing their own affairs. Nurses can encourage people to negotiate health care goals and practices, develop their own programs, contact their own resources (eg, support groups, transportation services), identify and implement lifestyle changes that promote wellness, and learn ways to monitor their own health.

Uses Aggregate Measurement and Analysis

Community health nursing uses aggregate measurement and analysis. The need to collect and examine data on the entire population under study before making intervention decisions is fundamental to community health nursing in a public health practice. Health states, environmental factors, health-related services, economic patterns, and social policy are among the many foci of community health research and evaluation, described further in Chapters 14 and 19.

Uses Principles of Organizational Theory

Community health nursing uses principles from organizational theory to provide effective administration of health care services. Public health has long been defined as the protection and improvement of community health through organized community efforts. It is the organization and administration of such services that enables practitioners to ultimately address community needs. Chapter 6 elaborates on this subject.

As community health nurses carefully assess group and community needs, establish priorities, and plan, implement, and evaluate services, they are using public health management and organizational principles. For example, Goldsmith (2001) writes about the role of communication technology in health care among professionals and consumers, bringing health information into every corner of the United States. The World Wide Web and other telecommunication devices contribute to access to care and information. Even by 1999, 70 million Americans used the Internet to seek health information. Today the numbers are much larger.

Community health nurses have used technology in rural areas for many years. For example, in Lawrence, Kansas, the Home-Based Electronic Link to Professionals allows nurses to use interactive televideo (ITV) to monitor chronically ill patients, guide caregivers in performing tasks, and educate and support patients and families without being physically present in the home. A hospice project uses low-end ITV equipment, which runs through a patient's television over regular telephone lines, to enable hospice nurses to be available for terminally ill patients and their families. Other programs use community education courses, delivered through ITV, to enhance participation from rural students in academic course work and for consumer health education. Consumers have access to programs on diabetes, Alzheimer disease, coping with cancer, attention deficit disorders, and weight management. Also, they can interact with health care professionals hundreds of miles away from their rural homes.

Involves Interprofessional Collaboration

Community health nurses must work in cooperation with other team members, coordinating services and addressing the needs of population groups. This interprofessional **collaboration** among health care workers, other professionals, and clients is essential for establishing effective services and programs. Individualized efforts and specialized programs, when planned in isolation, can lead to fragmentation and gaps in health services. For example, without collaboration, a well-child clinic may be started in a community that already has a strong early and periodic developmental screening and testing program, yet community prenatal services may be nonexistent. Interprofessional collaboration is important in individualized practice, because nurses need to plan with the client, family, physician, social worker, physical therapist, teacher, or counselor and must keep them informed of the client's health status; however, it is a greater necessity when working with population groups (Corrigan, 2000).

Effective collaboration requires team members who are strong individuals with various areas of expertise and who can make a commitment to team goals. Community health nurses who think and act interdependently make a great contribution to the team effort. In appropriate situations, community health nurses also function autonomously, making independent judgments. Collaboration involves working with members of other professions on community advisory boards and health planning committees to develop needs assessment surveys and contribute toward policy development efforts.

Interprofessional collaboration requires clarification of each team member's role, a primary reason for community health nurses to understand the nature of their practice. When planning a city-wide immunization program with a community group, for example, community health nurses need to explain the ways that they might contribute to the program's objectives. They can offer to contact key community leaders, with whom they have established relationships, to build community acceptance of the program. They can share their knowledge of the public's preference about times and locations for the program. They can help to organize and give the immunizations, and they can influence planning for follow-up programs. Collaboration is discussed further in Chapter 11.

Client participation is promoted when people serve as partners on the health care team. An aim of community health nursing is to collaborate with people rather than do things for them. As consumers of health services are treated with respect and trust and, as a result, gain confidence and skill in self-care—promoting their own health and that of their community—their contribution to health programs becomes increasingly valuable. The consumer perspective in planning and delivering health services makes those services relevant to consumer needs. Community health nurses encourage the involvement of health care consumers by soliciting their ideas and opinions, by inviting them to participate on health boards and committees, and by finding ways to promote their participation in decisions affecting their collective health.

SUMMARY

Community health nursing has opportunities and challenges to keep the nurse interested and involved in a community-focused career for a lifetime. Community health is more than environmental programs and large-scale efforts to control communicable disease. It is defined as the identification of needs and the protection and improvement of collective health within a geographically defined area. To comprehend the nature and significance of community health and to clarify its meaning for the specialty practice of community health nursing, it is important to understand the concepts of community and of health.

A community, broadly defined, is a collection of people who share some common interest or goal. There are three types: geographic, common-interest, and health problem-solving communities. Sometimes, a community such as a neighborhood, city, or county is formed by geographic boundaries. At other times, a community may be identified by its common interest; examples are a religious community, a group of migrant workers, or citizens concerned about air pollution. A community also is defined by a pooling of efforts by people and agencies toward solving a health-related problem.

Health is an abstract concept that can be understood more clearly by examining its distinguishing features. First, people are neither sick nor well in an absolute sense but have levels of illness or wellness. These levels may be plotted along a continuum ranging from optimal health to total disability or death. This is known as the health continuum. A person's state of health is dynamic, varying from day to day and even hour to hour.

Second, health is a state of being that includes all of the many characteristics of a person, family, or community, whether physical, psychological, social, or spiritual. These characteristics often indicate the degree of wellness or illness of an individual or community and suggest the presence or absence of vitality and well-being.

Third, health has both subjective and objective dimensions: the subjective involves how well people feel; the objective refers to how well they are able to function. Most often, functional performance diminishes dramatically toward the illness end of the health continuum.

Fourth, health care needs can be either continuing, as in developmental concerns that occur over a person's lifetime, or episodic, occurring unexpectedly once or twice in a lifetime. Community health nursing deals with continuing needs, whereas episodic needs are managed in acute care settings.

Community health practice incorporates six basic elements: (1) promotion of health, (2) prevention of health problems, (3) treatment of disorders, (4) rehabilitation, (5) evaluation, and (6) research.

The eight important characteristics of community health practice are the following: (1) it is a field of nursing; (2) it combines public health with nursing; (3) it is population focused; (4) it emphasizes prevention, health promotion, and wellness; (5) it promotes client responsibility and self-care; (6) it uses aggregate measurement and analysis; (7) it uses principles of organizational theory; and (8) it involves interprofessional collaboration.

ACTIVITIES TO PROMOTE CRITICAL THINKING

1. Identify a community of people about whom you have some knowledge. What makes it a community? What characteristics do this group of people share? Work on this activity in a group of peers or family members. Do they think as you do? Is there a difference between the views of family members and those of nursing student peers?

2. Select three populations for whom you have some concern, and place each group on the health continuum. What factors influenced your decision?

3. Describe three preventive actions (one primary, one secondary, and one tertiary) that might be taken to move each of your selected populations closer to optimal wellness.

4. Select a current health problem and identify the three levels of prevention and corresponding activities in which you as a community health nurse would engage in at each level.

5. Discuss how you might implement one health-promotion effort with each of your selected populations.

6. Browse the Internet for community health nursing research articles that focus on levels of prevention. Find one focusing on each level. For those involved in the articles focusing on secondary and tertiary prevention, what could you as a community health nurse have done to have kept the clients at the primary level of prevention?

7. Place yourself on the health continuum. What factors influenced your decision?

8. Using the eight characteristics of community health nursing outlined in this chapter, give examples of how a community health nurse might demonstrate meeting each characteristic.

REFERENCES

Allison, J., Kiefe, C., & Weissman, N.W. (1999). Can data-driven benchmarks be used to set the goals of Healthy People 2010? *American Journal of Public Health, 89*(1), 61–65.

American Nurses Association. (1999). *Scope and standards of public health nursing practice*. Washington, DC: American Nurses Publishing.

American Nurses Association. (2000). *Public health nursing: A partner for healthy populations*. Washington, DC: American Nurses Publishing.

Anderson, C.A. (2000). Revisiting the Parenting Profile Assessment to screen for child abuse. *Journal of Nursing Scholarship, 32*(1), 53.

Barton, P.L. (1999). *Understanding the U. S. health service system*. Chicago: AUPHA Press.

Beckerman, A.G. & Tappen, R. (2000). *It takes more than love: A practical guide to taking care of an aging adult*. Baltimore: Health Professions Press.

Berg, K., Hines, M., & Allen, S. (2002). Wheelchair users at home: Few home modifications and many injurious falls. *American Journal of Public Health, 92*(2), 48.

Berkman, A. (2001). Confronting global AIDS: Prevention and treatment. *American Journal of Public Health, 91*(9), 1348–1349.

Brownson, R.C., Baker, E.A., & Novick, L.F. (1999). *Community-based prevention: Programs that work*. Gaithersberg, MD: Aspen.

Clark, C.C. (2002). *Health promotion in communities: Holistic and wellness approaches*. New York: Springer.

Corrigan, D. (2000). The changing role of schools and higher education institutions with respect to community-based interagency collaboration and interprofessional partnerships. *Peabody Journal of Education, 75*(3), 176–195.

Cottrell, L.S., Jr. (1976). The competent community. In B.H. Kaplan, R.N. Wilson, & A.H. Leighton (Es.), *Further explorations in social psychiatry*. New York: Basic Books.

Davis, L.L., Broome, M.E., & Cox, R.P. (2001). Maximizing retention in community-based clinical trials. *Journal of Nursing Scholarship, 34*(1), 47–53.

Flynn, B.C. (1998). Communicating with the public: Community-based nursing research and practice. *Public Health Nursing, 15*(3), 165–170.

French, S.A., Jeffery, R.W., Story, M., Breitlow, K.K., Baxter, J.S., Hannan, P., et al. (2001). Pricing and promotion effects on low-fat vending snack purchases: The CHIPS Study. *American Journal of Public Health, 91*(1), 112–117.

Gaffney, K.F. (2001). Infant exposure to environmental tobacco smoke. *Journal of Nursing Scholarship, 33*(4), 343–347.

Galavotti, C., Pappas-DeLucca, K.A., & Lansky, A. (2001). Modeling and reinforcement to combat HIV: The MARCH approach to behavior change. *American Journal of Public Health, 91*(10), 1602–1607.

Gantt, C.J. (2001). The theory of planned behavior and postpartum smoking relapse. *Journal of Nursing Scholarship, 33*(4), 337–341.

Goldmith, J. (2001). How will the Internet change our health system? In E.C. Hein (Ed.), *Nursing issues in the 21st century: Perspectives from the literature* (pp. 295–308). Philadelphia: Lippincott, Williams & Wilkins.

Institute of Medicine. (2001). *Clearing the smoke: Assessing the science base for tobacco harm reduction.* Washington, DC: National Academy Press.

Jha, P., Dphil, M., Ranson, K., Nguyen, S.N., & Yach, D. (2002). Estimates of global and regional smoking revalence in 1995, by age and sex. *American Journal of Public Health, 92*(6), 1002–1006.

Keane, A., Houldin, A.D., Allison, P.D., Jepson, C., Shults, J., Nuamah, I.F., et al. (2002). Factors associated with distress in urban residential fire survivors. *Journal of Nursing Scholarship, 34*(1), 11–17.

Kriebel, D., & Tickner, J. (2001). Reenergizing public health through precaution. *American Journal of Public Health, 91*(9), 1351–1354.

McGrady, G.A., & Pederson, L.L. (2002). Do sex and ethnic difference in smoking initiation mask similarities in cessation behavior? *American Journal of Public Health, 92*(6), 961–965.

Moser, D., Dracup, K., & Doering, L. (2000). Factors differentiating dropouts from completers in a longitudinal, multicenter clinical trial. *Nursing Research, 49*(2), 9–116.

Neuman, B. (2001). The Neuman systems model. In B. Neuman (Ed.), *The Neuman systems model* (4th ed.). Norwalk, CT: Appleton & Lange.

Nightingale, F. (1859/1992). Notes on nursing: What it is, and what it is not [Commemorative edition]. Philadelphia: Lippincott.

Nordstrom, B.L., Kinnunen, T., Utman, C.H., Krall, E.A., Vokonas, P.S., & Garvey, A.J. (2000). Predictors of continued smoking over 25 years of follow-up in the normative aging study. *American Journal of Public Health, 90*(3), 404–406.

Orem, D. (2001). *Nursing concepts of practice* (6th ed.). St. Louis: Mosby-Year Book.

Pender, N.J. (2001). *Health promotion in nursing practice* (4th ed.). Norwalk, CT: Appleton & Lange.

Pickett, G.E., & Hanlon, J.J. (1990). *Public health administration and practice* (9th ed.). St. Louis: Times Mirror-Mosby.

Pollack, H.A. (2001). Sudden infant death syndrome, maternal smoking during pregnancy, and the cost-effectiveness of smoking cessation intervention. *American Journal of Public Health, 91*(3), 432–436.

Porter-O'Grady, T. (2001). Profound change: 21st century nursing. *Nursing Outlook, 49*(4), 182–186.

Roach, S.S. (2000). *Introductory gerontological nursing.* Philadelphia: Lippincott Williams & Wilkins.

Robbins, L.B., Pender, N.J., Conn, V.S., Frenn, M.D., Neuberger, G.B., Nies, M.A., et al. (2001). Physical activity research in nursing. *Journal of Nursing Scholarship, 33*(4), 315–321.

Rockhill, B., Willett, W.C., Manson, J.E., Leitzmann, M.F., Stampfer, M.J., Hunter, D.J., et al. (2001). Physical activity and mortality: A prospective study among women. *American Journal of Public Health, 91*(4), 578–583.

Segui-Gomez, M., Wittenberg, E., Glass, R., Levenson, S., Hingson, R., & Graham, J.D. (2002). Where children sit in cars: The impact of Rhode Island's new legislation. *American Journal of Public Health, 91*(2), 311–313.

Sorensen, G., Stoddard, A., Peterson, K., Cohn, N., Hunt, M.K., Stein, E., et al. (1999). Increasing fruit and vegetable consumption through worksites and families in the Treatwell 5-a-Day Study. *American Journal of Public Health, 89*(1), 54–60.

Spector, R.E. (2000). *Cultural diversity in health and illness* (5th ed.). Upper Saddle River, NJ: Prentice-Hall Health.

Stone, R.I. (2000). *Long-term care for the elderly with disabilities: Current policy, emerging trends, and implications for the twenty-first century.* New York: Milbank Memorial Fund.

Turnock, B.J. (1997). *Public health: What it is and how it works.* Gaithersburg, MD: Aspen.

U.S. Department of Health and Human Services. (2000). *Healthy People 2010* (Conference ed., in two volumes). Washington, DC: U.S. Government Printing Office.

Venes, D. (Ed.). (2001). *Taber's cyclopedic medical dictionary* (19th ed.). Philadelphia: F.A. Davis.

Wang, P.S., Demler, O., & Kessler, R.C. (2002). Adequacy of treatment for serious mental illness in the United States. *American Journal of Public Health, 92*(1), 92–98.

Williams, C. (1977). Community health nursing: What is it? *Nursing Outlook, 25*(4), 250–254.

Williams, C. (2000). Community-based population-focused practice: The foundation of specialization in public health nursing. In M. Stanhope & J. Lancaster (Eds.). Community health nursing: Process and practice for promoting health (5th ed.), St. Louis: Mosby.

Wurzbach, M.E. (2002). *Community health education and promotion: A guide to program design and evaluation.* Gaithersburg, MD: Aspen.

SELECTED READINGS

Baldwin, J.H., Conger, C.O., Abegglen, J.C., & Hill, E.M. (1998). Population-focused and community-based nursing: Moving toward clarification of concepts. *Public Health Nursing, 15*(1), 12–18.

Black, D.R., Tobler, N.S., & Sciacca, J.P. (1998). Peer helping/involvement: An efficacious way to meet the challenge of reducing alcohol, tobacco, and other drug use among youth? *Journal of School Health, 68*(3), 87–93.

Chaudry, R.V., Polivka, B.J., & Kennedy, C.W. (2000). Public health nursing directors' perceptions regarding interagency collaboration with community mental health agencies. *Public Health Nursing, 17*(2), 75–84.

Coile, R.C., & Trusko, B.E. (2001). Healthcare: Technology in the new millennium. In E.C.Hein (Ed.), *Nursing issues in the 21st century: Perspectives from the literature* (pp. 291–294). Philadelphia: Lippincott Williams & Wilkins.

Hinshaw, A.S. (2000). Nursing knowledge for the 21st century: Opportunities and challenges. *Journal of Nursing Scholarship, 32*(2), 117–123.

Hornsby, P.J. (2000). Cell transplantation and aging. *Generations, 24*(1), 54–57.

Keller, L.O., Strohschein, S., Lia-Hoagberg, B., & Schaffer, M. (1998). Population-based public health nursing interventions: A model from practice. *Public Health Nursing, 15*(3), 207–215.

Kiefe, C.I., Weissman, N.W., Allison, J.J., Farmer, R.M., Weaver, M., & Williams, O.D. (1998). Identifying achievable benchmarks of care (ABCs): Concepts and methodology. *International Journal of Quality Health Care, 10*, 443–447.

Khoury, M.J., Burke, W., & Thompson, E.J. (2000). *Genetics and public health in the 21st century: Using genetic information to improve health and prevent disease.* New York: Oxford University Press.

Jones, J., & Moore, S.M. (2001). Telehealth: Can nursing values be preserved? Point-Counterpoint. In H.R. Feldman (Ed.), *Nursing leaders speak out: Issues and opinions* (pp 55–61). New York: Springer.

Mo-Im, K. (2000). Meeting the challenges of the 21st century. *Journal of Nursing Scholarship, 32*(1), 7–9.

Novick, L.F., & Mays, G.P. (Eds.). (2000). *Public health administration: Principles for population-based management.* Gaithersburg, MD: Aspen.

Roberts, P. (2001). Electronic media and the tie that binds. *Generations, 25*(2), 96–98.

Schneiderman, N., Speers, M.A., Silva, J.M., Tomes, H., & Gentry, J.H. (Eds.). (2001). *Integrating behavioral and social sciences with public health.* Washington, DC: American Psychologial Association.

Sharpe, C.C. (2001). *Telenursing: Nursing practice in cyberspace.* Westport, CT: Auburn House.

Shinitzky, H.E., & Kub, J. (2001). The art of motivating behavior change: The use of motivational interviewing to promote health. *Public Health Nursing, 18*(3), 178–185.

Somerville, M.A. (1998). Making health, not war: Musings on global disparities in health and human rights. A critical commentary by Solomon R. Benatar. *American Journal of Public Health, 88*(2), 301–303.

Sullivan, M., & Kelly, J.G. (2001). *Collaborative research: University and community partnership.* Washington, DC: American Public Health Association.

The Future of Children (2000, Fall/Winter). Five commentaries: Looking to the future. *Children and Computer Technology, 10*(2), 168–180.

2

Evolution of Community Health Nursing

Key Terms

- Causal thinking
- Community-based nursing
- District nursing

Learning Objectives

Upon mastery of this chapter, you should be able to:

- Describe the four stages of community health nursing's development.
- Analyze the impact of societal influences on the development and practice of community health nursing.
- Recognize the contributions of selected nursing leaders throughout history to the advancement of community health nursing.
- Explore the academic and advanced professional preparation of community health nurses.

We believe that the story of the evolution of community health nursing—complete with its heroines, antagonists, battlefields, epidemics, plot twists, setbacks, and triumphs—is as exciting as any novel. And we hope that this brief overview of this fascinating story will inspire you to meet the challenges awaiting you in your own community health experience and to seize your opportunity to enrich the heritage of earlier public health nursing efforts.

This chapter examines the international roots of community health nursing as a specialty. The historical and philosophical foundations of community health nursing that undergird the dynamic nature of its practice are explored. First, the chapter traces community health nursing's historical development as a specialty practice, highlighting the contributions of several nursing leaders. Next, it describes the global societal influences that shaped early and evolving community health nursing practice. Finally, the chapter describes the academic and advanced professional preparation required of community health nurses today. Nursing's past influences its present, and both guide the future of community health nursing in the 21st century.

HISTORICAL DEVELOPMENT OF COMMUNITY HEALTH NURSING

Before the nature of community health nursing can be fully grasped or its practice defined, it is necessary to understand its roots and the factors that shaped its growth over time. Community health nursing is the product of centuries of responsiveness and growth. Its practice has adapted to accommodate the needs of a changing society, yet it has always maintained its initial goal of improved community health. Community health nursing's development, which has been influenced by changes in nursing, public health, and society, can be traced through several stages. This section examines these stages.

The history of public health nursing, since its recognized inception in Europe, and more recently in America, encompasses continuing change and adaptation (Hein, 2001). The historical record reveals a professional nursing specialty that has been on the cutting edge of innovations in public health practice and has provided leadership to public health efforts. A summary of public health nursing made in the early 1900s still holds true:

It is precisely in the field of the application of knowledge that the public health nurse has found her great opportunity and her greatest usefulness. In the nationwide campaigns for the early detection of cancer and mental disorders, for the elimination of venereal disease, for the training of new mothers and the teaching of the principles of hygiene to young and old; in short, in all measures for the prevention of disease and the raising of health standards, no agency is more valuable than the public health nurse

(Central Hanover Bank and Trust Company, 1938, p. 8).

In tracing the development of public health nursing and, later, community health nursing, the leadership role clearly has been evident throughout its history. Nurses in this specialty have provided leadership in planning and developing programs, in shaping policy, in administration, and in the application of research to community health.

Four general stages mark the development of public health/community health nursing: (1) the early home care nursing stage, (2) the district nursing stage, (3) the public health nursing stage, and (4) the community health nursing stage.

Early Home Care Nursing (Before Mid-1800s)

Within the historical development of home care nursing, the prototype of **community-based nursing** can be seen; the term is used to describe the setting for nursing care delivery. For many centuries, the sick were tended at home by female family members and friends. In fact, in 1837 Farrar (p. 57) reminded women, "You may be called upon at any moment to attend upon your parents, your brothers, your sisters, or your companions." The focus of this care was to reduce suffering and promote healing. The Bible cites numerous instances of visiting the sick and extols a woman of noble character as one who "opens her arms to the poor and extends her hands to the needy" (Proverbs 31:20) and who is "a helper of many," as Phoebe was described in the New Testament (Romans 16:2).

The early roots of home care nursing began with religious and charitable groups. Even emergency care was provided. In 1244, a group of monks in Florence, Italy, known as the Misericordia provided first-aid care for accident victims on a 24-hour basis. Another example is the Knights Hospitallers, who were warrior monks in western Europe. They protected and cared for pilgrims on their way to Jerusalem ("Men, Monasteries, Wars and Wards," 2001).

Medieval times saw the development of various institutions devoted to the sick, including hospitals and nursing orders. In England, the Elizabethan Poor Law, written in 1601, provided medical and nursing care to the poor and disabled. Another example was the Friendly Visitor Volunteers organized by St. Frances de Sales in the early 1600s in France. This association was directed by Madame de Chantel and assisted by wealthy women who cared for the sick poor in their homes (Dolan, 1978). In Paris, St. Vincent de Paul started the Sisters of Charity in 1617, an organization composed of nuns and lay women dedicated to serving the poor and needy. The ladies and sisters, under the supervision of Mademoiselle Le Gras in 1634, promoted the goal of teaching people to help themselves as they visited the sick in their homes. In their emphasis on preparing nurses and supervising nursing care, as well as determining causes and solutions for clients' problems, the Sisters of Charity laid a foundation for modern community health nursing (Bullough & Bullough, 1978).

Unfortunately, the years that followed these accomplishments marked a serious setback in the status of nursing and care of the sick. From the late 1600s to the mid-1800s, the social upheaval after the Reformation caused a decline in the number of religious orders, with subsequent curtailing of nursing care for the sick poor. Babies continued to be delivered at home by self-declared midwives, most of whom had little or no training. Concern over high maternal mortality rates prompted efforts to better prepare midwives and medical students. One midwifery program was begun in Paris in 1720 and another in London by Dr. William Smellie in 1741.

The Industrial Revolution created additional problems; among them were epidemics, high infant mortality, occupational diseases and injuries, and increasing mental illness in both Europe and America. Hospitals were built in larger cities, and dispensaries were developed to provide greater access to physicians. However, disease was rampant, mortality rates were high, and institutional conditions, especially in prisons, hospitals, and "asylums" for the insane, were deplorable. The sick and afflicted were kept in filthy rooms without adequate food, water, cover, or care for their physical and emotional needs (Bullough & Bullough, 1978). Reformers such as John Howard, an Englishman who investigated the spread of disease in prisons and hospitals in 1779, revealed serious needs that would not be addressed until much later.

Both Catholic and Anglican religious nursing orders, although few, continued their work of caring for the sick poor in their homes. For example, in 1812, the Sisters of Mercy organized in Dublin to provide care for the sick at home. Generally, however, with the status of women at an all-time low, often only the least respectable women pursued nursing. In 1844, in his novel *Martin Chuzzlewit,* Charles Dickens portrayed the nurse Sairy Gamp as an unschooled and slovenly drunkard, reflecting society's view of nursing at the time. It was in the midst of these deplorable conditions and in response to them that Florence Nightingale began her work.

Much of the foundation for modern community health nursing practice was laid through Florence Nightingale's remarkable accomplishments (Fig. 2–1). She has been referred to as a reformer, a reactionary, and a researcher (Palmer, 2001). Born in 1820 into a wealthy English family, her extensive travel, excellent education—including training at the first school for nurses in Kaiserwerth, Germany—and determination to serve the needy resulted in major reforms and improved status for nursing. Her work during the Crimean War (1854–1856) with the wounded in Scutari is well documented (Woodham-Smith, 1951; Florence Nightingale Museum, 1997). Conditions in the military hospitals during the war were unspeakable. Thousands of sick and wounded men lay in filth, without beds, clean coverings, food, water, or laundry facilities. Florence Nightingale organized competent nursing care and established kitchens and laundries that resulted in hundreds of lives being saved. Her work further demonstrated that capable nursing intervention could prevent illness and improve the health of a population at risk—

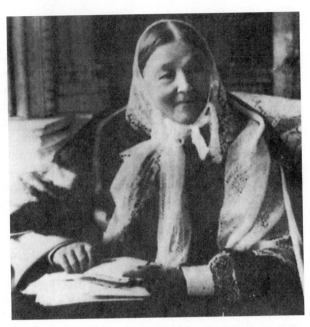

FIGURE 2–1. Florence Nightingale's concern for populations at risk as well as her vision and successful efforts at health reform provided a model for community health nursing today.

precursors to modern community health nursing practice. Her subsequent work for health reform in the military was supported by implementing another public health strategy: the use of biostatistics. Through meticulously gathered data and statistical comparisons, Miss Nightingale demonstrated that military mortality rates, even in peacetime, were double those of the civilian population because of the terrible living conditions in the barracks. This work led to important military reforms.

Miss Nightingale's concern for populations at risk included a continuing interest in the population of the sick at home. Her book, *Notes on Nursing: What It Is, and What It Is Not,* published in England in 1859, was written to improve nursing care in the home.

Florence Nightingale also became a skillful lobbyist for health care reform. Her exemplary influence on English politics and policy improved the quality of existing health care and set standards for future practice. Furthermore, she demonstrated how population-focused nursing works.

In her work to help establish the first nonreligious school for nurses in 1860 at St. Thomas Hospital in London, she promoted a standard for proper education and supervision of nurses in practice, known as the Nightingale Model. Principles she wrote about in *Notes on Nursing* relate directly to her early education and the notions held by Hippocrates in ancient Greece, which she had studied for years. Specifically, her concern with the environment of patients, the need for keen observation, the focus on the whole patient rather than the disease, and the importance of assisting nature to bring about a cure all reflect Hippocrates' teachings (Nightingale, 1859; Palmer, 2001).

Another great nurse and healer in her own right was Mary Seacole (1805–1881). She has been called the "Black Nightingale." She was the daughter of a well-respected "doctress" who practiced Creole or Afro-Caribbean medicine in Jamaica. She began by helping her mother at an early age and spent many years developing her skills. She helped populations who experienced tropical diseases, especially cholera, in Central America, Panama, and the Caribbean. She attempted, through many formal channels, to join Florence Nightingale in Scutari and was rejected again and again. Undaunted, she went to the Crimea on her own to open a hotel for sick and convalescing soldiers, where she met Miss Nightingale and many of the troops she had cared for in Jamaica. Many of the military commanders sought her out for her knowledge of healing, and she was affectionately known by the troops as "Mother Seacole." After the war and into her old age, she continued to provide nursing care in London and when visiting Jamaica. She focused her caregiving among high-risk clients of the day and did so in an innovative, entrepreneurial manner unique for women, especially for women of color in the 1800s (Florence Nightingale Museum, 1997).

District Nursing (Mid-1800s to 1900)

The next stage in the development of community health nursing was the formal organization of visiting nursing, or **district nursing**. In 1859, William Rathbone, an English philanthropist, became convinced of the value of home nursing as a result of private care given to his wife. He employed Mary Robinson, the nurse who had cared for his wife, to visit the sick poor in their homes and teach them proper hygiene to prevent illness. The need was so great, it soon became evident that more nurses were needed. In 1861, with Florence Nightingale's help and advice, Rathbone opened a training school for nurses connected with the Royal Liverpool Infirmary and established a visiting nurse service for the sick poor in Liverpool. Florence Lees, a graduate of the Nightingale School, was appointed first Superintendent-General of the District Nursing System (Mowbray, 1997). As the service grew, visiting nurses were assigned to districts in the city—hence the name, district nursing. Subsequently, other British cities also developed district nursing training and services. An example is the Nurse Training Institution for district nurses, founded in Manchester in 1864. Privately financed, the nurses were trained and then "dispensed food and medicine" to the sick poor in their homes; they were "closely supervised by various middle and upper class women who collected the necessary supplies" (Bullough & Bullough, 1978, p. 143).

Although Florence Nightingale is best remembered for her professionalization of nursing, she had a full understanding of the need for community health nursing. This was documented in her writings and recorded conversations:

Hospitals are but an intermediate stage of civilisation. At present hospitals are the only

place where the sick poor can be nursed, or, indeed often the sick rich. But the ultimate object is to nurse all sick at home (Nightingale, 1876).

The aim of the district nurse is to give first rate nursing to the sick poor at home (Nightingale, 1876 [cited in Mowbray, 1997, p. 24]).

The health visitor must create a new profession for women (conversation with Frederick Verney, 1891 [cited in Mowbray, 1997, p. 25]).

For years, Miss Nightingale studied the social and economic conditions of India (Nightingale, 1864). The plight of the poor and ill in India led her to become involved with Frederick Verney in a pioneering "health at home" project in England in 1892. She wrote a series of papers on the need for "home missioners" and "health visitors," endorsing the view that prevention was better than cure (Mowbray, 1997).

In the United States, the first community health nurse, Frances Root, hired by the Women's Board of the New York Mission in 1877, pioneered home visits to the poor in New York City. District nursing associations were founded in Buffalo in 1885 and in Boston and Philadelphia in 1886. These district associations served the sick poor exclusively, because patients with enough money had private home nursing care. However, the English model with its standards for visiting nurses' education and practice, established in 1889 under Queen Victoria, was not followed in the United States. Instead, visiting nursing organizations sprang up in many cities without common standards or administration. Twenty-one such services existed in the United States in 1890.

Although district nurses primarily cared for the sick, they also taught cleanliness and wholesome living to their patients, even in that early period. One example was the Boston program, founded by the Women's Educational Association, which "emphasized the teaching of hygiene and cleanliness, giving impetus to what was called instructive district nursing" (Bullough & Bullough, 1978, p. 144). This early emphasis on prevention and "health" nursing became one of the distinguishing features of district nursing and, later, of public health nursing as a specialty.

The work of district nurses in the United States focused mostly on the care of individuals. District nurses recorded temperatures and pulse rates and gave simple treatments to the sick poor under the immediate direction of a physician. They also instructed family members in personal hygiene, diet and healthful living habits, and the care of the sick. The problems of early home care patients in the United States were numerous and complex. Thousands of European and eastern European immigrants filled tenement housing in the poorest and most crowded slums of the large coastal cities during the late 1800s. Inadequate sanitation, unsafe and unhealthy working conditions, and language and cultural barriers added to poverty and disease. Nursing educational programs at that time did not prepare district nurses to cope with their patients' multiple health and social problems.

The sponsorship of district nursing changed over time. Early district nursing services in both England and the United States were founded by religious organizations. Later, sponsorship shifted to private philanthropy. Funding came from contributions and, in a few instances, from fees charged to patients on an ability-to-pay basis. Finally, visiting nursing began to be supported by public money. An early example occurred in Los Angeles where, in 1897, a nurse was hired as a city employee. Although one form of funding dominated, all three types of financing continued to exist, as they still do. Although the government was beginning to assume more responsibility for the public's health, most district nursing services during this time remained private.

In England, the establishment of "health visitors" in poor areas of London began early in the 19th century. These health care providers enhanced the English model of health visitor/district nurse/midwife as the backbone of the primary health care system in the second half of the 1800s. "The impact of early health visiting was clearly shown by the halving of infant mortality in the areas within two years" (Beine, 1996, p. 59). The main focus of the health visitor's work was giving advice to poor mothers and teaching hygiene to prevent infant diarrhea (Beine, 1996).

Public Health Nursing (1900 to 1970)

By the beginning of the 20th century, district nursing had broadened its focus to include the health and welfare of the general public, not just the poor. This new emphasis was part of a broader consciousness about public health. Robert Koch's demonstration that tuberculosis was communicable led the Johns Hopkins Hospital to hire a nurse, Reba Thelin, in 1903 to visit the homes of tuberculosis patients. Her job was to ensure that patients followed prescribed regimens of rest, fresh air, and proper diet and to prevent possible infection (Sachs, 1908). A growing sense of urgency about the interrelatedness of health conditions and the need to improve the health of all people led to an increased number of private health agencies. These agencies supplemented the often-limited work of government health departments. By 1910, new federal laws made states and communities accountable for the health of their citizens.

Specialized programs such as infant welfare, tuberculosis clinics, and venereal disease control were developed, causing a demand for nurses to work in these areas (Fig. 2–2). As Bullough and Bullough commented, "Although the hospital nursing school movement emphasized the care of the sick, a small but growing number of nurses were finding employment in preventive health care" (1978, p. 143). In

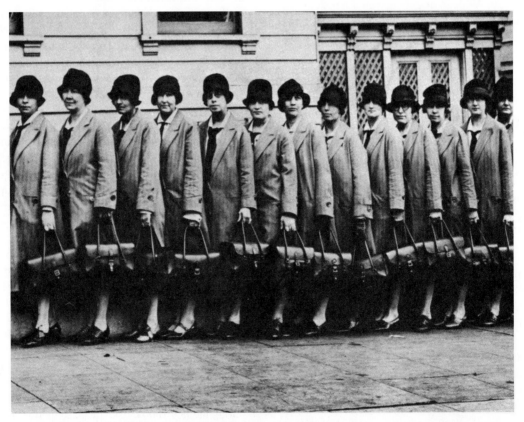

F I G U R E 2 - 2 .   Public health nurses—uniforms and symbols. (Photograph courtesy of Visiting Nurses and Hospice of San Francisco.)

1900, there were an estimated 200 public health nurses. By 1912, that number had grown to 3000 (Gardner, 1936). "This development was important: it brought health care and health teaching to the public, gave nurses an opportunity for more independent work, and helped to improve nursing education" (Bullough & Bullough, 1978, p. 143).

The role of the district nurse expanded during this stage. Lillian D. Wald (1867–1940), a leading figure in this expansion, first used the term "public health nursing" to describe this specialty (Bullough & Bullough, 1978). District nurses, while caring for the sick, had pioneered in health teaching, disease prevention, and promotion of good health practices. Now, with a growing recognition of familial and environmental influences on health, public health nurses broadened their practice even more. Nurses working outside of the hospital increased their knowledge and skills in specialized areas such as tuberculosis, maternal and child health, school health, and mental disorders.

Lillian Wald's contributions to public health nursing were enormous. A graduate of the New York Hospital Training School, she started teaching home nursing but quickly changed to a career of social reform and nursing activism (Christy, 1970). Appalled by the conditions of an immigrant neighborhood in New York's Lower East Side, she and a nurse-friend, Mary Brewster, started the Henry Street Settlement in 1893 to provide nursing and welfare services. Her books, *The House on Henry Street* (1915) and *Windows of Henry Street* (1934), portray her work and views on public health nursing. Nursing visits conducted through her organization were supervised by nurses, in contrast to earlier models, in which nursing services were administered by lay

boards and actual care was supervised by lay persons. Demonstrating that nursing could reduce illness-caused absenteeism, Wald convinced the New York City Board of Education in 1902 to hire the first school nurse in the United States, Lina Rogers. Her suggestion that nurse intervention could reduce death rates resulted in the Metropolitan Life Insurance Company's starting a visiting nurse service for policy holders in 1909 (Christy, 1970).

The legendary accomplishments of Lillian Wald reflect her driving commitment to serve needy populations. Through her efforts, the New York City Bureau of Child Hygiene was formed in 1908 and the Children's Bureau at the federal level in 1912 (Fig. 2–3). Wald's emphasis on illness prevention and health promotion through health teaching and nursing intervention, as well as her use of epidemiologic methodology, established these actions as hallmarks of public health nursing practice. She promoted rural nursing and family-focused nursing and encouraged improved coursework at the Teachers College of Columbia University (New York) to prepare public health nurses for practice. Through her work and influence with the legislature to establish health and social policies, improvements were made in child labor and pure food laws, tenement housing, parks, city recreation centers, immigrant handling, and teaching of mentally handicapped children. In 1912, she helped to found and was first president of the National Organization for Public Health Nursing (NOPHN), an organization that set standards and guided public health nursing's further development and impact on public health (Christy, 1970). Her exemplary accomplishments truly reflect a concern for populations at risk. They further demonstrate how nursing leadership, involve-

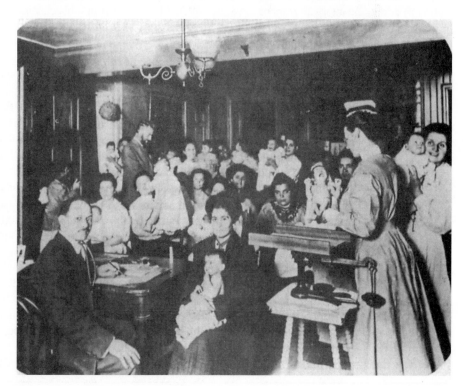

FIGURE 2–3. Examination of infants was part of early health department programs in which district nurses played a major role.

ment in policy formation, and use of epidemiology lead to improved health for the public.

By the 1920s, public health nursing was acquiring a more professional stature, in contrast to its earlier association with charity. Nursing as a whole was gaining professional status as a science in addition to being an art. National nursing organizations began to form during this stage and contributed to nursing's professional growth. The first of these emphasized establishing educational standards for nursing. Called the American Society of Superintendents of Training Schools for Nurses in the United States and Canada, it was started by Isabel Hampton Robb in 1893 and later became known as the National League of Nursing Education in 1912. This was the forerunner of the National League for Nursing (NLN), which was established in 1952 (Ellis & Hartley, 2000). In 1890, a meeting of nursing leaders at the World's Fair in Chicago initiated an alumnae organization of 10 schools of nursing to form the National Associated Alumnae of the United States and Canada in 1896, which was created to promote nursing education and practice standards. In 1899, the group was renamed the Nurses' Associated Alumnae of the United States and Canada. Canada was excluded

from the title in 1901 because New York, where the organization was incorporated, did not allow representation from two countries. In 1911, the organization went through a final name change to the American Nurses' Association (ANA), while Canadian nurses formed their own nursing organization (Ellis & Hartley, 2000) (see The Global Community). The previously mentioned NOPHN, founded by Lillian Wald and Mary Gardner, merged with the NLN in 1952. These three organizations, in particular, strengthened ties between nursing groups and improved nursing education and practice.

As nursing education became increasingly rigorous, collegiate programs began to include public health as essential content in basic nursing curricula. The first collegiate program with public health content to be accredited by the NLN began in 1944 (National Organization for Public Health Nursing, 1944). Previously, only postgraduate courses in public health nursing had been offered for nurses choosing this specialty. The first of such courses had been developed by Adelaide Nutting in 1912 at Teachers College in New York in affiliation with the Henry Street Settlement. A group of agencies met in 1946 to establish guidelines for public health nursing, and by

THE GLOBAL COMMUNITY

Mill, J.E., Leipert, B.D., & Duncan, S.M. (2002). A history of public health nursing in Alberta and British Columbia, 1918–1939. *Canadian Nurse, 98*(1), 18, 20–23.

Three doctoral students examined public health nursing (PHN) during the interwar years of 1918 to 1939 in Alberta and British Columbia. They reviewed PHN practice within provincial departments of health and the conditions contributing to their practice—geography, mobility, and disease.

In Alberta, the population was stable and was located both in urban centers and in sparsely populated and widely dispersed areas. In British Columbia, forestry, fishing, and mining played a big part in economic development and contributed to the creation of a mobile and transient population beset by individual and family problems. The establishment of PHN services met challenges in this environment.

To compound these geographic and population issues, the postwar effects of World War I, along with the pneumonia endemic of 1918–1919 and a receptive political climate, confirmed the need for more governmental support for PHN services in both provinces.

In addition, it was recognized that the public health nurses had a specialized role, which required more than just basic training. In 1918, the University of Alberta became the first Canadian university to offer a course in public health nursing, even if it was only 2 months in

length. Education for PHN was limited in the following years in Alberta due to a withdrawal of financial and political support following concerns about the government's excessive involvement in the lives of its citizens. In 1919, the University of British Columbia established the first baccalaureate degree program in nursing in Canada and in the British Empire. Support for PHN continued to grow in this province throughout the 1920s. By the 1930s, declining revenues to universities caused by the Great Depression had an impact on all educational programs.

The PHN role in these two provinces focused on school nursing, community education, maternal and infant mortality, the control of communicable diseases, and in the 1930s, social welfare. Throughout the first 20 years, the number of public health nurses in Alberta increased from 0 to 20; in the early 1920s, it dropped down to 5 for several years, and it never increased above 20 until after 1938. In British Columbia, where there was stronger political and financial support for PHN, the number of nurses increased slowly between 1919 and 1923 to 15 and then increased dramatically. By 1931 there were more than 70 public health nurses, and in 1937 the number again increased to more than 90. Both provinces were at the mercy of political and economic forces while having the same health care needs among their diverse populations.

How alike do you think these situations were to PHN in areas of the United States during the same years?

1963 public health content was required for NLN accreditation in all baccalaureate nursing programs. The nurse practitioner (NP) movement, starting in 1965 at the University of Colorado, initially was a part of public health nursing and emphasized primary health care to rural and underserved populations. The number of educational programs to prepare NPs increased, with some NPs continuing in public health and others moving into different clinical areas.

During this period, as a result of the influence of Lillian Wald and other nursing leaders, the family began to emerge as a unit of service (Fig. 2–4). The multiple problems faced by many families impelled a trend toward nursing care generalized enough to meet diverse needs and provide holistic services. Public health nurses gradually gained more autonomy in such areas as home care and instruction of good health practices to families and community groups. Their collaborative relationships with other community health providers grew as the need to avoid gaps and duplication of services became apparent. Public health nurses also began keeping better records of their services.

Industrial nursing, another form of public health nursing, also expanded during this period (see Chap. 29). The first known industrial nurse, Philippa Flowerday Reid, was hired in Norwich, England, by J. and J. Colmans in 1878. Her job was to assist the company physician and to visit sick employees and their families in their homes. In the United States, the Vermont Marble Company was first to begin a nursing service in 1895; other companies followed soon after. By 1910, 66 firms in the United States employed nurses. During World War I, the number of industrial nurses greatly increased with the recognition that nursing service reduced worker absenteeism (Bullough & Bullough, 1978). Early industrial nursing was the forerunner of modern occupational and environmental health nursing, which is explored in depth in Chapter 29.

During this stage, the institutional base for much of public health nursing shifted to the government. By 1955, 72% of the counties in the continental United States had local health departments. Public health nursing constituted the major portion of these local health services and emphasized health promotion as well as care for the ill at home (Scutchfield & Keck, 2003). Some of the district nursing services, known as visiting nurse associations (VNAs), remained privately funded and administered, offering their own home nursing care. In some places, city or county health departments joined administratively and financially with VNAs to provide a combination of services, such as home care of the sick and health promotion to families.

Rural public health nursing, which had already been organized around 1900 in Great Britain, Germany, and Canada, also expanded in the United States (see Chap. 31). Initially, starting in 1912, rural nursing was privately financed and largely administered through the Red Cross and the Metropolitan Life Insurance Company, but responsibility had shifted to the government by the 1940s (Bullough & Bullough, 1978). An innovative example of rural nursing was the Frontier Nursing Service, which was started by Mary Breckenridge (1881–1965) in 1925 to serve mountain families in Kentucky. From six outposts, nurses on horseback visited remote families to deliver babies and provide food and nursing services. Over the years, the service has expanded to provide medical, dental, and nursing care. The Frontier Nursing Service continues today, in its remarkable accomplishments of reducing mortality rates and promoting health among this disadvantaged population, as the parent holding company for the Frontier School of Midwifery and Family Nursing. It is the lagest nurse-midwifery program in the United States. In addition, Mary Breckinridge Healthcare, Inc., consists of a home health agency, two outpost clinics,

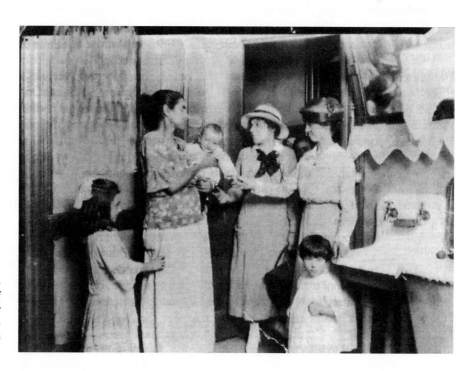

FIGURE 2–4. The public health nurse, carrying her bag of equipment and supplies, makes regular home visits to provide physical and psychological care as well as health lessons to families.

one primary care clinic, and the Kate Ireland Women's Healthcare Clinic (Simpson, 2000).

The public health nursing stage was characterized by service to the public, with the family targeted as a primary unit of care. Official health agencies, which placed greater emphasis on disease prevention and health promotion, provided the chief institutional base.

Community Health Nursing (1970 to the Present)

The emergence of the term *community health nursing* heralded a new era. While public health nurses continued their work in public health, by the late 1960s and early 1970s many other nurses, who were not necessarily practicing public health, were based in the community. Their practice settings included community-based clinics, doctors' offices, work sites, and schools. To provide a label that encompassed all nurses in the community, the ANA and others called them community health nurses.

This term was not universally accepted, however, and many people—including nurses and the general public—had difficulty distinguishing community health nursing from public health nursing. For example, nursing education, recognizing the importance of public health content, required course work in public health for all baccalaureate students. This meant that graduates were expected to incorporate public health principles such as health promotion and disease prevention into nursing practice, regardless of their sphere of service. Consequently, some people questioned whether public health nursing retained any unique content. Although leaders such as Carolyn Williams clearly stated that community health nursing's specialized contribution lay in its focus on populations (Williams, 1977), this concept did not appear to be widely understood or practiced.

To distinguish the domains of community and public health nursing, the U.S. Department of Health and Human Services, Bureau of Health Professionals, Division of Nursing, in 1984 convened a Consensus Conference on the Essentials of Public Health Nursing Practice and Education in Washington, D.C. (U.S. Department of Health and Human Services [USDHHS], Division of Nursing, 1984). This group concluded that *community health nursing* was the broader term, referring to all nurses practicing in the community, regardless of their educational preparation. *Public health nursing,* viewed as a part of community health nursing, was described as a generalist practice for nurses prepared with basic public health content at the baccalaureate level and a specialized practice for nurses prepared in public health at the masters level or beyond.

Confusion also arose regarding the question of whether community health nursing is a generalized or a specialized practice. Graduates from baccalaureate nursing programs were inadequately prepared to practice in public health; their education had emphasized individualized and direct clinical care and provided little understanding of applications to populations and communities. By the mid-1970s, various community health nursing leaders had identified knowledge and skills needed for more effective community health nursing practice (Roberts & Freeman, 1973). These leaders valued promoting the health of the community, but both education and practice continued to emphasize direct clinical care to individuals, families, and groups in the community (de Tornyay, 1980). Reflecting this view, the ANA's Division of Community Health Nursing developed *A Conceptual Model of Community Health Nursing* in 1980. This document distinguished generalized community health nursing preparation at the baccalaureate level and specialized community health nursing preparation at the masters or postgraduate level. The generalist was described as one who provides nursing service to individuals and groups of clients while keeping "the community perspective in mind" (American Nurses Association, 1980, p. 9).

Finally, confusion also arose regarding the changing roles and functions of community health nurses. Accelerated changes in health care organization and financing, technology, and social issues made increasing demands on community health nurses to adapt to new patterns of practice. Many new kinds of community health services appeared. Hospital-based programs reached into the community. Private agencies proliferated, offering home care and other community-based services. Other community health professionals assumed responsibilities that traditionally had been the domain of public health nursing. For example, some school counselors in Oregon began coordinating home visits previously done by school nurses, and health educators (who were part of a more recently developed discipline) took over large segments of client education. Social workers, too, provided services that overlapped with community health nursing roles. Health educators, counselors, social workers, epidemiologists, and nutritionists working in community health came prepared with different backgrounds and emphases in their practice. Their contributions were and still are important. Their presence, however, forced community health nurses to reexamine their own contribution to the public's health and incorporate stronger interdisciplinary and collaborative approaches into their practice (see Levels of Prevention Matrix).

The debate over these areas of confusion continued through the 1980s, and some issues are yet unresolved. Still, the direction in which public health and community health nursing must move remains clear: to care *for,* not simply *in,* the community. Public health nursing continues to mean the synthesis of nursing and the public health sciences applied to promoting and protecting the health of populations. Community health nursing, for some, refers more broadly to nursing in the community. In this text, the term *community health nursing* is used synonymously with *public health nursing* and refers to specialized, population-focused nursing practice, which applies public health science and nursing science. A possible distinction between the two terms might be to view community health nursing as a beginning level of specialization and public health nursing as an advanced level.

LEVELS OF PREVENTION MATRIX

SITUATION: Clarify and enhance the community health nurse's role to promote impact.

GOAL: Using the three levels of prevention, negative health conditions are avoided, or promptly diagnosed and treated, and the fullest possible potential is restored.

PRIMARY PREVENTION		SECONDARY PREVENTION		TERTIARY PREVENTION		
Health Promotion and Education	*Health Protection*	*Early Diagnosis*	*Prompt Treatment*	*Rehabilitation*	*Primary Prevention*	
					Health Promotion and Education	*Health Protection*
Proactively develop knowledge and skills to prevent misunderstanding and misuse of role	Stay current in the community health nursing field	Detect early signs of misuse and misunderstanding (eg, not working up to ability, weak collaboration with community members)	Select agencies where community health nurses can practice population-based nursing more fully	Minimize the impact of misunderstanding and misuse by clarifying the nurse's role and focusing the nurse's vision through education, staff development, and reassignment that helps to enlarge the community health nurse's role and impact on the health of populations	With successful rehabilitation, the community health nurse is able to participate again at the primary level of prevention	
Participate in policy formation		Develop measures to enhance the nurse's vision	Foster nurse involvement on community boards, in politics, and in policy formation, program development, research, and collaboration with colleagues and community members			
Be politically active		Promote aggregate-level interventions				
Work collaboratively to develop community health programs						
Conduct research on health and nursing outcomes to ensure theory-based practice						
Assist in acquiring funding for community health programs						

Clarification and consensus on the meaning of these terms help to avoid misconceptions and misuse and are explored more fully in Chapter 17. Whichever term is used to describe this specialty, the fundamental issues and defining criteria remain the same: (1) Are populations and communities the target of practice? and (2) Are the nurses prepared in public health and engaging in public health practice?

As community health nursing continues to evolve, many signs of positive growth are evident. Community health nurses are carving out new roles for themselves in primary health care. Collaboration and interdisciplinary teamwork are recognized as crucial to effective community nursing. Practitioners work through many kinds of agencies and institutions, such as senior citizen centers, ambulatory services, mental health clinics, and family planning programs. Community needs assessment, documentation of nursing outcomes, program evaluation, quality improvement, public policy formulation, and community nursing research are high priorities. This field of nursing is assuming responsibility as a full professional partner in community health.

Internationally, community nursing services are well established in England, although they may be an invisible service, as was implied in a London newspaper, which reported that "one of the possible memorials for Princess Diana might be a new nursing service based along the lines of the 'old nursing service' " (Birch, 1998, p. 19). Scandinavia, the Netherlands, and Australia have active community health services, but services are relatively underdeveloped in France and Ireland. Furthermore, there are relatively few professional nurses working in the community in central and eastern Europe and in the former USSR. Volunteers, lay providers, and paraprofessionals provide the bulk of community health services in China, Africa, and India.

In 1978, a joint World Health Organization (WHO) and

TABLE 2-1

Development of Community Health Nursing

Stages	Focus	Nursing Orientation	Service Emphasis	Institutional Base (Agencies)
Early home care (Before mid-1800s)	Sick poor	Individuals	Curative	Lay and religious orders
District nursing (1860–1900)	Sick poor	Individuals	Curative; beginning of preventive	Voluntary; some government
Public health nursing (1900–1970)	Needy public	Families	Curative; preventive	Government; some voluntary
Emergence of community health nursing (1970–present)	Total community	Populations	Health promotion; illness prevention	Many kinds; some independent practice

the United Nations Childrens' Fund International Conference in Alma-Ata, in the Soviet Union, adopted a declaration on primary health care as the key to attaining the goal of health for all by the year 2000. At this conference, delegations from 134 governments agreed to incorporate the concepts and principles of primary health care in their health care systems to reach this goal (WHO, 1978, 1998). This was adopted by the World Health Assembly and endorsed by the United Nations General Assembly in 1981. On paper, at least, everyone acknowledged the crucial need for nurses to be involved in reaching this goal. In practice, support has not been forthcoming in many countries. Policymakers and the public still need to be educated to realize that nursing's most effective contributions to the overall health of the population are based in the community.

Table 2–1 summarizes the most important changes that have occurred during community health nursing's four stages of development. It shows these changes in terms of focus, nursing orientation, service emphasis, and institutional base.

SOCIETAL INFLUENCES ON THE DEVELOPMENT OF COMMUNITY HEALTH NURSING

Many factors have influenced the growth of community health nursing. To better understand the nature of this field, the forces that began and continue to shape its development must be recognized. Six are particularly significant: advanced technology, progress in causal thinking, changes in education, demographic changes and the role of women, the consumer movement, and economic factors.

Advanced Technology

Advanced technology has contributed in many ways to shaping the practice of community health nursing. For example, technologic innovation has greatly improved health care, nutrition, and lifestyle and has caused a concomitant increase in life expectancy. Consequently, community health nurses direct an increasing share of their effort toward meeting the needs of the elderly population and addressing chronic conditions. As another example, the advances in technology in the home have been life-altering. Online communities for older adults have been developed, bringing the elderly out of loneliness and among a community of caring others through the computer (Furlong, 1997); online interfaith programs connect homebound people with religious leaders and fellow parishioners (Gunderson, 1997); and telecommunication technologies promote safety, independence, and social interaction for those with disabilities (Mann, 1997).

Advanced technology also has been a strong force behind industrialization, large-scale employment, and urbanization. We are now primarily an urban society, with approximately 75% of the world's population living in urban or suburban areas. Population density leads to many health-related problems, particularly the spread of disease and increased stress. Community health nurses are learning how to combat these urban health problems. In addition, changes in transportation and high job mobility have affected the health scene. As people travel and relocate, they are separated from families and traditional support systems; community health nurses design programs to help urban populations cope with the accompanying stress. New products, equipment, methods, and energy sources in industry also have increased environmental pollution and industrial hazards. Community health nurses have become involved in related research, occupational health, and preventive education. Technologic innovation has promoted complex medical diagnostic and treatment procedures, making illness-oriented care more dramatic and desirable, as well as more costly. Community health nurses face a challenge to demonstrate the physical and economic value of technology for wellness-oriented care.

Finally, innovations in communications and computer technology have shifted America from an industrial society to an "information economy." Our economy is built on information—the production and marketing of knowledge—making it global and around-the-clock. Community health nurses now are in the business of information distribution and use computer technologies to enhance the efficiency and effectiveness of their services. Telenursing, Telehealth, and nursing informatics are part of our professional activities as community health nurses. We communicate by e-mail, use computer-based applications to enhance education among peers and with clients, and comfortably use the computers that are found in all areas where nurses function (Saba, 2001). As we move deeper into the 21st century, we move to "mobile care," using handheld, wireless technology tools that are nurse-friendly and compatible with the nurse's role. We have the ability to "tele-visit" our clients, and we regularly use smaller and smaller laptop computers for video conferencing (Saba, 2001).

Progress in Causal Thinking

Relating disease or illness to its cause is known as **causal thinking** in the health sciences. Progress in the study of causality, particularly in epidemiology, has significantly affected the nature of community health nursing (Fos & Fine, 2000; Thomas & Weber, 2001). The *germ theory* of disease causation, established in the late 1800s, was the first real breakthrough in control of communicable disease. At that time, it was established that disease could be spread or transmitted from patient to patient or from nurse to patient by contaminated hands or equipment. Nurses incorporated the teaching of cleanliness and personal hygiene into basic nursing care.

A second advance in causal thinking was initiated by the tripartite view that called attention to the interactions among a causative agent, a susceptible host, and the environment. This information offered community health nurses new ways to control and prevent health disorders. For example, nurses could decrease the vulnerability of individuals (host) by teaching them healthier lifestyles. They could instigate measles vaccination programs as a means of preventing the organism (agent) from infecting children. They could promote proper disinfection of a neighborhood swimming pool (environment) to prevent disease.

Further progress in causal thinking led to the recognition that not just one single agent, but many factors—a multiple causation approach—contribute to a disease or health disorder. A food poisoning outbreak that is associated with a restaurant might be caused not only by the salmonella organism but also by improper food handling and storage, lack of adherence to minimum food preparation standards, and lack of adequate health department supervision and enforcement (see Chap. 8). A chronic condition such as coronary heart disease can be related to other kinds of multicausal factors, such as heredity, diet, lack of exercise, smoking, and personal and work stress.

Community health nurses can control health problems by examining all possible causes and then attacking strategic causal points. Efforts to prevent acquired immunodeficiency syndrome (AIDS) provide a dramatic case in point. Contact reporting, condom use, protection of health workers serving patients infected with the human immunodeficiency virus (HIV), screening for HIV infection, and public education about AIDS are examples of a multifaceted approach. Current causal thinking has led to a broader awareness of unhealthy conditions; in addition to disease, problems such as accidents and environmental pollution are major targets of concern. Work-related stress, environmental hazards, chemical food additives, and alcohol and nicotine consumption during pregnancy are all examples of concerns in community health nursing practice.

Nursing's contribution to public health adds a further application of causal thinking. That is, nursing seeks to identify and implement the causes, or contributing factors, of wellness. Community health nurses do more than prevent illness; they seek to promote health. By conducting research and applying research findings, community health nurses promote health-enhancing behaviors. Nurses promote healthier lifestyle practices such as eating low-fat diets, exercising, and maintaining social support systems; promote healthy conditions in schools and work sites; and design meaningful activities for adolescents and the elderly.

Changes in Education

Changes in education, especially those in nursing education, have had an important influence on community health nursing practice. Education, once an opportunity for a privileged few, has become widely available; it is now considered a basic right and a necessity for a vital society. When people's understanding of their environment grows, an increased understanding of health usually is involved. For the community health nurse, health teaching has steadily assumed greater importance in practice. For the learner, education has led to more responsibility. As a result, people believe that they have a right to know and question the reasons behind the care they receive. Community health nurses have shifted from planning for clients to collaborating with clients.

Education has had other effects. Scientific inquiry, considered basic to progress, has created a dramatic increase in knowledge. The wealth of information relevant to community health nursing practice means that nursing students have more content to assimilate, and practicing community health nurses have to make greater efforts to keep abreast of knowledge in their field. In contrast to earlier times, when nurses were trained to work as apprentices in hospitals or health agencies and to follow orders perfunctorily, today's educational programs, including continuing education, prepare nurses to think for themselves in the application of theory to practice. Community health nursing has always required a fair measure of independent thinking and self-reliance; now, community health nurses need skills in such areas as population assessment, policy making, political advocacy, research, management, collaborative functioning, and critical thinking. As the result of expanding education, community health nurses have had to reexamine their practice, sharpen their knowledge and skills, and clarify their roles.

Demographic Changes and the Role of Women

The changing demographics in the country and the changing role of women have profoundly affected community health nursing. In the 20th century, the women's rights movement made considerable progress; women achieved the right to vote and gained greater economic independence by moving into the labor force. Today, there are 131 million people employed in the United States, 46.2% of whom are female. In the decade between 1998 and 2008, the number of women in the labor force will increase by 15%, compared with 10% for men. In the same decade, the percentage of workers age 45 years or older will increase from 33% to 40% of the workforce.

Women nurses are aging in a women's profession. In 1980, 52.9% of nurses were younger than 40 years of age, and 26% were younger than 30. By the year 2000, the percentages had changed: only 31.4% of nurses were younger than 40 years of age, and fewer than 10% were younger than 30. Although most nursing schools remain full and many have a waiting list, the number of nurses staying active in their profession keeps dwindling. Those remaining in the profession are graying and retiring.

Salaries for nurses compare favorably with those for other workers who have four years of education in fields other than health care, such as education, human services (social work), and business. When compared with other workers in the health care field, nurses make a lower salary. For example, among the 2,317,980 practicing registered nurses in the United States in 2001, the average salary was $48,240. In comparison, the average salary for physical therapists was $59,210; for dental hygienists it was $56,770, and for occupational therapists it was $52,210 (U.S. Department of Labor, 2002).

More than 30 years after the peak of the women's movement, women continue to be paid less than men. For example, figures from the U. S. Department of Labor show that women earn 71% of a man's salary for the same job (U.S. Department of Labor, 2002). This discrepancy is most noticable in business; in nursing the difference is not as great, although men who go into nursing eventually move into management positions more often than female nurses do. They also are promoted faster and move into management earlier in their careers.

Changing demographics, such as shifting patterns in immigration, varying numbers of births and deaths, and a rapidly increasing population of elderly persons, affect community health nursing planning and programming efforts. Monitoring these changes is essential for relevant and effective nursing services.

In 2000, the U.S. Department of Health and Human Services predicted that the labor force share would decrease for whites, there would be little or no change for blacks, and the share would increase for Hispanics, Asians, and people of other races. This shift is reflected among registered nurses. In 1999–2000, 81% of all practicing nurses were white, 9.9% were black, 4.4% Asian, 3.9% Hispanic, and 0.8% American Indian. These precentages show slight shifts from 1990, with the Hispanic and Asian percentages increasing and the white

WHAT DO YOU THINK? I

Nurses are in good company, according to a Gallop Poll taken in 2002. When asked how they would rate the honesty and ethical standards of people in the following fields as either "very high," "high," "average," "low," or "very low," 84% of Americans reported that nurses have "very high" or "high" standards (Domrose, 2002). Here are the results for various professions:

- Firefighters   90
- Nurses   84
- U.S. military personnel   81
- Police officers   68
- Pharmacists   68
- Medical doctors   66
- Clergy   64

and black percentages lowering, while the percentage for Native Americans remained the same (USDHHS, 2002).

Although the diversity of career options and employment opportunities for women has been a positive factor, these gains have decreased the number of women entering nursing. As a profession, nursing's contributions and status have improved, but its ability to compete with careers offering higher pay and status remains problematic. Changes resulting from the women's movement continue. Nurses still struggle for equality—equality of recognition, respect, and autonomy, as well as job selection, equal pay for equal work, and equal opportunity for advancement in the health field (see What Do You Think? I). If community health nurses are to influence the field of community health, they need status and authority equal to that of their colleagues. This step requires nurses to demonstrate their competence and learn to be assertive in assuming roles as full professional partners. Although only 6.8% of registered nurses (RNs) in 2000 were men (up from 4.2% in 1983), they held more than one third of nursing administrative positions (U.S. Department of Labor, 2002). This finding may in part reflect a larger proportion of women in nursing who have less than full-time careers. The women's movement has contributed to community health nursing's gains in assuming leadership roles, but a need for greater influence and involvement remains.

Consumer Movement

The consumer movement also has affected the nature of community health nursing. Consumers have become more aggressive in demanding quality services and goods; they assert their right to be informed about goods and services and to participate in decisions that affect them regardless of sex, race, or socioeconomic level. This movement has stimulated some basic changes in the philosophy of community health nursing. Health care consumers are viewed as active members of the health team rather than as passive recipients of care. They may contract with the community health nurse for family care or group services, represent the community on the local health board, or act as ombudsmen by serving as representatives or advocates for their community constituents (eg, to investigate complaints and report findings to protect the quality of care in a local nursing home). This assumption of consumers' responsibility for their own health means that the community health nurse often supplements clients' services, rather than primarily supervising them.

The consumer movement also has contributed to increased concern for the quality of health services, including a demand for more humane, personalized health care. Dissatisfied with fragmented services offered by an array of health workers, consumers seek more comprehensive, coordinated care. For example, senior citizens in a high-rise apartment building need more than a series of social workers, nutritionists, recreational therapists, nurses, and other callers ascertaining a variety of specific needs and starting a variety of separate programs. Community health nurses seek to provide holistic care by collaborating with others to offer more coordinated, comprehensive, and personalized services—a case-management approach.

Economic Forces

Myriad economic forces have affected the practice of community health nursing. Unemployment and the rising cost of living, combined with mounting health care costs, have resulted in numerous people carrying little or no health insurance. With limited or no access to needed health services, these populations are especially vulnerable to health problems and further economic stress. Other economic forces affecting community health nursing are changing health care financing patterns (including prospective payment and Diagnosis-Related Groups); decreased federal, state, and local subsidies of public health programs; pressures for health care cost containment through managed care; and increased competition and managed competition among providers of health services (see Chap. 7).

Global economic forces also influence community health nursing practice. As the United States experiences increasing interdependence with foreign countries for trade, investment, and production of goods, the population has experienced a growing mobility and increased immigration, particularly among Hispanic and Asian groups. Under these conditions, the spread of communicable diseases poses a serious threat, as do problems associated with unemployment and poverty. Furthermore, the fastest-growing sector of the job market is in technical fields, which require new or retrained workers, and these jobs frequently are accompanied by health problems related to the stresses of ever-changing technology and financial and competitive pressures to produce.

Community health nursing has responded to these economic forces in several ways. One is by assuming new roles, such as health educators in industry or case managers for government and privately sponsored programs for the elderly. Another is by directly competing with other community health service providers, particularly in such areas as

ambulatory care or home care. Still another is by developing new programs and service emphases. Elder day care, respite care, senior fall-prevention programs, teen pregnancy and drug prevention projects, and programs for the homeless are a few examples of the response by community health nursing to the changing community needs created by demographic and economic forces. Yet another community health nursing response has been to develop new revenue-generating services, such as workplace wellness or health screening programs, to augment depleted budgets.

Economic factors continue to play a significant role in shaping community health nursing practice. Limited dollars for health promotion services and a continued need for home care have drawn some public health agencies into more illness-oriented rather than wellness-oriented services. Yet, community health nurses continue to be resourceful in finding ways to foster the community's optimal health while adapting to changing economic conditions (see What Do You Think? II).

WHAT DO YOU THINK? II

In July, 2002, the U. S. House and Senate passed the Nurse Reinvestment Act. "Unnoticed and uncelebrated by almost everyone outside the health care profession," this act was passed by "patient negotiation and sheer persistence."

This legislation is remarkable for two reasons. First, more than any bill in 2002, it bore the imprint of women legislators. And secondly, it has the potential to bring substantial benefits to untold millions of people during the decades ahead.

We are in the midst of a critical nursing shortage. Health care in the United States is being jeopardized by the convergence of three trends: a rapid increase in the number of elderly Americans, the retirement or dropout of an already aging and overworked generation of nurses, and a steep decline in the number of people entering the nursing profession. From 2010 forward, the situation will get steadily worse . . . a graying population . . . accompanied by a staggering decline and shortage of registered nurses.

This bill is designed to address the nursing shortage. Public service announcements will be designed to promote the nursing profession, scholarships will be offered for nursing students who agree, upon graduation, to work for a period of time in a facility facing a critical nursing shortage. It will cancel student loans for nurses who seek advanced degrees and agreee to join the faculties of nursing schools. It will give schools special grants to train nurses in geriatric care. It will also include strategies to attack the burnout and frustration that are driving many out of nursing and into less-demanding work.

PREPARATION FOR COMMUNITY HEALTH NURSING

The demands of community health nursing practice are significant, as described in Chapter 1, and are elaborated elsewhere in this textbook. The daily routine of the community health nurse may include organizing a flu clinic for seniors in the community, making home visits, giving a presentation on playground safety at a parent-teacher meeting, participating in a team meeting in the health department office, answering telephone calls, and charting. All of the skills learned in a basic baccalaureate nursing program are needed to effectively manage this type of day. Furthermore, this day may not represent the bigger picture of the community health nurse's role on community advisory panels, grant writing for new programs, or participation in or presentation of inservice programs. Academic preparation for this role is necessary, as is continuous professional development, and this training must meet the requirements expected by employers for people in this specialty in nursing and, in many instances, by state regulations.

Academic Preparation

The minimum preparation for community health nurses in many states has been graduation from a baccalaureate-level nursing program, a nursing major built on 2 years of liberal arts and sciences courses (Ellis & Hartley, 2000). This can be achieved in a variety of ways. Some students enter a baccalaureate program as their initial higher educational experience after high school or later. Others complete an associate degree program in nursing and continue on to a university to receive the baccalaureate degree. This requires additional courses in liberal arts and sciences, along with selected nursing courses, usually one or more courses in public health nursing and often critical care nursing and leadership-management courses as well. In some programs designed to extend an RN to a Bachelor of Science in Nursing (BSN), nurses with years of experience in acute care nursing can "challenge" the previously mentioned courses by taking a test to demonstrate clinical expertise or by presenting a portfolio of experience, or a combination of these. Nevertheless, whatever the initial entry into practice, a comprehensive nursing education that is rich in leadership, management, research, health maintenance and promotion, disease prevention, and community health nursing experience is needed to meet the demands of this specialty.

In some states, meeting criteria for entry into practice as a public health nurse is required by some employers. In California, the State Board of Registered Nursing (BRN) has established specific criteria, including completion of specific coursework (eg, child abuse and prevention information), which must be documented in undergraduate classes. On graduation, a school transcript, application, and fee are sent to the BRN to receive the public health nursing certificate. After they pass the RN license examination (NCLEX), these nurses can sign "RN, PHN" after their names. Only those who have completed a baccalaureate nursing program can apply for this certificate, and only people with the certificate can take jobs as community health nurses. In California, this means that employment as an RN in settings such as health departments, schools, and Native American health services requires a PHN certificate.

Professional Development

Completion of a baccalaureate education may not be sufficient educational preparation for the more demanding community health nursing settings. Furthermore, to maintain licensure in most states, it is mandated that nurses participate in continuing education programs and receive continuing education units (Ellis & Hartley, 2000). In the United States, courses on specific topics are offered by employers, nursing associations, nursing journals, and private programs that travel to various cities. These help nurses to remain current on topics covered by the courses; however, a community health nurse may consider more lengthy and formal professional development opportunities such as advanced nursing practice (NP) programs or certification opportunities.

To someone who is just finishing an undergraduate nursing program, the thought of continuing on in school may be overwhelming. However, within a few months or years after graduation, continuing in higher education may seem right. It can take time and experience to find a particular focus in nursing and to decide on specializing at an advanced level. When that time comes, a variety of course work and degree options are available. For example, short-term certificate programs specialize in a narrow focus of health care such as early recognition and prevention of child abuse, research, grant writing, or team management. These may or may not be offered for university credit, but, in any case, the content enhances a nurse's role in an agency.

Matriculation in an NP program or a master's degree program in nursing is a longer commitment and gives the nurse greater marketability. In some health departments, NPs run well-child clinics, and a school nurse with an NP license can direct a school-based clinic. Advanced practice in community health nursing can open doors into leadership positions in community health agencies. A master's degree in business, public health, education, or epidemiology can lead to management positions, private community health agency ownership, agency teaching, or research positions. A doctoral program may be the next educational step for those wanting tenure-track university teaching, research, or upper-level administrative positions.

The American Nurses Credentialing Center (ANCC) provides other opportunities by offering nurses certification in more than 45 specialty areas. There are two specialties in community health nursing: a generalist certificate as a community health nurse, and a clinical nurse specialist certificate in community health nursing. Related certifications as an NP or in nursing administration also exist. Each certificate is awarded after completion of a certain number of years of practice in the specialty, payment of a fee, and passage of an ANCC Certification Examination. When certification is awarded, the nurse can sign as "RN,C." Many employers reward the initiative required for certification with promotion or a higher salary accompanied by additional responsibilities and opportunities.

SUMMARY

The specialty of community health nursing developed historically through four stages. The early home care stage (before the mid-1800s) emphasized care to the sick poor in their homes by various lay and religious orders. The district nursing stage (mid-1800s) included voluntary home nursing care for the poor by specialists or "health nurses" who treated the sick and taught wholesome living to patients. The public health nursing stage (1900 to 1970) was characterized by an increased concern for the health of the general public. The community health nursing stage (1970 to the present) includes increased recognition of community health nursing as a specialty field with focus on communities and populations.

Six major societal influences have shaped the development of community health nursing. They are advanced technology, progress in causal thinking, changes in education, the changing demographics and role of women, the consumer movement, and economic factors such as health care costs, access, limited funds for public health, and increased competition among health service providers.

Academic preparation for community health nursing begins at the baccalaureate level. However, students beginning at the diploma or associate degree level can advance to a BSN completion program and then are prepared to enter this challenging specialty in nursing. The demands of community health nursing require additional courses in liberal arts and science, along with courses in community health nursing practice at the student level. Once students achieve an undergraduate degree, completion of additional educational programs is required to keep current and, in most states, to maintain licensure, advance in practice opportunities, or branch out into administration, teaching, or research.

ACTIVITIES TO PROMOTE CRITICAL THINKING

1. Select one societal influence on the development of community health nursing and explore its continuing impact. What other events are occurring today that shape community health nursing practice? Support your arguments with documentation. Use the Internet to find your documentation.

2. Using the Internet, seek out information about an historical public health nursing leader. Using this information, determine how this practitioner might deal with current population-based issues such as AIDS, sexually transmitted diseases, or child neglect and abuse.

3. Assume that you have been asked to make a home visit to a 75-year-old man living alone whose wife recently died. Besides assessing his individual needs, what additional factors should you consider for assessment and intervention that would indicate an aggregate or population-focused approach? What self-care practices might you encourage or teach?

4. Interview a community health nursing director to determine what population-based programs are offered in your locality. Explore nursing's role in the assessment, development, implementation, and evaluation of these programs. Discuss with the director how community health nurses might expand their population-focused interventions.

5. Go to your university, nursing college, or school and locate brochures for advanced degrees in nursing and related areas. Peruse them and see whether any of the programs appeal to you. Request more information from at least one of these programs through the mail or the Internet.

REFERENCES

American Nurses Association, Community Health Nursing Division. (1980). *A conceptual model of community health nursing* (Publication No. CH-10 2M 5/80). Kansas City, MO: Author.

Beine, J. (1996). Changing with the times. *Nursing Times, 92*(48), 59–62.

Birch, K. (1998). Speaking out. *Nursing Times, 94*(27), 19.

Broder, D. (2002, August 7). Reinvestment in nursing healthy decision. *The Fresno Bee*, B9.

Bullough, V., & Bullough, B. (1978). *The care of the sick: The emergence of modern nursing.* New York: Neale, Watson.

Central Hanover Bank and Trust Company, Department of Philanthropic Information. (1938). *The public health nurse.* New York: National Organization for Public Health Nursing.

Christy, T.W. (1970). Portrait of a leader: Lillian D. Wald. *Nursing Outlook, 18*(3), 50–54.

de Tornyay, R. (1980). Public health nursing: The nurse's role in community-based practice. *Annual Review of Public Health, 1,* 83.

Dickens, C. (1910). *Martin Chuzzlewit.* New York: Macmillan.

Dolan, J.A. (1978). *Nursing in society: A historical perspective.* Philadelphia: W.B. Saunders.

Domrose, C. (2002). Mending our image. *Nurseweek, 15*(14), 13–15.

Ellis, J.R., & Hartley, C.L. (2000). *Nursing in today's world: Challenges, issues, and trends* (7th ed.). Philadelphia: Lippincott Williams & Wilkins.

Farrar, E.W. (1837). *The young lady's friend—By a lady* (p. 57). Boston: American Stationer's Co.

Florence Nightingale Museum Trust. (1997). *The Florence Nightingale Museum's School Visit Pack.* London: Author.

Fos, P.J., & Fine, D.J. (2000). *Designing health care for populations: Applied epidemiology in health care administration.* San Francisco: Jossey-Bass.

Furlong, M. (1997). Creating online community for older adults. *Generations, 21*(3), 33–35.

Gardner, M.S. (1936). *Public health nursing* (3rd ed.). New York: Macmillan.

Gunderson, G. (1997). Spirituality, community, and technology: An interfaith program goes online. *Generations, 21*(3), 42–45.

Hein, E.C. (2001). *Nursing issues in the 21st century: Perspectives from the literature.* Philadelphia: Lippincott Williams & Wilkins.

Mann, W.C. (1997). Common telecommunications technology for promoting safety, independence, and social interaction for older people with disabilities. *Generations, 21*(3), 28–29.

Men, monasteries, wars, and wards. (2001). *Nursing Times, 97*(44), 25–26.

Mill, J.E., Leipert, B.D., & Duncan, S.M. (2002). A history of public health nursing in Alberta and British Columbia, 1918–1939. *Canadian Nurse, 98*(1), 18, 20–23.

Mowbray, P. (1997). *Florence Nightingale museum guidebook.* London: The Florence Nightingale Museum Trust.

National Organization for Public Health Nursing. (1944). Approval of Skidmore College of Nursing as preparing students for public health nursing. *Public Health Nursing, 36,* 371.

Nightingale, F. (1859). *Notes on nursing: What it is, and what it is not.* London: Harrison.

Nightingale, F. (1864). *How people may live and not die in India.* London: Longman, Green, Longman, Roberts, & Green.

Nightingale, F. (1876, April 14). [Letter to the editor]. *The Times* (London).

Palmer, I.S. (2001). Florence Nightingale: Reformer, reactionary, researcher. In E.C. Hein, *Nursing issues in the 21st century: Perspectives from the literature* (pp. 26–38). Philadelphia: Lippincott Williams & Wilkins.

Roberts, D., & Freeman, R. (Eds.). (1973). *Redesigning nursing education for public health: Report of the conference* (Publication No. HRA 75–75). Bethesda, MD: U.S. Department of Health, Education, and Welfare.

Saba, V.K. (2001). Nursing informatics: Yesterday, today, and tomorrow. *International Nursing Review, 48,* 177–187.

Sachs, T.B. (1908). The tuberculosis nurse. *American Journal of Nursing, 8,* 597.

Scutchfield, F.D., & Keck, C.W. (2003). *Principles of public health practice.* Albany, NY: Delmar.

Simpson, M.S. (2000). Nurses and models of practice: Then and now. *American Journal of Nursing, 100*(2), 82–83.

Thomas, J.C., & Weber, D.J. (2001). *Epidemiologic methods for the study of infectious diseases.* Oxford: Oxford University Press.

U.S. Department of Health and Human Services, Division of Nursing. (1984). *Consensus conference on the essentials of public health nursing practice and education: Report of the conference.* Rockville, MD: Author.

U.S. Department of Health and Human Services, National Center for Health Statistics. (2002). *Health, United States, 2002 with chartbook on trends in the health of America* (DHHS Publication No. 1232). Washington, DC: Author.

U.S. Department of Health and Human Services, National Institute for Occupational Safety and Health. (2000). *Worker Health Chartbook, 2000.* Washington, DC: Author.

U.S. Department of Labor, Bureau of Labor Statistics. (2002). Available: *www.dol.gov*

Wald, L.D. (1915). *The house on Henry Street.* New York: Holt.

Wald, L.D. (1934). *Windows of Henry Street.* Boston: Little Brown.

Williams, C.A. (1977). Community health nursing: What is it? *Nursing Outlook, 25,* 250–254.

Woodham-Smith, C. (1951). *Florence Nightingale.* New York: McGraw-Hill.

World Health Organization. (1978). *Primary health care: Report of the International Conference on Primary Health Care, Alma-Ata, USSR.* Geneva: Author.

World Health Organization. (1998). *The world health report: 1998.* Geneva: Author.

SELECTED READINGS

100 years in pictures. (2000). *American Journal of Nursing, 100*(10), 40–45.

Baer, E.D., D'Antonio, P., Rinker, S., & Lynaugh, J.E. (2001). *Enduring issues in American nursing.* New York: Springer.

Brink, S. (1997). The twin challenges of information technology and population aging. *Generations, 21*(3), 7–10.

Bullough, V.L., & Sentz, L. (2000). *American nursing: A biographical dictionary* (Vol. 3). New York: Springer.

Chaska, N.L. (2001). *The nursing profession: Tomorrow and beyond.* Thousand Oaks, CA: Sage.

Duffus, R.L. (1938). *Lillian Wald: Neighbor and crusader*. New York: Macmillan.

Fitzpatrick, M.L. (1975). Nursing and the Great Depression. *American Journal of Nursing, 75*(12), 2188–2190.

Hardin, S., & Langford, D. (2001). Telehealth's impact on nursing and the development of the interstate compact. *Journal of Professional Nursing, 17*(5), 243–247.

Hawkins, J.W., & Bellig, L.L. (2000). The evolution of advanced practice nursing in the United States: Caring for women and newborns. *Journal of Obstetric, Gynecologic, and Neonatal Nursing, 29*(1), 83–89.

Henderson, V. (1969/2000). Excellence in nursing: An AJN classic, October 1969. *American Journal of Nursing, 100*(10), *96I, 96K, 96M-96R*.

Heistand, W.C. (2000). Think different: Inventions and innovations by nurses, 1850–1950. *American Journal of Nursing, 100*(10), 72–77.

Jenkins, R.L., & White, P. (2001). Telehealth advancing nursing practice. *Nursing Outlook, 49*(2), 100–105.

Libster, M. (2001). *Demonstrating care: The art of integrative nursing*. Albany, NY: Delmar.

Lynaugh, J.E. (2002). *Nursing History Review: Official journal of the American Association for the History of Nursing*. New York: Springer.

Macrae, J.A. (2001). *Nursing as a spiritual practice: A contemporary application of Florence Nightingale's views*. New York: Springer.

Nichols, F.H. (2000). History of the women's health movement in the 20th century. *Journal of Obstetric, Gynecologic, and Neonatal Nursing, 29*(1), 56–64.

Sandelowski, M. (2000). Thermometers and telephones: A century of nursing and technology. *American Journal of Nursing, 100*(10), 82–86.

Sarnecky, M.T. (2001). Army nurses in "The Forgotten War." *American Journal of Nursing, 101*(11), 45–49.

U.S. Department of Health and Human Services. (2000). *Healthy people 2010* (Conference ed., Vols. 1 & 2). Washington, DC: Author.

Internet Resources

American Academy of Nursing: *http://www.nursingworld.org/aan*

American Assembly for Men in Nursing: *http://www.aamn.org*

American Nurses Association: *http://www.ana.org*

American Nurses Credentialing Center: *http://www.nursingworld.org/ancc/index.html*

American Nursing Informatics Association: *http://www.ania.org*

American Public Health Association: *http://www.apha.org*

National Association of Hispanic Nurses: *http://www.nahnhq.org*

National Center for Health Statistics: *http://www.cdc.gov/hchc*

National League for Nursing: *http://www.nln.org*

Sigma Theta Tau International Honor Society of Nursing: *http://www.nursingsociety.org*

U.S. Department of Labor. Bureau of Labor Statistics: *http://www.bls.gov*

3

Roles and Settings for Community Health Nursing Practice

Key Terms

- Advocate
- Assessment
- Assurance
- Case management
- Clinician
- Collaborator
- Conceptual skills
- Controller
- Educator
- Evaluator
- Human skills
- Leader
- Managed care
- Manager
- Organizer
- Planner
- Policy development
- Researcher
- Technical skills

Learning Objectives

Upon mastery of this chapter, you should be able to:

- Identify the three core public health functions basic to community health nursing.
- Describe and differentiate among seven different roles of the community health nurse.
- Discuss the seven roles within the framework of public health nursing functions.
- Explain the importance of each role for influencing people's health.
- Identify and discuss factors that affect a nurse's selection and practice of each role.
- Describe seven settings in which community health nurses practice.
- Discuss the nature of community health nursing, and the common threads basic to its practice, woven throughout all roles and settings.
- Identify principles of sound nursing practice in the community.

istorically, community health nurses have engaged in many roles. From the beginning, nurses in this professional specialty have provided care to the sick, taught positive health habits and self-care, advocated on behalf of needy populations, developed and managed health programs, provided leadership, and collaborated with other professionals and consumers to implement changes in health services. The settings in which these nurses practiced varied, too. The home certainly has been one site for practice, but so too have clinics, schools, factories, and other community-based locations. Today, the roles and settings of professional community health nursing practice have expanded even further.

This chapter examines how the conceptual foundations and core functions of community health nursing are integrated into the various roles and the settings in which community health nurses practice. It provides an opportunity to gain greater understanding about how and where community health nursing is practiced. Furthermore, it will expand awareness of the many existing and future possibilities for community health nurses to improve the public's health.

CORE PUBLIC HEALTH FUNCTIONS

Community health nurses work as partners within a team of professionals (in public health and other disciplines), non-professionals, and consumers to improve the health of populations. The various roles and settings for practice hinge on three primary functions of public health: assessment, policy development, and assurance. They are foundational to all roles assumed by the community health nurse and are applied at three levels of service: to individuals, to families, and to communities (Display 3–1). Regardless of role or setting of choice, these foundational responsibilities direct the work of all community health nurses.

Assessment

An essential first function in public health, **assessment**, means that the community health nurse must gather and analyze information that will affect the health of the people to be served. The nurse and others on the health team need to determine health needs, health risks, environmental conditions, political agendas, and financial and other resources, depending on the persons, community, or population targeted for intervention. Data may be gathered in many ways; typical methods include interviewing people in the community, conducting surveys, gathering information from public records, and using research findings.

The community health nurse usually is trusted and valued by clients, agencies, and private providers. This trust typically affords a nurse access to client populations that are difficult to engage, to agencies, and to health care providers. In the capacity of trusted professional, community health nurses gather relevant client data that enable them to identify strengths, weaknesses, and needs.

At the community level, assessment is done both formally and informally as nurses identify and interact with key community leaders. With families, the nurse can evaluate family strengths and areas of concern in the immediate living environment and in the neighborhood. At the individual level, people are identified within the family who are in need

DISPLAY 3–1

Public Health Nursing Within the Core Public Health Functions Model

The model includes assessment, policy development, and assurance surrounding the individual, family, and community. *Assessment* is the regular collection, analysis, and sharing of information about health conditions, risks, and resources in a community. *Policy development* uses the information gathered during assessment to develop local and state health policies and to direct resources toward those policies. *Assurance* focuses on the availability of necessary health services throughout the community. It includes maintaining the ability of both public health agencies and private providers to manage day-to-day operations as well as the capacity to respond to critical situations and emergencies (Conley & Dahl, 1993).

of services, and the nurse evaluates the functional capacity of these individuals through the use of specific assessment measures, using a variety of tools. Assessment of communities and families is described in detail in Chapters 18 and 23.

Policy Development

Policy development, defined in Display 3–1, is enhanced by the synthesis and analysis of information obtained during assessment. At the community level, the nurse provides leadership in convening and facilitating community groups to evaluate health concerns and develop a plan to address the concerns. Typically, the nurse recommends specific training and programs to meet identified health needs of target populations. This is accompanied by raising the awareness of key policy makers about factors such as health regulations and budget decisions that negatively affect the health of the community. With families, the nurse recommends new programs or increased services based on identified needs. Additional data may be needed to identify trends in groups or clusters of families so that effective intervention strategies can be used with these families. At the individual level, the nurse assists in the development of standards for individual client care, recommends or adopts risk-classification systems to assist with prioritizing individual client care, and participates in establishing criteria for opening, closing, or referring individual cases.

Assurance

Assurance activities—activities that make certain that services are provided—often consume most of the community health nurse's time. With the increase in programmatic funding and direct state reimbursement through Medicaid programs, community health nurses in many settings have been required to focus on direct service to individuals rather than on population-based services. Nonetheless, community health nurses perform the assurance function at the community level when they provide service to target populations, improve quality assurance activities, and maintain safe levels of communicable disease surveillance and outbreak control. In addition, they participate in research, provide expert consultation, and provide services within the community based on standards of care. Care is provided to clusters of families within a geographic setting or in one setting, such as a neighborhood clinic.

Individuals should receive nursing services based on standards developed by the American Nurses Association (ANA), such as the *Code for Nurses With Interpretive Statements* (1985), *Nursing's Social Policy Statement* (1995), *Standards of Clinical Nursing Practice* (2nd edition) (1998a), and *The Scope and Standards of Public Health Nursing Practice* (1999). The community health nurse consults with other health care providers and team members regarding the individual's plan of care and participates on quality assurance teams to measure the quality of care provided. The three core functions of assessment, policy development, and as-

surance are woven throughout all of the nurse's roles and the various community settings of practice.

ROLES OF COMMUNITY HEALTH NURSES

Just as the health care system is continually evolving, community health nursing practice evolves to remain effective with the clients it serves. Over time, the role of the community health nurse has broadened. This breadth is reflected in the definition of public health nursing from the American Public Health Association, Public Health Nursing Section (1996):

Public health nurses integrate community involvement and knowledge about the entire population with personal, clinical understandings of the health and illness experiences of individuals and families within the population. They translate and articulate the health and illness experiences of diverse, often vulnerable individuals and families in the population to health planners and policy makers, and assist members of the community to voice their problems and aspirations. Public health nurses are knowledgeable about multiple strategies for intervention, from those applicable to the entire population, to those for the family, and the individual. Public health nurses translate knowledge from the health and social sciences to individuals and population groups through targeted interventions, programs, and advocacy.

Public health nursing may be practiced by one public health nurse or by a group of public health nurses working collaboratively. In both instances, public health nurses are directly engaged in the interdisciplinary activities of the core public health functions of assessment, assurance and policy development. Interventions or strategies may be targeted to multiple levels depending on where the most effective outcomes are possible. They include strategies aimed at entire population groups, families, or individuals. In any setting, the role of public health nurses focuses on the prevention of illness, injury, or disability, the promotion of health, and maintenance of the health of populations.

Community health nurses wear many hats while conducting day-to-day practice. At any given time, however, one role is primary. This is especially true for specialized roles such as that of full-time manager. This chapter examines seven major roles: (1) clinician, (2) educator, (3) advocate, (4) manager, (5) collaborator, (6) leader, and (7) researcher. It also describes the factors that influence the selection and performance of those roles.

Clinician Role

The most familiar role of the community health nurse is that of clinician or care provider; however, the provision of nursing care takes on new meaning in the context of community health. The **clinician** role in community health means that the nurse ensures that health services are provided not just to individuals and families, but also to groups and populations. Nursing service still is designed for the special needs of clients; however, when those clients comprise a group or population, clinical practice takes different forms. It requires different skills to assess collective needs and tailor service accordingly. For instance, one community health nurse might visit elderly persons in a seniors' high-rise apartment building. Another might serve as the clinic nurse in a rural prental clinic that serves migrant farm workers. These are opportunities to assess the needs of entire aggregates and design appropriate services.

For community health nurses, the clinician role involves certain emphases that are different from those of basic nursing. Three clinician emphases, in particular, are useful to consider here: holism, health promotion, and skill expansion.

Holistic Practice

Most clinical nursing seeks to be broad and holistic. In community health, however, a holistic approach means considering the broad range of interacting needs that affect the collective health of the "client" as a larger system (Dossey, Keegan, & Guzzetta, 1999; Venes, 2001). Holistic nursing care encompasses the comprehensive and total care of the client in all areas, such as physical, emotional, social, spiritual, and economic. All are considered and cared for when the client is a large system, just as it should be with individual clients. The client is a composite of people whose relationships and interactions with each other must be considered in totality. Holistic practice must emerge from this systems perspective.

For example, when working with a group of pregnant teenagers living in a juvenile detention center, the nurse would consider the girls' relationships with one another, their parents, the fathers of their unborn children, and the detention center staff. The nurse would evaluate their ages, developmental needs, and peer influence, as well as their knowledge of pregnancy, delivery, and issues related to the choice of keeping or giving up their babies. The girls' reentry into the community and their future plans for school or employment also would be considered. Holistic service would go far beyond the physical condition of pregnancy and childbirth. It would incorporate consideration of pregnant adolescents in this community as a population at risk. What factors contributed to these girls' situations, and what preventive efforts could be instituted to protect other teenagers or these teens from future pregnancies? The clinician role of the community health nurse involves holistic practice from an aggregate perspective.

Focus on Wellness

The clinician role in community health also is characterized by its focus on promoting wellness. As discussed in Chapter 1, the community health nurse provides service along the entire range of the health continuum but especially emphasizes promotion of health and prevention of illness. Nursing service includes seeking out clients who are at risk for poor health and offering preventive and health-promoting services, rather than waiting for them to come for help after problems arise (Bracht, 1999; Wurzbach, 2002). People, programs, and agencies are identified who are interested in achieving a higher level of health, and the community health nurse works with them to accomplish that goal and then sustain the expected changed behavior. The nurse may help employees of a business learn how to live healthier lives or work with a group of people who want to quit smoking. The community health nurse may hold seminars with a men's group on enhancing fathering skills or assist a corporation with implementation of a health promotion program. Groups and populations are identified that may be vulnerable to certain health threats, and preventive and health-promoting programs can be designed. Examples include immunization of preschoolers, family planning programs, cholesterol screening, and prevention of behavioral problems in adolescents. Protecting and promoting the health of vulnerable populations is an important component of the clinician role and is addressed extensively in the chapters in Unit VII on vulnerable aggregates.

Expanded Skills

Many different skills are used in the role of the community health clinician. In the early years of community health nursing, emphasis was placed on physical care skills. With time, skills in observation, listening, communication, and counseling became integral to the clinician role as it grew to encompass an increased emphasis on psychological and sociocultural factors. Recently, environmental and community-wide considerations—such as problems caused by pollution, violence and crime, drug abuse, unemployment, poverty, homelessness, and limited funding for health programs—have created a need for stronger skills in assessing the needs of groups and populations and intervening at the community level. The clinician role in population-based nursing also requires skills in collaboration with consumers and other professionals, use of epidemiology and biostatistics, community organization and development, research, program evaluation, administration, leadership, and effecting change (Novick & Mays, 2000). These skills are addressed in greater detail in later chapters.

Educator Role

A second important role of the community health nurse is that of **educator** or health teacher. Health teaching, a widely recognized part of nursing practice, is legislated through nurse practice acts in several states and is one of the major functions of the community health nurse (Williamson & Drummond, 2000).

The educator role is especially useful in promoting the public's health for at least two reasons. First, community clients usually are not acutely ill and can absorb and act on health information. For example, a class of expectant parents, unhampered by significant health problems, can grasp the relationship of diet to fetal development. They understand the value of specific exercises to the childbirth process, are motivated to learn, and are more likely to perform those exercises. Thus, the educator role has the potential for finding greater receptivity and providing higher-yield results.

Second, the educator role in community health nursing is significant because a wider audience can be reached. With an emphasis on populations and aggregates, the educational efforts of community health nursing are appropriately targeted to reach many people. Instead of limiting teaching to one-on-one or small groups, the nurse has the opportunity and mandate to develop educational programs based on community needs that seek a community-wide impact. Community-wide antidrug campaigns, dietary improvement programs, and improved handwashing efforts among children provide useful models for implementation of the educator role at the population level and demonstrate its effectiveness in reaching a wide audience (MacIntosh, J., & McCormack, D., 2000; Rankin & Stallings, 2001; Redman, 2001).

One factor that enhances the educator role is the public's higher level of health consciousness. Through plans ranging from the President's Physical Fitness Program to local anti-smoking campaigns, people are recognizing the value of health and are increasingly motivated to achieve higher levels of wellness. When a middle-aged man, for example, is discharged from the hospital after a heart attack, he is likely to be more interested than before the attack in learning how to prevent another. He can learn how to reduce stress, develop an appropriate and gradual exercise program, and alter his eating habits. Families with young children often are interested in learning about children's growth and development; most parents are committed to raising happy, healthy children. Health education can affect the health status of people of all ages (Bomar & Baker-Wood, 2001; Floyd, 2000). Today, in more businesses and industries, nurses promote the health of employees through active wellness-education and injury-prevention programs. The companies recognize that improved health of their workers, which includes earning a living wage, means less absenteeism and higher production levels in addition to other benefits (Bhatia & Katz, 2001). Some companies even provide exercise areas and equipment for employees to use and pay for the cost of their participation or allow paid time off for the exercise.

Whereas nurses in acute care teach patients with a one-on-one focus about issues related to their hospitalization, community health nurses go beyond these topics to educate people in many areas. Community-living clients need and want to know about a wide variety of issues, such as family planning, weight control, smoking cessation, and stress reduction. Aggregate-level concerns also include such topics as environmental safety, sexual discrimination and harassment at school or work, violence, and drugs. What foods and additives are safe to eat? How can people organize the community to work for reduction of violence on television? What are health consumers' rights? Topics taught by community health nurses extend from personal and family health to environmental health and community organization.

As educators, community health nurses seek to facilitate client learning. Information is shared with clients both formally and informally. Nurses act as consultants to individuals or groups. Formal classes may be held to increase people's understanding of health and health care. Established community groups may be used in the nurse's teaching practice. For example, a nurse may teach parents and teachers at a parent-teacher meeting about signs of mood-modifying drug and alcohol abuse, discuss safety practices with a group of industrial workers, or give a presentation on the importance of early detection of child abuse to a health planning committee considering the funding of a new program. At times, the community health nurse facilitates client learning through referrals to more knowledgeable sources or through use of experts on special topics. Clients' self-education is facilitated by the nurse; in keeping with the concept of self-care, clients are encouraged and helped to use appropriate health resources and to seek out health information for themselves. The emphasis throughout the health teaching process continues to be placed on illness prevention and health promotion. Health teaching as a tool for community health nursing practice is discussed in detail in Chapter 12.

Advocate Role

The issue of clients' rights is important in health care. Every patient or client has the right to receive just, equal, and humane treatment. The role of nurse includes client advocacy, which is highlighted in the ANA's *Code for Nurses* (1985) and *Nursing's Social Policy Statement* (1995). Our current health care system often is characterized by fragmented and depersonalized services, and many clients—especially the poor, the disadvantaged, those without health insurance, and people with language barriers—frequently are denied their rights. They become frustrated, confused, degraded, and unable to cope with the system on their own. The community health nurse often acts as an **advocate** for clients, pleading their cause or acting on their behalf. Clients may need someone to explain which services to expect and which services they ought to receive, to make referrals as needed, and to write letters to agencies or health care providers for them. They need someone to guide them through the complexities of the system, to assure the satisfaction of their needs. This is particularly true for minorities and disadvantaged groups (Kumanyika, Morssink, & Nestle, 2001; Skinner, Arfken, & Waterman, 2000) (see What Do You Think?).

Advocacy Goals

There are two underlying goals in client advocacy. One is to help clients gain greater independence or self-determination. Until they can research the needed information and access health and social services for themselves, the community

WHAT DO YOU THINK?

As a community health nurse, you would like to enhance your health department's outreach services and ability to case-find. You brainstorm with colleagues. What creative, yet feasible settings can you imagine?

health nurse acts as an advocate for the clients by showing them what services are available, the ones to which they are entitled, and how to obtain them. A second goal is to make the system more responsive and relevant to the needs of clients. By calling attention to inadequate, inaccessible, or unjust care, community health nurses can influence change.

Consider the experience of the Merrill family. Gloria Merrill has three small children. Early one Tuesday morning, the baby, Tony, suddenly started to cry. Nothing would comfort him. Gloria went to a neighbor's apartment, called the local clinic, and was told to come in the next day. The clinic did not take appointments and was too busy to see any more patients that day. Gloria's neighbor reassured her that "sometimes babies just cry." For the rest of the day and night, Tony cried almost incessantly. On Wednesday, there was a 45-minute bus ride and a wait of 3½ hours in the crowded reception room, a wait punctuated by interrogations from clinic workers. Gloria's other children were restless, and the baby was crying. Finally, they saw the physician. Tony had an inguinal hernia that could have strangulated and become gangrenous. The doctor admonished Gloria for waiting so long to bring in the baby. Immediate surgery was necessary. Someone at the clinic told Gloria that Medicaid would pay for it. Someone else told her that she was ineligible because she was not a registered clinic patient. At this point, all of her children were crying. Gloria had been up most of the night. She was frantic, confused, and felt that no one cared. This family needed an advocate.

Advocacy Actions

The advocate role incorporates four characteristic actions: (1) being assertive, (2) taking risks, (3) communicating and negotiating well, and (4) identifying resources and obtaining results.

First, advocates must be assertive. Fortunately, in the Merrills' dilemma, the clinic had a working relationship with the City Health Department and contacted Tracy Lee, a community health nurse liaison with the clinic, when Gloria broke down and cried. Tracy took the initiative to identify the Merrills' needs and find appropriate solutions. She contacted the Department of Social Services and helped the Merrills to establish eligibility for coverage of surgery and hospitalization costs. She helped Gloria to make arrangements for the baby's hospitalization and the other children's care. Second, advocates must take risks—go out on a limb if need be—for

the client. The community health nurse was outraged by the kind of treatment received by the Merrills: the delays in service, the impersonal care, and the surgery that could have been planned as elective rather than as an emergency. She wrote a letter describing the details of the Merrills' experience to the clinic director, the chairman of the clinic board, and the nursing director. This action resulted in better care for the Merrills and a series of meetings aimed at changing clinic procedures and providing better telephone screening. Third, advocates must communicate and negotiate well by bargaining thoroughly and convincingly. The community health nurse helping the Merrill family stated the problem clearly and argued for its solution. Finally, advocates must identify and obtain resources for the client's benefit. By contacting the most influential people in the clinic and appealing to their desire for quality service, the nurse caring for the Merrill family was able to facilitate change.

Advocacy at the population level incorporates the same goals and actions. Whether the population is homeless people, battered women, or migrant workers, the community health nurse, in the advocate role, speaks and acts on their behalf. The goals remain the same: to promote clients' self-determination and to shape a more responsive system. Advocacy for large aggregates, such as the millions with inadequate health care coverage, means changing national policies and laws (see Chapter 16). Advocacy may take the form of presenting public health nursing data to ensure that providers deliver quality services. It may mean conducting a needs assessment to demonstrate the necessity for a shelter and multiservice program for the homeless. It may mean testifying before the legislature to create awareness of the problems of battered women and the need for more protective laws. It may mean organizing a lobbying effort to require employers of migrant workers to provide proper housing and working conditions. In each case, the community health nurse works with representatives of the population to gain their understanding of the situation and to ensure their input.

Manager Role

Community health nurses, like all nurses, engage in the role of managing health services. As a manager, the nurse exercises administrative direction toward the accomplishment of specified goals by assessing clients' needs, planning and organizing to meet those needs, directing and leading to achieve results, and controlling and evaluating the progress to ensure that goals are met. The nurse serves as a **manager** when overseeing client care as a case manager, supervising ancillary staff, managing caseloads, running clinics, or conducting community health needs assessment projects. In each instance, the nurse engages in four basic functions that make up the management process. The management process, like the nursing process, incorporates a series of problem-solving activities or functions: planning, organizing, leading, and controlling and evaluating. These activities are sequential and yet also occur simultaneously for managing service objectives (Cherry & Jacob, 2002; Swansburg & Swansburg, 1999). While performing these functions, community health nurses most often are participative managers; that is, they participate with clients, other professionals, or both to plan and implement services.

Nurse as Planner

The first function in the management process is planning. A **planner** sets the goals and direction for the organization or project and determines the means to achieve them. Specifically, planning includes defining goals and objectives, determining the strategy for reaching them, and designing a coordinated set of activities for implementing and evaluating them. Planning may be strategic, which tends to include broader, more long-range goals (Cherry & Jacob, 2002; Swansburg & Swansburg, 1999; U.S. Department of Health and Human Services, 2000). An example of strategic planning is setting 2-year agency goals to reduce teenage pregnancies in the county by 50%. Planning may be operational, which focuses more on short-term planning needs. An example of operational planning is setting 6-month objectives to implement a new computer system for client record keeping.

The community health nurse engages in planning as a part of the manager role when supervising a group of home health aides working with home care clients. Plans of care must be designed that include setting short-term and long-term objectives, describing actions to carry out the objectives, and designing a plan for evaluating the care given. With larger groups, such as a program for a homeless mentally ill population, the planning function is used in collaboration with other professionals in the community to determine appropriate goals for shelter and treatment and to develop an action plan to carry out and evaluate the program (Berkowitz, 2001; Grembowski, 2001). The concepts of planning with communities and families are discussed further in Chapters 19 and 24, respectively.

Nurse as Organizer

The second function of the manager role is that of **organizer**. This involves designing a structure within which people and tasks function to reach the desired objectives. A manager must arrange matters so that the job can be done. People, activities, and relationships have to be assembled to put the plan into effect. Organizing includes deciding the tasks to be done, who will do them, how to group the tasks, who reports to whom, and where decisions will be made (Cherry & Jacob, 2002). In the process of organizing, the nurse manager provides a framework for the various aspects of service so that each runs smoothly and accomplishes its purpose. The framework is a part of service preparation. When a community health nurse manages a well-child clinic, for instance, the organizing function involves making certain that all equipment and supplies are present, that required staff are hired and are on duty, and that staff responsibilities are clearly designated. The final responsibility as an organizer is to evaluate the effectiveness of the clinic. Is it providing the

needed services? Are the clients satisfied? Do the services remain cost-effective? All of these questions must be addressed by the organizer.

Nurse as Leader

In the manager role, the community health nurse also must act as a **leader**. As a leader, the nurse directs, influences, or persuades others to effect change so as to positively affect people's health and move them toward a goal. The leading function includes persuading and motivating people, directing activities, ensuring effective two-way communication, resolving conflicts, and coordinating the plan. Coordination means bringing people and activities together so that they function in harmony while pursuing desired objectives.

Community health nurses act as leaders when they direct and coordinate the functioning of a hypertension screening clinic, a weight control group, or a three-county mobile health assessment unit. In each case, the leading function requires motivating the people involved, keeping clear channels of communication, negotiating conflicts, and directing and coordinating the activities established during planning so that the desired objectives can be accomplished.

Nurse as Controller and Evaluator

The fourth management function is to control and evaluate projects or programs. A **controller** monitors the plan and ensures that it stays on course. In this function, the community health nurse must realize that plans may not proceed as intended and may need adjustments or corrections to reach the desired results or goals. Monitoring, comparing, and adjusting make up the controlling part of this function. At the same time, the nurse must compare and judge performance and outcomes against previously set goals and standards—a process that forms the **evaluator** aspect of this management function.

An example of the controlling and evaluating function was evident in a program started in several preschool day care centers in a city in the Midwest. The goal of the project was to reduce the incidence of illness among the children through intensive physical and emotional preventive health education with staff, parents, and children. The two community health nurses managing the project were pleased with the progress of the classes and monitored the application of the prevention principles in day-to-day care. However, staff became busy after several weeks, and some plans were not being followed carefully. Preventive activities were not being closely monitored, such as ensuring that the children covered their mouths if they coughed and washed their hands after using the bathroom and before eating. Several children who were clearly sick had not been kept at home. Including the lonely children in activities sometimes was overlooked. The nurses worked with staff and parents to motivate them and get the project back on course. They held monthly meetings with the staff, observed the classes periodically, and offered one-on-one instruction to staff, parents, and children. One activity was to establish competition between the centers for the best health record, with the promise of a photograph of the winning center's children and an article in the local newspaper. Their efforts were successful.

Management Behaviors

As managers, community health nurses engage in many different types of behaviors. These behaviors or parts of the manager role were first described by Mintzberg (1973). He grouped them into three sets of behaviors: (1) decision-making, (2) transferring of information, and (3) engaging in interpersonal relationships.

Decision-Making Behaviors

Mintzberg identified four types of decisional roles or behaviors: entrepreneur, disturbance handler, resource allocator, and negotiator. A manager serves in the entrepreneur role when initiating new projects. Starting a nursing center to serve a homeless population is an example. Community health nurses play the disturbance-handler role when they manage disturbances and crises—particularly interpersonal conflicts among staff, between staff and clients, or among clients (especially when being served in an agency). The resource-allocator role is demonstrated by determining the distribution and use of human, physical, and financial resources. Nurses play the negotiator role when negotiating, perhaps with higher levels of administration or a funding agency, for new health policy or budget increases to support expanded services for clients.

Transfer of Information Behaviors

Mintzberg described three informational roles or behaviors: monitor, information disseminator, and spokesperson. The monitor role requires collecting and processing information, such as gathering ongoing evaluation data to determine whether a program is meeting its goals. In the disseminator role, nurses transmit the collected information to people involved in the project or organization. In the spokesperson role, nurses share information on behalf of the project or agency with outsiders.

Interpersonal Behaviors

While engaging in various interpersonal roles, the community health nurse may function as figurehead, a leader, and a liaison. In the figurehead role, the nurse acts in a ceremonial or symbolic capacity, such as participating in a ribbon-cutting ceremony to mark the opening of a new clinic or representing the project or agency for news media coverage. In the leader role, the nurse motivates and directs people involved in the project. In the liaison role, a network is maintained with people outside the organization or project for information exchange and project enhancement.

Management Skills

What types of skills and competencies does the community health nurse need in the manager role? Three basic management skills are needed for successful achievement of goals: human, conceptual, and technical. **Human skills** refer to the ability to understand, communicate, motivate, delegate, and work well with people (Cherry & Jacob, 2002). An example is a nursing supervisor's or team leader's ability to gain the trust and respect of staff and promote a productive and satisfying work environment. A manager can accomplish goals only with the cooperation of others. Therefore, human skills are essential to successfully perform the manager role. **Conceptual skills** refer to the mental ability to analyze and interpret abstract ideas for the purpose of understanding and diagnosing situations and formulating solutions. Examples are analyzing demographic data for program planning and developing a conceptual model to describe and improve organizational function. Finally, **technical skills** refer to the ability to apply special management-related knowledge and expertise to a particular situation or problem. Such skills performed by a community health nurse might include implementing a staff development program or developing a computerized management information system.

Case Management

Case management has become the standard method of managing health care in the delivery systems in the United States, and managed care organizations have become an integral part of community-oriented care. **Case management** is a systematic process by which a nurse assesses clients' needs, plans for and coordinates services, refers to other appropriate providers, and monitors and evaluates progress to ensure that clients' multiple service needs are met in a cost-effective manner. **Managed care**, the broader umbrella under which case management exists, is a cost-containing system of health care administration (Powell, 2000). Managed care, as an approach to delivering health care, is discussed in detail in Chapter 7. As clients leave hospitals earlier, as families struggle with multiple and complex health problems, as more elderly persons need alternatives to nursing home care, as competition and scarce resources contribute to fragmentation of services, and as the cost of health care continues to increase, there is a growing need for someone to oversee and coordinate all facets of needed service (Harris, Ripperger, & Horn, 2000). Through case management, the nurse addresses this need in the community.

The activity of case management often follows discharge planning as a part of continuity of care. When applied to individual clients, it means overseeing their transition from the hospital back into the community and monitoring them to ensure that all of their service needs are met. Case management also applies to aggregates. In this context, it involves overseeing and ensuring that a group's or population's health-related needs are met, particularly for those who are at high risk of illness or injury. For example, the community health nurse may work with battered women who come to a shelter. First, the nurse must ensure that their immediate needs for safety, security, food, finances, and child care are met. Then, the nurse must work with other professionals to provide more permanent housing, employment, ongoing counseling, and financial and legal resources for this group of women. Whether

RESEARCH: BRIDGE TO PRACTICE

Parker, M.W., Bellis, J.M., Bishop, P., Harper, M., Allman, R.M., Moore, C., et al. (2002). A Multidisciplinary Model of Health Promotion incorporating spirituality into a successful aging intervention with African American and White elderly groups. *The Gerontologist, 42*(3), 406–415.

This interprofessional model of health promotion incorporates the skills of multitalented professionals with the needs of 500 seniors and their families. The design of this study used an expanded Rowe and Kahn model of successful aging (which includes positive spirituality as a core construct) to present a community-based initiative focusing on primary prevention. The planning between African-American and White community members was a first for this town. It included lay people from the community along with spiritual leaders, university professionals, and community medical personnel.

Topics for discussion during this conference focused on successful aging themes: the importance of elder leadership, spiritual growth, avoidance of disease and disability, active engagement with life, maintenance of high cognitive and physical fitness, intergenerational transfers of wisdom, awareness of services and programs for seniors, and late-life legal, health, and financial planning.

Evaluations by conference attendees were positive. Ninety-seven percent of the African-American and 80% of White attendees reported an intention to make changes as a result of the conference. Both ethnic groups rated the conference highly, with 98% rating their experience as either excellent or good.

The desired sequelae emerging from the conference were the establishment of continuing health promotion and the formation of life-affirming activities focused on older adults within these newly established faith-based coalitions. There also developed an ongoing relationship among the denominational and racial groups resulting in functional, proactive, ongoing coalitions that have planned and implemented further health promotion activities within the community.

The positive results of this intervention demonstrate a variety of roles and settings for the community health nurse: as a presenter (educator), as an initiator and planner (leader), and as a clinician for health screening services also offered at this conference. The setting was unique (a conference held at a religious center) and served a group of high-risk African-American elders, an often underserved group.

applied to families or aggregates, case management, like other applications of the manager role, uses the three sets of management behaviors and engages the community health nurse as planner, organizer, leader, controller, and evaluator (see Research: Bridge to Practice).

Collaborator Role

Community health nurses seldom practice in isolation. They must work with many people, including clients, other nurses, physicians, teachers, health educators, social workers, physical therapists, nutritionists, occupational therapists, psychologists, epidemiologists, biostaticians, attorneys, secretaries, environmentalists, city planners, and legislators. As members of the health team (Corrigan, 2000; Mulligan et al., 1999), community health nurses assume the role of **collaborator**, which means to work jointly with others in a common endeavor, to cooperate as partners. Successful community health practice depends on this multidisciplinary collegiality and leadership. Everyone on the team has an important and unique contribution to make to the health care effort. As on a championship ball team, the better all members play their individual positions and cooperate with other members, the more likely the health team is to win.

The community health nurse's collaborator role requires skills in communicating, in interpreting the nurse's unique contribution to the team, and in acting assertively as an equal partner. The collaborator role also may involve functioning as a consultant.

The following examples show a community health nurse functioning as collaborator. Three families needed to find good nursing homes for their elderly grandparents. The community health nurse met with the families, including the elderly members; made a list of desired features, such as a shower and access to walking trails; and then worked with a social worker to locate and visit several homes. The grandparents' respective physicians were contacted for medical consultation, and in each case the elderly member made the final selection. In another situation, the community health nurse collaborated with the city council, police department, neighborhood residents, and the manager of a senior citizens' high-rise apartment building to help a group of elderly people organize and lobby for safer streets. In a third example, a school nurse noticed a rise in the incidence of drug use in her schools. She initiated a counseling program after joint planning with students, parents, teachers, the school psychologist, and a local drug rehabilitation center.

Leadership Role

Community health nurses are becoming increasingly active in the leadership role, separate from leading within the manager role mentioned earlier. The leadership role focuses on effecting change (see Chapter 13); thus, the nurse becomes an agent of change. As leaders, community health nurses seek to initiate changes that positively affect people's health. They also seek to influence people to think and behave differently about their health and the factors contributing to it.

At the community level, the leadership role may involve working with a team of professionals to direct and coordinate such projects as a campaign to eliminate smoking in public areas or to lobby legislators for improved child day care facilities. When nurses guide community health decision-making, stimulate an industry's interest in health promotion, initiate group therapy, direct a preventive program, or influence health policy, they assume the leadership role. For example, a community health nurse started a rehabilitation program that included self-esteem building, career counseling, and job placement to help women in a halfway house who had recently been released from prison.

The community health nurse also exerts influence through health planning. The need for coordinated, accessible, cost-effective health care services creates a challenge and an opportunity for the nurse to become more involved in health planning at all levels: organizational, local, state, national, and international. A community health nurse needs to exercise leadership responsibility and assert the right to share in health decisions (Cherry & Jacob, 2002). One community health nurse determined that there was a need for a mental health program in his district. He planned to implement it through the agency for which he worked, but certain individuals on the health board were opposed to adding new programs because of the cost. The nurse's approach was to gather considerable data to demonstrate the need for the program and its cost-effectiveness. He invited individual key board members to lunch to convince them of the need. He prepared written summaries, graphs, and charts and, at a strategic time, presented his case at a board meeting. The mental health program was approved and implemented.

A broader attribute of the leadership role is that of visionary. A leader with vision develops the ability to see what can be and leads people on a path toward that goal. A leader's vision may include long-term and short-term goals. In one instance, it began as articulating the need for stronger community nursing services to an underserved population in an inner-city neighborhood served by a community health nurse. In this densely populated, tenant-occupied neighborhood, drugs, crime, and violence were commonplace. One summer, an 8-year-old boy was shot and killed. The enraged immigrant families in the neighborhood felt helpless and hopeless. Several families were visited by the nurse, and they shared their concerns with her. The nurse felt strongly about this blighted community and offered to work with the community to effect change. Volunteers from neighborhood churches were gathered by the community health nurse, and together they began to discuss the community's concerns. Together they prioritized their needs and began planning to make theirs a healthy community. The nurse organized her work week to provide health screening and education to families in the basement of

a church on one morning each week. Initially, only a few families accessed this new service. In a matter of months, it became recognized as a valuable community service, and it expanded to a full day, with an expanding volunteer group soon outgrowing the space. The community health nurse worked closely with influential community members and the families being served. They determined that many more services were needed in this neighborhood, and they began to broaden their outreach and think of ways to get the needed services.

Within a year, the group had written several grants to the city and to a private corporation in an effort to expand the voluntary services. The funding that they obtained allowed them to rent vacant storefront space, hire a part-time nurse practitioner, contract with the health department for additional community health nursing services, and negotiate with the local university to have medical, nursing, and social work students placed on a regular basis. The group, under the visionary leadership of the community health nurse, planned to add a one-on-one reading program for children, a class in English as a second language for immigrant families, a mentoring program for teenagers, and dental services. Even the police department had opened a substation in the neighborhood, making their presence more visible. This community health nurse's vision filled an immediate, critical need in the short term and developed into a comprehensive community center in the long term. Violence and crime diminished, and the neighborhood became a place where children could play safely.

Researcher Role

In the **researcher** role, community health nurses engage in systematic investigation, collection, and analysis of data for solving problems and enhancing community health practice. But how can research be combined with practice? Although research technically involves a complex set of activities conducted by persons with highly developed and specialized skills, research also means applying that technical study to real-practice situations. Community health nurses base their practice on the evidence found in the literature to enhance and change practice as needed. For example, the work of several researchers over 15 years supports the value of intensive home visiting to high-risk families (Olds et al., 1997, 1998). The outcomes of this research are changing practice protocol to high-risk families in many health departments today.

Research is an investigative process in which all community health nurses can become involved in asking questions and looking for solutions. Collaborative practice models between academics and practitioners combine research methodology expertise with practitioners' knowledge of problems to make community health nursing research both valid and relevant.

The Research Process

Community health nurses practice the researcher role at several levels. In addition to everyday inquiries, community health nurses often participate in agency and organizational studies to determine such matters as job satisfaction among public health nurses and risks associated with home visiting (Kendra & George, 2001). Some community health nurses participate in more complex research on their own or in collaboration with other health professionals (Navaie-Waliser et al., 2000). The researcher role, at all levels, helps to determine needs, evaluate effectiveness of care, and develop theoretic bases for community health nursing practice. Chapters 14 and 17 explain community health research in greater detail.

Research literally means to *search again*—to investigate, discover, and interpret facts. All research in community health, from the simplest inquiry to the most complex epidemiologic study, uses the same fundamental process. Simply put, the research process involves the following steps: (1) identify an area of interest, (2) specify the research question or statement, (3) review the literature, (4) identify a conceptual framework, (5) select a research design, (6) collect and analyze data, (7) interpret the results, and (8) communicate the findings (see Chapter 14).

Investigation builds on the nursing process, that essential dynamic of community health nursing practice, using it as a problem-solving process (Polit, Beck, & Hungler, 2001). In using the nursing process, the nurse identifies a problem or question, investigates by collecting and analyzing data, suggests and evaluates possible solutions, and selects a solution, or rejects them all and starts the investigative process over again. In a sense, the nurse is gathering data for health planning—investigating health problems to design wellness-promoting and disease-preventing interventions for community populations (see The Global Community).

Attributes of the Researcher Role

A questioning attitude is a basic prerequisite for good nursing practice. A nurse may have revisited a patient many times and noticed some change in his or her condition, such as restlessness or pallor; consequently, the nurse wonders what is causing this change and what can be done about it. In everyday practice, numerous situations are encountered that chal-

---

THE GLOBAL COMMUNITY

Hisama, K.K. (2000). Carrying your own lamp. *Reflections on Nursing Leadership, 26*(1), 30–32.

This article discusses the health care reforms implemented in Japan after World War II that improved nursing education through modeling United States pedagogy. Some nurses have taken the initiative to develop theories based on their own practices, which incorporate the characteristics of the Japanese people to improve nursing care. A nursing role, based on the population served and congruent with culturally competent care for practicing nurses, is needed in all countries.

The qualities of the Japanese people require the nurses' roles to accomodate cultural norms. For example, one characteristic among the Japanese is called *amae,* this is a child-like dependency or attachment that goes beyond childhood and is especially evident when people are sick or facing difficulties. Nursing practice based on Dorothea Orem's theory of self-care would not be appropriate in this culture. Another characteristic is the dominance of emotion over reason, which leads patients to prefer nurses' accomodating personalities instead of their scientific skills. Professionalism tends to not be recognized, or rewarded, as much as kindness. Because of such traits, nurses' roles are not clearly defined and they burn out quickly from overwork.

Through working with Western nursing theorists over the past 50 years, Japanese nurses have developed a style of nursing that focuses on four major forces: spiritual, scientific, humanistic, and social. Examples and leaders of these foci are as follows:

- Spiritual—Japan has a long tradition of respect for the dead, nurses perform elaborate nursing procedures after a death, which are best and most comfortably conducted at home. Sr. Matuno Teramoto is an expert in spirituality and nursing in the Japanese tradition.
- Scientific—Hiroko Usui conducted research over a 5-year period in order to argue that nursing is a true profession. She has written textbooks based on Nightingale's theory that rewrites traditional medical books on anatomy and physiology, disease, and recovery from the perspective of nursing.
- Humanistic—Masako Suzuki's major work concerns the communication between nurses and patients. Through her research, she discovered that many Japanese seldom tell nurses their needs even when their lives are at risk. The patients expect the nurse to understand their needs, just as a mother does for a baby and child. Her theory explains how nurses may bring out crucial medical information from patients by creating contexts favorable for communication.
- Social—Midori Kawashima was inspired by Virginia Henderson's theory on basic nursing and the importance of nurses' working conditions and wages. She became the leader of the grassroots movement to provide nurses with continuing education.

The author of this article has demonstrated that the nurse's role varies according to the client's culture and the setting in which nursing care is delivered; this is a lesson for all nurses working in a multicultural society.

lenge the nurse to ask questions. Consider the following examples.

- The newspaper reports that another group of children has been arrested for using illegal drugs. Is there an increase in the incidence of illegal drug use in the community?
- Several children attending a day care center appear to have excessive bruises on their arms and legs. What is the incidence of reported child abuse in this community? What could be done to promote earlier detection and improved reporting?
- Several elderly persons are living alone and without assistance in a neighborhood. How prevalent is this situation, and what are this population's needs?
- While driving through a particular neighborhood, the nurse notices that there is not a single playground. Where do the kids play?

Each of these questions places the nurse in the role of investigator. They express the fundamental attitude of every researcher: a spirit of inquiry.

A second attribute, careful observation, also is evident in the examples just given. The nurse needs to develop a sharpened ability to notice things as they are, including deviations from the norm and subtle changes suggesting the need for nursing action. Coupled with observation is openmindedness, another attribute of the researcher role. In the case of the bruises seen on day care children, a community health nurse's observations suggest child abuse as a possible cause. However, openmindedness requires consideration of other alternatives, and, as a good investigator, the nurse explores these possibilities as well.

Analytic skills also are used in this role. In the example of illegal drug use, the nurse already has started to analyze the situation by trying to determine its cause-and-effect relationships. Successful analysis depends on how well the data have been collected. Insufficient information can lead to false interpretations, so it is important to seek out the needed data. Analysis, like a jigsaw puzzle, involves studying the pieces and fitting them together until the meaning of the whole picture can be described.

Finally, the researcher role involves tenacity. The community health nurse persists in an investigation until facts are uncovered and a satisfactory answer is found. Noticing an absence of playgrounds and wondering where the children play is only a beginning. Being concerned about the children's safety and need for recreational outlets, the nurse gathers data about the location and accessibility of play areas as well as felt needs of community residents. A fully documented research report may result. If the data support a need for additional play space, the report can be brought before the proper authorities (see Research: Bridge to Practice).

SETTINGS FOR COMMUNITY HEALTH NURSING PRACTICE

The previous section examined community health nursing from the perspective of its major roles. The roles now can be placed in context by viewing the settings in which they are practiced. The types of places in which community health nurses practice are increasingly varied and include a growing number of nontraditional settings and partnerships with nonhealth groups. Employers of community health nurses range from state and local health departments and home health agencies to managed care organizations, businesses and industries, and nonprofit organizations. For this discussion, these settings are grouped into seven categories: (1) homes, (2) ambulatory service settings, (3) schools, (4) occupational health settings, (5) residential institutions, (6) parishes, and (7) the community at large.

Homes

For a long time, the most frequently used setting for community health nursing practice was the home. In the home, all of the community health nursing roles, to varying degrees, are performed. Clients who are discharged from acute care institutions, such as hospitals or mental health facilities, are regularly referred to community health nurses for continued care and follow-up. Here, the community health nurse can see clients in a family and environmental context, and service can be tailored to the clients' unique needs.

For example, Mr. White, 67 years of age, was discharged from the hospital with a colostomy. Doreen Levitz, the community health nurse from the county public health nursing agency, immediately started home visits. She met with Mr. White and his wife to discuss their needs as a family and to plan for Mr. White's care and adjustment to living with a colostomy. Practicing the clinician and educator roles, she reinforced and expanded on the teaching started in the hospital for colostomy care, including bowel training, diet, exercise, and proper use of equipment. As part of a total family care plan, Doreen provided some forms of physical care for Mr. White as well as counseling, teaching, and emotional support for both Mr. White and his wife. In addition to consulting with the physician and social service worker, she arranged and supervised visits from the home health aide, who gave personal care and homemaker services. She thus performed the manager, leader, and collaborator roles.

The home also is a setting for health promotion. Many community health nursing visits focus on assisting families to understand and practice healthier living behaviors. Nurses may, for example, instruct clients on parenting, infant care, child discipline, diet, exercise, coping with stress, or managing grief and loss.

The character of the home setting is as varied as the clients served by the community health nurse. In one day, the nurse may visit a well-to-do widow in her luxurious home, a middle-income family in their modest bungalow, an elderly transient man in his one-room fifth-story walk-up apartment, and a teen mother and her infant living in a group foster home. In each situation, the nurse can view the clients in perspective and, therefore, better understand their limitations, capitalize on their resources, and tailor health services to meet their needs. In the home, unlike most other health care settings, clients are on their own turf. They feel comfortable and secure in familiar surroundings and often are better able to understand and apply health information. Client self-respect can be promoted, because the client is host and the nurse is a guest.

Sometimes, the thought of visiting in clients' homes can cause anxiety for the nurse. This may be the nurse's first experience outside the acute care, long-term care, or clinic setting. Visiting clients in their own environment can make the nurse feel uncomfortable. The nurse may be asked to visit families in unfamiliar neighborhoods and must walk through those neighborhoods to visit the client. Frequently, fear of the unknown is the real fear, and often it has been enhanced by stories from previous nurses. This may be the same feeling as that experienced when caring for your first client, first entering the operating room, or first having a client in the intensive care unit. However, in the community there are more variables, and there are basic safety measures that should be used by all people when out in public. General guidelines for safety and making home visits are covered in detail in Chapter 23. Nevertheless, the specific instructions given during the clinical experience should be followed, and everyday, common-sense safety precautions should be used.

Changes in the health care delivery system, along with shifting health economics and service delivery (discussed in Chapter 7), are changing community health nursing's use of the home as a setting for practice. The increased demand for highly technical acute care in the home requires specialized skills that are best delivered by nurses with this expertise. With skills in population-based practice, community health nurses serve the public's health best by focusing on sites where they can have the greatest impact. At the same time, they can collaborate with various types of home care providers, including hospitals, other nurses, physicians, rehabilitation therapists, and durable medical equipment companies, to ensure continuous and holistic service. The nurse continues to supervise home care services and engage in case management. Chapter 37 further examines the nurse's role in the home care setting.

Ambulatory Service Settings

Ambulatory service settings include a variety of venues for community health nursing practice in which clients come for day or evening services that do not include overnight stays. Community health centers are an example of an ambulatory setting. Sometimes, multiple clinics offering comprehensive services are community based or are located in outpatient departments of hospitals or medical centers. They also may be based in comprehensive neighborhood health centers. A single clinic, such as a family planning clinic or a well-child clinic, may be found in a location that is more convenient for clients, perhaps a church basement or empty storefront. Some kinds of day care centers, such as those for physically disabled or emotionally disturbed adults, use community health nursing services. Additional ambulatory care settings include health departments and community health nursing

agencies where clients may come for assessment and referral or counseling.

Offices are another type of ambulatory care setting. Some community health nurses provide service in conjunction with a medical practice; for example, a community health nurse associated with a health maintenance organization sees clients in the office and undertakes screening, referrals, counseling, health education, and group work. Others establish independent practices by seeing clients in community nursing centers as well as making home visits.

Another type of ambulatory service setting includes places where services are offered to selected groups. For example, community health nurses practice in migrant camps, on Native American reservations, at correctional facilities, in children's day care centers, through churches as parish nurses, and in remote mountain and coal-mining communities. Again, in each ambulatory setting, all of the community health nursing roles are used to varying degrees. Several special ambulatory settings are explored in detail later: children's day care centers are discussed in Chapter 27; migrant health is explored in Chapter 33; correctional nursing is described in detail in Chapter 36; and parish nursing is discussed later in this chapter (Display 3–2).

Schools

Schools of all levels make up a major group of settings for community health nursing practice. Nurses from community health nursing agencies frequently serve private schools at elementary and intermediate levels. Public schools are served by the same agencies or by community health nurses hired through the public school system. The community health nurse may work with groups of students in preschool settings, such as Montessori schools, as well as in vocational or technical schools, junior colleges, and college and university settings. Specialized schools, such as those for the developmentally disabled, are another setting for community health nursing practice.

Community health nurses' roles in school settings are changing. School nurses, whose primary role initially was that of clinician, are widening their practice to include more health education, interprofessional collaboration, and client advocacy. For example, one school had been accustomed to using the nurse as a first-aid provider and record keeper. Her duties were handling minor problems, such as headaches and cuts, and keeping track of such events as immunizations. This nurse sought to expand her practice and, after consultation and preparation, collaborated with a health educator and some of the teachers to offer a series of classes on personal hygiene, diet, and sexuality. She started a drop-in health counseling center in the school and established a network of professional contacts for consultation and referral.

Community health nurses in school settings also are beginning to assume managerial and leadership roles and to recognize that the researcher role should be an integral part of their practice. The nurse's role with school-age and adolescent populations is discussed in detail in Chapter 28.

DISPLAY 3-2

Innovative Community Health Nursing Practice

In some community health nursing courses, students do not have access to an established agency such as a health department or community center from which to establish a client base. Student nurses and practicing community health nurses can provide outreach services and do case-finding in innovative settings such as these:

Settings	Clients	Roles of the Community Health Nurse
1. Senior centers when flu shots are given or commodities are distributed	Older adults	Educator, Clinician, Advocate
2. Outside of grocery stores, department stores, movie theaters, large pharmacies	People of all ages and families	Educator, Clinician, Advocate
3. At PTA meetings, sporting events, dances, and school registration (in collaboration with school nurses).	Young adults, children, and teenagers	Educator, Clinician, Advocate
4. Outside of concerts, plays, the circus, etc.	People of all ages	Educator, Clinician, Advocate
5. Other public gatherings: farmers markets, neighborhood yard sales, etc.	People of all ages	Educator, Clinician, Advocate
6. Conferences or seminars	People of all ages	Leader, Educator, Clinician
7. "On the street"	Homeless persons, passersby, transients, low-income urban dwellers	Educator, Clinician, Advocate
8. Truck stops	Predominently employed men	Educator, Clinician, Advocate

   Leader Role—initiate, plan, strategize, collaborate, and cooperate with community groups to present programs that are focused on specific population's needs (see Research: Bridge to Practice).

   Educator Role—teach nutrition, stress management, safety, exercise, prevention of sexually transmitted diseases, and other mens' and womens' health issues, child home/school/play and stranger safety, and child growth and development, and provide anticipatory guidance. Have pamphlets available to support verbal information on health and safety topics, specific diseases, Social Security, Medicare, and Medicaid.

   Clinician Role—perform blood pressure screening, height, weight, blood testing for diabetes and cholesterol, occult blood test, hearing and vision tests, scoliosis measurements, and administration of immunizations.

   Advocate Role—provide information regarding community resources as needed, cut "red tape" for those who need it, answer questions, and guide people to additional resources, such as Internet Web sites and "800" phone numbers.

Occupational Health Settings

Business and industry provide another group of settings for community health nursing practice. Employee health has long been recognized as making a vital contribution to individual lives, productivity of business, and the well-being of the entire nation. Organizations are expected to provide a safe and healthy work environment in addition to offering insurance for health care. More companies, recognizing the value of healthy employees, are going beyond offering traditional health benefits to supporting health promotional efforts. Some businesses, for example, offer healthy snacks such as fruit at breaks and promote jogging during the noon hour. A few larger corporations have built exercise facilities for their employees, provide health education programs, and offer financial incentives for losing weight or staying well.

   Community health nurses in occupational health settings practice a variety of roles. The clinician role was primary for many years, as nurses continued to care for sick or injured employees at work. However, recognition of the need to protect employees' safety and, later, to prevent their illness led to the inclusion of health education in the occupational health nurse role. Occupational health nurses also act as employee advocates, assuring appropriate job assignments for workers and adequate treatment for job-related illness or injury. They collaborate with other health care providers and company management to offer better services to their clients. They act as leaders and managers in developing new health services in the work setting, endorsing programs such as hypertension screening and weight control. Occupational health settings range from industries and factories, such as an automobile assembly plant, to business corporations and even large retail sales systems. The field of occupational health offers a challenging opportunity, particularly in smaller businesses, where nursing coverage usually is not provided. Chapter 29 more fully describes the role of the nurse serving the working adult population.

Residential Institutions

Any facility where clients reside can be a setting in which community health nursing is practiced. Residential institutions can include a halfway house in which clients live temporarily while recovering from drug addiction or an inpatient hospice program in which terminally ill clients live. Some residential settings, such as hospitals, exist solely to provide health care; others provide other services and support. Community health nurses based in a community agency maintain continuity of care for their clients by collaborating with hospital personnel, visiting clients in the hospital, and planning care during and after hospitalization. Some community health nurses serve one or more hospitals on a regular basis by providing a liaison with the community, consultation for discharge planning, and periodic inservice programs to keep hospital staff updated on community services for their clients. Other community health nurses with similar functions are based in the hospital and serve the hospital community.

A continuing care center is another example of a residential site providing health care that may use community health nursing services. In this setting, residents usually are elderly; some live quite independently, whereas others become increasingly more dependent and have many chronic health problems. The community health nurse functions as advocate and collaborator to improve services. The nurse may, for example, coordinate available resources to meet the needs of residents and their families and help safeguard the maintenance of quality operating standards. Chapter 30 discusses the community health nurse's role with elders aging in place. Chapter 37 discusses nursing services needed by clients after hospitalization through home care services or by families and clients in hospice programs. Sheltered workshops and group homes for mentally ill or developmentally disabled children and adults are other examples of residential institutions that serve clients who share specific needs; they are discussed in Chapters 34 and 35.

Community health nurses also practice in settings where residents are gathered for purposes other than receiving care. Health care is offered as an adjunct to the primary goals of the institution. For example, many nurses work with camping programs for children and adults offered by churches and other community agencies, such as the Boy Scouts, Girl Scouts, or YMCA. Other camp nurses work with children and adults who have chronic or terminal illnesses, through disease-related community agencies such as the American Lung Association, American Diabetes Association, and American Cancer Society. Camp nurses practice all available roles, often under interesting and challenging conditions.

Residential institutions provide unique settings for the community health nurse to practice health promotion. Clients are a "captive" audience whose needs can be readily assessed and whose interests can be stimulated. These settings offer the opportunity to generate an environment of caring and optimal-quality health care provided by community health nursing services.

Parishes

Parish nursing finds its beginnings in an ancient tradition. The beginnings of community health nursing can be traced to religious orders (see Chapter 2), and for centuries churches, temples, mosques, and other spiritual communities were important sources of health care. In parish nursing today, the practice focal point remains the faith community and the religious belief system provided by the philosophical framework (Clark & Olson, 2000; Hughes et al., 2001). Parish nursing may take different names, such as church-based health promotion (CBHP), faith community nursing, or primary care parish nursing practice (PCPNP). Whatever the service is called, it involves a large-scale effort by the church community to improve the health of its members through education, screening, referral, treatment, and group support. In the PCPNP program in Patterson, New Jersey, the focus of care is "aimed at promoting health and preventing disease among a vulnerable urban immigrant population" and "uses the talents of a family nurse practitioner and a nurse case manager to provide easy access to underserved populations, promote early recognition and treatment of disease, and encourage healthy behaviors and lifestyles" (Hughes et al., 2001, p. 46).

In some geopolitical communities, parish nurses are the most acceptable primary care providers. The role of the parish nurse can be broad, being defined by the needs of the members and the philosophy of the religious community. However, the goal is to enhance and extend services available in the larger community, not to duplicate them (see Display 3–2).

The ANA has written standards of care for parish nursing practice in collaboration with Health Ministries Association, Inc. (ANA, 1998b). The standards act as guidelines for faith communities that plan to offer or are offering parish nursing services. Parish nursing is guided by a variety of standards set up by several groups. Together they provide guidance and direction for caregiving within the faith community (Display 3–3).

When community health nurses work as parish nurses, they enhance accessibility to available health services in the community while meeting the unique needs of the members of that religious community, practicing within the framework of the tenets of that religion.

For instance, in a Roman Catholic community in which artificial forms of birth control are not acceptable, client education about family planning methods would incorporate methods approved by the clergy, and referrals to primary care providers would be limited to those with similar beliefs.

Working in an ashram-based program, the nurse might be asked to teach nutrition and stress reduction based on vegetarian meals and relaxation exercises grounded in Hindu tradition, such as meditation and yoga.

Most Muslims prefer health teaching from persons of the same gender and accept personal care only from people of the same gender. It is imperative to know this information so as to be culturally appropriate when making nursing care decisions on behalf of Muslim clients. When working with an Islamic faith community on nutrition, the nurse must recognize that Muslims avoid pork and alcohol. And when discussing death and dying, cremation of deceased Muslims is

DISPLAY 3 – 3

Assuring Congregational Health and Wholeness

Roles of the Parish Nurse
1. Counselor
2. Integrator of faith and health
3. Educator
4. Referral agent
5. Coordinator of volunteers
6. Collaborator

Accountability
1. ANA Standards of Clinical Nursing Practice
2. ANA Scope and Standards of Parish Nursing Practice
3. Congregational Standards
4. Institutional Standards
5. ANA Social Policy Statement
6. State Nurse Practice Act
7. Patient Rights (American Heart Association)

not practiced and is not a part of end-of-life discussions or decisions.

When conducting nutrition teaching, the nurse takes into account that Buddhists have restrictions against some food combinations, and dietary extremes are to be avoided. Considering these dietary choices, menus and meal planning would recognize the limitations. In addition, Buddhists believe in good and bad luck and have many superstitions about health and illness, some universal among Buddhists and others unique to individuals. If a Buddhist is dying, last-rite chanting at the bedside is common; accomodations for such religious practices should be encouraged with hospital staff or with family members at home. Buddhists believe in reincarnation, and cremation is preferred over burial (Spector, 2000).

A nurse working within a faith community must be cognizant of basic principles and practices of the religious group served. In most situations, the nurse is a practitioner of the same religious belief system.

Community at Large

Unlike the six settings already discussed, the seventh setting for community health nursing practice is not confined to a specific philosophy, location, or building. When working with groups, populations, or the total community, the nurse may practice in many different places. For example, a community health nurse, as clinician and health educator, may work with a parenting group in a church or town hall. Another nurse, as client advocate, leader, and researcher, may study the health needs of a neighborhood's elderly population by collecting data throughout the area and meeting with resource people in many places. Also, a nurse may work with community-based organizations such as an AIDS organization or a support group for parents experiencing the violent death of a child. Again, the community at large becomes the setting for practice of a nurse who serves on health care planning committees, lobbies for health legislation at the state capitol, runs for a school board position, or assists with flood relief in another state or another country.

Although the term "setting" implies a place, remember that community health nursing practice is not limited to a specific site. Community health nursing is a specialty of nursing that is defined by the nature of its practice, not its location, and it can be practiced anywhere (Williams, 2000).

SUMMARY

Community health nurses play many roles, including that of clinician, educator, advocate, manager, collaborator, leader, and researcher. Each role entails special types of skills and expertise. The type and number of roles that are practiced vary with each set of clients and each specific situation, but the nurse should be able to successfully function in each of these roles as the particular situation demands. The role of manager is one that the nurse must play in every situation, because it involves assessing clients' needs, planning and organizing to meet those needs, directing and leading clients to achieve results, and controlling and evaluating the progress to ensure that the goals and clients' needs are met. A type of comprehensive management of clients that has become known as case management is an integral part of community health nursing practice.

As a part of the manager role, the nurse must engage in three crucial management behaviors: decision-making, transferring information, and relationship building. Nurses also must use a comprehensive set of management skills: human skills that allow them to understand, communicate, motivate, and work with people; conceptual skills that allow them to interpret abstract ideas and apply them to real situations to formulate solutions; and technical skills that allow them to apply special management-related knowledge and expertise to a particular situation or problem.

There also are many types of settings in which the community health nurse must practice and in which these roles are enacted. "Setting" does not necessarily refer to a specific location or site, but rather to a particular situation. These situations can be grouped into seven major categories: homes; ambulatory service settings, where clients come for care but do not stay overnight; schools; occupational health settings, which serve employees in business and industry; residential institutions such as hospitals, continuing care facilities, halfway houses, or other institutions in which people live and sleep; parishes, where care is based on the philosophy of the religious organization; and the community at large, which encompasses a variety of expected and innovative locations (see Clinical Corner).

CLINICAL CORNER

ROLES AND SETTINGS OF COMMUNITY HEALTH NURSING PRACTICE

Scenario

You are a nurse working in the cardiac intensive care unit (CICU) in Capitol City Hospital. Your hospital recently has been purchased by a health maintenance organization. Rumors about downsizing of nursing staff are rampant among hospital employees. Realizing that many nurses have more seniority than you, you decide to make an appointment with your supervisor to discuss the rumors and assess your status with the hospital. Your supervisor advises you that layoffs are imminent and that, given your date of hire, there is a high likelihood that you are at risk of "termination."

Your situation is as follows:

You received an Associate of Arts (ADN) Degree in Nursing 10 years ago. You worked as a Registered Nurse on the medical-surgical unit for 6 years at Capitol City Hospital. Four years ago, you left your permanent position to work part-time on the evening shift to continue your education and receive a Bachelor of Science in Nursing (BSN). Your goal in returning to school was to prepare yourself for either a supervisory position in the hospital or future practice in the community setting. You completed your BSN 2 years ago and subsequently obtained your permanent position in the CICU.

During your BSN education, you studied under one of the administrators of the local managed care program and became interested in managed care. Your county has operated a managed care program for 2 years. Your preceptor encouraged you to apply for a position as a nurse liaison, but you decided to return to work at Capitol City Hospital because you believed that you lacked the necessary experience for a position in the community setting.

Recently, you were approached by a neighbor who volunteers for his daughter's school. He informed you of a vacancy in the position of school nurse. This position was appealing to you because of the proximity to your home and the flexible schedule. Once again, however, you gave it little serious consideration because of your perceived lack of experience.

Glancing in the classified section of the newspaper last Sunday, you noticed advertisements for the following nursing positions:

- Clinic nurse in the local health department
- Occupational health nurse for a computer company in Metropolis

You now have four possible community health nurse (CHN) employment avenues to pursue:

- Managed care
- School nursing
- Clinic nurse
- Occupational health nurse

Questions

1. List factors that must be considered when analyzing employment opportunities:
   - Salary
   - Job location
   - Flexibility in hours
   - Professional challenge
   - Opportunity for advancement
   - Personal comfort level with existing skills (versus challenge of learning new job)
   - Adequacy of personal skills and knowledge base

2. Given the scenario, brainstorm about actual and potential options:
   - Continue in present position and hope that position is not eliminated
   - Analyze options for advancement within Capitol City Hospital
   - Identify means of securing current position
   - Contact your preceptor to explore employment opportunities with managed care program
   - Apply for CHN position of
     - School nurse
     - Occupational health nurse
     - Clinic nurse

3. For each of the CHN roles, identify what clients you might be serving:
   - Individuals
   - Aggregates
   - Communities
   - Disease-focused
   - High-risk
   - Cultural
   - Ethnic
   - Geographic

4. Choose one of the CHN roles along with a setting and client base. Discuss potential issues related to:
   - Ethical considerations and dilemmas
   - Benefits of this CHN role
   - Drawbacks of working in this role
   - Job stability
   - Experience and education requirements
   - Social justice
   - Developing interdisciplinary partnerships

ACTIVITIES TO PROMOTE CRITICAL THINKING

1. Discuss ways for a community health nurse to make service holistic and focused on wellness with (a) preschool-age children in a day care setting; (b) a group of chemically dependent adolescents; or (c) a group of elders living in a senior high-rise building.

2. Select one community health nursing role and describe its application in meeting the needs of your friend or next-door neighbor.

3. Describe a hypothetical or real situation in which you, as a community health nurse, would combine the roles of leader, collaborator, and researcher (investigator). Discuss how each of these roles might be played.

4. If your community health nursing practice setting is the community at large, will your practice roles be any different from those of the nurse whose practice setting is the home? Why? What determines the roles played by the community health nurse?

5. Interview a practicing community health nurse and determine which roles are part of the nurse's practice over 1 month of caregiving. Describe the ways in which each role is enacted. How many instances of this nurse's practice were aggregate focused? In which of the settings does the nurse mostly practice? If you were a public health consultant, what suggestions might you make to expand this nurse's role into aggregate-level practice?

6. Search the Internet or go to the library and find two sources of health-related information for consumers. Was the information accurate?

7. Search the Internet or go to the library and find two research articles on community health nursing. In what settings did the research take place? Did the nursing authors collaborate with interdisciplinary team members on this research? If so, how do you think this collaboration helped the research? If you were to conduct research in the community, would you conduct it with only nurses on the team, or would your team be interdisciplinary? Why? What would be the benefits or limits of each approach? (see Clinical Corner).

8. This chapter briefly covers the role of the parish nurse. Search for information about this area of community health nursing in your community. Do you know a parish nurse? If so, plan to observe his or her practice for a few hours and explore what the role entails in this faith community.

REFERENCES

American Nurses Association. (1985). *Code for nurses with interpretive statements*. Kansas City, MO: American Nurses Publishing.

American Nurses Association. (1995). *Nursing's social policy statement*. Washington, DC: American Nurses Publishing.

American Nurses Association. (1998a). *The scope and standards of parish nursing practice*. Washington, DC: American Nurses Publishing.

American Nurses Association. (1998b). *Standards of clinical nursing practice* (2nd ed.). Washington, DC: American Nurses Publishing.

American Nurses Association. (1999). *Scope and standards of public health nursing practice*. Washington, DC: American Nurses Publishing.

American Public Health Association. (1996, March). *The definition and role of public health nursing: A statement of APHA* (Public Health Nursing Section 1–5). Washington, DC: Author. Retrieved 4/12/03 from American Public Health Association Web site: *http://www.apha.org/science/sections/phnrole.html*

Berkowitz, G. (2001). *Public health nursing leadership: A guide to managing the core functions*. Washington, DC: American Nurses Publishing.

Bhatia, R., & Katz, M. (2001). Estimation of health benefits from a local living wage ordinance. *American Journal of Public Health, 91*(9), 1398–1402.

Bomar, P.J., & Baker-Wood, P. (2001). Family health promotion. In S.M.H. Hanson (Ed.), *Family health care nursing: Theory, practice, and research* (2nd ed., pp. 197–219). Philadelphia: F.A. Davis.

Bracht, N. (1999). *Health promotion at the community level: New advances* (2nd ed.). Thousand Oaks, CA: Sage.

Cherry, B., & Jacob, S.R. (2002). *Contemporary nursing: Issues, trends, and management*. St. Louis: Mosby.

Clark, M.B., & Olson, J.J. (2000). *Nursing within a faith community*. Thousand Oaks, CA: Sage.

Conly, E., & Dahl, J. (1993). *Public health nursing within core public health functions: A progress report from public health nursing directors of Washington*. Olympia: Washington State Department of Health.

Corrigan, D. (2000). The changing role of schools and higher education institutions with respect to community-based interagency collaboration and interprofessional partnerships. *Peabody Journal of Education, 75*(3), 176–195.

Dossey, B.M., Keegan L., & Guzzetta, C.E. (1999). *Holistic nursing: A handbook for practice* (3rd ed.). Gaithersburg, MD: Aspen.

Floyd, J.M. (2000). The public's use of nurses for health care advice. *Journal of Nursing Scholarship, 32*(3), 220.

Grembowski, D. (2001). *The practice of health program evaluation*. Thousand Oaks, CA: Sage.

Harris, G.E., Ripperger, M.J., & Horn, H.G.S. (2000). Managed care at a crossroads. *Health Affairs, 18*(1), 157–163.

Hisama, K.K. (2000). Carrying your own lamp. *Reflections on Nursing Leadership, 26*(1), 30–32.

Hughes, C.B., Trofino, J., O'Brien, B.L., Mack, J., & Marrinan, M. (2001). Primary care parish nursing: Outcomes and implications. *Nursing Administration Quarterly, 21*(1), 45–59.

Kendra, M.A., & George, V.D. (2001). Defining risk in home visiting. *Public Health Nursing, 18*(2), 128–137.

Kumanyika, S.K., Morssink, C.B., & Nestle, M. (2001). Minority women and advocacy for women's health. *American Journal of Public Health, 91*(9), 1383–1388.

MacIntosh, J., & McCormack, D. (2000). An integrative review illuminates curricular applications of primary health care. *Journal of Nursing Education, 39*(3), 116–123.

Mintzberg, H. (1973). *The nature of managerial work.* New York: Harper & Row.

Mulligan, R.A., Gilroy, J., Katz, K., Rodan, M.F., & Subramanian, K.N. (1999). Developing a shared language: Interdisciplinary communication among diverse health care professionals. *Holistic Nursing Practice, 13*(2), 47–53.

Navaie-Waliser, M., Martin, S.L., Campbell, M.K., Tessaro, I., Kotelchuck, M., & Cross, A.W. (2000). Factors predicting completion of a home visitation program by high-risk pregnant women: The North Carolina maternal outreach worker program. *American Journal of Public Health, 90*(1), 121–124.

Novick, L.E., & Mays, G.P. (2000). *Public health administration: Principles for population-based management.* Gaithersburg, MD: Aspen.

Olds, D.L., Eckenrode, J., Henderson, C., Kitzman, H., Powers, J., Cole, R., et al. (1997). Long-term effects of home visitation on maternal life course and child abuse and neglect: Fifteen-year follow-up of a randomized trial. *Journal of the American Medical Association, 278,* 637–643.

Olds, D.L., Henderson, C., Cole, R., Ekenrode, J., Kitzman, H., Luckey, D., et al. (1998). Long-term effects of nurses' home visitation on children's criminal and antisocial behavior. *Journal of the American Medical Association, 280,* 1238–1244.

Parker, M.W., Bellis, J.M., Bishop, P., Harper, M., Allman, R.M., Moore, C., et al. (2002). A multidisciplinary model of health promotion incorporating spirituality into a successful aging intervention with African-American and White elderly groups. *The Gerontologist, 42*(3), 406–415.

Polit, D.F., Beck, C.T., & Hungler, B.P. (2001). *Essentials of nursing research: Methods, appraisal, and utilization* (5th ed.). Philadelphia: Lippincott Williams & Wilkins.

Powell, S.K. (2000). *Case management: A practical guide to success in managed care* (2nd ed.). Philadelphia: Lippincott Williams & Wilkins.

Rankin, S.H., & Stallings, K.D. (2001). *Patient education: Principles and practice* (4th ed.). Philadelphia: Lippincott Williams & Wilkins.

Redman, B.K. (2001). *The practice of patient education* (9th ed.). St. Louis: Mosby.

Skinner, C.S., Arfken, C.L., & Waterman, B. (2000). Outcomes of the learn, share & live breast cancer education program for older urban women. *American Journal of Public Health, 90*(8), 1229–1234.

Spector, R.E. (2000). *Cultural diversity in health & illness* (5th ed.). Upper Saddle River, NJ: Prentice-Hall Health.

Swansburg, R.C., & Swansburg, R.J. (1999). *Introductory management and leadership for nurses* (2nd ed.). Sudbury, MA: Jones & Bartlett Publishers.

U.S. Department of Health and Human Services. (2000). *Healthy people 2010.* (Conference ed., Vols. 1 & 2). Washington, DC: U.S. Government Printing Office.

Venes, D. (2001). *Taber's cyclopedic medical dictionary* (19th ed.). Philadelphia: F.A. Davis.

Williams, C. (2000). Community-based population-focused practice: The foundation of specialization in public health nursing. In M. Stanhope & J. Lancaster (Eds.), *Community health nursing: Process and practice for promoting health* (5th ed.). St. Louis: Mosby.

Williamson, D.L., & Drummond, J. (2000). Enhancing low-income parents' capacities to promote their children's health: Education is not enough. *Public Health Nursing, 17*(2), 121–131.

Wurzbach, M.E. (2002). *Community health education and promotion: A guide to program design and evaluation* (2nd ed.). Gaithersburg, MD: Aspen.

SELECTED READINGS

Baird, M., & Lafferty, S. (2001). *Tele-nurse: Telephone triage protocols.* Albany, NY: Delmar.

Buswell-Robinson, C. (2002). Street nursing. *American Journal of Nursing, 102*(1), 73, 75, 77.

Clampitt, P.G., & DeKoch, R.J. (2001). *Embracing uncertainty: The essence of leadership.* Armonk, NY: M.E. Sharpe.

Clark, C. (Ed.). (2001). *Adult day services and social inclusion: Better days.* Philadelphia: Jessica Kingsley Publishers.

Dossey, B.M., Quinn, J.A., Frisch, N., & Guzzetta, C.E. (2000). *AHNA standards of holistic nursing practice: Guidelines for caring and healing.* Gaithersburg, MD: Aspen.

Feldman, H.R. (2001). *Strategies for nursing leadership.* New York: Springer.

Flarey, D.L., & Travis, L.L. (2001). Case management: Is it improving health outcomes? In H.R. Feldman (Ed.). *Nursing leaders speak out* (pp. 3–10). New York: Springer.

Hale, W.D., & Bennett, R.G. (2000). *Building health communities through medical-religious partnerships.* Baltimore, MD: John Hopkins University Press.

Kearny, M.H., York, R., & Deatrick, J.A. (2000). Effects of home visits to vunerable young families. *Journal of Nursing Scholarship, 32*(4), 369–376.

Leininger, M.M. (2001). *Culture care, diversity, and universality: A theory of nursing.* Sudbury, MA: Jones & Bartlett.

Macrae, J.A. (2001). *Nursing as a spiritual practice: A contemporary application of Florence Nightingale's views.* New York: Springer.

McSherry, W. (2000). *Making sense of spirituality in nursing practice: An interactive approach.* Edinburgh, England: Churchill Livingstone.

Porter-O'Grady, T. (2001). Beyond the walls: Nursing in the entrepreneurial world. *Nursing Administration Quarterly, 25*(2), 61–68.

Powell, S.K. (2000). *Advanced case management: Outcomes and beyond.* Philadelphia: Lippincott Williams & Wilkins.

Solari-Twadell, P.A., & McDermott, M.A. (1999). *Parish nursing: Promoting whole person health within faith communities.* Thousand Oaks, CA: Sage.

Stewart, L.E. (2000). Parish nursing: Renewing a long tradition of caring. *Gastroenterology Nursing, 23*(3), 116–120.

Trofino, J., Hughes, C.B., O'Brien, B.L., Mack, J., Marrinan, M.A., & Hay, K.M. (2000). Primary care parish nursing: Academic, service and parish partnership. *Nursing Administration Quarterly, 25*(1): 59–74.

Wallace, D.C., Tuck, I., Voland, C.S., & Witucki, J.M. (2002). Client perceptions of parish nursing. *Public Health Nursing, 19*(2), 128–135.

Williams, C. A. (1977). Community health nursing: What is it? *Nursing Outlook, 25,* 250–254.

4

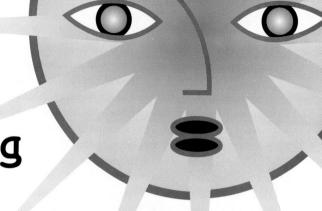

Transcultural Nursing
in the **Community**

Learning Objectives

Upon mastery of this chapter, you should be able to:

- Define and explain the concept of culture.

- Discuss the meaning of cultural diversity and its significance for community health nursing.

- Describe the meaning and effects of ethnocentrism on community health nursing practice.

- Identify five characteristics shared by all cultures.

- Contrast the health-related values, beliefs, and practices of selected culturally diverse populations with those of the dominant U. S. culture.

- Conduct a cultural assessment.

- Apply transcultural nursing principles in community health nursing practice.

American society values individuality. In fact, the United States was settled almost 400 years ago by people who wanted to be able to freely express their particular thoughts. It took powerful independence to pioneer the West in the 1800s. Partly because of this pioneer spirit, people from all nations have sought to live in America. Some came of their own free will as an adventure and opportunity. Others saw this land as a refuge from political, religious, or economic strife. Others were brought here against their will. Consequently, we have not become the ideal melting-pot once described, but an amalgamation of people who have different values, ideals, and behaviors.

You and I bring our differences to this country, yet we remain united. In the Western culture, there is joy in seeing children grow and develop in unique ways. An individual's creative achievements are applauded. There is also respect for one another's personal preferences about food, dress, or the vehicles one drives. The right to be yourself—and thereby to be different from others—is even protected by state and federal laws.

Although individuality is part of the dominant culture, there are limits to the range of differences most Americans find acceptable. People whose behavior falls outside the acceptable range are labeled as deviants or misfits. For example, the U. S. culture approves moderate social drinking but not alcoholism. The beliefs and sanctions of the dominant or majority culture are called **dominant values**. In the United States, the majority culture is made up largely of Anglo-Saxons whose dominant values include the work ethic, thrift, success, independence, initiative, respect for others, privacy, cleanliness, youthfulness, attractive appearance, and a focus on the future. However, in some regions and even in some states, Anglo-Saxons are not the majority. For example, in California more people come from Hispanic or Asian origins than from Western European countries, and the dominant culture is no longer Anglo-Saxon.

Dominant values are important to consider in the practice of community health nursing because they shape people's thoughts and behaviors. Why are some client behaviors acceptable to health professionals and others not? Why do nurses have such difficulty persuading certain clients to accept new ways of thinking and acting? Explanations can be found by examining the concept of culture, especially its influence on health and on community health nursing practice. For example, an emphasis on the need for milk in the diet may demonstrate cultural blindness, considering the number of people in diverse ethnic groups who are lactose intolerant. Regardless of their own cultural backgrounds, nurses are socialized throughout the educational process; the biomedical model is frequently the framework, and dominant social values are reinforced.

THE MEANING OF CULTURE

Culture refers to the beliefs, values, and behavior that are shared by members of a society and provide a design or "map" for living. It is culture that tells people what is acceptable or unacceptable in a given situation. It is culture that dictates what to do, say, or believe. Culture is learned. As children grow up, they learn from their parents and others around them how to interpret the world. In turn, these assimilated beliefs and values prescribe desired behavior.

Anthropologists describe culture as the acquired knowledge that people use to generate behavior and interpret experience (Spradley & McCurdy, 2000). This knowledge is more than simply custom or ritual; it is a way of organizing and thinking about life. It gives people a sense of security about their behavior; without having to consciously think about it, they know how to act. Culture also provides the underlying values and beliefs on which people's behavior is based. For example, culture determines the value placed on achievement, independence, work, and leisure. It forms the basis for the definitions of male and female roles. It influences a person's response to authority figures, dictates religious beliefs and practices, and shapes child-rearing. According to Giger and Davidhizar (2002, p. 80), "Culture is a patterned behavioural response that develops over time as a result of imprinting the mind through social and religious structures and intellectual and artistic manifestations."

Every community and social or ethnic group has its own culture. Furthermore, all of the individual members believe and act based on what they have learned within that specific culture. As anthropologist Edward Hall (1959) said a half-century ago, culture controls our lives. Even the smallest elements of everyday living are influenced by culture. For instance, culture determines the proper distance to stand from another person while talking. A comfortable talking distance for Americans is at least 2.5 feet, whereas Latin Americans prefer a shorter distance, often only 18 inches, for dialogue. Culture also influences one's perception of time. In American culture, when someone makes an appointment, he or she expects the other person to be on time or not more than a few minutes late; to keep a person waiting (or to be kept waiting) for 45 minutes or 1 hour is insulting and intolerable. Yet other cultural groups, including Native Americans and Asians, have a much more flexible response to time; their members think nothing of waiting or keeping someone else waiting for an hour or two. Culture is the knowledge people use to design their own actions and, in turn, to interpret others' behavior (Spradley & McCurdy, 2000).

Cultural Diversity

Race refers to biologically designated groups of people whose distinguishing features, such as skin color, are inherited; examples include Asian, Black, and White. An **ethnic group** is a collection of people who have common origins and a shared culture and identity; they may share a common geographic origin, race, language, religion, traditions, values, and food preferences (Spector, 2000). A person's **ethnicity** is that group of qualities that mark his or her association with a particular ethnic group. When a variety of racial or ethnic groups join a common, larger group, cultural diversity occurs. **Cultural diversity** (also called cultural plurality) means that a variety of cultural patterns coexist within a designated geographic area. Cultural diversity occurs not only between countries or continents, but also within many countries, including the United States (Spector, 2000). However, the term *culture,* used alone, has no single definition. We have defined it for use in this book at the beginning of this section. Others have described culture as meaning the total socially inherited characteristics of a group, comprising everything that one generation can tell, convey, or hand down to the next. Culture has also been described as "the luggage that each of us carries around for a lifetime" (Spector, 2000, p. 78).

Immigration patterns over the years have contributed to significant cultural diversity in the United States. Early settlers came primarily from European countries through the 1800s, peaking in numbers just after the turn of the century, with almost 9 million immigrants admitted in the first decade of the 20th century. During much of that time, especially during the late 1600s through the early 1800s, African slaves were brought to the United States against their will, mostly to southern states, where they were sold to plantation owners as laborers. Immigration stayed high during the early 1900s, and then dropped sharply from 1930 to 1950. Immigration from non-European regions such as Asia and South America then steadily increased. The total number of immigrants from all countries in the 1990s almost equaled the number who arrived during the 1910s, when immigration was at a peak (Table 4–1).

As shown in Table 4–2, immigrants come from all regions of the world, in greater numbers from some areas than others. Of the 849,807 people immigrating in 2000, almost half came from the Western Hemisphere: 20% from Mexico, 16% (138,100 immigrants) from Central and South America,

TABLE 4 – 1

Immigrants Admitted to the United States in the 20th Century

Decade	Number of Immigrants
1901–1910	8,795,386
1911–1920	5,735,611
1921–1930	4,107,209
1931–1940	528,431
1941–1950	1,035,039
1951–1960	2,515,479
1961–1970	3,322,677
1971–1980	4,493,314
1981–1990	7,338,062
1991–2000	9,095,417

From U. S. Department of Commerce. (2001). *Statistical abstract of the United States, 2001* (121st ed.). Washington, DC: Government Printing Office.

TABLE 4 – 2

Immigrants and Region of Birth (2000)

Origin	No. of Immigrants
All countries	849,807
Europe	132,480
Asia	265,400
North America	344,805
Central America	66,443
South America	56,074
Africa	44,731

From U. S. Department of Commerce. (2001). *Statistical abstract of the United States, 2001.* Washington, DC: Government Printing Office.

and 10% (85,875 immigrants) from the Caribbean, including Cuba, Dominican Republic, Haiti, Jamaica, Trinidad, and Tobago (U. S. Department of Commerce, 2001). Undocumented immigrants, mostly from Mexico, continue to stream into the United States. This is an emotionally charged situation, especially considering the economic and social differences between our two countries and the existence of a long border with very few official border crossings. According to the U. S. Committee for Refugees (USCR), in 2001 the United States hosted 492,500 refugees and asylum seekers, the greatest number coming from Mexico.

One devastating situation concerning undocumented immigrants from Mexico is the number of people who die while attempting to cross the Sonora Desert to enter the United States. In 2001, 350 immigrants died (USCR, 2002). Most died from exposure, because the temperature can reach greater than 110°F, and a person on foot can carry only enough water for a few miles. Some immigrants died in the care of the person hired to get them across the border; often they were hidden in trucks, with dozens of people crammed together, suffocating from the heat. Others died just after arriving in the United States. If you travel major highways near southern and western U. S. border cities, you will see universal signs showing three running people, an adult and two children, indicating that undocumented immigrants may be running across the highway, to escape capture, near this area. The issue of undocumented immigrants is a frustrating problem that continues to plague both countries and the border guards and rescue personnel involved.

The 2000 U. S. Census indicated that 33 million people were added to the total U. S. population between 1990 and 2000. The fastest growing racial/ethnic group is the Hispanic population, which increased by 13 million people in that decade (Table 4–3). Such numbers can be deceiving, however, because the 2000 Census was the first one in which individuals were able to indicate two or more races or ethnic groups. Four million people indicated multiple races or ethnic groups. Approximately 50% of these people indicated

TABLE 4-3

U. S. Population by Race, 1980–2000 (%)

Origin	1980	1990	2000
White	79.8	75.6	69.1
Black	11.5	11.7	12.1
Asian[a]	1.6	2.8	3.7
American Indian	0.6	0.7	0.7
Some other race	0.1	0.1	0.2
Hispanic[b]	6.4	9.0	12.5

[a]Includes native Hawaiians and other Pacific Islanders.

[b]Note that 2 million Hispanics marked two or more races in the 2000 Census.

From U. S. Bureau of Census. (n.d.). *The Hispanic population in the United States.* Retrieved November 11, 2003. From *http://www.census.gov*

DISPLAY 4-1

Hispanic Population Trend in the United States

A report conducted by the Pew Hispanic Center and the Brookings Institution Center on Urban and Metropolitan Policy and released in July 2002 indicated that the Hispanic population has spread out across the nation faster and farther than any previous wave of immigrants. Hispanics are moving from immigrant gateways into the heartland and suburbs at a rate possibly exceeding that of European immigrants in the early 20th century and of African Americans moving away from the Deep South in the years before World War II.

Although large metropolitan areas such as New York, Los Angeles, and Miami accounted for the largest increases in number of Hispanics between 1980 and 2000, smaller communities charted a faster rate of growth in their Hispanic populations.

More than half of Hispanics now live in suburbs, and many migrants are skipping metropolitan areas and heading straight to jobs and housing in outlying areas. Researchers indicate that this is not one trend replacing another, but several trends expanding at once.

Hispanic population spreads out. (2002, August 1). *The Fresno Bee,* p. A4.

Hispanic along with a second or third race or ethnic group (U. S. Department of Commerce, 2001).

People representing more than 100 different ethnic groups, more than half of them significant in size, live in the United States. Significant minorities include Hispanic-Americans, numbering more than 35 million in 2000 and representing approximately 12.5% of the population; African-Americans, numbering 34 million, or approximately 12.1% of the population; Asian-Americans, numbering slightly more than 10 million, or approximately 3.7% of the population; and American Indians, Eskimos, and Aleuts, numbering 2.5 million, or 0.7% of the population. In 2000, Hispanics surpassed the African-American population as the largest race/ethnic group in the United States (U. S. Department of Commerce, 2001). By 2050, number of Hispanic-Americans is projected to double, making up 24.5% of the population; Asian–Pacific Islanders will more than double their numbers, to 8.2% of the U. S. population; and the number of African-Americans will increase to 15.4% of the population. The American Indian, Eskimo, and Aleut population will probably stay at or near 0.7%. These changes, primarily resulting from immigration, are projected to result in 49.8% of the population of the United States in 2050 belonging to "minority" groups, and European-Americans/Whites may no longer be the majority. In some states, especially those bordering Mexico and some industrialized states in the eastern part of the country, this change already has occurred or will occur much sooner than 2050 (Display 4–1).

Immigration patterns are strongly influenced by immigration laws established since the 1800s. The Immigration Reform and Control Act of 1986 (Public Law 99–603) and the Immigration Act of 1990 (Public Law 101–649) set new limits on the number of immigrants admitted. These laws set annual numerical ceilings on certain immigrant groups while authorizing increases for highly skilled workers or family members of aliens who have recently achieved legal status. After the terrorist attacks on September 11, 2001, President Bush suspended all immigration for 2 months. Suspicion about people from Middle Eastern countries permeated the nation. This did not help the social climate for immigrants.

Immigrants and refugees in recent years have found themselves in a more confusing social climate than did those who came before them. This climate is characterized by ambivalence about whether immigrants should be accepted and ambiguity about their status. The newcomers find an environment that is both welcoming and hostile. On one hand, they may find tolerance of diversity in the United States, demonstrated by interest in ethnic food, cultural celebrations, and sensitivity to employees from different backgrounds. On the other hand, a backlash exists, demonstrated by a rise in hate crimes, national and local policies that curb services to undocumented immigrants, restriction in English as a second language (ESL) and bilingual education, and limits to potential class action suits challenging practices of the Immigration and Nationalization Service.

Although broad cultural values are shared by most large national societies, within those societies smaller cultural groups called subcultures exist. **Subcultures** are relatively large aggregates of people within a society who share separate distinguishing characteristics, such as ethnicity (e.g., African-American, Hispanic-American), occupation (e.g., farmers, physicians), religion (e.g., Catholics, Muslims), geographic area (e.g., New Englanders, Southerners), age (e.g., the elderly, school-age children), gender (e.g., women), or sexual preference (e.g., the gay community).

Within these subcultures are even smaller groups that anthropologists call microcultures. "**Microcultures** are systems of cultural knowledge characteristic of subgroups within larger societies. Members of a microculture usually share much of what they know with everyone in the greater society but possess a special cultural knowledge that is unique to the subgroup" (Spradley & McCurdy, 2000, p. 15). Examples of microcultures can range from a group of Hmong immigrants adopting selected aspects of the United States culture to a third-generation Norwegian-American community whose members share unique foods, dress, and values.

The members of each subculture and microculture retain some of the characteristics of the society from which they came or in which their ancestors lived (Mead, 1960). Some of their beliefs and practices—such as the food they eat, the language they speak at home, the way they celebrate holidays, or their ideas about sickness and healing—remain an important part of their everyday life. Native American groups have retained some aspects of their traditional cultures. Mexican-Americans, Irish-Americans, Swedish-Americans, Italian-Americans, African-Americans, Puerto Rican–Americans, Chinese-Americans, Japanese-Americans, Vietnamese-Americans, and many other ethnic groups have their own microcultures.

Furthermore, certain customs, values, and ideas are unique to the poor, the rich, the middle class, women, men, youth, or the elderly. Many deviant groups, such as narcotics abusers, transient alcoholics, gangs, criminals, and terrorist groups, have developed their own microcultures. Regional microcultures, such as that of the White Appalachian people living in the hills of Kentucky, also have distinctive ways of defining the world and coping with life. Other microcultures, such as those of rural migrant farm workers or urban homeless families, acquire their own sets of beliefs and patterns for dealing with their environments. Many religious groups have their own microcultures. Even occupational and professional groups, such as nurses or attorneys, develop their own special languages, beliefs, and perspectives.

Ethnocentrism

There is a difference between a healthy cultural or ethnic identification and ethnocentrism. Anthropologists explain that "**ethnocentrism** is the belief and feeling that one's own culture is best. It reflects our tendency to judge other people's beliefs and behavior using values of our own native culture" (Spradley & McCurdy, 2000, p. 16). It causes people to believe that their way of doing things is right and to judge others' methods as inferior, ignorant, or irrational. Ethnocentrism blocks effective communication by creating biases and misconceptions about human behavior. In turn, this can cause serious damage to interpersonal relationships and interfere with nurse effectiveness (Leininger, 2001).

People can experience a developmental progression along a continuum from ethnocentrism, feeling one's own culture is best to **ethnorelativism**, seeing all behavior in a cultural context. Some people may stop progressing and remain stagnated at one step, and others may move backward on the continuum. The left side of the continuum represents the most extreme reaction to intercultural differences: refusal or denial. On the right side is the characterization of people who show the most sensitivity to intercultural differences: incorporation (Figure 4–1).

CHARACTERISTICS OF CULTURE

In their study of culture, anthropologists and sociologists have made significant contributions to the field of community health. Their findings shed light on why and how culture influences behavior. Five characteristics shared by all cultures are especially pertinent to nursing's efforts to improve community health: (1) culture is learned, (2) it is integrated, (3) it is shared, (4) it is tacit, and (5) it is dynamic.

Culture Is Learned

Patterns of cultural behavior are acquired, not inherited. Rather than being genetically determined, the way people dress, what they eat, and how they talk are all learned.

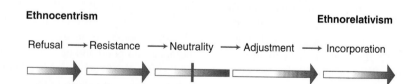

F I G U R E   4 – 1 . Cross-cultural sensitivity continuum. Being extremely ethnocentric (on the left of mid-point) and totally ethnorelative (on the far right) are reflected in the diagram. The steps toward ethnorelativism begin at the most ethnocentric view with refusal and resistance. Neutrality is mid-point, and adjustment and incorporation bring the person to an ethnorelative perspective.

Spradley and McCurdy (2000, p. 14) offered the following explanation:

> *At the moment of birth, we lack a culture. We don't yet have a system of beliefs, knowledge, and patterns of customary behavior. But from that moment until we die, each of us participates in a kind of universal schooling that teaches us our native culture. Laughing and smiling are genetic responses, but as infants we soon learn when to smile, when to laugh, and even how to laugh. We also inherit the potential to cry, but we must learn our cultural rules for when crying is appropriate.*

Each person learns his or her culture through socialization with the family or significant group, a process called **enculturation.** As a child grows up in a given society, she or he acquires certain attitudes, beliefs, and values and learns how to behave in ways appropriate to that group's definition of the female or male role; by doing so, children are learning their culture.

Although culture is learned, the process and results of that learning are different for each person. Each individual has a unique personality and experiences life in a singular way; these factors influence acquisition of culture. Families, social classes, and other groups within a society differ from one another, and this sociocultural variation has important implications. Because culture is learned, parts of it can be re-learned. People might change certain cultural elements or adopt new behaviors or values. Some individuals and groups are more willing and able than others to try new ways and thereby influence change.

Culture Is Integrated

Rather than being merely an assortment of various customs and traits, a culture is a functional, integrated whole. As in any system, all parts of a culture are interrelated and interdependent. The various components of a culture, such as its social mores or religious beliefs, perform separate functions but come into relative harmony with each other to form an operating and cohesive whole. In other words, to understand culture, single traits should not be described independently. Each part must be viewed in terms of its relationship to other parts and to the whole.

A person's culture is an integrated web of ideas and practices. For example, a nurse may promote the need for consuming three balanced meals a day, a practice tied to the beliefs that good nutrition leads to good health and that prevention is better than cure. These cultural beliefs, in turn, are related to the nurse's values about health. Health, the nurse believes, is essential for maximum energy output and productivity at work. Productivity is important because it enables people to reach goals. These values are linked to social or religious beliefs about hard work and taboos against laziness. Through such connections, these ideas and beliefs

about nutrition, health, economics, religion, and family are all interrelated and work to motivate behavior.

For example, parents who are Jehovah's Witnesses may refuse a blood transfusion for their child. Their actions might seem irrational or ignorant to those who do not understand the parents' religious beliefs. However, the couple's choice represents behavior consistent with their cultural values and standards. The single behavior of refusing blood transfusions, when viewed in context, is seen to be part of a larger religious belief system and a basic component of the parents' culture.

In some cultural groups (eg, Muslims), modesty for women may make it uncomfortable and perhaps traumatic to be examined by a person of the opposite sex. Asking certain Native American groups to comply with rigid appointment scheduling requires them to reframe their concept of time. It also violates their values of patience and pride. Before nurses attempt to change a person's or group's behavior, they need to ask how that change will affect the people involved through its influence on other parts of their culture. Extra time and patience or different strategies may be needed if change still is indicated. Nurses often may find, however, that their own practice system can be modified to preserve clients' cultural values.

Culture Is Shared

Culture is the product of aggregate behavior, not individual habit. Certainly, individuals practice a culture, but customs are phenomena shared by all members of the group. Thirty years ago, anthropologist G. Murdock explained (1972, p. 258):

> *Culture does not depend on individuals. An ordinary habit dies with its possessor, but a group habit lives on in the survivors and is transmitted from generation to generation. Moreover, the individual is not a free agent with respect to culture. He is born and reared in a certain cultural environment, which impinges on him at every moment of his life. From earliest childhood his behavior is conditioned by the habits of those around him. He has no choice but to conform to the folkways current in his group.*

A culture's values are among its most important elements. A **value** is a notion or idea designating relative worth or desirability. For example, some cultures place value on honesty, loyalty, and faithfulness more than other traits. Also, there may be strong values against lying, stealing, and cheating, behaviors to avoid. Each culture classifies phenomena into good and bad, desirable and undesirable, right and wrong. When people respond in favor of or against some practice, they are reflecting their culture's values about that practice. One person may eagerly anticipate eating a steak for dinner. Another, who believes that eating meat is sacrilegious or unhealthful, experiences revulsion at the idea. Some American subcultures think that loud, vocal expressions are a necessary way to deal with pain; others value silence and stoicism. Some have high regard for speed and efficiency, whereas others prefer patience and thoughtfulness. Either way, values serve a purpose. Shared values give people in a specific culture stability and security and provide a standard for behavior. From these values, members know what to believe and how to act. The normative criteria by which people justify their decisions are based on values that are more deeply rooted than behaviors and consequently more difficult to change.

Knowing that culture is shared helps nurses to understand human behavior. For example, a community health nurse tried unsuccessfully to persuade a mother to limit the amount of catnip tea she fed her infant. The infant was pacified with the tea and was not consuming a sufficient amount of infant formula, thus putting him at risk for nutritional deficiencies and developmental problems. The nurse discovered that the mother was acting in the tradition of her rural subculture, which held that catnip promoted good health (it acts as an antispasmodic, perhaps causing relaxation and resulting in a more contented infant with fewer symptoms of colic [Spector, 2000]). The fact that all of the other mothers in that group also used catnip with their babies proved a powerful deterrent to the change suggested by the nurse. Individual health behavior always is influenced by other people of the same culture. It is difficult for one person to eliminate a cultural practice when it is reinforced by other group members. Group acceptance and a sense of membership usually depend on conforming to shared cultural practices (Spradley & McCurdy, 2000).

Community health nurses may need to focus on an entire group's health behavior to affect individual practices. In the example described, the pattern of consuming large amounts of catnip tea was modified after the nurse worked with the entire rural community. She began with a well-recognized cultural strategy: working through formal or informal leaders. She contacted the oldest woman in the community and discussed the cultural practice. The elder shared the group's beliefs that catnip tea is vital to the well-being of infants for the first 6 months. When the nurse explained her concerns about low formula intake and low weight gain, the community leader clarified that only one or two ounces of the tea a day was needed. The nurse shared this information among the women, and as a result, the mothers gradually reduced the amount of tea they gave their infants. Consequently, the clients' infants drank more formula and gained weight appropriately. A cultural tradition was retained while the health of the infants was improved. The community health nurse could then use this new information and supportive information from the community leader to improve the health of other infants.

Culture Is Mostly Tacit

Culture provides a guide for human interaction that is **tacit**— that is, mostly unexpressed and at the unconscious level.

Members of a cultural group, without the need for discussion, know how to act and what to expect from one another. Culture provides an implicit set of cues for behavior, not a written set of rules. Spradley and McCurdy explained that culture often is "so regular and routine that it lies below a conscious level" (2000, p. 16). It is like a memory bank in which knowledge is stored for recall when the situation requires it, but this recall process is mostly unconscious. Culture teaches the proper tone of voice to use for each occasion. It prescribes how close to stand when talking with someone and how to respond to elders. Individuals learn to make responses that are appropriate to their sex, role, and status. They know what is right and wrong. All of these attitudes and behaviors are so ingrained, so tacit, that people seldom, if ever, need to discuss them.

Because culture is mostly tacit, realizing which of one's own behaviors may be offensive to people from other groups is difficult. It also is difficult to know the meaning and significance of other cultural practices. In some groups, such as Native American or Islamic women, silence is valued and expected but may make others uncomfortable. Offering food to a guest in many cultures is not merely a social gesture but an important symbol of hospitality and acceptance; to refuse it, for any reason, may be an insult and a rejection. Touching or calling someone by their first name may be viewed as a demonstration of caring by some groups but is seen as disrespectful and offensive by others. Consequently, community health nurses have a twofold task in developing cultural sensitivity: not only must they try to learn their clients' cultures, but they also must try to make their own culture less tacit and more explicit. Nurses bring both their professional and personal cultural history to the workplace, often developing unique values not shared with others who are not in the profession (Cherry & Jacob, 2001). Cross-cultural tension can be resolved through conscious efforts to develop awareness, patience, and acceptance of cultural differences (Display 4–2).

Culture Is Dynamic

Every culture undergoes change; none is entirely static. Within every cultural group, some individuals generate innovations. More important, some members see advantages in doing things differently and are willing to adopt new practices. Each culture, including our own, is an amalgamation of ideas, values, and practices from a variety of sources. This process depends on the extent of exposure to other groups. Nonetheless, every culture is in a dynamic state of adding or deleting components. Functional aspects are retained; less functional ones are eliminated.

When this adaptation does not occur, the cultural group may face serious difficulty. For example, Hmong teenagers from Southeast Asian refugee families in the United States are among the first generation to be raised in America. Their parents had hoped they could restore honor and pride to a displaced people, but the teens struggle to balance their American lifestyle with Hmong traditions. The stresses they feel as

DISPLAY 4-2

Culture Shock

An increasing number of immigrants and refugees from many different countries have been assimilated into American culture in recent years. Although they quickly adapt in many respects, such as learning the language and seeking housing and employment, they continue to operate within the framework of their own cultural beliefs and behaviors. The conflict between their culture and American culture often causes **culture shock**, "a state of anxiety that results from cross-cultural misunderstanding . . . and an inability to interact appropriately in the new context" (Spradley & McCurdy, 2000, p. 16). Immigrants and refugees find themselves in a strange setting with people who act in unfamiliar ways. Speaking their own language in their homes and retaining values and familiar practices all help to promote some sense of security in the new environment.

The same is true for nurses and others working in unfamiliar countries. No longer are the small but important cues available that orient a stranger to appropriate behavior. Instead, a person in a different culture may feel isolated and anxious and even become dysfunctional or ill. Immersion in the culture over time and learning the new culture are the major remedies. As adjustment occurs, old beliefs and practices that are still functional in the new setting can be retained, but others that are not functional must be replaced.

VOICES FROM THE COMMUNITY

"You are talking about parents who are medieval, coming to a country that is hundreds of years ahead of theirs. They're trying to catch up, but it's hard."—Mymee (college instructor)

"There is much research that shows people who stand in the middle of two cultures are really at risk of depression and anxiety."—Valerie (psychologist)

"The kids are constantly living between two cultures. At some point, they may give up."—Leng (psychologist, Southeast Asian adult services center)

"I think it's a topic that nobody wants to talk about. It's hard for me to say if the Hmong community is ready to deal with it."—Xong (social worker, Hmong suicide task force)

"We parents think we know only one way to raise our kids. We ignore that these children are living in America and are espousing everything that is American, good and bad."—Andy (Hmong parent)

Ellis, A.D. (2002, August 11). Hmong Teens: Lost in America [Special report]. *The Fresno Bee*, pp. 1–12.

---

a result of the generational and cultural gaps between themselves and their parents are overwhelming. Many have not been successful in balancing these stresses and have chosen suicide as a way to relieve their frustration and depression (Ellis, 2002). Hmong community leaders, community health workers, school districts, law enforcement, and Hmong families are working together to develop interventions that will bring this "trail of tears" to an end. Another example of cultural adaptation's not occurring successfully is in China. Because China is so densely populated, couples are limited to one child, and this rule is closely monitored by the government. In addition, in this culture male offspring are more highly valued than female. Therefore, couples who have a female infant frequently choose to place the baby in an orphanage and make her available for adoption. These babies have been adopted throughout the world, especially in the United States and Australia.

Community health nurses need to remember the dynamic nature of culture for several reasons. First, cultures and subcultures do change over time. Patience and persistence are key attributes to cultivate when working toward improving health behaviors. Second, cultures change as their members see greater advantages in the "new ways." Discussions of these advantages need to be done in a language understood by members and in the context of their own cultural value system. This is an important reason for nurses to develop an understanding of their clients' culture and to deliver culturally competent care (Callister, 2001; Giger & Davidhizar, 2002; Leininger, 2001). Third, change within a culture is usually brought about by certain key individuals who are receptive to new ideas and able to influence their peers. These key persons can adapt the change process so that "new" practices are culturally consistent and fit with group values. Tapping this resource becomes imperative for successful change. Finally, the health care culture is dynamic, too. Westerners are just beginning to appreciate the validity of many of non-Western cultures' health care practices, such as acupuncture, meditation, and the use of various therapeutic herbs and spices (eg, turmeric, fenugreek). Nurses can learn much from their clients and their cultures (Spector, 2000). While discovering more effective ways of working with clients, nurses may choose to modify their own practices.

ETHNOCULTURAL HEALTH CARE PRACTICES

Throughout history, people have relied on natural elements to treat various maladies that family, clan, tribe, or community members experience. Knowledge of culturally recognized practices or substances, such as berries, plants, barks, or rituals and incantations usually becomes the responsibility of one person in the community. This revered community leader is known as a medicine man/woman, healer, or shaman (Spector, 2000). As time passes this person teaches the skills of recognizing and treating ailments or performing rituals to an apprentice, thereby continuing the healing knowledge and traditions.

In the following sections, we discuss how various geographic or ethnocultural groups view health care, including the biomedical, magicoreligious, and holistic views. We then look at selected folk medicines and home remedies, such as herbs, over-the-counter (OTC) drugs, and patent medications. In addition to these forms of treatments, there are complementary or alternative therapies and various self-care practices. This section concludes with the community health nurse's role and responsibilities to provide culturally competent care in relation to caring for, respecting, teaching, and treating clients from different cultures.

The World Community

Beliefs about the causes and effects of illness, health practices, and health-seeking behaviors are all influenced by a person's, group's, or community's perception of what causes illness and injury and what actions will treat or cure the health problem. The three major views in the world community are biomedical, magicoreligious, and holistic health beliefs (Spector, 2000).

Biomedical View

Western societies in general have a biomedical view of health and illness. The biomedical view relies on scientific principles and sees diseases and injuries as life events controlled by physical and biochemical processes that humans can manipulate through medication, surgery, and other treatments. Examples of this view include the following beliefs:

- Specific elements, such as bacteria, fungi, or viruses, are causes of illness.
- The lack of certain elements, such as an adequate diet, calcium, or iron, causes other health problems, such as malnutrition, osteoporosis, or anemia.
- Surgery is an accepted treatment for many physical ailments, to remove diseased organs, or to treat injuries from falls or accidents.

People living in countries where Western medicine is practiced believe that theirs is the best and perhaps the only way to deal with illness or injury. The dominant values presume that science is value free and not constructed by the social norms of the cultural group. The same is true, however, where Western medicine is not practiced and the social norms of the cultural group support the healing practices of that group. Many people (including community health nurses) are not open to other ways of looking at a person's wellness capabilities. As a result, clients may not receive culturally competent care from their caregivers.

Magicoreligious View

Magicoreligious themes of health and illness, which focus on the control of health and illness by supernatural forces, are prominent in some cultural groups. Diseases occur as a result of "committing sins" or "going against God's will." Good health is a gift from God, and illness is a form of punishment that affords an opportunity to be forgiven and to realign oneself with God. Prayer to God or other religious figures is used to cope with illness, seek intervention for healing, and ask for forgiveness and entrance into heaven, if death be God's will.

Some cultures mix traditional folk beliefs with organized religious practices and participate in forms of magic or voodoo. In cultures that have such beliefs, a hex or spell can be placed on another person through the use of incantations, elixirs, or an object resembling the person. For some, illness results from a look or a touch from another person considered to have special powers or intent to harm. Later in this chapter, we discuss some specific health beliefs and practices common to cultural groups in North America.

Religious beliefs, an individual's spirituality, and how these factors interface with feelings of wellness and specific healing practices are personal and important to clients and cannot be separated from their culture. This makes it imperative for community health nurses to be familiar with folk beliefs commonly seen in their practice. Only then can culturally competent nursing care be considered.

Holistic View

Holistic health believers come from many different cultural groups and view the world as being in harmonious balance. If the principles guiding natural laws that maintain order are disturbed, an imbalance in the forces of nature is created, resulting in chaos and disease. For an individual to be healthy, all facets of the individual's nature—physical, mental, emotional, and spiritual—must be in balance.

Some cultural groups believe that all things in creation or the universe have a Spirit and therefore are considered equal in value, purpose, and contribution (Lowe, 2002). Individuals have universal connectedness and are viewed as holistic beings. Persons are extensions to and integrated with family, community, tribe, and the universe. For example, "mother and fetus are viewed as interrelated and as affecting each other: They are one, but also they are two. In the circle of life, each individual is believed to be on a journey experiencing a process of being and becoming" (Lowe, p. 6).

Folk Medicine and Home Remedies

Folk medicine is a body of preserved treatment practices that has been handed down verbally from generation to generation. It exists today as the first line of treatment for many individuals. Some clients may never plan to seek Western medical treatment but may share with you, the community health nurse, a practice they are using to treat a family member. Your response and actions may mean the difference between health and illness or injury. Some maternal-child health practices from the U. S. rural midwest that may be encountered in community health nursing practice include the following:

- Not reaching above your head if you are pregnant, because doing so will cause the umbilical cord to strangle the baby

- Pregnant women eating handfuls of clay, dirt, or cornstarch
- Taping coins over a newborn's umbilical area to prevent hernias
- Giving catnip tea to infants because it saves their lives
- Shaking a baby upside down while holding her by a heel to "wake up her liver"
- Not letting a cat in a room with a sleeping baby, because the cat will "suck the life" out of the baby

Home remedies are individualized caregiving practices that are passed down within families. Even individuals who routinely seek the guidance of a health care practitioner for diagnosis and treatment may try home remedies before seeking professional advice. Each of us has a set of home remedies our parents used on us that we are likely to use on our own children before or instead of calling the pediatrician. Examples include using baking soda paste on a bee sting, ice on a "cold sore," or cranberry juice to prevent a urinary tract infection.

Herbalism

Textbooks have been written on the many uses of medicinal herbs. The use of some herbs has waxed and waned in favor. Some continue to be much touted, whereas others have been designated as dangerous and to be avoided. Increasingly, the public is using herbal preparations in the form of self-selected OTC products for therapeutic or preventive purposes.

In an increasingly multicultural society, the source, form, and recognition of many herbs, roots, barks, and liquid preparations become impossible for most community health nurses to identify. The most astute among us may be familiar with herbs used by one cultural group while herbs used by another escape us. A book with pictures and descriptions, botanical form, purported indications and uses, and implications for nursing management is an important tool to keep handy when interacting with clients. Basic safety questions that community health nurses should answer about an herb when teaching or interacting with families include the following:

- Is the herb contraindicated with prescription medications the client is taking?
- Is the herb harmful? Does it have negative side effects?
- Is the client relying on the herb, without positive health changes, while neglecting to get effective treatment from a health care practitioner?

Herbs are not regulated as drugs and are not risk free. Dosages are not standardized and are left to the individual. Quality of the product may be suspect. For these reasons, herbs must be used in moderation and with caution, preferably with guidance by a health care practitioner.

Prescription and Over-the-Counter Drugs

The cautions mentioned about herbs can also apply to prescription and OTC medications. First, they are not risk free. Prescription drugs are tested by the U. S. Food and Drug Administration, and OTC drugs are reviewed by the Federal Office of OTC Drug Evaluation. However, many OTC drugs were once available only by prescription and remain powerful medicines. All drugs can have major side effects, may be contraindicated in people with certain conditions, and may not be safe to use in combination with certain other drugs. Medication instruction and review is an important part of the community health nurse's role on some home visits, especially with elderly clients.

Second, some new prescription medications are so expensive that clients cannot afford to take them as prescribed. Often, older, less expensive, and more frequently used drugs work as well as the newer, more expensive ones, which are heavily marketed to health care practitioners by drug companies. If you encounter clients who are unable to pay for drugs, you may need to advocate for them with health care providers to prescribe a less expensive medication or change to the generic form of the same drug, usually sold at a fraction of the cost. Some health care practitioners have samples of drugs available and may be able to use them for medically indigent clients.

Third, the efficacy of medications needs to be assessed. At times, the use of a new drug or an additional drug does not have the effect intended. As someone who sees the client managing at home over time, the community health nurse may be able to give the best information to the health care provider about the effectiveness of new medications for a client.

Complementary Therapies and Self-Care Practices

Complementary therapies (also called alternative medicine or alternative therapies) are practices that are used to complement contemporary Western medical and nursing care and are designed to promote comfort, health and well-being (Cleveland et al., 1999). The range of complementary therapies is broad and includes

- Diet therapies (cancer diets, juice diets, fasting)
- Gastrointestinal treatments (coffee enemas, high colonic enemas)
- Balance and exercise activities (t'ai-chi, yoga)
- Sensory exposure (aromatherapy, music therapy, light therapy)
- Therapeutic manipulation (acupuncture, acupressure, reflexology)

Books or videos are available on each technique, and new therapies are always being suggested.

Consumers need to be well informed regarding the efficacy and safety of complementary therapies and how they can be true complements to other treatment modalities. The community health nurse should be aware of the variety of therapies available and how to get information for clients while remaining objective and supportive of the client's choices. At times, if a therapy contradicts the recommendations of the client's health care practitioner, the nurse may be in a position to provide the pros and cons of continuing the complementary therapy. On the other hand, the nurse may be able to suggest therapy forms that would complement Western medicine for the client, such as music therapy to promote relaxation and reduce stress or biofeedback for chronic pain management.

Self-care activities include complementary therapies, medications, and spiritual and cultural practices. They are uniquely individual for each person as well as among different cultural groups. Chapter 23 includes a Self-Care Assessment Guide that may be helpful in assessing the self-care practices of families.

Role of the Community Health Nurse

When working with different cultural groups in the area of health care practices, the community health nurse can be an effective advocate for the client. First, however, the nurse must be prepared to speak knowledgeably about health care practices and choices. The nurse also must be able to assess the client or family adequately so as to know what belief system motivates their choices. Finally, the nurse must be prepared to teach clients about the limits and benefits of cultural health care practices. The community health nurse should always individualize assessment and caregiving for the client within his or her culture and should not generalize about the client based on cultural group norms.

Preparation of the Community Health Nurse

To be effective when working with clients in the area of cultural health care and spirituality, the nurse needs to be prepared. There are many ways to increase your cultural awareness and promote sensitivity to the differences among people from ethnocultural groups different from your own. You can acquire information from peers who are from the same cultural group as your clients; attend workshops or conferences on chosen cultural topics; read books on ethnocultural health care practices, herbalism, or complementary therapies; talk with clients about their views and practices and learn from them; keep an open mind and be curious about various practices; or attend community cultural events such as Native American powwows, ethnic food events held in some cities, or Cinco de Mayo celebrations. There are textbooks, novels, and articles about cultures in the community in which one practices. For example, *The Spirit Catches You and You Fall Down* (Fadiman, 1997) describes a Hmong child, her American doctors, and the collision of two cultures. Universities offer courses in transcultural nursing, ethnic studies programs or courses, and cultural events that can be valuable.

Assessment

When beginning to work with a group or family, it is important for the nurse to be as familiar with them as possible. In addition to a family assessment or an individual health assessment, your care of the group would be enhanced by doing an ethnocultural or self-care assessment. Such an assessment reveals information about day-to-day living, cultural/spiritual influences, traditional/cultural health care choices and practices, and cultural taboos. Often this type of information is the most useful as you work with clients on a regular basis. Tools that might be useful are the two cultural assessment tools at the end of this chapter (see Tables 4–7 and 4–8) and the self-care assessment tool in Chapter 23.

Teaching

Teaching is a most important community health nursing role. When working with families, it takes most of your time. It is something you have studied and prepared to do with all clients in acute care settings and at home. And it is what communities, groups, families, and clients need the most. Likewise, it is something that can be done in ways that are incomplete, culturally inappropriate, or inadequate. Becoming ethnoculturally focused and prepared to teach from the client's view of the world will start you in the right direction. The suggestions in Display 4–3 offer ideas for providing culturally competent care. Chapter 12 on Health Education will help prepare you as well.

DISPLAY 4–3

Developing Cultural Competence

First: Know that culture is dynamic.
It is a continuous and cumulative process.
It is learned and shared by people.
Cultural behaviors and values are exhibited by people.
Culture is creative and meaningful to our lives.
It is symbolically represented through language and interaction.
Culture guides us in our thinking, feeling, and acting.

Second: Become aware of culture in yourself.
Thought processes that occur within you also occur within others but may take on a different shape or meaning.
Cultural values and biases are interpreted internally.
Cultural values are not always obvious since they are shared socially with those you meet on a daily basis and are perceived through your senses.

Third: Become aware of culture in others, especially among client groups you serve.
This is best represented by the belief that there are many cultural ways that are correct, each in its own location and context.
It is essential to build respect for cultural differences and appreciation for cultural similarities.
Develop the ability to work within others' cultural context, free from ethnocentric judgments.

SELECTED CULTURAL COMMUNITIES

An examination of the meaning and nature of culture clearly underscores the need to recognize cultural differences and to understand clients in the context of their cultural backgrounds. Practically speaking, how can knowledge of cultural diversity be integrated into everyday community health nursing practice? Who are the diverse cultural communities served by community health nurses? What are their differences? Do they share some features? To provide insights and answers to these questions, this section describes five cultural communities. Three are dominant in the United States, and the other two represent populations native to North America and people from a Middle Eastern culture, an expanding group in the United States. These descriptions are brief and are not to be considered as a stand-alone guide to cultural competence. Each culture is complex and unique and deserves a more comprehensive study than is possible within the scope of this chapter. There are many good references on cultural diversity for nurses, especially Spector's *Cultural Diversity in Health and Illness* (2000). Also, remember that more than 100 different ethnic groups live in the United States, only 5 of which are described here. Four of the groups highlighted represent groups identified in *Healthy People 2010* (U. S. Department of Health and Human Services [USDHHS], 2000). The fifth group, Middle Easterners from Saudi Arabia, is presented because of the significant media attention Middle Easterners have received in recent years. Further information is provided by the references and selected readings.

WHAT DO YOU THINK?

Tobacco use is the leading preventable cause of death in the United States today, resulting in almost half a million deaths each year. Thirty-six percent of teens smoke, including 40% of white high school students, 34% of Hispanics, and 23% of African-American teens, as well as 24% of the adults. *Healthy People 2010* (USDHHS, 2000) set 2% as its target for smokers by 2010. Do you think we will reach it?

Healthy People 2010 (USDHHS, 2000) described significant disparities among members of some of the five groups highlighted here. Several of the disparities are displayed in Table 4–4. On the particular issue of smoking, see What Do You Think?

Native American Indians, Aleut, and Eskimo Communities

Native American Indians, Aleuts, and Alaska natives (Eskimo communities residing in Alaska), the first known settlers of this continent, form a large cluster of tribal groups whose members are descendants of the original Native Americans who were inhabiting this country when whites settled here. First, the Vikings came in about 1010 AD, and then Europeans "discovered" this continent in the 1500s

T A B L E   4 – 4

Healthy People 2010 and Disparities

Goal of Healthy People 2010	Baseline values				
	White	Native American	Hispanic	Black	Asian
Health insurance: 79% of population	89%	79%	70%	84%	83%
Cancer deaths/100,000: 158.7	202.2	131.8	125.5	262.1	127.2
End-stage renal disease/1 million: 217	218	586	N/A	873	344
Diabetes deaths/100,000: 45	68	107	86	130	62
CHD deaths/100,000: 166	214	134	151	257	125
Stroke deaths/100,000: 48	60	39	40	82	55
HIV/AIDS deaths/100,000: 0.8	2.8	2.5	8.9	26.6	0.9
Deaths from firearms/100,000: 4.9	10.4	11.4	10.7	22.9	5.0
Motor vehicle deaths/100,000: 9.0	15.8	31.5	15.2	17.0	10.6
Unintentional injury deaths/100,000: 20.8	34.3	62.7	30.1	40.9	20.9
Residential fire deaths/100,000: 0.6	1.1	2.2	0.8	3.4	0.8
Homicides/100,000: 3.2	4.3	10.4	9.9	25.2	4.1
Low-birth-weight babies: 7.6% of births	6.5	6.8	6.4	13.0	7.2
Suicides/100,000: 6.0	12.8	12.4	6.4	6.3	7.0
Drug induced deaths/100,000:1.0	5.7	6.6	6.0	9.0	1.6
Smokers: 12% of population	25%	34%	20%	26%	16%

CHD, coronary heart disease; HIV/AIDS, human immunodeficiency virus/acquired immunodeficiency syndrome; N/A, not available.
From U. S. Department of Health and Human Services. (2000). *Healthy people 2010* (Conference edition, Vols. 1 and 2). Washington, DC: Author.

(Spector, 2000). Native Americans, Aleuts, and Eskimos have adopted many Anglo-American values and practices, yet they preserve many aspects of their own culture.

Population Characteristics and Culture

Native American Indians and Alaska natives are a diverse group made up of different tribes and 561 federally recognized nations that speak approximately 250 languages. They make up just 0.9% of the U. S. population, or about 2.5 million people (U. S. Department of Commerce, 2001). In the 2000 Census, 4.1 million people said they were at least "part" Indian and 2.5 million identified themselves only as American Indian. Today, people are proud to identify themselves as being Native American, whereas in the past to claim to be part Indian was not a respectable acknowledgment. In addition to societal changes about being Indian, there are incentives for many American Indians who are recognized tribal members. More than 300 of the Indian Nations receive revenue from gambling casinos. In 1988, casinos owned by Native Americans made $212 million, and in 2000 they grossed $10 billion (U. S. Department of Commerce, 2001).

Native Americans mainly live in 26 states in the United States, including Alaska and the Aleutian Islands (Spector, 2000). Many live on reservations and in rural areas; however, just as many live in cities. Eskimos, Aleuts, and Indians living in Alaska are known as Alaska natives; those living in other states are known as American Indians. The largest numbers live in Oklahoma, Arizona, California, New Mexico, North Carolina, and Alaska, as a result of the forced westward migration (Spector, 2000). By 2050, the U. S. Census Bureau estimates there will be about 4.5 million American Indians, nearly double the number in 2000 (U. S. Department of Commerce, 2001). Some of this increase can be attributed to official recognition as tribal members of persons who can provide information linking them to a tribe or nation; if they are accepted, they can then declare themselves as Native Americans.

Each tribe or nation has its own distinct language, beliefs, customs, and rituals. The community health nurse cannot assume that knowledge of one group can be generalized to others. Knowledge of certain similarities among the various Native American cultures (Display 4–4) can assist nurses working with members of a specific tribe. For many Native American groups, large, extended family networks reinforce cultural standards and expectations and provide emotional support and practical assistance.

Health Problems

Health problems among Native Americans tend to be both chronic and socially related. One third of Native Americans live in abject poverty and experience the afflictions associated with poor living conditions, including malnutrition, tuberculosis (TB), and high maternal and infant death rates (Spector, 2000). The highest-ranking health problems in children include dysentery, impetigo, intestinal infectious diseases, skin diseases, staphylococcal infections, respiratory diseases, influenza, and pneumonia. For adults, trachomatous conjunctivitis poses a serious health threat that is not common in the

---

DISPLAY 4–4

Similarities Among Native American Cultures

All of creation/universe has Spirit and is considered equal in value.

Everything is considered alive with energy and importance.

People have universal connectedness.

Harmony is a way of life based on cooperation and sharing.

Dignity of the individual, family, and community is valued.

Respect for advancing age is valued; elders are leaders.

There is present-time orientation, grounded in what is happening at the moment.

Symbolic arts and crafts are valued.

Life is lived in the present, with little concern for the distant future.

Generosity, harmony, and sharing are valued.

Religion is integrated into everyday life.

Herbal medicines and traditional healing practices are used.

Rituals and ceremonies are valued.

Silence is used as a way to practice presence and strength.

Thoughtful speech is valued.

Patience is valued.

Adapted from Lowe, 2002; Lowe and Struthers, 2001; and Spector, 2000.

---

rest of the U. S. population. Diabetes, TB, and obesity all rank higher among Native Americans than in the general population. Poor sanitation, crowded housing, and low immunization levels contribute to the prevalence of a variety of communicable diseases. On the other hand, the prevalence of heart disease is lower in this population than among Whites.

Alcoholism is the major health problem of Native Americans. There are both traditional/cultural and medical explanations for the disproportionate number of health problems in American Indians. Tribal medicine men have attributed the problems of alcoholism to loosing "the opportunity to make choices," stating that until "people return to a sense of identification within themselves they will not rid themselves of this problem of alcoholism" (Spector, 2000, p. 186). Medically, it appears that Native Americans have a much lower tolerance for alcohol and therefore demonstrate the effects of alcohol with lower amounts consumed. When individuals are under the influence of alcohol, other health and safety problems occur. Instances of domestic violence, child abuse and neglect, traffic injuries and deaths, and homicides are higher because of the abuse of alcohol. Its destructive effects on families continue with a high incidence of fetal alcohol syndrome (FAS) and fetal alcohol effects (FAE), along with the high incidence of violence and injuries. Substance abuse is also prevalent among those living on reservations, and increasingly among children using inhalants.

Health Beliefs and Practices

Native Americans as a group prefer traditional healing practices and folk medicine over Western medicine. Most American Indians today still seek out a medicine man or rely on traditional remedies before going to a health clinic. Many of their beliefs about health and illness have common traditional roots, regardless of tribe or location. Health and dietary practices are closely tied to cultural and religious beliefs. Beliefs about health reflect living in total harmony with nature. The earth is considered a living organism that should be treated with respect, as should the body (Spector, 2000).

American Indians practice purification rituals such as immersion in water and the use of sweat lodges to maintain their harmony with nature and cleanse the body and spirit. The basis of therapy lies in nature, with herbal teas, charms, and fetishes used as preventive and curative measures.

Because of decades of racism and government paternalism, many Native Americans feel oppressed and dehumanized and carry considerable resentment and lack of trust toward Whites. As a result, many maintain a degree of separateness from overall American culture. Nurses must overcome these barriers through patience, acceptance, and respect for their clients' culture, as illustrated in the case study of the community health nurse, Sandra Josten, and her new client from a Native American community (see Clinical Corner I).

CLINICAL CORNER I

SANDRA'S NEW CLIENTS

As she drove up the dirt road and parked her car next to the community hall, Sandra Josten felt apprehensive. She had been alerted by the previous community health nurse about the difficulty of working with these Native American people: "This tribe is lazy and unappreciative. You can't get anywhere with them." Only through the urging of Mrs. Brown, an Indian community aide, had a group of the women reluctantly agreed to meet with the new nurse. They would see what she had to say.

Sandra's steps echoed hollowly as she walked across the wooden floor of the large room to the far corner where a group of women sat silently in a circle. Only their eyes turned; their faces remained impassive. Mrs. Brown rose slowly, greeted the nurse, and introduced her to the group. Swallowing her fear, Sandra smiled. She told them of her background and explained that she had not worked with Indian people before. There was a long silence. No one spoke. Sandra continued, "I'd like to help you if I can, maybe with problems about care of your children when they are sick or questions about how to keep them healthy, but I don't know what you need or want." Silence fell again. She would like to learn from them, she repeated. Would they help her? Again Sandra felt an uncomfortable silence.

Then one woman began to speak. Quietly, but with deep feeling, she described several bad experiences with the previous nurse and the county social worker. Then others spoke up: "They tell us what we should do. They don't listen. They say our way is not good." Seeing Sandra's interest and concern, the women continued. One of their main concerns was their children's health. Another was the high incidence of accidents and injuries on the reservation. They wanted to learn how to give first aid. Other concerns were expressed. The group agreed that Sandra could help them by teaching a first-aid class.

In the weeks that followed, Sandra taught several classes on first aid and emergency care. She then began a series of sessions on child health. Each time, she asked the women to choose a topic or problem for discussion and then elicited from them their accustomed ways of dealing with each problem; for example, how they handled toilet training or taught their children to eat solid foods. Her goal was to learn as much as she could about their culture and incorporate that information into her teaching, which preserved as many of their practices as possible. Sandra also visited informally with the women in their homes and at community gatherings.

She learned about their way of life, their history, and their values. For example, patience was highly valued. It was important to be able to wait patiently, even if a scheduled meeting was delayed as much as 2 hours. It also was important for others to speak, which explained the Indian women's comfort with silences during a conversation. Other values influenced their way of life. Courage, pride, generosity, and honesty all were important determinants of behavior. These also were values by which they judged Sandra and other professionals. Sandra's honesty in keeping her promises enabled the women to trust her. Her generosity in giving her time, helping them occasionally with some household task, and arranging for child care during classes won their respect.

The women came to accept her, and Sandra was invited to eat with them and share in tribal get-togethers. The women criticized and advised her on acceptable ways to speak and act. Her openness and patience to learn and her respect for them as a people had paved the way to improving their health. At first, Sandra felt that her progress was slow, but this slowness was an advantage. She had built a solid foundation of cross-cultural trust, and in the months that followed she saw many changes in her clients' health practices.

African-Americans

Some of the ancestors of black Americans, or African-Americans, originally came to this continent as free settlers as early as 1619, but most of the approximately 4 million who followed came as slaves in the 17th and 18th centuries, mostly from the west coast of Africa. Most African-Americans living today were born in the United States; some, however, have immigrated recently from African countries. Other immigrants or black Americans come from the West Indies, the Dominican Republic, Haiti, and Jamaica, often to escape poverty or political persecution. These people do not self-identify as African-Americans but as Hispanics. This can cause some difficulty for these populations when they identify with the Hispanic culture and others identify them as African-Americans. Similarly, some people from the Philippines have Hispanic surnames and skin tones similar to those of Mexicans. If there are people from the Philippines in parts of the country with large Mexican populations, they can be misidentified and misunderstood.

Population Characteristics and Culture

In 2000, African-Americans numbered 36.4 million and constituted 13% of the U. S. population; projections showed an increase to 15.4% by the year 2050 (U. S. Census Bureau, 2001; U. S. Department of Commerce, 2001). One third of the African-American population is younger than 18 years of age. Slightly more than 8% of African-Americans are older than 65 years, and most of them are women; in comparison, 13% of the total population is older than 65 years of age. Fifty-eight percent of black children live with their mothers only, compared with 21% of white children.

Despite improvements in the legal and social climate for African-Americans, great disparities exist between them and white Americans (Williams & Collins, 2001). Average family income for African-Americans is 62% of the income earned by white families. More than 26% of black Americans live in poverty, compared with 8.9% of whites. Although African-Americans make up only 13% of the population, more than 50% of prison inmates are black. A greater percentage of blacks use illicit drugs (7.7%), compared with whites (6.6%) or Hispanics (6.8%) (Antai-Otong, 2002). Approximately 36% of African-American families in households headed by women live below the poverty level. Unemployment among African-Americans is 8.9%, compared with 3.9% for whites (U. S. Department of Commerce, 2001).

Educational disparities also exist. Among people age 25 years and older, 76% of blacks and 83.7% of whites have a high school education. More than half of those African-Americans with less than a high school education are not in the workforce, compared with 36% of whites with a similar education. However, 89% of both blacks and whites with a college degree are employed; 14.7% of blacks and 25% of whites are college graduates (Williams & Collins, 2001). African-American women acquire more educational training than their black male counterparts do, but their earnings are lower than those of the men, as is also the case with white and Hispanic women compared with men in those groups.

Like Native Americans and Asian-Americans, African-Americans do not comprise a single culture; rather, this group forms a heterogeneous community. As with other large ethnic and racial groups, many factors influence their culture, resulting in much diversity within the African-American population. Among the variables determining specific microcultures within the African-American community are economic level, religious background, education, occupation, social class identity, geographic origin, and residence in an integrated or segregated neighborhood. For community health nurses, this means that specific groups of African-Americans have their own unique values, character, lifestyle, and health needs.

The primary language of most African-Americans is English. Recent black immigrants from Caribbean or other countries may retain the language of their country of origin but usually learn English as well. Many African-Americans speak variations of soul talk, also called Black English or Black Creole. It evolved from pidgin spoken during the era of slavery and has become a dynamic and meaningful language of its own. For some African-Americans, soul talk symbolizes racial pride and identity.

Health Problems

African-Americans have much higher mortality rates than white Americans, with a life expectancy of 71.1 years (U. S. Department of Commerce, 2001). This number is the same as the life expectancy of whites in 1966, revealing a 35-year lag for the Black population compared with the white population. This demonstrates the inequality in mortality and life expectancy, an outcome of health care, economic, and educational disparity (Levine et al., 2001). Life expectancy for whites in 2000 was 76.8 years (U. S. Department of Commerce, 2001). The major health problems for blacks include cardiovascular disease and stroke, cancer, diabetes mellitus, cirrhosis, a high infant mortality rate (twice that of whites), homicide, accidents, and malnutrition (Display 4–5).

Stress and discrimination, poverty, lack of education, high rates of teen pregnancy, inadequate housing, and inadequate insurance for health care are among the risk factors influencing the health of this population. In the last three decades, a dramatic increase in black households headed by women, single-parent births (most frequently among teenagers), and a limited presence of male role models has further exacerbated family vulnerability.

Mortality rates for communicable diseases, including the acquired immunodeficiency syndrome (AIDS), also are higher for blacks than for whites. The incidence of TB in this population also is rising, with many cases being diagnosed in conjunction with an AIDS diagnosis (see Chapter 9). Other infectious and parasitic diseases are three to six times more prevalent among African-Americans than among white Americans (U. S. Department of Health and Human Services, 2000). There are two areas in which blacks demonstrate a lower incidence than for whites: suicide is 50% less

DISPLAY 4-5

Mortality Data for African Americans

- African-American men die from strokes at almost twice the rate of White men.
- Coronary heart disease death rates are higher for African-American women than for White women.
- Black men experience a higher risk of cancer than White men do.
- Diabetes is 33% more common among African-Americans than among Whites.
- African-American babies are twice as likely as White babies to die before their first birthday.
- Homicide is the most frequent cause of death for male African-Americans between 15 and 34 years of age; the homicide rate for those between 25 and 34 years is seven times that for Whites.
- The rate of acquired immunodeficiency syndrome (AIDS) among male African Americans is more than triple that of White males; among women and children, the gap is even wider.

Adapted from Spector, R. E. (2000). *Cultural diversity in health and illness* (5th ed.). Stamford, CT: Appleton & Lange.

DISPLAY 4-6

Asian-Pacific Populations

Asian refers to:	Pacific Islander refers to:
Chinese	Polynesian
Filipino	Hawaiian
Japanese	Samoan
Asian Indian	Tongan
Korean	Micronesian
Vietnamese	Guamanian
Laotian	Melanesian
Thai	Fijian
Cambodian	Tahitian
Pakistan	Marshallese
Indonesian	Trilese
Hmong	
Mien	

prevalent among blacks, and rate of chronic obstructive pulmonary disease (COPD) is 20% to 30% less. All other leading causes of death are higher for black populations, much of which can be attributed to lifestyle and poverty.

Health Beliefs and Practices

Although African-Americans have absorbed most of the dominant culture in the United States, some retain aspects of their ancestors' traditional values and practices. Some, for example, hold traditional African beliefs about health being a sign of harmony with nature and illness being evidence of disharmony. Evil spirits, the punishment of God, or a hex placed on the person might account for this disharmony. Healers treat body, mind, and spirit. Prayer, laying on of hands, magic or other rituals, special diets, wearing of preventive charms or copper bracelets, ointments, and other folk remedies sometimes are practiced. Each African-American community has its own set of health beliefs and practices that must be determined by the community health nurse before any interventions are planned.

Asian-Americans

A third cultural cluster is composed of immigrants and refugees from various Pacific Rim countries, such as China, Korea, Japan, Thailand, Laos, the Philippines, Vietnam, and Cambodia (Display 4–6). Some have been transplanted fairly recently from their own cultures to an entirely different culture, whereas others may have lived here many years or were born in America.

Population Characteristics and Culture

In 2000, more than 11 million Asians and Pacific Islanders were living in the United States, representing 3.1% of the total population (U. S. Department of Commerce, 2001). The largest groups were Chinese and Filipinos, with more than 1.5 million persons from each country, and the Vietnamese people numbered a close second. Other fairly large groups came from Korea, India, Laos, and Cambodia. Each group represents a distinct culture with its own unique challenges for community health nurses, as illustrated in the case study of the Kim family (see Clinical Corner II).

Whereas each Asian culture is distinct in language, values, and customs, some general traits are shared by many Asians. Traditional Asian families tend to be patriarchal (the father is the head of the household) and patrilineal (the genealogy is carried through the male line). Male members are valued over female members. Elders are respected. The male role generally is that of provider, whereas the female role is that of homemaker. Traditional Asians value achievement because it brings honor to the family name. Saving face or preserving dignity and family pride is important. Cooperation is valued over competition (Spector, 2000).

Health Problems

Health problems for Asian-Americans include malnutrition, TB, mental illness, cancer, respiratory infections, arthritis, parasitic infestations, and chronic diseases associated with aging. Suicide rates and stress-related illness are particularly high among Asian refugee groups who have had to flee their countries under stressful conditions and among teens born in the United States to Asian immigrants having difficulty living between two cultures. However, Asians view mental illness as shameful, and the stigma attached to it prompts them to express the mental illness as a disturbed bodily function or to hide it as long as possible.

CLINICAL CORNER II

THE KIM FAMILY

Armed with enthusiasm and pamphlets on pregnancy and prenatal diet, Paula Morrow, the community health nurse, began home visits to the Kim family. Paula's initial plan was to discuss pregnancy and fetal development, teach diet, and prepare the mother for delivery. Mr. Kim, a graduate student, was present to interpret, because Mrs. Kim spoke little English. Their two boys, age 1½ and 3 years, played happily on the kitchen floor. The family offered tea to the nurse and listened politely as she explained her reasons for coming and asked, "How can I be most helpful to you? What would you like from my visits?"

The Kims were grateful for this approach. Hesitant at first, they hinted at Mrs. Kim's fears of American doctors and hospitals; her first two children had been born in Korea. None of the family had any experience with Western medicine. They shared some concerns about adjustment to living in the United States. It was difficult to shop in American food stores with their overwhelming variety of foods, many of which the Kims found unfamiliar. Mrs. Kim, who had come from a family whose servants prepared the food, was an inexperienced cook. Servants also had cared for the children, and her role had been that of an aristocrat in hand-tailored silk gowns.

Listening carefully, Paula began to realize the striking differences between her own culture and that of her clients. Her care plans changed. In subsequent visits, she determined to learn about Korean culture and base her nursing intervention on that knowledge. She learned about their traditional ways of raising children, the traditional male and female roles, and practices related to pregnancy and lactation. She respected their value of "saving face" and attempted never to offend their pride or dignity. As time went on, her interest and respect for their way of life won their trust. She inquired about their cultural practices before attempting any intervention. As a result, the Kims were receptive to her suggestions. Whenever possible, Paula adapted her teaching and suggestions to comply with the Kims' culture. For example, appropriate changes were made in Mrs. Kim's diet that were compatible with her food preferences and cultural eating patterns. Because she was not accustomed to drinking milk, she increased her calcium intake by learning to prepare custards (which disguised the milk flavor) and by eating more green, leafy vegetables. After 5 months, a strong, positive relationship had been established between this family and the nurse. Mrs. Kim delivered a healthy baby girl and looked forward to continued supportive visits from the community health nurse.

Health Beliefs and Practices

Asian health beliefs vary among subcultures. Many Asians believe in the Chinese concepts of yin (cold) and yang (hot), which do not refer to temperature but to the opposing forces of the universe regulating normal flow of energy. A balance of yin and yang results in qi (pronounced *chee*), which is the desired state of harmony. Illness results when there is an imbalance in these forces. If the imbalance is an excess of yin, then "cold" foods, such as vegetables and fruits, are avoided, and "hot" foods, such as rice, chicken, eggs, and pork, are offered. Some Asians view Western medicines as "hot" and Eastern folk medicines and herbal treatments as "cold," which explains why some groups practice both for balance. The Vietnamese have a similar hot-and-cold belief but call it Am and Dong. Other Asian groups, such as the Filipinos, view illness as an act of God and pray for healing, reflecting their strong religious beliefs as Catholics or Muslims. The Khmer of Cambodia believe that illness reflects a deviation from moral standards, and the Hmong consider illness to be a visitation by spirits.

Asian groups have traditional healers, who, depending on the culture, may include acupuncturists, herbalists, herb pharmacists, spirit and magic experts, or a shaman. Most Asian cultures also exercise traditional self-care practices,

including herbal medicines and poultices, types of acupuncture, and massage (Davis, 2001; Kim et al., 2002; Spector, 2000). Southeast Asians also practice dermabrasive techniques of cupping, pinching, rubbing, and burning. These methods are used to relieve symptoms such as headache, sore throat, cough, fever, and diarrhea by bringing toxins to the skin surface or compensating for heat lost. Because these techniques leave a bruise-like lesion on the skin, they can be mistaken for physical abuse. Each client requires careful **cultural assessment**, detailed data-gathering about the client's cultural practices, before nursing action is implemented (see Research: Bridge to Practice).

Hispanic-Americans

A fourth cultural cluster comprises groups who are of Hispanic origin and have immigrated to the United States, some many generations ago. More than half come from Mexico, followed by Puerto Rico, Cuba, Central and South America, and Spain (Spector, 2000). Those with Mexican and Central American backgrounds generally are referred to as Latinos (Holland & Courtney, 1998). Depending on the region of the country, socioeconomic status, immigration or citizenship status, or age, members of this large mi-

RESEARCH: BRIDGE TO PRACTICE

Yu, E.S.H., Chen, E.H., Kim, K.K., & Abdulrahim, S. (2002). Smoking among Chinese Americans: Behavior, knowledge, and beliefs. *American Journal of Public Health, 92(6)*, 1007–1012.

SMOKING AMONG CHINESE AMERICANS

This population-based study looked at smoking among a sample of 644 Chinese-Americans between the ages of 40 and 69 years, using a Chinese questionnaire from the National Health Interview Survey (NHIS); 93% of the participants, all from Chicago's Chinatown, had smoked regularly for 10 or more years. Smoking prevalence was 34% for men and 2% for women (17.4% among all participants)—a very different ratio from that within the total U. S. population, where the rates are only slightly higher for men than for women, but the overall smoking by adults is 24%. Among Asian adults in the United States, men smoke four times as frequently as women, according to *Healthy People 2010*. The population in this study was skewed, with male participants smoking 17 times more frequently than females.

Additional information gained from the participants revealed that, compared with the population as a whole, they had a lower education rate, used non-Western physicians or clinics more often for health care, and stated more frequently that they had no knowledge of early cancer warning signs and symptoms.

Conclusions from this study included a male smoking prevalence higher than that reported in national sources, such as the NHIS and the Behavioral Risk Factor Surveillance System (BRFSS) questionnaires. Chinese-American men smoke more than members of other minority groups, and their smoking rate is far above the *Healthy People 2010* target goal of less than 12%.

Recommendations included conducting multisite surveys and initiating smoking cessation campaigns in Chinese. This could include posters; word-of-mouth information shared in the Chinatown neighborhood, especially where Chinese men gather; and smoking cessation classes conducted by Chinese community health nurses and community health education workers.

---

nority group refer to themselves as Mexican-American, Spanish-American, Latin American, Latin, Latino, or Mexican (Spector, 2000).

The subgroups of Hispanics vary by their patterns of geographic distribution in the United States. Those from Mexico tend to live predominantly in the west (56.7%) and south (32.6%), Puerto Ricans are most likely to live in the northeast (63.9%), and Cubans are highly concentrated in the South (80.1%). Central and South Americans are concentrated in the northeast (32.3%), the south (34.6%), and the west (28.2%) (U. S. Bureau of Census, 2001).

Population Characteristics and Culture

Hispanics are the fastest growing and largest ethnic group in the United States, and people of Hispanic origin are predicted to number more than 58 million, or 17.5% of the population, by 2025 (U. S. Department of Commerce, 2001). In 2000, this group comprised more than 35 million people and accounted for 12.5% of the U. S. population.

The Hispanic population has Spanish as its common and primary language; nonetheless, its diverse cultural and linguistic backgrounds account for diversity in dialects. Hispanic people value extended, cohesive families. Families have been patriarchal, with male members perceived as superior and female members seen as a family-bonding life force. These traditional family structures are changing because of migration, urbanization, women in the work force, and social movements. Spousal roles are becoming more egalitarian. However, vestiges of the macho man and the self-sacrificing woman still are evident in the Hispanic culture and continue to shape behavior (see Clinical Corner III).

Health Problems

Health problems among the Hispanic population are complicated by experiences in their countries of origin as well as socioeconomic and lifestyle factors in this country. TB is high in this group, especially among those younger than 35 years of age. Hypertension, diabetes, and obesity are major concerns. Other problems include infectious diseases, particularly AIDS and pneumonia, parasitic infections, malnutrition, gastroenteritis, alcohol and drug abuse, accidents, and violence. Frequently, the most important health issues for Hispanics are related to the fact that the population is young and has a high birth rate. Posttraumatic stress disorder is a major problem among refugees from Central and South America who have experienced war and physical and emotional torture.

Health Beliefs and Practices

Religion plays an important part in Latino culture. For most Latinos, Catholicism is the dominant religion (95% of Mexican Americans, for example, are Catholic), but often it is a blend of both Catholicism and pre-Cartesian Indian beliefs and ideology along with magicoreligious practices. Latinos believe in submission to the will of God and that illness may be a form of "castigo," or punishment for sins. They cope

CLINICAL CORNER III

MARIA JUAREZ

Maria Juarez, a 53-year-old Mexican-American widow, was referred to a community health nursing agency by a clinic. Her married daughter reported that Mrs. Juarez was having severe and prolonged vaginal bleeding and needed medical attention. The daughter had made several appointments for her mother at the clinic, but Mrs. Juarez had refused at the last minute to keep any of them.

After two broken home visit appointments, the community health nurse made a drop-in call and found Mrs. Juarez at home. The nurse was greeted courteously and invited to have a seat. After introductions, the nurse explained that she and the others were only trying to help. Mrs. Juarez had caused a lot of unnecessary concern to everyone by not cooperating, she scolded in a friendly tone. Mrs. Juarez quickly apologized and explained that she had felt fine on the days of her broken appointments and saw no need "to bother" anyone. Questioned about her vaginal bleeding, Mrs. Juarez was evasive. "It's nothing," she said. "It comes and goes like always, only maybe a little more." She listened politely, nodding in agreement as the nurse explained the need for her to see a physician. Her promise to come to the clinic the next day, however, was not kept. The staff labeled Mrs. Juarez as unreliable and uncooperative.

Mrs. Juarez had been brought up in traditional Mexican-American culture that taught her to be submissive and interested primarily in the welfare of her husband and children. She had learned long ago to ignore her own needs and found it difficult to identify any personal wants. Her major concern was to avoid causing trouble for others. To have a medical problem, then, was a difficult adjustment. The pain and bleeding had caused her great apprehension. Many Mexican-Americans have a particular dread of sickness and especially hospitalization. Furthermore, Mrs. Juarez's culture had taught her the value of modesty. "Female problems" were not discussed openly. This cultural orientation meant that the sickness threatened her modesty and created intense embarrassment. Conforming to Mexican-American cultural values, she had first turned to her family for support. Often, only under dire circumstances do members of this cultural group seek help from others; to do so means sacrificing pride and dignity. Mrs. Juarez agreed to go to the clinic because refusal would have been disrespectful, but her fear of physicians and her reluctance to discuss such a sensitive problem kept her from going. Mrs. Juarez was being asked to take action that violated several deeply felt cultural values. Her behavior was far from unreliable and uncooperative. With no opportunity to discuss and resolve the conflicts, she had no other choice.

with illness through prayers and faith that God will heal. Their religion also determines the rituals used in healing. For example, "solito," a condition of depression in women similar to a midlife crisis in American culture, is treated by having the patient lie on the floor while her body is stroked by the curandero (native healer) until the depression passes. Latino culture includes beliefs that witchcraft ("brujeria") and evil eye ("mal de ojo") are supernatural causes of illness that cannot be treated by "Anglo" medicine. "Empacho," a stomach ache in children that occurs after a traumatic event, is treated by the curandero with herbal mixtures made into teas. After tender loving care and a bowel movement, the child is "healed" (Table 4–5). Like Asians, Latinos believe in "hot" and "cold" categories of foods that influence their diet during illness. Many Latinos tend to be oriented to the present and are not as concerned about keeping time schedules or preparing for the future.

Arab Populations and Muslims

The final cultural community selected for this discussion is made up of groups of people who come from Arabic countries, especially those who are Muslims. By comparison with the groups previously mentioned, the number of people from Arabic countries in the United States is small, but because of the terrorist attacks of September 11, 2001, increasing racial and religious animosity has been directed toward people from this part of the world and those who bear physical resemblances to members of these groups (Giger & Davidhizar, 2002). It is our desire that more information about these groups of people will dispel myths and alleviate fear.

About 4 million people of Arab descent are living in the United States. A common language (Arabic) and a common religion (Islam) unite them, yet only 18% of the followers of Islam in the world reside in Middle Eastern countries. Islam is the fastest-growing global religion, with more than 1 billion followers worldwide. Most Muslims live in Indonesia, the southern Philippines, and the United States. Eight million Americans are Muslim. In Britain it is estimated that Muslim worshippers will outnumber Anglicans within a few years, and the Christian Research Organization in England projected that, if current trends continue, by 2039 Muslims will surpass all British Christians in worship attendance (Baqi-Aziz, 2001). The tenets of Islam are interpreted more liberally in some nations and more strictly in others, but all prac-

TABLE 4 – 5

Hispanic Health Beliefs and Folk Diseases

Belief Name	Explanation/Treatment
Ataque	Severe expression of shock, anxiety, or sadness characterized by screaming, falling to the ground, thrashing about, hyperventilation, violence, mutism, and uncommunicative behavior. Is a culturally appropriate reaction to shocking or unexpected news, which ends spontaneously.
Bilis	Vomiting, diarrhea, headaches, dizziness, nightmares, loss of appetite, and the inability to urinate brought on by livid rage and revenge fantasies. Believed to come from bile pouring into the bloodstream in response to strong emotions and the person "boiling over."
Bilong (hex)	Any illness may be caused by this; proper diagnosis and treatment requires consulting with a santero or santera (priest or priestess).
Caide de mollera	A condition thought to cause a fallen or sunken anterior fontanel, crying, failure to nurse, sunken eyes, and vomiting in infants. Popular home remedies include holding the child upside down over a pan of water, applying a poultice to the depressed area of the head, or inserting a finger in the child's mouth and pushing up on the palate. (Note: According to Western medicine, these symptoms are indicative of dehydration and can be life-threatening. The community health nurse's role is imperative—to promoting hydration and definitive health care.)
Empacho	Lack of appetite, stomach ache, diarrhea, and vomiting caused by poorly digested food. Food forms into a ball and clings to the stomach, causing pain and cramping. Treated by strongly massaging the stomach, gently pinching and rubbing the spine, drinking a purgative tea (*estafiate*), or by administering *azarcon* or *greta,* medicines that have been implicated, in some cases, in lead poisoning. (Note: The community health nurse must assess family for the use of these "medicines" and initiate appropriate follow-up).
Fatigue	Asthma-like symptoms treated with western health care practices, including oxygen and medications.
Mal de ojo	A sudden and unexplained illness including vomiting, fever, crying, and restlessness in a usually well child (most vulnerable) or adult. Brought on by an admiring or covetous look from a person with an "evil eye." It can be prevented if the person with the "evil eye" touches the child when admiring him or her if the child wears a special charm. Treated by a spiritualistic sweeping of the body with eggs, lemons, and bay leaves accompanied by prayer.
Pasmo	Paralysis-like symptoms in the face and limbs treated by massage.
Susto	Anorexia, insomnia, weakness, hallucinations, and various painful sensations brought on by traumatic situations such as witnessing a death. Treatment includes relaxation, herb tea, and prayer.

Adapted from Spector, R. E. (2000). *Cultural diversity in health and illness* (5th ed.). Stamford, CT: Appleton & Lange.

ticing Muslims adhere to the five tenets of Islam in some fashion (Table 4–6.)

TABLE 4 – 6

The Five Pillars (Tenets) of Islam

1. The two testifications	To testify that there is no God save Allah and that Mohammad is the messenger of Allah
2. The prayers	A form of worship rites that involves specific movements and sayings performed five times a day
3. Almsgiving	To pay 2.5% of the wealth annually for the benefit of the needy in Muslim communities
4. The fasting	To abstain from eating, drinking, and sexual intercourse during daytime (from dawn to sunset) throughout the 9th lunar month (Ramadan)
5. The pilgrimage	The pilgrimage to Makkah once in a lifetime for those who are physically and financially able

Population Characteristics and Culture

An Arab is defined as "an individual who was born in an Arab country, speaks the Arabic language, and shares the values and beliefs of an Arab culture" (Kridli, 2002, p. 178). Arab-Americans are people who can trace their ancestry to the North African countries of Morocco, Tunisia, Algeria, Libya, Sudan, and Egypt, as well as the western Asian countries of Lebanon, Palestine, Syria, Jordan, Bahrain, Qatar, Oman, Saudi Arabia, Kuwait, United Arab Emirates, and Yemen. In general, the cultural practices of people from such different and distant countries cannot be folded into one culture. Some of these countries are more westernized, have natural resources such as crude oil and the riches that follow, and are more liberal in following traditional cultural practices.

Arabs are divided into two distinct religious groups: Muslims and Christians. Arabs value Western medicine and trust American health care workers. Several practices, however, are unfamiliar to most Americans. Many Arabic women stay at home and are not in the workforce. Families impose stricter rules for girls than for boys. After menarche, teenage girls may not socialize with boys. The adolescent female also begins to cover her head and perhaps wears *hijab*, which takes the form of the modest dress and veil designed to diminish attractiveness and appeal to the opposite sex. Some Arab groups take this outfit to extremes and not even a woman's eyes show out of the hijab. Modesty is one of the core values for Arabs; it is expressed by both genders, though more evidently by females (Al-Shahri, 2002).

Within the Arabic population, there are strict sexual taboos and social practices. All sexual contacts outside the marital bond are considered illegal. Those known to have been involved in such activities can be socially rejected, and the stigma of lost honor can continue with their families for generations to come. Another social practice, at times mistakenly related to the Islamic religion, is the practice of female genital mutilation. This is practiced in a few of the Arabic countries on the African continent and has spread to southern Egypt, but it is rare or nonexistent in other Arabic countries. This horrific practice may include the removal of a young woman's labia or clitoris, or both, and it sometimes includes closing the vaginal opening by suturing it closed (Kridli, 2002).

Health Problems

Health problems among Middle Easterners are most frequently lifestyle related. These include poor nutritional practices, resulting in obesity, especially among women; smoking among men; and lack of physical exercise (Al-Shahri, 2002). In some rural areas, especially in Saudi Arabia, men and women chew tobacco and an increase of oral cancers is seen. Major public health concerns for most Arabs are related to motor vehicle accidents, maternal-child health, TB, malaria, trachoma, typhus, hepatitis, typhoid fever, dysentery, and parasitic infections (Giger & Davidhizar, 2002).

Most social restrictions are directed toward women and can affect their health. Pregnancy can be complicated by genital mutilation, which results in infections and difficult deliveries. Child bearing continues up until menopause, and 30% of marriages in some Arabic countries are between first cousins; both factors contribute to the prevalence of genetically determined diseases (Giger & Davidhizar, 2002). The desire to have more sons than daughters often results in very large families and closely occurring pregnancies, without the benefit of family planning. (It is debated whether birth control methods are sanctioned by Islam or not.)

Health Beliefs and Practices

Traditional medicine is practiced in spite of a developmental boom in medical services in some of the richer Arab nations. Traditional health care practices are much more common in the poorer Middle Eastern countries and in rural areas of all Arabic countries.

Muslims believe in predestination, that life is determined beforehand, and they attribute the occurrence of disease to the will of Allah. However, this does not prevent people from seeking medical treatment. Islamic law prohibits the use of illicit drugs, which include alcohol. Users of such substances are liable to trial, and those convicted of smuggling substances into the country are sentenced to death in some cases.

Cleanliness is paramount and ritualistic, especially before prayers and after sexual intercourse. The bodies of both genders are kept free of axillary and pubic hair. The left hand is used for cleaning the genitals and the right one is reserved for eating, hand shaking, and other hygienic activities.

When caring for Arabs in clinics or at home, a nurse of the same sex as the client should be assigned. Many topics, such as menstruation, family planning, pregnancy, and childbirth, must be discussed only with the women, and only by women; men are not included in these discussions. Additional guidelines for nurses working with immigrant groups include the following:

- Do not make assumptions about a client's understanding of health care issues.
- Allow more time for interviewing; allow time to evaluate beliefs and provide appropriate interventions.
- Conduct educational programs to correct any misconceptions about health issues; this can occur in clinics, mosques, schools, or homes.
- Use an appropriate interpreter to improve communication with immigrants who do not speak English well.

TRANSCULTURAL COMMUNITY HEALTH NURSING PRINCIPLES

Culture profoundly influences thinking and behavior and has an enormous impact on the effectiveness of health care. Just as physical and psychological factors determine clients' needs and attitudes toward health and illness, so too does culture. Kark emphasized 30 years ago that "culture is perhaps the most relevant social determinant of community health" (1974, p. 149). Culture determines how people rear their children, react to pain, cope with stress, deal with death, respond to health practitioners, and value the past, present, and future. Culture also influences diet and eating practices. Partly because of culturally derived preferences, dietary practices are very difficult to change (Nakamura, 1999).

Despite its importance, the client's culture often is misunderstood or ignored in the delivery of health care (Leininger, 2001). The growth in non-White populations demands that "health care providers must be prepared for interactions with increasingly diverse health care team members and clients." (Giger & Davidhizar, 2002, p. 80). Nurses must avoid ethnocentric attitudes and must attempt to understand and bridge cultural differences when working with others. Nurses must develop knowledge and skill in serving multicultural clients and must put clients' responses to experiences within the context of their clients' lives; otherwise, their understanding and interpretation of their clients' experience will be limited.

Overcoming ethnocentrism requires a concerted effort on the nurse's part to see the world through the eyes of clients. It means being willing to examine one's own culture carefully and to become aware that alternative viewpoints are possible. It means attempting to understand the meaning of other people's culture for them and appreciating their culture as important and useful to them. Ignoring consideration of clients' different cultural origins often has negative results, as was illustrated in the Clinical Corner discussion about Maria Juarez.

Culture is a universal experience. Each person is part of some group, and that group helps to shape the values, beliefs, and behaviors that make up their culture. In addition, every cultural group is different from all others. Even within fairly homogeneous cultural groups, subcultures and microcultures have their own distinctive characteristics. Further differences, based on such factors as socioeconomic status, social class, age, or degree of acculturation, can be found within microcultures. These latter differences, called intraethnic variations, only underscore the range of culturally diverse clients served by community health nurses.

Given such diversity, community health nurses face a considerable challenge in providing service to cross-cultural groups. This kind of practice, known as **transcultural nursing**, means providing culturally sensitive nursing service to people of an ethnic or racial background different from the nurse's. Community health nurses in transcultural practice with client groups can be guided by several principles: (1) develop cultural self-awareness, (2) cultivate cultural sensitivity, (3) assess the client group's culture, (4) show respect and patience while learning about other cultures, and (5) examine culturally derived health practices.

Develop Cultural Self-Awareness

The first transcultural nursing principle focuses on the nurse's own culture. Self-awareness is crucial for the nurse working with people from other cultures (Leininger, 2001). Nurses must remember that their culture often is sharply different from the culture of their clients. **Cultural self-awareness** means recognizing the values, beliefs, and practices that make up one's own culture. It also means becoming sensitive to the impact of one's culturally based responses. The community health nurse who assisted Mrs. Juarez probably thought that she was being friendly, efficient, and helpful. In terms of her own culture, this nurse's behavior was intended to reassure clients and meet their needs. Unaware of the negative consequences of her behavior, the nurse caused damage rather than meeting needs.

To gain skill in understanding their own culturally based behavior, nurses can complete a cultural self-assessment by analyzing their own

- Ethnic and racial background influences
- Typical verbal and nonverbal communication patterns
- Cultural values and **norms**, or expected cultural practices or behaviors
- Religious beliefs and practices
- Health beliefs and practices

Start with a detailed list of values, beliefs, and practices relative to each point. Next, enlist one or more close friends to call attention to selected behaviors, to bring them to a more conscious level. Videotaping practice interviews with colleagues and actual interviews with selected clients creates further awareness of the nurse's unconscious culturally based responses. Finally, ask selected clients to critique nursing actions in the light of the clients' own culture. Feedback from clients' perspectives can reveal many of the nurse's own cultural responses.

Because culture is mostly tacit, as discussed earlier, it takes conscious effort and hard work to bring the nurse's own cultural biases or influence to the surface. Doing so, however, rewards the nurse with a more effective understanding of self and an enhanced ability to provide culturally relevant service to clients.

Cultivate Cultural Sensitivity

The second transcultural nursing principle seeks to expand the nurse's awareness of the significance of culture on behavior. Nurses' beliefs and ways of doing things frequently conflict with those of their clients. A first step toward bridging cultural barriers is to recognize those differences and develop cultural sensitivity. **Cultural sensitivity** requires recognizing that culturally based values, beliefs, and practices influence people's health and lifestyles and need to be considered in plans for service. Mrs. Juarez's values and health practices sharply contrasted with those of the clinic's staff. Failure to recognize these differences led to a breakdown in communication and ineffective care. Once differences in culture are recognized, it is important to accept and appreciate them. A nurse's ways are valid for the nurse; clients' ways work for them. The nurse visiting the Kim family avoided the dangerous ethnocentric trap of assuming that her way was best, and she consequently developed a fruitful relationship with her clients.

As a part of developing cultural sensitivity, nurses need to try to understand clients' points of view. They need to stand in their clients' shoes and try to see the world through their eyes. By listening, observing, and gradually learning other cultures, the nurse must add a further step of choosing to avoid ethnocentrism. Otherwise, the nurse's view of a different culture will remain distorted and perhaps prejudiced. The ability to show interest, concern, and compassion enabled Sandra Josten to win the trust and respect of the Native American women and told the Kims that their nurse cared about them. These nurses attempted to understand the feelings and ideas of their clients; in this way, they established a trusting relationship and opened the door to the possibility of their clients' adopting healthier behaviors.

Assess the Client Group's Culture

A third transcultural nursing principle emphasizes the need to learn clients' cultures. All clients' actions, like our own, are based on underlying culturally learned beliefs and ideas. Mrs. Kim did not like milk because her culture had taught her that it was distasteful. Also, many Asians are lactose intolerant. The Native American women's response to waiting or keeping someone else waiting was influenced by their value of patience. There usually is some culturally based reason that causes clients to engage in (or avoid) certain actions. Instead of making assumptions or judging clients' behavior, the nurse first must learn about the culture that guides that behavior (Al-Shahri, 2002). During a cultural assessment, the nurse obtains health-related information about the values, beliefs, and practices of a designated cultural group. Learning the culture of the client first is critical to effective nursing practice. The Giger and Davidhizar Transcultural Assessment Model (2002) considers six interrelated factors for assessing differences between people in cultural groups (Fig. 4–2). Understanding these phenomena is a first step toward appreciating the diversity that exists among people from different cultural backgrounds. Interviewing members of a subcultural group can provide valuable data to enhance understanding.

To fully understand a group's culture, it should be studied in depth, as Bernal maintains (1993, p. 231):

Although a general knowledge base and skills are applicable transculturally, immersion in a given culture is necessary to understand fully the patterns that shape the behavior of individuals within that group. Experience with one group can be helpful in understanding the concept of diversity, but each group must be understood within its own ecologic niche and for its own historical and cultural reality.

Practically speaking, however, it is not possible to study in depth all of the cultural groups that the nurse encounters. Instead, the nurse can conduct a cultural assessment by questioning key informants, observing the cultural group, and reading additional information in the literature. The data can be grouped into six categories:

1. *Ethnic or racial background:* Where did the client group originate, and how does that influence their status and identity?
2. *Language and communication patterns:* What is the preferred language spoken, and what are the group's culturally based communication patterns?
3. *Cultural values and norms:* What are the client group's values, beliefs, and standards regarding such things as family roles and functions, education, child rearing, work and leisure, aging, death and dying, and rites of passage?
4. *Biocultural factors:* Are there physical or genetic traits unique to this cultural group that predispose them to certain conditions or illnesses?
5. *Religious beliefs and practices:* What are the group's religious beliefs, and how do they influence life events, roles, health, and illness?
6. *Health beliefs and practices:* What are the group's beliefs and practices regarding prevention, causes, and treatment of illnesses?

The cultural assessment guide presented in Table 4–7 gives suggestions for more detailed data collection.

Many cultural assessment guides can be found throughout the nursing literature. Nonetheless, a thorough cultural assessment may be too time-consuming and costly. Instead, the two-phase assessment process is proposed, as outlined in Table 4–8. Categories to explore in the assessment include values, beliefs, customs, and social structure components. Two methods that have proved highly effective for in-depth study of cultural groups are ethnographic interviewing and participant observation. Classic models of these methods have been published by Spradley (1979, 1980).

Show Respect and Patience While Learning About Other Cultures

The fourth transcultural nursing principle emphasizes key behaviors for the nurse to practice during the cultural learning process. Respect is the first behavior, and it is shown in many ways. When Sandra Josten involved the Native American women in decisions and gave them choices, she was showing respect. When the nurse gave positive recognition to the importance of the Kims' culture, she was showing respect. Attentive listening is a way to show respect and to learn about a client's culture. Within the United States, people of minority groups particularly need respect. At times, for

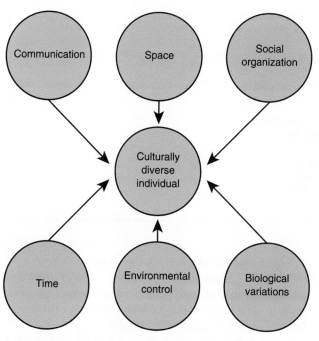

FIGURE 4–2. Components of the Giger and Davidhizar Transcultural Assessment Model, showing the culturally diverse individual through communication, space, social organization, time, environmental control, and biological variations. (Adapted from Giger, J.N., & Davidhizar, R. [2002] Culturally competent care: Emphasis on understanding the people of Afghanistan, Afghanistan Americans, and Islamic culture and religion. *International Nursing Review, 49,* 79–86.)

TABLE 4-7

Cultural Assessment Guide

Category	Sample Data
Ethnic/racial background	Countries of origin Mostly native-born or U.S. born? Reasons for emigrating if applicable Racial/ethnic identity Experience with racism or racial discrimination?
Language and communication patterns	Languages of origin Languages spoken in the home Preferred language for communication How verbal communication patterns affected by age, sex, other? Preferences for use of interpreters Nonverbal communication patterns (eg, eye contact, touching)
Cultural values and norms	Group beliefs and standards for male and female roles and functions Standards for modesty and sexuality Family/extended family structures and functions Values re: work, leisure, success, time Values re: education and occupation Norms for child-rearing and socialization Norms for social networks and supports Values re: aging and treatment of elders Values re: authority Norms for dress and appearance
Biocultural factors	Group genetic predisposition to health conditions (eg, hypertension, anemia) Socioculturally associated illnesses (eg, AIDS, alcoholism) Group attitudes toward body parts and functions Group vulnerability or resistance to health threats? Folk illnesses common to group? Group physical/genetic differences (eg, bone mass, height, weight, longevity)
Religious beliefs and practices	Religious beliefs affecting roles, childbearing and child-rearing, health and illness? Recognized religious healers? Religious beliefs and practices for promoting health, preventing illness, or treatment of illness Beliefs and rituals re: conception and birth Beliefs and rituals re: death, dying, grief
Health beliefs and practices	Beliefs re: causes of illness Beliefs re: treatment of illness Beliefs re: use of healers (traditional and Western) Health promotion and illness prevention practices Folk medicine practices Beliefs re: mental health and illness Dietary, herbal, and other folk cures Food beliefs, preparation, consumption Experience with Western medicine

groups with limited English skills and a community health nurse who is not bilingual, an interpreter who can assist with communication becomes a necessity (Display 4–7).

A **minority group** is part of a population that differs from the majority and often receives different and unequal treatment. Their ways contrast with those of the dominant culture. It is difficult for them to retain pride in their lifestyles, or in themselves, when the majority culture suggests that they are inferior. This message may be only implied or even unintentional, as was the case for Mrs. Juarez in the Clinical Corner. The clinic's routine and the manner of the staff were not intended to show disrespect. They did, nevertheless, and Mrs. Juarez was intimidated and was unable to

receive the help that she needed. Everyone needs respect to enhance pride, dignity, and self-esteem; it is an important contributor to good mental health. Showing respect also is an important means for breaking down barriers in cross-cultural communication. For community health nurses, culturally relevant care means practicing cultural relativism. **Cultural relativism** is recognizing and respecting alternative viewpoints and understanding values, beliefs, and practices within their cultural context.

In addition to respect, patience is essential. It takes time to build trust and effect cultural change. It can be difficult to establish the nurse-client relationship when it involves two different cultures. Trust must be won, and winning it may

TABLE 4–8

Two-Phased Cultural Assessment Process

Phase I—Data Collection

Stage 1	Assess values, beliefs, and customs (eg, ethnic affiliations, religion, decision-making patterns).
Stage 2	Collect problem-specific cultural data (eg, cultural beliefs and practices related to diet and nutrition). Make nursing diagnoses.
Stage 3	Determine cultural factors influencing nursing intervention (eg, child-rearing beliefs and practices that might affect nurse teaching toilet training or child discipline).

Phase II—Data Organization

Step 1	Compare cultural data with Standards of client's own culture (eg, client's diet compared with cultural norms) Standards of the nurse's culture Standards of the health facility providing service.
Step 2	Determine incongruities in above standards.
Step 3	Seek to modify one or more systems (client's, nurse's, or the facility's) to achieve maximum congruity.

take weeks, months, or years. Time must be allowed for both nurse and clients to learn how to communicate with one another, to test one another's trustworthiness, and to learn

DISPLAY 4–7

Interpreter Guidelines

1. Unless the community health nurse is thoroughly effective and fluent in the client's language, an interpreter should be used.
2. Meet with interpreters on a regular basis, since they provide both a window and a mirror when dealing with other clients.
3. Confidentiality must be maintained by the interpreter, who divulges nothing without the full approval of the client and community health nurse.
4. Evaluate the interpreter's style, approach to clients, and ability to develop a relationship of trust and respect. Try to match the interpreter to the client.
5. Be patient. Careful interpretation often requires that the interpreter use long, explanatory phrases.
6. Interpreters must interpret everything that is said by all of the people in the interaction but should inform the community health nurse if the content might be perceived as offensive, insensitive, or harmful to the dignity and well-being of the client.
7. When appropriate, encourage interpreters to explain cultural differences to the client and to yourself.
8. Interpretation conveys the content and spirit of what is said, with nothing omitted or added.
9. Volunteer interpreters receive no fee. Employed interpreters receive their fee or salary from the hiring agency. They should not accept money or favors from clients or the community health nurse. A sincere "thank you" is most appropriate (Kaufert & Putsch, 1997; Putsch, 1985).

about one another. Change in behavior (learned aspects of the culture) occurs gradually. Some aspects of both the nurse's and the clients' cultures can, and probably will, change. The Kims' nurse, Paula Morrow, for example, modified some of her usual practices and adapted them to the Kims' culture and needs. They, in turn, began to assume some American practices and values. However, the process took several months. Time, respect, and patience help to break down cultural barriers.

Examine Culturally Derived Health Practices

The final transcultural nursing principle involves scrutiny of the client group's cultural practices as they affect the group's health status. Once the community health nurse has assessed the culture of the client group, cultural practices affecting the health of the client group need to be examined. Are these behaviors preserving and enhancing the group's health, or are they harmful to their health? Some traditional practices, such as customary diet, birth rituals, and certain folk remedies, may promote both physical and psychological health. These can be considered healthful. Other practices may be neither harmful nor particularly health promoting but are useful in preserving the culture, security, and sense of identity of a particular ethnic group. And some traditional practices may be directly harmful to health. Examples include using herbal poultices to treat an infected wound or "burning" the abdomen to compensate for heat loss associated with diarrhea.

Cultural assessment and aggregate health assessment need to go hand in hand. If the group is experiencing a high incidence of low-birth-weight babies, pregnancy complications, skin infections, mental illness, or other evidence of health problems, these can be clues to prompt an examination of cultural health practices. Those that are clearly damaging to health can be discussed with group leaders and healers. It is in this situation that knowing the group's cultural norms for authority and decision making can be helpful.

CLINICAL CORNER IV

THE IMPORTANCE OF CULTURAL SENSITIVITY

In Australia, well-intentioned government officials, including representatives of the health ministry, identified problems related to substandard housing among a particular aggregate of aboriginal people. To assist this community, the officials spent a great deal of time, energy, and finances planning and building homes for the Aborigines. The homes were small but modern and offered many of the conveniences that officials believed would improve the quality of life for the community.

The Aborigines were appreciative of the group's efforts and moved into their new homes. Before long, however, officials realized that one by one the community members moving back to their "substandard" housing. When asked about their lack of appreciation for the improved lifestyle, the group informed the officials that their watering hole was their life-line and that the houses were not only uncomfortable to them but were too far from their watering hole. Soon, all of the aboriginal families had returned to living on the land, and the homes were part of a veritable ghost town in the middle of nowhere.

QUESTIONS

- What does the phrase *"globalization not gobbleization,"* mean to you?
- Was the aboriginal community truly "poor," as the officials seemed to think?
- Discuss your perception of the following issues:
    Cultural imposition
    Cultural poverty
    Dignity and spirit
- If you were part of an international health team assigned to return to the community to try again to improve their quality of life, what steps would you take to ensure that previous mistakes are not repeated?

Often, a cultural practice can be continued or modified and combined with Western medicine so that respect for the culture is maintained while full treatment efficacy is accomplished (see Clinical Corner IV).

SUMMARY

Community health clients belong to a variety of cultural groups. A culture is a design for living; it provides a set of norms and values that offer stability and security for members of a society and plays a major role in motivating behaviors. The increase in and great variety of cultural groups reinforce the need for community health nurses to understand and appreciate cultural diversity. Ethnocentrism is the bias that a person's own culture is best and others are wrong or inferior. It can create serious barriers to effective nursing care. Understanding cultural diversity and being sensitive to the values and behaviors of cultural groups often is the key to effective community health intervention.

Culture has five characteristics: it is learned from others; it is an integrated system of customs and traits; it is shared; it is tacit; and it is dynamic. Every culture preserves its integrity by deleting nonfunctional practices and acquiring new components that better serve the group. To gain acceptance, nurses must strive to introduce improved health practices that are presented in a manner consistent with clients' cultural values.

Five transcultural nursing principles, drawn from an understanding of the concept of culture, can guide community health nursing practice:
1. Develop cultural self-awareness.
2. Cultivate cultural sensitivity.
3. Assess the client group's culture.
4. Show respect and patience while learning other cultures.
5. Examine culturally derived health practices.

ACTIVITIES TO PROMOTE CRITICAL THINKING

1. Based on your own cultural background, how would you feel and what behaviors would you exhibit if you were
   a. A client sitting in a clinic waiting room in a foreign country whose language you did not know?
   b. Part of a nutrition class being told to eat foods you had never heard of before?
   c. Visited in your home by a nurse who told you to discipline your child in a way that contradicted everything you had been raised to believe about parenting?
2. Describe three tacit cultural rules that govern your own behavior. How might these affect your interactions with clients from another culture?
3. What does the term *ethnocentrism* mean to you? Have you ever experienced someone else's being ethnocentric in their attitude toward you? If so, describe that experience. Using the Cross-Cultural Sensitivity Continuum (see Fig. 4–1), explore where your own attitudes are on the continuum toward several of the cultural groups with which you regularly come in contact or from which you know people well.
4. Imagine that you are assigned to work with a Mexican-American migrant population. What are the steps that you would take to gather the appropriate information to provide culturally relevant nursing service? What sources might provide that information?
5. A Hmong father who severely beat his 12-year-old son with a belt, leaving cuts and bruises, is charged with child abuse. "If I can't discipline my son, how can he be a good child?" said the father. What nursing responses would show respect for this cultural group's norms and values and yet be constructive in resolving the cultural conflict?
6. Find Web sites that elaborate on transcultural nursing and cross-cultural health care concerns. Print materials of interest and develop a resource file for your professional use.
7. Interprofessional communication techniques among diverse health care disciplines are imperative to effective caregiving. How comfortable are you with knowing the linguistic style, practice, and research backgrounds of social workers, pharmacists, physical therapists, educators, psychologists, and others? Seek out a colleague from a different interprofessional discipline and discuss developing a shared language (Milligan et al., 1999).

REFERENCES

Al-Shahri, M. (2002). Culturally sensitive caring for Saudi patients. *Journal of Transcultural Nursing, 13*(2), 133–138.

Antai-Otong, D. (2002). Culturally sensitive treatment of African-Americans with substance-related disorders. *Journal of Psychosocial Nursing, 40*(7), 14–21.

Baqi-Aziz, M. (2001). Where does she think she is? *American Journal of Nursing, 101*(11), 11.

Bernal, H. (1993). A model for delivering culture-relevant care in the community. *Public Health Nursing, 10*(4), 226–232.

Callister, L.C. (2001). Culturally competent care of women and newborns: Knowledge, attitude, and skills. *JOGNN, 30*(2), 209–215.

Cherry, B., & Jacob, S.R. (2001). *Contemporary nursing: Issues, trends, & management* (2nd ed.). St. Louis: Mosby.

Cleveland, L., Aschenbrenner, D.S., Venable, S.J., & Yensenm, J.A.P. (1999). *Nursing management in drug therapy.* Philadelphia: Lippincott Williams & Wilkins.

Davis, R.E. (2001). The postpartum experience for Southeast Asian women in the United States. *The American Journal of Maternal Child Nursing, 26*(4), 208–213.

Ellis, A.D. (2002, August 11). Hmong teens: Lost in America [Special report]. *The Fresno Bee,* pp. 1–12.

Fadiman, A. (1997). *The spirit catches you and you fall down.* New York: Noonday Press.

Giger, J.N., & Davidhizar, R. (2002). Culturally competent care: Emphasis on understanding the people of Afghanistan, Afghanistan Americans, and Islamic culture and religion. *International Nursing Review, 49,* 79–86.

Hall, E.T. (1959). *The silent language.* Garden City, NY: Doubleday.

Hispanic population spreads out. (2002, August 1). *The Fresno Bee,* p. A4.

Holland, L., & Courtney, R. (1998). Increasing cultural competence with the Latino community. *Journal of Community Health Nursing, 15*(1), 45–53.

Kark, S.L. (1974). *Epidemiology and community medicine.* New York: Appleton-Century-Crofts.

Kim, M.J., Cho, H., Cheon-Klessig, Y.S., Gerace, L.M., & Camilleri, D.D. (2002). Primary health care for Korean immigrants: Sustaining a culturally sensitive model. *Public Health Nursing, 19*(3), 191–200.

Kridli, S.A. (2002). Health beliefs and practices among Arab women. *The American Journal of Maternal Child Nursing, 27*(3), 178–182.

Leininger, M. (2001). *Culture, care, diversity, and universality: A theory of nursing.* Boston: Jones & Bartlett.

Levine, R.S., Foster, J.E., Fullilove, R.E., Fullilove, M.T., Briggs,

N.C., Hull, P.C., et al. (2001). Black-White inequalities in mortality and life expectancy, 1933–1999: Implications for *Healthy People 2010*. *Public Health Reports, 116*(5), 474–483.

Lowe, J. (2002). Balance and harmony through connectedness: The intentionality of Native American nurses. *Holistic Nursing Practice, 6*(4), 4–11.

Lowe, J., & Struthers, R. (2001). A conceptual framework of nursing in the Native American culture. *Journal of Nursing Scholarship, 33*(3), 279–283.

McCarty, L.J., Enslein, J.C., Kelley, L.S., Choi, E., & Tripp-Reimer, T. (2002). Cross-cultural health eduction: Materials on the world wide web. *Journal of Transcultural Nursing, 13*(1), 54–60.

Mead, M. (1960). Cultural contexts of nursing problems. In F.C. MacGregor (Ed.), *Social science in nursing*. New York: Wiley.

Milligan, A., Gilroy, J., Katz, K.S., Rodan, M.F., & Subramamian, K.N. (1999). Developing a shared language: Interdisciplinary communication among diverse health care professionals. *Holistic Nursing Practice, 13*(2), 47–53.

Murdock, G. (1972). The science of culture. In M. Freilich (Ed.), *The meaning of culture: A reader in cultural anthropology* (pp. 252–266). Lexington, MA: Xerox College Publishing.

Nakamura, R.M. (1999). *Health in America: A multicultural perspective*. Boston: Allyn & Bacon.

Spector, R.E. (2000). *Cultural diversity in health and illness* (5th ed.). Stamford, CT: Appleton & Lange.

Spradley, J.P. (1979). *The ethnographic interview*. New York: Holt.

Spradley, J.P. (1980). *Participant observation*. New York: Holt.

Spradley, J.P., & McCurdy, D.W. (2000). *Conformity and conflict: Readings in cultural anthropology* (10th ed.). Boston: Allyn & Bacon.

U. S. Bureau of Census. (2001). *The Hispanic population in the United States*. Retrieved November 11, 2003, from *http://www.census.gov*.

U. S. Committee for Refugees (USCR). (2002). *World Refugee Survey 2002: The Americas and the Caribbean*. Washington, DC: Author.

U. S. Department of Commerce. (2001). *Statistical abstract of the United States, 2001* (121st ed.). Washington, DC: Government Printing Office.

U. S. Department of Health and Human Services. (2000). *Healthy people 2010* (Conference ed., Vols. 1 & 2). Washington, DC: Author.

Williams, D.R., & Collins, C. (2001). Racial residential segregation: A fundamental cause of racial disparities in health. *Public Health Reports, 116*(5), 404–416.

Yu, E.S.H., Chen, E.H., Kim, K.K., & Abdulrahim, S. (2002). Smoking among Chinese Americans: Behavior, knowledge, and beliefs. *American Journal of Public Health, 92*(6), 1007–1012.

SELECTED READINGS

Andrews, M.M., & Boyle, J.S. (1999). *Transcultural concepts in nursing care* (3rd ed.). Philadelphia: Lippincott Williams & Wilkins.

Bennett, L. (1962). *Before the Mayflower: A history of the black American, 1619–1962*. Chicago: Johnson.

Brown, S.A., Garcia, A.A., Kouzekanani, K., & Hanis, C.L. (2002). Culturally competent diabetes self-management education for Mexican Americans. *Diabetes Care, 25*(2), 259–268.

Coleman, K.J., & Gonzalez, E.C. (2001). Promoting stair use in a US-Mexico border community. *American Journal of Public Health, 91*(12), 2007–2009.

Engebretson, J. (2001). Alternative and complementary healing: Implications for nursing. In E.C. Hein, *Nursing issues in the 21st century: Perspectives from the literature* (pp. 150–167). Philadelphia: Lippincott Williams & Wilkins.

Foss, G.F. (2001). Maternal sensitivity, posttraumatic stress, and acculturation in Vietnamese and Hmong mothers. *The American Journal of Maternal Child Nursing, 26*(5), 257–263.

Gleeson-Kreig, J., Bernal, H., & Woolley, S. (2002). The role of social support in the self-management of diabetes mellitus among a Hispanic population. *Public Health Nursing, 19*(3), 215–222.

Greenspan, B. (2001). Health disparities and the U. S. health care system. *Public Health Reports, 116*(5), 417–418.

Jacobellis, J., & Cutter, G. (2002). Mammography screening and differences in stage of disease by race/ethnicity. *American Journal of Public Health, 92*(7), 1144–1150.

Johnson, S.K. (2000). Hmong health beliefs and experiences in the Western health care system. *Journal of Transcultural Nursing, 13*(2), 126–132.

Jonas, W.B. (2001). Alternative medicine: Value and risks. In E.C. Hein, *Nursing issues in the 21st century: Perspectives from the literature* (pp.145–149). Philadelphia: Lippincott Williams & Wilkins.

Jones, M.E., Bercier, O., Hayes, A.L., Wentrcek, P., & Bond, M.L. (2002). Family planning patterns and acculturation level of high-risk, pregnant Hispanic women. *Journal of Nursing Care Quality, 16*(4), 46–55.

Kumanyika, S.K., Morssink, C.B., & Nestle, M. (2001). Minority women and advocacy for women's health. *American Journal of Public Health, 91*(9), 1383–1388.

McGrady, G.A., & Pederson, L.L. (2002). Do sex and ethic differences in smoking initiation mask similarities in cessation behavior? *American Journal of Public Health, 92*(6), 961–965.

McLaughlin, D.K., & Stokes, S. (2002). Income inequality and mortality in U. S. counties: Does minority racial concentration matter? *American Journal of Public Health, 92*(1), 99–104.

Navaie-Waliser, M., Feldman, P.H., Gould, D.A., Levine, C., Kuerbis, A.N., & Donelan, K. (2002). The experiences and challenges of informal caregivers: Common themes and differences among Whites, Blacks, and Hispanics. *The Gerontologist, 41*(6), 733–741.

Nichols, F.H. (2000). History of the women's health movement in the 20th century. *JOGNN, 29*(1), 56–64.

Nolt, S. (1992). *A history of the Amish*. Intercourse, PA: Good Books.

Oppenheimer, G.M. (2001). Paradigm lost: Race, ethnicity, and the search for a new population taxonomy. *American Journal of Public Health, 91*(7), 1049–1055.

Pappas, G., Aktar, T., Gergen, P.J., Hadden, W.C., & Khan, A.Q. (2001). Health status of the Pakistani population: A health profile and comparison with the United States. *American Journal of Public Health, 91*(1), 93–98.

Parker, M.W., Bellis, J.M., Bishop, P., Harper, M., Allman, R.M., Moore, C., et al. (2002). A multidisciplinary model of health promotion incorporating spirituality into a successful aging intervention with African American and White elderly groups. *The Gerontologist, 42*(3), 406–415.

Phillips, J., & Grady, P.A. (2002). Reducing health disparities in the twenty-first century: Opportunities for nursing research. *Nursing Outlook, 50*(3), 117–120.

Portillo, C.J., Villarruel, A., Siantz, M.L., Peragallo, N., Calvillo, W.R., & Eribes, C.M. (2001). Research agenda for Hispanics in the United States: A nursing perspective. *Nursing Outlook, 49*(6), 263–269.

Satcher, D. (2000). Eliminating racial and ethnic disparities in health: The role of the ten leading health indicators. *Journal of the National Medical Association, 92*(6), 315–318.

Cross-Cultural Web Sites

AltaVista's Translator—translates any Web page to one of 8 languages: *http://abelfish.altavista.com*

American Diabetes Association, Facts and Figures: *http://www.diabetes.org*

American Immigration Resources on the Internet—general references for immigrants: *http://theodora.com*

Cultural Competence Compendium: *http://www.ama-assn.org*

Culture and Diversity: *http://www.amsa.org*

Ensuring Linguistic Access in Health Care Settings: Legal Rights and Responsibilities: *http://www.kff.org*

Indian Health Service—an agency within U. S. Department of Health and Human Services that provides health services and information about American Indians and Alaska Natives: *http://www.ihs.gov*

Multicultural Health Communication Service. The goal of this Australian site is to provide quality health care information to people of non–English-speaking backgrounds. Information is offered in 36 languages, including Arabic, Chinese, Russian, and Vietnamese: *http://www.mhcs.health.nsw.gov.au/*

The American Academy of Child and Adolescent Psychiatry (AACAP), Facts for Families (available in four languages): *http://www.aacap.org/publications/factsfam/index.htm*

The Association of Asian Pacific Community Health Organizations (AAPCHO). Health education information to improve the health status of Asians and Pacific Islanders in the United States. Available in 12 languages. *http://www.aapcho.org*

5

Values and Ethics in Community Health Nursing

Key Terms

- Autonomy
- Beneficence
- Distributive justice
- Egalitarian justice
- Equity
- Ethical decision-making
- Ethical dilemma
- Ethics
- Fidelity
- Instrumental values
- Justice
- Moral
- Moral evaluations
- Nonmaleficence
- Respect
- Restorative justice
- Self-determination
- Self-interest
- Terminal values
- Value
- Value systems
- Values clarification
- Veracity
- Well-being

Learning Objectives

Upon mastery of this chapter, you should be able to:

- Describe the nature of values and value systems and their influence on community health nursing.
- Identify personal and professional values that you bring to decision-making with and for community health clients.
- Articulate the impact of key values on professional decision-making.
- Discuss the application of ethical principles to community health nursing decision-making.
- Use a decision-making process with and for community health clients that incorporates values and ethical principles.

In the United States, community health nurses face an expanding number of ethical dilemmas every day. Imagine, for example, that you are providing health care to a population of migrant vineyard workers whose housing lacks toilets, heating, and equipment for cooking and refrigerating food. You report the situation to your supervisor, but you are told to ignore the conditions because the wineries that employ the workers contribute heavily to a much-publicized clinic for all of the region's children. What would you do? Or what if you were working in a homeless shelter and were told to evict someone who would not agree to take a tuberculin test? Would your decision change if the resident were elderly or the mother of a newborn?

Within the United States, many marginalized people are failed by the public health care system or go without any health care at all. At the same time, affluent individuals enjoy a wide variety of health care options, including preventive screenings and health promotion classes. Community health nurses often are confronted by this disparity when making ethical decisions about client care.

In addition to these dilemmas within U. S. borders, progress in the United States often is linked to exploitation of people in less-developed countries and contributes to widening disparities in health, wealth, and human rights. Failure to respond to such global challenges only leads to greater poverty and deprivation, continuing conflict, escalating migration, and the spread of infectious disease, all adding to our ethical dilemmas (see The Global Community).

Not only disparity but also advances in technology contribute to ethical dilemmas. For example, computerized record-keeping systems make client information readily accessible, raising issues of confidentiality, clients' rights, and informed consent (Torrance, Lasome, & Agazio, 2002). Technology also forces nurses to confront the issues of human cloning, assisted suicide, and euthanasia (Spears & Warren, 2002). Organ, tissue, and limb transplants and the question of who is to receive them are further ethical questions.

Underlying every issue and influencing every ethical and professional decision are values. Ethics and values are inextricably intertwined in professional decision-making, because values are the criteria by which decisions are made. This chapter explores (1) the nature and function of values and value systems, (2) the role of values and value systems in ethical decision-making, (3) the central values related to health care choices and their potential conflicts, and (4) the implications of values and ethics for community health nursing decision-making and practice.

VALUES

What are values? A **value** is something that is perceived as desirable or "the way things ought to be" (Ellis & Hartley, 2000; Husted & Husted, 2001). A value motivates people to behave in certain ways that are personally or socially preferable. As seen in Chapter 4, a group's culture often is defined by its members' common or shared values.

THE GLOBAL COMMUNITY

The Globalization of Public Health: An Ethical Mandate

Communicable diseases, bioterrorist attacks, and other health care concerns know no national boundaries. Contaminated exported feedstuff transmits bovine spongiform encephalopathy ("mad cow disease") to cattle herds in many European countries; the weakness of national policies and actions for health affect residents in the United States who consume winter fruits and vegetables grown and inspected under questionable conditions in South or Central America in the midst of a political uprising; the sneezing and coughing passenger on an international flight may have some unknown disease, which then is passed to unsuspecting contacts; and suicide bombers attacking buses, shopping areas or buildings with civilians going about their day-to-day business. There is a need for global awareness, analysis, and action of public health authorities to eliminate, interrupt, or contain the potential risks to international public health in the global community.

Nations cannot remain isolated. Efficient information and well-developed surveillance systems must be a top priority. It is imperative for all health professionals and the general public to be informed regularly about the health consequences of globalization in order to keep everyone aware of the transnational dimensions of health.

In this new millennium, the world is increasingly confronted with problems that could affect future generations. The globalization of the dangers and challenges of war, terrorism, and the international marketplace call for addressing international policy issues. It is ethically imperative that policy development move beyond its myopic view and provincialism.

Standards for Behavior

In general, values function as standards that guide actions and behavior in daily situations. Once internalized by an individual, a value such as honesty becomes a criterion for that individual's personal conduct. Values may function as criteria for developing and maintaining attitudes toward objects and situations or for justifying a person's own actions and attitudes. Values also may be the standard by which people pass moral judgments on themselves and others.

Values have a long-term function in giving expression to human needs. The strong motivational component of values helps people to adjust to society, defend egos against threat, and test reality (Thompson, Melia, & Boyd, 2000). In addition, values are used as standards to guide presentation of the self to others, to ascertain personal morality and competency, and to persuade and influence others by indicating which beliefs, attitudes, and actions of others are worth trying to reinforce or change. As a practitioner, values act as a compass to direct the nurse when working with clients.

Qualities of Values

The nature of values can be described according to five qualities: endurance, hierarchical arrangement, prescriptive-proscriptive belief, reference, and preference.

Endurance

Values remain relatively stable over time and persist to provide continuity to personal and social existence. Enduring religious beliefs, for example, offer stability to many people. This is not to say that values are completely stable over time; values do change throughout a person's life. Yet social existence in the community requires standards within the individual as well as an agreement on standards among groups of individuals. As Kluckhohn (1951, p. 400) once pointed out, without values, "the functioning of the social system could not continue to achieve group goals; individuals . . . could not feel within themselves a requisite measure of order and unified purpose." A group's culture, as discussed in the previous chapter, provides such a set of enduring values. By adding an element of collective purpose in social life, values most often guarantee endurance and stability in social existence.

Hierarchical System

Isolated values usually are organized into a hierarchical system in which certain values have more weight or importance than others. For instance, in a team sport such as baseball, values regarding individual performance, batting and running records, speed, and throwing and catching all fall into a hierarchy, with the values of team and winning being at the top. As an individual confronts social situations throughout life, isolated values learned in early childhood come into competition with other values, requiring a weighing of one value against another. Concern for others' welfare, for instance, competes with self-interest. Through experience and maturation, the individual integrates values learned in different contexts into systems in which each value is ordered relative to other values.

Prescriptive-Proscriptive Beliefs

Rokeach (1973) described values as a subcategory of beliefs. He argues that some beliefs are descriptive or capable of being true or false (eg, the chair on which I am sitting will hold me up). Other beliefs are evaluative, involving judgments of good and bad (eg, that was an excellent lecture). Still other beliefs are prescriptive-proscriptive, determining whether an action is desirable or undesirable (eg, this music is too loud, those baseball fans shouldn't yell when the pitcher is winding up). Values, Rokeach says, are prescriptive-proscriptive beliefs. They are concerned with desirable behavior or what ought to be. Parents' values about child behavior, for example, determine how they choose to discipline their children. Values have cognitive, affective, and behavioral components. According to Rokeach, to have a value, it is important

(1) to know the correct way to behave or the correct end state for which to strive (cognitive component); (2) to feel emotional about it—to be affectively for or against it (affective component); and (3) to take action based on it (behavioral component).

Reference

Values also have a reference quality. That is, they may refer to end states of existence called **terminal values**, such as spiritual salvation, peace of mind, or world peace, or they may refer to modes of conduct called **instrumental values**, such as confidentiality, keeping promises, and honesty. The latter can have a moral focus or a nonmoral focus, and these values may conflict. For example, a nurse may experience a conflict between two moral values, such as whether to act honestly (tell a client about a fatal diagnosis) or to act respectfully (honor the family's request not to tell the client). Similarly, the nurse may experience conflict between two nonmoral values, such as whether to plan logically (design a traditional group intervention for mental health clients) or to plan creatively (design an innovative field experience). The nurse also may experience conflict between a nonmoral value and a moral value, such as whether to act efficiently or to act fairly when establishing priorities for funding among community health programs.

Adults generally possess only a few—perhaps no more than 20—terminal values, such as peace of mind or achievement. These are influenced by complex physiologic and social factors. The needs for security, love, self-esteem, and self-actualization, proposed by Maslow (1969), are believed to be the greatest influences on terminal values. Although an individual may have only a few terminal values, the same person may possess as many as 50 to 75 instrumental values. Any single instrumental value, or several instrumental values combined, also may help to determine terminal values. For example, the instrumental values of acceptance, taking it easy, living one day at a time, and not being concerned about the future can shape the terminal value of peace of mind, or the instrumental values of hard work, driving oneself to compete, and not letting anyone get in the way can influence the terminal value of achievement. Figure 5–1 illustrates the influence of instrumental values and human needs on the development of terminal values.

Preference

A value may show preference for one mode of behavior over another, such as exercise over inactivity, or it may show a preference for one end state over another, such as trimness over obesity. The preferred end state, or mode of behavior, is located higher in the personal value hierarchy.

Value Systems

Value systems generally are considered organizations of beliefs that are of relative importance in guiding individual behavior (Rokeach, 1973). Instead of being guided by single or isolated values, however, behavior at any point in time (or

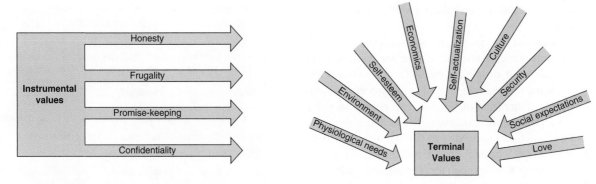

FIGURE 5-1.   Factors influencing personal values.

over a period of time) is influenced by multiple or changing clusters of values. Therefore, it is important to understand how values are integrated into a person's total belief system, how values assume a place in a hierarchy of values, and how this hierarchical system changes over time.

Hierarchical System of Values

Learned values are integrated into an organized system of values, and each value has an ordered priority with respect to other values (Rokeach, 1973). For example, a person may place a higher value on physical comfort than on exercising. This system of ordered priority is stable enough to reflect the continuity of someone's personality and behavior within culture and society, yet it is sufficiently flexible to allow a re-ordering of value priorities in response to changes in the environment or social setting or changes based on personal experiences. Behavioral change would be regarded as the visible response to a reordering of values within an individual's hierarchical value system.

Conflict Between Values in a System

When an individual encounters a social situation, several values within the person's value system are activated, rather than just a single value. Because not all of the activated values are compatible with one another, conflict between values occurs. This conflict between values is a part of the decision-making process, and resolving these value conflicts is crucial to making good decisions. Community health nurses face conflicting values when they seek to promote the well-being of certain individuals, a result that may come at the expense of the public good. Even within a single community agency, nurses may find that they prioritize client service or programming values differently.

Some values seem to consistently triumph over others and seem to be stronger directives for individual behavior; an example is the value placed on high achievement in the United States. It is this persistence on the part of some values (eg, individualism versus community) that makes universal coverage and other issues so controversial in health care reform (Emanuel, 2000). Other values lose their positions of importance in a value hierarchy. It is this changing

arrangement of values in a hierarchical system that determines, in part, how conflicts are resolved and how decisions are made. In this way, people's value systems function as a learned organization of principles and rules that helps them to choose among alternative courses of action to reach decisions.

Values Clarification

One way to understand the influence and priority of values in your own behavior as well as that of community health clients is to use various values-clarification techniques in decision-making. **Values clarification** is a process that helps to identify the personal and professional values that guide your actions by prompting you to examine what you believe about the worth, truth, or beauty of any object, thought, or behavior and where this belief ranks compared with your other values (Catalano, 2000; Thompson, Melia, & Boyd, 2000). Because individuals are largely unaware of the motives underlying their choices, values clarification is important for understanding and shaping the kind of decisions people make. Only by understanding your values and their hierarchy can you ascertain whether your choices are the result of rational thinking or of external influences, such as cultural or social conditioning. Values clarification by itself does not yield a set of rules for future decision-making and does not indicate the rightness or wrongness of alternative actions. It does, however, help to guarantee that any course of action chosen by people is consistent and in accordance with their beliefs and values (Redman, 2001).

Process of Valuing

Before values clarification can take place, it must be understood how the process of valuing occurs in individuals. In 1977, Uustal listed the following seven steps, which remain useful today:

1. Choose the value freely and individually.
2. Choose the value from among alternatives.
3. Carefully consider the consequences of the choice.
4. Cherish or prize the value.
5. Publicly affirm the value.

6. Incorporate the value into behavior so that it becomes a standard.
7. Consciously use the value in decision-making.

These steps provide specific actions for the discovery and identification of people's values. They also assist the decision-making process by explicating the process of valuing itself. For example, some people may choose to value honesty in a presidential candidate. They choose this over other values, such as knowledge of foreign affairs or public-speaking ability, because, considering the consequences, they want a leader who will deliver on promises made, who will be the person represented to the public during campaigning. They prize this value of honesty, affirm it publicly, and consciously use it as a standard when deciding whom to vote into office or reject.

Values-Clarification Strategies

In 1978, Uustal offered several strategies of values clarification that are ultimately useful to the decision-making process in community health nursing practice today. Strategy 1 is a way for nurses to come to know themselves and their values better (Fig. 5–2). Strategy 2 assists in discovering value clusters and the priority of values within personal value systems (Fig. 5–3). Strategy 3 can be used to examine personal responses to selected issues in nursing practice. Each response helps to establish priorities of values by asking the nurse to choose among the alternatives presented or to indicate degree of agreement or disagreement (Fig. 5–4). Other values-clarification strategies are included in the critical thinking activities at the end of this chapter to assist in understanding personal ordering of values and to help when considering directions for change. These strategies also help the nurse to assist community health clients to become clearer about their own values.

All of these strategies can be used to analyze and understand how values are meaningful to people and ultimately influence their choices and behavior. Clarification of a person's

---

Patterns

Which of the following words describe you? Draw a circle around the seven words that best describe you as an individual. Underline the seven words that most accurately describe you as a professional person. (You may circle and underline the same word.)

ambitious   reserved   assertive   opinionated
    concerned   generous   independent
easily hurt   outgoing   reliable   indifferent
    capable   self-controlled   fun-loving
suspicious   solitary   likable   dependent
    intellectual   argumentative   dynamic   unpredictable
compromising   thoughtful   affectionate   obedient
    logical   imaginative   self-disciplined
moody   easily led   helpful   slow to relate

Reflect on the following questions:

1. What values are reflected in the patterns you have chosen?
2. What is the relationship between these patterns and your personal values?
3. What patterns indicate inconsistencies in attitudes or behavior?
4. What patterns do you think a nurse should cultivate?

FIGURE 5–3.   Values clarification strategy 2.

Forced Choice Ranking

How do you order the following alternatives by priority? (There is no correct set of priorities.) What values emerge in response to each question?

1. With whom on a nursing team would you become most angry? The nurse who
    _____ never completes assignments.
    _____ rarely helps other team members.
    _____ projects his or her feelings on clients.

2. If you had a serious health problem, you would rather
    _____ not be told.
    _____ be told directly.
    _____ find out by accident.

3. You are made happiest in your work when you use
    _____ your technical skills in caring for adults with complex needs.
    _____ your ability to compile data and arrive at a nursing diagnosis.
    _____ your ability to communicate easily and skillfully with clients.

4. It would be most difficult for you to
    _____ listen to and counsel a dying person.
    _____ advise a pregnant adolescent.
    _____ handle a situation of obvious child abuse.

FIGURE 5–4.   Values clarification strategy 3.

Name Tag

Take a piece of paper and write your name in the middle of it. In each of the four corners, write your responses to these four questions:

1. What two things would you like your colleagues to say about you?
2. What single most important thing do you do (or would you like to do) to make your nurse-client relationships positive ones?
3. What do you do on a daily basis that indicates you value your health?
4. What are the three values you believe in most strongly?

In the space around your name, write at least six adjectives that you feel best describe who you are.

Take a closer look at your responses to the questions and to the ways in which you described yourself. What values are reflected in your answers?

FIGURE 5–2.   Values clarification strategy 1.

values is the first step in the decision-making process and affects the ability of people to make ethical decisions. Values clarification also promotes understanding and respect for values held by others, such as community health clients and other health care providers. As pointed out by Uustal (1977, p. 10), "Nurses cannot hope to give optimal, sensitive care to any patient without first understanding their own opinions, attitudes, and values." This values-clarification process provides a backdrop for next exploring the role of values in ethical decision-making.

ETHICS

Values are central to any consideration of ethics or ethical decision-making. Yet it is not obvious at first what counts as an ethical problem in health care or in the practice of community health nursing. Most nurses easily recognize the moral crisis in some kinds of decisions—for example, whether to let seriously deformed newborn infants die, whether to terminate pregnancies resulting from rape, or whether to provide universal health care coverage. However, there are other, less obvious moral dilemmas that are faced in the routine practice of community health nursing that often are not considered to be ethical in nature.

What is "ethics" and what is "ethical"? *Webster's American Dictionary* (2000) defines **ethics** as "a system or set of moral principles; the rules of conduct recognized in respect to a particular class of human actions or governing a particular group, culture, etc." Ethics, Catalano explains, "are declarations of what is right or wrong, and of what ought to be"

(2000, p. 113). **Ethical decision-making**, then, means making a choice that is consistent with a moral code or that can be justified from an ethical perspective. Of necessity, the decision-maker must exercise moral judgment. Remember that the term **moral** refers to conforming to a standard that is right and good. Community health nurses become "moral agents" by making decisions that have direct and indirect consequences for the welfare of themselves and others. The next section examines how a nurse makes these moral decisions.

Identifying Ethical Situations

Ethics involves making evaluative judgments. To be ethically responsible in the practice of nursing, it is important to develop the ability to recognize evaluative judgments as they are made and implemented in nursing practice. Nurses must be able to distinguish between evaluative and nonevaluative judgments. Evaluative statements involve judgments of value, rights, duties, and responsibilities. Examples are, "Parents should never strike their children," and "It is the duty of every citizen to vote." Among the words to watch for are verbs such as *want, desire, refer, should,* or *ought* and nouns such as *benefit, harm, duty, responsibility, right,* or *obligation.*

Sometimes, the evaluations are expressed in terms that are not direct expressions of evaluations but clearly are functioning as value judgments. For example, the American Nurses Association (ANA) *Code for Nurses with Interpretive Statements* (2001), in its nine statements, has several that actually refer to "the nurse's obligation" or "owing the same duties to self as to others" and "nursing values" (see Code of Ethics for Nurses—Provisions).

Code of Ethics for Nurses—Provisions, Approved as of June 30, 2001

1. The nurse, in all professional relationships, practices with compassion and respect for the inherent dignity, worth, and uniqueness of every individual, unrestricted by considerations of social or economic status, personal attributes, or the nature of health problems.
2. The nurse's primary commitment is to the patient, whether an individual, family, group, or community.
3. The nurse promotes, advocates for, and strives to protect the health, safety, and rights of the patient.
4. The nurse is responsible and accountable for individual nursing practice and determines the appropriate delegation of tasks consistent with the nurse's obligation to provide optimum patient care.
5. The nurse owes the same duties to self as to others, including the responsibility to preserve integrity and safety, to maintain competence, and to continue personal and professional growth.

6. The nurse participates in establishing, maintaining, and improving health care environments and conditions of employment conducive to the provision of quality health care and consistent with the values of the profession through individual and collective action.
7. The nurse participates in the advancement of the profession through contributions to practice, education, administration, and knowledge development.
8. The nurse collaborates with other health professionals and the public in promoting community, national, and international efforts to meet health needs.
9. The profession of nursing, as represented by associations and their members, is responsible for articulating nursing values, for maintaining the integrity of the profession and its practice, and for shaping social policy.

From American Nurses Association. (2001). *Code of ethics for nurses with interpretive statements.* Washington, DC American Nurses Publishing, with permission.

Another important step is to distinguish between moral and nonmoral evaluations. **Moral evaluations** refer to judgments that conform to standards of what is right and good. Moral evaluations assess human actions, institutions, or character traits rather than inanimate objects such as paintings or architectural structures. They are prescriptive-proscriptive beliefs having certain characteristics that separate them from other evaluations such as aesthetic judgments, personal preferences, or matters of taste. Moral evaluations also have distinctive characteristics (Thompson, Melia, & Boyd, 2000):

1. The evaluations are ultimate. They have a preemptive quality, meaning that other values or human ends cannot, as a rule, override them.
2. They possess universality or reflect a standpoint that applies to everyone. They are evaluations that everyone in principle ought to be able to make and understand, even if some individuals, in fact, do not.
3. Moral evaluations avoid giving a special place to a person's own welfare. They have a focus that keeps others in view, or at least considers one's own welfare on a par with that of others.

Resolving Moral Conflicts and Ethical Dilemmas

When judgments involve moral values, conflicts are inevitable. In clinical practice, the nurse may be faced with moral conflicts such as the choice between preserving the welfare of one set of clients over that of others. For example, the nurse may have to choose whether to keep a promise of confidentiality to persons who are infected by the human immunodeficiency virus (HIV) when these individuals continue to have unprotected sex with unknowing partners. Nurses may have to choose between protecting the interests of colleagues or the interests of the employing institution. They may have to decide whether to serve future clients by striking for better conditions or to serve present clients by refusing to strike. Each decision involves a potential conflict between moral values and is called an **ethical dilemma**. An ethical dilemma occurs when morals conflict with one another, causing the nurse to face a choice with equally attractive or equally undesirable alternatives (Thompson, Melia, & Boyd, 2000). It can create a decision-making problem, even in ordinary nursing situations.

Decision-Making Frameworks

To resolve ethical dilemmas or the conflict between moral values in community health nursing practice, and to provide morally accountable nursing service, several frameworks for ethical decision-making have been proposed. Among these frameworks, three key steps are considered as fundamental to choosing alternative courses of action that reflect moral reasoning: (1) separate questions of fact from questions of value, (2) identify both clients' and nurse's value systems, and (3) consider ethical principles and concept.

The identification of clients' values and those of other persons involved in conflict situations is an important part of ethical decision-making. In the example given in Clinical Corner I, what are Mr. Bell's values? What are the values of neighbors who are concerned but feel that they can no longer care for him? What are the nurse's values? What are the values of the nurse's employing agency?

CLINICAL CORNER I

MR. BELL

Community health nurses encounter value differences every day, and value differences, in turn, create ethical problems. Consider, for example, the dilemma faced by one nurse in Seattle on her first home visit to an elderly man, Mr. Bell. Referred by concerned neighbors, this 82-year-old gentleman was homebound and living alone with severe arthritis under steadily deteriorating conditions. Overgrown shrubs and vines covered the yard and house, making access impossible except through the back door. A wood-burning stove in the kitchen was the sole source of heat, and that room, plus a corner of the dining room, were Mr. Bell's living quarters. The remainder of the once-lovely three-bedroom home, including the bathroom, was layered with dust, unused. His bed was a cot in the dining room; his toilet, a two-pound coffee can placed under the cot. Unbathed, unshaven, and existing on food and firewood brought by neighbors, Mr. Bell seemed to be living in deplorable conditions. Yet he prized his independence so highly that he adamantly refused to leave.

The conflict of values between Mr. Bell's choice to live independently and the nurse's value of having him in a safer living situation raises several ethical questions. When do health practitioners or family members have the right or duty to override an individual's preferences? When do neighbors' rights (Mr. Bell's home was an eyesore and his care was a source of anxiety for his neighbors) supersede one homeowner's rights? Should the nurse be responsible when family members can help but won't take action? Mr. Bell had one son living in a neighboring state.

In this case, the nurse entering Mr. Bell's home applied her values of respect for the individual and his right to autonomy even at the risk of public safety. Not until he fell and broke a hip did he reluctantly agree to be moved into a nursing home.

DISPLAY 5-1

A Framework for Ethical Decision-Making

1. *Clarify the ethical dilemma:* Whose problem is it? Who should make the decision? Who is affected by the decision? What ethical principles are related to the problem?
2. *Gather additional data:* Have as much information about the situation as possible. Be up to date on any legal cases related to the ethical question.
3. *Identify options:* Brainstorm with others to identify as many alternatives as possible. The more options identified, the more likely it is that an acceptable solution will be found.
4. *Make a decision:* Choose from the options identified and determine the most acceptable option, the one more feasible than others.
5. *Act:* Carry out the decision. It may be necessary to collaborate with others to implement the decision and identify options.
6. *Evaluate:* After acting on a decision, evaluate its impact. Was the best course of action chosen? Would an alternative have been better? Why? What went right and what went wrong? Why?

An ethical decision-making framework that is referred to as the DECIDE model is a practical method of making prudent value judgments and ethical decisions (Thompson, Melia, & Boyd, 2000). It includes the following steps:

D—*Define the problem (or problems):* What are the key facts of the situation? Who is involved? What are their rights and duties and your rights and duties?

E—*Ethical review:* What ethical principles have a bearing on the situation, and which principle or principles should be given priority in making a decision?

C—*Consider the options:* What options do you have in the situation? What alternative courses of action exist? What help, means, and methods do you need to use?

I—*Investigate outcomes:* Given each available option, what consequences are likely to follow from each course of action open to you? Which is the most ethical thing to do?

D—*Decide on action:* Having chosen the best available option, determine a specific action plan, set clear objectives, and then act decisively and effectively.

E—*Evaluate results:* Having initiated a course of action, assess how things progress, and when concluded, evaluate carefully whether or not you achieved your goals.

Other frameworks can be used. The framework for ethical decision-making shown in Display 5–1 helps to organize thoughts and acts as a guide through the decision-making process. The steps help to determine a course of action, with heavy responsibility at the evaluation level: here the outcomes need to be judged and decisions repeated or rejected in future situations. Figure 5–5 summarizes several views in the field on ethical decision-making. This framework advocates keeping multiple values in tension before resolution of conflict and action on the part of the nurse. It suggests that value conflict is not capable of resolution until all possible alternative actions have been explored. Final resolution of the ethical conflict occurs through conscious choice of action even though some values would be overridden by other stronger, presumably moral values. The triumphant values would be those values located higher in the decision-maker's hierarchy of values.

Basic Values That Guide Decision-Making

When applying a decision-making framework, certain values influence community health nursing decisions. Three basic human values are considered key to guiding decision-making in the provider–client relationship: self-determination, well-being, and equity.

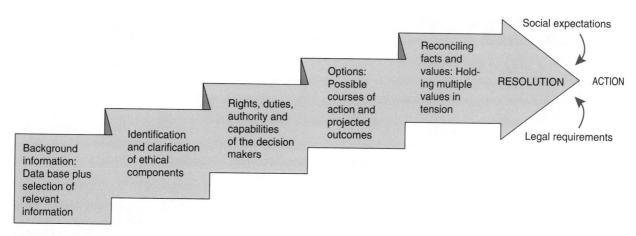

FIGURE 5–5. An ethical decision-making framework. Although legal requirements or social expectations may sway a decision one way or another, they are extrinsic to the ethical analysis and should not be confused with right and wrong. What is legal and what is expected are not necessarily right and wrong.

Self-Determination

The value of **self-determination** or individual autonomy is a person's exercise of the capacity to shape and pursue personal plans for life. Self-determination is instrumentally valued because self-judgment about a person's goals and choices is conducive to an individual's sense of well-being. Respecting self-determination is based on the belief that better outcomes will result when self-determination is respected. The outcomes that could be maximized by respecting self-determination include enhanced self-concept, enhanced health-promoting behaviors, and enhanced quality of care. Self-determination is a major value in the United States but does not receive the same emphasis in all societies or ethnic groups.

In health care contexts, the desire for self-determination has been of such high ethical importance in U. S. society that it overrides practitioner determinations in many situations. Client empowerment is an approach that differs from the paternalistic approach to health care in which decisions are made for, rather than with, the client; instead, it enables patients and professionals to work in partnerships (Williams, 2002). Many physicians and other health providers, including community health nurses, fail to recognize the high value attributed to self-determination by many consumers or the differences in views of self-determination among ethnic groups.

The conflict between provider and consumer may be broader. When self-determination deteriorates into self-interest, it poses a major road block to equitable health care. **Self-interest** is the fulfillment of one's own desires without regard for the greater good. Consumers mostly have to fend for themselves when they encounter the world of for-profit health care, just as they do in other commercial markets, where "buyer beware" is the standard (Drevdahl, 2002; Williams, 2002).

Self-determination and taking personal responsibility for health care decisions should be nourished when providing health care. This includes informing clients of options and the reasoning behind all recommendations. Yet self-determination and personal autonomy at times are impermissible or even impossible. For example, society must impose restrictions on unacceptable client choices, such as child abuse and other abusive behaviors, or situations in which clients are not competent to exercise self-determination, as is true for certain levels of mental illness or dementia. There are two situations in which self-determination should be restricted: (1) when some objectives of individuals are contrary to the public interest or the interests of others in society, and (2) when a person's decision-making is so defective or mistaken that the decision fails to promote the person's own values or goals. In these situations, self-determination is justifiably overridden on the basis of the promotion of one's own well-being or the well-being of others, another important value in health care decision-making.

Well-Being

Well-being is a state of positive health. Although all therapeutic interventions by health care professionals are intended to improve clients' health and promote well-being, well-intended interventions sometimes fall short if they are in conflict with clients' preferences and needs. Determining what constitutes health for people and how their well-being can be promoted often requires a knowledge of clients' subjective preferences. It is generally recognized that clients may be inclined to pursue different directions in treatment procedures based on individual goals, values, and interests. Community health nurses, who are committed not only to helping clients but also to respecting their wishes and avoiding harming them, must understand each client group's needs and develop reasonable alternatives for service from which clients may choose (see Clinical Corner II). In addition, when individuals are not capable of making a choice, the nurse or other surrogate decision-maker is obliged to make health care decisions that promote the value of well-being. This may mean

---

CLINICAL CORNER II

A FAMILY LIVING IN POVERTY

Contrasting value systems may be seen in many community health practice settings. Andrea Varga, a community health nurse, experienced such a contrast on her first home visit to a family living in poverty. Referred by a school nurse for recurring problems with head lice and staphylococcal infections, the family was living in the worst conditions that the nurse had ever seen. Papers, moldy food, soiled clothing, and empty beer cans covered the floor. Andrea recoiled in dismay. The children, home from school, were clustered around the television. Their mother, a divorced, single parent, unkempt and obese, sat smoking a cigarette with a can of beer in her hand. Although she worked as a waitress part time, she had been unable to earn enough money to support herself and the children, so the family was now temporarily receiving state aid. The mother's main pleasure in life was watching soap operas on television. The nurse interpreted the situation through the framework of her own value system in which health and cleanliness were priorities. Yet the mother, who might have shared those values in the past, appeared to prize freedom and pleasurable diversion, perhaps as a way to cope with her situation. In this instance, it is possible that environmental influences reordered the family's value-system priorities. Rather than imposing her own values, Andrea chose to determine the priorities of the family, assessed their needs, and began where they were.

that the alternatives presented by the nurse for choice are only the alternatives that will promote well-being. With shared decision-making, the nurse not only seeks to understand clients' needs and develop reasonable alternatives to meet those needs, but also to present the alternatives in a way that enables clients to choose those they prefer. Well-being and self-determination are two values that are intricately related when providing community health nursing service.

Equity

The third value that is important to decision-making in health care contexts is the value of **equity**, which means being treated equally or fairly. The principle of equity implies that it is unjust (or inequitable) to treat people the same if they are, in significant respects, unlike. In other words, different people have different needs in health care, but all must be served equally and adequately. Equity generally means that all individuals should have the same access to health care according to benefit or needs (see Levels of Prevention Matrix).

The major problem with this definition of equity, of course, is that it assumes that an adequate level of health care can be economically available to all citizens. In times of lim-

ited technical, human, and financial resources, however, it may be impossible to fully respect the value of equity (Drevdahl, 2002; Ross, 2000). Choices must be made and resources allotted while the value obligations of professional practice create conflicts of values that seem impossible to resolve. Many of these conflicts are reflected in current health care reform efforts that focus on access to services, quality of services, and ways to control rising costs. However, the following list represents the most pressing aggregate health problems related to inequities in the distribution of and access to health and illness care facing our nation:

Too many women go without preventive care. The overall rate of infant mortality (all infant deaths before 1 year of age, per 1000 births) in the United States remains among the highest in the industrialized world (U.S. Department of Health and Human Services [USDHHS], 2000). The rates for some people of color—African-Americans (13.7), Native Hawaiian and other Pacific Islanders (7.9), and Native Americans (8.7) specifically—are higher than those for European-Americans (6.0) or Hispanic-Americans (6.0) (USDHHS, 2000). Forty percent of the pregnancies among White and Hispanic females are unintended, as are 70% of

---

LEVELS OF PREVENTION MATRIX

SITUATION: Provide distributive justice for battered women and children by changing a proposed state law that would eliminate funding for shelters for battered women and children to a law that preserves resources for this population.

GOAL: Using the three levels of prevention, negative health conditions are avoided, or promptly diagnosed and treated, and the fullest possible potential is restored.

PRIMARY PREVENTION		SECONDARY PREVENTION		TERTIARY PREVENTION		
Health Promotion and Education	*Health Protection*	*Early Diagnosis*	*Prompt Treatment*	*Rehabilitation*	*Primary Prevention*	
					Health Promotion and Education	*Health Protection*
Advocacy Active lobbying against the bill Garnering community support in favor of the revised bill		Recognition that the proposed bill is going to pass	Advocate for amendments to the proposed bill to preserve limited funding for shelters	(If unable to stop the proposed law:) Seek volunteer services to fill the gaps in funding paid employees Seek donations to support existing shelter buildings	Educate the public regarding the need for lost/limited services using various forms of media and/or venues	Seek private resources to fund shelters Propose a new bill to match private funding for shelters at the next legislative session

the pregnancies among African-American females. Poverty is strongly related to difficulty in accessing family planning services.

Immunization rates for some diseases are at dangerously low levels. For example, only 43% of children between the ages of 19 and 35 months were immunized for varicella (chickenpox) in 1998 (USDHHS, 2000).

The uninsured are likely to go without physician care. Differences in access to expensive, discretionary procedures emerge according to health insurance status, race, and other sociodemographic factors of the client. The poor are only two thirds as likely as others to obtain needed services.

Evidence of excess mortality rates for fetuses and perinatal infants continues among members of certain races. African-Americans experience a rate of 12.5 and 13.4 fetal and perinatal deaths, respectively, per 1000 births. The rates are lower and very similar for White and Hispanic fetuses (5.8 and 5.9) and perinatal infants (6.4 and 6.5). Asian-Americans experience even lower rates, 4.8 and 4.6 (USDHHS, 2000).

Social Security, without supplements, limits access. The elderly find themselves paying higher out-of-pocket costs and higher insurance premiums, often with forced choices. Prescription drug coverage and provisions for long-term care are not available for most, and basic entitlements continue to be reduced.

Environmental hazards threaten global health. Global trade, travel, and changing social and cultural patterns make the population vulnerable to diseases that are endemic to other parts of the world as well as to previously unknown diseases. Pollution of air, water, and soil to support industry contributes to pathogen mutations and threatens public health.

International terrorism and fear of terrorist attacks affects people in all countries. This "newest" hazard to the well-being of nations has taken many governments and populations by surprise. It has them responding with mixed feelings of anger and fear along with a level of unpreparedness in the decision-making needed for appropriate responses.

To promote the achievement of equity, self-determination, and clients' well-being, certain conclusions drawn from the literature can enhance community health nursing practice (Catalano, 2000; Des Jardin, 2001):

1. Society has an ethical obligation to ensure equitable access to health care for all. This obligation rests on the special importance of health care and is derived from its role in relieving suffering, preventing premature death, restoring functioning, increasing opportunity, providing information about an individual's condition, and giving evidence of mutual empathy and compassion.

2. The societal obligation is balanced by individual obligations. Individuals ought to pay a fair share of the cost of their own health care and take reasonable steps to provide for such care when they can do so without excessive burdens.

3. Equitable access to health care requires that all citizens can secure an adequate level of care without excessive burdens. Equitable access also means that the burdens borne by individuals in obtaining adequate care ought not to be excessive or to fall disproportionately on particular individuals. Communities need to be empowered to address distribution problems.

4. When equity occurs through the operation of private forces, there is no need for government involvement. However, the ultimate responsibility for ensuring that society's obligation is met—through a combination of public and private sector arrangements—rests with the federal government.

5. The cost of achieving equitable access to health care ought to be shared fairly. The cost of securing health care for those who are unable to pay ought to be spread equitably at the national level and should not fall more heavily on the shoulders of particular practitioners, institutions, or residents of different localities.

6. Efforts to contain rising health care costs are important but should not focus on limiting the attainment of equitable access for the least-served portion of the public. Measures designed to contain health care costs that exacerbate existing inequities or impede the achievement of equity are unacceptable from a moral standpoint. Aggregates in the community should be involved in planning and problem-solving to increase the distribution of resources where those resources are most needed.

Ethical Decision-Making in Community Health Nursing

The key values described in this chapter of self-determination, well-being, and equity influence nursing practice in many ways. The value of self-determination has implications for how community health nurses

- Respect the choices of clients
- Protect privacy
- Provide for informed consent
- Protect diminished capacity for self-determination

The value of well-being has implications for how community health nurses

- Reduce or prevent harm and provide benefits to client populations
- Measure the effectiveness of nursing services
- Balance costs of services against real client benefits

The value of equity has implications for community health nursing in terms of its priorities for

- Broadly distributing health goods (macroallocation issues)
- Deciding which populations will obtain available health goods and services (microallocation issues)

Decisions based on one value mean that this value often will conflict with other values. For example, deciding primarily on the basis of client well-being may conflict with deciding on the basis of self-determination or equity. How community health nurses balance these values may even conflict with their own personal values or the values of the

VOICES FROM THE COMMUNITY

Four community health nurses describe some ethical issues or dilemmas they have encountered in the community (Oberle & Tenove, 2000):

1. "With health care so political as it is right now, . . . every sort of little agency or sometimes even programs within an agency are . . . wanting to get all the glory or credit and forgetting about the client, . . . losing sight of what we're doing."

2. "Where my [problem] comes in is there just isn't enough of me to do the kind of job to meet the need that's there, and, you know, at what point do you draw the line and say 'I have to stop here, I can't do any more.' "

3. "Our clients see us as a helper, but that in a way makes us more likely to be caught into . . . ethical issues, because we're like a confidante: they sometimes tell us things that they wouldn't tell other people. So that means that we're always wrestling with that whole idea of 'Now whose rights are highest here? Gee, a doctor should know this' — but on the other hand, they'd asked me not to tell."

4. "It's their right to choose [but] there is a great deal of language barriers and . . . I don't really think they understand what it is that the risks are. . . . They are smiling and say, 'Yes, yes, yes,' and you know they're not [understanding], and you go ahead and do the vaccination."

nursing profession. In these situations, values-clarification techniques used with an ethical decision-making process may assist in making decisions that promote the greatest well-being for clients without substantially reducing their self-determination or ignoring equity (see Voices from the Community).

Ethical Principles

Seven fundamental ethical principles provide guidance in making decisions regarding clients' care: respect, autonomy, beneficence, nonmaleficence, justice, veracity, and fidelity (Husted & Husted, 2001; Thompson, Melia, & Boyd, 2000).

Respect

The principle of **respect** refers to treating people as unique, equal, and responsible moral agents. This principle emphasizes people's importance as members of the community and of the health services team. To apply this principle in decision-making is to acknowledge community clients as valued participants in shaping their own and the community's health outcomes. It includes treating them as equals on the health team and holding them and their views in high regard.

Autonomy

The principle of **autonomy** means freedom of choice and the exercise of people's rights. Individualism and self-determination are dominant values underlying this principle. As nurses apply this principle in community health, they promote individuals' and groups' rights to and involvement in decision-making. This is true, however, only so long as those decisions enhance these people's well-being and do not harm the well-being of others (Catalano, 2000). When applying this principle, nurses should make certain that clients are fully informed and that the decisions are made deliberately, with careful consideration of the consequences.

Beneficence

The ethical principle of **beneficence** means doing good or benefiting others. It is the promotion of good or taking action to ensure positive outcomes on behalf of clients. In community health, the nurse applies the principle of beneficence by making decisions that actively promote community clients' best interests and well-being. Examples are developing a seniors' health program that ensures equal access to all in the community who need it and supporting programs to encourage preschool immunizations.

Nonmaleficence

The principle of **nonmaleficence** means avoiding or preventing harm to others as a consequence of a person's own choices and actions. This involves taking steps to avoid negative consequences. Community health nurses can apply this ethical principle in decision-making by actions such as encouraging physicians to prescribe drugs with the fewest side effects, promoting legislation to protect the environment from pollutants emitted from gasoline even if it raises prices, and lobbying for lower speed limits or gun controls to save lives.

Justice

The principle of **justice** refers to treating people fairly. It means the fair distribution of both benefits and costs among society's members. Decisions about equal access to health care, equitable distribution of services to rural as well as urban populations, not limiting amount or quality of service because of income level, and fair distribution of resources all draw on the principle of justice.

Within this principle are three different views on allocation, or what constitutes the meaning of "fair" distribution. One, **distributive justice**, says that benefits should be given first to the disadvantaged or those who need them most (see Levels of Prevention Matrix). Decisions based on this view particularly help the needy, although it may mean withholding good from others who also are deserving but less in need. The second view, **egalitarian justice**, promotes decisions based on equal distribution of benefits to everyone, regardless of need. The third, **restorative justice**, says that benefits should go primarily to those who have been wronged by prior injustice, such as victims of crime or racial discrimination. Programs are in place to compensate victims for their injury or families for their loss—a beginning to restore justice. Another example is the funds that were set up by several agencies, corporations, and groups to assist the families of victims of the September 11, 2001, terrorist attacks. The principle of justice seeks to promote equity, a value that was discussed in the previous section.

Veracity

The principle of **veracity** refers to telling the truth. Community clients deserve to be given accurate information in a timely manner. To withhold information or not tell the truth can be self-serving to the nurse or other health care provider and hurtful as well as disrespectful to clients. Truth-telling treats clients as equals, expands the opportunity for greater client involvement, and provides needed information for decision-making (Catalano, 2000).

Fidelity

The final ethical principle, **fidelity**, means keeping promises. People deserve to count on commitments being met. This principle involves the issues of trust and trustworthiness. Nurses who follow through on what they have said earn their clients' respect and trust. In turn, this influences the quality of the nurse's relationship with clients, who then are more likely to share information, leading to improved decisions. Conversely, when a promise (eg, a commitment to institute child care during health classes) is not kept, community members may lose faith and interest in participation.

Ethical Standards and Guidelines

As the number and complexity of ethical decisions in community health increase, so too does the need for ethical standards and guidelines to help nurses make the best choices possible. The ANA's *Code for Nurses with Interpretive Statements* (2001) provides a helpful guide. Some health care organizations and community agencies, using the ANA code or a similar document, have developed their own specific standards and guidelines.

More health care organizations are using ethics committees or ethics rounds to deal with ethical aspects of client services (Holstein & Mitzen, 2002). These committees are common in the acute care setting and in senior and long-term care settings and focus on such issues as caregiving dilemmas that may involve practitioner negligence or poor client outcomes and the related health care decisions. However, these committees also function in a variety of community health care settings. In long-term care and home care settings, such a committee may consider conflicts in client care issues that involve family members. In public health agencies, clients with complicated communicable disease diagnoses and health care provider concerns are discussed as they relate to policy, protocols, and the health and safety of the broader population.

SUMMARY

Values and ethical principles have significance for our global community as well as our local community. They strongly influence community health nursing practice and ethical decision-making. Values are lasting beliefs that are important to individuals, groups, and cultures. A value system organizes these beliefs into a hierarchy of relative importance that motivates and guides human behavior. Values function as standards for behavior, as criteria for attitudes, and as standards for moral judgments, and they give expression to human needs. The nature of values can be understood by examining their qualities of endurance, their hierarchical arrangement, and their function as prescriptive-proscriptive beliefs and by examining them in terms of reference and preference.

The nurse often is faced with decisions that affect client's values and involve conflicting moral values and ethical dilemmas. Understanding what personal values are and how they affect behavior assists the nurse in making ethical evaluations and addressing ethical conflicts in practice. Various strategies can guide the nurse in making these decisions; one example is values clarification, which clarifies what values are important. Several frameworks for ethical decision-making that include the identification and clarification of values impinging on the making of ethical decisions were discussed in this chapter.

Three key human values influence client health and nurse decision-making: the right to make decisions regarding a person's health (self-determination), the right to health and well-being, and the right to equal access and quality of health care. At times, these values are affected by the value of self-interest on the part of another person or a system. Seven fundamental principles guide community health nurses in making ethical decisions: respect, autonomy, beneficence, nonmaleficence, justice, veracity, and fidelity.

ACTIVITIES TO PROMOTE CRITICAL THINKING

1. Describe where you stand on the following issues. For each statement, decide whether you strongly agree, agree, disagree, strongly disagree, or are undecided.
   a. Clients have the right to participate in all decisions related to their health care.
   b. Nurses need a system designed to credit self-study.
   c. Continuing education should not be mandatory to maintain licensure.
   d. Clients always should be told the truth.
   e. Standards of nursing practice should be enforced by state examining boards.
   f. Nurses should be required to take relicensure examinations every 5 years.
   g. Clients should be allowed to read their health record on request.
   h. Abortion on demand should be an option available to every woman.
   i. Critically ill newborns should be allowed to die.
   j. Laws should guarantee desired health care for each person in this country.
   k. Organ donorship should be automatic unless a waiver to refuse has been signed.

2. In a grid similar to the one shown, write a statement of belief in the space provided and examine it in relation to the seven steps of the process of valuing. Areas of confusion and conflict in nursing practice that should be examined are peer review, accountability, confidentiality, euthanasia, licensure, clients' rights, organ donation, abortion, informed consent, and terminating treatment. To the right of your statements, check the appropriate boxes to indicate when your beliefs reflect one or more of the seven steps in the valuing process. Is your belief a value according to the valuing process?

3. Rank in order the following 12 potential nursing actions, using "1" to indicate the most important choice in a client–community health nurse relationship and "12" to indicate the least important choice.

Touching clients
Empathetically listening to clients
Disclosing yourself to clients
Becoming emotionally involved with clients
Teaching clients
Being honest in answering clients' questions
Seeing that clients conform to professionals' advice
Helping to decrease clients' anxiety
Making sure that clients are involved in decision-making
Following legal mandates regarding health practices
Remaining "professional" with clients
(Add an alternative of your own)
Examine your ordering of these options. What values can be identified based on your responses in this exercise? How do these values emerge in your behavior?

4. Request to attend two or three sessions of an ethics committee meeting of a community health agency. Observe and make notes on (a) what values are evident in the discussion, (b) what ethical principles are used, (c) what decision-making framework is used, and (d) what you would have liked to contribute if you had been a member of the committee.

5. Search the World Wide Web on the Internet for activities in your state legislature or the national legislature on bills that might affect the health and well-being of clients. How do you feel about the pieces of legislation? What could a community health nurse do regarding the impending legislation? What could you do right now?

Statement	Freely chosen	Alternatives	Consequences	Cherished	Affirmed	Incorporated	Employed
	1	2	3	4	5	6	7

REFERENCES

American Nurses Association. (2001). *Code for nurses with interpretive statements*. Washington, DC: Author.

Catalano, J.T. (2000). *Nursing now! Today's issues, tomorrow's trends* (2nd ed.). Philadelphia: F.A. Davis.

Des Jardin, K. (2001). Political involvement in nursing: Politics, ethics, and strategic action. *AORN Journal, 74*(5), 614–626.

Drevdahl, D. (2002). Social justice or market justice? The paradoxes of public health partnerships with managed care. *Public Health Nursing, 19*(3), 161–169.

Ellis, J.R., & Hartley, C.L. (2000). *Nursing in today's world: Challenges, issues, and trends* (7th ed.). Philadelphia: Lippincott Williams & Wilkins.

Emanuel, E.J. (2000). Justice and managed care: Four principles for the just allocation of health care. *Hastings Center Report, 30*(3), 8–16.

Holstein, M.B., & Mitzen, P. (2002). *Ethics in community-based elder care*. New York: Springer.

Husted, G.L., & Husted, J.H. (2001). *Ethical decision making in nursing and healthcare* (3rd ed.). New York: Springer.

Kluckhohn, C. (1951). Values and value-orientations in the theory of action: An exploration in definition and classification. In T. Parsons & E.A. Shils (Eds.), *Toward a general theory of action* (pp. 388–433). Cambridge, MA: Harvard University Press.

Maslow, A. (1969). *Toward a psychology of being* (2nd ed.). New York: Van Nostrand.

Oberle, K. & Tenove, S. (2000). Ethical issues in public health nursing. *Nursing Ethics, 7*(5), 425–437.

Redman, B.K. (2001). *Measurement tools in clinical ethics*. Thousand Oaks, CA: Sage.

Rokeach, M. (1973). *The nature of human values*. New York: Free Press.

Ross, E.C. (2000). Will managed care ever deliver on its promises? Managed care, public policy, and consumers of mental health services. *Administration and Policy in Mental Health, 28*(1), 7–22.

Spears, V.H., & Warren, J. (2002, August 7). U.S. pair to try cloning [*Lexington Herald-Leader*]. *The Fresno Bee*, A5.

Thompson, I.E., Melia, K.M., & Boyd, K.M. (2000). *Nursing ethics* (4th ed.). Edinburgh: Churchill Livingstone.

Torrance, R.J., Lasome, C.E.M., & Agazio, J.B. (2002). Ethics and computer-mediated communication: Implications for practice and policy. *JONA: The Jounal of Nursing Administration, 32*(6), 346–353.

U.S. Department of Health and Human Services. (2000). *Healthy people 2010* (Cconference ed., Vols. 1 & 2). Washington, DC: Author.

Uustal, D.B. (1977). The use of values clarification in nursing practice. *Journal of Continuing Education in Nursing, 8*, 8–13.

Uustal, D.B. (1978). Values clarification in nursing. *American Journal of Nursing, 78*, 2058–2063.

Webster's American dictionary (College ed., 2000). New York: Random House.

Williams, T. (2002). Patient empowerment and ethical decision making. *Dimensions of Critical Care Nursing, 21*(3), 100–104.

SELECTED READINGS

Bandman, E., & Bandman, B. (2002). *Nursing ethics through the life span*. Upper Saddle River, NJ: Prentice-Hall Health.

Beauchamp, D.E. (1976). Public health as social justice. *Inquiry, 13*, 3–14.

Callahan, D., & Jennings, B. (2002). Ethics and public health: Forging a strong relationship. *American Journal of Public Health, 92*(2), 169–176.

Couto, R.A. (2000). Community health as social justice: Lessons on leadership. *Family and Community Health, 23*(1), 1–17.

Daly, B.J. (2002). Moving forward: A new code of ethics. *Nursing Outlook, 50*(3), 97–99.

Guido, G.W. (2001). *Legal and ethical issues in nursing* (3rd ed.). Upper Saddle River, NJ: Prentice-Hall Health.

Iyer, P.W. (2003). *Legal nurse consulting: Principles and practice* (2nd ed.). Boca Raton, FL: CRC Press.

Kaler, M.M., & Ravella, P.C. (2000). Staying on the ethical high ground with complementary and alternative medicine. *The Nurse Practitioner, 27*(7), 38–42.

Kapp, M.B. (2001). *Ethics, law, and aging review. Vol. 7: Liability issues and risk management in caring for older persons*. New York: Springer.

Kapp, M.B. (2002). *Ethics, law, and aging review. Vol. 8: Conducting research with and about older persons: Ethical and legal issues and implications*. New York: Springer.

Kass, N.E. (2001). An ethics framework for public health. *American Journal of Public Health, 91*(11), 1776–1782.

Pies, C., & Samuels, S. (1999). *Using incentives in reproductive health programs: An ethical framework*. Berkeley: University of California Berkeley, School of Public Health.

Porter-O'Grady, T. (1999). *Leading the revolution in healthcare: Igniting performance, advancing systems*. Rockville, MD: Aspen.

Roberts, M.J., & Reich, M.R. (2002). Ethical analysis in public health. *Lancet, 359*, 1055–1059.

Rodriguez-Garcia, R., & Akhter, M.N. (2000). Human rights: The foundation of public health practice. *American Journal of Public Health, 90*(5), 693–694.

Thomas, J.C., Sage, M., Dillenberg, J., & Guillory, V.J. (2002). A code of ethics for public health. *American Journal of Public Health, 92*(7), 1057–1059.

Volbrecht, R.M. (2002). *Nursing ethics: Communities in dialogue*. Upper Saddle River, NJ: Prentice-Hall Health.

Internet Resources

American Nurses Association: *http://www.ana.org*

Healthy People 2010: *http://www.health.gov/healthypeople*

International Council of Nurses: *http://www.icn.ch/index.html*

United Nations: *http://www.un.org*

U.S. Department of Health and Human Services: *http://www.os.dhhs.gov*

World Health Organization: *http://www.who.int*

6

Structure and Function of Community Health Services

Learning Objectives

Upon mastery of this chapter, you should be able to:

- Trace historic events and philosophical developments leading to today's health services delivery systems.

- Outline the current organizational structure of the public health care system.

- Examine the three core functions of public health as they apply to health services delivery.

- Differentiate between the functions of public versus private sector health care agencies.

- Explain the influence of selected legislative acts in the United States on shaping current health services policy and practice.

- Examine the public health services provided by selected international health organizations.

- Explore how the structure and functions of community health services affect community health nursing practice.

Nurses preparing for population-based practice need to be familiar with how the health care delivery system is organized and operates, because it is through this system that community health services are delivered (see Chapter 3). This system forms an organizing framework for the design and implementation of programs aimed at improving the health of communities and vulnerable groups. It is within this system or framework that community health nurses work. Furthermore, through the vehicle of this system, community health nurses have the opportunity to shape the future of health services and develop innovative and more effective means of improving community health.

Service delivery systems directed at restoring or promoting the public's health have evolved over centuries. The structure, function, and financing of health care systems have changed dramatically during that time. These changes have come about in response to evolving societal needs and demands, scientific advancements, the development of more effective methods of service delivery, new technologies, and varying approaches to resource acquisition and allocation (Barton, 1999). Considerable progress has been made toward a healthier global society. At the same time, many problems remain, particularly those of controlling health care costs, assuring equitable distribution and effectiveness of health services, and assuring the quality of and access to those services (Pan American Health Organization, 2001; U.S. Department of Health and Human Services, 2000).

This chapter examines the current structure and functions of community health services in the United States and reviews historical and legislative events that have influenced the planning for and the delivery of those services.

HISTORICAL INFLUENCES ON HEALTH CARE

Health care has changed dramatically from previous centuries. Yet personal and community hygiene and health care seem to have been practiced from the beginning of time. Many primitive tribes engaged in sanitary practices such as burial of excreta, removal of the dead, and isolation of members with certain illnesses. In addition, treatment of the sick included use of a variety of therapeutic agents administered by a "healer." Whether these activities were superstitious, derived from survival needs, or primarily tied to religious beliefs is unknown. Nonetheless, records show that in Egypt and the Middle East, as early as 3000 BC, people were building drainage systems, using toilets and systems for water flushing, and practicing personal cleanliness (Scutchfield & Keck, 2003). The **Hebrew hygienic code**, described in the Bible in Leviticus circa 1500 BC, probably was the first written code in the world and was the prototype for personal and community sanitation. It emphasized bodily cleanliness, protection against the spread of contagious diseases, isolation of lepers, disinfection of dwellings after illness, sanitation of campsites, disposal of excreta and refuse, protection of water and food supplies, and maternity hygiene (Scutchfield and

Keck, 2003). Even more advanced were the Athenians, circa 1000 to 400 BC, who emphasized personal hygiene, diet, and exercise in addition to a sanitary environment, albeit for the benefit of the wealthy. Their successors, the Romans, added more community health measures, such as laws regulating environmental sanitation and nuisances and construction of paved streets, aqueducts, and a subsurface drainage system.

The Middle Ages (from about 500 to 1500 AD) marked a distinct change in health beliefs and practices in Europe based on the philosophy that to pamper the body was evil. Neglected personal hygiene, improper diets, and accumulation of refuse and body wastes soon led to widespread epidemics and pandemics of disease, including cholera, plague, and leprosy (Hecker, 1839). Increased trade between Europe and Asia, military conquests, and Christian crusades to the Middle East only furthered the spread of disease. Bubonic plague, known as the Black Death, was the most devastating of pandemics, reportedly killing more than 60 million people in the mid-1300s—half the population of the known world (Hecker, 1839). In response to the Black Death, in 1348, Venice banned entry of infected ships and travelers—a form of quarantine. **Quarantine** is a period of enforced isolation of persons exposed to a communicable disease, during the incubation period of the disease, to prevent its spread should infection occur. The first known official quarantine measure was instituted in 1377 at the port of Ragusa (now Dubrovnik in Croatia, formerly Yugoslavia) where travelers from plague areas were required to wait 2 months and to be free of disease before entry. Marseilles, in 1383, passed the first quarantine law (Scutchfield and Keck, 2003). During this regressive period in history, health care was scarce, private, and reserved for the wealthy few, whereas public health problems were rampant but only minimally and ineffectively addressed.

By the end of the Middle Ages, more enlightened Europeans began to challenge the prevailing beliefs and conditions. They no longer believed that disease was a punishment for sin. However, traces of stigma regarding such conditions as leprosy and tuberculosis still can be found today, and sexually transmitted diseases and acquired immunodeficiency syndrome (AIDS) are regarded by some as punishment for immoral conduct. During the late 18th century, new efforts at reform were influenced by a growing emphasis on human dignity, human rights, and the search for scientific truth. These efforts continued through the 19th and 20th centuries.

Despite such signs of improvement, during the 17th and 18th centuries serious problems persisted and new ones developed. Industrialization, masses of people moving to cities, and low regard for human life all contributed to deplorable living and working conditions. Hundreds of pauper children died in England's abusive but socially approved workhouses and apprentice slavery system. Most of Europe continued in unspeakable misery and filth. Householders dumped their refuse from windows or doors into the streets. Stinking rivers and water supplies were seriously contaminated. Numerous diseases, including cholera, typhus, typhoid, smallpox, and tuberculosis, took a tremendous toll on human life.

Around the turn of the 19th century, England's leaders

became increasingly concerned about social and sanitary reform. The term **sanitation** refers to the promotion of hygiene and prevention of disease by maintenance of health-enhancing (sanitary) conditions. The first sanitary legislation, passed in 1837, established vaccination stations in London. One of the most notable reformers, Edwin Chadwick, published his *Report on an Inquiry into the Sanitary Conditions of the Laboring Population of Great Britain* in 1842 (Richardson, 1887). Chadwick, the father of modern public health, believed that disease and poverty were related and could be changed. His efforts resulted in passage of the English Public Health Act and establishment of a General Board of Health for England in 1848, as reported by Lewis more than a century later (1952). An epidemiologist and anesthetist, John Snow (1813–1858) worked on the cholera outbreak in London in 1854. His investigations of cholera outbreaks and conclusions led to changes in sewage dumping practices into the Thames River, improving London's morbidity and mortality from cholera. His 1855 work, *On the Mode of Communication of Cholera* (2nd ed.), was a public health contribution. Conditions improved and scientific study advanced in England and, concurrently, in France, Germany, Scandinavia, and other European countries. England, however, set the pace for application of research, particularly with reference to public health measures, through steadily improved legislation. British laws subsequently became the pattern for American sanitary ordinances.

HEALTH CARE SYSTEM DEVELOPMENT IN THE UNITED STATES

Today's relatively organized health care system was long in developing. Most health-related services in the United States were initially reactive, responding to the pressure of immediate needs and uncoordinated from one locality to another. Over time, events and insights contributed to a gradually improving system of programs and services, along with recognition that the health of individuals was affected by the health of the wider community (Table 6–1).

T A B L E   6 – 1

Changes in Health Status and Health Care Services

Turn of the 20th Century	Turn of the 21st Century
MORBIDITY AND MORTALITY	
Then	**Now**
High communicable disease and mortality	High chronic disease morbidity and mortality
Little prevention	Old and new sexually transmitted diseases
Infrequent cure	Resurgence of tuberculosis
Life span of 47 yr	Life span of 76 yr
High infant mortality	Significant infant mortality
High maternal mortality	High teenage pregnancy
Alcohol abuse	Multiple substance abuse
Many undiagnosed and untreated conditions	New strains of multidrug-resistant diseases, long-term chronicity, and disability
ACCESS TO HEALTH CARE	
Then	**Now**
Access primarily for those who could pay a fee	Access for those with health insurance
No health insurance	Insurance with copayments shifting to managed care
Public health clinics for poor and underserved	Free health clinics for medically indigent (especially children)
Limited treatments available	Multitude of treatments with regular new advances
HEALTH CARE DELIVERY SYSTEM	
Then	**Now**
Extended hospital stays	Short-term, acute-care hospitalizations
Discharge on recovery	Recovery occurs at home or in a transitional setting
Extended maternal and newborn hospitalization	Short-stay maternal and newborn care
Many home deliveries with lay assistance	Few home deliveries with skilled assistance
Home care through not-for-profit agencies	Home care through not-for-profit and proprietary agencies
PHN begun in health departments	Shifting PHN role in health deparments
Health departments provide personal care services for poor and underserved	Health department's personal care services a part of managed care systems

PHN, public health nursing.

(Adapted from Erickson, G.P. [1996]. To pauperize or empower: Public health nursing at the turn of the 20th and 21st centuries. *Public Health Nursing, 13*[3], 163–169.)

Precursors to a Health Care System

Early health care in the American colonies consisted of private practice with occasional (but infrequent) governmental action for the public good. Action usually was in the form of isolated local responses to specific dangers or nuisances, such as the 1647 regulation to prevent pollution of Boston Harbor or the 1701 Massachusetts law requiring ship quarantine and isolation of smallpox patients. New York City, in the late 1700s, formed a public health committee to monitor, among other public concerns, water quality, sewer construction, marsh drainage, and burial of the dead.

The U.S. Constitution, adopted in 1789, made no direct reference to public health, nor was the federal government active in health matters. It was the responsibility of each sovereign state to manage its own health affairs. The first federal intervention for health problems was the Marine Hospital Service Act of 1798. It subsidized medical and hospital care for sick and injured merchant seamen, with the first marine hospital being located in Boston. During the early years, a scourge of epidemics, especially smallpox, cholera, typhoid, and typhus, caused deaths throughout the colonies and decimated the Native American population (Woodward, 1932). Slave trade further threatened the lives of colonists by introducing diseases such as yaws (an infectious nonvenereal disease caused by a spirochete), yellow fever, and malaria (Marr, 1982). Quarantine efforts under local control proved ineffective. In 1837, Congress finally instituted the national port quarantine system, which was regulated and enforced by the Marine Hospital Service. Epidemics were quickly brought under control, causing society to recognize the benefits of uniform central government policy. However, improvements in public health and sanitation generally throughout the states were held back by delayed progress in coping with other competing needs, such as police and fire protection (Table 6–2).

T A B L E 6 – 2

Societal Events and Situations Affecting Health Care Needs

Turn of the 20th Century	Turn of the 21st Century
SOCIETAL AND POPULATION SHIFTS	
Then	**Now**
Industrial society focusing on production	Postindustrial, service and information oriented
Rural to urban	Urban to suburban
Limited violence	Rampant violence and terrorism
Wide gaps between rich and poor	Widening gaps between rich and poor
Growing philanthropy	Declining support for charitable health care
Intense immigration from eastern Europe	Moderate immigration—Mexico, Carribean, Middle East, and Asia
ENVIRONMENT	
Then	**Now**
Overcrowded, unsanitary housing	Deteriorating inner-city neighborhoods
Unsafe workplaces, lack of worker safeguards	Environmental hazards in some workplaces
Rampant child labor	Homelessness
Poor public sanitation	Good public sanitation
Multiple health risks	Increasing environmental and behavioral risks
SKILL CHANGES AND EMPLOYMENT	
Then	**Now**
Farm to factory	Factory to service and information
Low wages	Improving wages, limited benefits
Dramatic disparity in wages between men and women	Slowly resolving disparity in male/female wage differences
Not enough jobs	Downsizing, layoffs, corporate streamlining, failing companies
PEOPLE LIVNG IN POVERTY	
Then	**Now**
Women and children	Women, children, the aged
Immigrants—European	Immigrants—Hispanic, Caribbean, Middle Eastern, and Asian
Migration—south to north	Seasonal migration of farm workers

(Adapted from Erickson, G.P. [1996]. To pauperize or empower: Public health nursing at the turn of the 20th and 21st centuries. *Public Health Nursing, 13*[3], 163–169.)

The Shattuck Report

The **Shattuck Report**, a landmark document, made a tremendous impact on sanitary progress. Lemuel Shattuck, a layman and legislator, chaired a legislative committee that studied health and sanitary problems in the commonwealth of Massachusetts. In 1850, he produced the "Report of the Sanitary Commission of Massachusetts" (Shattuck et al., 1850). It described public health concepts and methods that form the base for current public health practice. Among his recommendations, Shattuck advocated the establishment of state and local boards of health, environmental sanitation, collection and use of vital statistics, systematic study of diseases, control of food and drugs, urban planning, establishment of nurses' training schools (there were none before this time), and preventive medicine. Unfortunately, almost 25 years passed before the recommendations were appreciated and implemented. A similar report by John C. Griscom, conducted about the same time, concluded that illness, premature death, and poverty were directly related. He also recommended sanitary reform.

Official Health Agencies

The beginnings of an organized health care system in the United States came in the form of **official health agencies**, later called public health agencies. These were publicly funded and operated by state or local governments with a goal of providing population-based health services. Development occurred initially at the local level. Many cities established local boards of health in the late 1700s and early to middle 1800s. Among the earliest were those in Baltimore, Maryland (1798); Charleston, South Carolina (1815); and Philadelphia, Pennsylvania (1818). As their efforts expanded from handling public "nuisances" to dealing with epidemics and complex public health problems, local health boards recognized that employment of full-time staff was needed, and thus health departments were formed. The first full-time county health departments were established in 1911 in the states of North Carolina and Washington. Louisiana formed the nation's first state board of health in 1855, followed by Massachusetts in 1869. A few years later, Massachusetts created the first state department of health. Congress formed a National Board of Health to combat yellow fever in 1878. However, because of poor organization, it existed for only 10 years. Again at the national level, the Marine Hospital Service, now with a broader function, became the Public Health and Marine Hospital Service in 1902. Congress gave it a more clearly defined organizational structure and specific functions for its director, the Surgeon General. In 1912, it was renamed the United States Public Health Service (PHS).

Rapidly expanding through World War I and the Great Depression, the PHS strengthened its research activity through the National Institutes of Health (NIH, founded in 1912), added demonstration projects, and initiated greater cooperation with the states. Responding to increasingly complex needs, the NIH added programs significant to public health, such as the Children's Bureau (1912); the National Leprosarium at Carville, Louisiana (1917); examination of arriving aliens (1917); the Division of Venereal Diseases (1918); the Food and Drug Administration (1927); and the Narcotics Division (1929), which later became the Division of Mental Hygiene. Title VI of the 1935 Social Security Act promoted stronger federal support of state and local public health services, including health manpower training.

As health, welfare, and educational services proliferated, the need for consolidation prompted the creation of the Federal Security Agency in 1939. In 1953, it was enlarged and renamed the Department of Health, Education and Welfare (DHEW), established under President Eisenhower. In 1979, education was made a separate cabinet-level department, and the DHEW was renamed the Department of Health and Human Services (DHHS). Other significant events include the establishment during World War II of the Communicable Disease Center in Atlanta, currently known as the National Centers for Disease Control and Prevention (CDC), and the development after World War II of the National Office of Vital Statistics, now called the National Center for Health Statistics (NCHS).

Voluntary Health Agencies

The private sector responded first to America's health problems and continues to complement and supplement the government's role in providing health services. By the late 1800s, **voluntary health agencies** (later called private agencies) began to emerge. They were privately funded and operated to address specific health needs. The first of these was the Anti-Tuberculosis Society of Philadelphia, which was formed in 1892 to educate the public and the government about tuberculosis, then causing 10% of all deaths. Other agencies followed: the National Society to Prevent Blindness was formed in 1908, the Mental Health Association in 1909, the American Cancer Society in 1913, the National Easter Seal Society for Crippled Children and Adults in 1921, and the Planned Parenthood Federation of America, also in 1921. In the late 1800s, organized charities such as the Red Cross, previously denounced for promoting dependent poverty, began to be recognized for their contributions to health and welfare. Philanthropy, too, became respected with the establishment of the Rockefeller Foundation in 1913, followed by the Carnegie-Mellon, Kellogg, and Robert Wood Johnson Foundations.

Health-Related Professional Associations

Many health-related professional associations have influenced the quality and type of community health services delivery. Among these, the National Organization for Public Health Nursing from 1912 to 1952 significantly influenced early preparation for and quality of public health nursing services (Fitzpatrick, 1975). The American Public Health Association (APHA), founded in 1872, maintains a prominent role in the dissemination of public health information, influence on health policy, and advocacy for the nation's health. Other nursing and community health organizations that have promoted quality efforts in community health include the Association of State and Territorial Directors of Nursing, the Association of State and Territorial Health Officers, the National League for Nursing (NLN), the American Nurses Association (ANA), and the Association for Community Health Nursing Educators (ACHNE).

HEALTH ORGANIZATIONS IN THE UNITED STATES

The historical record demonstrates that people have attempted to address community health needs for centuries. Responsibility has shifted between private groups and governing institutions. Each arm, public and private, offers a unique perspective, different skills, and different resources. However, lack of coordination between them, coupled with the lack of a method for comprehensive planning and delivery of health services, left huge gaps in some areas and duplication in others. Only within the last century have the two arms gradually begun to work together to create a loosely structured "system" of health care.

Barton spoke of the growing interdependence of the public and private sectors (1999). How does that system work today? What are its strengths and weaknesses? To answer these questions, its structure must first be examined. Structure is important because it becomes the operational base for assessment, diagnosis, planning, implementation, and evaluation of services and because it provides a framework for intersystem and intrasystem communication and coordination.

Health services occur at four levels: local, state, national, and international. Like ever-widening concentric circles, these levels encompass broader populations. The organization of health services at each level can be classified as one of two types: public or private.

Public Sector Health Services

Government health agencies, the tax-supported arm of the public health effort, perform a vital function in community health practice. They are the official public health agencies whose areas of jurisdiction and types of service are dictated by law. They coordinate and administer activities that often can be carried out only by group or community-wide action: for example, proper sewage disposal, the provision of sanitary water systems, or regulation of toxic wastes. Many community health activities require an authoritative legal backing to ensure enforcement (another useful function of public health agencies) of control in areas such as environmental pollution, highway safety practices, and proper handling of food. Official or public health agencies provide important record-keeping services, including the collection and monitoring of vital statistics. They also conduct research, provide consultation, and sometimes financially support other community health efforts.

Core Public Health Functions

Public health services encompass a wide variety of activities, but all can be grouped under one of three **core public health functions**. They are assessment, policy development, and assurance (Fig. 6–1). As discussed in Chapter 3, public health nurses practice as partners with other public health professionals within these core functions.

Assessment refers to measuring and monitoring the health status and needs of a designated community or population. As a core function, it is a continuous process of collecting data and disseminating information about health, diseases, injuries, air and water quality, food safety, and available resources. This function helps to identify trends in morbidity, mortality, and causative factors. It identifies available health resources, unmet needs, and community perceptions about health issues.

Policy development is the formation of a guide for action that determines present and future decisions affecting the public's health. As a core public health function, good public policy development builds on data from the assessment function and incorporates community values and citizen input. It provides leadership and administration for the development of sound health policy and planning.

Assurance is the process of translating established policies into services. This function ensures that population-based services are provided, whether by public health agencies or private sources. It also monitors the quality of and access to those services. The specific functions of assessment, policy development, and assurance are described in Table 6–3.

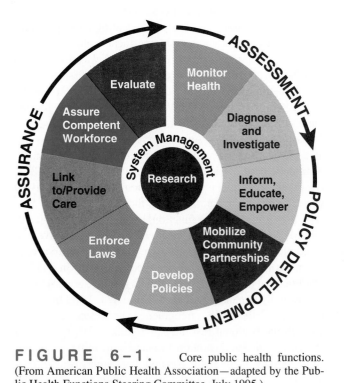

FIGURE 6–1. Core public health functions. (From American Public Health Association—adapted by the Public Health Functions Steering Committee, July 1995.)

TABLE 6-3

Core Public Health Functions applied to Populations and People at Risk

Population-Wide Services

Assessment

Health status monitoring and disease surveillance

Public Policy

Leadership, policy, planning, and administration

Assurance

Investigation and control of diseases and injuries
Protection of environment, workplaces, housing, food, and water
Laboratory services to support disease control and environmental protection
Health education and information
Community mobilization for health-related issues
Targeted outreach and linkage to personal services
Health services quality assurance and accountability
Training and education of public health professionals

Personal Services and Home Visits for People at Risk

Primary care for unserved and underserved people
Treatment services for targeted conditions
Clinical preventive services
Payments for personal services delivered by others

The roles of public health agencies vary by level, with each level carrying out the core functions in different ways to form a partnership in protecting the public's health (Williams & Torrens, 1999). International health agencies focus on issues of global concern, setting policy, developing standards, and monitoring health conditions and programs. At the national level, government health agencies engage in similar functions aimed at regional or nationwide concerns. The federal level provides funds (eg, through the Medicaid program) and develops policy (eg, air pollution policy) but depends on the states to implement them. Agencies at the federal level also develop facilities and programs for special groups, such as Native Americans, migrant workers, inmates of federal prisons, and military personnel and veterans, whose health care is not the direct responsibility of any one state or locality. State government health agencies function fairly autonomously while working within federal guidelines. They assess, develop, and monitor statewide health needs and services. At the local level, one may find a city government health agency, a county agency, or a combination of both to assess, plan, and serve the health needs of that locality.

Unlike private organizations that tend to have a specific focus, government health agencies exist to accomplish a broad goal of protecting and promoting the health of the total population under their jurisdiction. Such a task requires a wide range of services and the combined talents of many types of professional disciplines. Among them are nurses, physicians, health educators, sanitarians, epidemiologists, statisticians, engineers, administrators, accountants, computer programmers, planners, sociologists, nutritionists, laboratory technicians, chemists, physicists, veterinarians, dentists, pharmacists, demographers, and meteorologists. Furthermore, public health agencies must function not only on an interdisciplinary basis but on an interorganizational one as well. Other government services (eg, education) can meet their goals fairly autonomously, but public health cannot accomplish its important objectives without the collaboration of many agencies and organizations, both public and private (Barton, 1999; Williams & Torrens, 1999). A case in point is the working together of many organizations with public health to manage the AIDS epidemic, including educational institutions, welfare agencies, mental health programs, home care services, Medicaid, and private groups.

Many different government agencies contribute to the health of a community. Most obvious are the local and state health departments, which provide a variety of direct and indirect health services, including community health nursing. Other tax-supported agencies that sponsor health care or health-related services include welfare departments, departments of public works, public schools and hospitals, police departments, county agricultural services, and local housing authorities.

Local Public Health Agencies

At the grassroots level, government health agencies vary considerably in structure and function from one locality to the next. This partly results from variations in local needs and size of the community. For example, a rural community served by a county or state health department may have widely differing needs and services than a densely populated urban community. Differing health care standards and regulations, as well as the type and stipulations of funding sources, also contribute to variations in the structure and function of health agencies. Nonetheless, each local governmental health agency shares some commonly held responsibilities, functions, and structural features.

The primary responsibilities of the local health department are (1) to assess its population's health status and needs, (2) to determine how well those needs are being met, and (3) to take action toward satisfying unmet needs (Scutchfield & Keck, 2003). Specifically, local government health agencies should fulfill the core functions as follows:

- Assess and monitor local health needs and the resources for addressing them.
- Develop policy and provide leadership in advocating equitable distribution of resources and services, both public and private.
- Ensure availability, accessibility, and quality of health services for all members of the community.
- Keep the community informed on how to access public health services.

The local health agency is a critical level of health services' provision because of its closeness to the ultimate recipients: health care consumers.

The structure of the local health department varies in complexity with the setting. Rural and small urban agencies need only a simple organization, whereas large metropolitan agencies require more complex organizational structures to support the greater diversity and quantity of work. A local board of health generally holds the legal responsibility for the health of its citizens. Health board members may be appointed by the mayor if the board of health serves a city, or by a board of supervisors if the board of health serves a county, or they may be publicly elected. In turn, the board of health appoints a health officer, usually a physician with public health training, who employs the remaining staff of the health department, including public health nurses, environmental health workers, health educators, and office personnel. Others, such as nutritionists, statisticians, epidemiologists, social workers, physical therapists, veterinarians, or public health dentists, may be added as needs and resources dictate.

Revenue to support local health department expenditures comes from a variety of sources. State and county general appropriations make up the largest share of the local health department's budget, with additional funds provided through special levies and programs such as school health, Headstart, air pollution, toxic substance control, primary care, immunizations, fees, and private foundation grants. Federal funds provide another source of revenue targeted at specific efforts,

such as AIDS research and services, family planning, child health, environmental protection, and hypertension and nutrition programs. Fees, reimbursements, and additional miscellaneous sources, such as state laboratory revenues and food supply supplements, make up the remaining portion of the budget. Figure 6–2 depicts the organization of one local health department serving a population of approximately 300,000.

State Public Health Agencies

State-level government health agencies also vary in structure and in how they carry out the core functions. Each state, as a sovereign government, establishes its own state health department, which in turn determines its goals, actions, and administrative structure. The state health department is responsible for providing leadership in and monitoring of comprehensive public health needs and services in the state. It establishes statewide health policy standards, assists local communities, allocates funds, promotes state-level health planning, conducts and evaluates state-level health programs, promotes cooperation with voluntary (private) health agencies, and collaborates with the federal government for health planning and policy development (Scutchfield & Keck, 2003). Of the various levels of government health agencies, the states recently have played the most pivotal role in health policy formation.

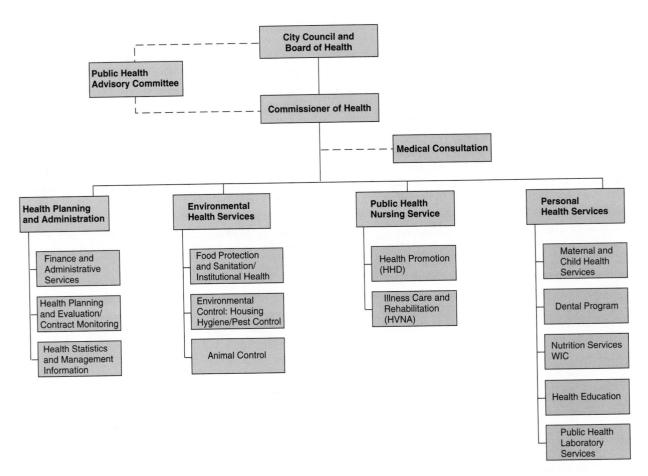

FIGURE 6–2. Organizational chart of a city public health department.

General functions of state health departments include the following (Scutchfield & Keck, 2003):

1. Statewide health planning
2. Intergovernmental and other agency relations
3. Intrastate agency relations
4. Certain statewide policy determinations
5. Standards setting
6. Health regulatory functions

Specifically, the Institute of Medicine (1988) described the role of state government related to health. Summarized, it includes the following:

- Collect data statewide to assess health needs.
- Ensure an adequate statutory base for state health activities.
- Establish statewide health objectives (holding localities accountable where power for implementation has been delegated).
- Ensure statewide development and maintenance of essential personal, educational, and environmental health services.
- Solve problems that threaten the health of the state.
- Support local health services (when needed to achieve adequate service levels) through subsidies, technical and administrative assistance, or direct action.

State public health agencies face a challenge in addressing the health-related issues confronting them. Health insurance, long-term care, organ transplants and donations, AIDS, care of the **medically indigent** (those who are unable to pay for and totally lack medical services), malpractice, and certificates of need for new health services are among the problems faced by most states. Clearly, state health departments must collaborate closely with other agencies, such as social services, education, public works, the legislature, and the housing bureau, to effectively solve such problems. Thus, the solution of state health problems and delivery of health services requires the functioning of an interdependent network of organizations, many of which are not health agencies per se.

Budgetary sources for operating a state health department include state-generated funds, federal grants and contracts, and fees and reimbursements. A large source of federal monies to the states comes through the Department of Agriculture, which has supported the Women, Infants, and Children (WIC) Program, a supplemental nutrition program.

Each of the 50 state health departments in the United States has developed its own unique structure. Some are strongly centralized organizations, and others are decentralized. All are overseen by a director of public health, but titles vary. Under the director are several divisions or bureaus. Those most commonly found in state health department organizational structures are environmental health, disease prevention and control, community health services, maternal and child health, health systems and technical services, laboratory services, and state center for health statistics. Figure 6–3 shows the organizational chart of a state health department.

National Public Health Agencies

The national level of public health organization consists of many government agencies. They can be clustered into four groups. First and most directly focused on health is the **Public Health Service** (PHS). It is an umbrella organization concerned with the broad health interests of the country and is directed by the Assistant Secretary for Health. The PHS is made up of six functional branches: the CDC, the Food and Drug Administration, the NIH, the Substance Abuse and Mental Health Services Administration, the Health Resources and Services Administration, and the Agency for Toxic Substances and Disease Registry. One of its major functions through these six branches is the administration of grants and contracts with other government agencies, private organizations, and individuals. In some instances, the PHS provides hospital, clinical, and other types of health services, such as for Native Americans on reservations and for Eskimos through the Indian Health Service. Through the CDC and the NIH, it provides epidemiologic surveillance and numerous research programs. The Food and Drug Administration of the PHS monitors the safety and usefulness of various food and drug products as well as cosmetics, toys, and flammable fabrics.

Through its staff offices, the PHS offers other services. It has responsibility for the formation, planning, and evaluation of health policy; health promotion; health services management; health research and statistics; intergovernmental affairs; legislation; population affairs; and international health. It provides financial assistance to the states through grants-in-aid—monies raised by Congress through taxes for specific purposes. It also offers consultation through a National Advisory Health Council and special advisory committees made up of lay experts. The PHS maintains 10 regional offices to make its services more readily available to the states. These offices are located in New York, Boston, Philadelphia, Atlanta, Chicago, Kansas City, Dallas, Denver, Seattle, and San Francisco. Figure 6–4 portrays the PHS organizational structure.

At the federal level, the primary agencies concerned with health are organized under the **Department of Health and Human Services** (DHHS). The PHS is one of five major units in this department. The other four are the Office of Human Development Services, the Health Care Financing Administration, the Family Support Administration, and the Social Security Administration. Within the DHHS, clusters of federal agencies deal with the needs of special population groups such as the elderly (Administration on Aging), farmers (Agricultural Extension Service), Native Americans (Bureau of Indian Affairs), and the military (Veterans Administration). Another cluster addresses special programs or problems. Examples are the Bureau of Labor Standards, the Office of Education, the Bureau of Mines, the Department of Agriculture, and the Bureau of Labor Statistics. A final cluster of federal agencies focuses on international health concerns of interest to the nation. Two important ones are the Office of International Health, part of the PHS, and the U.S. Agency for International Development (USAID), under the Department of State.

Private Sector Health Services

The nongovernmental and voluntary arm of the health care delivery system includes many types of services. Privately

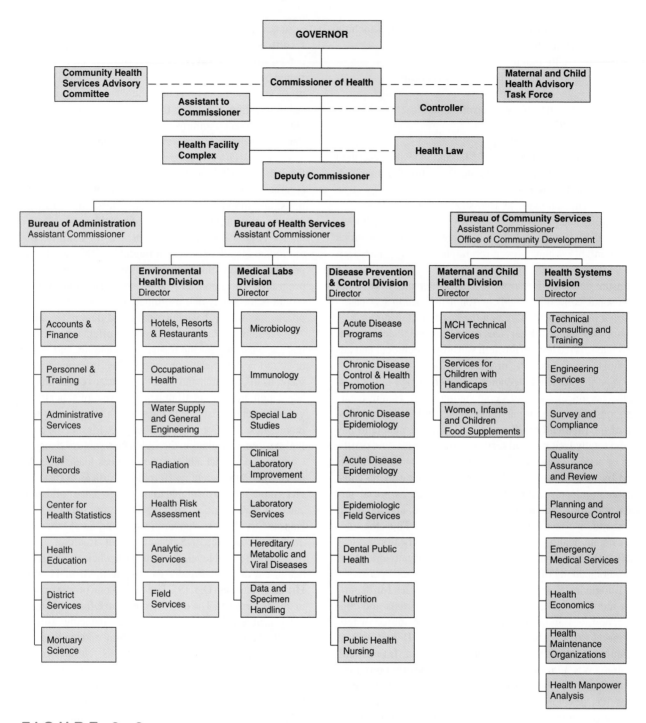

FIGURE   6–3.   Organizational chart of a state public health department.

owned, nonprofit health agencies, which includes most hospitals, and welfare agencies make up one large group. Privately owned (proprietary), for-profit agencies are another. Private professional health care practice, composed largely of physicians in solo practice (about two fifths) or group practice (three fifths), forms a third group. These make up the nontax-supported, nongovernmental dimension of community health care.

Private health services are complementary and supplementary to government health agencies. They often meet the needs of special groups, such as those with cancer or heart disease; they offer an avenue for private enterprise or philanthropy; they are freer than government agencies to develop innovations in health care; and they have been spurred to development, in part, by impatience or dissatisfaction with government programs. Their financial

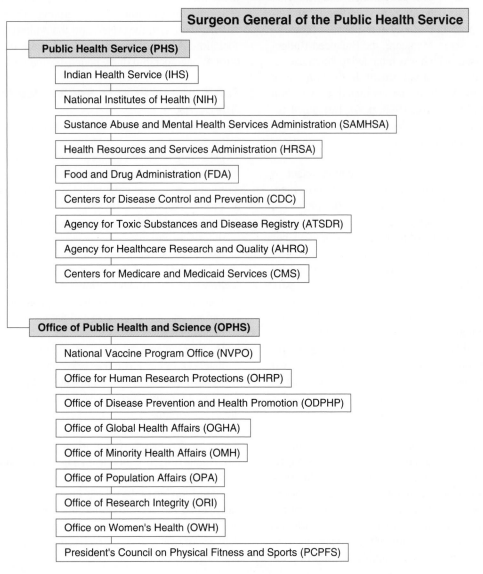

FIGURE 6–4.   Office of the Surgeon General—The United States Public Health Service and Office of Public Health and Science.

support comes from voluntary contributions, bequests, or fees.

For-Profit and Not-for-Profit Health Agencies

Proprietary health services are privately owned and managed. They may be nonprofit or for-profit. Many hospitals and nursing homes offer nonprofit services but must generate sufficient revenues to keep ahead of operating costs. Often, one or more special services offered by a hospital generate enough income to cover the drain from more expensive programs or uncompensated care. As more hospitals have merged or been integrated into larger health conglomerates, the practice often has been to establish a separate, for-profit corporation that generates revenues so that the basic organization can retain its nonprofit, tax-exempt status.

Examples of for-profit health services include a wide range of private practices by physicians, nurses, social workers, psychologists, and laboratory and radiation technologists. With the greater demand for home care services since the 1980s, the number of new, for-profit services such as home care agencies, nursing personnel pools, and durable medical equipment supply companies increased well into the 1990s. Medicare's annual costs for home care services per enrollee went from $4 in 1969 to more than $300 by the late 1990s. When all personal health expenditures are considered (hospital care, physician services, and home health), it costs Medicare almost $5000 per year per enrollee, and Medicare barely covers 50% of total health care spending by the elderly (Tyson, 2001, p. 459). Partially in response to these escalating home care costs to Medicare, the Balanced Budget Act of 1997 was passed, which was intended to "increase efficiency, reduce fraud, and curtail growth in the home care industry while saving Medicare an estimated $1.6 billion during the first year" (Flaherty, 1998, p. 6). Instead, it reduced Medicare reimbursement by 31% to the for-profit home care agencies, causing 10% of them to close nationwide, placing some clients in jeopardy.

Although Medicare entered the 21st century intact, it offered very limited outpatient prescription drug coverage, limited services in many areas (eg, chiropractic, physician second opinions, immunosuppressive drug therapy for transplant patients, and the number of home care home visits per spell-of-illness), and increasing premiums for the optional Medicare Part B. In 2003, Medicare Part B increased by 8.7%, whereas Social Security benefits increased modestly with a 1.4% cost-of-living adjustment (COLA)—the smallest in 4 years. This amounts to an even lower COLA when the higher cost of Medicare Part B is considered (U.S. Departmnt of Health and Human Services, 2002). The federal legislature passed a complex Medicare law in 2003 designed to overhaul the burdened program. The new law will assist many elders but will do little to rein in drug prices. Chapter 7 covers the financing of health care in the United States in greater detail.

Not-for-profit private health agencies are organizations that are established and administered by private citizens for a specific health-related purpose. Often, this purpose is seen as a special need either not addressed or served inadequately by government. An example is visiting nurse associations, which were formed to provide care for the sick in their homes. The contribution of the private, not-for-profit health agency then becomes complementary to public health services.

Three types of private, not-for-profit health agencies have specialized interests. Some, such as the American Cancer Society and the American Diabetes Association, are concerned with specific diseases. Others, such as the National Society for Autistic Children, Planned Parenthood Federation of America, and the National Council on Aging, focus on the needs of special populations. A third group, including agencies such as the American Heart Association and the National Kidney Foundation, are concerned with diseases of specific organs. All of these agencies are funded through private contributions.

Another group of private, not-for-profit agencies affecting health and health care includes the many foundations that support health programs, research, and professional education. Examples include the W.K. Kellogg Foundation, the Pew Charitable Trusts, the Robert Wood Johnson Foundation, and the Bush Foundation. Some agencies, such as the United Way, exist to fund other voluntary efforts. Another group includes professional associations that work to improve the public's health through the promotion of standards, research, information, and programs. Examples are the APHA, the NLN, the ANA, and the American Medical Association (AMA). These organizations are funded primarily through membership dues, bequests, and contributions.

Functions of Private-Sector Health Agencies

The general functions of private-sector health agencies are as follows:

1. Detecting unserved needs or exploring better methods for meeting needs already addressed
2. Piloting or subsidizing demonstration projects
3. Promoting public knowledge
4. Assisting official agencies with innovative programs not otherwise possible
5. Evaluating official programs and assuming a public advocacy role
6. Promoting health legislation
7. Planning and coordinating to promote collaboration among voluntary services and between voluntary and official agencies
8. Developing well-balanced community health programs that seek to make services relevant and comprehensive

Future functions of both private and public sectors most likely will remain much the same. However, the structure of the organizations within both sectors is changing dramatically and will continue to do so as managed care organizations blur the lines between private and public sectors. The movement toward national managed care and its effect on health care delivery are discussed in Chapter 7.

The blurring of the private and public health care sectors has opened the doors to emerging creative health care services. An example of public and private cooperation in the delivery of health care is described in Display 6–1.

INTERNATIONAL HEALTH ORGANIZATIONS

On October 12, 1999, the United Nations announced that the global population had reached the 6 billion mark, just 12 years after passing 5 billion. According to the most recent projections of the United Nations Population Division, the world's population could reach 7 billion as early as 2011 or as late as 2015 (Population Reference Bureau, 2002).

The health of countries around the world cannot be ignored. Besides important humanitarian and moral concerns, there are pragmatic reasons for addressing health issues at the international level. Today, health—along with politics and economics—has become a global issue. Health care among 65% to 80% of the world's population, or about 4 billion people, continues to be based on traditional medicine. At the same time, the ever-changing global electronic

DISPLAY 6-1

Community Partnerships

Community partnerships are emerging between cities, communities, and other groups, such as businesses, governmental agencies, academic institutions, and voluntary organizations, to meet the health and related needs of citizens. Both government and foundations are encouraging these as an answer to unmet needs.

The Kentucky Partnership for Farm Family Health and Safety began with funds from the Kellogg Foundation but now is a nonprofit, independent, community-based organization. Farm wives have been identified and trained in health education and health-related services and serve as the health "officers" for farm and rural families. This type of community-based organization is being replicated in various counties in Kentucky and in other states to meet the needs of rural farm families.

Organizations such as these highlight the weaknesses and gaps in the U.S. system. They also provide direction for the future of primary care in the United States while assisting all involved to understand the value of interprofessional collaboration. This type of partnering in an organization is becoming more common as they link the private and public sectors and create many new and exciting roles for the professional nurse in the community.

information technologies are revolutionizing health practices with distance education, training, and telemedicine, allowing the transmission of health information to create a more level field for the delivery of health services in all countries. The nations of the world are dependent on one another for goods and services, and, as in any set of interdependent systems, a problem in one nation has repercussions on others.

The Director-General of the World Health Organization (WHO) stated that "all countries, their governments, their civil societies, and their individuals . . . can be partners who are willing to share and exchange the life-enhancing information and technology that is already at the fingertips of the rich but as yet beyond the reach of the poor" (WHO, 1998, p. 6); such is the political vision of theWHO. Furthermore, the constitution of the WHO considers that the health of all people is fundamental to the attainment of peace and security (WHO, 1998).

As stated in the 2002 executive summary of the PAHO, *Health in the Americas,* "new information technologies have played an invaluable role in improving access to and the quality of health care, as well as in the organization, administration, and operation of new health services models being introduced in the Region [the Americas—Canada, the United States, Central and South America]" (p. 14).

It may not seem possible that the health of a resident of a country 9000 miles away can affect that of a student from the United States. However, when taking a transnational flight for a school holiday to Mazatlan, Mexico, to Jamaica in the Caribbean, or to Bermuda in the Atlantic, the student will be seated among groups of tourists and business people from many nations of the world. There is close scrutiny of airline passengers for passports, visas, customs regulations, weapons, and drugs, but does anyone know whether a passenger from a developing country—who is sitting next to the student for a 6-, 8-, or 10-hour flight—has an airborne communicable disease that is resistant to known antibiotics? (See Table 6–4.)

International cooperation in health dates back to early concerns for epidemics. In 1851, representatives from 12 countries met in Paris for the First International Sanitary Conference. They later established a more permanent organization, the Office Internationale d'Hygiene Publique in 1907. Epidemics on the American continent also prompted representatives from 21 American republics to meet for the First International Sanitary Conference in Mexico City in 1902. In that same year, they formed the International Sanitary Bureau, later renamed the Pan American Health Organization (PAHO). After World War I, the League of Nations

TABLE 6-4

Drug Resistance Levels in Microbes Causing Infectious Diseases

Disease	Causative Agent	Antimicrobial Drug	Drug Resistance Level (%)
Acute respiratory illness	S. pneumoniae	Penicillin	12–55
AIDS	HIV	Antiretrovirals	N/A
Diarrheal diseases	S. dysenteriae	Cotrimoxazole	5–95
Tuberculosis	M. tuberculosis	Isoniazid	2–39
Malaria	P. falciparum	Chloroquine	30–50
Gonorrhea	N. gonorrhoeae	Penicillin	Up to 98

N/A, not available.

(From World Health Organization reports in U.S. Agency for International Development. (2001). Child survival and disease programs fund progress report, fiscal year 2001. Washington, DC: Author.)

in 1921 formed a health organization, which merged with the Office Internationale d'Hygiene Publique.

World Health Organization

The **World Health Organization** (WHO), an agency of the United Nations, was developed to direct and coordinate the promotion of health worldwide. It was formed after World War II, in 1948, and assumed the functions of the League of Nation's health organization. The PAHO remained separate but became WHO's regional office for the Americas. The WHO began its existence with 61 member nations, one of which was the United States. By 1998, it had expanded its membership to 191 nations and two associate members (WHO, 1998).

The mission of the WHO is to serve as the one directing and coordinating authority on international health. From its inception, the WHO has influenced international thinking with its classic definition of health as "a state of complete physical, mental, and social well-being and not merely the absence of disease or infirmity" (WHO, 1998). WHO's primary function is to help countries improve their health status and services by assisting them to help themselves and each other. To accomplish this, it provides member countries with technical services, information from epidemiology and statistics, advisory and consulting services, and demonstration teams.

For 20 years, WHO had a realistic expectation that by the year 2000, no individual citizen in any country would have a level of health below an acceptable minimum, and that the global community would later adopt a new strategy to take people further toward the goal of health for all in the future (WHO, 1998). The target date of the year 2000 was intended as a challenge to the member nations. Although the goal has not been met entirely, the WHO continues to emphasize sustaining primary health care, environmental health, control of infectious and diarrheal diseases, maternal and child health care, nutrition, injury prevention, and occupational health (WHO, 1998). These emphases point to a change in focus from primarily reactive programs (eg, stopping epidemics, instituting quarantines) to a more positive stance of promoting the health status of the world community (Display 6–2).

In addition to its headquarters in Geneva, Switzerland, the WHO has six regional offices. The office for the Americas, the PAHO, is located in Washington, DC. The other regional offices are in Copenhagen (Europe), Alexandria (eastern Mediterranean), Brazzaville (Africa), New Delhi (southeast Asia), and Manila (western Pacific). Its funding comes from member countries and from the United Nations. It holds an annual World Health Assembly to discuss international health policies and programs.

The WHO publishes several periodicals of interest to the global community, which are available through subscription for a fee and in partial text through WHO's various Web sites:

Bulletin of the World Health Organization—bimonthly
International Digest of Health Legislation—quarterly
Weekly Epidemiological Record—weekly

DISPLAY 6–2

The 21st Century Goals of the International Community

By 2005
End gender discrimination in education.
Implement strategies that will reverse current losses of environmental resources by 2015.
Build capacity for democratic and accountable governing, protection of human rights, and respect for the rule of law.

By 2015
Cut extreme poverty in half.
Secure universal primary education for all.
Reduce infant mortality rates by two thirds.
Cut the number of mothers who die giving birth by 75%.
Make family planning services available to all who want them.

(From U.S. Agency for International Development. [1998]. *Making a world of difference: Celebrating 30 years of development progress.* Washington, DC: Author.)

WHO Drug Information—quarterly
World Health—bimonthly
World Health Forum—quarterly
World Health Statistics Quarterly—quarterly

Pan American Health Organization

The **Pan American Health Organization** (PAHO) serves as the central coordinating organization for public health in the Western Hemisphere. Founded in 1902, it is the oldest continuously functioning international health organization in the world. Its budget comes from assessments contributed by the American Republics member countries, augmented by funds from WHO, the United Nations, and a variety of other sources, including private donations.

As WHO's regional office for the Americas, PAHO disseminates epidemiologic information, provides technical assistance, finances fellowships, and promotes cooperative research and professional education. An annual conference convened by PAHO provides an opportunity for delegates from all of the member nations to discuss issues of concern and plan strategies for addressing health needs. Periodicals published by PAHO include *Perspectives in Health*, published biannually, and *Bulletin of the Pan American Health Organization*, published quarterly.

United Nations International Children's Emergency Fund

Organized in 1946, the United Nations Children's Fund, now called the **United Nations International Children's Emer-**

gency Fund (UNICEF), was established initially as a temporary emergency program to assist children of war-torn countries. That focus has broadened, and it has become a permanent agency. It now promotes child and maternal health and welfare globally through a variety of programs and activities, including provision of food and supplies to underdeveloped countries, immunization programs in cooperation with the WHO, disease control, prevention demonstrations, and, in particular, promotion of family planning in developing countries. Its International Children's Center, opened in the 1940s, has made a significant international impact through teaching, research, publications, and cooperation on projects related to the health and welfare of children.

United States Agency for International Development

The USAID has been in existence for more than 30 years and is committed to the goals of improving the health, education, and well-being of the populations of developing countries. "To achieve the goals of reducing poverty and creating economic growth, developing countries need healthy citizens who have the skills provided by basic education" (USAID, 2001). This agency is also working with countries of the developing world to achieve the Education for All goals by 2015 (see The Global Community I).

Other International Health Organizations

Many other organizations deal with health concerns at the international level. The United Nations Educational, Scientific, and Cultural Organization (UNESCO) offers assistance on international health matters. The Southeast Asia Treaty Organization (SEATO) and the North Atlantic Treaty Organization (NATO) both have health components. The World Bank addresses health problems through funding and technical assistance. The Food and Agricultural Organization works to improve world food supplies.

In addition to these international organizations, most developed countries have agencies that provide assistance, some in major proportions, to underdeveloped countries. The United States has many agencies, both within the federal government and the private sector, that provide other countries with health-related assistance. Government examples include the USAID, the Office of International Health in DHHS, the CDC, the Fogarty International Center in the NIH, and the Peace Corps. Examples of private agencies include Project HOPE, International Planned Parenthood Federation, CARE (the Cooperative for Assistance and Relief Everywhere), International Women's Health Coalition, and private foundations and missionary groups.

A description of a fascinating public health agency in Australia is provided in The Global Community II. For a more comprehensive view of world health and international health concerns, see Chapter 21.

THE GLOBAL COMMUNITY I

The developing world consists of 90 countries that were seen as presenting the most difficult development challenges in the 1960s and have been reviewed since then based on developmental statistics. Broad changes over the last 30 years have benefited these nations and the world as a whole. "Conditions in the developing world have improved more in the second half of the 20th century than in the previous 500 years" (U.S. Agency for International Development, 1998, p. 6).

THE DEVELOPING WORLD:

1968	1998
53% of the people were illiterate	Literacy has risen by almost 50%
62% of these illiterate people were women	Girls and women have significantly closed the gap in gender disparity in education
The average woman had six children	The average woman now has three children
More than one in eight of those children did not live to see their first birthday	Infant mortality has been halved
Nearly 12 million infants died each year, mostly from preventable diseases	5 million fewer children die every year
40% of the people were malnourished	17% of the people were malnourished
75% of the people did not have access to clean water or sanitation	The percentage of population with access to clean water has tripled, and access to sanitation has doubled
Life expectancy was just over 50 years	Life expectancy has risen by more than 10 years
80% of the countries were not democracies	71 more nations have become free or partly free
Annual per capita income was about $700	Annual per capita income has risen more than 60%
More than half of the people lived on less than a dollar a day	The percentage of people living in absolute poverty has been cut almost in half

SIGNIFICANT LEGISLATION

During the 20th century in the United States, an ever-widening sense of responsibility for health in the public sector led to passage of an increasing amount of health-related legislation. Some acts are of particular significance to the financing and delivery of community health services.

The Shepard-Towner Act of 1921

The Shepard-Towner Act of 1921 provided federal grant-in-aid funds to the states for administration of programs to promote the health and welfare of mothers and infants. The act ex-

THE GLOBAL COMMUNITY II

THE ROYAL FLYING DOCTOR SERVICE: THE OUTBACK, ALICE SPRINGS, AUSTRALIA

The story of the Royal Flying Doctor Service (RFDS) began with one man's frustration. John Flynn was a young Presbyterian minister working in the remote Outback and felt helpless and dismayed that so many people died or suffered because they were too far from medical help. He was a man of vision and saw the possibilities of two new industries that were in their infancy in the 1920s: radio and aviation. Together with Alf Traeger, who devised a transmitter for use in remote areas with no power supply to bring communications to the Outback (an area almost the size of the United States of America and larger than all of Europe), and Hudson Fysh, a young aviator (who later founded Qantas Airlines), they set up the fledgling Flying Doctor Service, which had its first mercy flight in 1928.

The service now is world famous and serves people living in remote communities in some of the harshest conditions on earth. The Central Station, located in the heart of Australia in Alice Springs, provides nearly 30,000 patient contacts a year, including field clinics and remote medical consultations. This station's 10 aircraft make nearly 10,000 flights, about half of which are evacuation flights. Over 150 nurses work for the RFDS. They practice in remote field clinics and are team members with physicians on rescue flights. The flights rarely land at an official airport; most likely, it is the airstrip of a sheep station (a large ranch the size of some small states), with the ill or injured person brought by four-wheel drive vehicle to the airplane. The distances are too great and too remote for the rescue team to get directly to the victim in most cases. If the rescue is for people involved in an automobile crash, the pilot will use the road as a landing strip.

This is a different type of population-based health care that encompasses predominantly public health nursing along with emergency flight nursing and obstetrics. The caregivers (doctors, nurses, Aboriginal health workers, and allied health professionals) refer to the *Central Australian Rural Practitioners Association* (CARPA) *Standard Treatment Manual* for caregiving (CARPA, 1997). Since 98% of the RFDS's clients are Aboriginal, the treatment manual includes protocols that best represent practice for the common presenting problems in remote areas among native people, while highlighting the role of native healers. The manual provides due consideration for the cultural aspects of therapy and recognition of the need to facilitate self-management when possible, since the clients may be hundreds of kilometers from

a town large enough to support health care services and the RFDS' remote field clinic may meet at the end of a landing strip on a large sheep station only once a month.

The daily operating costs of the RFDS are covered by a combination of federal, state and territory government grants, as well as donations from corporations and the public. They serve anyone in need. A tourist may be visiting the Australian Outback and become injured while hiking up Ayres' Rock (Ularu); the RFDS would assist that person in the same way that they would respond to an Aboriginal woman who needs help during a complicated delivery but who is living 600 km from the nearest health care practitioner.

Because the work environment is so stressful, a 24-hour, confidential Bush Crisis Line has been established. The personal support telephone network assists remote-area health professionals and their families in dealing with normal responses to difficult situations and helps them to maintain the well-being of themselves and their families by effectively managing cumulative and traumatic stress.

(CARPA, 1997; Royal Flying Doctor Service, 1999)

pired in 1929, but it set a pattern for maternal and child health programs that later was revived and strengthened through the successful and far-reaching efforts of the Children's Bureau, housed in the Department of Labor. Through the leadership of this bureau, many programs were instituted that enhanced children's health. Among them were services targeting prematurity, perinatal mortality, nutrition, mental retardation, audiology, rheumatic fever, cerebral palsy, epilepsy, dentistry, juvenile delinquency, and the problems of migrant workers' children (Elliot, 1962). The Children's Bureau maintained its impact through several administrative changes (it was moved to the Federal Security Agency in 1946 and to the DHEW in 1953, becoming the Office of Child Development) but was phased out in 1972. For several years, federal advocacy for maternal and child health per se was considerably weakened.

The Social Security Act of 1935

The Social Security Act of 1935 had tremendous consequences for public health. In addition to its revolutionary welfare insurance and assistance programs, which particularly benefited high-risk mothers and children, Title VI of the act financially assisted states and localities in providing public health services. These funds were and still are allocated on the basis of population, public health problems, economic need, and need for training of public health personnel. Many of the grants had to be matched by the states or localities. This served to increase their knowledge of and commitment to health programs. The act strengthened local health departments and health programs in most states (Scutchfield & Keck, 2003; Williams & Torrens, 1999).

The Hill-Burton Act (Hospital Survey and Construction Act) of 1946

The Hill-Burton Act of 1946 was an important breakthrough in nationwide health facilities planning. It marked the first real effort to link health planning with population needs on a comprehensive basis. The act provided federal funds to states for hospital construction. Allocation of funds, however, was contingent on the states' forming planning councils to survey and document needs for new facilities and other capital expansion. The Hill-Harris Amendments in 1954 shifted the emphasis from purely construction to broader health planning based on needs assessment (Hyman, 1982).

The Maternal and Child Health and Mental Retardation Planning Amendments of 1963

The Maternal and Child Health and Mental Retardation Planning Amendments of 1963 opened the door for improved services to selected mothers and children. Recognizing the nation's high perinatal mortality rate and the accompanying problems of premature births, handicapping conditions, and mental retardation, Congress, through this law, authorized grants to fund projects offering comprehensive care to high-risk, low-income mothers and children. It also provided grants to states to design comprehensive programs addressing mental retardation.

The Heart Disease, Cancer, and Stroke Amendments of 1965 (Pub L No. 89–239)

The Heart Disease, Cancer, and Stroke Amendments of 1965 are noteworthy for their establishment of regional medical programs, one of the first real efforts at comprehensive health planning. Fifty-six regions in the United States were designated, and each was charged with the responsibility to evaluate the overall health needs of its region and cooperate with other regions for program development. Although the amendments initially were categoric (limited to heart disease, cancer, and stroke), amendments in 1970 expanded the focus. The act was important for two additional reasons: it encouraged local participation in health planning, which was previously done at federal and state levels, and it funded program operations and planning.

The Social Security Act Amendments of 1965 (Pub L No. 89–97)

The Social Security Act Amendments of 1965 addressed a concern for some type of national health insurance. Title XVIII, Medicare, provided federally funded health insurance for the elderly (65 years and older) and for disabled persons. Title XIX, Medicaid, is a joint federal-state welfare assistance program that serves the blind, certain families with dependent children, the disabled, and eligible elderly. These two pieces of legislation have enabled many of the poor, disabled, and elderly to receive quality health care, which otherwise would not be available to them (Scutchfield & Keck, 2003; Williams & Torrens, 1999). More information on Medicare and Medicaid can be found in Chapter 7.

The Comprehensive Health Planning and Public Health Service Amendments Act (Partnership for Health Act) of 1966 (Pub L No. 89–749)

The Partnership for Health Act of 1966 promoted further advances in comprehensive health planning. It established comprehensive health planning agencies and coordinated the many categoric health and research efforts into an integrated system. It emphasized comprehensive health planning and cost containment at local, state, and regional levels. Its goals were improved efficiency and effectiveness of health care. Many problems, including unclear expectations, uncertain funding, and limited authority, prevented full accomplishment of these goals.

The Health Manpower Act of 1968 (Pub L No. 90–490)

The Health Manpower Act of 1968 increased the supply of health personnel by providing federal money to educational institutions for construction, training, special projects, student loans, and scholarships. The act replaced several previous acts that had similar goals but resulted in only fragmentary efforts to address the problem. Among them were the Nurse Training Act (1966) and the Allied Health Professions Personnel Training Act (1966). In 1976, Congress passed the Health Professions Education Assistance Act (Pub L No. 94–484) to effect a better balance between the country's health needs and the supply of available health professionals. One of its major emphases was to address the problem of physician maldistribution between underserved (rural) and overserved (urban) areas through educational incentive programs.

The Occupational Safety and Health Act of 1970 (Pub L No. 91–956)

The Occupational Safety and Health Act of 1970 provided protection to workers against personal injury or illness resulting from hazardous working conditions. This and other acts affecting the working population, such as workers' compensation, toxic substance control, access to employee exposure and medical records, and "right-to-know" legislation, are discussed in Chapter 29.

The Professional Standards Review Organization Amendment to the Social Security Act of 1972 (Pub L No. 92–603)

The Professional Standards Review Organization (PSRO) Amendment to the Social Security Act of 1972 had two goals: cost containment and improved quality of care. PSRO legislation created autonomous organizations, external to hospitals and ambulatory care agencies, to monitor and review objectively the quality of care delivered to Medicare and Medicaid patients. The PSRO review boards, composed mostly of physicians, examined such things as need for care, length of stay, and quality of care against predetermined standards developed locally. Failure to meet standards could mean denial of federal funding. The PSRO concept created considerable controversy, partly because the two mandated goals, cost containment and quality of care, are potentially incompatible. The federal government's primary emphasis on costs frequently clashed with local concerns for quality. Also, the lack of criteria or standards for review and the fact that governing was performed primarily by physicians made it hard to evaluate the program's success. Some studies, however, indicated a substantial cost saving in Medicare expenditures (Hyman, 1982).

The Health Maintenance Organization Act of 1973 (Pub L No. 93–222)

The Health Maintenance Organization Act of 1973 added federal support to the concept of prepayment for medical care. Congress authorized funding for feasibility studies, planning, grants, and loans to stimulate growth among qualifying health maintenance organizations (HMOs). In addition, this act requires a business employing 25 people or more to offer an HMO health insurance option, if such an option is available locally.

The National Health Planning and Resource Development Act of 1974 (Pub L No. 93–641)

The National Health Planning and Resource Development Act of 1974 was a major breakthrough in comprehensive health planning. Replacing the Partnership for Health Act, it combined Hill-Burton, comprehensive health planning agencies, and regional medical programs into a single, new program. It fostered not only comprehensive health planning but regulation and evaluation, and it promoted collaborative efforts among regional, state, and federal governments. An important contribution of this act was its emphasis on consumer involvement in health planning. The act was divided into two titles. Title XV, National Health Planning and Development, established national health priorities and assisted the development of area-wide and state planning through health systems agencies and state health planning and development

agencies. Title XVI, Health Resources Development, coordinated health facilities planning with health planning, replacing the Hill-Burton Act (Hyman, 1982).

The National Center for Health Statistics (Pub L No. 93–353)

The NCHS, established in 1974, arose from the earlier National Office of Vital Statistics and became part of the CDC under the PHS in 1987. The NCHS operates data collection systems that provide vital information for public health planning and service delivery. Display 6–3 lists the data collection systems presently used.

The Omnibus Budget Reconciliation Act of 1981 (Pub L No. 97–35)

The Omnibus Budget Reconciliation Act (OBRA) of 1981 had a profound effect on public health. In this act, Congress halted the progress made in most of the public health laws of the previous 45 years, substantially reducing their funding authorization. To shift more power to the states and cut the budget, the Reagan administration consolidated categoric grants into four block grants. The first block grant targeted general preventive health services; the second addressed alcohol, drug abuse, and mental health; the third focused on maternal and child health; and the fourth addressed primary care, which covered federal support for community health centers. Although block grants provide some advantages, these came with limiting restrictions on the amount and use of the funds. The result was a significant reduction in funding for state and local health programs. Under OBRA, new legislation was introduced in 1987 to increase quality control in nursing homes and home care.

The Social Security Amendments of 1983 (Pub L No. 98–21)

The Social Security Amendments of 1983 became law in response to accelerating health care costs. The act represented a major reform in health care financing from retrospective to prospective payment. It introduced a billing classification system consisting of 467 diagnosis-related groups (DRGs), with Medicare payments provided to hospitals based on a fixed rate set in advance (Scutchfield & Keck, 2003; Williams & Torrens, 1999). The fixed payment could not be increased if hospital costs for care exceeded that amount. Conversely, if costs were less than the paid amount, the hospital could keep the difference. Thus, a positive incentive was introduced to reduce hospital costs and promote timely patient discharge.

The Consolidated Omnibus Budget Reconciliation Act of 1985

The Consolidated Omnibus Budget Reconciliation Act (COBRA) of 1985 required employers to provide extended (up to

DISPLAY 6-3

The National Center for Health Statistics (NCHS) Data Collection Systems

Some collection systems of the NCHS are ongoing annual systems, and others are conducted periodically. There are two major types of data systems: those based on populations, which are collected by personal interview and examination, and those based on records, collected from vital and medical records.

National Health Interview Survey
National Health Interview Survey on Disability: a continuous nationwide survey of illness and disability—their amount, distribution, and affects—in the United States

National Health and Nutrition Examination Survey (NHANES)
NHANES I Epidemiologic Followup Study: provides physical, physiologic, and biochemical data related to nutrition of national population samples

National Health Care Survey
Ambulatory Health Care Data (NAMCS/NHAMCS): gathers data from physicians on ambulatory services by specialty and target population
    Hospital Discharge and Ambulatory Survey Data: provides annual data on such things as length of stay, diagnosis, procedures performed, and patient use patterns

National Home and Hospice Care Survey
National Nursing Home Survey: collects data from nursing home residents and staff regarding need, level of care, costs, and use patterns
    National Employer Health Insurance Survey

National Vital Statistics System
Birth Data
Mortality Data
Fetal Death Data
Linked Birth/Infant Deaths
National Mortality Followback Survey
    National Survey of Family Growth: consists of fertility, family planning practices, family formation and dissolution, and matters affecting maternal and child health
    National Maternal and Infant Health Survey

National Immunization Survey
State and Local Area Intergrated Telephone Survey

From National Center for Health Statistics Web site: www.cdc.gov/nchs, accessed 10/30/03.)

36 months) group-rate insurance coverage for laid-off workers and their dependents. This proved to be expensive for employers. The act also expanded Medicaid services and permitted states to offer hospice services to terminally ill Medicaid recipients.

Omnibus Budget Reconciliation Act Expansion of 1986

The OBRA Expansion of 1986 promoted a prospective payment system for hospital outpatient services. In 1989, a further OBRA expansion regulated fee schedules for physicians, encouraging less use of "high-tech" methods. Also under OBRA, the Agency for Health Care Policy and Research was established in 1989 to study the effectiveness of health care services.

The Medicare Catastrophic Coverage Act of 1988 (Pub L No. 100–360)

The Medicare Catastrophic Coverage Act (MCCA) of 1988 expanded Medicare benefits significantly. Coverage was extended to include a portion of outpatient prescription drug costs and greater posthospital extended care facility and home health benefits. Also, the MCCA set limits on beneficiary liability and provided increased inpatient hospital benefits.

The Family Support Act of 1988

The Family Support Act of 1988 reformed the federal welfare system to emphasize work and child support. It established child support programs, work opportunities, and basic skill and training programs. It included a requirement that recipients seek employment and that states establish an education, training, and work program.

The Health Objectives Planning Act of 1990 (Pub L No. 101–582)

The Health Objectives Planning Act of 1990 was significant for its support of the report by the Institute of Medicine, *Healthy People 2000,* with funding to improve the health status of the nation. Funding for health promotion and disease prevention was added in the 1991 legislative session. Ten years later, *Healthy People 2010* followed.

Preventive Health Amendments of 1992

The Preventive Health Amendments of 1992 placed a focus by the federal government on preventive health and primary prevention initiatives. It changed the name of the Centers for Disease Control to the Centers for Disease Control and Prevention. It enhanced services to Migrant Health Centers, especially in maternal and child health and community education. It promoted international exchange programs for public health officials from around the world who are interested in working in another country.

Personal Responsibility and Work Opportunity Reconciliation Act of 1996

The Personal Responsibility and Work Opportunity Reconciliation Act of 1996 is commonly known as the "Welfare Reform Bill." It amended the Social Security Act to reform the federal welfare system, imposing a 5-year lifetime limit on welfare benefits. It also changed Aid to Families with Dependent Children (AFDC) to Temporary Assistance to Needy Families (TANF). Finally, it restricted benefits to legal immigrants.

Nurse Reinvestment Act of 2002

The Nurse Reinvestment Act of 2002 addresses the nation's critical shortage of nurses. Developed with support and input from female legislators, the bill is well designed to address several issues contributing to the nursing shortage. It includes a media campaign to promote the nursing profession; offers scholarships for nursing students who agree to work on graduation in an agency facing a critical shortage of nurses; cancels student loans; provides grants to hospitals and other medical facilities that are willing to offer career incentives to nurses to advance in their field and to take on larger responsibilities in oganizing and directing patient care; and includes strategies to attack the burnout and frustration that are driving many people out of nursing.

IMPLICATIONS FOR COMMUNITY HEALTH NURSING

The structure and functions of the health care delivery system, as well as particular legislative acts, have had a significant impact on community health nursing. Community health nurses have had to learn to adapt to a constantly changing system. They have developed innovative modes of service delivery, such as community-based nursing centers for health education, counseling, and screening of low-income populations. They have learned to practice in a variety of settings extending beyond homes, worksites, schools, churches, clinics, and voluntary agencies. They have acquired skills in teamwork, leadership, and political activism. They have recognized the importance of outcomes research to document the value of nursing interventions with at-risk populations.

Community health nurses incorporate the three core public health functions while providing care to aggregates in the community (ANA, 2000), as the following activities for each core function demonstrate:

Assessment
- Assess the health needs of aggregates
- Collect data on health and safety hazards in the community
- Determine unmet community health needs
- Identify available health resources

Policy Development
- Incorporate community values and input in agency policy formation
- Formulate plans and policies that address community health needs
- Advocate for the health of the public and promote interprofessional collaboration

Assurance
- Translate intent of agency policies into needed services
- Assure access to services by community members
- Implement and provide services through programs

At the national, state, and local level, community health nursing has important ties to both private and public health agencies. Community health nurses may be employed by either type of organization. When serving in the public sector, they often provide consultation, serve on boards, volunteer their services, or collaborate with private-sector health organizations to ensure quality and access of care to the broader community. Examples include joint efforts to promote certain types of health legislation and collaboration to produce and disseminate health education materials targeting specific populations. Sometimes, community health nursing services operate within a single organization that combines public- and private-sector organization and funding. An example is the Metropolitan Visiting Nurse Association of Minneapolis, Minnesota, which is a combined public-private agency supported by taxes and voluntary funds.

Community health nurses also have many opportunities to serve in international health. Some work with WHO, PAHO, or other agencies to assist in direct-care projects such as famine relief, immunization efforts, or nutritional screening and education programs. Other nurses serve as health planners, assist with policy development, conduct collaborative needs-assessment projects and research efforts, or engage in program development.

SUMMARY

Many factors and events have influenced the current structure, function, and financing of community health services. Understanding this background gives the community health nurse a stronger base for planning for the health of community populations.

Historically, health care has progressed unevenly, marked by numerous influences. Primitive practices of early centuries were replaced with more advanced sanitary measures by the Greeks and Romans. The Middle Ages saw a serious health decline in Europe, with raging epidemics leading to extensive 19th-century reform efforts in England and later in the United States.

Organized health care in the United States developed slowly. Public health problems, such as the need for isolation of persons with communicable diseases and control of environmental pollution, prompted the gradual development of official interventions. For example, quarantines to control the spread of communicable disease were imposed in the late 1700s. Sanitary reform was pursued more vigorously during the 1800s. Local and then state health departments were formed starting in the late 1700s. By the early 1900s, the federal government had assumed a more active role in public health with a proliferation of health, education, and welfare services.

For years, efforts to address community health needs have been made by private individuals and public agencies. These two arms of service were not coordinated in the past.

ACTIVITIES TO PROMOTE CRITICAL THINKING

1. Interview someone at your local health department. How do the services offered compare with those listed in this chapter? How does the role of the community health nurse incorporate the core public health functions?
2. Make an on-site visit to your state health department or visit their Web site. Compare its functions with the core public health functions described in this chapter. Identify areas where improvement may be needed.
3. Conduct an interview on site with someone at a private health agency, voluntary agency, or community-based organization. Compare their functions with those listed in this chapter for private health agencies. Describe how this agency works collaboratively with public health agencies and other community organizations. What is the role of the nurse in this agency?
4. Look up various international health agencies on the Internet and explore Web sites that discuss current international health care issues. What topics are of concern currently? Are new epidemics or emerging strains of a virus being highlighted? What could (or should) a community health nurse in your local community do with this information?
5. With your classmates, debate the pros and cons of a strong federal role in health care provision, as opposed to decentralized (state and local) control.
6. Interview two consumers about their perception of the problems and strengths of our health care system. Select people who represent distinctly different age groups and life situations, such as a 25-year-old mother of three children and a 75-year-old widower.

Only gradually and recently have they begun to work together to form an emerging health care system.

The public arm of health services includes all government, tax-supported health agencies and occurs at four levels: local, state, national, and international. Each level deals with the health needs of the population encompassed by its boundaries. Each level has a different structure and set of functions. Public health services include three core public health functions: assessment, policy development, and assurance.

Private health services are the unofficial arm of the community health system. They include voluntary nonprofit agencies as well as privately owned (proprietary) and for-profit agencies. Their financial support comes from voluntary contributions, bequests, or fees. Private health organizations often supplement and complement the work of official agencies.

The delivery and financing of community health services has been significantly affected by various legislative acts. These acts have prompted such innovations as health insurance and assistance for the poor, the elderly, and the disabled; money to train health personnel and conduct health research; standards for health planning and delivery; health protection for workers on the job; and the financing of health services.

REFERENCES

American Nurses Association. (2000). *Public health nursing: A partner for healthy populations.* Washington, DC: American Nurses Publishing.

Barton, P.L. (1999). *Understanding the U.S. health service system.* Chicago: AUPHA Press.

Central Australian Rural Practitioners Association (CARPA). (1997). *Central Australian Rural Practitioners Association standard treatment manual* (3rd ed.). Alice Springs, Australia: Author.

Elliot, M. (1962). The Children's Bureau: Fifty years of public responsibility for action in behalf of children. *American Journal of Public Health, 52,* 576.

Erickson, G.P. (1996). To pauperize or empower: Public health nursing at the turn of the 20th and 21st centuries. *Public Health Nursing, 13*(3), 163–169.

Fitzpatrick, M.L. (1975). *The National Organization for Public Health Nursing, 1912–1952: Development of a practice field.* New York: National League for Nursing.

Flaherty, M. (1998). Close to closure: Home care agencies feel the budget squeeze. *Nurseweek, 11*(19), 1, 6.

Hecker, J.F.C. (1839). *The epidemics of the Middle Ages.* London: Trubner and Company.

Hyman, H. (1982). *Health planning: A systematic approach* (2nd ed.). Rockville, MD: Aspen Systems.

Institute of Medicine. (1988). *The future of public health.* Washington, DC: National Academy Press.

Lewis, R.A. (1952). *Edwin Chadwick and the public health movement, 1832–1854.* New York: Longman's.

Marr, J. (1982, Winter). Merchants of death: The role of the slave trade in the transmission of disease from Africa to the Americas. *Pharos,* 31.

Pan American Health Organization. (2001). *Equity & Health: Views from the Pan American Sanitary Bureau.* Washington, DC: Author.

Pan American Health Organization. (2002). *Executive Summary: Health in the Americas*. Washington, D.C.: Author.

Population Reference Bureau. (2002). *2002 World population data sheet*. Washington, D.C: Author.

Richardson, B.W. (1887). *The health of nations: A review of the works of Edwin Chadwick* (Vol. 2). London: Longmans, Green.

Royal Flying Doctor Service. (1999). Alice Springs, Australia: Central Station.

Scutchfield, F.D., & Keck, C.W. (2003). *Principles of public health practice*. Albany, NY: Delmar.

Shattuck, L., et al. (1850). *Report of the Sanitary Commission of Massachusetts*. Cambridge, MA: Harvard University Press (Original work published by Dutton & Wentworth in 1850)

Snow, J. (1855). *On the mode of communication of cholera* (2nd ed.). London: John Churchill.

Tyson, L.D. (2001). Healing Medicare. In E. C. Hein (Ed.), *Nursing issues in the 21st century: Perspectives from the literature* (pp. 459–468). Philadelphia: Lippincott Williams & Wilkins.

U.S. Agency for International Development. (1998). *Making a world of difference: Celebrating 30 years of development progress*. Washington, DC: Author.

U.S. Agency for International Development. (2001). *Child survival and disease programs fund progress report, fiscal year 2001*. Washington, DC: Author.

U.S. Department of Health and Human Services. (2000). *Healthy people 2010* (Conference ed., Vols. 1 & 2). Washington, DC: Author.

U.S. Department of Health and Human Services. (2002). *Medicare & you 2003*. Washington, DC: Author.

Williams, S.J., & Torrens, P.R. (1999). *Introduction to health services* (5th ed.). Albany, NY: Delmar.

Woodward, S.B. (1932). The story of smallpox in Massachusetts. *New England Journal of Medicine, 206*, 1181.

World Health Organization. (1998). *World health report 1998: Life in the 21st century. A vision for all*. Geneva: Author.

Howard, G., Bogh, C., Goldstein, G., Morgan, J., Pruss, A., Shaw, R., et al. (2002). *Healthy villages: A guide for communities and community health workers*. Geneva:World Health Organization.

Institute of Medicine. (2002). *Unequal treatment: What healthcare providers need to know about racial and ethnic disparities in healthcare* (pp. 1–8). Washington, DC: National Academy of Sciences.

Jonas, S. & Kovner, A.R. (2002). *Health care delivery in the United States* (7th ed.). New York: Springer.

Log on to mobilize political power. (2002). *American Journal of Nursing, 102*(9), 24.

Longest, B.B., Rakish, J.S., & Darr, K. (2000). *Managing health services organizations and systems* (4th ed.). Baltimore: Health Professions Press.

Lopez, A.D., Ahmad, O.B., Gulliot, M., Ferguson, B.D., Salomon, J.A., Murray, C.J.L., et al. (2002). *World mortality in 2000*. Geneva: World Health Organization.

Mays, G.P., Miller, C.A., & Halverson, P.K. (2000). *Local public health practice: Trends and models*. Washington, DC: American Public Health Association.

McCarthy, M. (2002). What's going on at the World Health Organization? *The Lancet, 360*, 1108–1112.

McDonald, R. (2002). *Using health economics in health services: Rationing rationally*. Independence, KY: Open University Press.

McKelvey, N. (2002). Building on the past, preparing for the future. *Reflections on Nursing Leadership (Sigma Theta Tau International), 28*(3), 28–31.

Health in the Americas (Vols. I & II). (2002). Washington, DC: Pan American Health Organization.

Pol, L.G. (2001). *The demography of health and health care* (2nd ed.). Norwell, MA: Kluwer Plenum.

Warren, M. (2000). *A chronology of state medicine, public health, welfare and related services, 1066–1999*. London: Faculty of Public Health Medicine of the Royal Colleges of Physicians of the United Kingdom.

SELECTED READINGS

American Public Health Association. (1999). President's proposal gives public health short shrift. *The Nation's Health, 1*, 6.

Boykin, A., & Schoenhofer, S. (2001). The role of nursing leadership in creating caring environments in health care delivery systems. *Nursing Administration Quarterly, 25*(3), 1–7.

Drevdahl, D. (2002). Social justice or market justice? The paradoxes of public health partnerships with managed care. *Public Health Nursing, 19*(3), 161–169.

Elder, J.P. (2001). *Behavior change and public health in the developing world*. Thousand Oaks, CA: Sage.

Gebbie, K.M., & Hwang, I. (2000). Preparing currently employed public health nurses for changes in the health system. *American Journal of Public Health, 90*(5), 716–721.

Gebbie, K.M., Wakefield, M., & Kerfoot, K. (2000). Nursing and health policy. *Journal of Nursing Scholarship, 32*(3), 307–315.

Internet Resources

American Nurses Association: *http://www.NursingWorld.org/ gova.politicalpower*

CARE: *http://www.care.org*

Central Australian Rural Practitioners Association: *carpastm@ taunet.net.au*

Department of Health and Human Services, Health Resources and Services Administration: *www.hrsa.gov*

National Center for Health Statistics: *http://www.cdc.gov/nchs/*

Pan American Health Organization: *http://www.paho.org*

Population Reference Bureau: *http://www.prb.org*

Rollins School of Public Health InfoLinks: Reference Resources— The History of Public Health: *http://www.sph.emory.edu/PHIL/ history.html*

United Nations Association of the United States of America: *http://uuu.unausa.org*

U.S. Agency for International Development: *http://www.info. usaid.gov*

World Health Organization: *http://www.who.org*

7

Economics of Health Care

Learning Objectives

Upon mastery of this chapter, you should be able to:

- Define the concept of health care economics.
- Describe three sources of health care financing.
- Compare and contrast retrospective and prospective health care payment systems.
- Analyze the issues and trends influencing health care economics and community health services delivery.
- Explain the causes and effects of health care rationing.
- List the pros and cons of managed competition as opposed to a single-payer system.
- Explain the philosophical implications of health care financing patterns on community health nursing's mission and values.

Nurses concerned with the delivery of needed community health services also must understand how those services are financed. In an era when health care resources are limited and provider organizations are competing for scarce dollars, it is essential for nurses to be knowledgeable about the issues related to health care financing and about ways to obtain funding to address identified health needs in the community.

Behind the financing of health care lies the science of **health care economics**. The field of economics, as a whole, is a science that describes and analyzes the production, distribution, and consumption of goods and services. It also is concerned with a variety of related problems, such as finance, labor, and taxation. It studies and seeks to promote the best use of scarce resources for the greatest good of society. The science of health care economics describes and analyzes the production, distribution, and consumption of health care goods and services to maximize the administration of scarce resources to benefit the most people. The goal of health economics—similar in some ways to that of public health—is to promote the greatest good for the greatest number using available resources and knowledge.

This chapter summarizes the changing picture of health care economics and its financial incentives and disincentives for enhancing the public's health. More extensive treatment of these subjects is found in the Selected Readings section.

ECONOMIC THEORIES AND CONCEPTS

Health economics can be better understood by examining the two basic theories underlying the science of economics. The first is microeconomics, and the second is macroeconomics. In addition, concepts of health care payment are discussed.

Microeconomics

Microeconomic theory is concerned with supply and demand. Economists using microeconomic theory study the supply of goods and services as these relate to consumer income allocation and distribution. They further study how this allocation and distribution affects consumer demand for these goods and services. Supply and demand influence each other and, in turn, affect prices. An increase in or oversupply of certain products leads to less overall consumption (decreased demand) and lowered prices. The opposite also is true. Limited availability of desired products means that supply does not meet demand, and prices increase. Microeconomic theory is useful for understanding price determination, resource allocation, consumer income, and spending distribution at the level of individuals and organizations.

Macroeconomics

Macroeconomic theory is concerned with the broad variables that affect the status of the total economy. Economists using macroeconomics study factors influencing employment, income, prices, and economic growth rates. Their focus is on the larger view of economic stability and growth. Macroeconomic theory is useful for providing a global or aggregate perspective of the variables affecting the total economic picture.

The economics of health care encompasses both microeconomics and macroeconomics, examining an intricate and complex set of interacting variables. It is concerned with supply and demand: Is the supply of available resources sufficient to meet the demand for use by consumers? It examines costs and benefits, cost-effectiveness, and cost efficiency: Are the resources expended achieving the desired outcomes? It studies the allocation of scarce resources for health care: Where should resources, such as funding for health programs and services for at-risk populations, be applied when there are insufficient resources to address all of the needs?

Health economics is a major field of study in and of itself. Health economists draw on economic theory to study and develop an understanding of the factors influencing the financing and delivery of health services. Macroeconomic theory has been useful in providing a large-scale perspective on health care financing that has resulted in various proposals for national health plans, health care rationing, competition, and managed care. These concepts are described later in the chapter. Microeconomic theory may prove more useful if health care competition increases, because the success of the supply-and-demand concept depends on a competitive market. The pros and cons of competition also are examined later in this chapter. Issues such as cost containment, competition between providers, accessibility of services, quality, and need for accountability continue to be targets of major concern in the 21st century.

Payment Concepts in Health Care

Reimbursement for health care services generally has been accomplished through one of two approaches: retrospective or prospective payment. Conceptually, these approaches are opposite each other. It is helpful to understand their differences and their meaning for the financing and delivery of health services, past and present.

Retrospective Payment

A traditional form of reimbursement for any kind of service, including health care, is **retrospective payment**, which means to reimburse for a service after it has been rendered. A fee may be established in advance. However, payment of that fee occurs after the fact, or retrospectively. This is known as the fee-for-service (FFS) approach.

In health care, limited accountability in the use of retrospective payment has created several problems. With third-party payers serving as intermediaries, neither consumers nor providers of health services were accountable for containing costs. Patients and providers alike often insisted on expensive or unnecessary tests and treatments. Because reimbursement was made retrospectively by the insuring agency, there was no incentive to keep a lid on this spending. Third-party reimbursement increased, along with rising physician fees, to create an inflationary spiral of escalating costs. Abuse of the FFS system made it more difficult to develop retrospective payment for other health care providers, including nurses.

A further problem associated with the FFS concept was its tendency to encourage sickness care rather than wellness services. Physicians and other providers were rewarded financially for treating illness. There were few incentives for prevention or health promotion in an industry that reaped its revenues from keeping hospital beds full and caring for the sick and injured. Although retrospective payment worked well in other industries, from a cost containment as well as a public health perspective, it was problematic in health care.

Prospective Payment

Prospective reimbursement, although not a new concept, was implemented for inpatient Medicare services in 1984 in response to the health care system's desperate need for cost containment. It has since influenced the Medicaid program as well as private health insurers. The prospective payment form of reimbursement has essentially eliminated the retrospective payment system (Longest, Rakich, & Darr, 2000). **Prospective payment** is a payment method based on rates derived from predictions of annual service costs that are set in advance of service delivery. Providers receive payment for services according to these fixed rates set in advance. Payments may be in the form of premiums paid before receipt of service or in response to fixed rate (not cost) charges. To correct unlimited reimbursement patterns and counteract disincentives to contain costs, prospective payment involves four classic steps (Dowling, 1979):

1. An external authority is empowered (by statute, market power, or voluntary compliance by providers) to set provider charges, third-party payment rates, or both.
2. Rates are set in advance of the prospective year during which they will apply and are considered fixed for the year (except for major, uncontrollable occurrences).
3. Patients, third-party payers, or both pay the prospective rates rather than the costs incurred by providers during the year (or charges adjusted to cover these costs).
4. Providers are at risk for losses or surpluses.

The concept of prepayment, or consumers paying in advance of health care, has existed for many years. As far back as 1933, prepaid medical groups were advocated to reduce costs and make services more accessible (Hyman, 1982). This pattern of prepayment for comprehensive services has since continued in a variety of forms. Examples of early plans were the Health Insurance Program of Greater New York City and the Kaiser Plan. The success of these two plans helped to influence the growth of the health maintenance organization (HMO), a type of managed care discussed later in this chapter.

Prospective payment imposes constraints on spending and gives incentives for cutting costs. The Federal government therefore enacted a prospective payment plan (Social Security Amendments Act) in 1983. The plan, called **diagnosis-related groups** (DRGs), is a billing classification system based on 23 major diagnostic categories and 467 DRGs that provides fixed Medicare reimbursement to hospitals. This system was enacted to curb Medicare spending in hospitals and to extend the program's solvency period. The regulatory approach of DRGs changed Medicare hospital reimbursement from a cost-based retrospective payment system, in which a hospital was paid its costs, to a fixed-price prospective payment system. It was designed to create incentives for hospitals to be efficient in the delivery of services.

Indeed, the prospective payment system has reduced Medicare's rate of increase in inpatient hospital spending and increased hospital productivity (Conger, 1999). It also has reduced hospital stays and unnecessary admissions and created a boom in home health care (D'Angelo & D'Angelo, 1999). A spinoff, however, was fierce competition among providers and mounting concern about quality of care—in hospitals, ambulatory settings, and home care.

The prospective payment concept also has proved useful from a public health perspective. Prepaid services create incentives for providers to keep their enrollees healthy, thus reducing provider costs. A potential, indirect benefit from fixed rates and reduced costs is that more of the health care dollar is available for spending on prevention programs.

Further understanding of health economics and its impact on community health and community health nursing can be obtained by examining methods of health care financing, issues and trends influencing health care economics, and the effects of financing patterns on community health practice.

SOURCES OF HEALTH CARE FINANCING: PUBLIC AND PRIVATE

Financing of health care significantly affects community health and community health nursing practice. It influences the type and quality of services offered as well as the ways in which those services are used. Sources of payment may be clustered into three categories: third-party payments, direct consumer payment, and private or philanthropic support.

Third-Party Payments

Third-party payments are monetary reimbursements made to providers of health care by someone other than the consumer who received the care. The organizations that administer these funds are called third-party payers because they are a third party, or external, to the consumer-provider relationship. Included in this category are four types of payment sources: private insurance companies, independent health plans, government health programs, and claims payment agents (Harrington & Estes, 2001).

Private Insurance Companies

Private insurance companies market and underwrite policies aimed at decreasing consumer risk of economic loss because of a need to use health services. No private insurer directly delivers health services, although some, such as John Hancock, have a history of subsidiary proprietary home health agencies. Private health insurers have been experiencing decelerating growth for more than a decade as the result of a shift by employees to lower-cost managed-care plans offered through the workplace. Even with this change, in bad economic times companies downsize and lay off workers and many people "feel they are only a pink slip away from being uninsured" (Brink, 2002, p. 63) (see What Do You Think? I).

There are three types of private insurers. First are commercial stock companies that sell health insurance, usually as a sideline. They are private, stockholder-owned corporations that sell insurance nationally; examples are Aetna, Travelers, and Connecticut General. Mutual companies, a second type of insurer that operates in the national marketplace, are owned by their policyholders. Examples are Mutual of Omaha, Prudential, and Metropolitan Life. The third type, nonprofit insurance plans, include companies such as Blue Cross, Blue Shield, and Delta Dental. These operate under special state-enabling laws that give them an exclusive franchise to the whole state (or a part of it) and to a specific type of insurance. For example, Blue Cross, in most instances, sells only hospital coverage; Blue Shield, only medical insurance; and Delta Dental, only dental insurance. Because they are nonprofit, they are tax exempt and at the same time subject to tighter state regulation than the commercial health insurance companies are. Combined, the nonprofit and commercial carriers have sold most of the private health insurance in the United States recently (Lee & Estes, 2001).

Independent Health Plans

Independent or self-insured health plans underwrite the remaining private health insurance in the United States. These plans have been offered through several hundred smaller organizations, such as businesses, unions, consumer coopera-tives, and medical groups. The HMOs and various companies' self-insured plans also are included in this category. Usually they may sell only health insurance; in some cases, they also may provide health services. They focus on a localized population. As a group, they generate a large amount of premium revenues but still only a small percentage of the amount generated by the nonprofit and commercial health insurance companies. In the late 1980s, the United States had more than 1000 for-profit, commercial health insurers and 85 Blue Cross and Blue Shield plans. The managed care movement since has become one of the most common and rapidly expanding forms of health insurance, with many companies dropping private insurer choices. Between 1997 and 2002, 93% of Fortune 500 companies reduced the number of health plans they offered their workers, and none increased their options (Hellander, 2002).

Government Health Programs

Government health programs make up the largest source of third-party reimbursement in the United States. The government's four major health insurance programs are Medicare, Medicaid, the Federal Employees Health Benefits Plan, and the Civilian Health and Medical Program of the Uniformed Services (CHAMPUS). As a whole, government funding is responsible for a lower portion of health care financing in the United States than in other countries in the world. In 1999, 432 billion dollars was spent on Medicare and other social welfare health programs, which is less than 50% of the actual health care costs. In comparison, almost 100% of actual health care costs were funded by the government in Norway, more than 85% in the United Kingdom, and about 75% in Canada and Australia (U.S. Department of Commerce, 2001). Of the government's health insurance programs, Medicare and Medicaid constitute the largest.

Medicare

Medicare, known as Title XVIII of the Social Security Act Amendments of 1965, has provided mandatory federal health insurance since July 1, 1966, for adults age 65 years and older who have paid into the Social Security system and for certain disabled persons. Medicare is the largest health insurer in the United States, covering about 16% of the population. Of the approximately 40 million beneficiaries, about 12% are younger than 65 years of age and permanently disabled or chronically ill with end-stage renal disease, and another 9% are 85 years of age and older (www.cms.gov, 2002). The Medicare population is projected to grow to 44.5 million by 2008 and to more than 63 million by 2027 (Figs. 7–1 and 7–2).

Medicare is administered by the Health Care Financing Administration (HCFA) of the U. S. Department of Health and Human Services. Part A of Medicare, the hospital insurance program, covers inpatient hospitals, limited-skilled nursing facilities, and home health and hospice services to participants eligible for Social Security. It is financed through trust funds derived from employment payroll taxes. Part B, the supplementary and voluntary medical insurance

WHAT DO YOU THINK? I

The increasing unemployment trends in the first years of the 21st century caused the number of uninsured persons to increase. In 1999, the National Institute for Health Care Management Foundation "calculated that for each half-percentage-point increase in the unemployment rate, an estimated 1 million people lose health insurance coverage" (Brink, 2001, p. 63). "More than 13 million uninsured people live in a household with income of at least $50,000 a year" (p. 58). Where are these people going to get their health care?

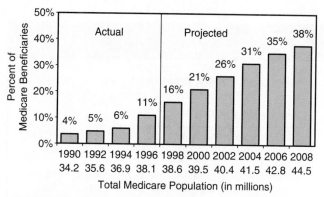

SOURCE: Health Care Financing Administration, *Medicare managed care contract report summary,* December 1990, 1992, 1994, 1996; Congressional Budget Office, *The economic and budget outlook: fiscal years 1999–2008,* January, 1998.

FIGURE 7-1. Enrollment in Medicare HMOs and other Medicare + Choice plans, 1990–2008.

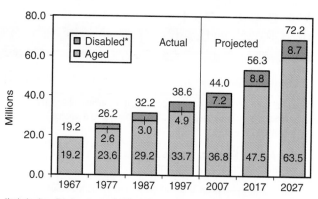

*Includes beneficiaries whose eligibility is based solely on end-stage renal disease (96,000 in 1997).
SOURCE: Health Care Financing Administration, Office of the Actuary, April 1998.

FIGURE 7-2. Number of Medicare beneficiaries, fiscal years 1967–2027.

program, primarily covers physician services but also covers home health care for beneficiaries not covered under part A. It is funded through enrollee monthly premiums (about 25%) and a tax-supported federal subsidy (about 75%).

Medicare was managed in the same manner for more than 30 years until August 1997, when President Clinton signed the Balanced Budget Act (Pub L No. 105–33). This act, which took effect in 1998, provided Medicare beneficiaries with markedly different options. In addition, the National Bipartisan Commission on the Future of Medicare was established by Congress in 1997 to consider options to preserve the fiscal integrity of the program while sustaining health coverage for an aging "baby boom" generation. One of the plans being considered by this committee is an increase in the eligibility age for Medicare, from 65 to 67 years, over a 24-year span that would coincide with the increasing age requirements for full Social Security benefits beginning to take effect. This could save $620 billion over 30 years and would affect the entire baby boom generation. Decisions on this plan have not been made. Financing Medicare benefits into the future while maintaining or improving coverage for elderly and disabled beneficiaries remains the major challenge facing the program (Firshein, 1999).

Among the most significant alterations brought about by the Balanced Budget Act are those to the fast-growing managed-care side of Medicare, which in 2002 covered about 30% of enrollees. To control Medicare costs while expanding the range of available health care options, beneficiaries are offered a relativity new program called Medicare Plus Choice Plans. This program seeks to accelerate the migration of patients away from Medicare's traditional and more expensive FFS program into various managed care options. Enrollees opting to remain in traditional Medicare will continue to be covered by the traditional FFS program, which gives patients unlimited choice of doctors, hospitals, and other providers. Those moving to the Medicare Plus Choice plans have a limited choice of providers but, in return, will be offered options such as joining coordinated care plans, includ-

ing HMOs, preferred provider organizations (PPOs), provider-sponsored organizations, private FFS plans, and on a limited basis, medical savings account plans. With this new law, Medicare has changed from an FFS, when-you-are-sick program to a preventive and wellness program (U.S. Department of Health and Human Services, 2002).

Although Medicare attempts to meet a need among the elderly in the United States, it has significant gaps. The original Medicare program has high deductibles, no cap on out-of-pocket expenditures, and no outpatient prescription drug coverage. As a result, it covers less than half of total health spending by the elderly and is less generous than health plans typically offered by large employers. Medicare Plus Choice Plans, however, provide extra benefits such as coverage for prescription drugs and more preventive and wellness services (www.cms.gov, 2002). These plans are paid for out-of-pocket by the enrollee or are covered as part of prior employer retirement benefits (Table 7–1).

With increased choices and options that provide more comprehensive coverage come higher costs for managed care organizations. Employer benefits and enrollee copay amounts alone do not cover the higher health care costs that older adults incur. As a result, many managed care organizations began dropping out of Medicare Plus Choice plans early in the 21st century. Those plans that remained committed to the Medicare Plus Choice Plan program increased enrollee copayments. In addition to these changes, Medicare cut payments to doctors by 5.4% in January 2002 and were expected to announce a further cut of 4.4% in January 2003, but it was overturned (ASTRO, 2004). If cuts continue in future years, it will only further increase physician or managed care organization withdrawal from the Medicare Plus Choice Plan program. Medicare's administrator described the likely effects: "You'll have mad doctors, there will be access problems, and seniors will feel it" (Pear, 2002, p. A4) (see Voices from the Community).

Medicare funding, drawn primarily from working people's taxes to benefit the elderly, will need to find new revenue sources in the future. As the population of elderly in-

T A B L E   7 – 1

Medicare and Medicare + Choice Plans, 2003

Original Medicare

Enrollee can go to any doctor, specialist, or hospital that accepts Medicare. In general, a fee is charged each time a service is provided.

Part A (Free) Enrollees receive all of the Medicare Part A covered services, which include

Hospital stays—with $876 deductible per benefit period (2004).
Skilled nursing facility care—limited to skilled care, not custodial care
Home health care—part-time skilled care from a nurse, physical or occupational therapist, or speech-language therapist, as well as durable medical equipment and medical supplies
Hospice care—for terminally ill patients; includes drugs for symptom control and pain relief at home, inpatient respite care, and short-term hospital care
Blood—for blood given at a hospital or skilled nursing facility

Part B (Monthly Premiums, Which Increase Yearly) Enrollees (who pay $66.60 in 2004) receive all of the Medicare Part B covered services, which include

Medical and other services—doctors' services, outpatient services and supplies, some diagnostic tests, and durable medical equipment
Clinical laboratory services—blood tests, urinalysis, and more
Home health care—part-time skilled care, as for Part A
Outpatient hospital services—hospital services and supplies received as an outpatient as part of a doctor's care
Blood—blood received as an outpatient

Medicare + Choice Plans

Medicare-Managed Care Plan

Enrollees receive services from doctors and hospitals that join the plan and receive most of their care and services from the plan's network.
Enrollees are asked to choose a primary care doctor; if the doctor leaves the plan or the enrollee desires a different doctor, the enrollee chooses another.
Enrollees can join or leave Medicare Managed Care Plan at any time.
Special rules might apply in emergencies or for urgently needed care.
The enrollee needs a referral to see a specialist, and if the services are from a provider outside of the plan's network, they may cost more.
Yearly, Medicare Managed Care Plans may leave the Medicare program, but other plans remain available.
Benefits/Drawbacks: Enrollees are provided with seam-free care but have limited provider and hospital choices. At some point a provider may leave the program and a new provider or hospital must be chosen. No paperwork is involved other than showing an identification card when receiving care.

Medicare Private Fee-for-Service Plan

The plan pays the doctor or hospital for the care the enrollee gets; enrollees may be required to pay a premium and other costs (copayments).
Enrollees may receive services from any doctor or hospital that is willing to give care and accepts the terms of the plan's payment.
Enrollee pays a fee (copayment) for the services received; there is very limited paperwork for enrollees.
Yearly, Medicare Private Fee-for-Service Plans may leave the Medicare program, but other plans remain available.
Benefits/Drawbacks: Enrollees can select their health care provider and hospital, but at some point they may leave the program and a new provider or hospital must be chosen. Care may be more fragmented than in Managed Care Plans. Limited paperwork is involved.

creases, fewer workers will be available to support the program. When Medicare began, there were five workers for each Medicare beneficiary. Projections for the year 2040 indicate that there will be fewer than 2 workers for each beneficiary.

Medicaid

Medicaid, known as Title XIX of the Social Security Act Amendments of 1965, provides medical assistance for children; for those who are aged, blind, or disabled; and for people who are eligible to receive federally assisted income maintence payments (www.cms.gov, 2002). It is jointly funded between federal and state governments to assist the states in the provision of adequate medical care to these eligible needy persons. The states have some discretion in determining which groups their Medicaid programs will cover and the financial criteria for Medicaid eligibility. To be eli-

gible for federal funds, however, states are required to provide Medicaid coverage for most individuals who receive federally assisted income maintenance payments, as well as for related groups not receiving cash payments. The states determine the type, amount, duration, and scope of services. The following are examples of mandatory Medicaid eligibility groups:

- Recipients of federally assisted income maintence, including Supplemental Security Income recipients
- Infants born to Medicaid-eligible pregnant women
- Children younger than 6 years of age and pregnant women who meet the state's assisted income maintence requirements or whose family income is at or below 133% of the federal poverty level
- Recipients of adoption assistance and foster care under title IV-E of the Social Security Act

VOICES FROM THE COMMUNITY

"My rent, my malpractice insurance premiums, my nurses' wages—indeed, all our expenses have gone up, but Medicare payments are going down. How can we make ends meet? Who will want to do this job? It will be harder for Medicare patients to find physcians willing to treat them."

Dr. Harold M. Sokol, Albany, NY (Pear, 2002, p. A4)

- Certain Medicare beneficiaries (qualified disabled workers and certain poor Medicare recipients)
- Special protected groups who lose cash assistance because of the cash programs' rules

Coverage includes preventive, acute, and long-term care services. Potential Medicaid recipients must apply for coverage and prove their eligibility in terms of category and limited income.

In 2002, 36 million low-income Americans were enrolled in Medicaid (www.cms.gov, 2002). This is 5 million citizens lower than in the mid-1990s. Many Americans were affected by dramatic changes in the scope and limits of federally supported income maintence programs and no longer meet the financial requirements for the Medicaid program. As with Medicare, Medicaid programs moved to a managed care concept, following mandates within the Balanced Budget Act of 1997.

The move has not been without its problems for those receiving Medicaid. Medicaid beneficiaries are economically disadvantaged, frequently reside in medically underserved areas, and often have more complex health and social needs than do Americans with higher incomes. Early evidence on the implementation of Medicaid managed care showed some improvement in access to a regular provider but more difficulties in obtaining care and dissatisfaction with care compared with those in Medicaid FFS. In recent years, many people who were never before eligible for Medicaid benefits have become eligible due to downward national economic trends, company downsizing, and corporate scandals. Subsequently, families have lost the health care benefits that were employer subsidized and now find themselves among those eligible for Medicaid managed care programs.

Medicaid's use of managed care has grown dramatically. The percentage of Medicaid recipients enrolled in a broad array of managed care arrangements increased from 10% in 1991 to 37% in 1996 and is projected to continue to increase. The future success of Medicaid managed care depends on the adequacy of the **capitation rates** (fixed amounts of money paid per person by the health plan to the provider for covered services) and the ability of state and federal governments to monitor access and quality. Quality performance standards are evolving, and ensuring access and quality of care in a managed care environment will require

fiscally solvent plans, established provider networks, education of providers and beneficiaries about managed care, and awareness of the unique needs of the Medicaid population. The success of managed care programs depends on adequate financial support through enrollee premiums, a focus on wellness and prevention, and corporate solvency enhanced by good management practices, moderate enrollee usage, and a stable economic environment.

Other Government Programs

A federal health insurance program known as the Consolidated Omnibus Budget Reconciliation Act, which was developed in 1985 and designated to be self-financing, protects unemployed workers who have lost their benefits. Another workers' compensation program is state administered and requires employers to pay health care costs of workers who sustain illness or injury associated with their jobs. In addition to third-party reimbursement, the government offers some direct health services to selected populations, including Native Americans, military personnel, veterans, merchant marines, and federal employees.

Claims Payment Agents

Claims payment agents administer the claims payment process of government third-party payments. That is, the government contracts with private agents to handle the claims payment process. More than 80% of the government's third-party payments have been handled by these private contractors, who sometimes are known as fiscal intermediaries (when processing Medicare hospital claims), carriers (when dealing with insurance under Medicare), or fiscal agents (as applied to Medicaid programs). As an example, Blue Cross, in addition to being a private insurance company, also is a claims payment agent for Medicare.

Direct Consumer Reimbursement

A second major source of health care financing comes from direct fees paid by consumers. This refers to individual out-of-pocket payments made for several different reasons. One is payments made by individuals who have no insurance coverage so that fees must be paid directly for health and medical services. Another is payments for limited coverage and exclusions (services for which the consumer must bear the entire expense). For example, many individuals carry only major medical insurance and must pay directly for physician office visits, prescriptions, eye glasses, and dental care. In other instances, the insurance contract may include a deductible amount that must be paid by the insuree before reimbursement begins (eg, the first day of hospital care under Medicare must be paid by the patient—$876 per benefit period in 2004). The contract may be established on a copayment basis, which determines a percentage to be paid by the insurer and the rest by the individual. Or, the individual may pay the remainder of a health service bill after the insurer has paid a previously agreed-on fixed amount, such as a fixed coverage for labor and delivery. Direct consumer payment has accounted for approximately one third of total personal health care expenditures in the United States.

Private Support

Private or philanthropic support, a third source, contributes both directly and indirectly to health care financing. Many private agencies fund programs, underwrite research, and provide benefits for people who otherwise would go without services. In addition, volunteerism, the efforts of numerous individuals and organizations who donate their time and services, provides tremendous cost savings to health care institutions. It also enables many individuals to receive services, such as home-delivered meals or transportation to health care facilities, at no charge. Philanthropic financing of health care has significantly decreased in the last two decades. However, continued private support is essential, particularly when federal and state monies for health and social programs have been severely restricted (Harrington & Estes, 2001).

TRENDS AND ISSUES INFLUENCING HEALTH CARE ECONOMICS

Cost Control

Control of rapidly rising costs has been one of the largest driving forces behind health care reform in the 1980s and 1990s. Despite a variety of cost-control strategies tried by public- and private-sector payers, health care costs have continued to rise. In 2000, health care costs rose 7.2%, the biggest jump in a decade, and employer-based health premiums were expected to rise 13% to 16% in 2002, the largest increase since 1990 (Hellander, 2002). Health expenditures in 1980 accounted for 9.1% of the **gross national product** (GNP), which is the total value of all goods and services produced in the United States economy in 1 year. Health expenditures rose to 12.6% of the GNP by 1990, to 14.1% in 1994, and then modified somewhat to 14% in 1997, but rose again and by 2000 were greaer than 15% (U.S. Department of Commerce, 2001). In 1999, HCFA (now called the Center for Medicare and Medicaid Servces) estimated that health expenditures would rise to $2.1 trillion by the year 2007; this prediction may hold true or be exceeded, but with managed care, the impact of HMOs, and the general concern about health care costs held by all members of the health care community, it may, hopefully, turn out to be an overestimation. Overall, our health care economic situation as a country is not as positive as it could be. Many groups are underserved; prescription medication coverage is not common in health care plans and is coming into the Medicare program in a limited way in 2006; and the poorest of the poor gain in numbers and go without any health care coverage (see Bridging Financial Gaps).

Health care costs in the United States remain high; however, in the 1990s they decelerated from the escalation experienced during the 1970s and 1980s, when costs were spiraling out of control. Nonetheless, in the early 2000s there was again a dramatic rise. A major factor contributing to the high health care costs of those two decades was that health care providers were rewarded for focusing on the tertiary level of preventative care—the highest level of health care services and the most expensive—rather than focusing on the less-expensive primary and secondary health care practices. Areas that saw increases included nursing home care, medications, and dental care costs.

A focus on primary prevention demands a paradigm shift in thinking about the practice and delivery of health care. It is one that fits more closely with the mission of public health. It expects that citizens are involved in their health care, are knowledgeable about their health status, manage self-care practices, and modify lifestyle behaviors to promote wellness. This creates a rich environment for community health nurses to work in collaboration with primary care practitioners and other health care professionals to keep the cost of health care under control while providing quality care focusing on primary prevention.

Cost sharing is a cost-containment strategy in which consumers pay a portion of health care costs. Insurance deductibles of $100 to $500 per person per year are typical, as are coinsurance rates of 20% per service. Cost sharing has successfully reduced utilization of health services without having negative health effects. Utilization review techniques have further enhanced utilization and cost control. However, when considering coverage for low-income and some elderly persons, cost sharing appears to have limited usefulness (Sultz & Young, 2001).

Global Cost Control

Internationally, health care expenditures also are of concern. Health care costs consumed a greater percentage of the Unites States' GNP than that of most of the 15 countries in the Organization for Economic Cooperation and Development (OECD) between 1980 to 1997. Health care expenditures remained the same over those 17 years in Turkey and Sweden and decreased in Denmark. Public health expenditures rose 60% in the United States during those years; in other countries, the increase was more modest, and in four countries—Denmark, Ireland, Italy, and Sweden—expenditures decreased. It seems likely that the health of citizens in the countries that have been spending less on health care over the last 20 years or that have spent a smaller share of their GNP might be poorer; however, this is not necessarily true. In life expectancy, women in the United States rank below 18 other countries and men rank below 24 countries, including Italy and Sweden (Display 7–1). Using health care dollars wisely, promoting health through primary prevention, and combining other factors such as heredity, diet, exercise, attitude, and a moderate pace of life all contribute to longevity.

BRIDGING FINANCIAL GAPS

Hellander, I. (2002). A review of data on the health sector of the United States, January 2002. *International Journal of Health Services, 32(3),* 579–599.

The U. S. health care delivery system has problems with accessibility, inequalities, increasing costs for health care and health insurance, and at times the questionable role of corporate involvement in the development, marketing, and patenting of pharmaceuticals. Highlights of these issues include the following.

- In 2000, 38.7 million Americans were uninsured for the entire year.
- Hispanic full-time workers are less likely to be offered employer-sponsored health insurance (69%) than are non-Hispanic workers (87%).
- One-third of immigrant Hispanics remain uninsured after 15 years in the United States.
- Eighty percent of the uninsured live in working families.
- Almost 12 million women of child-bearing age were uninsured in 1999.
- Approximately 4.3 million low-income mothers of school-age or younger children lack health insurance.
- Among private-sector workers under age 65, employer-sponsored health insurance dropped from 66% to 54% between 1979 and 1998.
- Almost 50% of companies that offer their employees prescription drug benefits have increased copayments and instituted tiers—lower copay for generic drugs versus a higher copay for brand-name drugs

and even a higher cost for "expensive top-of-the-line drugs."

- Some 37% of people who apply for insurance in the private insurance market are turned down, even with a $500 deductible and a $20 copay for doctor's visits.
- Elderly African-Americans receive flu vaccinations less frequently than white seniors (46.1% versus 67.7%).
- Only 4.1% of Medicare patients without drug coverage were receiving statins, although as many as 60% could benefit from their use.
- Over the past 5 years, 93% of Fortune 500 companies have reduced the number of health plans they offer their workers, and none have increased their options.
- Hospitals charge uninsured Latino patients almost five times as much as they charge health maintenance organizations (HMOs); in California, 40% of Latinos are uninsured.
- For-profit nursing homes are more likely to provide poor care than are not-for-profit nursing homes.
- Drug companies overcharged Medicare $1.9 billion for 24 common prescription drugs in 2001.
- The pharmaceutical industry had 625 lobbyists and spent $262 million on lobbying and campaign contributions in 1999 and 2000.
- Medicare HMOs dropped coverage for 536,000 elderly and disabled people on January 1, 2002; Medicare HMOs are also cutting benefits and raising premiums nationwide.

Access to Health Services: The Uninsured and Underinsured

A growing segment of the U. S. population has limited or no access to health care because they are without coverage for health services. The consequences of not getting needed medical care are not trivial and can result in unnecessary hospitalization and serious health problems. In 2000, 38.7 million Americans were uninsured for the entire year, a drop from 39.3 million in 1999 (Hellander, 2002, p. 579). These figures represent a revised Census Bureau survey methodology, which reduced the baseline figure of the number of uninsured in 1999 by 8%. Before the revision, the Census Bureau reported that more than 42 million persons lacked coverage in 1999. Who are the uninsured? They are predominantly workers and their families, many of whom have low incomes.

The poor and the elderly are among the most vulnerable to access problems. Although the prospective payment sys-

tem has cost-saving benefits, it also has negative effects. The prospective payment system has shortened hospital length of stays, on average by 24%. But researchers from RAND-University of California, Los Angeles, found that under the prospective payment system elderly patients were much more likely to be discharged in an unstable condition than before and that the risk of dying for these patients was much higher than before. This situation is only made worse by the crisis-level nursing shortage presently being experienced around the country. Measures were taken to reduce risks to discharged patients with a broadening array of home care services, which have been expanding since the 1980s (see Chapter 37). To control costs in the health care setting, the Balanced Budget Act also affected home care services. A benefit of the act was to decrease federal government spending on health care, by making numerous changes to the way programs operate (Harris, 1998). This is another example of reducing costs at the more expensive tertiary level of pre-

DISPLAY 7-1

Life Expectancy by Selected Countries

Life Expectancy by Country

Female		Male	
Country	**Years of life expectancy**	**Country**	**Years of life expectancy**
Japan	82.9	Japan	76.4
France	82.6	Sweden	76.2
Switzerland	81.9	Israel	75.3
Sweden	81.6	Canada	75.2
Spain	81.5	Switzerland	75.1
Canada	81.2	Greece	75.1
Australia	80.9	Australia	75.0
Italy	80.8	Norway	74.9
Norway	80.7	Netherlands	74.6
Netherlands	80.4	Italy	74.4
Greece	80.3	England and Wales	74.3
Finland	80.3	France	74.2
Austria	80.1	Spain	74.2
Germany	79.8	Austria	73.5
Belgium	79.8	Singapore	73.4
England and Wales	79.6	Germany	73.3
Israel	79.3	New Zealand	73.3
Singapore	79.0	Northern Ireland	73.1
United States	78.9	Belgium	73.0
		Cuba	73.0
		Costa Rica	73.0
		Finland	72.8
		Denmark	72.8
		Ireland	72.5
		United States	72.5

U.S. Department of Health and Human Services. (2000). *Healthy people 2010* (Conference ed., Vols. 1 & 2). Washington, DC: Author.

vention. As a result, real people with disease processes in progress are affected.

Medicare Plus Choice Plans, created in 1997, were intended to increase beneficiary participation in HMOs and other private plans. The Medicaid program, too, depends on managed care to deliver services to the 36 million Americans enrolled in 2001. Tight budget constraints on Medicaid operations have resulted in provider payment rates that often are substantially below market rates, contributing to access

problems. Capitation rates need to be sufficient to ensure that plans are able to care for Medicaid enrollees. The future success of Medicaid managed care depends on the adequacy of the capitation rates and the ability of state and federal governments to monitor access and quality.

In the private sector, numerous firms do not offer health insurance to their employees; almost 80% of the uninsured are employees of these firms or are their dependents (Hellander, 2002). Self-employed individuals also find it difficult to pay the higher costs of insurance premiums without the benefit of group rates. Consequently, many of the self-employed can access health services only by making expensive out-of-pocket payments.

Managed Care

The term **managed care** became popular in the late 1980s and early 1990s. It refers to systems that coordinate medical care for specific groups to promote provider efficiency and control costs. Although the term is relatively new, the concept has been practiced for many years through a variety of models of alternative health care delivery. It is a cost-control strategy used in both public and private sectors of health care. Care is "managed" by regulating the use of services and levels of provider payment. This approach includes the use of HMOs and PPOs. In contrast to FFS models, managed care plans operate on a prospective payment basis and control costs by managing utilization and provider payments. The managed care model encourages the provision of services within fixed budgets, thus avoiding cost escalation. However, if a system rewards increased FFS billings, managed care can provide only a partial solution to controlling utilization. These are issues that various managed care organizations (MCOs) are trying to eliminate.

Health Maintenance Organizations

A **health maintenance organization** (HMO) is a system in which participants prepay a fixed monthly premium to receive comprehensive health services delivered by a defined network of providers to plan participants. The HMOs are the oldest model of coordinated or managed care. Several HMOs have existed for decades, but many have developed recently. Enrollees benefit from lower costs, less cost-sharing, and minimal billing paperwork.

From 1930 to 1965, the HMO movement, supported initially by the private sector, gradually gained federal backing. Group plans were included as a part of Medicare and Medicaid legislation as well as the Partnership for Health Act. The HMO Act of 1973 demonstrated stronger federal support. Amendments to this act in 1976 lifted restrictions and further encouraged HMO growth. Currently, there are numerous HMOs with much internal diversity in the industry. However, HMOs continue to claim unique properties (Harrington & Estes, 2001):

- There is a contract between the HMO and the beneficiaries (or their representative), the enrolled population.
- The HMO absorbs prospective risk.
- A regular (usually monthly) premium to cover specified (typically comprehensive) benefits is paid by each enrollee of the HMO; few additional charges are levied, because the payment mechanism is not FFS.
- HMOs have an integrated delivery system with provider incentives for efficiency. The HMO contracts with professional providers to deliver the services due the enrollees; the basis for reimbursing those providers varies among HMOs.

Official encouragement, government subsidies, and the pressures for cost control spurred the growth of HMOs. Some HMOs follow the traditional model, employing health professionals (eg, physicians, nurses), building their own hospital and clinic facilities, and serving only their own enrollees. Other HMOs provide some services while contracting for the rest. Variations of the HMO model include solo practice physicians (some also continuing FFS medicine) who affiliate with hospitals. Americans enrolled in HMOs—whether through government programs (eg, Medicare), employer-based programs, or private insurers—number more than 130 million people. The HMOs have been viewed as a positive alternative delivery system because of their potential for conserving costs, which results from their emphasis on prevention, health promotion, and ambulatory care, with a concomitant reduction in hospital and medical care utilization. However, there are questions as to whether the cost savings might result partly from favorable selection of enrollees. Quality concerns also have been raised about the danger of underserving enrollees to stay within payment limits (Sultz & Young, 2001). Nevertheless, since the expanding years of HMOs in the early 1990s, many individuls have chosen a managed care plan.

The American Public Health Association has significant concerns about the ongoing changes in the organization and financing of medical care and health services and the impact of these changes on public health. While managed care arrangements hold the promise of providing affordable, quality health care for our nation, reports of financial considerations taking precedence over patients' health deserve attention. Specific issues of concern include denials of necessary care, underfunding of public health and prevention services, lack of accountability, loss of choice of health care provider, inadequate access to care (especially specialists), lack of comparable and consumer-friendly information and data about health plans, and abuses in marketing (American Public Health Association, 1998a).

These concerns have not gone unattended. The Health Insurance Portability and Accountability Act of 1996 and the Newborns' and Mothers' Health Protection Act of 1996 were passed by the 104th Congress of the United States and signed into law by the President. Both significant pieces of legislation addressed health care concerns among the nation's citizens and official organizations such as the American Public Health Association (APHA). The Health Insurance Portability and Accountability Act assured people that they would not lose health care coverage if they changed jobs. In addition, for a while in the United States, insurance for labor and delivery hospitalization covered only 24 hours or less after the delivery. Infants and mothers were being sent home in unstable postdelivery conditions. Newborns would go home when younger than 1 day of age, in some cases so soon after birth that body temperature was not stabilized and the ability to suck and take the breast or formula was not established. The Newborns' and Mothers' Health Protection Act eliminated such "drive-by deliveries," ensuring that mothers and newborns would have the right to remain in the acute care setting for at least 48 hours, covered by their insurance plan.

Furthermore, in 1998, Congress considered the Patients' Bill of Rights, modeled after recommendations from the Advisory Commission on Consumer Protection and Quality, which stipulated that managed care plans (APHA, 1998a):

- Provide emergency services
- Are legally liable for medical malpractice
- May not use "gag" clauses in provider contracts
- Offer sufficient access to specialists, including direct access to specialists for ongoing treatment and obstetricians-gynecologists for women
- Offer an external, accessible, independent appeals process for service denials
- May not retaliate against "whistle blowers"
- May not offer financial incentives to providers to discourage service utilization by patients
- Incorporate quality assurance programs
- Reimburse for approved clinical trials

APHA policy supports all of these reforms as they address, at the federal level, some of the problems occurring in the HMO plans during the years of significant growth.

Preferred Provider Organizations

A **preferred provider organization** (PPO) is another model of managed or coordinated care that developed earlier than the HMO. A PPO is a network of physicians, hospitals, and other health-related services that contracts with a third-party payer organization to provide comprehensive health services to subscribers on a fixed FFS basis. Because of contractual fixed costs, employing organizations who subscribe can offer medical services to their employees at discounted rates. In PPOs, consumer choice exists. Enrollees have a choice among providers within the plan and contracted providers out of the plan. The PPOs practice utilization review and use formal standards for selecting providers.

Enrollment in PPOs grew from about 10 plans in 1981 to more than 700 plans in the 1990s. The number of people enrolled in PPOs also increased, from an estimated 10.4% of individuals with private insurance in 1988 to 40% by the late 1990s, with the numbers leveling off as the decade came to a close. Early use of PPOs appeared to promote cost savings, but the long-range cost effectiveness of this model has yet to be proved, especially with the expansion of HMOs.

Other variations on managed care models continue to appear. One is the point-of-service network, which combines HMO cost containment with PPO freedom to choose providers. Enrollees may use their HMO's physicians or may select outside physicians by paying a higher coinsurance charge. Issues of cost, quality, extent of coverage, and freedom to choose providers remain dominant in discussions of the managed care concept.

Health Care Rationing

The concept of **rationing** in health care refers to limiting the provision of adequate health services to save costs, but in so doing jeopardizing the well-being of some groups of people. Rationing implies that resources are limited and therefore must be used sparingly. Its effect is to restrict people's choices and deny access to beneficial services. Although some consumer choice is involved, mostly it is the providers and insurers of health services who are unilaterally making rationing decisions to contain costs. When rationing occurs, there always is the danger of compromising what is acceptable to consumers and the quality of services that they receive.

Rationing in health care has been practiced for many years. With limited resources for health services delivery, government programs have had to establish strict eligibility levels and monitor the use of these resources sparingly to ensure their most equitable distribution. Private insurers, to maintain organizational viability and some kind of profit margin, have engaged in rationing to exclude enrollees who are at greatest risk for health problems (Sultz & Young, 2001) (see Bridging Financial Gaps). Advances in knowledge and technical capabilities through research and technology compound rationing decisions. When several individuals need an organ transplant and only one organ is available, what criteria should be used to select the recipient? Now that it is known that certain lifestyle behaviors, such as smoking or driving without restraints, create health risks, should people who engage in these activities pay a higher price for health care or be excluded from certain services? Should a younger person needing specialized surgery take priority over an elderly person needing similar care? There are no easy answers. Providers and insurers have struggled with these difficult policy issues for years. In today's health economics, the problems are even more complex.

Competition and Regulation

Competition and regulation in health economics often have been viewed as antagonistic and incompatible concepts. **Competition** means a contest between rival health care organizations for resources and clients. **Regulation** refers to mandated procedures and practices affecting health services delivery that are enforced by law. In a society where freedom of choice and individualism have long been valued, competition provides opportunities for entrepreneurism, free enterprise, and scientific advancement. Yet to promote the public good, oversee equitable distribution of health services, and foster community-wide participation, regulation also serves an important role.

Health care incorporates four major kinds of regulation: (1) laws, (2) regulations, (3) programs, and (4) policies (Sultz & Young, 2001). Laws that regulate health care include any legislation that governs financing or delivery of health services, such as legislation regulating Medicare reimbursement to hospitals. Regulations guide and clarify implementation; they are issued under the authority of law and are part of most federal health care programs. Examples include regulations governing project grants such as HMO development, formula grants such as Hill-Burton, and entitlements such as Medicare and Medicaid (Jacobs & Rapoport, 2002). Regulatory programs are created from free-standing legislative enactments and are designed to accomplish specific goals, such as accreditation and licensing rules for hospitals, public health agencies, and other health service providers. Regulatory policies have a broader focus and involve decisions that shape the health care system by channeling the flow of resources into it and setting limits on key players' actions. Examples of regulatory policies are found by reviewing state or federal budget proposals for funding programs such as health manpower training, research, and technology development.

From the 1950s through the 1970s, the federal government assumed a strong role in the regulation of health services. First, federal subsidy of health care costs increased, and there was greater federal control of state programs. Health services became regionalized and more comprehensive. Federal appropriations supported operational as well as capital and planning costs. There was greater federal support for health research and the training of health professionals. Group medical practice multiplied as a cost-saving measure. More than 60% of the population was covered by some form of prepaid health insurance, largely because of the effects of Medicare and Medicaid. There was an increase in interagency health planning cooperation and improved health program evaluation. Neighborhood health centers, community mental health centers, and other programs were developed to improve health care access for everyone. Although costs were rising, it was a period of relative economic stability that emphasized quality of care. During this period, the federal government assumed a major role, regulating the planning, use, and reimbursement of health care services.

In the early 1980s, the passage of the Omnibus Budget Reconciliation Act caused dramatic changes affecting health care. The federal government, having failed to contain rising health care costs, shifted responsibility for the public's health and welfare back to state and local governments. Large amounts of federal funding for health research, health manpower training, and public health programs were withdrawn. Continued escalation of health care costs prompted a concentrated effort among public and private providers alike to find cost-containment measures. From all this grew the competition-versus-regulation debate.

Competition, its proponents say, offers wider consumer choice and positive incentives for cost containment and enhanced efficiency (Sultz & Young, 2001); that is, consumers are free to select among various health plans on the basis of cost, quality, and range of services. Competing providers must develop efficient production and distribution methods to stay in business, and consumers, because of the required cost sharing that is part of the competition model, are more likely to use only necessary services. Examples of competition are increas-

WHAT DO YOU THINK? II

Managed care organizations and preferred provider organizations require a large pool of potential enrollees from which to chose. Selecting "healthy" subscribers helps to keep their costs down. Enrollees with preexisting health problems are expensive, and healthy enrollees help keep costs down. There are moral and ethical issues when such practices are instituted, but they are a reality and regularly occur. Similar practices are seen when people seek out life insurance policies. Many are rejected because they have high-risk lifestyle practices or chronic illnesses. What do you think about these practices? Do you think they are appropriate and "part of business," or should they be stopped?

ingly evident as more health plans, including HMOs and PPOs, vie with insurance companies for subscribers (see What Do YouThink? II). Many hospitals, too, compete aggressively for patients. For example, some hospitals now promote their services with advertisements depicting a new mother and father having a candlelight dinner in the hospital with their newborn infant in the bassinet beside them, or surgical centers promote the "hotel guest" concept with dramatically appointed rooms including meals and lodging for a guest.

Although it appears that competition offers the best service for the least cost, regulation advocates have for almost 20 years argued that there are at least four problems associated with the competition model: (1) consumers often do not make proper health care choices because of limited knowledge of health services; (2) competition may discriminate against enrolling certain consumers, especially high-risk, high-cost patients, thus excluding those who may need services the most; (3) the competition model may not encourage enough teaching and research—expensive elements of our present system; and (4) quality may be sacrificed to keep costs down. Regulation advocates conclude that standardization and controls are needed to guarantee quality and equal access. Leaders in the field have concluded that both competition and regulation are needed (APHA, 1998b; Sultz & Young, 2001; Kongstvedt, 2002). With foresight, McNerney wrote in 1980, "It is rapidly becoming apparent that what we need is a proper balance between competition and regulation with more effective links [and] regulation [should be] used as a force to keep the market honest" (p. 1091).

HEALTH CARE REFORM POSSIBILITIES

HMOs and PPOs have become the accepted methods of delivering health care in the United States in the past 25 years.

During recent decades, other methods have been considered, yet not passed by legislation and adopted. Two plans seriously considered by our nation that are worth exploring are managed competition and universal coverage with a single-payer system. We have come close to adopting the latter, and the benefits and drawbacks of each are important to discuss here.

Managed Competition

The idea of managed competition, as a health care delivery method, was born from the controversy regarding competition versus regulation and was driven by the need for health care reform. **Managed competition**, it was hoped, would combine market competition to achieve cost savings with government regulation to achieve expanded coverage. This idea, whose origin is credited to economist Alain C. Enthoven of Stanford University, has played a major part in debates on health care reform. It sought to address the two fundamental issues driving reform: cost containment and universal access to health care (Geyman, 2002).

Managed competition was seen as a market-based solution that placed accountability for resolving the health care crisis with the insurance industry. Insurers would be required to accept all applicants, without excluding those at poorer risk, and at the same time must control costs. Consumers would choose among competing health insurance plans in the form of "super-HMOs" (operated for profit and privately owned). These plans would compete for managed care contracts from large employers and group purchasers known as "health insurance purchasing cooperatives" (HIPCs). The HIPCs would be mostly geographically based (region or state), quasigovernmental organizations that would consolidate purchasing power in the health care market. The HIPCs would contract only with insurers whose plans both meet federal guidelines and include a mandated package of basic benefits—hence, the "managed" or regulated segment. Other common features of managed competition proposals include regulations that prevent screening-out of high-risk enrollees, penalties for companies that try to achieve better risk pools, community ratings to prevent companies from setting rates by risk pool, and guaranteed coverage for all who apply (Sultz & Young, 2001).

Proponents of managed competition cite many advantages. Managed competition would encourage insurance companies to compete on price and quality of services to attract enrollees. It would also offer consumers tax incentives to purchase the lowest-cost plans that meet minimum benefit requirements. Managed competition, although market driven, would be highly regulated to ensure quality and access. Besides HIPCs, some managed care proposals include the formation of two additional government bodies: a National Health Board to set the minimum benefits package, and an Outcomes Management Standards Board to set standards for the health plans' reporting on the quality of their care. Managed competition, as a reform concept, would have the potential for reducing expenditures and improving access to health care coverage.

There are problems, however, with the managed competition concept. It remains untested anywhere in the world, and many believe that it would fail to achieve the needed cuts in the growth of health care spending. Similar models, such as HMOs and the Federal Employee Health Benefits Program, have failed to slow health care inflation (Sultz & Young, 2001).

Some argue that managed care networks, which enhance managed competition and enable health insurance plans to control cost and quality, also would limit consumers' choices in selecting their own providers and hospitals. Consumers would have to pay out of pocket if they chose services from outside the network. Cost-saving incentives built into managed competition networks still have the potential for reduced quality of services and denial of care to enrollees.

Another major criticism of managed competition is its potential failure to provide equitable and universal coverage. It is possible that large employers would benefit financially under managed competition, but small businesses would find the cost burden heavy, and many individuals, such as the self-employed, would remain uninsured. A basic benefits package, critics argue, must address the special concerns affecting such groups as women and the elderly, including coverage for long-term care, home care, mental health, abortions, and prescriptions. Competition among providers would be inefficient in rural areas with fewer providers, such as county nursing agencies and isolated small-town hospitals scattered over great distances.

Although the private insurance industry and many physicians endorsed the managed competition concept, a number of respectable groups in the United States strongly oppose it. Among the organizations that oppose managed competition and support some kind of single-payer plan are the American Nurses Association, the National League for Nursing, the National Women's Health Network, the APHA, Physicians for a National Health Program, the American Association for Retired Persons, and the Older Women's League. Dissatisfaction with managed competition as a reform solution has spurred a host of different proposals, all addressing cost savings and access issues.

Universal Coverage and a Single-Payer System

A different approach to health care reform emphasizes universal health insurance coverage through a stronger role played by government. This so-called **single-payer system** would replace the almost 1500 health insurance companies in the United States with a single, public-sector insurer that would entitle all citizens to **universal coverage**. Efforts to accomplish this approach have been evident for many years.

Growing concern over the cost and accessibility of health services in the 1960s and again in the mid-1970s led to a renewed focus on **national health insurance** (NHI) as a solution; in this scheme, health insurance coverage would be provided for all citizens through a single-payer system. Since 1912, NHI has been debated while its proponents have sought comprehensive health care protection, in particular, for the aged and needy. Numerous attempts to pass some form of NHI resulted in piecemeal legislation that added various benefits for Social Security recipients. The Kerr-Mills bill (1960) set a precedent of public financing for elderly persons who were "medically needy" but not receiving public assistance. Medicare (1965) was the first compulsory NHI program in the United States. By 2001, it reached some 40 million people—only 16% of the population (www.cms.gov, 2002).

In the 1970s, the debate over NHI revived in full force. Many proposed NHI bills were considered by Congress. The seeming consensus over the need for government to ensure access to needed health services for the total population was misleading. Divergent interests and conflicting philosophies led to heated debate, with four issues emerging as core areas of controversy. First was the public-private mix: What should be the amount and nature of private health insurance involvement in the public program? Second was the cost-sharing issue: To what extent should consumers share in the cost of the coverage? Third, What should be the amount and nature of cost and quality controls built into the program? And fourth, Should an NHI program be used as a vehicle for reform of the health care provision system? Resolution depends, in part, on reconciling the major roles of large private health insurers, hospitals, and the medical profession along with the nation's inherent aversion to direct government intervention.

In the 1980s, study of NHI as an important concept continued. In 1977, Somers and Somers recommended that NHI in its ideal form should include the following aspects, and the intents remain current.

1. Universal coverage regardless of income
2. Equitable financing using multiple sources but channeled through one mechanism
3. Comprehensive and balanced benefit structure
4. Incentives for efficient and effective use of resources and discouragement of health care price inflation
5. Controlled competition in the underwriting and administration of the program
6. Appropriate and feasible consumer options
7. Administrative simplicity
8. Flexibility
9. Acceptability to providers and consumers

These recommendations continue to be viable and have permeated discussions on health care reform in the 1990s and into the 21st century.

Some proponents of universal coverage point to Canada's health care system as a model to emulate (see The Global Community).

As a strategy for health care reform, a major advantage of the single-payer approach is that accountability for cost-saving, quality, and access lies with a single payer, most likely the government. This contrasts with accountability resting in multiple, competing insurers under managed competition. Other advantages include its more comprehensive approach to reform, its limited role for private insurance, and elimination of the tie between health insurance and employ-

ment. Furthermore, a single-payer approach would significantly reduce administrative expenditures by eliminating the overhead costs of multiple private insurers. Supporters of a single-payer system, including the nursing and public health professions who are concerned for at-risk populations, believe that it offers the best approach for getting rid of inequities in the system, providing universal access, and reducing soaring costs.

Health Care Reform: Making the Change

Consumers and professionals agree that health care reform is needed in the United States. The disagreement lies in the form that it should take. At issue is a fundamental conflict in values between advocates of the managed competition model and advocates of the universal coverage or single-payer plan. On the one hand are those who strongly value the competition model, which ensures a free market, individualism, and the right to choose the type of health care desired.

On the other hand, proponents of universal coverage argue that more comprehensive benefits are needed to include the unemployed and those who are physically or economically disadvantaged and cannot afford health care. Furthermore, they argue that universal coverage emphasizes prevention and primary health care as key factors in reducing long-range health care costs and, more importantly, in ensuring improved levels of health for the public. *Nursing's Agenda for Health Care Reform* (American Nurses Association, 2002) supports this emphasis by promoting nurses as primary providers of health care. Nursing's agenda proposes a "core of care" that involves restructuring of the health care system, a federally-defined standard package of essential health care services, planned change to anticipate the needs of a population with changing demographics, steps to decrease costs, insurance reform, case management, assured access to health care for all, and establishment of public/private sector review. This plan is enthusiastically endorsed by more than 60 nursing organizations and 4 non-nursing organizations.

Designers of health reform have faced a difficult challenge in reconciling these conflicting views. As a result, elements of both models have been used to shape an improved system. Reform proposals include an incremental plan that allows for a flexible transition and opportunities for states to experiment with both approaches. Sultz and Young (2001) pointed out the importance of separating the task of financing (how insurance funds are collected) from that of disbursement (how providers receive payment). Financing might be tried through an income-based premium that would go into a publicly administered health insurance fund. The methods of collection and administration are undecided. Japan and Germany have used a payroll-collection method for years to successfully finance their health care systems. Supplemental financing (to adjust for low-income or no-income households) might come from an extra tax on the affluent or from a tax on products that are known to contribute

THE GLOBAL COMMUNITY

HISTORY OF THE CANADIAN HEALTH CARE SYSTEM

Canada's present health care system is modeled after the 1944 depression-born program proposed by Tommy Douglas, leader of Canada's Socialist Party. The party won a spectacular election, Mr. Douglas became Minister of Health and began immediately to plan a hospital service plan. It was to be (1) universal and compulsory; (2) comprehensive, providing all medically necessary hospitalization; and (3) premium financed, supported by those who could pay. It became effective in Saskatchewan in 1947.

In 1949, 80% of Canada's residents reported in a Gallop Poll that they wanted a government health plan. With Saskatchewan as a successful model, the federal government offered to finance 50% of each provincial hospital's operating costs.

In 1957, Canada's Parliment passed the Hospital Insurance and Diagnosis Services Act (HIDS). By 1961, all provinces were in the system. It was well received and was a huge success. However, Saskatchewan passed the Medical Care Insurance Act to take effect in 1962 — a modification of HIDS. Physicians were not happy and protested. The government gave them four choices: accept the Act and practice as the government dictated; test the Act in the courts (which was unlikely to be successful); leave the province; or withdraw services. Mediation and compromise with the physicians enabled them to practice under a plan that not all were happy with, and many physicians did leave the province. British physicians were recruited and stayed in the province. Surprisingly, salaries rose and the new doctors replaced the old.

Saskatchewan showed how a successful plan could be feasable, effective, desirable, affordable, and popular. Canada passed the Medical Care Insurance bill, which was adopted by all provinces between 1968 and 1972. Twenty years later, Canada's federal government could no longer afford the 50% of hospital costs it was paying. Presently, the government reimburses to the provinces based on the gross national product and a percentage of income tax revenues; this puts more costs on the provincial governments.

The Canadian Health Act of 1984 modified the 1966 bill. Each provincial government was to be responsible for providing health care to all citizens and for developing a plan that met the following criteria:
1. Provide universal coverage that does not interfere with reasonable access.
2. Make benefits transferable between provinces.
3. Provide insurance for all medically necessary services.
4. Provide a plan that is administered and nonprofit.

Today, Canada's health system is known as Medicare. Physicians are paid on a fee-for-service basis, with no deductibles, copayments, or dollar limits. Hospitals are paid according to global budgets, and drugs, dental care, appliances, and vision care are outside the national plan.

Rising costs are an ongoing problem for Canada, with health care accounting for one third to one half of provincial budgets. Canada is threatened with a high national debt, a soaring budget deficit, and 50% of all health care dollars being spent on an aging population. Still, the principle of spreading the financial risk for health care over the entire population has worked. Philosophically, "Canadians are endeavoring to develop a health care system directed to health needs — not a competitive system to serve an illness market."

Cumming, B. (1999). *Canada's health system today*. Retrieved October 3, 2003, from http://www.medinfo. ufl.edu

directly to health care costs, such as alcohol and tobacco. Disbursement of health insurance funds could occur in at least two ways. First, a strictly federal program could enroll all Americans who are not privately insured and disburse funds through a program similar to Medicare. A second option could be to disburse capitated funds from the federal government to the states for payment to providers. In some cases, state funds could supplement federal disbursement. Forms of either the single-payer or the managed competition models could be tried to accomplish disbursement, allowing states to adjust for local preferences and existing delivery systems (Sultz & Young, 2001).

Another aspect of health care reform that has been considered is a global budget. In this system, a single, nation-wide health budget, funding for which might come from income-based premiums (mentioned earlier) plus supplemental sources, would help to control certain aspects of national health spending. The amount of money in this budget would help to determine the size of disbursements to federal programs (eg, Medicare) and to the states. States could choose to spend more on health care out of their own resources.

A standard set of benefits, set by law and enjoyed by the entire population, regardless of age, health, income, and employment status, is an important health care reform element. Many countries have successfully implemented such a package under a plan called a "statutory" model. Various versions of this model have worked well in Austria, France, Belgium, Japan, Germany, the Netherlands, and Switzerland. In this model, health insurance falls under the rubric of social security and is funded through government-mandated payroll premiums or taxes. Payment is made to private-sector health insurers, called "sickness funds" in some countries. Individuals select among nationwide plans and choose their doctor and hospital. Reimbursement for services is made directly by insurers to providers. This model eliminates the need for separate programs such as Medicaid and Medicare. It also provides uniform and comprehensive benefits (Harrington & Estes, 2001).

Other issues to be addressed in health reform include making the FFS system more accountable, eliminating adverse risk selection, and providing informed choices to consumers. Although reform is underway, there continues to be a need for advocates of universal access and cost containment to influence the process. Furthermore, health reform proposals must be encouraged to focus on the central question: Do they fund the promotion of health and prevention of illness or simply pay for the diagnosis and treatment of those who are already ill? World Bank evaluations show that public health interventions repeatedly have been found to be more cost-effective than medical services, yet health reform proposals have paid minimal attention to this critical issue. In addition, "the current emphasis on managing medical care for cost containment disregards the social and environmental genesis of many health problems" (McIntosh, 2002, p. 85). Community health nurses can play an influential role in emphasizing the importance of incorporating health promotion services into future health reform efforts through political involvement and policy development. An example of such policy development is the international effort to control population expansion

The need for health care reform, however, is not new. Perkins examined the work of the 1927 to 1932 Committee on the Costs of Medical Care. More than 70 years ago, the committee defined *costs* as the major problem and *business models of organization* as the major solution (Perkins, 1998).

EFFECTS OF HEALTH ECONOMICS ON COMMUNITY HEALTH PRACTICE

Health economics has significantly affected community health and community health practice by advancing (1) disincentives for efficient use of resources, (2) incentives for illness care, and (3) conflict with public health values.

Disincentives for Efficient Use of Resources

All of the system structures that directly or indirectly promote cost escalation and prevent cost containment contribute to disincentives for efficient use of resources. For example, retrospective financial reimbursement, with its lack of setting limits, encourages spending on nonessential tests and treat-

ments and drives up costs. Tax-deductible employer contributions for health care coverage and nontaxable employee health benefits encourage unnecessary use of services and drive up costs. Lack of cost sharing by consumers and no financial risk for decisions made by providers create further disincentives to keep costs down.

Community health has been affected in several ways. Abuse of resources in some parts of the system means a depletion in other areas. Community and public health programs recently have experienced diminished federal and state allocations and severe budget cuts affecting even basic community health services. Competition from the private sector in home care and other community services, such as health education programs, has forced traditional public health agencies to reexamine their programs and seek new avenues for service and new revenue sources. Costs indirectly affect even appropriate use of nursing personnel in community health. Failing to recognize the differences in skills of community health nurses and less-prepared personnel, proliferating agencies in community health often have hired persons who are underqualified to give the needed high-caliber and comprehensive care. Finally, the advent of prospective payment and limits on lengths of stay have encouraged early hospital discharge, resulting in more acutely ill people needing home care services. The immediate effect has been an increase in the demand for highly skilled and more expensive home care services, which requires changes in provision patterns of community health care. The long-range effects of this phenomenon on family stress and caregiver health, on community health care reimbursement, and on the nature and structure of community health services, including the role of the community health nurse, have yet to be determined.

Incentives for Illness Care

The traditional American health care system inadvertently tends to promote illness because health care providers have primarily been rewarded for treating problems, not for preventing them. Hospitals have had more income when their beds stayed full of sick or injured people. The bulk of most reimbursable health services has centered on treating illness or disability in hospitals, nursing homes, and ambulatory care facilities, using physicians or skilled nursing care in the home—situations in which the individual must play the role of patient. Health promotional nursing activities such as comprehensive prenatal, maternal, and infant care; health education; childhood immunizations; and home services to enable the elderly to live independently have not been covered by most insurers.

A system that financially supports illness care affects community health practice in several ways. The number and severity of health problems in a community increase when individuals postpone care because they cannot afford visits to the doctor or clinic. It has been more difficult to encourage community clients to assume responsibility for their own health and to engage in self-care and prevention. Furthermore, such illness-oriented incentives create a basic societal valuing of illness care that, conversely, devalues wellness care. Health promotion and disease prevention efforts become second-ranked priorities in the competition for scarce resources. In communities where a greater proportion of community health practice is spent on treatment of disorders and rehabilitation, resources are limited for prevention and health promotion. Prepayment methods and the growth of managed care have been positive moves in the direction of a more wellness-oriented financial incentive structure. An HMO has the incentive to offer preventive and health-promoting services such as early detection and treatment of symptoms, regular physical examinations, and health teaching. Health care reform proposals show promise of greater recognition of the cost-saving value of prevention efforts.

Managed care has evolved but remains a "system of business strategies employed to make health care services efficient and cost-effective" with the "highest priority to market principles" (Drevdahl, 2002, p. 163). This makes individual rights significant, whereas societal obligations are pushed to the background. "Freedom of choice and action take precedence over issues of equality and equity" (p. 163). The MCOs have business-focused goals which are given more consideration than is equal access to health care.

Initially, MCOs focused on event-driven cost avoidance. Strategies included decreasing inpatient days, decreasing specialty physician use, using physician extenders, and implementing provider discounting. This evolved into a second stage, in which the principal objective was to control resource intensity and improve the delivery process. Strategies used to meet this objective included capitation of specialist costs, controls on units of service, patient-focused redesign, clinical pathways, and total quality management.

The emphasis, however, is now shifting to a focus on community-based health status improvement that goes beyond just measuring utilization of care or mortality outcomes. This focus calls for new strategies, such as community health assessments, identification of high-risk individuals, targeted interventions, case management, and management of illness episodes across the continuum (Weiss, 1997, p. 28).

Weiss (1997) believed that community health assessments will become standard quality tools for MCOs. Community assessments establish the baseline health status of a community and measure changes in the health of the community over time. Community health assessments must include source information that is both primary (health status assessment surveys, focus groups, and satisfaction surveys) and secondary (data collected by public health agencies and state agencies, such as birth rates, mortality rates, and incidence of communicable diseases in the community).

Improving the health status of a community mandates that the MCO—the organization providing health care services through managed care agencies, such as an HMO or PPO—be actively involved in accurately assessing the community's health status and the major issues facing the community. This would involve "informing health care consumers of how to care for themselves and empowering them to do so, and developing a community action plan that fosters collaboration among organizations and focuses on preventive service strategies" (Weiss, 1997, p. 29). Are these not the proposals that public health advocates have been making for more than a century?

In 2002, Drevdahl expressed concerns regarding the paradoxical missions of public health and managed care. One relies on partnerships for fostering health care equity and creating healthy communities and populations as it embraces a social justice mission, whereas the other "falls more along the line of market justice" (p. 163). Perhaps the incentive to keep costs down will be the motivation needed to work with clients at the primary prevention level of care. Although public health proponents have advocated preventive care as the best care for the individual, family, and community as long as the goal of community health is reached, the motivating factor becomes insignificant. If the community health approach is embraced by MCOs, the conflict with public health can be minimized and perhaps eliminated.

Managed Care and Public Health Values

Competition in health care is a reality with which community health practice must cope. Although competition offers several benefits, it poses some dilemmas for community health that may be difficult to resolve. Values underlying the competition model can be in direct conflict with several basic public health values (Drevdahl, 2002). Competition for the healthier and younger enrollee, for example, encourages MCOs to develop market strategies that entice the client to choose one over another. This is a win-lose situation for the MCO: one MCO wins while another loses. Public health, however, operates on the basis of collaboration and cooperation. Competition among MCOs serves a selected market partly determined by those who are able to purchase products or services.

Public health is committed to serving all persons in need, regardless of ability to pay. Traditionally, the competition model has focused on individuals and has been oriented to the present; public health is concerned with aggregates and is future oriented, emphasizing prevention. Competition establishes relatively fixed limits for service, whereas public health must remain flexible if it is to respond to the health needs of the entire population. These dramatic differences between MCOs and public health are beginning to blur and out of necessity will continue to be less adversarial and more collegial. By shifting their focus to community health as a systems outcome, MCOs can create several positive changes, including a safe environment, wholesome nutrition, healthy lifestyle, adequate education, sufficient income, meaningful spirituality, challenging work, recreation, and functional families (Weiss, 1997).

If enrollees in health insurance programs from Medicare, Medicaid, or other MCOs become empowered to assume responsibility for their own self-care and well-being, a cooperative and collaborative relationship can be achieved between MCOs and public health. Healthy competition may remain between MCOs for enrollees, but this level of competition will help to decrease costs and improve quality of care, as has occurred with telephone services and utility companies. Consumers can select their service providers, choosing the one that best fits their needs. Competition always has improved services and lowered costs in other markets, such as among retailers, and should do the same in the health care industry.

There are philosophical differences as well as constraints, such as civil service restrictions and political influences, under which most public health agencies must operate, that make it difficult for them to compete. Likewise, MCOs have stockholders, boards of directors, employees, and state and federal regulations that they must satisfy. Public health agencies must remain committed to providing the health promotion and disease prevention services that are their public trust. This may become the commitment of MCOs as they see the cost savings and health benefits of disease prevention. Yet some aspects of competition seem necessary if both forms of health care delivery are to stay in business. Exclusion from health care competition, freedom from unreasonable constraints, and dependable financial support are needed to maintain the organizational viability of many public health agencies. Competition also may stimulate new and innovative community health services and the introduction of new roles and revenue sources for traditional public health agencies. The evolution of the reform of health care implementation may see developing public and private health care partnerships, with MCOs contracting with public health agencies for certain services and MCOs more effectively expanding the reach of public health agencies into the suburbs or rural areas. Reform will need to continue to address issues affecting the delivery of public health services.

SUMMARY

Health care economics studies the production, distribution, and consumption of health care goods and services to maximize the use of scarce resources to benefit the most people. This science underlies the financing of the health care system. It is influenced by microeconomics as well as macroeconomics.

Health care is funded through public and private sources, which fall into three categories: third-party payers, direct consumer payment, and private support. Health care services have been reimbursed either retrospectively, typical of FFS plans, or prospectively, typical of most HMOs.

Several issues and trends have influenced community health care financing and delivery and are important to understanding health care economics and helping to improve community health. They include cost control, financial access, managed care, health care rationing, competition and regulation, managed competition, universal coverage and a single-payer system, and health care reform.

The changing nature of health care financing has adversely affected community health and its practice in three important ways: (1) retrospective payment without limiting costs, tax-deductible employer contributions for health care coverage and nontaxable employee health benefits, together with a lack of consumer involvement in cost sharing, have created disincentives for efficient use of resources; (2) because the health care system traditionally has reimbursed only for treatment of the ill or disabled, with no reward for health promotion and prevention efforts, it has promoted incentives to focus only on illness care; and (3) the competition model, which has long driven up health care costs and eliminated many from being able to afford health care services, has generated a conflict with the basic public health values of health promotion and disease prevention for all persons. Health care reform efforts in the 1990s focused on reversing these patterns by combining positive elements of competition, free enterprise, and regulation to allow all individuals access to adequate health care and to bring MCOs more in line with the goals of public health. However, unexpected challenges to homeland security and international crises bringing us to the brink of war have kept the concerns for rising health care costs off federal agendas as legislators deal with other pressing issues.

ACTIVITIES TO PROMOTE CRITICAL THINKING

1. Compare and contrast the goal of public health with the goal of health care economics.
2. Interview a community nursing administrator to determine the impact that managed care has had on community health and the delivery of community health nursing services.
3. Discuss the pros and cons of prospective payment versus retrospective reimbursement. How has each influenced community health and health care?
4. Form two teams with your classmates and debate the advantages and disadvantages of managed competition as opposed to universal coverage and a single-payer system.
5. On the Internet or in the library, locate recent articles on health care reform, managed care, and the public health response. What are the current thoughts on health care reform and managed care? What are the effects on public health services and the agencies?
6. Visit the APHA Web site (*http://www.apha. com*) on the Internet and read the most recent position statements or legislation affecting public health. What are some of the concerns? What can you do about the issues as a student?

REFERENCES

American Nurses Association (2002). *Nursing's Agenda for Health Care Reform.* Retrieved October 14, 2003, from *http://nursingworld.org/readingroom/magenda.htm*

American Public Health Association. (1998a). *Managed care reform: Fact sheet.* Washington, DC: Author.

American Public Health Association. (1998b). *Regulatory reform: Fact sheet.* Washington, DC: Author.

ASTRO (American Society for Therapeutic Radiology and Oncology). (2004). Healthcare economics. Retrieved February 14, 2004, from *http://www.astro.org/healthcare_economics/ medicare_reimbursement_and_coverage/PhysicianPayment Cut.htm*

Brink, S. (2002). Living on the edge. *U. S. News & World Report, 133*(14), 58–64.

Center for Medicare and Medicaid Services. (2002). Retrieved October 3, 2003, from *http://www.cms.gov*

Conger, M.M. (1999). *Managed care: Practice strategies for nursing.* Thousand Oaks, CA: Sage.

Cumming, B. (1999). Canada's health system today [Slide 34]. In *History of Canada's health plan* [On-line slide/RealPlayer lecture]. Retrieved October 3, 2003, from *http://www.medinfo. ufl.edu/other/histmed/cumming/slide34.html*

D'Angelo, F.G., & D'Angelo, A.M. (1999). Financial, legal, and ethical issues when providing health care for elderly clients at home. In S. Zang & J.A. Allender (Eds.), *Home care of the elderly* (pp. 17–33). Philadelphia: Lippincott Williams & Wilkins.

Dowling, W.L. (1979). Prospective rate setting: Concept and practice. *Topics in Health Care Financing, 3*(2), 35–42.

Drevdahl, D. (2002). Social justice or market justice? The paradoxes of public health partnerships with managed care. *Public Health Nursing, 19*(3), 161–169.

Firshein, J. (1999). Medicare panel weights higher eligibility age. *AARP Bulletin, 40*(2), 6, 17.

Geyman, J.P. (2002). *Health care in America: Can our ailing system be healed?* Boston: Butterworth-Heinemann.

Harrington, C., & Estes, C.L. (2001). *Health policy and nursing: Crisis and reform in the U.S. health care delivery system* (3rd ed.). Boston: Jones & Bartlett.

Harris, M.D. (1998). The impact of the Balanced Budget Act of 1997 on home healthcare agencies and nurses. *Home Healthcare Nurse, 16*(7), 435–437.

Hellander, I. (2002). A review of data on the health sector of the United States, January 2002. *International Journal of Health Services, 32*(3), 579–599.

Hyman, H. (1982). *Health planning: A systematic approach* (2nd ed.). Rockville, MD: Aspen.

Jacobs, P., & Rapoport, J. (2002) *The economics of health and medical care* (5th ed.). Boston: Jones & Bartlett.

Kongstvedt, P.R. (2002). *Managed care: What it is and how it works* (2nd ed.). Boston: Jones & Bartlett.

Lee, P.R., & Estes, C.L. (2001). *The nation's health* (6th ed.). Boston: Jones & Bartlett.

Longest, B.B., Rakich, J.S., & Darr, K. (2000). *Managing health services organizations and systems* (4th ed.). Baltimore, MD: Health Professions Press.

McIntosh, M.A.E. (2002). The cost of healthcare to Americans. *JONA's Healthcare Law, Ethics, and Regulation, 4*(3), 78–89.

McNerney, W.J. (1980). Control of health care costs in the 1980s. *The New England Journal of Medicine, 303,* 1088–1095.

Pear, R. (2002, October 25). Medicare cuts likely to reduce care access. *The Fresno Bee,* p. A4.

Perkins, B.B. (1998). Economic organization of medicine and the Committee on the Costs of Medical Care. *American Journal of Public Health, 88*(11), 1721–1726.

Somers, A.R., & Somers, H. (1977). *Health and health care: Policies in perspective.* Germantown, MD: Aspen.

Sultz, H.A., & Young, K.A. (2001). *Health care USA: Under-standing its organization and delivery* (3rd ed.). Boston: Jones & Bartlett.

U.S. Department of Commerce. (2001). *Statistical abstract of the United States, 2001* (121st ed.). Washington, DC: U.S. Government Printing Office.

U.S. Department of Health and Human Services. (2000). *Healthy people 2010* (Conference ed., Vols. 1 & 2). Washington, DC: Author.

U.S. Department of Health and Human Services, Centers for Medicare and Medicaid Services. (2002). *Medicare & you, 2003.* Washington, DC: Author.

Weiss, M. (1997). The quality evolution in managed care organizations. *Journal of Nursing Care Quality, 11*(4), 27–31.

SELECTED READINGS

Andrulis, D.P. (2000). Community, service, and policy strategies to improve health care access in the changing urban environment. *American Journal of Public Health, 90*(6), 858–862.

Cunningham, P.J., & Trude, S. (2001). Does managed care enable more low income persons to identify a usual source of care? Implications for access to care. *Medical Care, 39*(7), 716–726.

Drummond, M., & McGuire, A. (2002). *Economic evaluation in health care: Merging theory with practice.* New York: Oxford University Press.

Emanuel, E.J. (2000). Justice and managed care: Four principles for the just allocation of health care. *Hastings Center Report, 30*(2), 8–16.

Federwisch, A. (1999). Runaway costs: How can we rein in healthcare expenses? *NurseWeek, 12*(4), 1, 10.

Finkelman, A.W. (2001). *Managed care: A nursing perspective.* Upper Saddle River, NJ: Prentice-Hall Health.

Goody, B., Mentnech, R., & Riley, G. (2002). Changing nature of public and private health insurance. *Health Care Financing Review, 23*(3), 1–7.

Institute of Medicine. (2001). *Coverage matters: Insurance and health care.* Washington, DC: National Academy Press.

Langner, B.E. (2001). The uninsured—A chronic American problem: Finding the elusive solution. *Journal of Professional Nursing 17*(6), 277.

Leavitt, J.K., & Beacham, T.B. (2002). Policy perspectives: The effects of September 11 on health policy. *American Journal of Nursing, 102*(9), 99–102.

Loewy, E.H., & Loewy, R.S. (2001). *Changing health care systems from ethical, economic, and cross cultural perspectives.* Norwell, MA: Kluwer Plenum.

Longest, B.B., Jr. (2001). *Contemporary health policy.* Washington, DC: Health Administration Press.

Mays, G.P., Halverson, P.K., & Stevens, R. (2001). The contributions of managed care plans to public health practice: Evidence from the nation's largest local health departments. *Public Health Reports, 116*(1 Suppl. 2001), 50–67.

McDonald, R. (2002). *Using health economics in health services: Rationing rationally?* Philadelphia: Open University Press.

Mechanic, D. (2000). Managed care and the imperative for a new professional ethic. *Health Affairs, 19*(5), 100–111.

Mossialos, E., Dixon, A., & Figueras, J. (Eds.). (2002). *Funding health care: Options for Europe.* Philadelphia: Open University Press.

Mufti, M.H. (2000). *Healthcare development strategies in the Kingdom of Saudi Arabia.* Norwell, MA: Kluwer Plenum.

Novic, L., & Mays, G.P. (2001). *Public health administration: Principles for population-based management.* Gaithersburg, MD: Aspen.

Nunn, P., Harries, A., Godfrey-Faussett, P., Gupta, R., Maher, D., & Raviglione, M. (2002). The research agenda for improving health policy, systems performance, and service delivery for tuberculosis control: A WHO perspective. *Bulletin of the World Health Organization, 80,* 471–476.

Oleske, D.M. (2001). *Epidemiology and the delivery of health care services: Methods and applications* (2nd ed.). Norwell, MA: Kluwer Plenum.

Pol, L.G., & Thomas, R.K. (2001). *The demography of health and health care* (2nd ed.). Norwell, MA: Kluwer Plenum.

Stone, P.W., Curran, C.R., & Bakken, S. (2002). Economic evidence for evidence-based practice. *Journal of Nursing Scholarship, 34*(3), 277–282.

Walshe, K. (2002). *Regulating healthcare: A prescription for improvement?* Philadelphia: Open University Press.

Internet Resources

American Nurses Association: *http://www.nusingworld.org/readingroom/rnagenda.htm*

Center for Medicare and Medicaid Services: *http://www.cms.hhs.gov*

Joint Commission on Accreditation of Healthcare Organizations: *http://www.jcaho.org*

Kaiser Family Foundation: *http://www.kff.org*

Medicaid: *http://www.medicaid.gov*

Medicare: *http://www.medicare.gov*

National Committee for Quality Assurance: *http://www.ncqa.org*

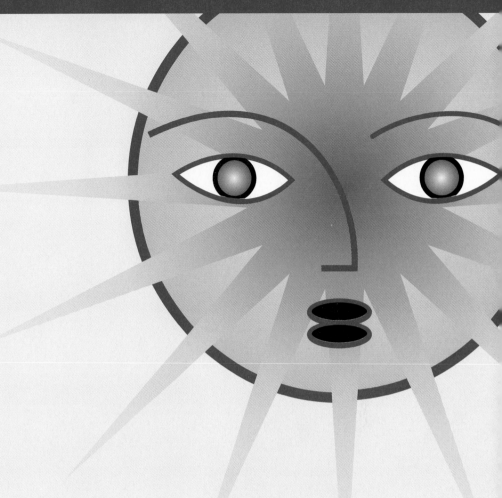

Public Health Principles in Community Health Nursing

8

Epidemiology in Community Health Care

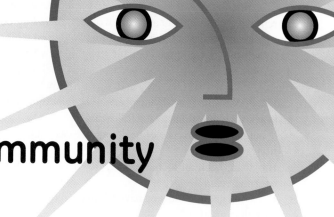

Learning Objectives

Upon mastery of this chapter, you should be able to:

- Explore the historical roots of epidemiology.
- Explain the host, agent, and environment model.
- Describe theories of causality in health and illness.
- Explain a "web of causation" matrix that assists you with recognition of multicausal factors in disease or injury occurrences.
- Define immunity and compare passive immunity, active immunity, cross-immunity, and herd immunity.
- Explain how epidemiologists determine populations at risk.
- Identify the four stages of a disease or health condition.
- List the major sources of epidemiologic information.
- Distinguish between incidence and prevalence in health and illness states.
- Use epidemiologic methods to describe an aggregate's health.
- Discuss the types of epidemiologic studies that are useful for researching aggregate health.
- Use the seven-step research process when conducting an epidemiologic study.

Epidemiology is the study of the determinants and distribution of health, disease, and injuries in human populations. It is a specialized form of scientific research that can provide health care workers, including community health nurses, with a body of knowledge on which to base their practice and methods for studying new and existing problems. The term is derived from the Greek words *epi* (upon), *demos* (the people), and *logos* (knowledge): the knowledge or study of what happens to people. Epidemiologists ask such questions as the following:

- What is the occurrence of health and disease in a population?
- Has there been an increase or decrease in a health state over the years?
- Does one geographic area have a higher frequency of disease than another?
- What characteristics of people with a particular condition distinguish them from those without the condition?
- What factors need to be present to cause disease or injury?
- Is one treatment or program more effective than another in changing the health of affected people?
- Why do some people recover from a disease and others do not?

The ultimate goals of epidemiology are to determine the scale and nature of human health problems, identify solutions to prevent disease, and improve the health of the entire population (Fos & Fine, 2000).

Epidemiology offers community health nurses a specific methodology for assessing the health of aggregates. Furthermore, it provides a frame of reference for investigating and improving clinical practice in any setting. For example, if a community health nursing goal is to lower the incidence of sexually transmitted diseases (STDs) in a given community, such a prevention plan requires information about population groups. How many STD cases have been reported in this community in the past year? What is the expected number of STD cases (the morbidity rate)? Which members of the community are at highest risk of contracting STDs? Any program of screening, treatment, or health promotion regarding STDs must be based on this kind of information about population groups to be effective. Whether the community health nurse's goals are to improve a population's nutrition, control the spread of human immunodeficiency virus (HIV), deal with health problems created by a flood, protect and promote the health of battered women, or reduce the number of automobile crash injuries and fatalities at a specific intersection, epidemiologic data are essential.

HISTORICAL ROOTS OF EPIDEMIOLOGY

The roots of epidemiology can be traced to Hippocrates, a Greek physician who lived from about 460 to 375 BC and who is sometimes referred to as the first epidemiologist. Hippocrates and other members of the Hippocratic School be-

lieved that disease not only affects individuals but is a mass phenomenon. This was one of the earliest associations of the occurrence of disease with lifestyle and environmental factors, specifically geographic location (Lawson & Williams, 2001). It was not until the late 19th century, however, that modern epidemiology came into existence.

An **epidemic** refers to a disease occurrence that clearly exceeds the normal or expected frequency in a community or region. In past centuries, epidemics of cholera, bubonic plague, and smallpox swept through community after community, killing thousands of people, changing the community structure, and altering the lifestyle of masses of people. When an epidemic, such as the bubonic plague (also called pneumonic plague, the plague, or the Black Death) or acquired immunodeficiency syndrome (AIDS), is worldwide in distribution, it is called a **pandemic**.

Epidemic and pandemic diseases clearly prompted the development of epidemiology as a science. It became a distinct branch of medical science through its concern with massive waves of infectious diseases. In 1348, the Black Death (caused by the bacillus *Yersinia pestis*) swept through continental Europe and England, killing millions of people and lowering life expectancy to 20 years from 30 to 35 years (see What Do You Think?). In England alone, approximately one fourth of the population died from the plague.

The plague continued in Europe, but with less force, for three centuries and then waned, only to reappear in an epidemic in Hong Kong in 1896. Shibasaburo Kitasato (1852–1931), a Japanese bacteriologist, discovered the plague bacillus during this Hong Kong epidemic; within 10 years, epidemiolo-

WHAT DO YOU THINK?

IMPACT OF THE PLAGUE

When the plague appeared in the 14th century and periodically returned throughout the next two centuries, it crystallized the interest in public health that had begun with the isolation of lepers in the 13th century. In some cities, "books of the dead" were kept. They amounted to comprehensive mortality records used to identify epidemics and follow their course. Mortality rates in the early plague epidemics were staggering, with up to half of the population dying. In response to the first plague pandemic, city-states in Northern Italy instituted a series of public health measures designed to protect the health of the elite, such as quarantining ships suspected of carrying disease for 40 days.

Beaglehole, R., & Bonita, R. (1997). *Public health at the crossroads: Achievements and prospects.* Cambridge, England: Cambridge University Press.

gists had traced its life cycle from rats to their infected fleas that bit humans. Now intervention was possible, and public health officials declared war on rats, seeking to make ships and wharf buildings ratproof. The first major campaign against rats that took place in California, after an outbreak of plague in 1900, was successful. However, wild rodents, especially ground squirrels, as well as rabbits and domestic cats, remained a natural reservoir of the plague bacillus. Cases still occur occasionally in the western half of the United States, and there are periodic outbreaks in large areas of South America; north-central, eastern, and southern Africa; and central and Southeast Asia (Chin, 1999). The continuing presence of a disease or infectious agent in a given geographic area, such as plague in Vietnam or malaria in the tropics of Brazil and Indonesia, means that the disease is **endemic** to that area.

As the threat of the great epidemic diseases declined, epidemiologists began to focus on other infectious diseases, such as diphtheria, infant diarrhea, typhoid, tuberculosis, and syphilis. They also studied diseases linked to occupations, such as scurvy among sailors and scrotal cancer among chimney sweeps. In recent years, epidemiologists have turned to the study of major causes of death and disability, such as cancer, cardiovascular disorders, AIDS, violence, mental illness, accidents, arthritis, and congenital defects.

Nursing's epidemiologic roots can be traced to Florence Nightingale (1820–1910). Nightingale often obtained advice on issues related to hospital statistics and disease classification from her close friend William Farr, who established the field of medical statistics as chief statistician of England's General Register Office for health and vital statistics. Her detailed records, morbidity (sickness) statistics, and careful description of the health conditions among the soldiers in the Crimean War represent one of the first systematic descriptive studies of the distribution and patterns of disease in a population. She used wedge-shaped graphs, circles, and squares that were shaded and colored to illustrate preventable deaths of the hospitalized Crimean soldiers, compared with hospitalized soldiers in England at the time. The sophisticated level of detail in her studies heralded her as the first nursing researcher. Changes made according to her suggestions, which seem common knowledge now—such as establishing a clean environment, providing edible foods, cleaning wounds and using new bandages, and separating infectious soldiers from injured soldiers—brought dramatic proof of the authenticity of her observations and knowledge. Forty out of every 100 British troops were dying in the Crimea before Nightingale instituted environmental and nutritional changes in the hospital and field. When her work was finished, the mortality (death) rate was only 2%.

Nightingale's use of statistical data along with her commitment to environmental reform strongly influenced nursing's evolution into a profession whose service addressed public health problems as well as hospital care (Kopf, 1978). As nursing has evolved, community health nurses have been increasingly challenged to intervene at the aggregate level, using epidemiologic approaches to address the needs of high-risk groups and populations.

Eras in the Evolution of Modern Epidemiology

Modern epidemiology can be described as having four distinct eras, each based on causal thinking; sanitary statistics, infectious-disease epidemiology, chronic-disease epidemiology, and, emerging now, eco-epidemiology.

Early causal thinking was dominated by the *miasma theory,* which had its origins in the work of the Hippocratic School and was formally developed in the early 1700s. This theory held that a substance called miasma was composed of malodorous and poisonous particles generated by the decomposition of organic matter and was the cause of disease. Prevention based on this theory attempted to eliminate the sources of the miasma or polluted vapors. Despite its faulty reasoning, this type of prevention had positive consequences because it made people aware that decaying organic matter can be a source of infectious diseases. This theory dominated until the first half of the 19th century.

The era of infectious-disease epidemiology was dominated by the *contagion theory* of disease, which had developed by the mid-18th century. Prompted by the development of increasingly sophisticated microscopes, this theory attempted to identify the microorganisms that cause diseases as a first step in prevention. It inspired various theories of immunity and even some initial attempts at vaccination against smallpox. Additionally, once an agent had been identified, measures were taken to contain its spread. Fumigating ships to kill rats, protecting wharf buildings and human habitations against rats, and removing rat food supplies from easy access were all measures taken to protect the public by further preventing the spread of plague bacilli. Based on the work of Jacob Henle, Louis Pasteur, and Robert Koch (Kerns, 2001), the contagion theory was refined and became best known as the germ theory of disease, which was predominant from the late 19th century through the first half of the 20th century (Lawson & Williams, 2001).

In the era of infectious-disease epidemiology, scientists viewed disease in terms of a simple cause-and-effect relationship. Finding a single cause (plague bacilli) and attacking it (eliminating rats) seemed to be the solution for preventing many diseases. In the case of bubonic plague, this approach appeared to be quite effective. However, scientific research eventually revealed that disease causation was much more complex than first suspected. For example, although most members of a group might be exposed to the plague, many did not contract it. With bubonic plague, as with many other infectious diseases, the characteristics of the host can determine the spread of the disease. Not everyone in a population is at risk; it is now known that untreated bubonic plague has a case-fatality rate of only 50% to 60%. Furthermore, the agent and course of transmission can be quite complex. Although a flea carries the bacilli from rat to human in bubonic plague, many infectious diseases spread directly from one human being to another. Finally, the environment must be considered as part of the cause of disease. Evidence suggests that the plague originated in the high steppes of Asia and spread to other parts of the world. However, questions remain as to whether the bacillus spread from rats to ground squirrels or had always been part of the squirrels' ecology.

After World War II, the causative agents of major infectious diseases were identified, methods of prevention were recognized, and antibiotics and chemotherapy were added to the arsenal to fight communicable diseases. The focus then became understanding and controlling the new chronic disease epidemics. The researchers such as R. Doll, A. B. Hill, J. Morris, and T. McKeown completed case-control and cohort studies (discussed later) that linked the causative factors of cholesterol levels and smoking with coronary heart disease and associated smoking with lung cancer. Today, the major causes of mortality are noninfectious diseases. Chronic diseases of the heart, cancer, and stroke alone account for more than 60% of deaths; accidents, including road traffic injuries, suicide, and homicide, account for another 6%. These major health problems are not caused by infectious agents (Krug, Sharma, & Lozano, 2000; Wimbush & Peters, 2000).

We are entering a new era of eco-epidemiology, distinguished by transforming global health patterns and technological advances. **Global health patterns**, the route, form, and virulence in which diseases appear in countries around the world, with consideration of environmental, ecologic, human, technologic, and political factors, are in transformation. The West Nile virus, severe acute respiratory syndrome (SARS), and the HIV epidemic illustrate this transformation.

In most cases, causative organisms and critical risk factors are known, yet diseases occur, spread, and suddenly appear in countries or regions previously free of them. We know which social behaviors need to change, but we are at a loss for how to create a climate of permanent change, even when entire populations are at stake. For example, we know how to prevent the transmission of HIV, yet thousands of new cases are reported each year. How can we promote preventive practices in populations at risk for communicable diseases? The same is true for many current chronic diseases. How many nurses smoke? Do you exercise as you know you should? Do you know your cholesterol level and eat appropriate foods accordingly? What are we missing to effectively change social behaviors?

Developments in technology drive research primarily in biology and biomedical techniques and in information system capabilities. For example, possibilities now exist through DNA studies to recognize both viral and genetic components in insulin-dependent diabetes; to track HIV, tuberculosis, and other infections from person to person through molecular specificity of the organisms; and to track and mark a breast cancer gene. The possibilities of learning through technology have just begun as we enter this fourth epidemiologic era. Table 8–1 summarizes the four eras in the evolution of modern epidemiology.

CONCEPTS BASIC TO EPIDEMIOLOGY

The science of epidemiology draws on certain basic concepts and principles to analyze and understand patterns of occurrence among aggregate health conditions.

T A B L E   8 – 1

Eras in the Evolution of Modern Epidemiology

Era	Paradigm	Analytic Approach	Prevention Approach
Sanitary statistics (1800–1850)	Miasma: poisoning from foul emanations	Clustering of morbidity and mortality	Drainage, sewage, sanitation
Infectious disease epidemiology (1850–1950)	Germ theory: single agent related to specific disease	Laboratory isolation and culture from disease sites and reproduce lesions	Interrupt transmission (vaccines, isolation, and antibiotics)
Chronic disease epidemiology (1950–2000)	Exposure related to outcome	Risk ratio of exposure to outcome at individual level in populations	Control risk factors by modifying lifestyle (diet), agent (guns), or environment (pollution)
Eco-epidemiology (emerging)	Relations within and between localized structures organized in a hierarchy of levels	Analysis of determinants and outcomes at different levels of organization using new information systems and biomedical techniques	Apply both information and biomedical technology to find leverage at efficacious levels

(Adapted from Susser, M., & Susser, E. [1996a]. Choosing a future for epidemiology: I. Eras and paradigms. *American Journal of Public Health, 86* [5], 668–673; and Susser, M., & Susser, E. [1996b]. Choosing a future for epidemiology: II. From black box to Chinese boxes and eco-epidemiology. *American Journal of Public Health, 86* [5], 674–677.)

Host, Agent, and Environment Model

Through their early study of infectious diseases, epidemiologists began to consider disease states generally in terms of the epidemiologic triad, or the *host, agent, and environment model*. Interactions among these three elements explained infectious and other disease patterns.

Host

The **host** is a susceptible human or animal who harbors and nourishes a disease-causing agent. Many physical, psychological, and lifestyle factors influence the host's susceptibility and response to an agent. Physical factors include age, sex, race, and genetic influences on the host's vulnerability or resistance. Psychological factors, such as outlook and response to stress, can strongly influence host susceptibility. Lifestyle factors also play a major role. Diet, exercise, sleep patterns, and healthy or unhealthy habits all contribute to either increased or decreased vulnerability to the disease-causing agent.

The concept of resistance is important for community health nursing practice. People sometimes have an ability to resist pathogens called *inherent resistance*. Typically, these people have inherited or acquired characteristics, such as the various factors mentioned earlier, that make them less vulnerable. For instance, people who maintain a healthful lifestyle may not contract influenza even if exposed to the flu virus. Resistance can be promoted through preventive interventions.

Agent

An **agent** is a factor that causes or contributes to a health problem or condition. Causative agents can be factors that are present (eg, bacteria that cause tuberculosis, rocks on a mountain road that contribute to an automobile crash) or factors that are lacking (eg, lack of iron in the body that causes anemia; lack of seat belt use that contributes to the extent of injury during an automobile crash).

Agents vary considerably and include five types: biologic, chemical, nutrient, physical, and psychological. Biologic agents include bacteria, viruses, fungi, protozoa, worms, and insects. Some biologic agents are infectious, such as influenza virus or HIV. Chemical agents may be in the form of liquids, solids, gases, dusts, or fumes. Examples are poisonous sprays used on garden pests and industrial chemical wastes. The degree of toxicity of the chemical agent influences its impact on health. Nutrient agents include essential dietary components that can produce illness conditions if they are deficient or are taken in excess. For example, a deficiency of niacin can cause pellagra, and too much vitamin A can be toxic. Physical agents include anything mechanical (eg, chainsaw, automobile), material (rockslide), atmospheric (ultraviolet radiation), geologic (earthquake), or genetically transmitted that causes injury to humans. The shape, size, and force of physical agents influence the degree of harm to the host. Psychological agents are events that produce stress leading to health problems.

Agents may also be classified as either infectious or noninfectious. Infectious agents cause diseases, such as AIDS or tuberculosis, that are communicable—that is, the disease can be spread from one person to another. Certain characteristics of infectious agents are important for community health nurses to understand. Extent of exposure to the agent, the agent's pathogenicity (ability to produce pathologic changes and disease), its infectivity (ability to cause pathogenic organisms to be present), its virulence (severity of disease), and its structure and chemical composition all influence the effects of the agent on the host. Chapter 9 examines the subject of communicable disease in greater depth. Noninfectious agents have similar characteristics in that their relative abilities to harm the host vary with type of agent and intensity and duration of exposure.

Environment

The **environment** refers to all the external factors surrounding the host that might influence vulnerability or resistance. The physical environment includes factors such as geography, climate, weather, safety of buildings, water and food supply, and presence of animals, plants, insects, and microorganisms that have the capacity to serve as reservoirs (storage sites for disease-causing agents) or vectors (carriers) for transmitting disease. The psychosocial environment refers to social, cultural, economic, and psychological influences and conditions that affect health, such as access to health care, cultural health practices, poverty, and work stressors, which can all contribute to disease or health.

Host, agent, and environment interact to cause a disease or health condition. For example, the agent responsible for Lyme disease is the spirochete *Borrelia burgdorferi;* humans of all ages are susceptible hosts, along with dogs, cattle, and horses. Ticks that feed on wild rodents and deer transfer the spirochete to human hosts after feeding on them for several hours. Environmental factors, such as working or playing in tick-infested areas, influence host vulnerability. The host, agent, and environment model, shown in Figure 8–1, offered the epidemiologists who first studied Lyme disease in 1982

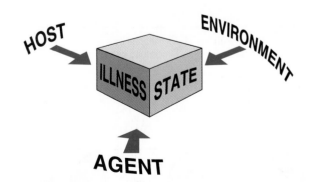

FIGURE 8–1. Epidemiologic triad. Epidemiologists study the causal agent, the susceptible host, and environmental factors that contribute to an illness, injury, or a wellness state. Intervention may focus on any of these three to prevent the spread of illness or to improve health in a population.

a plan for intervention. As soon as the agent was identified, measures could be taken to keep the spirochete from infecting human hosts, such as wearing protective clothing or tick repellent in tick-infested areas and promptly removing surface or attached ticks (Chin, 1999).

In another example, the West Nile virus, which was widespread in Africa and the Middle East, arrived in the United States in 1999 and began to spread. The first reported cases were in New York, where 45 people were infected. In that year, the region experienced a total of 59 hospitalized cases of West Nile disease, resulting in 7 deaths. By the summer of 2002, the disease had spread to 32 states and had infected 1800 people. The encephalitis-causing disease is transmitted by a mosquito bite. The virus survives winter in the body of the adult *Culex* mosquito. The infected mosquito bites a bird and infects it. Other mosquitos bite the bird and in turn become infected. The infected mosquitos pass the virus on to birds, humans, or horses. Many dead birds in an area may mean that the virus is circulating between the bird and mosquito populations and should be reported. In humans and animals with intact immune systems, the virus is usually destroyed in the bloodstream. If the virus survives in the body, it can infect membranes around the spinal cord and brain and cause encephalitis. Those at highest risk are the elderly, children, and people with impaired immune systems.

Prevention includes avoiding mosquito bites by applying insect repellent containing *N,N*-diethyl-*m*-toluemide (DEET) when outdoors; wearing long-sleeved clothing and long pants treated with DEET-containing repellents; staying indoors at dawn, dusk, and in the early evening; eliminating standing water sources where mosquitos lay their eggs; reporting dead birds; and ensuring that there is an organized mosquito control program in the area (Centers for Disease Control and Prevention [CDC], 2002).

Causality

Causality refers to the relationship between a cause and its effect. A purpose of epidemiologic study has been to discover causal relationships, so as to understand why conditions develop and offer effective prevention and protection. Over the years, however, as scientific knowledge of health and disease has expanded, epidemiology has changed its view of causality.

Chain of Causation

As the scientific community's thinking about disease causation and the tripartite model has grown more complex, epidemiologists have used the idea of a chain of causation (Fig. 8–2). The chain begins by identifying the reservoir (ie, where the causal agent can live and multiply). With plague, that reservoir may be other humans, rats, squirrels, and a few other animals. With malaria, infected humans are the major reservoir for the parasitic agents, although certain nonhuman primates also act as reservoirs (Chin, 1999). Next, the agent must have a portal of exit from the reservoir as well as some mode of transmission. For example, the bite of an *Anopheles* mosquito provides a portal of exit for the parasites, which spend part of their life cycle in the mosquito's body; the mosquito in this case is the mode of transmission. The next link in the chain of causation is the agent itself. Malaria, for instance, actually consists of four distinct diseases caused by four kinds of microscopic protozoa. The next link is the portal of entry. In the case of malaria, the mosquito bite provides a portal of exit as well as a portal of entry into the human host.

The box surrounding the chain of causation in Figure 8–2 represents the environment, which can have a profound influence at almost any point along the chain. Consider the impact of environmental factors in the malaria epidemic in Ceylon (an island country in the Indian Ocean off southern India) in 1934 and 1935. Historically, malaria occurred frequently in the dry northern area, where sparse vegetation allowed pools of water to be exposed to the sun, providing excellent breeding grounds for the *Anopheles* mosquito. In contrast, the more populous southwestern area usually had heavy monsoon rains and was relatively free from malaria. In 1934, however, a severe drought changed this environment drastically; throughout Ceylon, rivers almost dried up, leaving stagnant pools of water for mosquito breeding.

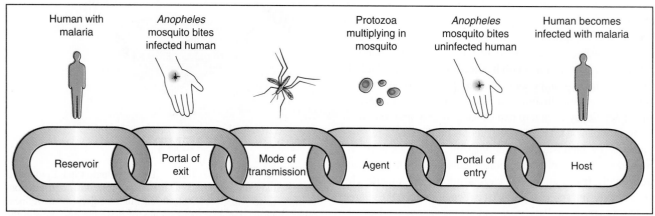

FIGURE 8-2.   Chain of causation in infectious disease.

Widespread crop failure caused the population to become badly undernourished, which added to the conditions that would foster a malaria epidemic. The epidemic hit in October 1934, affecting 2 to 3 million people and causing 80,000 deaths. The environment must certainly be seen as a major part of this causal chain (Burnet, 1962). A similar tragedy occurred in the African country of Rwanda in July of 1994. Civil war caused a large percentage of the population to flee an unfriendly regime. Hundreds of thousands of people filled refugee camps to overflowing. Conditions of squalor and poor sanitation led to contaminated water and resulted in a large-scale epidemic of cholera, a severe form of bacterial dysentery. Relief workers had limited supplies of intravenous or oral rehydration solutions and could do little to help. Uncounted thousands lost their lives. The unstable political environment, unsanitary conditions, and malnourishment were all part of the causal chain.

Multiple Causation

A more advanced concept of multiple causation has emerged to explain the existence of health and illness states and to pro-

vide guiding principles for epidemiologic practice (Valanis, 1999). Dever's Epidemiological Model considers the health status of the host and how it is impacted by human biology, life-style, environment, and the health care system (Poremba, 2003). Sometimes referred to as a "web of causation," this model attempts to identify all possible influences on the health and illness processes. Figure 8–3 shows the web of causation for myocardial infarction; such a health problem cannot be explained in single causal terms. Conditions that lead up to this critical situation exist for years and come from many factors, including heredity, lifestyle, environment, and the health care system. Recognition of multiple causes provides many points of intervention for prevention, health promotion, and treatment. For example, Figure 8–3 suggests interventions such as directly attacking significant coronary atherosclerosis (bypass surgery), reducing the incidence of obesity, helping people stop smoking, developing an exercise program, and making dietary modifications.

Figure 8–4 depicts the web of causation for infant mortality. Data from birth and death certificates were used to identify the complex interactions among multiple causal fac-

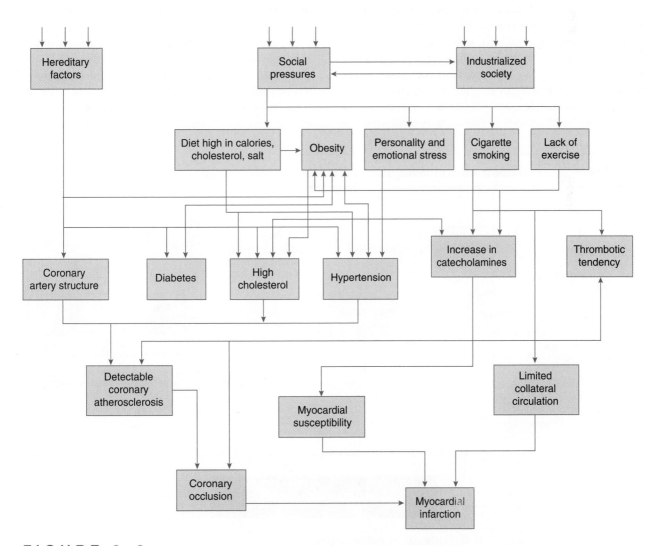

FIGURE 8–3.   Web of causation for myocardial infarction.

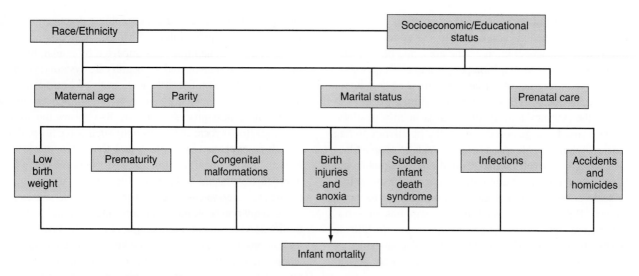

F I G U R E   8 – 4 .   A web of causation for infant mortality, based on information available from birth and death certificates. (From Anderson, E. T., & McFarlane, J. [2003]. *Community as partner* [4th ed.]. Philadelphia: Lippincott Williams & Wilkins.)

tors that produce a negative health condition leading to infant mortality. Figure 8–5 shows a web of causation for automobile crashes. All of the numerous factors involved must be considered when diagramming a web of causation. Speed, faulty equipment, heavy traffic, confusing traffic patterns, road construction, poor visibility, weather conditions, driver inexperience, and drinking or drug use, in any combination, can cause an automobile crash. All health conditions can be diagramed to depict a matrix of causation. A communicable

disease with one clearly identified organism as the agent has the ability to be diagramed based on factors in Dever's model.

Association is a concept that is helpful in determining multiple causality. Events are said to be associated if they appear together more often than would be the case by chance alone. Such events may include risk factors or other characteristics affecting disease or health states. Examples are the frequent association of cigarette smoking with lung cancer, obesity with heart disease, and severe prematurity with infant

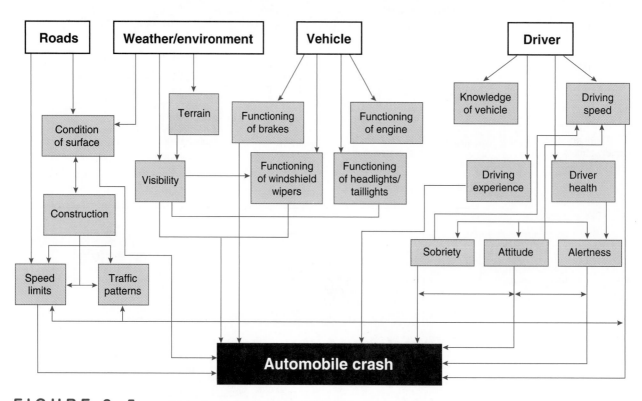

F I G U R E   8 – 5 .   Web of causation for automobile crashes.

mortality. The study of associated factors suggests possible causality and points for intervention. Contemporary epidemiologists continue to explore new and more comprehensive ways of viewing health and illness. The associations among lifestyle, behavior, environment, and stress of all kinds and the ways in which they affect health states are gaining importance in epidemiology.

In the host, agent, and environment model, a shifting emphasis of investigation over time may be noted. Early epidemiologists worked to identify and manage the causative agent; the focus of concern was the disease state. The emphasis then shifted to the host: Who was susceptible? What characteristics led to susceptibility? Through immunization and health promotion, efforts were made to improve host resistance. Increasingly, however, community health workers came to realize the limitations imposed on individual control of health. Even individuals who are in the best of health cannot withstand toxic agents in the workplace, nuclear wastes in the atmosphere from power plant accidents, or other debilitating conditions created by modern society. More and more, public health professionals are turning to a study of the environment and looking for methods to change environmental conditions that contribute to illness.

Immunity

Immunity refers to a host's ability to resist a particular infectious disease–causing agent. This occurs when the body forms antibodies and lymphocytes that react with the foreign antigenic molecules and render them harmless. For community health nursing, this concept has significance in determining which individuals and groups are protected against disease and which may be vulnerable. Four types of immunity are important in community health: passive immunity, active immunity, cross-immunity, and herd immunity.

Passive Immunity

Passive immunity refers to short-term resistance that is acquired either naturally or artificially. Newborns, through maternal antibody transfer, have natural passive immunity that lasts about 6 months. Artificial passive immunity is attained through inoculation with a vaccine that gives temporary resistance. Immune globulin (IGIM or IGIV) is used to boost a susceptible person's immunity and must be repeated periodically to maintain immunity levels. It is used to provide passive immunity against certain infectious diseases or to modify their severity; examples include rubeola, rubella, varicella-zoster, and type A hepatitis. Immune globulin is also used as an alternative to hepatitis B specific immune globulin (HBIG) to provide passive immunity in hepatitis B infection.

Active Immunity

Active immunity is long-term and sometimes lifelong resistance that is acquired either naturally or artificially. Naturally acquired active immunity comes through host infection. That is, a person who contracts a disease often develops long-

lasting antibodies that provide immunity against future exposures. Artificially acquired active immunity is attained through vaccine inoculation. Such vaccines are prepared from killed, living-attenuated, or living-virulent organisms administered to artificially produce or increase immunity to a particular disease. The concept of active immunity underlies public health immunization programs that have successfully kept polio, diphtheria, smallpox, and other major diseases under control worldwide.

Cross-Immunity

Cross-immunity refers to a situation in which a person's immunity to one agent provides immunity to another related agent as well. The immunity can be either passive or active. Sometimes, infection with one disease, such as cowpox, gives immunity to a related disease, such as smallpox. The concept of cross-immunity has also been useful in the development and administration of vaccines. Inoculation with a vaccine made from one disease-causing organism can provide immunity to a related disease-causing organism. Field trials in Uganda and Papua New Guinea and a study in India in the 1990s examined the administration of bacille Calmette-Guérin (BCG) vaccine, which is used to prevent tuberculosis, to people who had been exposed to Hansen's disease (leprosy). The vaccine against *Mycobacterium tuberculosis* appeared to provide these individuals with a degree of cross-immunity to the related infectious agent, *Mycobacterium leprae,* and prevented their contracting the disease (Chin, 1999).

Herd Immunity

Herd immunity describes the immunity level that is present in a population group (Chin, 1999). A population with low herd immunity is one with few immune members; consequently, it is more susceptible to the disease. Nonimmune people are more likely to contract the disease and spread it throughout the group, placing the entire population at greater risk. Conversely, a population with high herd immunity is one in which the immune people in the group outnumber the susceptible people; consequently, the incidence of the disease is reduced. High herd immunity (80% or more) provides a population with greater overall protection because nonimmune people are at less risk of disease exposure. Mandatory preschool immunizations and required travel vaccinations are applications of the herd immunity concept.

Risk

To determine the chances that a disease or health problem will occur, epidemiologists are concerned with **risk**, or the probability that a disease or other unfavorable health condition will develop. For any given group of people, the risk of developing a health problem is directly influenced by their biology, environment, lifestyle, and system of health care. A person's inherited health capacity, the environment lived in, the person's lifestyle choices, and the quality and accessibility of the health care system either negatively or positively affect health, thereby increasing or decreasing the likelihood that a health problem will occur. Negative influences are called *risk factors*. For example, low-birth-weight babies (biology, environment, and system of health care) tend to be at greater risk for health problems, as are people who smoke cigarettes, have diets high in cholesterol, and are sedentary (lifestyle). The degree of risk is directly linked to susceptibility or vulnerability to a given health problem.

Epidemiologists study populations at risk. A population at risk is a collection of people among whom a health problem has the possibility of developing because certain influencing factors are present (eg, exposure to HIV) or absent (eg, lack of childhood immunizations, lack of specific vitamins in the diet), or because there are modifiable risk factors (eg, with cardiovascular disease). A population at risk has a greater probability of developing a given health problem than other groups do. Epidemiologists measure this difference using the *relative risk ratio,* which statistically compares the disease occurrence in the population at risk with the occurrence of the same disease in people without that risk factor.

$$\text{Relative risk ratio} = \frac{\text{Incidence in exposed group}}{\text{Incidence in unexposed group}}$$

If the risk of acquiring the disease is the same regardless of exposure to the risk factor studied, the ratio will be 1:1, and the relative risk will be 1.0. A relative risk greater than 1.0 indicates that those with the risk factor have a greater likelihood of acquiring the disease than do those without it; for instance, a relative risk of 2.54 means that the exposed group is 2.54 times as likely to acquire the disease than the unexposed group. This statistic may be used, for example, to compare the incidence of heart disease among smokers (smoking is a risk factor) with the incidence among nonsmokers, assuming that all other factors are the same. The relative risk ratio assists in determining the most effective points for community health intervention in regard to particular health problems.

Natural History of a Disease or Health Condition

Any disease or health condition follows a progression known as its **natural history**; this refers to events that occur before its development, during its course, and during its conclusion. This process involves the interactions among a susceptible host, the causative agent, and the environment (Valanis, 1999). The natural progression of a disease occurs in four stages as they affect a population—two stages referred to as prepathogenesis (before the detectability of the disease or condition) and two referred to as pathogenesis (while the disease or condition is present). The four stages (Valanis, 1999) are susceptibility, adaptation, early pathogenesis, and clinical disease (Fig. 8–6).

The first stage is *susceptibility.* During this state, the disease is not present and individuals have not been exposed.

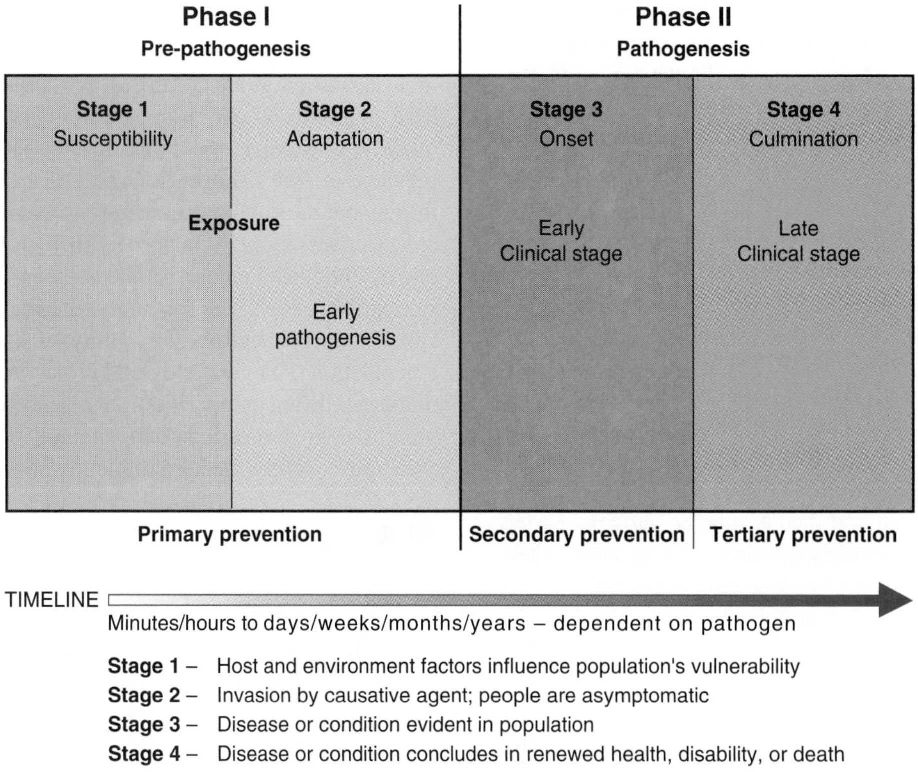

Phase I Pre-pathogenesis		Phase II Pathogenesis	
Stage 1 Susceptibility	**Stage 2** Adaptation	**Stage 3** Onset	**Stage 4** Culmination
Exposure		Early Clinical stage	Late Clinical stage
	Early pathogenesis		
Primary prevention		**Secondary prevention**	**Tertiary prevention**

TIMELINE
Minutes/hours to days/weeks/months/years – dependent on pathogen

Stage 1 –   Host and environment factors influence population's vulnerability
Stage 2 –   Invasion by causative agent; people are asymptomatic
Stage 3 –   Disease or condition evident in population
Stage 4 –   Disease or condition concludes in renewed health, disability, or death

FIGURE 8–6.   Natural history stages of a disease or health condition.

However, host and environmental factors could very likely influence people's susceptibility to a causative agent and lead to development of the disease. For example, college students with poor eating habits and fatigue from lack of sleep during final examinations present risk factors that promote the occurrence of the common cold. "If exposure to an agent occurs at this time, a response will take place. Initial responses reflect the normal adaptation response of the cell or functional system (eg, the immune system). If these adaptation responses are successful, then no disease occurs and the process is arrested in the second stage of prepathogenesis, adaptation" (Valanis, 1999, p. 22). In 1994, the overcrowded conditions and poor sanitation of Rwandan refugee camps in Africa, described earlier, as well as refugees' stress, fatigue, and malnutrition, made them extremely vulnerable to contracting cholera and other diseases. However, in a later tragedy in Kosovo in 1999, the thousands of refugees fleeing for their lives from Yugoslavian Serbs were housed in refugee border camps with adequate supplies and services, and many found temporary or permanent refuge in other countries, including the United States. They endured a shorter period of stress and fatigue with better nutrition than the refugees in Rwanda; as a result, malnutrition was not as rampant. Because improved conditions in refugee camps eliminated major outbreaks of cholera and other diseases, susceptibility to disease in the group as a whole was reduced. Nevertheless, the psychological trauma from the attempts at "ethnic cleansing" of the people in Kosovo remained an existing health problem for years.

The *exposure stage* occurs when individuals have been exposed to a disease but are asymptomatic. It is followed by an *incubation period*, during which the organism multiplies to sufficient numbers to produce a host reaction and clinical symptoms. Vulnerable children who have been exposed to chickenpox (varicella) but do not yet display signs of fever or lesions are in this stage. For diseases caused by infectious agents, the incubation period is relatively short, hours to months. In other conditions caused by noninfectious agents, the time from exposure to onset of symptoms, known as the *induction period* or *latency period*, is often years to decades. For example, children exposed to radiation may have a 5-year latency period for leukemia. Lung cancer caused by exposure to asbestos may have a latency period of 40 years between exposure and detection of the disease (Valanis, 1999).

During the *early pathogenesis or onset stage,* signs and symptoms of the disease or condition develop. In the early phase of this period, the signs may be evident only through laboratory tests, such as tubercular lesions on radiographs or premalignant cervical changes evident on Papanicolaou (Pap) smears. Later in this stage, acute symptoms are clearly visible, as in the case of widespread enterocolitis in a salmonellosis (food poisoning) outbreak. In this *early clinical stage* or *early discernible lesions stage,* evidence of the disease or condition is present and diagnosis occurs.

In the *clinical disease stage,* which includes the *culmination stage,* the disease or health condition causes sufficient anatomic or functional changes to produce recognizable signs and symptoms. Disease severity may vary from mild to severe. The disease may conclude with a return to health, a residual or chronic form of the disease with some disabling limitations, or death. This can also be called the *advanced disease stage,* because the disease or condition has completed its course.

Community health nurses can intervene at any point during these four stages to delay, arrest, or prevent the progression of the disease or condition. Primary, secondary, and tertiary prevention can be applied to the stages (see Levels of Prevention Matrix).

Epidemiology of Wellness

The public health science of epidemiology has traditionally studied the occurrence of disease and health problems. Because of their devastating effect on the health of populations, infectious diseases such as the plague, cholera, and AIDS, as well as chronic illnesses such as heart disease or cancer and fatal or debilitating injuries all require a continued epidemiologic focus. Nonetheless, the need to examine the epidemiology of wellness grows increasingly urgent, for if we continually examine and uncover new health promotion practices and encourage them we can focus on wellness at the ideal primary level of prevention. For example, in 2003 scientists discussed the production of a daily pill that people could begin taking at mid-life. It would include a mild blood pressure medication, a cholesterol-lowering drug, vitamin E, calcium, and a low dose of aspirin. The scientists believed that most of the chronic and life-threatening illnesses could be avoided or postponed, adding 10 to 12 healthy years to a person's life span.

Epidemiology has moved from concentrating only on illness to examining how host, agent, and environment are involved in wellness at various levels. In response to an escalating need for improved methods of health planning and health policy analysis, epidemiology has developed more holistic models of health. These newer epidemiologic models are organized around four attributes that influence health: (1) the physical, social, and psychological environment; (2) lifestyle with its self-created risks; (3) human biology and genetic influences; and (4) the system of health care organization. In the United States, *Healthy People 2010* (U. S. Department of Health and Human Services, 2000) and greater recognition of the importance and cost-effectiveness of illness prevention and health promotion are driving new efforts to develop policy and research initiatives for public health.

Wellness models that at first focused on individual behavior now include approaches that encompass aggregates. A variety of wellness models can be found for groups of seniors (see Chapter 30), in occupational health settings (see Chapter 29), at innovative schools where wellness programs for children and teens are initiated (see Chapter 28), and throughout the services provided for beginning and growing families (see Chapters 26 and 27). Programs designed for ag-

LEVELS OF PREVENTION MATRIX

SITUATION: Apply the levels of prevention during the four stages of the natural history of a disease to eradicate or reduce risk factors (examples of possible conditions provided).

GOAL: Using the three levels of prevention negative health conditions are avoided, or promptly diagnosed and treated, and the fullest possible potential is restored.

PRIMARY PREVENTION		SECONDARY PREVENTION		TERTIARY PREVENTION			
Health Promotion and Education	*Health Protection*	*Early Diagnosis*	*Prompt Treatment*	*Rehabilitation*	*Primary Prevention*		
					Health Promotion and Education	*Health Protection*	
May include • Nutrition counseling —diabetes • Sex education— pregnancy • Smoking cessation —lung cancer	May include • Improved housing and sanitation— waterborne diseases • Immunizations— communicable diseases • Removal of environmental hazards—accidents	The third stage in the natural history of disease, the early pathogenesis or onset stage: • Screening programs—breast and testicular cancer, vision and hearing loss, hypertension, tuberculosis, diabetes	• Initiate prompt treatment • Arrest progression • Prevent associated disability	• Reduce the extent and severity of a health problem to minimize disability • Restore or preserve function	• Training for employment —homeless population • Group treatment and rehabilitation —adolescent drug users • Food, shelter, rest/sleep, exercise	• Health services • Immunizations as needed	

gregates focus on a wellness approach to growth and development: examples include programs for pregnant teens and infant and child development programs (eg, Healthy Start, Head Start) that are funded by state and federal monies. Societal changes, such as the growing elderly population, the communication revolution, the global economy, environmental threats, technology development, and the holism and wellness movements are driving these new approaches.

The four stages of the natural history of disease can apply to an understanding of any health condition, including wellness states. In stage one, susceptibility, people can become amenable to healthier practices and improved health system organization. In stage two, adaptation/exposure, a community can learn about these health-promoting behaviors. Stage three, early onset, could be a period of trying out the beneficial policies and activities, and stage four, culmination, could encompass full adoption and a higher level of well-being for the community. This approach has important implications for community health nursing preventive and health-promotion practice.

Community health nursing can play a primary role in the investigation and identification of factors that not only prevent illness but also promote health. This means sharpening skills in epidemiologic research to uncover the factors that contribute to a full measure of healthful living. The time for an epidemiology of wellness has come.

Causal Relationships

One of the main challenges to epidemiology is to identify causal relationships in disease and health conditions in populations. As was previously suggested, the assessment of causality in human health is difficult at best; no single study is adequate to establish causality. Causal inference is based on consistent results obtained from many studies. Frequently, the accumulation of evidence begins with a clinical observation or an educated guess that a certain factor may be causally related to a health problem.

A **cross-sectional study** (which explores a health condition's relation to other variables in a specified population at a specific point in time) can show that the factor and the problem coexist. For example, one study compared the incidence of gonorrhea in a 55-block area in urban New Orleans with a "broken window index," which measured housing quality, abandoned cars, graffiti, trash, and public school deterioration (Cohen et al., 2000). The broken window index predicted the variance for gonorrhea rates more accurately than did a poverty index measuring income, unemployment, and low education.

A **retrospective study** (which looks backward in time to find a causal relationship) allows a fairly quick assessment of whether an association exists. Looking back at the use of lead in interior paint in the United States, history shows that even though the particular dangers to children were documented in English language literature as early as 1904, the U. S. lead industry did nothing to discourage the use of lead paint on interior walls and woodwork. In fact, some paint companies (eg, Dutch Boy Paint) used children in their advertising through the 1920s (Markowitz & Rosner, 2000). Not until the 1950s did the industry adopt a voluntary standard limiting the amount of lead in interior paints, and then only under increasing pressure.

A **prospective study** (which looks forward in time to find a causal relationship) is crucial to ensure that the presumed causal factor actually precedes the onset of the health problem. The prospective approach is concerned with current information and provides a direct measure of the variables in question. For example, scientists are looking at causative factors of Parkinson's disease: "Agrochemicals, organic gardening, identical twins, intravenous drug users, your cotton Levis, rhubarb pie, a pot of coffee and a carton of cigarettes—all play a role in the increasingly complicated search for a cure for Parkinson's disease" (Kleyman, 2001).

Finally, if ethically possible, an **experimental study** (in which the investigator controls or changes factors suspected of causing the condition and observes results) is used to confirm the associations obtained from observational studies (in which the investigator merely observes data or people without controlling or changing any factors). It often requires many years to accumulate enough evidence to suggest a causal relationship.

Epidemiologically, a causal relationship may be said to exist if two major conditions are met: (1) the factor of interest (causal agent) is shown to increase the probability of occurrence of the disease or condition as observed in many studies in different populations, and (2) evidence suggests that a reduction in the factor decreases the frequency of the given disease. The synthesis of data begins by selecting as many as of the various types of epidemiologic studies of the problem as possible. After those studies that are not methodologically sound are discarded, the studies are reviewed. The better the data meet the following six criteria, the more likely it is that the factor of interest is one of several causes of the disease:

1. *Temporal relationship:* Exposure to the suspected factor must precede the onset of disease.

2. *Strength of the association:* This refers to the ratio of disease rates in those with and without the suspected causal factor. A strong association would be noted if disease rates are much higher in the group with the factor than in the group without it.
3. *Dose–response relationship:* This relationship is demonstrated if, with increasing levels of exposure to the factor, there is a corresponding increase in occurrence of the disease.
4. *Consistency:* An association is demonstrated in varying types of studies among diverse study groups.
5. *Biological plausibility and coherence of the evidence:* The hypothesized cause makes sense based on current biologic knowledge.
6. *Lowering of disease risk:* Interventions that decrease exposure result in a lowering of disease risk (relative risk).

The goal of any epidemiologic investigation is to identify causal mechanisms that meet these six criteria and to develop measures for preventing illness and promoting health. The community health nurse may need to gather new data for this type of investigation, but pertinent existing data should be thoroughly examined first. This type of information can be obtained by the community health nurse from a variety of sources, which are discussed in the next section.

SOURCES OF INFORMATION FOR EPIDEMIOLOGIC STUDY

Epidemiologic investigators may draw data from any of three major sources: existing data, informal investigations, and scientific studies. The community health nurse will find all three sources useful in efforts to improve the health of aggregates.

Existing Data

A variety of information is available nationally, by state, and by section, such as county, region, or urbanized area. This information includes vital statistics, census data, and morbidity statistics on certain communicable or infectious diseases. Local health departments often can provide these data on request. Community health nurses seeking information on communities may find local health system agencies helpful. These agencies collect health information for groups of counties within states and interact with health planning authorities at the state level. They have access to many types of information and can give advice on specific problems raised by nurses.

Vital Statistics
Vital statistics refers to the information gathered from ongoing registration of births, deaths, adoptions, divorces, and marriages. Certification of births, deaths, and fetal deaths are the most useful vital statistics in epidemiologic studies. The community health nurse can obtain blank copies of a state's

birth and death certificates to become familiar with the information contained in each (Display 8–1). Much more information is recorded than the fact and cause of death on the death certificate. Birth certificates also can provide helpful information (eg, weight of the infant, amount of prenatal care received by the mother), which can be used to identify high-risk mothers and infants.

Sources for vital statistical information include state Web sites on the Internet, local and state health departments, city halls, and county halls of records (see list of Internet resources at the end of this chapter). Statistics regarding general morbidity and mortality for specific states are located in the aggregate from the CDC at the national level. State statistics are obtained from state health departments, and county information (specific cities or census tracts) can be obtained from either the state or the county health department.

Census Data

Data from population censuses taken every 10 years in many countries are the main source of population statistics. This information can be a valuable assessment tool for the community health nurse who is taking part in health planning for aggregates. Population statistics can be analyzed by age, sex, race, ethnic background, type of occupation, income gradient, marital status, educational level, or other standards, such as housing quality. Analysis of population statistics can provide the community health nurse with a better understanding of the community and help identify specific areas that may warrant further epidemiologic investigation. Data from the U. S. Census Bureau is found on their Web site.

Reportable Diseases

Each state has developed laws or regulations that require health organizations and practitioners to report to their local health authority cases of certain communicable and infectious diseases that can be spread through the community (Chin, 1999). This reporting enables the health department to take the most appropriate and efficient action. All states require that diseases subject to international quarantine regulations be reported immediately. However, these diseases (plague, cholera, yellow fever, and smallpox) are virtually unknown now in developed countries. Health care professionals have not had experience identifying smallpox, because no cases have been reported since 1978 (Sibley, 2002). In 1980, the World Health Organization (WHO) declared the global eradication of smallpox after more than 10 years of international effort. Numerous other diseases under surveillance by the WHO (eg, louse-borne typhus fever and relapsing fever, paralytic poliomyelitis, malaria, viral influenza) must also be reported. Other reportable diseases (numbering between 20 and 40 in each state) are usually classified according to the speed with which the health department should be notified. Some should be reported by phone or electronic mail, others weekly by regular mail. They vary in potential severity from chickenpox to rabies and include AIDS, encephalitis, meningitis, syphilis, and toxic shock syndrome.

Community health nurses should obtain the list of reportable diseases from their local or state health department office. Following up on occurrences of these diseases is a task frequently assigned to community nursing services.

Disease Registries

Some areas or states have disease registries or rosters for conditions with major public health impact. Tuberculosis and rheumatic fever registries were more common when these diseases occurred more frequently. Cancer registries provide useful incidence, prevalence, and survival data and assist the community health nurse in monitoring cancer patterns within a community. Community health nurses can access these registries through state health department Web sites.

Environmental Monitoring

State governments, through health departments or other agencies, now monitor health hazards found in the environment. Pesticides, industrial wastes, radioactive or nuclear materials, chemical additives in foods, and medicinal drugs have joined the list of pollutants (see Chapter 10 for a detailed discussion). Concerned community members and leaders view these as risk factors that affect health at both community and individual levels. Community health nurses can also obtain data from federal agencies such as the Food and Drug Administration, the Consumer Product Safety Commission, and the Environmental Protection Agency.

National Center for Health Statistics Health Surveys

On the national level, the National Center for Health Statistics (NCHS) furnishes valuable health prevalence data from surveys of Americans. Published data are also frequently available for regions. The National Health Survey was established by Congress in 1956 and provides a continual source of information about the health status and needs of the entire nation. It has been operated as part of the CDC since the 1980s (Thomas & Weber, 2001). The Health Interview Survey includes interviews from approximately 40,000 households each year and provides information about the health status and needs of the entire country. The National Nursing Home Survey primarily samples institutional records of hospitals and nursing homes; it provides information on those who are using these services along with diagnoses and other characteristics. The Health Examination Survey reports physical measurements on smaller samples of the population and augments the information provided by interviews. It also provides prevalence information on injuries, diseases, and disabilities that appear frequently in the population. The National Family Growth Survey focuses on fertility and family planning. Other studies investigate vital statistics events and characteristics of ambulatory patients in physicians' community practices.

Each of these nationally sponsored efforts suggests ways in which community health nurses can examine health problems or concerns affecting their communities. Inter-

D I S P L A Y   8 – 1

Standard Death Certificate

Birth No. _____   File No. 117_____

Name of decedent: for use by physician or institution

DECEDENT

1A. LAST NAME OF DECEDENT	1B. FIRST NAME	1C. MIDDLE NAME	2A. DATE OF DEATH (Month, Day, Year)

| 2B. HOUR OF DEATH | 3. SEX | 4. RACE (Specify White, Black, etc.) | 5. MARITAL STATUS (Specify Married, Never Married, Widowed, Divorced) | 6. SURVIVING SPOUSE (If Wife, give Maiden Name) |

7. DATE OF BIRTH (Month, Day, Year) | 8A. AGE YEARS | 8B. UNDER 1 YEAR MONTHS / DAYS | 8C. UNDER 1 DAY HOURS / MINUTES | 9. BIRTHPLACE (City and State or Foreign Country)

10. USUAL OCCUPATION (Kind of work done most of working life, NEVER specify retired) | 11. KIND OF BUSINESS/INDUSTRY | 12. OF HISPANIC ORIGIN?

13. EVER IN U.S. ARMED FORCES? (YES or NO) | 14. SOCIAL SECURITY NUMBER | 15. DECEDENT'S EDUCATION (Specify ONLY HIGHEST or age completed) ELEMENTARY/SECONDARY (0-12) / COLLEGE (1-4, 5+)

PLACE OF DEATH

16A. PLACE OF DEATH (Check ONLY one. If death in NON-LISTED facility check OTHER and specify on line BELOW)

HOSPITAL   1 ☐ INPATIENT   2 ☐ ER/OUTPATIENT   3 ☐ DOA   NON-HOSPITAL   4 ☐ NURSING HOME   5 ☐ RESIDENCE   6 ☐ OTHER

16B. NAME OF FACILITY (If not in Facility, give street address or location) | 16c. PLACE OF DEATH IN CITY LIMITS? (YES or NO)

17A. CITY, TOWN OR LOCATION OF DEATH | 17B. PARISH OF DEATH

RESIDENCE

18A. STREET ADDRESS (If rural specify rural route number or location) | 18B. PARISH OF RESIDENCE | 18C. STATE OF RESIDENCE

18D. USUAL RESIDENCE OF DECEDENT (City, town or location) | 18E. ZIP CODE | 18F. RESIDENCE INSIDE CITY LIMITS? (YES or NO)

PARENTS

19A. FATHER'S LAST NAME   FIRST   MIDDLE | 19B. FATHER'S PLACE OF BIRTH | 19C. STATE

20A. MOTHER'S LAST NAME   FIRST   MIDDLE | 20B. MOTHER'S PLACE OF BIRTH | 20C. STATE

INFORMANT

21A. TYPE OR PRINT NAME OF INFORMANT | 21B. INFORMANT'S ADDRESS | 21C. DATE (Month, Day, Year)

DISPOSITION

22A. METHOD OF DISPOSITION   1 ☐ BURIAL   2 ☐ CREMATION   3 ☐ REMOVAL   4 ☐ OTHER | 22B. DATE THEREOF (Month, Day, Year) | 22C. NAME AND LOCATION OF CEMETERY OR CREMATORIUM

23A. SIGNATURE AND ADDRESS OF FUNERAL DIRECTOR | 23B. FACILITY NUMBER | 23C. LICENSE NUMBER

24. ALTERATIONS

REGISTRAR

25A. BURIAL TRANSIT PERMIT | 25B. PARISH OF ISSUE | 25C. DATE OF ISSUE | 26. SIGNATURE OF LOCAL REGISTRAR

MANNER OF DEATH

27. MANNER OF DEATH   1 ☐ NATURAL   2 ☐ ACCIDENT   3 ☐ SUICIDE   4 ☐ HOMICIDE   5 ☐ PENDING INVESTIGATION   6 ☐ UNDETERMINED

28A. DATE OF INJURY (Month, Day, Year) | 28B. TIME OF INJURY | 28C. INJURY AT WORK (YES or NO) | 28D. DESCRIBE HOW INJURY OCCURRED

28E. PLACE OF INJURY (Specify at home, farm, factory, street, etc.) | 28F. LOCATION (Street Number or Rural Route, City, Parish, State)

CERTIFIER

29A. I CERTIFY THAT I ATTENDED THE DECEDENT   FROM   TO | AND THAT DEATH OCCURRED ON THE DATE AND HOUR STATED ABOVE DUE TO THE CAUSES AND IN THE MANNER SO STATED. | 29B. SIGNATURE OF PHYSICIAN OR CORONER | 29C. DATE (Month, Day, Year)

29D. TYPE OR PRINT NAME AND TITLE OF PHYSICIAN OR CORONER | 29E. ADDRESS OF PHYSICIAN OR CORONER

CAUSE OF DEATH

30.   PART I.   ENTER THE DISEASES, INJURIES OR COMPLICATIONS THAT CAUSED THE DEATH. DO NOT ENTER THE MODE OF DYING SUCH AS CARDIAC OR RESPIRATORY ARREST OR HEART FAILURE. LIST ONLY ONE CAUSE ON EACH LINE. | APPROXIMATE INTERVAL BETWEEN ONSET AND DEATH

IMMEDIATE CAUSE (Final disease or condition resulting in death.)   a. _____
DUE TO (OR AS A CONSEQUENCE OF)

Sequentially list conditions, if any, leading to immediate cause.   b. _____
DUE TO (OR AS A CONSEQUENCE OF)

Enter UNDERLYING CAUSE (Disease or injury that initiated events resulting in death) LAST.   c. _____
DUE TO (OR AS A CONSEQUENCE OF)

d. _____

30.   PART II.   OTHER SIGNIFICANT CONDITIONS CONTRIBUTING TO DEATH BUT NOT RESULTING IN THE UNDERLYING CAUSE IN PART I. | 31. IF DECEASED WAS FEMALE 10–49, WAS SHE PREGNANT IN THE LAST 90 DAYS? | 32A. WAS AN AUTOPSY PERFORMED? | 32B. WERE AUTOPSY FINDINGS AVAILABLE PRIOR TO COMPLETION OF CAUSE OF DEATH?

☐ Tobacco   ☐ Other | ☐ YES ☐ NO ☐ UNK. | ☐ YES ☐ NO | ☐ YES ☐ NO

views, physical examinations of subsets of community members, and surveillance of institutions, clinics, and private physicians' practices can be carried out locally after needs are identified and funds made available. Other sources may be found in data kept routinely but not centrally on the health problems of workers in local industries or the health problems of schoolchildren, a key issue to many community health nurses. Existing epidemiologic data can be used to plan parent education programs, health promotion among students, and almost any other type of service.

Another service of the CDC is its important publication, the *Mortality and Morbidity Weekly Report (MMWR)*. This publication presents weekly summaries of disease and death data trends for the nation. It includes reports on outbreaks or occurrences of diseases in specific regions of the country and international trends in disease occurrences that may affect the U. S. population. Most health departments subscribe to this publication, which provides important information for both epidemiologists and community health nurses.

Informal Observational Studies

A second information source in epidemiologic study is informal observation and description. Almost any client group encountered by the community health nurse can trigger such a study. If, for example, the nurse encounters an abused child at a clinic, a study of the clinic's records to screen for additional possible instances of child abuse and neglect could lead to more case findings. If several cases of diabetes come to the attention of a nurse serving on a Navajo reservation, a widespread problem might come to light through informal inquiries about the incidence and age at onset of the disease among this Native American population. In a study of culture, sexuality, and women's agency in the prevention of HIV/AIDS, two researchers explored the awareness among women in southern Africa of the HIV epidemic and methods they might use to protect themselves from the virus. Interviews and informal field observations were carried out over a 7-year period at five sites "that were selected to reflect urban and rural experiences, various populations, and economic and political opportunities for women at different historical moments over the course of the HIV epidemic" (Susser & Stein, 2000, p. 1042). The findings indicated that most women saw themselves as active participants in the search for a way to protect themselves in sexual situations and were not helpless victims. At all sites over the 7 years, women desired to control their own bodies and felt they had the right to use the female condom. However, political and economic concerns, combined with historically powerful patterns of gender discrimination and neglect of women's sexuality, were considered to be the main barriers to the development and distribution of methods that women could control. Collecting such information and complementing it with existing data about a population served by a community health nurse could lead to improved women's health promotion practices to prevent HIV/AIDS in the United States. Informal observational study often raises questions and suggests hypotheses that form the basis for designing larger-scale epidemiologic investigations, such as this study in Africa.

Scientific Studies

The third source of information used in epidemiologic inquiry involves carefully designed scientific studies. The nursing profession has recognized the need to develop a systematic body of knowledge on which to base nursing practice. Already, systematic research is becoming an accepted part of the community health nurse's role. Findings from epidemiologic studies conducted by or involving nurses are appearing more frequently in the literature. For example, concern about testicular cancer and the patterns of testicular self-examination (TSE) among young adult men was the impetus for a nurse to conduct a study between 1999 and 2001 among 191 men attending occupational health fairs in the American Midwest (Wynd, 2002). She learned that 64% rarely or never performed TSE and 36% practiced TSE monthly or every few months. Those who infrequently performed TSE more often were African-American or Hispanic and had less than a college education. Factors associated with infrequent TSE practice included less satisfaction with job assignment and with life in general; greater worries interfering with daily life; more serious family problems involving spouse, children, or parents; and fewer people to turn to for support. In another study, conducted in Baltimore, Maryland, researchers examined whether interventions aimed at aggressive and disruptive classroom behavior and poor academic achievement would also reduce the incidence of smoking initiation (Kellam & Anthony, 1998). The epidemiologically based, randomized, preventive study involved 2311 first- and second-grade boys in 19 urban Baltimore schools. Students were randomly assigned by classroom to one of two intervention groups or to the control group. Smoking initiation was reduced at the final assessment age of 14 years in both cohorts for boys who were assigned to the behavioral intervention. The researchers concluded that targeting early risk antecedents such as aggressive behavior appears to be an important smoking-prevention strategy. Systematic studies such as these, as well as informal studies and existing epidemiologic data, can provide the community health nurse with valuable information that can be used to positively affect aggregate health.

METHODS IN THE EPIDEMIOLOGIC INVESTIGATIVE PROCESS

The goals of epidemiologic investigation are to identify the causal mechanisms of health and illness states and to develop measures for preventing illness and promoting health. Epidemiologists employ an investigative process that involves a sequence of three approaches that build on one another: descriptive, analytic, and experimental studies. All three approaches have relevance for community health nursing (see Chapter 14 for a more detailed description).

Descriptive Epidemiology

Descriptive epidemiology includes investigations that seek to observe and describe patterns of health-related conditions that occur naturally in a population. For example, a community health nurse might seek to learn how many children in a school district have been immunized for measles, how many home births occur each year in the county, how many cases of STDs have occurred in the city in the past month, or how many automobile crashes have occurred near the community high school. At this stage in the epidemiologic investigation, the researcher seeks to establish the occurrence of a problem. Data from descriptive studies suggest hypotheses for further testing. Descriptive studies almost always involve some form of broad-based quantification and statistical analysis.

Counts

The simplest measure of description is a count. For example, an epidemiologic study of varicella deaths among all age groups tracked varicella deaths through hospital discharge records and death certificates in New York State (Galil et al., 2002). Since the varicella vaccine licensure in 1995, varicella incidence has decreased markedly. However, it is predicted that vaccination will shift the peak incidence of disease to older ages as the incidence declines. Therefore, monitoring of varicella mortality is important for evaluating the impact of a national vaccination program. One of the first steps in the research was to search death certificates and the Statewide Planning and Research Cooperative System database (SPARCS), a hospital discharge database in New York, for the period 1989–1995. The investigators discovered that the death certificates produced more reliable data, because the SPARCS database is from nonfederal hospitals. However, when both sources were accessed, the reliability increased and the total number of varicella deaths were revealed (Galil et al., 2002) (Table 8–2). Obtaining a count of this type always depends on the definition of what is being counted. This particular count, for example, could become contaminated if deaths are complicated by immunodeficiency and other underlying conditions. In addition, hospital records are often lost or provide incomplete data, so that some varicella deaths may not be counted. An important outcome of this study was the determination that availability of data influences the count. This is significant information for researchers who might plan to use a single database for their study. However, before making use of any statistics, whether from official state offices, the Census Bureau, or a health agency, it is necessary to determine what the information represents.

TABLE 8-2

Numbers of Potential Varicella Deaths in New York State (Excluding New York City) by Data Source (1989–1995)

Number (Total = 30)	Percent	Data Source
9	30	Death certificates
4	13	SPARCS
17	57	From both sources

SPARCS, Statewide Planning and Research Cooperative System database.

(From Galil, K., Pletcher, M. J., Wallace, B. J., Seward, J., Meyer, P. A., Baughman, A. L., et al. [2002]. Tracking varicella deaths: Accuracy and completeness of death certificates and hospital discharge records, New York State, 1989–1995. *American Journal of Public Health, 92*[8], 1248–1249.)

Rates

Rates are statistical measures expressing the proportion of people with a given health problem among a population at risk. The total number of people in the group serves as the denominator for various types of rates. To express a count as a proportion, or rate, the population to be studied must first be identified. If 30 varicella deaths are considered in relation to the total number of children in New York State, there will be one rate; if they are considered in relation to the total population of children in the country, there will be a different rate.

In epidemiology, the population represents the universe of people defined as the objects of a study. Because it is often difficult, if not impossible, to study an entire population, most epidemiologic studies draw a sample to represent that group. For example, in the Baltimore study dealing with behavioral interventions to decrease smoking initiation, the investigators selected a random sample of 2311 children in 19 classrooms to include as study subjects or controls out of a much larger urban school population (Kellam & Anthony, 1998). Sometimes, it is important to seek a random sample (in which everyone in the population has an equal chance of selection for study and choice is made without bias); at other times, a sample of convenience (in which study subjects are selected because of their availability) is sufficient. In many small epidemiologic studies, it may be possible to study almost every person in the population, eliminating the need for a sample.

Several rates have wide use in epidemiology. Those most important for the community health nurse to understand are the prevalence rate, the period prevalence rate, and the incidence rate.

Prevalence refers to all of the people with a particular health condition existing in a given population at a given point in time. The *prevalence rate* describes a situation at a specific point in time (Yassi et al., 2001). If a nurse discovers 50 cases of measles in an elementary school, that is a simple count. If that number is divided by the number of students in the school, the result is the prevalence of measles. For instance, if the school has 500 students, the prevalence of measles on that day would be 10% (50 measles/500 population).

$$\text{Prevalence rate} = \frac{\text{Number of persons with a characteristic}}{\text{Total number in population}}$$

In the study of varicella deaths, on the other hand, the investigators had a count for a 7-year period, 1989 to 1995. Rather than portraying only 1 day, this number covered an extended period of time. The prevalence rate over a defined period of time is called a *period prevalence rate:*

$$\text{Period prevalence rate} = \frac{\text{Number of persons with a characteristic during a period of time}}{\text{Total number in population}}$$

Not everyone in a population is at risk for developing a disease, incurring an injury, or having some other health-related characteristic. The *incidence rate* recognizes this fact. **Incidence** refers to all new cases of a disease or health condition appearing during a given time. Incidence rate describes a proportion in which the numerator is all new cases appearing during a given period of time and the denominator is the population at risk during the same period. For example, some childhood diseases give lifelong immunity. The children in a school who have had such diseases would be removed from the total number of children at risk in the school population. Three weeks after the start of a measles epidemic in a school, the incidence rate describes the number of cases of measles appearing during that period in terms of the number of persons at risk:

$$\frac{200}{1000} \text{ or } \frac{200 \text{ new cases}}{1000 \text{ persons at risk}}$$

The health literature is not always consistent in the use of the term *incidence;* sometimes, this word is used synonymously with *prevalence rates,* and the reader must take this into consideration.

$$\text{Incidence rate} = \frac{\text{Number of persons developing a disease}}{\text{Total number at risk per unit of time}}$$

Another rate that describes incidence is the attack rate. An *attack rate* describes the proportion of a group or population that develops a disease among all those exposed to a particular risk. This term is used frequently in investigations of outbreaks of infectious diseases such as influenza. If the attack rate changes, it may suggest an alteration in the population's immune status or that the disease-causing organism is present in a more or less virulent strain.

Computing Rates

To make comparisons between populations, epidemiologists often use a common base population in computing rates. For example, instead of merely saying that the rate of an illness is 13% in one city and 25% in another, the comparison is made per 100,000 people in the population. This population base can vary for different purposes from 100 to 100,000. To describe the **morbidity rate**, which is the relative incidence of disease in a population, the ratio of the number of sick individuals to the total population is determined. The **mortality rate** refers to the relative death rate, or the sum of deaths in a given population at a given time. Display 8–2 includes formulas for computing rates commonly used in community health.

The goal of descriptive studies is to identify the patterns of occurrence of any health-related condition. They can be retrospective (identify cases and controls, then go back to review existing data) or prospective (identify groups and exposure factors, then follow them forward in time). In a descriptive study of child abuse, for example, the investigator would note the age, sex, race or ethnic group, and physical and emotional conditions of the children affected. In addition, data would be collected that described the economic status and occupation of parents, the location and setting of abusive behavior, and the time and season of the year when abuse occurred. In the retrospective study on reported varicella deaths in New York State, the investigators described the age, sex, and ethnic background of victims and other information such as comorbidity and availability and completeness of hospital records. Describing facets of these deaths provided information for further study and suggested avenues for intervention or prevention. For another example of a descriptive study, see Research: Bridge to Practice.

Analytic Epidemiology

A second type of investigation, **analytic epidemiology**, goes beyond simple description or observation and seeks to identify associations between a particular human disease or health problem and its possible causes. Analytic studies tend to be more specific than descriptive studies in their focus. They test hypotheses or seek to answer specific questions and can be retrospective or prospective in design. For example, in a prospective analytic study, a researcher set out to address the question of whether involving youth in HIV prevention program development would improve the use of prevention methods and reduce HIV risk behaviors (Quander, 2001). The researcher reviewed several youth-driven programs throughout the nation: Chicago; Washington, D.C.; Maryland; Virginia; Santa Cruz, California; and Jackson, Mississippi. She went where the youth were. She did not find them on playgrounds or basketball courts: "Most are seen in urban clothing stores, record stores, barber shops, nail salons, hair braiding boutiques, mom-and-pop corner stores, and even McDonald's," (Quander, 2001, p. 2).

Analytic studies fall into three types: prevalence studies, case-control studies, and cohort studies.

Prevalence Studies

When examining prevalence, it is helpful to remember that the health condition may be new or may have affected some

DISPLAY 8-2

Common Epidemiologic Rates

General Mortality Rates

Crude Mortality Rate =

$$\frac{\text{Number of Reported Deaths During 1 Year}}{\begin{array}{c}\text{Estimated Population as of}\\\text{July 1 of Same Year}\end{array}} \times 100,000$$

Cause-Specific Mortality Rate =

$$\frac{\begin{array}{c}\text{Number of Deaths From a}\\\text{Stated Cause During 1 Year}\end{array}}{\begin{array}{c}\text{Estimated Population as of}\\\text{July 1 of Same Year}\end{array}} \times 100,000$$

Case Fatality Rate =

$$\frac{\text{Number of Deaths From a Particular Disease}}{\text{Total Number With the Same Disease}} \times 100$$

Proportional Mortality Ratio =

$$\frac{\begin{array}{c}\text{Number of Deaths From a Specific}\\\text{Cause Within a Given TIme Period}\end{array}}{\text{Total Deaths in the Same Time Period}} \times 100$$

Age-Specific Mortality Rate =

$$\frac{\begin{array}{c}\text{Number of Persons in a Specific Age}\\\text{Group Dying During 1 Year}\end{array}}{\begin{array}{c}\text{Estimated Population of the Specific Age}\\\text{Group as of July 1 of Same Year}\end{array}} \times 100,000$$

Specific Rates for Maternal and Infant Populations

Crude Birth Rate =

$$\frac{\text{Number of Live Births During 1 Year}}{\text{Estimated Population as of July 1 of Same Year}} \times 1,000$$

General Fertility Rate =

$$\frac{\text{Number of Live Births During 1 Year}}{\begin{array}{c}\text{Number of Females Aged 15–44}\\\text{as of July 1 of Same Year}\end{array}} \times 1,000$$

Maternal Mortality Rate =

$$\frac{\begin{array}{c}\text{Number of Deaths From}\\\text{Puerperal Causes During 1 Year}\end{array}}{\text{Number of Live Births During Same Year}} \times 100,000$$

Infant Mortality Rate =

$$\frac{\begin{array}{c}\text{Number of Deaths Under}\\\text{1 Year of Age for Given Year}\end{array}}{\text{Number of Live Births Reported for Same Year}} \times 1,000$$

Perinatal Mortality Rate =

$$\frac{\begin{array}{c}\text{Number of Fetal Deaths Plus Infant Deaths}\\\text{Under 7 Days of Age During 1 Year}\end{array}}{\begin{array}{c}\text{Number of Live Births Plus Fetal Deaths}\\\text{During Same Year}\end{array}} \times 1,000$$

---

people for many years. **Prevalence studies** describe patterns of occurrence, as in the study of varicella deaths in New York. They may examine causal factors, but a prevalence study always looks at factors from the same point in time and in the same population. Hypothesized causal factors are based on inferences from a single examination and most likely need further testing for validation.

Case-Control Studies

Case-control studies compare people who have a health or illness condition (number of cases with the condition) with those who lack this condition (controls). These studies begin with the cases and look back over time for presence or absence of the suspected causal factor in both cases and controls. In the study of early antecedents to prevent smoking initiation, 1604 students remained in the Baltimore City public schools and were found for follow-up 7 years later. Of that number, 700 had participated as study subjects (cases); the 904 other children, who had not experienced the interventions, were the controls. This study then reviewed the history of cases and controls for the presence of aggressive or disruptive behavior among the 1604 students who originally

participated in the study and were still in the school system. In a case-control study, the two groups should share as many characteristics as possible, to isolate possible causes; randomly selecting first- and second-grade classrooms helps to ensure this. A comparison between one group of children in first grade with another group in their late teens would have invalidated the conclusion in a study on the effects of behavioral interventions.

Cohort Studies

A **cohort** is a group of people who share a common experience in a specific time period. Examples are a group of elders or the employees of an industry. In epidemiology, a cohort of people often becomes a focus of study. Cohort studies, rather than measuring the relationship of variables in existing conditions, study the development of a condition over time. A cohort study begins by selecting a group of people who display certain defined characteristics before the onset of the condition being investigated. In studying a disease, the cohort might include individuals who are initially free of the disease but are known to have been exposed to a particular factor. They would be observed over time to evaluate which

RESEARCH: BRIDGE TO PRACTICE

Appel, S.J., Harrell, J.S., & Deng, S. (2002). Racial and socioeconomic differences in risk factors for cardiovascular disease among Southern rural women. *Nursing Research, 519*(3), 140–147.

RISK FACTORS FOR CARDIOVASCULAR DISEASE AMONG SOUTHERN RURAL WOMEN

It has been observed that African American women who live in the southeastern portion of the United States experience higher mortality related to cardiovascular disease (CVD) than their white counterparts. It is not clear whether their vulnerability to CVD is related to race, socioeconomic status, or health behaviors.

The researchers in this study sought to examine the disparities in cardiac health between Southern rural, African-American, and white women to determine whether a CVD Risk Index differed by race, education, or income levels and whether differences remained after controlling for body mass index (BMI).

The population used in this descriptive, comparative study consisted of 1110 women (27% African-American and 73% white) who lived in North Carolina and responded to mailed questionnaires. There were three research questions:

1. Is there a difference in the CVD Risk Index between African-American and white women residing in the rural Southeast?
2. To what extent does obesity affect the CVD Risk Index of these rural-dwelling women?
3. To what extent do the contextual factors of income and educational levels affect the CVD Risk Index?

Data collected were analyzed using analysis of variance (ANOVA) and analysis of covariance (ANCOVA).

The results showed that African-American women had significantly lower education and income than whites, a higher BMI, and a greater prevalence of hypertension, angina, and diabetes. In a three-way ANOVA that included race, income, and education, education and race were significant predictors of the CVD Risk Index. But after adjustment for BMI, race was no longer significant; the only significant predictors were BMI and educational level.

What this suggests is that women with the least education had the highest risk for CVD, regardless of race. These findings demonstrate the need to focus risk-reduction interventions on all Southern rural women with limited education, not just African-American women. The study results support the current view in the literature suggesting that race should be a risk marker rather than a risk factor.

---

variables were associated with the development or nondevelopment of the disease.

Recently concluded was a national longitudinal, experimental, cohort study involving thousands of nurses called the Brigham and Women's Hospital/Harvard Medical School Women's Health Study (Women's Health Study, 2003). It consisted of a randomized trial evaluating the balance of benefits and risks of low-dose aspirin and vitamin E in the prevention of cancer and cardiovascular disease. Depending on the random assignment of the nurses, participants took 100 mg of aspirin or placebo and 600 IU of vitamin E or placebo per day. Originally, 50 mg/day of β-carotene or placebo was also included, but after additional β-carotene was associated in other studies with a higher risk of lung cancer, it was removed from the Women's Health Study in the mid-1990s. This was a double-blind study: neither the participants nor the researchers knew which subjects were taking the study drugs or placebos. Nurses were selected for this major study because as an aggregate they are accessible through RN registry, and because it was assumed that nurses, who know the value of research, would have a higher rate of follow-through in taking the test drugs routinely than would the general public. Data on the health status of the participants

was gathered every 6 months, and the study was funded through 2004. Follow-up is planned on the health of these women for years to come. In addition, the women are being told which group they were in. Based on cohort ages, the findings will support or not support the use of aspirin and/or vitamin E supplements for reduction of heart disease and cancer risk. If findings are positive, regular supplementation with aspirin or vitamin E may be recommended for healthy women at specific ages.

In practice, the various types of studies just discussed are frequently mixed. A case-control study may include description and analysis with a retrospective focus; a cohort study may be conducted prospectively or retrospectively. The study of early antecedents to prevent tobacco smoking (Kellam & Anthony, 1998) was a case-control study, a cohort study, and an experimental study. Flexibility is essential to allow the investigator as much freedom as possible in choosing the most useful methodology.

Experimental Epidemiology

Experimental epidemiology follows and builds on information gathered from descriptive and analytic approaches. It is used to study epidemics, the etiology of human disease, the value of preventive and therapeutic measures, and the evaluation of health services (Valanis, 1999). In an experimental study, the investigator actually controls or changes the factors suspected of causing the health condition under study and observes what happens to the health state. In human populations, experimental studies should focus on disease prevention or health promotion rather than testing the causes of disease, which is done primarily on animals.

Experimental studies are carried out under carefully controlled conditions. The investigator exposes an experimental group to some factor thought to cause disease, improve health, prevent disease, or influence health in some way (as in the Women's Health Study). Simultaneously, the investigator observes a control group that is similar in characteristics to the experimental group but without the exposure factor.

The community health nurse should be alert for opportunities to conduct experimental studies in the course of working with groups. A study need not be elaborate to provide important data for future nursing practice. For example, a community health nurse can provide focused instruction to 20 new mothers encouraging them to breast feed and then compare the health of their infants with infants of 20 mothers in the same service area who use formula. A nurse can look at the number of automobile crashes at an intersection where there is a traffic light compared with a similar intersection that has stop signs. Based on the results of the investigation, the nurse may bring the information to the city council and petition for a stop light at the intersection. Study results can be used to bring about change in the community and are not limited to communicable or chronic diseases. Improving community safety is also an essential outcome.

An expanding area of experimental epidemiology involves the use of computers to simulate epidemics. With mathematical models, it is possible to determine the probabilities of various aspects of disease occurrence. This approach is making an increased contribution to epidemiologists' knowledge of etiology and prevention.

Occasionally, an experiment occurs naturally in which conditions offer the researcher the chance to make important discoveries. John Snow discovered such a "natural experiment" in London in 1854. In his seminal study of an epidemic of cholera, he observed one group that contracted the disease and another that did not. Closer inspection revealed that the major difference between these groups was their water supply. Eventually, the spread of cholera was traced to the water supply of the group with the high morbidity rate. In addition, Snow developed a theory of disease communication. As early as 1849, he promoted frequent hand-washing by those attending patients (Valanis, 1999).

A *community trial* is a type of experimental study done at the community level. Geographic communities are assigned to intervention (experimental) or nonintervention (control) groups and compared to determine whether the intervention produces a positive change in the community.

Community trials can be extremely expensive and are not undertaken unless there is substantial evidence that the intervention will make a difference at the aggregate level. A major community trial occurred in the 1950s in Kingston and Newburgh, New York. These were two cities of similar size and population make-up that had separate water supplies. Fluoride was added to Newburgh's water but not to Kingston's. A decrease in the incidence of dental caries was found in the city with the added fluoride. Because of this major community trial, fluoride began to be added to our nation's water supplies and toothpastes. Interestingly, more recent studies have shown that the fluoride does not provide the protection once thought. In fact, in recent years Newburgh has been found to have more cavities than the never-fluoridated Kingston. There is a backlash from dentists and activists to remove fluoride from general sources, such as water supplies and toothpaste (Traubman & Aroya, 2003).

CONDUCTING EPIDEMIOLOGIC RESEARCH

The community health nurse who engages in an epidemiologic investigation becomes a kind of detective. First, there is a problem to solve, a puzzle to unravel, or a question to answer. The nurse begins to search for basic information, for clues that might help answer the question. Information is never self-explanatory, and, like a detective, the nurse must analyze and interpret every additional clue. Slowly, there is a narrowing of possible suspects until the causes of a disease, the consequences of a prevention plan, or the results of treatment are identified. On the basis of this investigation, the nurse can draw further conclusions and make new applications to improve health services.

As discussed previously, epidemiologic studies are a form of research. The steps outlined here are similar to those discussed in Chapter 14, Research in Community Health Nursing. Epidemiologic research involves seven steps. Everything from an informal study in the course of nursing practice to the most comprehensive epidemiologic research project can be undertaken with these steps:

1. Identify the problem.
2. Review the literature.
3. Design the study.
4. Collect the data.
5. Analyze the findings.
6. Develop conclusions and applications.
7. Disseminate the findings.

Each of these steps is considered here in the context of a single nursing study that examined the negative effects of in utero drug exposure for a group of infants and children. Although research as a community health nursing role is covered in a separate chapter, the analysis of one epidemiologic study here reinforces the integration of research in the nurse's role.

Identify the Problem

Community health nurses are constantly confronted with threats to the health and well-being of the community. Almost daily, questions are raised, puzzles presented, and problems identified. Pregnant women who smoke or use cocaine threaten the health of their unborn children; what can be done to reduce this behavior? Rape is increasing; what can be done to prevent such violence or to bring aid to victims? Children are injured and die from bicycle accidents; why do these occur and how can they be prevented? Many farm workers have been killed or injured in farm equipment accidents; what can be done to prevent them? Any threat to the health of a group offers fertile ground for epidemiologic investigation.

One team of nurse researchers was concerned with responsiveness between mothers with depressive symptoms and their infants (Horowitz et al., 2001). They used an experimental design with 117 postpartum women who were randomly assigned either to the treatment or the control group. Both groups received home visits three times during the first 18 weeks after delivery. However, the treatment group received a coached behavioral intervention designed to promote maternal-infant responsiveness. As hypothesized, the treatment group showed significantly higher maternal-infant responsiveness after the intervention. Intensive home-based coached behavioral interventions provided by registered nurses proved an effective method to improve maternal-infant responsiveness, supporting the view that such interventions should be incorporated into the discharge planning of new mothers who demonstrate depressive symptoms.

Review the Literature

All too often, after identifying a problem, health professionals rush to take immediate action without reviewing solutions that have been tried previously. Every epidemiologic investigation should begin with a review of the literature. Even discovering that little research has been done on the problem can be valuable information. Conversely, if many studies have already been conducted in the area, this information can help narrow the study to areas not previously investigated or allow researchers to replicate earlier studies to confirm findings in a different setting. One of the most valuable sources in the literature is the review article, which essentially summarizes all the research that has been conducted on a subject.

A review of the literature often suggests hypotheses from discoveries made in other studies. In the home intervention program for new mothers with depressive symptoms, a review of the literature provided helpful background information. The literature review also revealed that interventions had proved to be an effective method in many other settings with different populations.

Design the Study

The first step in designing a study is to formulate one or more specific questions to answer or hypotheses to test. Some-times, the question or hypothesis emerges from the review of the literature; it also may be developed through the researcher's own analysis and hunches. It is a good idea to write out one or more hypotheses to test or questions to answer. The researchers in the postpartum intervention study formulated the hypothesis that the treatment group would exhibit significantly higher maternal-infant responsiveness after the intervention. As a framework for this study, A. Beck's cognitive model of depression was used along with two developmental models, a transactional model of child development and a model of developmental risk and resilience (Horowitz et al., 2001).

The next step is to plan what study type (descriptive, analytic, or experimental) or combination of study types best suits the goals of the research and how the study will be conducted. Will the data be collected retrospectively from existing records, or will new data be collected? Who will conduct interviews? What kinds of data will be needed to measure the outcomes of intervention? The mothers with depressive symptoms study used an experimental design. Eligible participants were randomly assigned to either the treatment or the control group, and to between-subjects or within-subjects measures (Munro, 2001).

Collect the Data

Data in the mothers with depressive symptoms study were collected from home visits conducted for the study. The research team of nurses who made the treatment home visits were trained in coaching techniques and kept scoring sheets and field notes. The team met regularly to review their participation activities. Women in the control group received standard postpartum primary care and also could receive additional psychiatric treatment for depression as needed.

It is useful to perform a pilot study that pretests an interview guide, questionnaire, or treatment. If one wishes to interview women about battering during pregnancy, it might be useful to prepare a guide and interview one or two people, then revise the guide on the basis of the experience. If development of a questionnaire to assess the nutritional needs of elderly people living alone is part of the study design, it would be helpful to test the survey on some volunteers to determine its clarity and relevance. And if the study is to provide a specific treatment such as coaching, teaching, or demonstration, it is important to practice it on a small group of people with characteristics similar to those of the subjects.

In community health nursing, data collection often can occur as part of ongoing practice. Unless the study has been carefully designed, however, data may be collected for months or years, only to discover that important questions have been omitted.

Analyze the Findings

In most epidemiologic studies, data analysis consists of summarizing the findings, computing rates and ratios, and displaying the findings in tables and graphs. At this stage, the data are used to address the original question or test the original hypothesis. Was the hypothesis supported or not supported by the data? Summarized data can also generate more questions or indicate areas that warrant further investigation. For example, data accumulated in the mothers with depressive symptoms study explored housekeeping behaviors observed on the three home visits, but this was not a main focus of the study. Did these behaviors change from before to after delivery? Did the mothers report signs and symptoms of depression before their pregnancies? How large are their social support systems? It is unusual for a study to not generate more questions, which then become the material for future research.

Develop Conclusions and Applications

Stating conclusions is an outcome of analysis and interpretation. The investigators summarize the results and their meaning for the purpose of making this information useful to other health services providers. Many times, research has direct practical application for improving health services, continuing or discontinuing services, or conducting future research. It is also important to describe mistakes made and lessons learned about study design and other aspects of the research, to assist future investigators.

In Horowitz's study of mothers with depressive symptoms, the researchers stated that future research directions should "include testing additional interventions designed to diminish depression and to reverse effects of maternal depression and dysphoria on child and family health" (2001, p. 328). In addition, the researchers indicated that future studies should include increased diversity of samples, matching of field researchers' ethnic and racial backgrounds with those of the study population; that future studies should include partners or other family members in research designs, which would expand knowledge about family processes in relation to maternal depression; and, finally, that qualitative research designs that explore women's interpretations of postpartum adjustment and depressive disorders would provide additional information.

Disseminate the Findings

Finally, research findings should be shared. Information gained from epidemiologic studies must be disseminated throughout the professional community to strengthen the knowledge base for improved practice and to promote future research. The authors of the mothers with depressive symp-

toms study disseminated their findings in a nursing journal article.

SUMMARY

Epidemiology is the study of the distribution and determinants of health, health conditions, and disease in human population groups. It shares with community health nursing the common focus of the health of populations. It is a specialized form of scientific research that can provide public health professionals with a body of knowledge on which to base their practice and methods for studying new and existing problems. To understand epidemiology, one must first understand some basic epidemiologic concepts: the host, agent, and environment model; causality; immunity; the natural history of disease or health conditions; risk; and prevention strategies.

Community health nurses can use three sources of information when conducting epidemiologic investigations: existing epidemiologic data, informal investigations, and carefully designed scientific studies.

Epidemiology employs three investigative approaches: descriptive studies, analytic studies, and experimental studies. Although studies can be either retrospective or prospective, some merely describe existing conditions (descriptive studies), whereas others seek to explain causes (analytic studies). Experimental studies seek to confirm causal relationships identified in descriptive and analytic studies. Analytic studies can be of three types: prevalence, case-control, or cohort. In practice, all these types of studies often become combined in various ways. They also make use of quantitative concepts such as count, prevalence rate, incidence rate, mortality rate, and various types of morbidity (sickness) rates.

Epidemiologic research includes seven steps:
1. Identify the problem, which is usually a threat to the population's health.
2. Review the literature to determine what other studies have found.
3. Carefully design the study.
4. Collect the data.
5. Analyze the findings.
6. Develop conclusions and applications.
7. Disseminate the findings.

Thinking epidemiologically can significantly enhance community health nursing practice. Epidemiology provides both the body of knowledge—information on the distribution and determinants of health conditions—and methods for investigating health problems and evaluating services.

ACTIVITIES TO PROMOTE CRITICAL THINKING

1. Identify an aggregate-level health problem in your community. Using the host, agent, and environment model, explain who is the host, what are the causative agents, and what environmental factors have promoted or delayed the development of the problem.

2. Select an aggregate health (wellness) condition, such as preschoolers' normal growth and development or elders' healthy aging, and list all the causal factors that might contribute to this healthy state. Now, plot these schematically in a diagram (such as those in Figs. 8–3, 8–4, or 8–5) to show the web of causation for this condition.

3. Using the same health condition that you selected in the previous exercise, describe the natural history of this condition, outlining its four stages. Identify three preventive nursing interventions, one for each level of prevention, that could apply to this condition.

4. Select an article that reports an epidemiologic study from a recent nursing or public health journal, and record your responses to the following questions:
   a. What prompted the study, and what was its purpose?
   b. Was it descriptive, analytic, or experimental research?
   c. Was the study design retrospective or prospective?
   d. Why did the investigators choose this design?
   e. What existing sources of epidemiologic data did this study use? List all sources specifically, such as *Morbidity and Mortality Weekly Report* or incomes by household in census data.
   f. What were the study findings? Identify the population group that will benefit from this research.

5. Interview one or more practicing public health nurses in your community, and identify an aggregate-level problem that needs epidemiologic investigation. Propose a rough draft study design to research this problem.

6. A major portion of the end of this chapter was devoted to the steps of the epidemiologic process using as an example Horowitz's study of women with depressive symptoms after delivery. Search the Internet for data on similar or related studies. In addition, search a topic of interest to you to see whether there is any current research being conducted by community health nurses or related community professionals on that topic.

REFERENCES

Appel, S.J., Harrell, J.S., & Deng, S. (2002). Racial and socioeconomic differences in risk factors for cardiovascular disease among southern rural women. *Nursing Research, 51*(3), 140–147.

Beaglehole, R., & Bonita, R. (1997). *Public health at the crossroads: Achievements and prospects.* Cambridge, England: Cambridge University Press.

Burnet, M. (1962). *Natural history of infectious diseases* (3rd ed.). Cambridge, England: Cambridge University Press.

Centers for Disease Control and Prevention, Division of Vector-borne Diseases. (2002). West Nile Virus Basics [online]. Retrieved November 11, 2003 from *http://www.cdc.gov/ncidod/dvbid/westnile/index.htm*

Chin, J.E. (Ed.). (1999). *Control of communicable diseases. manual* (17th ed.). Washington, DC: American Public Health Association.

Cohen, D., Spear, S., Scribner, R., Kissinger, P., Mason, K., & Wildgen, J. (2000). "Broken Windows" and the risk of gonorrhea. *American Journal of Public Health, 90*(2), 230–236.

Fos, P.J., & Fine, D.J. (2000). *Designing health care for populations: Applied epidemiology in health care administration.* San Francisco: Jossey-Bass.

Galil, K., Pletcher, M.J., Wallace, B.J., Seward, J., Meyer, P.A., Baughman, A.L., et al. (2002). Tracking varicella deaths: Accuracy and completeness of death certificates and hospital discharge records, New York State, 1989–1995. *American Journal of Public Health, 92*(8), 1248–1249.

Horowitz, J.A., Bell, M., Trybulski, J., Munro, B.H., Moser, D., Hartz, S.A., et al. (2001). Promoting responsiveness between mothers with depressive symptoms and their infants. *Journal of Nursing Scholarship, 33*(4), 323–329.

Kellam, S.G., & Anthony, J.C. (1998). Targeting early antecedents to prevent tobacco smoking: Findings from an epidemiologically based, randomized field trial. *American Journal of Public Health, 88*(10), 1490–1495.

Kerns, T. (2001). *Environmentally induced illnesses: Ethics, risk assessment and human rights.* Jefferson, NC: McFarland & Company.

Kleyman, P. (2001). Scientists link Parkinson's and pesticides in search for cure. *Aging Today, 22*(3), 1, 4.

Kopf, E.W. (1978). Florence Nightingale as statistician. *Research in Nursing and Health, 1*(3), 93–102.

Krug, E.G., Sharma, G.K., & Lozano, R. (2000). The global

burden of injuries. *American Journal of Public Health, 90*(4), 523–526.

Lawson, A.B., & Williams, F.L.R. (2001). *An introductory guide to disease mapping*. Chichester, UK: John Wiley & Sons.

Markowitz, G., & Rosner, D. (2000). Public health then and now. "Cater to the children": The role of the lead industry in a public health tragedy, 1900–1955. *American Journal of Public Health, 90*(1), 36–46.

Munro, B.H. (2001). *Statistical methods for health care research* (4th ed.). Philadelphia: Lippincott Williams & Wilkins.

Pormeba, B. (2003). Epidemiology. Available: *http://www.salemstate.edu~6porembia/epi99/*. Accessed March 15, 2004.

Quander, L. (2001, Spring). HIV/AIDS prevention programs: What's working with our youth? *HIV Impact, A Closing the Gap Newsletter of the Office of Minority Health*, pp. 1, 2, 4. Washington, DC: U. S. Department of Health and Human Services.

Sibley, C.L. (2002). Smallpox vaccination revisited. *The American Journal of Nursing 102*(9), 26–32.

Susser, I., & Stein, Z. (2000). Culture, sexuality, and women's agency in the prevention of HIV/AIDS in southern Africa. *American Journal of Public Health, 90*(7), 1042–1048.

Thomas, J.C., & Weber, D.J. (2001). *Epidemiologic methods for the study of infectious diseases*. New York: Oxford University Press.

Traubman, T., & Aroya, A.B. (2003). Dentists show fluoridation is a failure: No benefit to the majority. Available: *http://www.rense.com/general/24/fail.htm*. Accessed March 15, 2004.

U. S. Department of Health and Human Services. (2000). *Healthy people 2010* (Conference ed., Vols. 1 & 2). Washington, DC: Author.

Valanis, B. (1999). *Epidemiology in health care* (3rd ed.). Stamford, CT: Appleton & Lange.

Wimbush, F.B., & Peters, R.M. (2000). Identification of cardiovascular risk: Use of a cardiovascular-specific genogram. *Public Health Nursing, 17*(3), 148–154.

Women's Health Study. (2003). Boston: Brigham Women's Hospital.

Wynd, C.A. (2002). Testicular self-examination in young adult men. *Journal of Nursing Scholarship, 34*(3), 251–255.

Yassi, A., Kjellstrom, T., de Kok, T., & Guidotti, T.L. (2001). *Basic environmental health*. New York: Oxford University Press.

SELECTED READINGS

Allukian, M. (2000). The neglected epidemic and the Surgeon General's report: A call to action for better oral health. *American Journal of Public Health, 90*(6), 843–845.

Anderson, C.T., & McFarlane, J. (2000). *Community as partner* (3rd ed.). Philadelphia: Lippincott Williams & Wilkins.

Chatterjee, N., & Leonard, L. (2001). Partners-in-health: A new front line for disease prevention and health promotion in the community. *American Journal of Health Education, 32*(1), 52–55.

Centers for Disease Control and Prevention. (2001). *Sexually transmitted disease surveillance, 2000*. Atlanta, GA: U. S. Department of Health and Human Services.

Centers for Disease Control and Prevention. (2002). Trends in sexual risk behaviors among high school students—United States, 1991–2001. *MMWR Morbidity and Mortality Weekly Report, 51*(38), 856–859.

Cruz, M.A., Katz, D.J., & Suarez, J.A. (2001). An assessment of the ability of routine restaurant inspections to predict foodborne outbreaks in Miami Dade County, Florida. *American Journal of Public Health, 91*(5), 821–823.

Cubbin, C., LeClere, F.B., & Smith, G.S. (2000). Socioeconomic status and the occurrence of fatal and nonfatal injury in the United States. *American Journal of Public Health, 90*(1), 70–77.

Fleming, P.L., Wortley, P.M., Karon, J.M., DeCock, K.M., & Janssen, R.S. (2000). Tracking the HIV epidemic: Current issues, future challenges. *American Journal of Public Health, 90*(7), 1037–1041.

Friis, R.H., & Sellers, T.A. (1999). *Epidemiology for public health practice*. Gaithersburg, MD: Aspen Publishing.

Hench, C., & Simpkins, S. (2002). Hepatitis C: Risk factors, assessment and diagnosis. *Nurseweek, 15*(12), 19–21.

Karon, J.M., Fleming, P.L., Steketee, R.W., & DeCock, K.M. (2001). HIV in the United States at the turn of the century: An epidemic in transition. *American Journal of Public Health, 91*(7), 1060–1068.

Last, J.M. (2001). *A dictionary of epidemiology* (4th ed.). New York: Oxford University Press.

Mendez, D., & Warner, K.E. (2000). Smoking prevalence in 2010: Why the Healthy People goal is unattainable. *American Journal of Public Health, 90*(3), 401–403.

Sekikawa, A., & Kuller, L.H. (2000). Striking variation in coronary heart disease mortality in the United States among black and white women, ages 45–54, by state. *Journal of Women's Health and Gender-Based Medicine, 9*(5), 545–558.

Teutsch, S.M., & Churchill, R.E. (2000). *Principles and practice of public health surveillance*. New York: Oxford University Press.

Tomes, N. (2000). The making of a germ panic, then and now. *American Journal of Public Health, 90*(2), 191–198.

Vynnycky, E., & Fine, P.E. (2000). Lifetime risks, incubation period, and serial interval of tuberculosis. *American Journal of Epidemiology, 1*(52), 247–263.

Weisskopf, M.G., Anderson, H.A., Foldy, S., Hanrahan, L.P., Blair, K., Torok, T.J., et al. (2002). Heat wave morbidity and mortality, Milwaukee, Wisconsin, 1999 vs 1995: An improved response? *American Journal of Public Health, 92*(5), 830–833.

Internet Resources

Association for Professionals in Infection Control and Epidemiology, Inc.: *http://www.apic.org*

Centers for Disease Control and Prevention: *http://www.cdc.gov*

Certification Board of Infection Control and Epidemiology, Inc.: *http://www.cbic.org*

Environmental Protection Agency: *http://www.epa.gov*

Immunization Action Coalition: *http://www.immunize.org*

March of Dimes, perinatal statistics: *http://www.peristats.modimes.org/*

National Health Statistics: *http://www.health.gov*

Safety and Health Statistics: *http://www.bls.gov/iif/*

University of California at Los Angeles Center for Health Policy Research: *http://www.healthpolicy.ucla.edu/*

9

Communicable Disease Control

Key Terms

- **Acquired immunodeficiency syndrome (AIDS)**
- **Active immunity**
- **Communicable disease**
- **Direct transmission**
- **Fomites**
- **Herd immunity**
- **Human immunodeficiency virus (HIV)**
- **Immunization**
- **Incubation period**
- **Indirect transmission**
- **Infectious**
- **Isolation**
- **Passive immunity**
- **Quarantine**
- **Reservoir**
- **Ring vaccination**
- **Screening**
- **Surveillance**
- **Vaccine**
- **Vector**

Learning Objectives

Upon mastery of this chapter, you should be able to:

- Discuss the global and national trends and issues in communicable disease control.
- Describe the three modes of transmission for communicable diseases.
- Explain the strategies used for the three levels of prevention in communicable disease control.
- Explain the significance of immunization as a communicable disease control measure.
- Describe major issues that affect the control and elimination of tuberculosis.
- Differentiate between human immunodeficiency virus (HIV) infection and acquired immunodeficiency syndrome (AIDS).
- Discuss specific ways to prevent sexually transmitted diseases, including HIV/AIDS.
- Identify six globally emerging communicable diseases.
- Discuss the consequences of biologic terrorism with weapons such as anthrax and smallpox.
- Describe the nurse's role in communicable disease control.
- Discuss ethical issues affecting communicable disease and infection control.

Communicable diseases pose a major threat to public health and are of significant concern to community health nurses. A **communicable disease** is one that can be transmitted from one person to another. It is caused by an agent that is **infectious** (capable of producing infection) and is transmitted from a source, or **reservoir**, to a susceptible host.

Knowledge of communicable diseases is fundamental to the practice of community health nursing because these diseases typically spread through communities of people. Understanding of the basic concepts of communicable disease control, as well as the numerous issues arising in this area, helps a community health nurse work effectively to prevent and control communicable disease in populations and groups. It also helps nurses teach important and effective preventive measures to community members, advocate for those affected, and protect the well-being of uninfected persons (including the nurses themselves).

Several issues and circumstances have emerged during the last quarter-century that are important areas of concern to community health nurses:

- Despite significant declines in mortality, communicable diseases are responsible for persistently high morbidity among various age and population groups.
- Rates of some communicable diseases, especially tuberculosis (TB) and sexually transmitted diseases (STDs), remain disproportionately high in selected population groups (in some cases, shockingly high), a fact often masked when statistics are aggregated.
- Diseases that were once little-known in the United States, such as West Nile virus, are making an appearance.
- The development of resistant (MDR) strains of bacteria and viruses poses a significant occupational health challenge as well as a practice issue for health workers.
- New fears of terrorist attacks using anthrax, botulilinum (botulism), and smallpox create areas in which community health nurses must play a role. They can educate the public and help reduce fears and vulnerability as they remain knowledgeable regarding infrequently seen communicable diseases that might be potential terrorist weapons.
- Current research reveals that infectious agents may be responsible for a number of the chronic diseases, including some forms of cancer, that have occupied the interest of health care providers in the last few decades.

This chapter provides community health nurses with information to assess the communicable disease burden in a community. It describes ways to plan appropriate prevention interventions, including immunization of children and adults, environmental interventions, community education, screening programs, and case-finding and contact investigation. Ethical issues of communicable disease control are also discussed. A list of communicable disease information sources useful to the nurse is given at the end of this chapter.

BASIC CONCEPTS REGARDING COMMUNICABLE DISEASES

Evolution of Communicable Disease Control

Communicable diseases have challenged health care providers for centuries. They have led to the development of countless nursing and medical preventive measures, from simple procedures such as hand-washing, sanitation, and proper ventilation to the research and development of vaccines and antibiotics. Because these preventive measures have greatly reduced the spread of communicable diseases, many people consider communicable diseases to be a threat of the past. Yet this is not so. Communicable diseases, particularly those of epidemic and pandemic proportions, such as TB and acquired immunodeficiency syndrome (AIDS), continue to cost millions of lives and billions of dollars to the global human society every year.

As mentioned in Chapter 8, the first documented global threat from a communicable disease began in the 13th century in the form of bubonic plague. It was responsible for killing 25% of the population in some European countries in the years after the Crusades and during the years of exploration and trade by ship, in the 1400s to 1600s.

As commerce and industry continued to grow, people migrated from rural areas to towns and cities. However, health and hygiene practices that worked in remote areas did not transfer to the new urban settings. In tenements and overcrowded parts of towns, water for drinking easily became contaminated with human waste; mounting garbage and trash, unable to be composted or buried as was done in farming communities, created a rich habitat for rodents and other animals and insects, encouraging them to breed and act as vectors for many communicable diseases.

It was not until the 1700s and 1800s that the causative organisms for various infectious diseases were recognized through the assistance of increasingly sophisticated microscopes. With these discoveries came early attempts to create ways to prevent the spread of such organisms, either by decreasing their power or by eliminating them. Pasteurization of milk was invented, and efforts to eliminate rats from ships and food storage areas began. These measures began a global effort to eliminate communicable diseases.

One disease, smallpox, is a classic example of a communicable disease control success story. For centuries, smallpox, an infectious disease, killed millions of people and scarred survivors for life. It first responded to a crude vaccine that was developed, almost accidentally, in the 1800s. Notable people of the time withstood the months-long after-effects of the smallpox vaccine, including the family of our second president, John Adams (McCullough, 2001). The vaccine was studied and perfected and was used globally for decades. A major worldwide eradication campaign began in 1967. The last naturally acquired case of smallpox in the world occurred in October, 1977;

global eradication was certified 2 years later by the World Health Organization (WHO) and confirmed by the World Health Assembly in May 1980. Since then, no cases of small-pox have been identified in any country (Chin, 1999; WHO, 1998). However, the threat of biologic warfare using smallpox or other disease organisms raises concerns about how to pre-pare for the future. In fact, a new and controversial smallpox immunization program began in 2002 with President George Bush being immunized. The plan was to follow with military personnel, health care providers, and then voluntary immu-nization among the general population. In 2002, the Centers for Disease Control and Prevention (CDC) issued guidelines for state and local smallpox response, calling for "mass voluntary vaccinations to be performed together with **ring vaccination** in the event of an outbreak. Ring vaccination involves vaccinat-ing people who have been in close contact with an infected in-dividual" and initially was used successfully in the eradication of smallpox (Wright, 2002, p.1). The 2002 immunization pro-gram did not extend to the general population, as smallpox threats to our nation declined in 2003–2004, as did our fears.

Global Trends

During the last several decades, substantial progress has been made in controlling some major infectious diseases around the world, although other diseases have not been managed as well. The following are some of the major accomplishments:

- The WHO's Expanded Program on Immunization (EPI) was launched in 1974. As a result, by 1995, more than 80% of the world's children had been immunized against *diphtheria, tetanus, whooping cough, poliomyelitis, measles,* and *TB,* compared with fewer than 5% in 1974 (WHO, 1998).
- Global eradication of *smallpox* was achieved in 1980.
- The tropical disease *yaws* has virtually disappeared. The first yaws campaign was launched in Haiti in 1950, and by 1965, 46 million people in 49 countries had been suc-cessfully treated with penicillin. The disease is no longer a significant problem in most of the world.
- Because of improved sanitation and hygiene, outbreaks of *relapsing fever,* transmitted by lice, are rare today.
- In 1988, a campaign for global eradication of *poliomyelitis* by the year 2000 was launched. Reported cases worldwide have declined by 99% since the campaign began, with only 537 new cases in the world in 2001. The poliovirus has dis-appeared from the Americas, and Europe was declared free of polio in 1998, with its last case in Turkey (Olsen, 2002). However, polio remains endemic in 10 countries: India, Pakistan, and Nigeria are major reservoirs, cases are also reported from Afghanistan, Niger, Somalia, Egypt, Angola, Ethiopia, and Sudan ("Polio at All-time Low," June/July 2002).
- The global threat of *plague* has declined in the last 40 years, largely as a result of the use of antibiotics and in-secticides. However, there is evidence of plague in ro-dents spreading in parts of the western United States.

- *Leprosy* (Hansen disease), once a major communicable dis-ease, is almost eliminated. In 1966, there were 10.5 million reported cases worldwide. Through the use of multidrug therapy, the numbers were reduced to 5.4 million in 1985, and in 1999 there were 1.4 cases per 10,000 population. The WHO will no longer consider leprosy a public health prob-lem when there is less than 1 case per 10,000 population.

Some major problem communicable diseases and areas remain, including the following:

- *Malaria* remains a major threat, even though the mortality rate has improved in the last 25 years. In 1954, there were 2.5 million deaths annually and 250 million cases of malaria worldwide; in 2002, there were an estimated 1.5 to 2.7 million deaths and 300 to 500 million cases. Tropical Africa has 90% of the cases, and malaria is endemic in 92 countries. The Pan American Health Organization (PAHO) Global Strategy for Malaria Control is to collaborate with affected countries to reduce the incidence of the disease.
- *Cholera* was mainly confined to Asia in the early 20th century through improvements in sanitation elsewhere. However, a series of pandemics have affected much of the world since 1960 and have become more widespread and more frequent in Africa since the 1970s. A new strain, *Vibrio cholerae O139,* was identified in India in 1992. Cholera is endemic in 80 countries and is of concern in all parts of the world. Along with other diarrheal diseases, it ranked as the third leading cause of death worldwide in 1999, mostly among children younger than 5 years of age (Gannon, 2000).
- *TB* has made a powerful resurgence in the last 3 decades as many countries let their control programs become com-placent. WHO declared TB a global emergency in 1993. One third of the incidence in the last 5 years can be at-tributed to human immunodeficiency virus (HIV) infec-tion. Drug-resistant strains of the TB bacillus have in-fected up to 50 million people worldwide. Each year, 8 million people develop TB, and 1.8 million die of the dis-ease. The highest incidence rates are found in Africa and southeast Asia (Borgdorff, Floyd, & Broekmans, 2002).
- *Yellow fever* causes about 30,000 deaths each year among 200,000 annual cases. Since the late 1980s, there has been a dramatic resurgence of the disease in Africa and the Americas. It is endemic in 34 countries in Africa, where immunization programs are weak in the 14 poorest African countries. In 1995, Peru experienced the largest yellow fever outbreak reported from any country in the Americas since 1950.
- *Sleeping sickness* (African trypanosomiasis) cases have doubled in the past few years (WHO, 1998).

Global successes and failures to control communicable diseases are affected by a bevy of factors. First, the geopo-litical nature of an area influences who can respond when a communicable disease occurs in a country. Second, the nat-ural and manmade resources of an area influence the health status of the population before a disease strikes, contribut-ing to both disease resistance and the ability to survive once a communicable disease is contracted. This is one reason that poorer nations have higher incidences and greater numbers of deaths from communicable diseases. Finally, weather and climatic factors can influence health and illness. For example, both droughts and floods can lead to crop failure and subsequent famine. Other such factors include hurricanes, monsoons, earthquakes, tornadoes, floods, and fire.

National Trends

At the turn of the millennium in the United States, we are faced with the emergence of new and newly virulent diseases. The set of revised health objectives in *Healthy People 2010* (United States Department of Health and Human Services [USDHHS], 2000) was written in part to address this challenge in communicable disease control.

New, Emerging, and Resurging Diseases

At the national level, for several decades in the late 20th century, medical research and funding focused on major chronic diseases such as arteriosclerosis and cancer. During those years, it seemed that the war against communicable disease was being won, and the nation became complacent about communicable diseases. When HIV/AIDS emerged in the early 1980s, valuable time was lost because of unwillingness or inability to recognize its potential as a major killer among all people. At the same time, it was discovered that many children were not being immunized against communicable diseases at rates as high as those in poorer nations. Also,

some diseases, such as *Escherichia coli*–induced diarrhea and TB, were coming back with a vengeance, and current prevention or treatment regimens were not effective.

It now appears likely that we will always be challenged by communicable diseases. Pathogens that are considered to be under control because they respond well to current treatment can mutate and produce new, virulent strains; diseases that have been almost eliminated can emerge again if public health efforts slacken; and diseases that are eradicated in the United States can revisit this country on any one of the hundreds of international flights arriving each day. As a result, present concerns focus on three types of communicable disease: new diseases, emerging diseases, and resurging diseases.

Some communicable diseases have been affecting us for centuries or millennia, but a major new disease, HIV/AIDS, which is covered in detail later in this chapter, was first recognized only in 1981. Legionnaires' disease was first detected in Philadelphia in 1976; it has occurred sporadically in other countries since then. In 1999, West Nile virus was first diagnosed in the United States in New York City; in subsequent years more cases were confirmed. In 2002, there were 2946 cases with 160 fatalities by October of that year as the disease spread across the country (Chettle, 2002). These diseases are disturbing reminders that new threats to public health are always on the horizon (Fig. 9–1).

Emerging diseases are diseases rarely or never before seen in the United States. These diseases may also be new to public health officials in other countries. Emerging diseases occurring in the United States include the hantavirus, seen in the southwestern United States in 1993; dengue fever, ac-

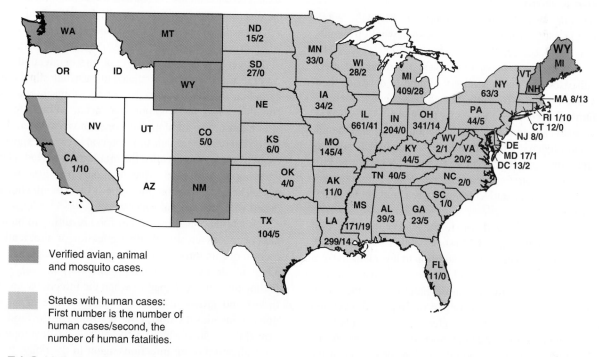

FIGURE 9–1. Areas reporting West Nile virus activity as of mid-October 2002.

quired from travel outside the United States and first seen among people in Texas in the 1980s; and typhoid, seen in a native Nigerian in New York City in 1994. Typically, diseases that are uncommon in the United States, such as malaria, plague, Lassa fever, cholera, and yellow fever, accompany people as they travel from one country to another on airlines and cruise ships. Dr. Mohammad Akhter, executive director of the American Public Health Association, said, "The [CDC] is just like the Justice Department before 9/11. It only comes in to investigate once a crime has been committed" (Mullins, 2002).

Resurging diseases are those communicable diseases that have been endemic in some parts of the world but are now endemic in more countries and are increasing to epidemic proportions in others. Often, the resurgence is caused by the emergence of new, drug-resistant strains of a familiar organism, such as the MDR TB bacillus. *Staphylococcus aureus* infections have some strains so powerful that they are not responding to vancomycin any longer; they still respond to two new antibiotics, but those could also lose effectiveness. This is a watershed moment in the fight to stay ahead of communicable diseases. In addition to *S. aureus* and the TB bacillus, the list of antimicrobial-resistant organisms includes strains of *Haemophilus influenzae, Neisseria gonorrhoeae, Bordetella pertussis,* and *Streptococcus pneumoniae.* TB is currently the communicable disease that affects the greatest number of people in the United States with strains of drug-resistant microbes. Hepatitis B, C, and D have resurged and are now seen in increasing numbers because of intravenous drug abuse.

Healthy People: The Prevention Agenda for the Nation

The *Healthy People 2010* document (USDHHS, 2000) groups the nation's health objectives somewhat differently from its predecessor, *Healthy People 2000* (USDHHS, 1991). Nevertheless, many objectives still focus on infectious diseases and immunizations, aiming to decrease morbidity and mortality from infectious diseases and to increase the number of children and adults immunized. In addition, the document attempts to guide the nation toward health with goals and objectives that include new focus areas such as arthritis, osteoporosis, chronic back conditions, chronic kidney diseases, respiratory diseases, vision and hearing, medical product safety, health communication, and public health infrastructure.

Healthy People 2010 was formulated with input from more than 350 national and 250 state public health, medical, and environmental agencies, in addition to lay advisors from around the country. These collaborators began to meet in 1996 to design the structure and content of the document. During its development, the Office of Disease Prevention and Health Promotion accepted electronic comments at its Web site and in writing, making this truly a document of the people. With so many people involved, achievement of the document's goals is more likely.

Modes of Transmission

As discussed in Chapter 8, the reservoir of infection can be a person, animal, insect, or inanimate material in which the infectious agent lives and multiplies and which serves as a source of infection to others. Transmission of a communicable disease can occur by direct or indirect methods.

Direct Transmission

Direct transmission occurs by immediate transfer of infectious agents from a reservoir to a new host. It requires direct contact with the source, through touching, biting, kissing, or sexual intercourse, or by the direct projection of droplet spray onto the conjunctiva or onto the mucous membranes of the eye, nose, or mouth during sneezing, coughing, spitting, laughing, singing, or talking. Direct transmission is limited to a distance of 1 meter or less.

Indirect Transmission

Indirect transmission occurs when the infectious agent is transported within contaminated inanimate materials such as air, water, or food. It is also commonly referred to as *vehicle-borne transmission.* Chapter 10 describes both the government's role and the nurse's role in helping to prevent food and water contamination by infectious agents.

People may be affected by certain communicable diseases merely through carrying on the normal activities of eating food and drinking beverages. Foodborne illnesses frequently reported to the CDC in the last few years include salmonellosis, a bacterial agent; hepatitis A, a viral agent; and shigellosis, a bacterial agent. The most commonly reported waterborne illness is infection by *Giardia lamblia,* a protozoan. *Giardia* can also occur as a food contaminant. Most of the disease-causing agents typically found in foods also survive in water to cause disease, although water may provide a less nutritive environment and result in lower concentrations of the agent. Most commonly, exposure to infectious food or water results in symptoms related to gastrointestinal function, including diarrhea, nausea, vomiting, stomach cramps, and jaundice. Onset of symptoms may occur within a few hours after exposure or not until days or even weeks later, depending on the organism. This time interval between exposure and onset of symptoms is called the **incubation period**. Note that waterborne pathogens affect not only the gastrointestinal tract. The CDC also compiles reports on skin infections associated with recreational water use.

Bacterial contamination of food resulting in human illness occurs as a result of either infection or intoxication. Infection occurs through ingestion of food contaminated with adequate doses of *Salmonella, Shigella, E. coli,* or other pathogens. The cycle begins when the infectious agent multiplies and grows in the food medium. The agent subsequently invades the host, after ingestion of the food. Infection then occurs, which is the entry and development or multiplication of an infectious agent in the body. It is usually accompanied by an immune response, such as the production of antibodies with or without clinical manifestation. The infectious organism produces illness by direct irritation of the normal gastrointestinal mucosa. In contrast, intoxication is caused by the production of toxins as a byproduct of the normal bacterial life cycle. This commonly occurs when cooked food is left standing at room temperature. It is ingestion of the toxin, rather than the microbe itself, that produces the illness.

The distinction between infection and intoxication is relevant for a number of reasons. Toxins may be difficult to isolate and identify, particularly in the absence of the bacteria; some suspected foodborne illnesses go unidentified for this reason. Although the bacteria may be killed after heating of foodstuffs before consumption, some bacteria-produced toxins are stable at normal cooking temperatures, so the food cannot be rendered safe. A bacteria that establishes itself in the human gastrointestinal system may require medical treatment to be eradicated. In contrast, individuals with food intoxication typically require essentially supportive care while in the process of ridding themselves of the toxin.

The most important aspects of foodborne and waterborne diseases for nurses in community health may be in recognizing, first of all, that outbreaks of illness affecting large numbers of people continue to occur fairly regularly, despite well-recognized standards for decontamination of water supplies and safe commercial food preparation. Second, such outbreaks may not be detectable by usual surveillance means because of individuals' mobility. For example, an outbreak of illness in Minnesota in the 1990s was associated with food served on an international airline. Had a large group of the affected travelers not communicated among themselves and with providers, the outbreak might never have been identified. Third, such outbreaks can serve to remind all community health practitioners that there continues to be a need to teach and observe the most basic methods for preventing food and water contamination. Display 9–1 summarizes correct methods for preserving the safety and cleanliness of food.

When transmission occurs through a **vector**, which is a nonhuman carrier such as an animal or insect, it is known as vector-borne transmission. Common vectors include bats, fleas, lice, mosquitoes, raccoons, rats, skunks, squirrels, and ticks. During vector-borne transmission, the infectious agent may be transported mechanically without multiplication or change, or the infectious agent may develop biologically before passage to a susceptible host.

Diseases transmitted through vectors prove challenging in communicable disease control, because individuals who become infected typically have no direct personal contact with other infected persons. Rather, isolated cases occur within areas inhabited by the vector. Nevertheless, human history has been significantly affected by vector-borne diseases. Louse-borne typhus and flea-borne plague together were responsible for a majority of the devastating epidemics that occurred over the last 600 years. Currently, mosquito-borne malaria and snail-borne schistosomiasis cause major human suffering to hundreds of millions of people in tropi-

---

DISPLAY 9–1

Correct Methods for Preserving the Safety and Cleanliness of Food

Before handling food:
- Wash hands and all food preparation surfaces and utensils thoroughly with soap and water.

When preparing food:
- Wash foods that are to be eaten raw and uncooked thoroughly in clean water. This includes foods that are to be peeled that grow on the ground or come in contact with soil.
- Cook all meat products thoroughly.
- Do not allow cooked meats to come in contact with dishes, utensils, or containers used when the foods were raw and uncooked.

When storing leftover foods:
- Cool cooked foods quickly; store under refrigeration in clean, covered containers.

When reheating leftover foods:
- Heat foods thoroughly. Bacteria contaminating food grow and multiply in a temperature range between 39°F and 140°F.

---

cal settings every year. The fact that most of these diseases are endemic to certain areas suggests the need for tight controls for prevention and intervention.

Control strategies directed toward vector-borne diseases typically involve, in addition to community education, complex environmental measures to hinder the vector from reaching the host (see Chapter 10). These strategies may include

- Reducing the population of insect vectors (eg, by spraying insecticides to kill mosquitoes)
- Treating the natural habitat of the vector to reduce the population density
- Reducing the population of other animal hosts that harbor the vector, as when rats are exterminated to reduce the risk of plague
- Erecting barriers between the susceptible human and the vector, such as use of mosquito nets or screened windows to control malaria or protective clothing and sprays against tick-borne diseases
- Educating the public about preventive and protective measures, including actions to take when attacked by the vector to prevent disease from developing

In the United States, vector-borne illnesses have received renewed attention with accumulating information about Lyme disease, a viral disease transmitted to humans by a tick vector. It results in symptoms of varying severity, including rash, joint pain, progressive weakness, vision changes, and other neuromuscular dysfunctions. Other vector-borne diseases receiving attention in the 1990s included tick-borne fevers, such as Rocky Mountain spotted fever and relapsing fever, and rabies, whose vector usually is a domestic animal, bat, skunk, or raccoon. As mentioned earlier, West Nile virus was first seen in the United States in 1999. Occasionally, imported vector-borne tropical diseases, including malaria and dengue fever, are reported. The return of military personnel from southeast Asia through the 1960s and 1970s had a significant effect on the numbers of imported cases of malaria reported in the United States.

Airborne Transmission

Airborne transmission occurs through droplet nuclei—the small residues that result from evaporation of fluid from droplets emitted by an infected host. They may also be created purposely by atomizing devices or accidentally in microbiology laboratories. Because of their small size and weight, they can remain suspended in the air for long periods before they are inhaled into the respiratory system of a host.

Airborne transmission can also occur in dust. Small particles of dust from soil containing fungus spores may cling to clothing, bedding, or floors. Alternatively, the spores may become separated from dry soil by the wind and then be inhaled by the host.

PRIMARY PREVENTION

In the context of communicable disease control, two approaches are useful in achieving primary prevention: (1) education using mass media and targeting health messages to aggregates and (2) immunization.

Education

Health education in primary prevention is directed both at helping at-risk individuals understand their risk status and at promoting behaviors that decrease exposure or susceptibility. Chapter 12 deals more extensively with the concepts of learning theory and the variety of health education approaches and materials available to community health nurses today.

Use of Mass Media for Health Education

All people need to be informed about the risks of communicable diseases. Often, use of the mass media is the most effective way to reach the largest number of people. Additionally, many target groups, such as low-income and racially and ethnically diverse communities at high risk for communicable diseases, are very hard to reach one on one. One way to reach them is through the media. To disseminate public health information to large numbers of people, there are four major roles of mass media:

1. Use the media as a primary change agent; community education programs can successfully increase knowledge about communicable diseases and preventive measures.
2. Use the media as a complement to other disease prevention efforts; the media can effectively model preventive behaviors, such as condom use and drug abstinence.

3. Use the media as a promoter of communicable disease control programs; the media can help to increase participation of community members in primary prevention services.
4. Use the media to promote disease prevention messages; the media can contribute to the creation of a social environment that promotes health (eg, increasing acceptance of regular condom use in the prevention of STDs).

The body of literature on mass communication for promoting health and preventing disease through the voluntary adoption of healthy behaviors is growing rapidly. Television, as a significant medium, reaches into most American homes, and public health campaigns are creatively designed to reach the target audiences.

The urgency to combat AIDS, as well as other life-threatening diseases, provides a strong rationale and impetus for developing effective disease prevention and control messages for dissemination through the media. Messages need to be tailored to the specific characteristics of target audiences and the media channels to which the audiences are exposed. Disadvantaged or stigmatized groups, such as the poor, ethnic minorities, gay men, injection drug users, and prostitutes, are more vulnerable to infectious diseases and need mass media messages targeted to them (Fig. 9–2). Those people who watch more television and listen to more radio respond to

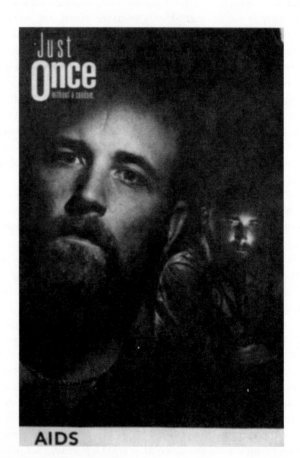

FIGURE 9-2.   This poster conveys a powerful message about AIDS.

health promotion messages received through these media more often than groups who do not. A behavior change is essential to control the spread of communicable diseases, and that change depends on successful communication between community health providers and target audiences, using the most appropriate media possible. Participation in media and education efforts depends on the awareness of target groups (eg, injection drug users) about available programs and how to access them. Carefully and thoughtfully designed disease prevention messages disseminated through the media are a reliable and effective way of reaching hard-to-reach populations. However, the mass media have the potential to undermine traditional customs and beliefs and may serve to sever individuals from their community (Mackenzie, 1998). This reinforces the need to screen selected media with community leaders for effectiveness and appropriateness before use and to plan, together with them, educational efforts that meet community needs.

Targeting Meaningful Health Messages to Aggregates

To effectively deliver a communicable disease prevention message, the message must reach the target (at-risk) population. This requires correct identification of the characteristics of the target audience, in terms of educational level, salience of the issue, involvement of the target audience with the issue, and access of the target audience to the media channels used. Cultural issues affect people's interpretation of messages and must be considered in the presentation of a disease-prevention message to ethnic and racial minority groups. There are principles for adapting health messages to specific population subgroups:

1. Develop educational materials from the community perspective, reflecting respect for community values and traditions, relevance to community needs and interests, and participation of the community in the preparation and use of the materials.
2. Ensure that materials are an integral part of a health education program, supported by other components of intervention, not standing alone as the educational program in itself.
3. Materials must be related to the delivery of health services that are available, accessible, and acceptable to the target population.
4. All materials must be pretested and have demonstrated attractiveness, comprehension, acceptability, ownership, and persuasiveness.
5. Materials must be distributed with instructions for their use (ie, how, when, and with whom they are to be used).

Immunization

Control of acute communicable diseases through immunization has been a common practice since the 19th century in the United States. **Immunization** is the process of introducing some form of disease-causing organism into a person's sys-

tem to cause the development of antibodies that will resist that disease. In theory, this process makes the person immune to that particular infectious disease (ie, able to resist a specific infectious disease-causing agent). That immunization requirements are acceptable in American society today is evidenced by high levels of immunization in school children and the fact that aggressive enforcement of school immunization requirements, starting in the late 1970s, has not met with widespread opposition. This is true even during the last decade, when common immunizations have been changed and the number of immunizations has increased. The schedule for administration of vaccines officially changes every January. In 2001, the CDC conducted the National Immunization Survey. Overall, 77.2% of children 18 to 35 months of age at the time of the survey had received all of the recommended immunizations (Neumann, 2002). This is not unlike the coverage rates over the last several years when our nation's immunization coverage rate was reported at an all time high of 79% (Institute of Medicine, 2000). Adolescent vaccination has lagged behind the rates achieved by younger children in the last decade. Barriers that must be overcome include lack of parental knowledge, inadequate access to medical care, and inadequate or no insurance coverage (Word, 2002). With adults, good progress has been made. Influenza vaccine coverage rates increased from 42% in 1991 to 63% in 2001 and pneumococcal vaccine coverage rates increased from 21% to 34% over the same period (Neumann, 2002).

The statutes that exist to ensure adequate immunization levels by the time of school entry place the school in the role of controlling agency, whereas public health departments and private health care providers are authorized to administer the required vaccines. An emerging drawback of this mechanism is the fact that many parents delay immunizations until the child's fifth year (Scutchfield & Keck, 2001). Preschool-age children represent a major proportion of all cases of immunizable diseases and are the group at highest risk for infection. Vaccines provide significant cost benefits. For example, for every dollar spent on the diphtheria, tetanus, and pertussis (DTaP) vaccine, $24 is saved, and $2 is saved per dollar for the more recently approved *H. influenzae* (Hib) vaccine (USDHHS, 2000).

The national objective stated in *Healthy People 2000* (USDHHS, 1991) was for 90% of American children to be vaccinated by their second birthday with four doses of DTaP, three doses of oral polio, and one dose of the combined measles, mumps, and rubella vaccine. *Healthy People 2010* (USDHHS, 2000) reinforced this goal by including an objective of reducing or eliminating all indigenous cases of vaccine-preventable disease (Table 9–1).

Although childhood immunization rates historically have been lower in minority populations compared with the White population, rates for minority preschool children have been increasing at a more rapid pace, and the gap has significantly narrowed (USDHHS, 2000). The National Immunization Survey has documented substantial progress toward

T A B L E 9 – 1

Healthy People 2010 Vaccine-Preventable Disease Objective

Disease	1997	2010 Target
Congenital rubella syndrome	4	0
Diphtheria (people <35 years of age)	4	0
Haemophilus influenzae type b	165	0
Hepatitis B (people <25 years of age)	8693	0
Measles	135	0
Mumps	612	0
Pertussis (children <7 years of age)	2633	2000
Polio (wild-type virus)	0	0
Rubella	161	0
Tetanus (among people <35 years of age)	10	0
Varicella (chickenpox)	4 million*	400,000

*Estimated from the National Health Interview Survey (NNHIS), 1990–1994.

(From U. S. Department of Health and Human Services. [2000]. *Healthy people 2010* [Conference ed., Vols. 1 & 2]. Washington, DC: U. S. Government Printing Office.)

achieving 1996 Childhood Immunization Initiative coverage goals by racial and ethnic groups. However, efforts to increase vaccination coverage need to be intensified, particularly for children living in poverty (USDHHS, 2000). It is critical to discover the social and cultural characteristics affecting health status, attitudes about preventive measures, behaviors in seeking services, acceptability of interventions, and perceptions of health care providers that determine parental action in having a child immunized in a regular and timely fashion. This is a unique area of health care delivery, where nurses must rely on parental initiative to obtain a form of care for the well child that may be perceived as producing pain and temporary illness for no observable benefit.

Vaccine-Preventable Diseases

Vaccine-preventable diseases (VPD), such as hepatitis B, *H. influenzae* type b, measles, polio, diphtheria, pertussis, and chickenpox, are diseases that can be prevented through immunization. Immunity may be either passive or active. **Passive immunity** is short-term resistance to a specific disease-causing organism; it may be acquired naturally (as with newborns through maternal antibody transfer) or artificially through inoculation with a vaccine that gives temporary resistance. Such immunizations must be repeated periodically to sustain immunity levels. An example is the influenza vaccination. **Active immunity** is long-term (sometimes lifelong) resistance to a specific disease-causing organism; it also can be acquired naturally or artificially. Naturally acquired active immunity occurs when a person contracts a disease and develops long-lasting antibodies that provide immunity against future exposure. Artificially acquired active

immunity occurs through inoculation with a vaccine, such as the diphtheria, pertussis, tetanus vaccination series given to children. A **vaccine** is a preparation made from killed, living attenuated, or living fully virulent organisms that is administered to produce or artificially increase immunity to a particular disease.

Because of the success of immunization strategies, few practicing nurses today have treated clients with tetanus or diphtheria (although some have cared for clients with residual polio disabilities). However, immunizable diseases still exist in force in the developing world, and outbreaks occur in the United States in groups of unimmunized or susceptible populations. For example, certain people are constitutionally exempt from immunization, others decline immunization for religious or personal reasons, and certain refugee populations can be especially vulnerable. Even with global and national efforts at reducing and eliminating VPD, some national goals have not been met. In fact, statistics for some diseases have gotten worse. Immunization rates of coverage have declined in some areas, with subsequent increases in VPDs (eg, pertussis).

Before the introduction of pertussis vaccine in the 1940s, more than 200,000 cases were diagnosed yearly in the United States, with 5000 to 10,000 deaths each year. Today, pertussis (whooping cough) claims 10 to 15 lives per year. After the introduction and widespread use of the DTaP vaccine, whooping cough infections dropped to 3417 cases in 1998; the goal is a reduction to 2000 cases by 2010 (USDHHS, 2000). With an intensified VPD effort among the families at highest risk, this goal should be achievable. However, outbreaks occur in areas where adult immunity levels have dropped and families neglect getting very young infants immunized. During 2001–2002, a total of 55 cases of pertussis were diagnosed at one children's hospital in California, a sharp rise from the usual 1 or 2 cases the hospital treats each month. Most of the patients were infants younger than 6 months of age (Aleman-Padilla, 2002).

Schedule of Recommended Immunizations

An annual schedule for the administration of childhood vaccinations is published based on recommendations by the Advisory Committee on Immunization Practices (ACIP), the American Academy of Pediatrics (AAP), the American Academy of Family Physicians (AAFP), and the CDC (Table 9–2). The CDC also provides schedules for children not receiving their first immunization at birth according to the standard schedule. Current recommendations call for a child to receive ten different vaccines or toxoids (many in combination form and all requiring more than one dose) in six or seven visits to a provider between birth and school entry, with boosters in the preteen to early teen years (CDC, 2003).

Factors influencing the recommended age at which vaccines are administered include the age-specific risks of the disease, the age-specific risks of complications, the ability of

T A B L E   9 - 2

Recommended Childhood and Adolescent Immunization Schedule: United States, January–June 2004

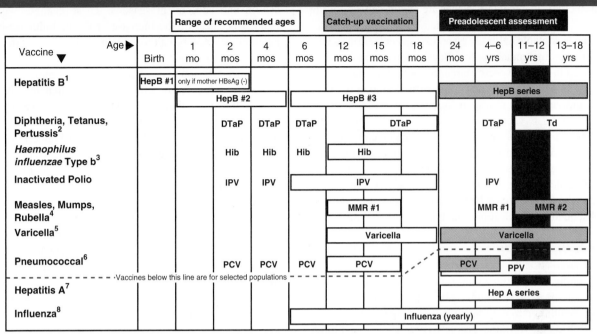

Vaccine ▼ / Age ▶	Birth	1 mo	2 mos	4 mos	6 mos	12 mos	15 mos	18 mos	24 mos	4–6 yrs	11–12 yrs	13–18 yrs
											Range of recommended ages / Catch-up vaccination / Preadolescent assessment	
Hepatitis B[1]	HepB #1 (only if mother HBsAg (-))										HepB series	
		HepB #2			HepB #3							
Diphtheria, Tetanus, Pertussis[2]		DTaP	DTaP	DTaP		DTaP			DTaP	Td	
Haemophilus influenzae Type b[3]		Hib	Hib	Hib	Hib						
Inactivated Polio		IPV	IPV		IPV				IPV		
Measles, Mumps, Rubella[4]					MMR #1				MMR #1	MMR #2	
Varicella[5]					Varicella				Varicella		
Pneumococcal[6]		PCV	PCV	PCV	PCV				PCV / PPV		
Hepatitis A[7]										Hep A series	
Influenza[8]					Influenza (yearly)						

Vaccines below this line are for selected populations

This schedule indicates the recommended ages for routine administration of currently licensed childhood vaccines, as of December 1, 2003, for children through age 18 years. Any dose not given at the recommended age should be given at any subsequent visit when indicated and feasible. ▨ Indicates age groups that warrant special effort to administer those vaccines not previously given. Additional vaccines may be licensed and recommended during the year. Licensed combination vaccines may be used whenever any components of the combination are indicated and the vaccines's other components are not contraindicated. Providers should consult the manufacturers' package inserts for detailed recommendations.

1. Hepatitis B vaccine (HepB). All infants should receive the first dose of HepB vaccine soon after birth and before hospital discharge; the first dose may also be given by age 2 months if the infant's mother is HBsAg-negative. Only monovalent HepB vaccine can be used for the birth dose. Monovalent or combination vaccine containing HepB may be used to complete the series. Four doses of vaccine may be administered when a birth dose is given. The second dose should be given at least 4 weeks after the first dose, except for combination vaccines which cannot be administered before age 6 weeks. The third dose should be given at least 16 weeks after the first dose and at least 8 weeks after the second dose. The last dose in the vaccination series (third or fourth dose) should not be administered before age 6 months.

Infants born to HBsAg-positive mothers should receive HepB and 0.5 mL Hepatitis B immune globulin (HBIG) within 12 hours of birth at separate sites. The second dose is recommended at age 1–2 months. The last dose in the vaccination series should not be administered before age 6 months. These infants should be tested for HBsAg and anti-HBs at 9–15 months of age.

Infants born to mothers whose HBsAg status is unknown should receive the first dose of the HepB vaccine series within 12 hours of birth. Maternal blood should be drawn as soon as possible to determine the mother's HBsAg status; if the HBsAg test is positive, the infant should receive HBIG as soon as possible (no later than age 1 week). The second dose is recommended at age 1–2 months. The last dose in the vaccination series should not be administered before age 6 months.

2. Diphtheria and tetanus toxoids and acellular pertussis vaccine (DTaP). The fourth dose of DTaP may be administered at age 12 months, provided that 6 months have elapsed since the third dose and the child is unlikely to return at age 15–18 months. Tetanus and diphtheria toxoids (Td) is recommended at age 11–12 years if at least 5 years have elapsed since the last dose of tetanus and diphtheria toxoid-containing vaccine. Subsequent routine Td boosters are recommended every 10 years.

3. Haemophilus influenzae type b (Hib) conjugate vaccine. Three Hib conjugate vaccines are licensed for infant use. If PRP-OMP (PedvaxHIB® or ComVax® [Merck]) is administered at age 2 and 4 months, a dose at age 6 months is not required. DTaP/Hib combination products should not be used for primary immunization in infants at age 2, 4, or 6 months but can be used as boosters following any Hib vaccine.

4. Measles, mumps, and rubella vaccine (MMR). The second dose of MMR is recommended routinely at age 4–6 years but may be administered during any visit, provided that at least 4 weeks have elapsed since the first dose and that both doses are administered beginning at or after age 12 months. Those who have not previously received the second dose should complete the schedule by the age 11–12 year old visit.

5. Varicella vaccine. Varicella vaccine is recommended at any visit at or after age 12 months for susceptible children, i.e. those who lack a reliable history of chickenpox. Susceptible persons age ≥13 years should receive two doses given, at least 4 weeks apart.

6. Pneumococcal vaccine. The heptavalent pneumococcal conjugate vaccine (PCV) is recommended for all children aged 2–23 months . It is also recommended for certain children aged 24–59 months. Pneumococcal polysaccharide vaccine (PPV) is recommended in addition to PCV for certain high-risk groups. See *MMWR* 2000;49(No. RR-9):1–38.

7. Hepatitis A vaccine. Hepatitis A vaccine is recommended for children and adolescents in selected states and regions, and for certain high-risk groups; consult your local public health authority. Children and adolescents in these states, regions, and high-risk groups who have not been immunized against hepatitis A can begin the hepatitis A vaccination series during any visit. The two doses in the series should be administered at least 6 months apart. See *MMWR* 1999;48(No. RR-12):1–37.

8. Influenza vaccine. Influenza vaccine is recommended annually for children aged ≥6 months with certain risk factors (including but not limited to asthma, cardiac disease, sickle cell disease, HIV, disabetes, and household members of persons in groups at high risk (see *MMWR* 2002;51(RR-3):1–31), and can be administered to all others wishing to obtain immunity. In addition, healthy children age 6–23 months are encouraged to receive influenza vaccine if feasible because children in this age group are at substantially increased risk for influenza-related hospitalizations. Children aged ≤12 years should receive vaccine in a dosage appropriated for their age (0.25mL if 6–35 months or 0.5 mL if ≥3 years). Children aged ≤8 years who are receiving influenza vaccine for the first time should receive two doses separated by at least 4 weeks.

For additional information about vaccines, including precautions and contraindications for immunization and vaccine shortages, please visit the National Immunization Program Website at www.cdc.gov/nip or call the National Immunization information Hotline at 800-232-2522 (English) or 800-232-0233 (Spanish).

Approved by the Advisory Committee on Immunization Practices (www.cdc.gov/nip/acip), the American Academy of Pediatrics (www.aap.org), and the American Academy of Family Physicians (www.aafp.org).

persons of a given age to produce an adequate and lasting immune response, and the potential for interference with the immune response acquired from passively transferred maternal antibodies. In general, vaccines are recommended for the youngest age group at risk whose members are known to develop an acceptable antibody response to vaccination (CDC, 2000a). Recommendations for vaccine administration may be revised in light of specific circumstances. For example, in response to a rising incidence of hepatitis B among sexually active individuals, it is now recommended that infants receive hepatitis B vaccine in doses that vary depending on whether their mothers have a positive or negative response to the hepatitis B surface antigen (CDC, 2000a). In addition, the rotavirus vaccine was eliminated from the 2000 immunization schedule because it caused too many serious illnesses in infants who received it in 1999. It has not been reintroduced in subsequent immunization schedule recommendations.

Assessing Immunization Status of the Community

Determining the immunization status of children in a community can be a time-consuming but worthwhile task. Community health nurses may consider assessing groups of children with some common characteristics such as children served by the Women, Infants and Children program (WIC), those served by private medical providers, or those attending public schools in various neighborhoods. Because all children attending school in the United States must show proof of immunization upon school entry, review of immunization records at school can provide a means of retrospectively determining the proportion of these children whose immunizations were up to date at age 3 months or at age 2 years. The CDC strongly promotes the retrospective school vaccination record survey as a means of estimating current levels and monitoring trends over time in immunization status. If no unusual immunization events occur in the intervening period, this retrospective record review gives a reasonable estimate of current immunization status of those age groups in the community. In addition, such a record review targeting children who were not up to date on their immunizations before school entry helps identify younger siblings who may also not be up to date.

With increasing numbers of children entering day care services in the preschool years, more states now require immunization for preschool children, often including immunization against influenza, which is not presently required for older age groups. Preschool or day care center operators now obtain information about immunization status of this younger cohort, a group that previously often escaped surveillance and immunization initiative.

Of interest to community health nurses, in 2002 the ACIP expanded the group of children eligible for influenza vaccine coverage under the Vaccines for Children (VFC) program. The resolution extends VFC coverage for influenza vaccine to all VFC-eligible children aged 6 to 23 months, as well as VFC-eligible children aged 2 to 18 years who are household contacts of children younger than 2 years of age. This resolution became effect in March, 2003, for vaccine to be administered during the 2003–2004 influenza vaccination season and subsequent seasons. These changes were expanded because of the increased risk for influenza-related hospitalizations among those younger than 23 months of age (CDC, 2002a).

Other community settings where community health nurses may identify underimmunized children include homeless shelters and other public service settings used by families and children, including local religious centers. A family with one underimmunized child may have underimmunized children of other ages as well as any number of other unmet preventive health care needs, which the community health nurse might help address.

Understanding disease rates and immunization status by race or ethnicity requires population data accurately showing the multicultural composition of the community. Such data can be obtained from census figures and augmented by refugee or immigration records. Noting the racial or ethnic heritage of the underimmunized child may lead to valuable insights about unique barriers for the group that must be addressed to reduce disease rates and increase healthy resilience.

Herd Immunity

Herd immunity is central to understanding immunization as a means of protecting community health. As described in Chapter 8, it is the immunity level present in a particular population of people (Chin, 1999). If there are few immune persons within a community, there is low herd immunity and the spread of disease is more likely. Vaccination of more individuals in the community, so that a high proportion have acquired resistance to the infectious agent, contributes to high herd immunity. High herd immunity reduces the probability that the few unimmunized persons will come in contact with one another, making spread of the disease less likely. Outbreaks may occur if the immunization rate falls to less than 85% (Scutchfield & Keck, 2001) or if unimmunized susceptible persons are grouped together rather than dispersed throughout the immunized community. An example of lack of herd immunity is presented in The Global Community.

Barriers to Immunization Coverage

Improving immunization coverage requires examination of reasons that children are not immunized. Many barriers exist. They include religious, financial, social, and cultural factors; philosophical objections; and provider limitations that form barriers to adequate immunization.

Religious Barriers. The right to religious freedom gives some groups of individuals in the United States the constitutional right to exemption from immunization if they object to vaccination on religious grounds. Children from these families are identified at school entry. Such exemptions must be specifically enacted by law, and, although it is not necessary to belong to a specific denomination, courts have required

Provider Limitations. Another barrier to immunization coverage is provider limitations. Health care providers may have contact with an eligible child, yet fail to offer vaccination. This occurs when providers see children for different reasons and do not review their immunization records, missing the opportunity to provide vaccination services at what may be a very convenient time for parents. Sometimes, children come for immunization services and receive some vaccines but not others, although the safety and efficacy of administering multiple vaccines on the same occasion are well established and recommended by the CDC. Providers may erroneously defer administration of a vaccine based on a condition (eg, symptom of illness) that is not a true contraindication to immunization. To address this particular issue, the CDC has developed guidelines for providers showing misconceptions concerning contraindications to vaccination (Table 9–3). Another provider limitation or barrier to timely immunization coverage is that few providers have the initiative and resources to establish a uniform system for recall and notification when the next immunization is due. In the United States, even clients of private providers often are not encouraged or assisted to maintain their own copies of personal written medical records.

T A B L E   9 – 3

General and Specific Guide to Contraindications and Precautions to Vaccinations*

True contraindications and precautions	Not contraindications (vaccines may be administered)
General for all vaccines (DTP/DTaP, OPV, IPV, MMR, Hib, Hepatitis B)	
CONTRAINDICATIONS Anaphylactic reaction to a vaccine contraindicates further doses of that vaccine Anaphylactic reaction to a vaccine constituent contraindicates the use of vaccines containing that substance Moderate or severe illnesses with or without a fever	NOT CONTRAINDICATIONS Mild to moderate local reaction (soreness, redness, swelling) following a dose of an injectable antigen Mild acute illness with or without low-grade fever Current antimicrobial therapy Convalescent phase of illnesses Prematurity (same dosage and indications as for normal, full-term infants) Recent exposure to an infectious disease History of penicillin or other nonspecific allergies or family history of such allergies
DTP/DTaP	
CONTRAINDICATIONS Encephalopathy within 7 days of administration of previous dose of DTP PRECAUTIONS† Fever of ≥40.5°C (105°F) within 48 h after vaccination with a prior dose of DTP Collapse or shocklike state (hypotonic-hyporesponsive episode) within 48 h of receiving a prior dose of DTP Seizures within 3 days of receiving a prior dose of DTP§ Persistent, inconsolable crying lasting ≥3 h within 48 h of receiving a prior dose of DTP	NOT CONTRAINDICATIONS Temperature of <40.5°C (105°F) following a previous dose of DTP Family history of convulsions§ Family history of sudden infant death syndrome Family history of an adverse event following DTP administration
OPV¶	
CONTRAINDICATIONS Infection with HIV or a household contact with HIV Known altered immunodeficiency (hematologic and solid tumors; congenital immunodeficiency; and long-term immunosuppressive therapy) Immunodeficient household contact PRECAUTION† Pregnancy	NOT CONTRAINDICATIONS Breast-feeding Current antimicrobial therapy Diarrhea
IPV	
CONTRAINDICATION Anaphylactic reaction to neomycin or streptomycin PRECAUTION† Pregnancy	

TABLE 9-3

General and Specific Guide to Contraindications and Precautions to Vaccinations* (continued)

True contraindications and precautions	Not contraindications (vaccines may be administered)
MMR¶	
CONTRAINDICATIONS Anaphylactic reactions to egg ingestion and to neomycin** Pregnancy Known altered immunodeficiency (hematologic and solid tumors; congenital immunodeficiency; and long-term immunosuppressive therapy)	NOT CONTRAINDICATIONS Tuberculosis or positive PPD skin test Simultaneous TB skin testing†† Breastfeeding Pregnancy of mother of recipient Immunodeficient family member or household contact
True contraindications and precautions PRECAUTION† Recent immune globulin administration	**Not contraindications (vaccines may be administered)** Infection with HIV Nonanaphylactic reaction to eggs or neomycin
Hib	
CONTRAINDICATION None identified	NOT CONTRAINDICATION History of Hib disease
Hepatitis B	
CONTRAINDICATION Anaphylactic reaction to common baker's yeast	NOT CONTRAINDICATION Pregnancy

(From Advisory Committee on Immunization Practices. [1994]. Guide to contraindications and precautions to vaccinations. *Morbidity and Mortality Weekly Report, 43* [RR-1], 24–25.)

*This information is based on the recommendations of the Advisory Committee on Immunization Practices (ACIP) and those of the Committee on Infectious Diseases (Red Book Committee) of the American Academy of Pediatrics (AAP). Sometimes these recommendations vary from those contained in the manufacturer's package inserts. For more detailed information, providers should consult the published recommendations of the ACIP, AAP, and the manufacturer's package inserts.

†The events or conditions listed as precautions, although not contraindications, should be carefully reviewed. The benefits and risks of administering a specific vaccine to an individual under the circumstances should be considered. If the risks are believed to outweigh the benefits, the vaccination should be withheld; if the benefits are believed to outweigh the risks (eg, during an outbreak or foreign travel), the vaccination should be administered. Whether and when to administer DTP to children with proven or suspected underlying neurologic disorders should be decided on an individual basis. It is prudent on theoretical grounds to avoid vaccinating pregnant women. However, if immediate protection against poliomyelitis is needed, OPV is preferred, although IPV may be considered if full vaccination can be completed before the anticipated imminent exposure.

§Acetaminophen given before administering DTP and thereafter every 4 hours for 24 hours should be considered for children with a personal or family history of convulsions in siblings or parents.

¶No data exist to substantiate the theoretical risk of a suboptimal immune response from the administration of OPV and MMR within 30 days of each other.

**Persons with a history of anaphylactic reactions following egg ingestion should be vaccinated only with caution. Protocols have been developed for vaccinating such persons and should be consulted. (*Journal of Pediatrics,* 196–199; 1983; 102. *Journal of Pediatrics,* 1988;113:504–506.)

††Measles vaccination may temporarily suppress tuberculin reactivity. If testing cannot be done the day of MMR vaccination, the test should be postponed for 4 to 6 weeks.

Planning and Implementing Immunization Programs

Immunization programs targeting specific subgroups can be effective if they include the following: (1) community assessment parameters by race or other cultural groupings in the planning phase; (2) assessment of specific characteristics of the groups such as language, child care practices, preventive health behaviors, extreme poverty, or high illiteracy; and (3) appropriate planning decisions to deal with these potential barriers. Successful outreach efforts are motivated by the desire to reach the target population, even if specific or unusual ac-commodations must be made. Clinics are scheduled and held at times and places specifically intended to make the service more accessible and convenient to the target group. Materials are designed and presented with the needs and abilities of target parents in mind. Interpreters are provided as needed. Display 9–2 outlines the necessary steps and considerations for administering immunization clinics in community settings.

Adult Immunization

Many people erroneously assume that vaccinations are for children only. Well-advertised influenza vaccination cam-

DISPLAY 9-2

Administrative Aspects of Immunization Programs

Study the Target Community
Assess disease incidence and level of immunization coverage.
Identify the target group.
Assess conditions in the community: Is the target group scattered or localized?
Assess level of community involvement and awareness of the problem.
Identify means of communicating with target group: Through the media or through leaders or other.
Consider political and social structure of the community. Identify important leaders.
Identify sites for immunization clinics that are appropriate, accessible, and available.

Plan the Immunization Program
Review budget for immunization services.
Determine goals for clinic performance or outcome measures.
Communicate with target group to notify them of need and promote involvement and participation.
Estimate needs for vaccines and supplies and obtain them. Plan care of vaccines before, during, and after clinic.
Develop team coordination among staff.
Plan clinic logistics: Available supply of needed materials; medical waste disposal; anaphylaxis supplies; records and means of clinic registration; staffing; floor plan for traffic control and efficient management of crowds.
Prepare staff with information regarding objectives for clinic; criteria for who shall not be immunized; mechanisms for referral of clients with other health needs.

Publicity
Inform target group of date, location, and times of immunization clinic.
Provide information on reasons for and benefits of (and contraindications to) immunization.
Encourage parents to bring existing immunization records to clinic.
Provide contact information for those with questions or inquiries.

Immunization Clinic
Registration system and records (for parent and clinic) ready.
Registrar or assistant(s) ready to assist parents not familiar with language of paperwork.
Parent education: informed consent; reporting of adverse reactions; date next vaccine due.
System for call-back, follow-up.
System for dealing with other health issues and/or adverse events.

Evaluation of Program
Assess numbers of immunizations given in relation to goals.
Assess suitability of approach in identification of target group, selection of sites, means of communication with group, availability of resources, and so forth.
Invite parental as well as community and staff feedback.
Evaluate results in relation to expenditures.

---

paigns in recent years have helped somewhat to correct this notion. However, media coverage about the adverse effects of such vaccination has done little to increase either community or provider enthusiasm about adult vaccination in general. Adults are at increased risk for many VPDs, and approximately 45,000 adult deaths each year are associated with complications from pneumococcal disease and influenza (USDHHS, 2000). As the nation's population ages, increasing numbers of adults will be at risk for these major causes of death and illness.

Adults may require vaccination for a variety of reasons. Occupational exposure to blood, blood products, or other potentially contaminated body fluids provides the basis for Occupational and Safety Health Administration (OSHA) requirements for hepatitis B vaccine. All persons should receive tetanus vaccine every 10 years unless they experience major or contaminated wounds. If such a wound is sustained, the individual should receive a single booster of a tetanus toxoid on the day of the injury if more than 5 years has elapsed since the last tetanus toxoid dose. In addition to influenza and pneu-

monia vaccinations, already mentioned, adult immunizations may also include adult diphtheria/tetanus (DT). Other reasons for adult vaccination include a history of high-risk conditions, such as heart disease, diabetes, and chronic respiratory diseases; international travel; and suspected failure of earlier vaccines to produce lasting immunity. Table 9–4 displays the *Healthy People 2010* objective for influenza and pneumonia vaccines for people older than 18 years of age (USDHHS, 2000).

A substantial portion of VPDs still occur among adults despite the availability of safe and effective vaccines. At least six factors contribute to low vaccination levels among adults:

1. Limited comprehensive vaccine delivery systems are available in the public and private sectors.
2. Although statutory requirements exist for vaccination of children, no such requirements exist for all adults.
3. Vaccination schedules are complicated because of detailed recommendations that may vary by age, occupation, lifestyle, or health condition.

TABLE 9-4

Healthy People 2010 Target for Influenza and Pneumonia Immunization in Adults

Objective: Increase to 90% the rate of immunization coverage among adults 65 years of age or older; 60% for high-risk adults 18 to 64 years of age.

Recommended Immunization	1995	Target 2010
Noninstitutionalized adults 65 years of age or older		
Influenza vaccine	58%	90%
Pneumococcal vaccine	32%	90%
Noninstitutionalized high-risk adults 18 to 64 years of age		
Influenza vaccine	30%	60%
Pneumococcal vaccine	15%	60%
Institutionalized adults (persons in long-term or nursing homes)		
Influenza vaccine	62%	90%
Pneumococcal vaccine	23%	90%

(U. S. Department of Health and Human Services. [2000]. *Healthy people 2010* [Conference ed., Vols. 1 & 2]. Washington, DC: U. S. Government Printing Office.)

4. Health care providers frequently miss opportunities to vaccinate adults during contacts in offices, outpatient clinics, and hospitals.
5. Comprehensive vaccination programs have not been established in settings where healthy adults congregate (eg, the workplace, senior centers).
6. Clients and providers may fear adverse effects after vaccination.

International Travelers, Immigrants, and Refugees

As Americans interact more and more with their neighbors in other parts of the world, the incidence of Americans with tropical or imported diseases also rises. Within 36 hours of beginning a trip, any destination in the world can be reached. That amount of time is within the incubation period of most infectious diseases, and microbial agents are rapidly spread around the globe.

Information necessary for a potential traveler to go to new and exotic places, remain healthy, and return healthy is available from a number of sources. At a minimum, all international travelers must take steps to be adequately immunized as required by international health practices. These steps include being immunized with immunoglobulin to prevent hepatitis A, having the necessary chemical prophylaxis on hand (and taking it regularly as instructed) if the traveler is to be in a malarious area, and being knowledgeable about food and water hygiene precautions as well as basic first aid

for the care of simple injuries. Every year during the 1990s, between 1000 and 1500 cases of malaria occurred among poorly prepared and careless international travelers from the United States. In many major cities of the United States, one finds tropical medicine or travelers' medicine specialists who can assist in adequate preparation for travel. The CDC offers a travelers' hotline with up-to-date recommendations regarding malaria prophylaxis. Health departments and large libraries usually offer materials on international travel, including those listed in this book.

Refugees and international travelers who arrive in the United States are often unfamiliar with its health systems, health precautions, and practices. Refugees and immigrants must follow prescribed guidelines for their acculturation, including extensive health screening mandated by U. S. immigration laws. More than ever before, community health nurses have professional contact with these new Americans, whether close to their time of arrival or later, in schools, immunization clinics, or other locations. Visitors from other countries may also require the assistance of community health professionals. For this reason, community health nurses are encouraged to develop and maintain a global perspective on communicable diseases.

SECONDARY PREVENTION

There are two approaches to secondary prevention of communicable disease: (1) screening and (2) contact investigation, partner notification, and case-finding.

Screening

The term **screening** is used in community health and disease prevention to describe programs that deliver a testing mechanism to detect disease in groups of asymptomatic, apparently healthy individuals. Familiar examples include (1) nontreponemal tests such as the rapid plasma reagin (RPR) test or Venereal Disease Research Laboratory (VDRL) test and (2) treponemal tests that can confirm a syphilis diagnosis, such as the fluorescent treponemal antibody absorbed (FTA-ABS) test and the *T. pallidum* particle agglutination (TP-PA) test (CDC, 2002c). The tine and Mantoux tuberculin tests for TB are common screening measures. For HIV, the HIV-1/HIV-2 antibody tests or a sensitive screening test such as the enzyme immunoassay (EIA), confirmed by a supplemental test such as the Western blot or an immunofluorescence assay (IFA) are used (CDC, 2002c). All screening tests are discussed later in this chapter. Screening is a secondary prevention method because it discovers those who may have already become infected in order to initiate prompt early treatment.

It is important to remember that the screening itself is not diagnostic but rather seeks to identify those persons with positive or suspicious findings who require further medical evaluation or treatment. Any community health nurse working with clients in a screening setting must be prepared to clearly and correctly explain to individuals that screening tests are not definitive and that positive findings require subsequent investigation before diagnostic conclusions can be drawn.

Criteria for Screening Tests

There are some important criteria for deciding whether to carry out a screening intervention in a community.

Validity and Reliability. The screening test must be valid and reliable. *Validity* refers to the test's ability to accurately identify those with the disease. *Reliability* refers to the test's ability to give consistent results when administered on different occasions by different technicians.

Predictive Value and Yield. The *predictive value* of a screening test is important for determining whether the screening intervention is justified. *Yield* refers to the number of positive results found per number tested. The predictive value and the yield of screening tests become important in planning screening programs for communicable disease detection and prevention because they can help planners locate screening efforts in areas or within population groups that are known to be at high risk for the disease. The predictive value of screening tests increases as the prevalence of the disease increases. For example, a screening test for syphilis targeted at the population associated with crack houses in a particular city would have greater predictive value and yield than a screening test for syphilis given to the city population at large.

Epidemiologic criteria for screening interventions for the detection of health problems are as follows:
1. Is the disease an important public health problem?
2. Is there a valid and reliable test?
3. Is there an effective and tolerable treatment that favorably influences the early stages of the disease?
4. Are facilities for diagnosis and treatment after a positive screening result available and accessible?
5. Is there a recognizable early asymptomatic or latent stage in the disease?
6. Do clear guidelines for referral and treatment exist?
7. Is the total cost of the screening justifiable compared with the costs of treating the disease if left undiscovered?
8. Is the screening test itself acceptable?
9. Will screening be ongoing?

The ethics or values represented by these statements include a clear and unwavering respect for the dignity and worth of individuals across racial, gender, religious, sexual, tribal, ethnic, and geographic lines (Satcher, 1996). They include a commitment to ensuring that resources are allocated to areas where they will have the most benefit in preventing disease and premature death. They speak to respect for the individual receiving the screening service, in that the person should take on the burden of diagnosis only if access to acceptable further intervention exists. Socioeconomically disadvantaged persons are often at greatest risk for disease, yet they are the least likely to receive screening services, because of financial barriers including lack of health insurance coverage for preventive care. Correction of this type of disparity in health care services is an objective of *Healthy People 2010* (USDHHS, 2000).

Contact Investigation, Partner Notification, and Case-Finding

Another secondary prevention approach is known as contact investigation, partner notification, and case-finding. In this approach, the community health nurse seeks to discover and notify those who have had contact with a person diagnosed with a communicable disease such as with TB and to notify partners in the case of STDs. The objective of contact investigation and partner notification is specifically to reach contacts of the *index case* (diagnosed person) before the contacts, in turn, become infectious (CDC, 2002c). Therefore, the rapidity with which contact investigation can be accomplished is a concern.

Healthy People 2010 (USDHHS, 2000) differentiates between two types of partner notification. *Patient referral* describes those clients who voluntarily advise their partners of the risk of disease and the need for contact with a health provider. *Provider referral* describes the community health workers who contact individuals exposed to the index case and encourage them to receive appropriate medical care. In both types of notification, clients need information and encouragement as well as assurance of confidentiality.

It is a fact that not all individuals who have a disease can accurately identify the persons with whom they have had close or intimate contact. This is particularly the case with STDs associated with drug abuse and the selling of sex for drugs. It is also true in situations involving highly mobile or transient people whose lifestyles preclude establishing relationships that can be traced or followed. These problems lead to the need for alternative approaches in case-finding, including the provision of screening activities in locations where people with similar risky lifestyle behaviors are likely to congregate. It further points to the critical need for tests that provide reliable results very rapidly, because it may not be possible to locate the person 24 hours or 2 weeks later for follow-up.

Contact investigation is most commonly practiced today in STD and TB control programs. It is also used with some types of foodborne illness outbreak-control efforts. Rapidly evolving diseases and those that produce acute, identifiable symptoms are not of concern in contact investigation so much as diseases with incipient onset and long periods of infectiousness. The latter allow infected persons to reside and interact extensively in the community in an infectious state without being aware of their illness.

Tertiary Prevention

The approaches to tertiary prevention of communicable disease include isolation and quarantine of the infected person and safe handling and control of infectious wastes.

Isolation and Quarantine

Communicable disease control includes two methods for keeping infected persons and noninfected persons apart to prevent the spread of a disease. **Isolation** refers to separation of the infected persons (or animals) from others for the period of communicability to limit the transmission of the infectious agent to susceptible persons. **Quarantine** refers to restrictions placed on healthy contacts of an infectious case for the duration of the incubation period to prevent disease transmission if infection should develop (Chin, 1999).

Transmission by Health Care Workers

The problem of MDR organisms has been increasing since the 1960s, when the first strains of methicillin-resistant *Staphylococcus aureus* (MRSA) were identified in the United Kingdom. Clients who are colonized with a MDR strain (ie, have organisms living in the host with no deleterious effects to the host) or infected with it (ie, have organisms in large enough numbers to cause deleterious effects) are discharged into and admitted from the community, reinforcing the problem. This is a special concern for nurses, not only because of the potential for the nurse to carry the infectious agent from client to client, but also because there is considerable uncertainty about the implications for practice of the nurse who becomes colonized with drug-resistant bacteria in the course of caring for clients.

Although there is no definitive evidence implicating colonized health care workers in outbreaks of drug-resistant infections, some agencies furlough colonized workers or limit their practice to infected patients. Studies have shown that effective decolonization may take 3 weeks to 1 year. Employee health care programs must include infection control policies that address this problem, provide recommendations to the nurse for the prevention of both infection and colonization, and provide agency policies regarding care of the infected or colonized nurse. Although this problem is more prevalent in hospitals, community health nurses who work in close contact with clients in occupational, school, or home health settings are also at risk for becoming infected or colonized.

Safe Handling and Control of Infectious Wastes

Also important to the control of infection in community health is the proper disposition of contaminated wastes. The CDC has developed universal precautions, which encourage health care workers to think of all blood and body fluids, and materials that have come in contact with them, as potentially infectious (Chin, 1999). The universal precautions include the following:

- Basic hand-washing after contact with the client or with potentially contaminated articles and before care of other clients
- Appropriate discarding or bagging and labeling of articles contaminated with infectious material before it is sent for decontamination and reprocessing

- Appropriate isolation based on the mode of transmission of the specific disease, which may include strict isolation, contact isolation, respiratory isolation, TB isolation (AFB isolation), enteric precautions, or drainage/secretion precautions

The Environmental Protection Agency (EPA) defines infectious waste as "waste capable of producing an infectious disease." The agency notes that for waste to be infectious, it must contain pathogens with sufficient virulence and quantity so that exposure to the waste by a susceptible host could result in an infectious disease. EPA requirements for medical waste disposal are for waste to be segregated into categories of (1) sharps; (2) toxic, hazardous, regulated, or infectious fluids of greater than 20 mL; and (3) other materials. Although incineration has long been recognized as an efficient method for disposing safely of sharps and other contaminated medical waste, fewer incinerators are available now, with increasing regulation of emissions, particularly regulations related to the burning chemical wastes.

Four key elements of an infectious waste management program are applicable to community practice:

1. Health professionals must be able to correctly distinguish waste that poses a significant infection hazard from other biomedical waste that poses no greater risk than general municipal waste, and such infectious waste must be clearly defined.
2. The waste management program must have administrative support and authority to institute practice guidelines and provide the containers and other resources needed for safe disposal of infectious wastes.
3. Handling of the infectious wastes must be minimized. Containers should be rigid, leak resistant, and impervious to moisture; they should have sufficient strength to prevent rupture or tearing under normal conditions; and they should be sealed to prevent leakage. Containers for sharps must also be puncture resistant.
4. There must be an enforcement or evaluation mechanism in place to ensure that the goal of reducing the potential for exposure to infectious waste in the community is met.

MAJOR COMMUNICABLE DISEASES IN THE UNITED STATES

There are several communicable diseases that community health nurses encounter in their practice. They are frequently diagnosed and treated in the community. Chlamydia, genital herpes, hepatitis, HIV/AIDS, influenza, pneumonia, syphilis, TB, and viral warts are discussed here. These common diseases are presented alphabetically and not by virulence or prevalence.

Chlamydia

Chlamydia trachomatis infections are the most commonly reported notifiable disease in the United States. Since 1994, they have comprised the largest proportion of all STDs reported to the CDC. In women, chlamydial infections, which are usually asympotmatic, may result in pelvic inflammatory disease (PID), which is a major cause of infertility, ectopic pregnancy, and chronic pelvic pain (CDC, 2000a). Chlamydia is a sexually transmitted bacterial infection, with 702,093 cases reported to the CDC in 2000, 436,350 in 1997, and 226,557 in 1990. The number of cases has increased primarily because of an increase in recognition, testing, and mandatory reporting by the states in the past 2 decades (CDC, 2000a; Chin, 1999; Mertz et al., 2001).

Until recently, chlamydia was probably the least recognized of the STDs. Only since 2000 has reporting of chlamydia been required by all states, including the District of Columbia; in 1984, only five states required it (CDC, 2000a). People with uncomplicated infection are quite often symptom free until late and serious complications occur. Women and children typically are the most adversely affected, particularly in terms of sequelae, including PID, ectopic pregnancy, infertility, infant conjunctivitis, and infant pneumonia (Chin, 1999; USDHHS, 2000).

Screening programs have been extremely effective in reducing the chlamydia burden in groups that are screened regularly. In one area, it was reduced by 65% within 7 years after the introduction of screening, and chlamydia complications such as PID were reduced by as much as 56% within 1 year after introduction. One of the goals of *Healthy People 2010* is to reduce the prevalence of *C. trachomatis* infections among young people (15 to 24 years of age) to no more than 3.0%. In 1997, for all races and ethnic groups, the percentage was 4.4% for females in family planning clinics and 12.2% and 15.7% for females and males, respectively, in STD clinics (USDHHS, 2000). In 2000, the overall reported rate of chlamydial infection among women in the United States (404.0 cases per 100,000) was 4 times higher than the reported rate among men (102.8 cases per 100,000); this difference probably reflects a greater number of women being screened for this disease (2002d). The lower rate among men suggests that many of the

sex partners of women with chlamydia are not diagnosed or reported. However, with the advent of the new, highly sensitive nucleic acid amplification tests that can be performed on urine, symptomatic and asymptomatic men are increasingly being diagnosed with chlamydial infection.

Control of chlamydial infections of the cervix is considered key to effective reduction in the rates of PID, particularly among teenage women. A recent investigation of people in a health maintenance organization (HMO) demonstrated that screening and treatment of cervical infection can reduce the likelihood of PID (CDC, 2002c). Although chlamydia can be successfully treated with relatively inexpensive therapy, efforts to identify infected asymptomatic people were initially slow, although they increased throughout the 1990s (Ku et al., 2002). As a result, reported rates of chlamydia continued to increase (Fig. 9–3). In one study of teen and young adult men who had their urine screened for chlamydia (Ku et al., 2002), 3.1% of the teenagers (age 15 to 19 years) and 4.5% of the young adults (age 22 to 26 years) had chlamydial infections, although the great majority of the participants were asymptomatic.

There are barriers to successful prevention, diagnosis, and treatment of chlamydia. Many people who are diagnosed with chlamydia are asymptomatic. They self-report use of prophylactic protection during sexual intercourse as sporadic. In Ku's study (2002), the number of reported partners per year was about 3 for both age groups. Another major barrier to effective control is lack of compliance with the required 7-day treatment regimen of doxycycline, 100 mg twice a day, or tetracycline four times a day. However, azithromycin, 1g in a single dose, is also effective (Chin, 1999). To minimize the risk for reinfection, clients should be instructed to abstain from sexual intercourse until all of their sex partners have been treated. Clients do not need to be retested for chlamydia after completion of treatment with doxycycline or azithromycin unless symptoms persist or reinfection is suspected. A test of cure may be considered 3 weeks after completion of treatment with erythromycin (CDC, 2002c).

Rate (per 100,000 population)

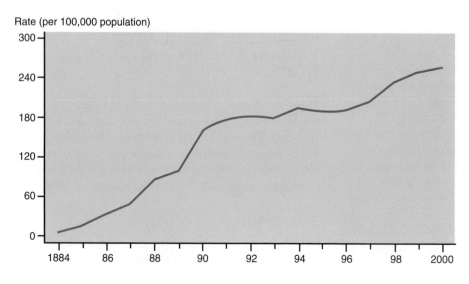

FIGURE 9–3.
Chlamydia rates—1984 to 2000.

As a primary prevention method, it is recommended that condom use be vigorously promoted and that condoms be made available at no cost at STD clinics, along with health education about the risk of STDs. STD screening should be incorporated into existing components of physical examinations for sports, school, or employment. Annual screening of all sexually active women age 20 to 25 years is also recommended, as is screening of older women with risk factors (eg, a new sex partner, multiple sex partners) (CDC, 2002c). If chlamydia is diagnosed, prophylactic treatment of sexual partners is recommended. The availability of new DNA-based methods now make STD testing possible in primary care settings.

Prenatal screening of pregnant women can prevent chlamydial infection among neonates. Initial *C. trachomatis* perinatal infection involves the mucous membranes of the eye, oropharynx, urogenital tract, and rectum. It is most often recogized by the presence of conjunctivitis, which develops 5 to 12 days after birth. Chlamydia is the most frequent indentifiable infectious cause of opthalmia neonatorum. Chlamydia also is a common cause of subacute, afebrile pneumonia with onset at 1 to 3 months of age. Either of these conditions may by observed by the community health nurse who makes a home visit for postdelivery follow-up of the family.

Genital Herpes

Genital herpes is caused by infection with the herpes simplex virus (HSV). Two serotypes of HSV have been identified: HSV-1 and HSV-2. Most of 50 million people in the United States diagnosed with herpes have HSV-2 genital infections. However, these numbers are misleading, because most people infected with HSV-2 have not been diagnosed (CDC, 2002c). Primary and recurrent infections occur, with or without symptoms. In women, sites of primary disease are the cervix and the vulva. Recurrent disease generally involves the vulva, perineal skin, legs, and buttocks. In men, lesions appear on the penis, and in the anus and rectum of those engaging in anal sex.

Since the late 1970s, the prevalence of genital herpes has increased by 30%. Approximately 1 in 5 adult Americans has serologic evidence of infection with genital herpes (HSV-2). The prevalence is increasing most dramatically among young white teens. The HSV-2 prevalence among 12- to 19-year-old Whites is now five times higher than it was 20 years ago. Seventeen percent of young adults age 20 to 29 years have HSV-2 (USDHHS, 2000). The *Healthy People 2010* goal is to reduce this percentage to 14%.

Control efforts for genital herpes are hampered because as many as three fourths of genital herpes infections are transmitted by people who are unaware of their own infection and because no cure for the condition exists. Symptomatic management is usually accomplished by antiviral chemotherapy treatment of the primary and recurrent episodes of genital herpes when used as daily suppressive therapy. The drugs available neither eradicate latent virus nor affect the risk, frequency, or severity of recurrences after the drug is discontinued. There are three antiviral medications that provide clinical benefit for genital herpes: acyclovir, valacyclovir, and famciclovir. Each is given orally for 7 to 10 days for a first clinical episode; for recurrent genital herpes, similar doses given twice a day is the recommended regimen. The drugs have been shown to reduce shedding of the virus, diminish pain, and accelerate healing. Intravenous acyclovir therapy is provided for clients who have severe disease or complications that necessitate hospitalization, such as disseminated infection, pneumonitis, hepatitis, or complications of the central nervous system (eg, meningitis, encephalitis) (CDC, 2002c).

When community health nurses counsel clients with genital herpes, the messages should include the following (CDC, 2002c):

- The natural history of the disease, with emphasis on recurrence, asymptomatic viral shedding, and risks of sexual transmission.
- Suppressive and episodic antiviral therapy is available and is effective in preventing or shortening the duration of recurrent episodes.
- The necessity of informing their current sex partners that they have genital herpes and of informing future partners before initiating a sexual relationship.
- Genital herpes can be transmitted during asymptomatic periods.
- The need to abstain from sexual activity with uninfected partners when lesions or prodromal symptoms are present.
- Latex condoms can reduce the risk for genital herpes when used consistently and correctly (ie, when the infected areas are covered or protected by the condom).
- Sex partners of infected persons should be advised that they might be infected even if they have no symptoms.
- The risk for neonatal HSV infection (which should be explained to all clients, including men).

Gonorrhea

The U. S. gonorrhea rate decreased by 56% between 1990 and 1997, from 278 to 122.7 cases per 100,000. The 1997 rate was the lowest ever reported in the United States. However, there are an estimated 600,000 new gonorrhea infections each year. Its causative agent is the gonococcus bacteria, *Neisseria gonorrhoeae*. Among women, those age 15 to 19 years had the highest rate, whereas among men, 20- to 24-year-olds had the highest rate. However, even in this group, gonorrhea decreased by 49% between 1990 and 1997. The incidence decreased in all ethnic and racial groups, from a high of 468 cases per 100,000 in 1975. By 1997, the nation as a whole had reached the *Healthy People 2000* target of 100 cases per 100,000. Nevertheless, among African-Americans, even with a 58% decrease in cases, the reported rate was 812 per 100,000 in 1997. The target for 2010 is 19 cases per 100,000 (Chin, 1999; USDHHS, 2000).

Antimicrobial resistance continues to be a concern in the treatment of gonorrhea. Overall, 29% of isolates collected in the United States in 1996 were resistant to penicillin, tetracycline, or both. Globally, the prevalence patterns for gonorrhea in developing countries are 10 to 15 times greater than those in developed countries, and drug-resistant strains of gonococcal infections provide added concern (WHO, 1998).

Frequently, the numbers of cases of gonorrhea are influenced by disease recurrence in the same individual, which is usually related to sexual lifestyle choices. Successful interventions in people with repeat infections could prove to be the most cost-effective way of managing the disease. Helping people to avoid repeat infections begins with a thorough personal history, including partner characteristics and willingness to also be treated. It also requires a more comprehensive, multiagency approach focusing on some of the other social, economic, and environmental issues that demand attention, for successful, lasting behavior change.

Gonorrhea commonly manifests in men as a purulent drainage from the penis, accompanied by painful urination, within 2 to 7 days after an infecting exposure. In women, the symptoms may be so mild as to go unnoticed. Progression of untreated gonorrhea can lead to serious reproductive system involvement causing PID and subsequent infertility. The recommended treatment regimen for gonorrhea has been ceftriaxone, ciprofloxacin 500 mg, ofloxacin 400 mg, or cefixime 400 mg orally in a single dose, followed by a regimen that is effective against concurrent chlamydial infection, doxycycline 100 mg twice daily orally for 7 days. This therapy also cures incubating syphilis and inhibits the emergence of antimicrobial-resistant gonococci (CDC, 2002c; Chin, 1999). Because treatment failure with the combined ceftriaxone/doxycycline regimen is rare, a follow-up test of cure is not considered essential except for pregnant women, who should have a culture performed as a test of cure.

Hepatitis

Five viral hepatitis infections are discussed in this section—hepatitis A, B, C, D, and E. Each constitutes a serious liver disease caused by a different hepatitis virus. Progress is being made to develop immunizations against various types of hepatitis. Nevertheless, the number of people being infected with hepatitis is globally epidemic. Nationally, substantial progress is being made in the elimination of some hepatitis viruses through the primary prevention practices of education and immunization for forms A and B.

Hepatitis A

Hepatitis A, caused by infection with the hepatitis A virus (HAV), occurs worldwide and is sporadic and epidemic, with cyclic recurrences affecting children and young adults most frequently. Most recent major U. S. epidemics cycled in 1961, 1971, and 1989. Case rates are high in Central and South America, the Caribbean, Mexico, Asia (except Japan), Africa, and southern and eastern Europe.

Hepatitis A is identified by the presence of immunoglobulin M (IgM) antibodies against HAV in the serum of acutely or recently ill clients. Approximately 33% of the U. S. population has serologic evidence of prior HAV infection; this percentage increases directly with age and reaches 75% among persons older than 70 years of age (CDC, 2002c). The disease is transmitted from person to person by the fecal-oral route and is characterized by the abrupt onset of symptoms including fever, malaise, anorexia, nausea, and abdominal discomfort, followed by jaundice in more severe cases. Mild illnesses last 1 to 2 weeks, but more severe cases last 1 month or longer. It is generally a self-limited disease that does not result in chronic infection or chronic liver disease. The case-fatality rate in the United States is low (less than 1/1000), but higher rates have been reported among those younger than 5 years of age (1.5/1000) and those older than 50 years of age (27/1,000) (Chin, 1999). The *Healthy People 2010* target for hepatitis A is to reduce new cases to no more than 4.5 per 100,000 (USDHHS, 2000).

Where environmental conditions are poor, infection is common and occurs at an early age. In the United States, most cases are transmitted in day care centers among diapered children, to household and sexual contacts of acute cases, and among travelers to countries where the disease is endemic. At times, there are common-source outbreaks related to contaminated water, food contaminated by infected food handlers, raw or undercooked shellfish from contaminated water, or contaminated produce such as lettuce or strawberries. Inactivated hepatitis A vaccines are prepared from formalin-inactivated, cell-culture–derived HAV and have been available in the United States since 1995 for people older than 2 years of age (CDC, 2002c). Administered in a two-dose series, these vaccines induce protective antibody levels in virtually all adults, providing the opportunity to eliminate this disease as a pubic health problem in the United States. The vaccine is recommended for high-risk groups and for children older than 2 years of age who are living in communities with high rates of HAV. Only 15% of hepatitis A cases are found in high-risk groups, and until the vaccine strategy is used on a wider scale (eg, routine vaccinations for all children), this disease will not be eliminated. A combined hepatitis A and B vaccine has been developed for adults.

Community health nurses have an important role in the prevention and control of this disease, including case-finding, education, and identifying at-risk populations for hepatitis A vaccination (eg, international travelers).

Hepatitis B

Hepatitis B is a global problem, with 66% of the world's population living in areas where there are high levels of infection by the hepatitis B virus (HBV). More than 2 billion people (one third of the world's population) have evidence of past or current HBV infection, and 350 million are chronic carriers of the virus. HBV causes 60% to 80% of all cases of primary liver cancer, which is one of the three top causes of cancer deaths in east Asia, southeast Asia, the Pacific Basin, and sub-Saharan Africa.

In the United States, cases of HBV are related to exposures common in certain high-risk groups, including injection drug users, homeless youth (Beech, Myers, & Beech, 2002), heterosexuals with multiple partners, homosexual men, incarcerated populations, and clients and staff in institutions for the developmentally disabled (Charuvastra et al., 2002). Occupationally acquired HBV can be traced to exposure to contaminated blood or serous fluids among health care workers such as surgeons, dentists, employees in hemodialysis centers, and operating room and emergency room staff.

The symptoms of HBV range from unnoticeable to fulminating and include anorexia, vague abdominal discomfort, nausea and vomiting, and rash, often progressing to jaundice. Diagnosis is confirmed by specific antigens or antibodies (or both) in serum.

Vaccination is the most effective way of preventing HBV transmission. (See Research: Bridge to Practice) Following WHO recommendations, 90 countries have integrated hepatitis B vaccine into their national immunization programs. By these means, the WHO's target is to reduce the incidence of new HBV carriers in children by 80% by the year 2001. Even at $1.50 for the three-dose series, vaccination is more expensive than the combined cost of required vaccines for six other diseases. WHO and the United Nations Children's Fund (UNICEF) have sought means to help the poorest and neediest countries to procure the vaccine. Effective implementation of this strategy could effectively eliminate transmission of hepatitis B by the year 2025 (WHO, 1998).

Healthy People 2010 targets hepatitis B in five objectives: (1) reduce incidence of chronic HBV infections in infants to no more than 400 per year (as a baseline there were 1682 chronic infections in 1995); (2) reduce the rate of hepatitis B in people younger than 25 years of age to 2.4 cases per 100,000; (3) reduce the number of hepatitis B cases among adults age 25 to 39 years to 5.1 per 100,000, and among adults 40 years and older to 3.8 per 100,000; (4) reduce hepatitis B cases in high-risk groups by 75%; and (5) decrease deaths from hepatitis B–related cirrhosis and liver cancer (USDHHS, 2000).

Community health nurses have an important role in the prevention and control of hepatitis B. Most importantly, this role includes teaching that encourages immunization compliance and consistent adherence to universal precautions (discussed earlier), especially for people in high-risk lifestyles or occupations.

Hepatitis C

Hepatitis C was first identified in 1989 and has already become a major public health problem. It causes a complex infection of the liver and is the most common bloodborne infection in the United States and in many other parts of the world. The incidence is not well known, but prevalence studies have led the WHO to estimate that 200 million people worldwide and 4 million people in the United States are infected with the hepatitis C virus (HCV) (Mee, 2001). Hepatitis C is more widespread than AIDS, and many infected people are unaware that they are infected (Lauer & Walker, 2001). About 170 million people are chronic carriers at risk for development of liver cirrhosis and liver cancer. In the United States, four times as many people have contracted HCV as have contracted HIV infection. Approximately 30,000 new acute infections and 8,000 to 10,000 deaths occur each year, and hepatitis C has become a leading reason

---

RESEARCH: BRIDGE TO PRACTICE

Hagan, H., Thiede, H., McGough, J.P., & Alexander, E.R. (2002). Hepatitis B vaccination among research participants, Seattle, Washington. *American Journal of Public Health, 92*(11), 1756.

This study reported on a protocol to increase hepatitis B virus (HBV) vaccination in participants in two research studies in Seattle in 1997 and 1998.

In a 1997 study, injection drug users were screened and those who were negative for the antibody to hepatitis B core antigen (anti-HBc) were given a voucher for a no-cost series of HBV vaccinations at a public health clinic in downtown Seattle. Those with vouchers were seen on a drop-in basis with little waiting. Of the 120 with vouchers, 91 (76%) did not complete any vaccinations; 6 (5%) completed 1 vaccination, and 5 (4%) completed 2; only 18 (15%) completed the series of 3 HBV vaccinations.

In the 1998 study, a similar HBV protocol was implemented for men age 15 to 22 years attending Seattle same-sex venues. Participants were tested for human immunodeficiency virus (HIV) and HBV infection, and 5% were anti-HBc positive. At the posttest visit, 285 HBV susceptible participants were given a voucher for free vaccinations, in a system similar to the prior study. Only the first vaccination was recorded by health department staff. Of those offered vouchers, only 9 (3%) initiated vaccination.

Providing financial incentives ($10) has increased vaccination rates in other studies, as has on-site vaccination at needle exchanges, drug treatment centers, and HIV counseling and testing programs. The voucher system in these two studies did not provide the incentive needed to contribute to a high vaccination rate.

for liver transplantation (Sarbah & Younossi, 2000). "Because most deaths result from chronic infection, the number is predicted to continue to rise as patients infected 20 or more years ago develop symptoms. Without intervention to stop this disease, that number may triple in the next 10 to 20 years" (Hench & Simpkins, 2002, p. 19).

Symptoms are similar to those of hepatitis A and B and may be unrecognizably mild to fulminating. Diagnosis depends on the demonstration of antibody to HCV, and a screening test for blood donors was established in 1992 (Chin, 1999). Before this test, HCV was the most common cause of posttransfusion hepatitis worldwide, accounting for approximately 90% of cases of this disease in the United States. The incidence of hepatitis C in the United States is highest in injection drug users (approximately 60%), hemophilia patients, and hemodialysis patients; it is also more frequently found among heterosexuals with multiple sexual partners, homosexual men, and health care workers than in the general public. Tattooing and body piercing provide an additional source of HCV transmission, and the exact role of tattooing is being studied. HCV testing is recommended for the following groups (Hench & Simpkins, 2002):

- People who inject illegal drugs, including those who injected once or a few times in the past and do not consider themselves drug users
- Recipients of transfusions or organ transplants before 1992 and recipients of blood from a positive donor
- People with selected medical conditions, including recipients of clotting factors before 1987, people undergoing chronic hemodialysis, and those with persistently elevated alanine aminotransferase levels
- People exposed to HCV-positive sources, such as needlesticks, sharps, or mucosal exposures, and children born to HCV-positive women

Healthy People 2010 objectives target two areas of improvement for hepatitis C: (1) increase the percentage of people with chronic HCV infection who are identified by state and local health departments, and (2) decrease the number of new cases to 1 per 100,000 (from 2.4 per 100,000 in 1996). Chronic liver disease is the tenth leading cause of death among adults in the United States, with 40% to 60% of the deaths related to HCV (8,000 to 12,000 deaths a year) (USDHHS, 2000).

A community health nurse's role includes case-finding, encouraging testing for people who received blood transfusions before 1992, and reinforcing universal precautions (see earlier discussion), along with strong nursing assessment skills and compassion. There is no vaccine, and chronic hepatitis C is a life-altering event; clients need emotional support. The nurse must build trust, and that begins with being nonjudgmental. Some of the hardest factors for many clients are the social stigma and others' fears that they can "catch" the disease. Community health nurses can provide education for clients and families. New drugs and clinical trials are being continually introduced, and nurses can provide up-to-date information.

Hepatitis D

Hepatitis D, caused by the hepatitis D virus (HDV), occurs worldwide, with variable prevalence. Sometimes called delta hepatitis, it occurs epidemically or endemically in populations at high risk for hepatitis B. The highest incidence occurs in parts of Russia, Romania, southern Italy, Africa, and South America. Severe epidemics have been observed in tropical South America, the Central African Republic, and in the United States in Massachusetts (Chin, 1999).

Diagnosis is made by detection of total antibody to HDV. Symptoms resemble those of hepatitis B, may be severe, and are always associated with a coexisting HBV infection. Delta hepatitis may be self-limited, or it may progress to chronic hepatitis. The role of the community health nurse is similar to that for hepatitis B.

Hepatitis E

Outbreaks of hepatitis E have occurred widely, primarily in developing countries with inadequate environmental sanitation, as waterborne epidemics. The hepatitis E virus (HEV) is transmitted by way of contaminated water and from person to person by the fecal-oral route. The attack rate is highest in young adults, and the disease is uncommon in children and the elderly. In the United States and most other developed countries, hepatitis E has been documented only among people traveling to HEV-endemic areas, such as India, Myanmar, Iran, Bangladesh, Ethiopia, Nepal, Pakistan, Central Asian republics of the former Soviet Union, Algeria, Libya, Somalia, Mexico, Indonesia, and China.

This disease runs a clinical course similar to that of hepatitis A, with a similar case-fatality rate, except in pregnant women, where the mortality rate may reach 20% among those infected during the third trimester of pregnancy. Education for primary prevention is the greatest role of the community health nurse, but epidemiologic investigation of suspected cases is an important activity if needed.

HIV/AIDS

The **human immunodeficiency virus (HIV)** is a retrovirus that attacks the body's immune system. Two types have been identified: type 1 (HIV-1) and type 2 (HIV-2). These viruses are relatively distinct serologically and geographically, but they have similar epidemiologic characteristics. The pathogenicity of HIV-2 appears to be less than that of HIV-1 (Chin, 1999).

In recent years, the incidence of HIV infection among heterosexuals has grown. In the 1980s, most HIV infections occurred in men who had sex with men and in injection drug users. When HIV entered the country's blood supply, it affected transfusion patients, hemophiliacs, and other persons who received infected blood or blood products. As more women of child-bearing age become infected, newborns were at increased risk for acquiring HIV infection. Today, almost all infections in infants and children are caused by transmission from the mother before or during birth. Today, most new cases of HIV/AIDS are transmitted through heterosexual or homosexual contact, the sharing of HIV-contaminated needles and syringes, or during the perinatal period from mother to child.

Acquired immunodeficiency syndrome (AIDS) is a severe, life-threatening condition, representing the late clinical stage of infection with HIV, in which there is progressive damage to the immune and other organ systems, particularly the central nervous system. Most people infected with HIV remain symptom free for long periods, but viral replication is active during all stages of infection. AIDS eventually develops in almost all HIV-infected people who are not receiving antiretroviral therapy (ART) or highly active antiretroviral therapy (HAART), from months to 17 years after infection, with a median of 10 years (CDC, 2001a, 2002c).

The early diagnosis of HIV infection is important so that treatment with ART or HAART can begin, to slow the declining function of the immune system. ART and HAART regimens have extended the length and improved the quality of life for many HIV-infected people in industrialized countries, but these therapies have not been widely used in resource-poor nations because of their cost and the need for an adequate health care infrastructure to administer and monitor complex therapeutic regimens of toxic agents. However, in 2001, momentum grew to provide options for the use of ART in these regions (NIH Office of AIDS Research, 2001). A compounding problem even in resource-rich countries such as the United States is that some people find it difficult or impossible to comply with the arduous treatment regimens, develop toxicities and side effects, or cannot afford the high cost of approximately $15,000 per year. Others fail to obtain a satisfactory reduction in viral load even while adhering to treatment regimens. In addition, metabolic complications, including insulin resistance, and body composition changes, such as deforming deposits of abdominal adipose tissue, have emerged in individuals on long-term antiretroviral regimens. Finally, an increasing number of treatment failures are linked to the emergence of drug-resistant HIV (NIH Office of AIDS Research, 2001).

ART regimens are designed to address opportunistic infections, cancers, and other conditions that have been shown to be associated with HIV infection. Preventive measures for *Pneumocystis carinii* pneumonia (PCP), toxoplasmis of the central nervous system, disseminated *Mycobacterium avium* complex (MAC) disease, TB, and bacterial pneumonia are available through ART and other related drugs, and HIV clients need to be aware of this. Because of its effect on the immune system, HIV affects the diagnosis, evaluation, treatment, and follow-up of such concurrent diseases.

The disenfranchised in marginalized communities in the United States, such as members of racial and ethnic minority groups, the poor, and substance and alcohol abusers, have less access to these life-extending therapies, regardless of the tribulations of treatment regimens.

Incidence and Prevalence

HIV/AIDS was recognized as an emerging disease less than 25 years ago, and it has rapidly established itself throughout the world, creating a global pandemic. It is now prevalent in virtually all parts of the world (WHO, 1998). An estimated 36 million adults and children were living with HIV/AIDS in 2000, and more than 22 million deaths had been recorded, with 5.8 million new HIV infections in 2000 (NIH Office of AIDS Research, 2001). Current estimates based on various studies are that more than 1 million people in the United States are infected with HIV, and 670,000 have been diagnosed with AIDS since the first reported case in 1981 (NIH Office of AIDS Research, 2001). The number of AIDS cases in the United States climbed each year until 1996, when it dropped into second place among leading causes of death in the 25- to 44-year-old age group for the first time in 4 years (USDHHS, 2000).

Annual costs of HIV/AIDS care in the United States have been in the billions of dollars. Because more people are being drawn into the health care system at an earlier point for interventions of long duration, it is expected that AIDS-related care costs will continue to grow. Combination therapy with at least three antiretroviral drugs was introduced in 1995 and became widespread in 1996 (NIH Office of AIDS Research, 2001). It is not yet known how long these therapies will prolong life, and they do not work for everyone, but their use is having a visible impact on AIDS incidence and AIDS mortality. The new antiviral drugs have delayed the onset of AIDS and have improved the quality of life for many HIV-infected people in North America (WHO, 1998).

The diversity of the spread of HIV throughout populations is striking: 16 countries (all in sub-Saharan Africa) report an overall adult HIV prevalence greater than 10%, 8 countries (also all in sub-Saharan Africa) report a rate between 5% and 10%, 28 countries have between 1% and 5%, and the remaining 119 countries of the world have a prevalence of less than 1% among adults (United States Agency for International Development [USAID], 2001a). More than two thirds of all the people now living with HIV—almost 25 million men, women, and children—live in Africa south of the Sahara desert. Also, 83% of the world's AIDS deaths have been in this region (USAID, 2001b). Four out of five HIV-positive women in the world live in Africa, and 87% of the affected children live there. This is happening for several reasons: more women of child-bearing age live in Africa than elsewhere; African women have more children on average that those on other continents; almost all children in Africa are breastfed, which is a way to transmit HIV; and the new drugs are far less readily available in developing countries.

In the United States, the HIV/AIDS epidemic continues to evolve. The rate of new HIV infections has been constant at approximately 40,000 new cases each year since 1990, meaning that the overall epidemic is continuing to expand (NIH Office of AIDS Research, 2001). AIDS disproportionately affects African-Americans and Hispanic-Americans; they accounted for 48% and 20%, respectively, of all persons diagnosed with AIDS in 1999 (NIH Office of AIDS Research, 2001). Eighty-three percent of women with AIDS in the United States are members of minority groups, as are 66% of the men with AIDS. Addressing these racial disparities is a high priority for the NIH and *Healthy People 2010.*

Populations at Risk

AIDS was first recognized as a distinct syndrome in 1981, and during the early years it was seen as a disease of male homosexuals, intravenous drug abusers, and people with a history of multiple blood transfusions. The at-risk population for AIDS now includes people with a large number of sexual partners, adolescents, injection drug users and their sexual partners, homosexual men and their male or female partners, people who exchange sex for drugs or money, and people already infected with HIV (USDHHS, 2000). Sexual transmission of HIV is closely associated with other STDs, particularly those that have an ulcerative phase, including syphilis. With belated but growing awareness of the AIDS epidemic on a global scale, it is becoming recognized as a universal threat to the health and well-being of individuals and of populations. AIDS is seen in the United States as a potential health threat to all sexually active people and their offspring. The number of cases of heterosexually acquired AIDS increased significantly in the 1990s, especially among women and minority populations, with Blacks and Hispanics accounting for 65% of AIDS cases reported in 1997 (Brooks, 1999; Chin, 1999) (Fig. 9–4).

Adolescents and young adults are considered to be at particular risk for HIV infection because many of them engage in high-risk behaviors, believing themselves to be invulnerable to infection. In addition to the considerable risks posed by potential HIV infection, other adverse outcomes related to early initiation of sexual activity include higher levels of all STDs (Quander, 2001; WHO, 1998).

Prevention and Intervention

National HIV prevention and intervention efforts depend on two important factors: (1) self-perception of risk and (2) adoption of risk-reducing behaviors in response to awareness of the risk. Consequently, education about HIV/AIDS, including safe sex and injection drug use behaviors, has become the key to prevention. Public health workers seek to identify and intervene with the at-risk population, providing counseling and prevention education as well as testing services. The primary purposes of counseling are to prevent further spread of HIV infection and, whenever possible, to slow the progression of HIV infection to AIDS. HIV counseling can help uninfected people initiate and sustain behaviors to reduce their risk of infection; help infected people adopt behaviors to reduce the risk of transmission to others; encourage spouses and partners of infected people to adopt safe behaviors; and help infected people take better care of themselves. Properly using condoms, reducing the number of sexual partners, and abstaining from injection drug use decrease, but do not eliminate, the risk of HIV infection (USDHHS, 2000).

HIV infection and AIDS are important topics of concern to community health nurses for a number of reasons. They present an intriguing service delivery problem that requires complex and sophisticated multidisciplinary interventions. Sexual behaviors, illegitimate drug use, end-of-life issues, and other psychosocial aspects provide very human dimensions to a problem that is also demanding of nursing, medical, social, epidemiologic, political, and economic resources.

Care of people with HIV infection presents a special opportunity for community health nurses to meet an important and visible challenge in modern society. People with HIV/AIDS are living longer, requiring nursing care that is widely integrated with other community services. This population requires knowledgeable, skilled, often aggressive therapeutic and preventive nursing services for acute as well as chronic illness, supported by an interdisciplinary network of providers. Three major goals of care with this population are (1) promoting general health and resilience, (2) preventing infections of all sorts, and (3) delaying the onset of clinical symptoms with antiviral therapy. To meet these goals, the community health nurse's role involves getting HIV-positive clients engaged in wellness programs, such as programs promoting nutritional health, exercise, drug management, and prevention of opportunistic infections. Stress reduction is essential for these clients; the nurse can facilitate relaxation activities, client and family counseling, and support groups to assist clients' coping abilities. An important part of nursing care with these clients is the use of universal precautions (discussed earlier), which refers to the CDC recommendations to prevent infections that are transmitted by direct or indirect contact with infected blood or body fluids (bloody body secretions, semen, vaginal secretions, tissue, cerebrospinal fluid, and synovial, pleural, peritoneal, pericardial, and amniotic fluids). Nurses can also make important contributions to the evolution of HIV/AIDS care and services by participating in the debates that occur and are likely to continue regarding the ethical dimensions of the AIDS crisis, including HIV screening, contact investigation, and AIDS-related discrimination (discussed later).

The therapeutic management of HIV infection and AIDS is evolving and is, in fact, largely experimental. Attempts at vaccine development are ongoing and include experimentation with vaccines for those already infected, to increase resistance to multiplication of the viral agent and development of clinical symptoms. The WHO reviews and approves HIV/AIDS drugs in an attempt to make them available to as many people as possible. A list released by the WHO in March, 2002, contained 40 drugs (including 11 antiretrovirals and 5 products for opportunistic infections), and another 100 products from 13 additional manufacturers were under review ("WHO Reviews," 2002, p. 14). Nurses who wish timely updates on clinical and medical aspects of AIDS case management may refer to recent issues of the CDC's *Morbidity and Mortality Weekly Report,* as well as profes-

New HIV Infections

There are an estimated 800,000 to 900,000 people currently living with HIV in the U.S., with approximately 40,000 new HIV infections occurring in the U.S. every year.

■ **By gender,** 70% of new HIV infections each year occur among men, although women are also significantly affected.

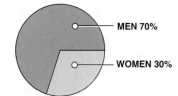

Estimates of annual new infections by gender (N = 40,000)

■ **By risk,** men who have sex with men (MSM) represent the largest proportion of new infections, followed by men and women infected through heterosexual sex and injection drug use (IDU).

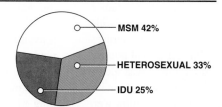

Estimates of annual new infections by risk (N = 40,000)

■ **By race,** more than half of new HIV infections occur among blacks, though they only represent 13% of the U.S. population. Hispanics, who make up about 12% of the U.S. population, are also disproportionately affected.

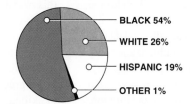

Estimates of annual new infections by race (N = 40,000)

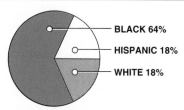

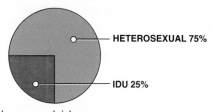

Estimates of annual new infections in women, U.S., by race and risk

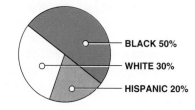

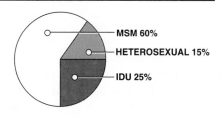

Estimates of annual new infections in men, U.S., by race and risk

FIGURE 9–4.
A glance at the HIV epidemic. (Centers for Disease Control and Prevention. [2001]. *HIV/AIDS update.* Atlanta: CDC.)

sional journals devoted to disseminating information to practitioners working with AIDS patients.

Influenza

Influenza derives its importance from the rapidity with which epidemics evolve, the widespread morbidity, and the seriousness of complications, namely pneumonias (Chin, 1999).

Influenza, an Italian word that means *influence of the cold*, has been recognized since 412 BC and was first described by Hippocrates. It existed throughout the early centuries, and about 30 possible pandemics have been documented in the past 400 years. Three have occurred in the 20th century—in 1918, 1957, and 1968. The 1918 "Spanish flu" was the most devastating, killing more than 20 million people worldwide from 1918 to 1920 (WHO, 1998). This pandemic occurred because the new virus was easily transmitted from person to person.

Influenza infections occur primarily in the winter months, affecting individuals in all age groups and causing approximately 20,000 deaths and 110,000 hospitalizations annually in the United States (Prisco, 2002).Children have the highest rates of infection, but individuals age 65 years and older and those with medical conditions who are at risk for complications have the highest rates of serious morbidity and mortality. Older adults account for more than 90% of the deaths attributed to influenza and pneumonia (Prisco, 2002).

The WHO Network for Global Influenza Surveillance, which involves 110 national influenza centers worldwide, maintains constant vigilance for new influenza viruses. Sources of influenza virus include swine, birds, and poultry. In 1997, a new influenza virus called A(H5N1) was identified in chickens in Hong Kong before it could emerge in humans. As a precautionary measure, the infected poultry were destroyed to eliminate the risk of further transmission. Globally, an expected pandemic event did not materialize.

FluNet is a prototype site on the World Wide Web for the electronic submission of influenza data from participating national laboratories. Only designated users can submit data, but the results—graphics, maps, and tables of influenza activity on a global scale—are available to the general public. As new data arrive and are verified, the maps and tables are revised to give users an up-to-date overview of the influenza situation. FluNet has speeded up the sharing of information on influenza patterns and virus strains and is becoming an essential tool in preparing for and preventing influenza pandemics. It is unknown when or where the next flu epidemic or pandemic will occur, but the emergency response plans have to be prepared in advance, and the recent Hong Kong scare became a practice event. Collaborating Influenza Surveillance Centers have created a task force of experts on influenza to develop a plan for the global management and control of a pandemic. The world's public health leaders are trying to prevent another 1918 pandemic of influenza.

Influenza is identified as an acute communicable viral disease of the respiratory tract characterized by fever, headache, myalgia, prostration, coryza, sore throat, and cough. When a new subtype appears, all children and adults are equally susceptible, except those who have lived through earlier epidemics caused by the same subtype. Influenza A virus causes the most severe and widespread disease (pandemics); influenza B causes milder disease outbreaks, and influenza C is connected with only sporadic cases of milder respiratory disease (Malhotra & Krilov, 2000).

Influenza immunization is available that has been closely matched to the circulating strains of the virus. Children younger than 2 years of age are at substantially increased risk for influenza-related hospitalizations. As a result, as mentioned earlier in this chapter, the VFC program has expanded coverage for influenza vaccine to all VFC-eligible children age 6 to 23 months and VFC-eligible children aged 2 to 18 years who are household contacts of children younger than 2 years of age (CDC, 2002a). Killed-virus vaccines provide 70% to 90% protection in healthy young adults (CDC, 2002b). In the elderly, immunization may be less effective in preventing illness, but they reduce the severity of disease. With vaccination, the incidence of complications among the elderly is reduced by 50% to 60% and death by approximately 80% (Chin, 1999).

The vaccine should be given every year *before* influenza is expected in the community (November to March in the United States). For those living or traveling outside the United States, timing of the immunization should be based on the seasonal patterns of influenza where they are traveling.

Community health nurses have a major role in primary prevention. Influenza vaccination clinics are frequently planned and organized by or with the local public health agency, with the injections administered by community health nurses. People can get immunized at worksites, shopping malls, pharmacies, and senior centers. Private physicians and HMOs provide immunization for their patients or members. Often, the community health nurse participates in this primary prevention activity during the fall of each year.

It is extremely important for older adults and people with chronic illnesses, respiratory diseases, or suppressed immune systems to get immunized each year. People working in critical professions, such as the health care industry, and people in congregate living situations, such as assisted living centers or skilled nursing facilities, also should be immunized.

In 1997, the immunization rate for influenza among noninstitutionalized adults, although only 25%, continued to increase toward the *Healthy People 2010* goal of 60%. Among noninstitutionalized adults aged 65 years and older, the goal is 90% and the total in 1997 was 63%. The year 2010 target rates for the African-Americans and Hispanic-American populations remain substantially below that of the general population, at 45% and 53%, respectively (USDHHS, 2000). *Healthy People 2010* has set an objective to monitor the national impact of influenza vaccinations on influenza-related hospitalizations and mortality among high-risk populations by annually collecting, analyzing, and reporting data from at least one medical care organization in all nine influenza surveillance regions of the country. If the immunization approach is successful, a dramatic decline should be seen in the rates of influenza-related morbidity requiring hospitalization and influenza-related mortality.

Pneumonia

Community-acquired pneumonia is a significant cause of morbidity and mortality. It is the sixth leading cause of death and the first leading cause of infectious death in the United States. An increased incidence of pneumonia often accompanies epidemics of influenza. There are an estimated 3 million cases per year, with approximately 20% requiring hospital admission, and 50,000 deaths per year from bacterial pneumonia (Schultz, 2002). Pneumonia hospital admissions and mortality are far more common among people older than

65 years of age; the mortality rate is approximately 50%. In the 1980s, acute respiratory infections in developing countries, mainly pneumonia, were the major killers of children younger than 5 years of age. These children often suffered several conditions at once, such as being dehydrated from diarrhea, being malnourished, and acquiring pneumonia. The WHO and UNICEF worked out clinical guidelines to approach these conditions collectively, and this integrated case management approach seems to be improving the plight of children in developing countries.

The incidence of pneumonia is highest in winter. It is spread by droplets, by direct oral contact, and through **fomites**, which are any inanimate objects freshly soiled with respiratory discharges. People most susceptible to pneumonia are the elderly and people with a history of chronic diseases, a compromised immune system, or any condition affecting the anatomic or physiologic integrity of the lower respiratory tract.

Pneumonia is a pulmonary infection that causes inflammation of the lobes of the lungs, bronchial tree, or interstitial space. The causative organism can be viral (50% of all cases), bacterial, or fungal (Schultz, 2002). Symptoms of pneumonia include sudden onset with a shaking chill, fever, pleural pain, dyspnea, a productive cough of "rusty" sputum, and tachypnea. The onset is less abrupt in elderly individuals, and the diagnosis may need to be confirmed by radiographic studies. In infants and young children, fever, vomiting, and convulsions may be the initial symptoms.

Primary prevention is the best course of action and includes a pneumonia vaccine, especially for the high-risk groups. *Healthy People 2010* targeted 90% as the goal for pneumococcal vaccinations among noninstitutionalized adults age 65 years and older and 60% among noninstitutionalized high-risk adults age 18 to 64 years; the corresponding 1997 values were 43% and 11%, respectively. Reimmunization is recommended every 6 years to these groups. The vaccine is not effective in children younger than 2 years of age and is not recommended for the healthy population age 2 to 65

years. For these people, education about preventing pneumonia is a major part of the community health nurse's role.

Secondary prevention includes the early diagnosis and prompt treatment of affected individuals. Antimicrobial agents such as penicillin and erythromycin are the first drugs of choice for treating pneumonia.

Syphilis

Syphilis is the first STD for which control measures were developed and tested. The incidence in the United States has decreased in recent years, from more than 50,000 cases in 1990 to 5979 cases in 2000; the latter value exceeds the *Healthy People 2000* target of 4.0 cases per 100,000 and is the lowest yearly number of cases ever reported (Fig. 9–5). In the United States, syphilis and congenital syphilis are highly focal both geographically and demographically. Syphilis contributes to HIV transmission in those parts of the country where rates of both infections are high (CDC, 2000b). In 1997, 75% of U. S. counties reported no cases of syphilis. Rates have decreased by more than 80% for all racial and ethnic groups. Only in the South do rates remain higher than the year 2000 target, with 6.6 cases per 100,000 people. The target for 2010 is 0.2 cases per 100,000, and the opportunity exists to eliminate syphilis within the U. S. borders.

> *Elimination of syphilis would have far-reaching public health implications because it would remove two devastating consequences of the disease—increased likelihood of HIV transmission and compromised ability to have healthy babies due to spontaneous abortions, stillbirths, and multi-system disorders caused by congenital syphilis acquired from mothers with syphilis (USDHHS, 2000, Section 25, p. 18).*

However, there remains a major disparity in the populations with syphilis. The secondary syphilis rate for non-Hispanic Blacks is 44 times greater than that for non-Hispanic Whites.

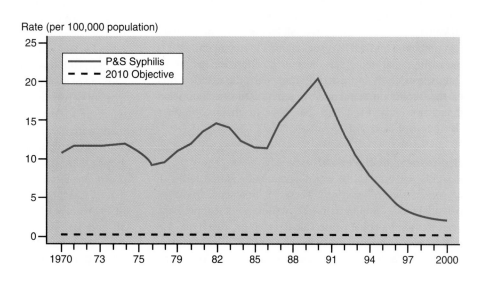

FIGURE 9–5.
Primary and secondary syphilis, 1970 to 2000, and *Healthy People 2010* objectives.

Syphilis, a genital ulcerative disease, manifests in several forms during the life cycle of the disease. Approximately 3 weeks after exposure, a primary lesion called a *chancre* characteristically appears as a painless ulcer at the site of initial invasion of the causative organism, *Treponema pallidum,* a spirochete. After 4 to 6 weeks, the chancre heals without treatment, to be replaced by the development of a more generalized secondary skin eruption, classically appearing on the soles of the feet and palms of the hands, often accompanied by constitutional symptoms. Secondary manifestations resolve spontaneously, and a latent period follows, which may last from weeks to years. Unpredictably, severe, systemic involvement with disability or even death may occur (Chin, 1999).

Treatment of early primary, secondary, and early latent syphilis is generally accomplished through antibiotic therapy. The specific treatment is a long-acting penicillin G (benzathine penicillin), 2.4 million units given in a single intramuscular dose on the day of diagnosis. Clients should be reexamined serologically at 3 and 6 months after treatment to ensure cure; however, the single-dose treatment is effective therapy even if the client fails to return (Chin, 1999).

Community health nurses need to provide the same level of support to clients diagnosed with syphilis as they give to other clients diagnosed with STDs. Occasionally, older clients may recall the horrors of untreated syphilis and the significant numbers of cases before the 1970s. They will need added assurance of the effectiveness of their treatment and education about the changes in the prevalence of this STD.

Tuberculosis

TB, once almost eradicated, has reemerged as a serious public health problem. In 2001, the CDC reported that the number of cases had decreased for the ninth straight year, to 15,991 cases of active TB. Although this is good news, there is evidence of sharply disparate rates among minority populations, with 54% of active TB cases in 1999 occurring among African-American and Hispanic-American individuals, and 20% among Asian-Americans (NIAID, 2002). In addition, the worldwide TB situation has worsened over the past 2 decades, especially in Africa because of the HIV/AIDS epidemic (there is a fatal association of TB with HIV infection and AIDS). The rate of TB among children is increasing, and there has been a proliferation of MDR strains, especially in Eastern Europe since the deterioration of the health infrastructure, which presents a significant threat not only to clients but also to their caregivers (Borgdorff, Floyd, & Broekmans, 2002).

Incidence and Prevalence

Roughly one third of the world's population is infected with *Mycobacterium tuberculosis.* These 2 billion people have the potential for developing active TB at some point in time. Each year, 8 million people worldwide develop active TB and 1.8 million people die. Approximately 80% of TB cases are found in 23 countries; the highest incidence rates are in Africa and

southeast Asia (Borgdorff, Floyd, & Broekmans, 2002). In the United States, 10 to 15 million people are infected with *M. tuberculosis* without displaying symptoms (latent TB) and about 1 in 10 of these individuals will develop active TB at some time in their lives. This makes TB the leading infectious killer of adults, despite the fact that effective anti-TB treatment has existed since the 1940s (WHO, 1998). TB is also a leading cause of death among people infected with HIV.

Exposure to TB does not lead to actual disease in all cases. A long latent period may persist for many years (even for a lifetime) before the infected person develops disease and becomes infectious. The probability of becoming infected depends primarily on the amount of exposure to air contaminated with *M. tuberculosis,* the proximity to the infectious person, and the degree of ventilation. The majority of individuals exposed to infectious cases do not become infected. Of those who do, all but about 5% to 10% will remain disease free, perhaps for a lifetime. The remaining 90% harbor the organism; although they are not infectious (capable of spreading infection to others), they represent a persistent pool of potential cases in a population. The likelihood of being among the 10% who develop clinical infectious disease is variable, depending on the initial dose of infection and certain other risk factors. Groups at increased risk include children younger than 3 years of age, adolescents, young adults, the aged, and the immunosuppressed (Chin, 1999). Unlike some other infectious diseases that spread rapidly in a susceptible community, immunizing or killing large numbers of people, TB can be maintained at endemic levels in populations for generations. Endemic levels are those at which the disease or infectious agent is habitually present in a geographic area but disease outbreaks are contained to a minimum.

Surveillance

Variably called *consumption, wasting disease,* and the *white plague,* TB has been one of the greatest scourges since times before recorded history. It was the leading cause of death in the United States through the 1930s because no cure was available. A diagnosis of TB was a slow death sentence, and the best chance of recovery was rest, sunshine, and plenty of food. Consequently, sanatoriums—rest homes where patients followed a prescribed routine every day—were built and were occupied for months until recovery or death (Fig. 9–6).

Surveillance of a disease refers to the continuous scrutiny of all aspects of occurrence and spread of the disease that are pertinent to effective control (Chin, 1999). In 1953, when uniform national surveillance for TB was initiated, there were more than 84,000 TB cases in the United States. With the introduction of effective antibiotics in the 1940s to 1960s, there was a 73% decline in the number of TB cases, and it was thought that the problem of TB had been solved. From 1953 through 1984, the number of TB cases decreased by an average of 6% each year, and in 1985 they reached an all-time low of 22,201. The decrease in the number of TB cases contributed to medical and political complacency that resulted in a lack of progress in the development of new ap-

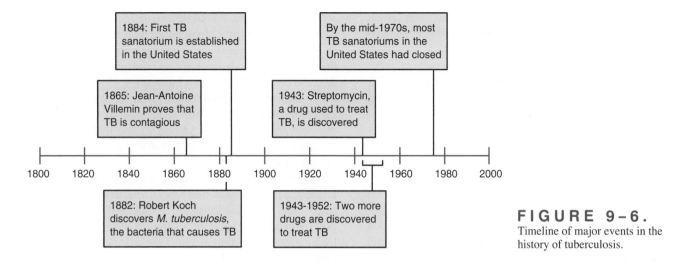

FIGURE 9–6.
Timeline of major events in the history of tuberculosis.

proaches and tools to control TB, and the disease is now resurging (Cowie, Field, & Enarson, 2002). In fact, TB was already dramatically increasing in developing countries, prompting the WHO in 1993 to declared TB a "global emergency" at a time when many Western countries were anticipating the impending elimination of the disease.

The number of TB cases in the United States increased by 20% between 1985 and 1992. At that time renewed efforts to combat the resurgence included improving laboratories, strengthening surveillance and expanding directly observed therapy, and expediting investigation of close contacts of TB patients (USDHHS, 2000). These efforts allowed the country to experience several years of declining TB cases to a new low of 18,361 cases in 1998, a rate of 6.8 cases per 100,000 (CDC, 1999). *Healthy People 2010* has a target of 1.0 new cases per 100,000 (USDHHS, 2000). However, the 1989 Strategic Plan for the Elimination of Tuberculosis in the United States set a TB elimination goal of 1 case per million people by 2010 (CDC, 1999).

Although the TB numbers were decreasing in those years, numbers being reported among members of racial and ethnic minorities, children, and foreign-born persons living in the United States were increasing. Compounding the effects of these demographic changes was the appearance of MDR TB strains. The rising incidence of TB and MDR TB has changed the TB situation considerably over the past decade and continues to offer a major public health challenge.

Populations at Risk

Minority populations tend to be at greater risk for TB. An increasing percentage of U. S. cases are occurring among people who were born in Asian, African, or Latin American countries, where TB rates are 5 to 30 times higher than in the United States. In the 1990s, TB cases among U. S.-born individuals declined 38%, whereas the number of TB cases among foreign-born persons in the United States increased by 6%. The TB case rate for foreign-born individuals has remained at least 4 to 5 times higher than for the U.S.-born, and the proportion of U.S. cases occurring in foreign-born

persons has increased steadily since the mid-1980s, reaching 46% in 2000 (Saraiya et al., 2002). TB disease cases occur predominantly among the following groups: foreign-born persons (46%), the elderly (23%), homeless people (5%), and individuals infected with HIV (8%). Higher incidences of TB are found among low-income people, persons with alcohol or drug abuse problems, the underserved, the malnourished, people in correctional facilities, people with other medical conditions, and individuals working where people at risk for TB are grouped together (eg, homeless shelters, drug treatment centers, health care facilities). TB rates are highest among refugees and immigrants, and noncompliance with treatment in all groups is a major factor in continued transmission of the disease and development of MDR organisms.

HIV infection is the strongest known risk factor for the development of TB. Immune-suppressed individuals such as those with AIDS can develop fulminant active TB within weeks after exposure to the mycobacterium, and the disease progresses much faster than in those with normal competent immune systems. Consequently, a suspected case of TB in a person with AIDS is usually treated immediately without waiting for the results of a sputum test or chest radiography. During the last 20 years, the incidence of HIV infection has shifted from a predominantly homosexual, White, middle-class male population to a more impoverished, heterosexual, inner-city minority population with a high prevalence of *M. tuberculosis* infection. Consequently, the incidence of HIV-related TB mortality has risen (Desvarieux, Hyppolite, Johnson, & Pape, 2001).

The risk of HIV-infected clients for TB infection is further complicated by false-negative reactions (anergy) of the tuberculin skin test resulting from the client's impaired immunity. Anergy testing seems to be the recommended next step, but the appropriate antigens for anergy testing are unclear and in individual patients the results can be very misleading. Therefore, anergy testing is not recommended in tuberculin-negative HIV-infected individuals (Reichman & Andriote, 2002).

Increasing numbers of TB cases among children are especially worrisome because they point to escalated transmission in the United States. Cases in children most often result from recent infection, in contrast to cases among older adults, which may develop as a result of infection occurring many years previously. TB among children suggests rising case rates among persons of reproductive age, who have contact with and transmit infection to susceptible children. This underscores the need to investigate the household and community contacts of the child for untreated disease. Likewise, when adult active TB cases are identified, it is essential to evaluate child contacts of the case.

Among children with active TB, minority groups account for a vast majority of the cases. Girls have a much higher incidence during elementary and high school years than do boys of the same age. Susceptibility in children and adolescents peaks during infancy and again in puberty. Infants show decreased ability to localize infection and have limited stores of acquired antibodies. It is unclear whether the increased susceptibility in adolescents is the result of increased contacts with infected persons, rapid hormonal changes and growth spurts, suboptimal diets, or a combination of all of these. The occurrence of TB infection and disease in children provides important information about its spread in homes and communities. For example, if a child has TB infection or disease, it must have been transmitted relatively recently; therefore, the person who transmitted the TB may still be infectious, other adults and children in the household or community have probably been exposed, and, if infected, others may develop TB disease in the future.

Prevention and Intervention

Tuberculin testing, the standard method for evaluating TB infection, is a simple skin test that measures by visible reaction whether the body has had immunologic experience with *M. tuberculosis* (Table 9–5). From there, evaluation procedures determine the classification status of the disease, ranging from 0 to 5. The two most used terms are infected without current disease (classification 2) and with current TB disease (classification 3) (Table 9–6). The skin test itself is not diagnostic of disease.

There are two widely available skin test products. The tine test, a multiple-puncture type of test, delivers a premeasured dose of purified protein derivative (PPD) under the skin by puncture. The Mantoux test delivers 0.1 mL of PPD by intradermal injection. Because the dose is measured at the time of injection, the Mantoux test is considered to be more reliable; the dose administered in the tine test and the technique of administration may be highly variable (Reichman & Andriote, 2002).

Interpretation of the tuberculin test is critical to subsequent evaluation of the client's status. The interpretation of this screening method must be as sensitive as possible while maintaining specificity for exposure.

The Committee on Infectious Disease of the American Academy of Pediatrics in 1988 developed guidelines based on cost-effectiveness for routine periodic skin testing only in high-risk populations. Such populations include children of American Indians and native Alaskans; children in neighborhoods where case rates are higher than the national average; children of immigrants from Asia, Africa, the Middle East, Latin America, and the Caribbean; and children from

T A B L E   9 – 5

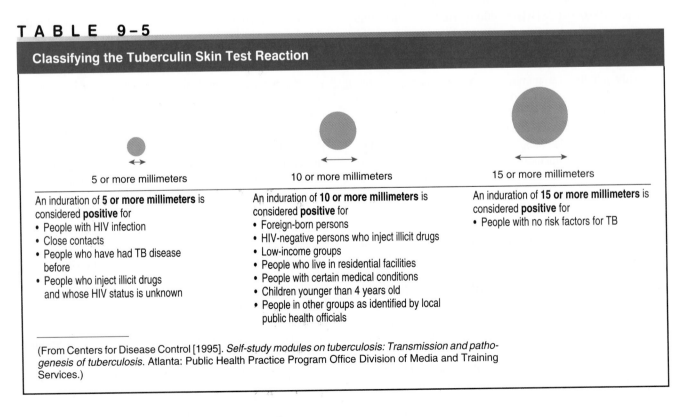

Classifying the Tuberculin Skin Test Reaction

5 or more millimeters	10 or more millimeters	15 or more millimeters
An induration of **5 or more millimeters** is considered **positive** for • People with HIV infection • Close contacts • People who have had TB disease before • People who inject illicit drugs and whose HIV status is unknown	An induration of **10 or more millimeters** is considered **positive** for • Foreign-born persons • HIV-negative persons who inject illicit drugs • Low-income groups • People who live in residential facilities • People with certain medical conditions • Children younger than 4 years old • People in other groups as identified by local public health officials	An induration of **15 or more millimeters** is considered **positive** for • People with no risk factors for TB

(From Centers for Disease Control [1995]. *Self-study modules on tuberculosis: Transmission and pathogenesis of tuberculosis.* Atlanta: Public Health Practice Program Office Division of Media and Training Services.)

TABLE 9-6

Classification System for TB

Class	Type	Description
0	No exposure to TB Not infected	No history of exposure, negative reaction to the tuberculin skin test
1	Exposure to TB No evidence of infection	History of exposure, negative reaction to a tuberculin skin test given at least 10 weeks after exposure
2	TB infection No TB disease	Positive reaction to the tuberculin skin test, negative smears and cultures (if done), no clinical or x-ray evidence of TB disease
3	Current TB disease	Positive culture for *M tuberculosis* (if done), **or** A positive reaction to the tuberculin skin test and clinical or x-ray evidence of current TB disease
4	Previous TB disease (not current)	Medical history of TB disease, **or** Abnormal but stable x-ray findings for a person who has a positive reaction to the tuberculin skin test, negative smears and cultures (if done), and no clinical or x-ray evidence of current TB disease
5	TB suspected	Signs and symptoms of TB disease, but evaluation not complete

(From: Centers for Disease Control and Prevention. [1995]. *Self-study modules on tuberculosis: Transmission and pathogenesis of tuberculosis.* Atlanta, GA: Public Health Practice Program Office Division of Media and Training Services.)

households with one or more cases of active TB. Routine periodic screening was recommended for all of these children at 12 to 16 months of age, 4 to 6 years, and at 14 to 16 years. Adults should be tested periodically once negative status has been determined. Frequency of testing depends on risk of exposure and symptoms, if any. Once a person is known to be a positive reactor to a skin test, the tuberculin test is not a valid means of assessing TB infection, and subsequent evaluation calls for a chest radiograph to identify tuberculous lesions.

Community health nurses working with ethnically diverse populations may meet clients who, after relating a history of vaccination or TB, have records or recall receiving bacille Calmette-Guérin (BCG) vaccination. BCG is an anti-TB vaccination, first developed in 1906, that has been widely used on a global scale since 1921 in all countries except the Netherlands and the United States. Through collaborative efforts with the nations of the world, the WHO in 1990 was able to meet its goal of immunizing 80% of the world's infants with the BCG vaccine. This rate was approximately 90% in 1997. BCG boosters for children at ages 5 to 7 years and 11 to 14 years are recommended in many countries (WHO, 1998).

The BCG vaccine is an attenuated strain of *M. bovis* and may induce a positive TB skin test, although skin test reactivity tends to diminish with time. It is not used in the United States because it destroys this country's only control measure (a positive PPD test) to identify individuals in classification 2 who should receive treatment for the TB infection. The efficacy of the BCG vaccine is also questionable. Protection begins to wane by 5 years, and by 10 years after vaccination most recipients do not have protection or measurable reactions. Another reason BCG has not been used in this country is that it has never been cloned, and vaccine products made in different locations may vary widely in effectiveness, providing from 0% to 80% effective protection for inoculated individuals. Because of these shortcomings, BCG is recommended in the United States *only* for infants and children with negative skin tests who (1) are at high risk for intimate and prolonged exposure to persistently untreated or ineffectively treated people with infectious pulmonary TB and cannot be removed from the source of exposure or placed on long-term preventive therapy, or (2) are continuously exposed to persons with TB who have bacilli resistant to both isoniazid and rifampin. Ideally, the development of a vaccine against TB with remarkably improved efficacy (similar to the efficacy currently achieved by other vaccines combating infectious diseases, 90% or greater) is needed to eliminate this disease.

In 1989, the CDC and the Advisory Council for the Elimination of Tuberculosis issued a Strategic Plan for the Elimination of Tuberculosis in the United States (CDC, 1999). This council established a national goal of TB elimination, defined as a case rate of less than 1/1,000,000 population by the year 2010. As a part of this effort, the CDC published guidelines for eliminating TB and for preventing TB transmission in health care facilities through a three-pronged strategy: (1) more effective use of existing prevention and control methods, especially among high-risk populations; (2) development and evaluation of new technologies for TB diagnosis, treatment, and prevention; and (3) rapid transfer of newly developed technologies into clinical and public health practice.

Between 1989 and 1999 this plan provided the framework for the nation's TB control efforts, including a successful mobilization against the resurgence of TB associated with deterioration of the public health infrastructure, increasing cases among foreign-born persons, HIV infection, and transmission of MDR TB in institutional settings. To continue toward accomplishing this goal, specific populations must be protected against the potential of exposure to people with latent infection. Public education and outreach need to develop positive working relationships with the target communities, involving them in successful program planning and implementation.

Successful interventions also require TB control programs to focus resources on high-risk people, including contacts of people recently diagnosed as having TB disease. Also targeted for prevention efforts are members of racial and ethnic minorities and people born in countries where TB prevalence is high. People with TB infection who have conditions placing them at increased risk for active TB (eg, HIV infection) also require special attention. The American Nurses Association has developed two position statements, on Tuberculosis and Public Health Nursing (1997b) (Display 9–3) and Tuberculosis and HIV (1997a) (Display 9–4), which support the management of TB and TB/HIV.

A well-functioning TB control program is the best way to prevent TB and to prevent the emergence of drug resistance. As stated by Horsburgh (1998), such programs:

- Follow standard public health practices
- Achieve prompt sputum conversion in people with active disease
- Investigate contacts of people with active TB to identify and treat other cases and people recently exposed
- Achieve a high completion-of-therapy rate within 1 year after diagnosis
- Have adequate funding and a dedicated TB control infrastructure
- Avoid block grants or "privatization" of public health disease control functions (despite supporters of such change)

Three model TB programs were established in 1994 as national educational resources to provide TB services, expert consultation, and training for health care providers. In 1999, these centers worked with the CDC to develop the *Strategic Plan for Tuberculosis Education and Training* to guide efforts in this area during the next 5 years (CDC, 1999).

One of the most effective ways to achieve a high completion-of-therapy rate is through the WHO-supported treatment strategy for detection and cure known as the directly observed treatment short-course (DOTS), frequently referred to as DOT (WHO, 1998). It has become clear that the DOTS strategy can achieve high cure rates in any country that is determined to succeed. The treatment success rate of cases in DOTS global areas was 78%, compared with 45% in non-DOTS areas. The use of DOTS expanded almost 10-fold between 1993 and 1997, cure rates nearly doubled, and drug resistance was lower in places where DOTS had been used (WHO, 1998). The American Thoracic Society and the CDC propose treating all patients with directly observed therapy because it reduces the sources of infection in the community.

This labor-intensive approach has proved effective for the most difficult of TB cases in the United States. The more difficult clients are those who do not realize their personal or social responsibility for health and those who do not have the resources to focus on health when there are

---

DISPLAY 9–3

The American Nurses Association Position Statement on Tuberculosis and Public Health Nursing—Summary

The ANA advocates a nursing care management model as a proven strategy for TB control and supports:

- The use of a nursing case management model in TB control to coordinate patient services; facilitate the safe delivery of TB medications to patients in the community; ensure completion of therapy; and limit the transmission of the disease by identifying newly infected and diseased persons through contact investigation procedures.
- The utilization of unlicensed assistive personnel working under the supervision and direction of nurses.
- The enhancement of nursing's role in surveillance, assessment, treatment, and evaluation activities with priority given to nursing management of patients on treatment, education, and infection control practices that will promote prevention in the community and among health care workers.
- Collaboration with other agencies to encourage research on the development and implementation of different treatment models of care to provide a full range of available treatment options for clients with TB.
- Nursing research initiatives on the effectiveness of different treatment modalities in improving treatment outcomes, including the use of directly observed therapy and other adherence strategies.
- Innovative demonstration projects to document effective strategies for surveillance and screening methods with at-risk populations.
- Accelerated research to document the most effective control measures that will prevent the transmission of TB to nurses providing treatment.

(From American Nurses Association [1997b]. Position statement—Tuberculosis and public health nursing. Retrieved November 10, 2003, from *http://www.nursingworld.org/readroom/position/blood/bltbhl.htm.*)

---

other stressors or diversions in their life. For these reasons, clients such as alcohol and drug abusers, transient homeless people, and low-income people may be the source cases for new cases of TB. DOTS therapy ensures that clients take a daily or intermittent dose of prescribed medication, locating them wherever they may be—in neighborhood bars, sleeping on the sidewalk, in a homeless shelter, or in a drug rehabilitation center. Most health departments and TB control programs have a percentage of their clients receiving DOTS therapy, with licensed staff or community health workers used to administer the TB drug regimen. These ancillary staff members are often former program participants, trained and supervised by professional health workers (American Nurses Association, 1997b). A program like

DISPLAY 9-4

The American Nurses Association Position Statement on Tuberculosis and Human Immunodeficiency Virus—Summary

The ANA supports:

- Closely monitoring the HIV-infected person for TB symptoms and screening for TB. All individuals found to be HIV positive should be offered an appropriate TB test.
- Policy development to support linkages of TB with HIV, primary care and substance abuse screening, education, and treatment in accessible and convenient programs.
- The provision of joint testing services for TB and HIV which employ confidentiality and pre- and post-test counseling services.
- The ethical responsibility of nurses to engage in ongoing assessment related to communicable diseases, such as TB.
- Education for all nurses about the epidemiology, transmission, prevention strategies, and symptoms of TB.
- Employers' provision of protective equipment and appropriate safe work environment for nurses to prevent the transmission of communicable diseases such as TB.
- Federal and state resources being applied to alleviate conditions of social deprivation.
- Funding for increased research to expand knowledge of HIV/TB transmission and treatment.
- Increased participation of nurses in research for safe workplace protective equipment and technology to reduce the risk of communicable disease transmission.
- Continued nursing input into federal, state and local agencies and legislative processes about TB and HIV disease concerns.
- The HIV positive nurse to:
  —Know their TB status by following CDC-recommended guidelines for ongoing assessment,
  —Self-limit their nursing practice based on a case-by-case assessment of their TB status,
  —Self-restrict their contact with patients, coworkers, and visitors if symptoms associated with airborne communicable disease are present,
  —Adhere to prescribed medication regimen for TB to decrease the opportunity for transmission of the disease.

(From American Nurses Association [1997a]. Position statement—Tuberculosis and HIV. Retrieved November 10, 2003, from *http://www.nursingworld.org/readroom/position/blood/blhvtb.htm*)

DOTS needs sustained political commitment, with the governments of nations recognizing the long-term benefits of providing the resources and staff necessary to ensure its proper implementation.

Commitment and flexibility on the part of health care providers and services can substantially enhance medication compliance. Significant improvement in compliance has been demonstrated with programs designed to provide DOTS therapy for all clients, using community-based health workers who meet with clients in residences, at job sites, and at other local venues. In addition, new variations on the standard treatment regimens are being researched. Approaches include allowing individuals to take larger medication doses on a twice-weekly schedule, or providing an observed medication program for a limited period, followed by a course of self-administered medication with periodic reevaluation by health care providers.

Multidrug-Resistant Tuberculosis

Epidemiologists and communicable disease specialists cite a number of factors that contribute to the development and spread of TB strains resistant to one or more of the standard arsenal of TB drugs. Strains now exist that are resistant to as many as 9 of 11 standard anti-TB drugs (see The Global Community). Chief among the factors contributing to drug resistance seems to be the political and social response to declining rates of TB over past decades, which has resulted in cuts in funding for surveillance, treatment, and research and a premature sense that TB was beaten. On an individual case basis, noncompliance with therapy for the full recommended period is the most common means by which resistant organisms are acquired. Public health services with limited resources have been unable to provide the intensive follow-up necessary to ensure that people who essentially feel well continue taking their medication (which may produce unpleasant although usually mild and manageable side effects) for the length of time considered necessary to achieve cure. Public health officials face a challenge to network effectively to provide continuous case management for highly mobile and often disenfranchised infected minority populations.

The reality of drug-resistant strains of TB significantly complicates the crisis of AIDS. When candidates for drug therapy are identified, it is essential to provide program support to ensure that the maximum number of individuals comply with their medication regimen for the full duration of therapy. Isoniazid therapy for individuals who are infected with TB but have no evidence of active disease has been shown to be highly effective in preventing progression to infectiousness and clinical symptoms. Isoniazid is also a key component of the treatment for active disease. Adverse effects of isoniazid therapy are often overestimated, leading to inappropriate withdrawal of therapy.

Clients with HIV and Tuberculosis

HIV infection is associated with an increased possibility of developing primary TB after exposure to a source. Someone with latent TB infection and HIV infection is up to 800 times more likely to develop active TB disease during his or her lifetime than someone without HIV (CDC, 2001b). The connection between TB and HIV/AIDS is dramatic, with one third of the incidence of TB in the last 5 years attributed to HIV. The weakened immune system makes an HIV-positive person infected with the tubercle bacillus 30 times more likely to become ill with TB. For example, 60% to 80% of people with AIDS in India, Myanmar, Nepal, and Thailand develop TB (WHO, 1998).

People with HIV infection should be given high priority for preventive therapy, regardless of their age. For HIV-infected people, preventive therapy consists of isoniazid daily for up to 1 year (the usual regimen for preventive therapy is 6 months). These clients must be monitored closely for effectiveness of the preventive therapy and for tolerance to isoniazid. This drug has the capacity to develop adverse reactions or negative side effects. Isoniazid can cause hepatitis or damage the liver. Close monitoring and regular follow-up are necessary to detect early symptoms, such as nausea, vomiting, abdominal pain, fatigue, and dark urine. Any combination of these symptoms would be sufficient to initiate liver function tests.

As mentioned earlier, HIV-positive clients may not have the ability to react to a skin test for TB because of a weakened immune system. Therefore, other methods to determine TB status are employed. If it is determined that TB disease is present, HIV-infected clients should begin a regimen of drugs according to the schedule used by their physicians or clinics. The clients should be closely monitored for response to treatment; if they do not seem to be responding, they should be reevaluated.

Community health nurses have a responsibility to help HIV-infected clients experience a successful TB treatment regimen. Caregiving includes observing for adherence to treatment, administering medications (either directly through DOTS or through DOTS supervision by ancillary staff), observing for signs and symptoms of adverse reactions, monitoring for overall health and well-being, educating, and making referrals as needed.

Viral Warts

Condyloma acuminata, verruca vulgaris, papilloma venereum, and the common wart are all forms of a viral disease manifested by a variety of mucous membrane and skin lesions (Chin, 1999). All are transmitted by direct contact, but condyloma acuminata, or genital warts, caused by the human papillomavirus (HPV) are usually sexually transmitted.

Researchers have identified more than 70 types of papilloma viruses, and at least 20 of these types of the virus commonly infect the anogenital area. Several of the subtypes of HPV (HPV-16, -18, -31, and -45) are associated with cervical dysplasia and genital cancers, which can occur 5 to 30 years after the initial infection, accounting for 80% of cervical cancers (WHO, 1998). The CDC estimates that 20 million Americans carry the virus and that as many as 1 million new cases are diagnosed each year, accounting for approximately 5% of all STD clinic visits. Reduction of HPV infection remains an objective in the *Healthy People 2010* document (USDHHS, 2000).

Among college populations, HPV is epidemic, with outbreaks usually occurring after vacation and semester breaks. As many as half of all sexually active college women may be infected with HPV. Most cases occur in the 20- to 24-year-old population, and more often in women than in men. People who are sexually active by about 15 years of age have double the risk of HPV than those who become sexually active after age 20 years. Genital HPV infection can be transmitted to newborns during passage through the birth canal, causing a sometimes fatal respiratory papillomatosis if lesions develop in the lungs. Many people believe that pregnant women with HPV should have cesarean deliveries to prevent this possibility.

Many people infected with HPV are asymptomatic and transmit the infection unknowingly. Genital HPV infections are difficult to treat and commonly reoccur. No culture method is available to diagnose HPV, so the diagnosis is commonly made based on the clinical presentation. HPV's telltale cauliflower-like, fleshy growths occur in and around the genitalia, around the anus, and within the anal canal, and are usually painless. The warts usually regress within months to years. Treatment (which is not recommended for pregnant women) involves treating visualized warts with a topical solution of podophyllin or by cryotherapy. If the genital lesions are widespread, 5-fluorouracil has been found to be helpful. The goal of therapy is removal of the warts and relief of symptoms (Chin, 1999).

Sexually Transmitted Disease Prevention and Control

Human history has been shaped by disease, and all historical events have played a part in creating the preconditions for epidemics. Of all the communicable diseases, perhaps none are as closely interrelated with human activities and attitudes than STDs. Many have occurred in epidemic proportions, and most have existed for centuries. They are mentioned in the Bible and in ancient Chinese and Greek medical texts. Gonorrhea was the most common STD until the 15th century, when a new and deadly disease called syphilis invaded Europe. It spread to the New World and remained a major problem through the 1940s. Since then, other STDs, such as chlamydia, genital herpes, HPV, and hepatitis, have taken over the headlines. Most likely, new STDs will continue to emerge in the new millennium.

STDs are those infections that are spread by transfer of organisms from person to person during sexual contact. STDs are of critical importance in any discussion of communicable disease control because, as a single class of disease, they include more than 25 infectious organisms and account for 87% of all cases among the top 10 most frequently reported diseases to the CDC and state health departments. Each year, 15 million Americans are infected with an STD, including 3 million teenagers (USDHHS, 2000). The total direct and indirect costs to society of the principal STDs are estimated to be $17 billion annually.

The U.S. STD rate exceeds that of all other industrialized countries in the world, indicating that national attempts to control STDs have not gone fast enough or far enough. The STDs discussed in this section included gonorrhea, syphilis, chlamydia, genital herpes, and HPV (genital warts). AIDS, of course, is an STD, as is hepatitis B, although transmission of these diseases can also occur through intravenous drug use, transfusion of blood products before 1986, or needlestick injury.

Of further concern to community health nurses is the fact that women and children suffer an inordinate amount of the STD burden. Aside from the risk of AIDS and subsequent death, the most serious complications of STDs are PID, sterility, ectopic pregnancy, blindness, cancer associated with HPV, fetal and infant death, birth defects, and mental retardation. The medically underserved, particularly the poor and marginalized and ethnic and racial minorities, shoulder a disproportionate share of this problem, experiencing higher rates of disability and death than the population as a whole. Some notable disproportionately affected groups are sex workers, adolescents and adults in detention, and migrant workers (USDHHS, 2000). Sexual violence and sexual coercion are significant problems for America's young women. Studies show that not all sexually experienced young females enter a sexual relationship as a willing partner (Hanson, 2002).

Healthy People 2010 identifies the availability and quality of public services for STD as key factors in reducing the spread of STDs and preventing complications (USDHHS, 2000). Effective health promotion approaches in the community must include STD prevention in the curricula of middle and secondary schools. The initiation of sexual activity early in life results in an increased number of sexual partners over a person's lifetime, establishing the behavioral link to higher levels of STDs.

In addition to the need for more innovative and effective sexual health promotion approaches in school settings, a number of recommendations have been made for improvements in current delivery systems (USDHHS, 2000). The number of clinics offering STD screening, diagnosis, treatment, counseling, and referral services should increase substantially to improve access to comprehensive services. Certainly, consideration, planning, and the allocation of resources should be directed to the quality-of-life issues that operate in young adults' lives and contribute to inappropriately early initiation of unprotected sexual activity. Case management by providers often does not conform to the CDC recommendations in regard to the nature of medical treatment, follow-up strategies to confirm cure, or notification and treatment of sexual partners. This failure may, in turn, contribute to inadequate treatment, continued transmission, higher risk of complications, and the increase in drug-resistant strains of gonorrhea and other diseases. *Healthy People 2010* (USDHHS, 2000) strongly recommends expansion of contact-tracing efforts. Treatment of individuals who present with symptoms is only half the job.

The partner or partners of infected people must be notified and also require treatment for effective and lasting "cure" of the case.

Adolescent and young adult women and men who have multiple sex partners over a specified period (eg, several months) are at increased risk for gonorrhea, syphilis, and chlamydia. Increased numbers of sex partners over a lifetime are associated with a greater cumulative risk of acquiring viral infections such as hepatitis B, genital herpes, HPV, and HIV. Nineteen of the national health objectives for the year 2010 (USDHHS, 2000) focus on activities, services, and behaviors to reduce STDs.

Changes in behavior require diverse and multidisciplinary interventions over an extended period. Such interventions must integrate the efforts of parents, families, schools, religious organizations, health departments, community agencies, and the media. The goals of educational programs should be to provide adolescents with the knowledge and skills they need to refrain from sexual intercourse, and to increase the use of condoms as well as other contraceptive measures among those unwilling to postpone onset of sexual activity (USDHHS, 2000). Studies have suggested that parent-child conversations about sexual matters are associated with delays in initiation of sexual activity and with increased use of contraceptives by adolescents who engage in sexual intercourse. Additional recommendations to promote sexual health in adolescent populations include (1) innovations for early detection and treatment of STDs among teenagers, (2) specialized training for clinicians providing health services for adolescents, (3) school education combined with accessible clinical services, and (4) behavioral interventions to prevent exposure to and acquisition of STDs.

Infectious Diseases of Bioterrorism

Information about anthrax and smallpox is presented here because of the threat these diseases present to the community as weapons of terrorism. Community health nurses are in the community and in the homes of people who express their fears perhaps to no other professional. This places the nurse in a position of responsibility to allay fears, provide correct information, and help people in the decision-making process regarding immunization. Other disease organisms may be used by terrorists in the future, but for now anthrax and smallpox are diseases that have been used as terrorist weapons or are clearly possible weapons.

Anthrax

Shortly after the terrorist attacks of September 11, 2001, the U. S. population was further terrorized by anthrax. Several people who handled or delivered mail inhaled and touched anthrax spores concealed in envelopes. Many acquired anthrax, and deaths were reported. The pervasiveness of the fear this act created was felt nationwide. No person or country has yet claimed responsibility or has been accused with spreading the causative organism.

In nature, anthrax is primarily a disease of herbivores, with humans and carnivores as incidental hosts. There are infrequent and sporadic human infections in most industrialized countries. It is an occupational hazard among workers who process hides, hair, bone and bone products, and wool in some countries. In fact, it has been called woolsorter disease and ragpicker disease.

In humans, anthrax is an acute bacterial disease that affects mainly the skin or respiratory tract. The two main forms—cutaneous anthrax and inhalation anthrax—account for most human anthrax cases. The case-fatality rate for cutaneous anthrax is 5% to 20%. Skin becomes itchy where exposed, a lesion becomes papular and then vesicular, and in 2 to 6 days a depressed black eschar surrounded by extensive edema develops. The infection may spread to the lymph system and cause septicemia. With inhalation anthrax, the initial symptoms are mild and nonspecific but progress to respiratory distress. Fever and shock follow in 3 to 5 days, and death is the expected outcome (Chin, 1999). Human anthrax is endemic in agricultural regions of the world where anthrax in animals is common, including countries in South and Central America, southern and eastern Europe, Asia, and Africa.

The causative organism, *Bacillus anthracis* is a gram-positive, encapsulated, spore-forming agent with livestock and wildlife as the main reservoirs. The incubation period is short (hours to 1 week), and most cases occur within 48 hours after exposure. Transmission from person to person is very rare, but articles and soil contaminated with spores may remain infective for decades. The longevity of the spores compounds fears, clean-up involvement, and control when anthrax is used as a bioterrorist weapon.

An anthrax vaccine exists, and all lots are owned by the Department of Defense. Troublesome side effects (fatigue, muscle or joint pains, and mental impairment) are experienced by 5% to 35% of recipients, and six doses are required over an 18-month period in addition to yearly booster doses. The vaccine was approved in 1970 for the treatment of cutaneous anthrax and has been administered primarily to members of the armed forces. However it is not licensed to be used with aerosol exposure, the form of anthrax that would be faced in a terrorist attack (Nass, 2002). Until a new vaccine is developed, what we have is not well tolerated and has never been proved to be safe.

Smallpox

Smallpox is a disease from our history books. In fact, the last case of smallpox was reported in 1978, and in 1980 the WHO declared the disease eliminated worldwide. However, as recently as 1966, the disease was widespread in 31 countries. Some 10 to 15 million people were contracting smallpox annually, 2 million people died each year, and millions more were permanently disfigured or blinded (Sibley, 2002). By the late 1970s, just over 1 decade later, the global eradication campaign had pushed smallpox to the brink of extinction. The last known naturally occurring case of smallpox was in Somalia in 1977. Officially, the smallpox virus presently ex-

ists at only two places: the CDC in Atlanta and the State Research Centre of Virology and Biotechnology, Koltsovo, Novosibirsk Region, Russian Federation (Chin, 1999; Sibley, 2002).

Routine vaccination against smallpox ended in 1972 in the United States, and the smallpox vaccine has not been available for general distribution since May 1983. Few health care practitioners today have seen cases of smallpox or have administered the vaccine. Currently, community health nurses are becoming involved in the primary prevention of smallpox and are learning the intricate techniques of smallpox vaccination and treatment of vaccine side effects as the nation prepares to immunize large portions of the population. Smallpox vaccinations have been resumed for the first time in 3 decades (Spake, 2002). Initially, key military units were inoculated, beginning in 2001, followed by "first responders" such as emergency health care providers and health department personnel. The general public is not targeted for immunization at this time, but if people insist, they can receive the vaccination.

The plan for smallpox preparedness will most likely rely on ring vaccination—containing an outbreak by rapidly isolating and vaccinating people who have had close, face-to-face contact with the victim. Nonetheless, it is not clear whether any groups other than the United States and Russia possess the virus; furthermore, the rate of transmission of variola is complex and is contingent on many social and biological factors. "Therefore, it's difficult both to determine how real the threat is and to calculate a meaningful risk-benefit ratio in regard to compulsory mass vaccination," (Veenema, 2002, p. 35). However, one bright spot with smallpox prevention is that people who come in contact with a victim can receive protection if they are vaccinated within as long as 7 days after exposure. This is unlike other VPDs and provides a window of time to reach exposed people.

There are risks to the smallpox vaccination. It is not a benign vaccine, and some experts allege that the morbidity associated with the vaccine has been understated (Veenema, 2002). One to 2 deaths per 1 million recipients of the vaccine can be expected, in addition to hundreds of cases of generalized vaccinia, eczema vaccinatum, and postvaccinal encephalitis (Henderson, 1999). Less severe but more common side effects include the formation of satellite lesions, regional lymphadenopathy, fever, headache, nausea, muscle aches, fatigue, and chills. In addition, the vaccine is contraindicated in the immunosuppressed, those with eczema, pregnant women, and infants younger than 1 year of age (see Voices from the Community) (Bicknell, 2002).

The variola virus causes smallpox and is transmitted from person to person. Initial infection begins with a febrile prodromal period that occurs 1 to 4 days before rash onset. Fever is 101°F or higher, and victims experience at least one of the following: prostration, headache, backache, chills, vomiting, and severe abdominal pain. This is followed by the classic smallpox lesions. They are deep-seated, firm/hard, round, well-circumscribed vesicles or pustules. On any one part of the body, all of the lesions are in the same stage of development. Practitioners must prepare to recognize and differentiate smallpox from other diseases. The smallpox lesion can be confused with other conditions, such as varicella, disseminated herpes zoster, impetigo, drug eruptions, contact dermatitis, scabies, or disseminated HSV. Accurate diagnosis depends on the practitioner's skill to clearly recognize the classic smallpox lesion, identify that the lesions are in the same stage of development, and get an accurate history of prodromal symptoms.

Community health nurses must raise their awareness and bioterrorism preparedness. As advocates for clients, families, groups, aggregates, and populations, community health nurses can do the following (Veenema, 2002):

- Prepare yourself with information about those infectious agents that pose the most significant threats of being used in cases of bioterrorism (eg, anthrax, botulism, plague, smallpox).
- Develop and implement educational programs designed to inform the public of the potential consequences of the smallpox vaccine and of mass vaccination.
- Keep current on evolving vaccination policies, evaluating their potential impact on community health.
- Get involved in the national smallpox vaccination policy debate.
- Participate in designing bioterrorism disaster response plans within your professional organizations and at the state and local level; anticipate the challenges associated with the plans.
- Help your facility prepare for the responsibilities it would assume in the event of a change in national policy mandating universal smallpox vaccination.
- Be ready to participate in the design and implementation of large-scale immunization programs.
- Consider voluntary vaccination if you work in a high-risk (first-response) clinical practice such as an outpatient clinic or health department.

GLOBAL ISSUES IN COMMUNICABLE DISEASE CONTROL

Our small planet has many common concerns, and communicable disease control is one of them. A new issue is the increasing number of emerging communicable diseases occurring globally. New diseases bring new challenges in case-finding, surveillance, and control. To conquer these challenges, community health nurses are assisted by the steps of the nursing process.

Globally Emerging Communicable Diseases

Emerging diseases are those that either have newly appeared or are rapidly increasing in incidence or geographic range. Most emerging diseases are not caused by genuinely new pathogens; rather, ecologic, environmental, and demographic factors place nonimmune people in increased contact with a pathogen or its host or promote the pathogen's dissemination. As mentioned earlier in this chapter, the current volume, speed, and reach of international travel make the emergence of communicable diseases truly a global problem. The following is a brief profile of some old and new emerging infectious diseases.

Ebola hemorrhagic fever, a severe acute viral illness with sudden onset of fever, malaise, myalgia, headache, pharyngitis, vomiting, diarrhea, and a maculopapular rash, has been confined to countries in tropical Africa. It was first identified in 1976, in the Democratic Republic of the Congo, where the case-fatality rate has ranged from 50% to 90%. Person-to-person transmission occurs by direct contact with infected blood, secretions, organs, or semen. People of all ages are susceptible.

Legionnaires' disease (legionellosis) is a form of a potentially fatal pneumonia caused by bacteria that contaminate water in air-conditioning systems. It was first identified in Philadelphia, Pennsylvania, in 1976. It is characterized by anorexia, malaise, myalgia, and headache; within 1 day, there is a rapidly rising fever associated with chills, a nonproductive cough, abdominal pain, and diarrhea. The case-fatality rate has been as high as 39% in hospitalized clients and higher among those with compromised immune systems. The disease occurs more frequently with increasing age, with most patients being older than 50 years of age. Primary prevention is easily accomplished by draining cooling towers when not in use, mechanically cleaning them, and using appropriate biocides.

Hantavirus is an old virus with a newly recognized clinical illness. It first occurred in Manchuria before World War II. In 1951, it was recognized in Korea. It is considered a major, expanding public health problem in China, with 40,000 to 100,000 cases reported annually. It was first seen in the United States in 1993 in the area where Utah, Colorado, New Mexico, and Arizona meet, and 28 people died. Since 1993, 217 cases have been identified in 30 states (Leslie et al., 1999). The severe form of the disease is endemic in Eurasia and Scandinavia. Deer mice appear to be the reservoir, and transmission is by way of aerosolization of infected droppings. It is an acute viral disease characterized by abrupt onset of fever, low back pain, varying degrees of hemorrhagic manifestations, renal involvement, hypotension, and shock. Prevention is focused on rodent control and surveillance for the infection in wild rodents.

E. coli O157:H7 was first identified as a pathogen in 1982 in the United States. An outbreak of severe bloody diarrhea was traced to contaminated hamburgers. In January 1993, a large outbreak caused by this *E. coli* strain affected 700 people who ate undercooked hamburgers in the Puget Sound area of Washington. Other outbreaks have been caused by unpasteurized milk and by apple cider made from apples contaminated by cow manure. Children younger than 5 years of age are most susceptible and are at greatest risk of developing hemolytic-uremic syndrome as a complication. *E. coli* infections are recognized to be an important problem in Europe, South Africa, Japan, South America, and Australia. Humans may serve as a reservoir for person-to-person transmission. Primary prevention can be accomplished by following federal guidelines, which require commercially prepared meat to be cooked to an internal temperature of 140°F, and by safe and hygienic cooking practices at home. Raw meats should be kept separated from fruits, vegetables, and cooked meats during preparation; separate cutting boards should be used, and they should be cleaned with hot soap and water and rinsed using a bleach solution.

Lyme disease was first discovered in the United States in the 1970s when an unusually high incidence of children developed rheumatoid arthritis in Lyme, Connecticut. It is an infection caused by a spirochete called *Borrelia burgdorferi* and is characterized by a distinctive skin lesion, systemic symptoms, and neurologic, rheumatologic, and cardiac involvement occurring over a period of months to years. A bite from a tick that can be carried by dogs and cats passes the disease to humans. All 48 mainland states have reported cases, but it is most prevalent in the Northeast. It is the most common tick-borne disorder in the United States. The number of cases soared each year until 1996, then decreased in the dryer year, 1997. Lyme disease is treatable and is not communicable from person to person. Two different vaccines for Lyme disease are being tested. Primary prevention includes educating the public about the mode of transmission, being aware of high-risk areas. In wooded, bushy, and tall-grass areas, people should walk in the middle of trails, wear a long-sleeved shirt, wear a hat, spray tick repellent on clothes and shoes, and wear long pants tucked into high socks. They should check for ticks after an outing. Light-colored clothing makes it easier to see ticks. If a tick is found, it should be removed with forceps (tweezers), trying not to crush the tick's body so that no fluid escapes.

Dengue fever, an acute febrile viral condition, is not transmitted from person to person but through the bite of an infected mosquito. Symptoms include sudden onset beginning with fever, severe headache, myalgia, arthralgia, retro-orbital pain, anorexia, gastrointestinal disturbances, and rash. Children have milder symptoms than adults do. The prevalence has increased as a result of increasing worldwide urbanization during the last few decades. Dengue and dengue hemorrhagic fever (DHF) have been reported from more than 100 countries in the world, but not in Europe. These two diseases often occur in massive epidemics, most recently in 1996, when severe epidemics were reported in 27 countries in the Americas and in southeast Asia. Outbreaks of DHF have recently been reported in Brazil, Cuba, India, and Sri Lanka. The WHO strategy of control is based on prevention of transmission by controlling the vector mosquito. Such measures start with eliminating areas for breeding, such as small pools of stagnant water, even in empty flowerpots or abandoned tires.

Other: In 1996, England reported the first cases of new-variant Creutzfeldt-Jakob disease (a fatal neurologic conditon), probably related to eating contaminated beef. In 1997, cases of *S. aureus* with reduced susceptibility to vancomycin occurred in Japan and the United States, raising concern for a return to the preantibiotic era. In that same year, an outbreak of avian influenza in Hong Kong raised concerns about a potential pandemic; it was the first time an avian influenza virus had infected humans (Binder, Levitt, & Hughes, 1999). In 2002 SARS (severe acute respiratory syndrome), an atypical pneumonia with a 10% fatality rate, was recorded in mainland China, Taiwan, and Hong Kong. By June of 2003 there were over 8400 cases with 772 deaths in 13 countries/regions of the world (WHO, 2004). Time will tell how this emerging disease will affect our small planet.

Global Response to Communicable Diseases

Communicable diseases are not limited to specific regions of the world; they are the problem of all people. In 1996, WHO focused on completing the unfinished business of eradication and elimination of specific diseases; tackling "old" diseases, such as TB and malaria, and the problem of antimicrobial resistance; and combating newly emerging diseases. WHO continues to focus on safeguarding the gains already achieved, which depends largely on sharing health and medical knowledge, expertise, and experience on a global scale. During the 50 years of its existence, WHO has taken a three-pronged approach to communicable diseases: case-finding, surveillance and control, and elimination and eradication.

Case-finding is an important beginning to communicable disease control and eventual eradication. Because of the changing nature of the world's demographics, use of space, and accelerating technology, old or once unknown diseases are reemerging and others are being seen on our planet for the first time. Differentiation of one set of symptoms from those of another disease is an essential first step in case-finding. Once a disease has been identified, all cases need to be found through the traditional case-finding methods of contact investigation. Each contact leads to another piece of information and becomes part of communicable disease detective work.

Once a disease has been identified and is known to exist in a particular community, the steps of surveillance and control begin. Questions need to be answered and acted upon: How is the disease spread? What needs to be done to reduce the impact of the source? Do infected persons need to be isolated? Does the disease respond to antimicrobial therapy? Weekly, monthly, and yearly documentation of disease frequency and distribution is gathered and shared globally. Control measures then begin. Some developing countries may need more technical and financial support to achieve control. The cost of locating cases, eliminating vector pools, and providing immunizations and/or treatment can be a burden beyond the capabilities of poorer nations.

Effective surveillance and control can lead to the goal of elimination and eradication of a disease in many cases. We have been successful with smallpox and are closing in on polio. Within the next 25 years, other diseases, such as measles and TB, have the potential for elimination. Global collaboration, using the strengths from all nations, is needed to achieve these goals.

USING THE NURSING PROCESS FOR COMMUNICABLE DISEASE CONTROL

As mentioned in Chapters 8 and 14, the nursing process has steps similar to the research process and the epidemiologic process when approaching any health problem or condition. Therefore, using the nursing process to achieve communicable disease control should be an important and natural process for community health nurses.

Assessment

The first step of the nursing process, assessment, aligns itself with case-identification and case-finding in communicable disease control. The community health nurse must use all assessment skills and tools available during contact with clients, so as not to overlook the possibility of a communicable disease. Assessment must be comprehensive, including physical, social, and environmental data. There is no place for assumption. At times, a nurse can become "lulled" into usual patterns of inquiry, and the oversight may prove fatal to the client.

"Baby Josephine is irritable," says the mother. "Well, babies sometimes are," the nurse says. "How are you feeding her? Show me how you hold her. Does she sleep well? Rock her in the rocking chair before bedtime. Burp her more frequently. I'll check back with you in 2 weeks." Does the nurse record the baby's temperature, look at her for a rash, compare present weight with last weight, ask about bowel habits or vomiting, inquire about illnesses in the family, check on breast-feeding technique or watch while the mother demonstrates formula preparation, inspect the family's water source, ask about other foods the baby is eating, and so forth?

Broader inquiry into a simple statement from the mother may lead to the discovery of a life-threatening, undiagnosed communicable disease.

Assessment in the broader community health nursing role may involve assessing a community's need for communicable disease surveillance and new or improved control programs. Nurses are in the community and can get a feel for the increasing or decreasing numbers of communicable diseases. They are often the first ones to know of a new outbreak of communicable disease in the community.

Planning

The planning step in the nursing process involves different activities depending on whether the planning is for an individual, family, group, or entire community. At the individual level, the nurse may assist a client with a communicable disease to get immunizations or definitive treatment. Or the nurse may assist the client in ways to care for the communicable disease symptoms that provide relief and comfort and reduce the chance of transmitting the disease to others in the family or community. When working with families, the nurse's actions are similar to those with individual clients and include assisting the family in getting available and needed immunizations, controlling the disease if present, limiting it to the people already exposed, and getting appropriate treatment and meaningful rehabilitation, if needed. With groups and communities, planning includes the collaboration of many different groups. Whether an immunization clinic is proposed or a flu shot day for senior citizens planned, there are location, staff, and supplies to prepare, which may include writing grants, establishing contracts, and training and orienting staff, before implementation can begin.

Implementation

During the implementation step, the nurse actually takes the action that was identified as being needed during assessment and planned for with clients and others in collaboration. In the implementation step, the nurse may actually deliver the service or may supervise other staff or volunteers. On a large scale, such as with the implementation of a new immunization clinic, the fact that this will be an ongoing service has to be considered in an agency's budget, staff turnover issues, relief when there is absence, and continuous formative (during the implementation process) evaluation of the services so that minor changes to improve day-to-day operation can be introduced. Implementing plans with small groups or families may involve arranging for transportation to get several people immunized or seen by a primary care provider. It may include gathering stool samples to bring to a laboratory from a family recovering from a *Salmonella* infection. Education on primary prevention of future infections is an essential part of the implementation phase. Agency record keeping, state-required contact investigation, and reporting cases of communicable diseases are essential in this phase. Figure 9–7 provides an example of a reporting form.

Evaluation

Evaluation is an essential step in the nursing process with all conditions, diseases, and services community health nurses provide. When dealing with communicable diseases, it is most important to determine whether actions have achieved the established goals. Have the outcomes been accomplished? Are people in the families immunized? Are all family members free of the disease? Do families know how to prevent this and other diseases from occurring or recurring? Does the community have the communicable disease services it needs? Is the community free of the disease? What needs to be done now to keep the community safe from communicable diseases? Are there funding issues, programs nearing completion that need support, or growth of services needed that can be addressed before there is a critical need? These are examples of questions that need answers during evaluation. The community health nurse who is concerned with the health and safety of the community follows the steps of the nursing process to achieve healthy community goals.

ETHICAL ISSUES IN COMMUNICABLE DISEASE CONTROL

When working to effectively control communicable diseases in communities and population groups, it is important to ensure that the activities undertaken are ethically sound and justified. It is important in communicable disease control to consider the ethical aspects of access to disease prevention and treatment services; enforced compliance with preventive measures; screening programs; privacy, confidentiality, and discrimination; and issues involving the health worker employee who is infected with or is a carrier of an infectious agent.

On a larger scale, there are ethical dimensions to the cause and elimination of barriers to accessibility of drugs in developing countries. Making the inexpensive measles vaccine available to children in African villages, providing effective malaria treatment for people in South Asia, applying DOTS research for use in rural Brazil, and making ART and HAART drugs available to people with HIV/AIDS in developing countries (USAID, 2001a) are examples of these issues (see Chap. 21 for further discussion).

Health Care Access in Communicable Disease Control

Access to health care means that people needing services find them available, acceptable, and appropriate, unrestricted by barriers to use. Such access has been advocated as an essential public health value, yet the global economy has been experiencing rising inequality, with income gaps between countries and within countries continuing to widen (WHO, 1998).

It would be misleading to say that rates of communicable diseases in population subgroups provide reliable indicators of health care access. The issue is significantly compounded when health care providers miss opportunities to vaccinate and when parents who have the means fail to seek out services to ensure that immunizations are up to date. It is clear that, in the absence of access to health care services, opportunities for people to receive the information and services necessary to prevent transmission and progression of infectious diseases are sharply curtailed.

Enforced Compliance

Legally, the responsibilities of public health officials in communicable disease control include the police power to enforce compliance with treatment or restrict the activity of infectious people to protect the welfare of others (Chin, 1999). In disease prevention, completely voluntary measures to encourage healthier lifestyles tend to be ineffective.

Regulations that enforce compliance with disease prevention strategies are a justifiable restriction if the measures proposed are demonstrably effective and grounded in ethical principles. Coercion must be of the mildest sort compatible with achieving the goals of the regulation. Information must be provided to allow consumers to see the consequences of deleterious habits and the value choices that must be made. Inducements should be favored over disincentives. Remediable conditions that make choice less than free should be ameliorated—through education, by restraints on misleading advertisement, reducing peer or group pressure, treating emotional problems, and so on. Regulation should be confined to actions with direct public impact and should be limited severely in matters that are personal and private.

Screening for Communicable Diseases

As discussed earlier in this chapter, screening programs for communicable diseases are conducted to detect existing or potential public health problems. One can argue that they are morally and ethically justified if they protect and serve infected people as well as those who might be at risk for exposure. However, other issues arise that must be addressed. Are screening resources allocated to areas where they will have the most benefit in preventing disease and premature death? Should people receiving the screening service take on the burden of diagnosis if treatment is unavailable because of cost or access? Are screening costs justified in light of scarce health care dollars?

Until recently, there was no ethical justification for an HIV screening program. Since the development of combinations of drugs that postpone the development of AIDS in the HIV-positive population and improve the quality of life, determining one's HIV status has become of immense value. Prevention of transmission of the virus continues to require voluntary changes in behavior of infected people, and there has always been an ethical justification for HIV screening for that reason. If screening were to become mandatory, identification of the estimated 1 million or more HIV-infected people in the United States would exceed the capacity of the health care system to provide services. However, people who

CONFIDENTIAL MORBIDITY REPORT

NOTE: For STD, Hepatitis, or TB, complete appropriate section below. Special reporting requirements and reportable diseases on back.

DISEASE BEING REPORTED: _____

Patient's Last Name

Social Security Number ___ – ___ – ___

Ethnicity (✔ one)
- ☐ Hispanic/Latino
- ☐ Non-Hispanic/Non-Latino

First Name/Middle Name (or initial)

Birth Date
Month   Day   Year   Age

Race (✔ one)
- ☐ African-American/Black
- ☐ Asian/Pacific Islander (✔ one)
  - ☐ Asian-Indian   ☐ Japanese
  - ☐ Cambodian   ☐ Korean
  - ☐ Chinese   ☐ Laotian
  - ☐ Filipino   ☐ Samoan
  - ☐ Guamanian   ☐ Vietnamese
  - ☐ Hawaiian   ☐ Other _____

Address: Number, Street   Apt./Unit Number

City/Town   State   Zip Code

- ☐ Native American/Alaskan Native
- ☐ White _____
- ☐ Other _____

Area Code   Home Telephone   ___ – ___ – ___

Gender ☐ M ☐ F

Pregnant? ☐ Y ☐ N ☐ Unk

Estimated Delivery Date
Month Day Year

Area Code   Work Telephone   ___ – ___ – ___

Patient's Occupation/Setting
- ☐ Food service   ☐ Day care   ☐ Correctional Facility
- ☐ Health care   ☐ School   ☐ Other _____

DATE OF ONSET
Month Day Year

Reporting Health Care Provider

Reporting Health Care Facility

REPORT TO

DATE DIAGNOSED
Month Day Year

Address

City   State   Zip Code

DATE OF DEATH
Month Day Year

Telephone Number ( )   Fax ( )

Submitted By   Date Submitted (Month/Day/Year)

(Obtain additional forms from your local health department.)

SEXUALLY TRANSMITTED DISEASES (STD)

Syphilis
- ☐ Primary (lesion present)
- ☐ Secondary
- ☐ Early latent < 1 year
- ☐ Latent (unknown duration)
- ☐ Neurosyphilis
- ☐ Late latent > 1 year
- ☐ Late (tertiary)
- ☐ Congenital

Syphilis Test Results
- ☐ RPR   Titer: _____
- ☐ VDRL   Titer: _____
- ☐ FTA/MHA: ☐ Pos. ☐ Neg.
- ☐ CSF-VDRL ☐ Pos. ☐ Neg.
- ☐ Other _____

Gonorrhea
- ☐ Urethral/Cervical
- ☐ PID
- ☐ Other _____

Chlamydia
- ☐ Urethral/Cervical
- ☐ PID
- ☐ Other _____

- ☐ PID (Unknown Etiology)
- ☐ Chancroid
- ☐ Non-Gonococcal Urethritis

STD TREATMENT INFORMATION
- ☐ Treated (Drugs, Dosage, Route)   Date Treatment Initiated
  Month Day Year
  _____
  _____

- ☐ Untreated
- ☐ Will treat
- ☐ Unable to contact patient
- ☐ Refused treatment
- ☐ Referred to _____

VIRAL HEPATITIS

		Pos.	Neg.	Pend	Not Done
☐ Hep A	anti-HAV IgM	☐	☐	☐	☐
☐ Hep B	HBsAg	☐	☐	☐	☐
☐ Acute	Anti-HBc	☐	☐	☐	☐
☐ Chronic	anti-HBc IgM	☐	☐	☐	☐
	anti-HBs	☐	☐	☐	☐
☐ Hep C	anti-HCV	☐	☐	☐	☐
☐ Acute	PRC-HCV	☐	☐	☐	☐
☐ Chronic					
☐ Hep D (Delta)	anti-Delta	☐	☐	☐	☐
☐ Other _____		☐	☐	☐	☐

Suspected Exposure Type
- ☐ Blood Transfusion
- ☐ Other needle exposure
- ☐ Sexual contact
- ☐ Household contact
- ☐ Child care
- ☐ Other _____

TUBERCULOSIS (TB)

Status
- ☐ Active Disease
  - ☐ Confirmed
  - ☐ Suspected
- ☐ Infected, No Disease
  - ☐ Convertor
  - ☐ Reactor

Site(s)
- ☐ Pulmonary
- ☐ Extra-Pulmonary
- ☐ Both

Mantoux TB Skin Test
Month Day Year
Date Performed _____
☐ Pending
Results _____ mm ☐ Not Done

Chest X-Ray
Month Day Year
Date Performed _____
☐ Normal ☐ Pending ☐ Not Done
☐ Cavitary ☐ Abnormal/Noncavitary

Bacteriology
Month Day Year
Date Specimen Collected _____
Source _____
Smear: ☐ Pos. ☐ Neg. ☐ Pending ☐ Not Done
Culture: ☐ Pos. ☐ Neg. ☐ Pending ☐ Not Done
Other test(s) _____

TB TREATMENT INFORMATION
- ☐ Current Treatment
  - ☐ INH   ☐ RIF   ☐ PZA
  - ☐ EMB   ☐ Other _____

Date Treatment Initiated
Month Day Year _____

- ☐ Untreated
  - ☐ Will treat
  - ☐ Unable to contact patient
  - ☐ Refused treatment
  - ☐ Referred to _____

REMARKS

F I G U R E   9 – 7.   Communicable disease reporting form—contact investigation.

engage in high-risk behaviors owe it to themselves to be screened for HIV so that the life-prolonging drugs can be started and precautions can be taken to not infect others.

Confidentiality, Privacy, and Discrimination

To carry out communicable disease interventions, client needs for confidentiality and privacy must be ensured. Screening and other interventions must take place in a physical setting that does not allow overt differentiation between those clients with positive and negative results. As agency and national data systems and programs continue to evolve, it is essential to make confidentiality and data protection measures clear priorities. Studies have reported that 60 to 100 people have access to an average hospital record. Anonymity is frankly incompatible with early intervention. Two areas of current practice that may benefit from closer ethical scrutiny in regard to protection of privacy are contact investigation in STD programs and school-based screening for pediculosis.

Human society has had a long-standing aversion to infectious diseases that is still true today. Ostracism in the past of people with leprosy and other contagious conditions has shifted to discrimination against people with TB, AIDS, head lice, and other current forms of communicable disease. Such discrimination should be of as much concern in the public health field as in the legal sector.

Passage of the Americans with Disabilities Act in 1990 has resulted in legal protections for people diagnosed with communicable diseases who suffer discrimination regardless of status of infectiousness. The objectives of *Healthy People 2010* encourage community-based agencies to expand communicable disease services, among other strategies, by offering expanded contact follow-up services (USDHHS, 2000). Such expansion should occur only in conjunction with careful planning for the ethical standards that will spell out the protections due each individual client while still effectively advancing the cause of disease prevention.

The issue of confidentiality has always been a major concern in contact investigation. It continues to be a source of debate in balancing the values of protection of the individual with protection of the public's health. Not only must the identity of the individual be protected to the maximum extent possible, but any breaches of confidentiality must be clearly justified on the basis of a threat to the safety of an individual. That is, failure to provide essential information must jeopardize the well-being of the exposed person or contact. It is important to ensure that accessible services exist for the exposed partner or contact in the event that, as a result of screening intervention, they are burdened with the emotional, physical, and financial consequences of diagnosis.

Infected Health Care Workers

Health workers have historically been at high risk when caring for clients with communicable diseases, be it plague, typhus, or TB. However, advances in treatment strategies for these clients have consistently resulted in a safer working environment for their caregivers and for those exposed to body fluids and various contaminated fomites. Trends in increasing community-based rather than inpatient care for communicable diseases have further contributed to equalizing the risk faced by health workers and the general population.

Yet the pendulum swings. HIV infection, MDR TB, and nosocomial infections, particularly MRSA, now threaten caregivers in significant ways, and the ethical implications of these issues are considerable and evolving. Legislation is proliferating to require health care workers who are known to be HIV positive to report to their local and state health authorities. MRSA is a growing problem in many facilities; health care workers are undergoing screening for colonization by the organisms, patients with MRSA are being refused admittance, and the work activities of colonized workers are being curtailed. Strategies for health care workers' protection and disease prevention must be mandated and enforced to a greater extent (see Clinical Corner).

SUMMARY

Communicable diseases pose a major threat to the public's health and have done so since the beginning of humankind. Such diseases are transmitted globally as the result of mobile populations, increased urbanization, and international travel. These diseases are transmitted through direct contact from one person to another or indirectly through contaminated objects (air, water, food) or a vector (animal or insect). Communicable diseases affect large groups of people and have worldwide significance.

Ideally, prevention of communicable diseases is accomplished through the primary prevention methods of mass media, one-on-one education, and immunization. Knowledge of the VPDs, the schedule of vaccinations, a community's immunization status, herd immunity, barriers to immunization coverage, planning and implementing immunization programs, adult immunizations, and the immunization needs of international travelers, immigrants, and refugees have been discussed. Secondary prevention activities of screening and contact investigation and case-finding are the steps to be taken when primary prevention activities have failed. Tertiary prevention is needed to ensure additional people are not infected. This is accomplished through isolation and quarantine, universal precaution practices among health care workers, and the safe handling and control of infectious wastes.

Becoming familiar with major communicable diseases affecting our nation is essential baseline information for community health nurses. TB, resurging since the 1980s, may be the biggest public health problem in the new millennium. Nurses need to be aware of the populations at risk, how the disease is prevented, appropriate interventions during diagnosis, and treatment. Issues compounding the control of TB are twofold: there are increasing infections with MDR strains, and the number of people with TB and HIV/AIDS is increasing, making diagnosis and treatment more complicated.

CLINICAL CORNER

SALMONELLA: A CULTURAL CONFLICT

You are a nurse working for the Brownsville Department of Health. One of your responsibilities is epidemiologic follow-up on reports of communicable disease. Today, you will be performing your second visit on the following clients:

- Tai: a 17-year-old boy
- Nguyen: a 15-year-old girl

Tai and Nguyen are cousins. Both clients became infected with *Salmonella* from undercooked pork, after a church picnic. Both are from Vietnamese families who immigrated to the United States 7 years ago.

During your initial visit, you spoke with the parents of Tai and Nguyen and educated them about the following:

1. Medication administration
2. Strict handwashing
3. Proper bowel habits
4. Food preparation and handling
5. Treatment of gastrointestinal sequelae
6. Collection of stool specimens
7. Modes of transmission
8. Assessment indicating exacerbation of signs and symptoms

The information you presented related to *Salmonella* was taken from recommendations from the Board of Health. In your education of the parents, you were careful to impress on them the potential deleterious consequences of non-compliance with these standards. You warned them that other family members would be placed at risk if there was deviation from the recommended practices.

Upon your return visit today, you are presented with the following scenarios:

Tai

Tai's family has followed your directions meticulously. His father tells you that the family has declined an invitation to an upcoming church social "because they're the ones who made my boy sick . . . they don't cook things right and I'm not taking my family there any more," he states. The parents also advise you that they have stopped giving Tai herbal teas and are instead providing him with rehydration drinks as recommended by his physician.

Additionally, Tai's parents have prohibited their children from visiting their cousins "because they don't take good care of themselves." Tai's mother tells you, "Their kids don't even wash their hands after using the toilet and you said that would make us all sick."

Nguyen

Your visit with Nguyen and her parents reveals the following information. Nguyen has refused to provide a stool specimen. Her parents speak little English and rely on Nguyen for interpretation. "They think you were mad at them last time," Nguyen informs you. "They got upset and scared." Nguyen goes on to tell you that "We're not drinking that stuff you told us about . . . my mom says that the tea has worked for our people for generations, so it's good enough for me." Nguyen adds that her parents have used spooning techniques to provide her with relief from gastrointestinal problems.

Questions

1. Is there a "good" and a "bad" client in this scenario?
2. Did you achieve desired nursing outcomes based on your intervention with Tai's family? Why or why not?
3. What might you have done differently to ensure the provision of culturally appropriate education with these families?
4. How might mutual goals have been developed?
5. What issues does this scenario elicit regarding:
   Fears and anxiety in this role
   Lack of immediate resources (eg, supervisor)
   Social justice
   Building partnerships within your communities
   Globalization of public health
6. In your role as the community health nurse, what activities might you be involved with in the prevention as well as reduction of the spread of communicable diseases within the aggregate of Vietnamese immigrants in your community?

A second major disease, HIV/AIDS, was first identified in the 1980s. In just over 20 years, 36 million people worldwide have become infected. With the success of antiviral drugs, this disease is becoming almost a chronic disease for clients in industrialized nations, and they can experience 10 to 15 years of life after diagnosis. Africa is being deeply affected by the massive numbers of women and children who are HIV positive, without access to the life-prolonging drugs available to people in developed nations.

STDs threaten the health and lives of millions of citizens. At risk are the sexually active, particularly adolescents and young adults, as well as minorities, women of child-bearing age, and children. Control of STDs can be accomplished through effective screening, treatment, contact investigation, and aggressive public education. Several common STDs were discussed, including gonorrhea, syphilis, chlamydia, genital herpes, and anogenital viral warts.

Five hepatitis viruses were discussed in this chapter. Hepatitis is more common than HIV and can lead to life-threatening events, such as cirrhosis and liver cancer. Yet these diseases do not get the attention they need. Most of the public is unaware of the types of hepatitis, prevention, transmission, and treatment. Vaccines for two of the forms are now available, and hepatitis B vaccine is required in the routine childhood vaccine schedule.

Influenza and pneumonia are "old" diseases that are causing increased morbidity and mortality in the United States. These diseases cause the most morbidity and mortality in the frailest citizens, the very young and the very old, although there are vaccines to prevent them. A national objective for 2010 is to increase the immunized population, achieving a herd immunity to prevent such preventable diseases.

Smallpox, an eradicated disease, and anthrax have been identified as potential diseases of bioterrorism. The community health nurse has several areas of responsibility in regard to bioterrorism. First, the nurse needs to know the signs and symptoms of potential infectious diseases used as weapons. Also, the nurse has a responsibility to the community to allay fears about bioterrorism and to provide information about prevention. Finally, community health nurses and other nurses are becoming technically skilled in providing smallpox vaccine as the nation prepares for possible bioterrorism at home or during war.

Several emerging or new diseases are occurring globally. Such diseases as Ebola, hantavirus, *E. coli,* Legionnaires' disease, Lyme disease, dengue fever, Creutzfeldt-Jakob disease, antibiotic resistant *S. aureus*, SARS, and avian influenza sound very new; however, they are occurring in increasingly alarming numbers. It may not be unusual for community health nurses to come across these diseases in their practice.

Internationally, WHO has been working for 50 years to make the world a healthier place to live. By providing all nations with the technical support, resources, and education they need, WHO is aggressively tackling communicable diseases. Case-finding, surveillance, control, elimination, and eradication are the steps toward meeting the WHO goals for communicable diseases.

Community health nurses use the nursing process in their important role with regard to all populations at risk for communicable diseases. Nurses concerned with communicable disease control must recognize who is at risk, where the potential reservoirs and sources of infectious disease agents are located, what environmental factors promote their spread, and what are the characteristics of vulnerability of community members and groups—particularly those subject to intervention. Community health nurses must work collaboratively with other public health professionals to establish immunization and education programs, to improve community infection control policies, and to develop a broad range of services to populations at risk.

Ethical issues in communicable disease and infection control include access to health care, enforced compliance, the justifiability of screening, preservation of confidentiality and privacy, avoidance of discrimination against infected people, and problems posed by infected health workers.

ACTIVITIES TO PROMOTE CRITICAL THINKING

1. Interview a professional in your local or state health department who works in communicable disease control. Determine (a) how he or she conducts communicable disease surveillance, (b) what diseases must be reported in your state, and (c) which communicable diseases are posing the greatest threat to the health of your state's citizens.

2. Compare a recent issue of *Mortality and Morbidity Weekly Report* with the same issue published a year earlier in terms of cases of specific notifiable diseases in the United States. Which diseases appear to be increasing? Decreasing? Select one disease and read at least one recent publication on this subject to determine the reasons for its rise or decline.

3. Determine through your local health department what percentage of preschool children are immunized in your city or county. Is this a safe level of herd immunity? Propose some recommendations for preserving or raising this level.

4. Select one high-risk population discussed in this chapter and list the factors that make this group vulnerable to communicable disease. Use at least one other published source to enhance your understanding. Propose one nursing intervention (such as a specific screening or educational program) and outline how it might be accomplished.

5. Interview a professional who works in STD services or with the HIV-infected population. Determine what methods he or she uses for contact investigation. How does this health care worker preserve privacy and confidentiality? What measures have proved most effective in reaching contacts? What is your evaluation of the success?

6. Bioterrorism is a new area of concern and study for nursing students. Discuss your feelings about the nation's attempts to prepare its population for the possibility of a terrorist attack using a biologic agent. Explore preparations against bioterrorism being put into place by your local health department. Discuss the plan with your peers and share thoughts in the group.

7. Access the CDC through the Internet (*http://www.cdc.gov*) and browse the site to learn about its various services. Are there special travelers' warnings in certain countries at this time? What are some of the CDC's current concerns regarding communicable diseases? Select a communicable disease and identify the number of cases presently reported. Return to the same Web site 1 month later. Has the incidence of the disease increased or decreased? (see Clinical Corner.)

REFERENCES

Aleman-Padilla, L. (2002, June 27). Whooping cough cases rise. *The Fresno Bee*, pp. B1, B2.

American Nurses Association. (1997a). *Position statement: Tuberculosis and HIV*. Retrieved November 10, 2003, from *http://www.nursingworld.org/readroom/position/blood/blhvtb.htm*.

American Nurses Association. (1997b). *Position statement: Tuberculosis and public health nursing*. Retrieved November 10, 2003, from *http://www.nursingworld.org/readroom/position/blood/bltbhl.htm*.

Beech, B.M., Myers, L., & Beech, D.J. (2002). Hepatitis B and C infections among homeless adolescents. *Family Community Health, 25*(2), 28–36.

Bicknell, W. (2002). The case for voluntary smallpox vaccine. *New England Journal of Medicine, 346*(17), 1275–1280.

Binder, S., Levitt, A.M., & Hughes, J.M. (1999). Preventing emerging infectious diseases as we enter the 21st century: CDC's strategy. *Public Health Reports, 114*(2), 130–134.

Borgdorff, M.W., Floyd, K., & Broekmans, J.F. (2002). Interventions to reduce tuberculosis mortality and transmission in low- and middle-income countries. *Bulletin of the World Health Organization, 80*, 217–227.

Brooks, J. (1999). *The minority AIDS crisis: Closing the gap* (pp. 1–3). Washington, DC: U.S. Department of Health & Human Services, Office of Minority Health.

Centers for Disease Control and Prevention. (1995). *Self-study modules on tuberculosis: Transmission and pathogenesis of tuberculosis*. Atlanta, GA: Public Health Practice Program Office Division of Media and Training Services.

Centers for Disease Control and Prevention. (1999). Strategic plan for the elimination of tuberculosis in the United States. *Morbidity and Mortality Weekly Report, 48* (RR-09), 1–13.

Centers for Disease Control and Prevention. (2000a). *STD surveillance 2000: National profile chlamydia*. National STD Surveillance Report. Retrieved November 10, 2003 *http://www.cdc.gov/std/stats/chlamydia2000/*.

Centers for Disease Control and Prevention. (2000b). *STD surveillance 2000: National profile syphilis*. National STD Surveillance Report. Retrieved November 10, 2003 from *http://www.cdc.gov/std/stats/Syphilis2000/*.

Centers for Disease Control and Prevention. (2001a). *HIV/AIDS update*. Atlanta, GA: Author.

Centers for Disease Control and Prevention. (2001b). *TB and HIV coinfection*. Atlanta, GA: Author.

Centers for Disease Control and Prevention. (2002a). Notice to readers: Expansions of eligibility for influenza vaccine through the Vaccines for Children Program. *Morbidity and Mortality Weekly Report, 51*(38), 864, 875.

Centers for Disease Control and Prevention. (2002b). Prevention and control of influenza: Recommendations of the advisory committee on immunization practices. *Morbidity and Mortality Weekly Report, 51*(RR-3), 1–32.

Centers for Disease Control and Prevention. (2002c). Sexually transmitted diseases treatment guidelines, 2002. *Morbidity and Mortality Weekly Report, 51*(RR-6).

Centers for Disease Control and Prevention. (2002d). Surveillance 2000: Special focus profiles STDs in women and infants. Available: *http://www.cdc.gov/std/stats/2000sfwomen&inf.htm*. Accessed on September 30, 2002.

Centers for Disease Control and Prevention. (2003). *Recommended childhood immunization schedule—United States, January–June 2004*. Atlanta, GA: Author.

Charuvastra, A., Stein, J., Schwartzapfel, B., Spaulding, A., Horowitz, E., Macalino, G., et al. (2001). Hepatitis B vaccination practices in state and federal prisons. *Public Health Reports, 116*(3), 203–209.

Chettle, C.C. (2002). West Nile virus: Spread of the mosquitoborne illness. *Nurseweek, 15*(22), 24–26.

Chin, J.E. (Ed.). (1999). *Control of communicable diseases manual* (17th ed.). Washington, DC: American Public Health Association.

Cowie, R.L., Field, S.K., & Enarson, D.A. (2002). Tuberculosis in immigrants to Canada: A global problem which requires a global solution. *Canadian Journal of Public Health, 93*(2), 85–86.

Desvarieux, M., Hyppolite, P., Johnson, W.D., & Pape, J.W. (2001). A novel approach to directly observed therapy for tuberculosis in an HIV-endemic area. *American Journal of Public Health, 91*(1), 138–141.

Donnelly, J., & Montgomery, D. (1999, March 18). Drug-resistant TB could be "principal epidemic of the next decade." *The Fresno Bee*, pp. A7, A8.

Gannon, J.C. (2000). The global infectious disease threat and its implication for the United States. NIE99-17D. Retrieved on November 21, 2003, from *www.odci.gov/cia/reports/nie/report/nie99-17d.html*.

Hagan, H., Thiede, H., McGough, J.P., & Alexander, E.R. (2002). Hepatitis B vaccination among research participants, Seattle, Washington. *American Journal of Public Health, 92*(11), 1756.

Hanson, R.F. (2002). Adolescent dating violence: Prevalence and psychological outcomes. *Child Abuse & Neglect, 25*, 449–453.

Hench, C., & Simpkins, S. (2002, June 17). Hepatitis C. *Nurseweek*, 1921.

Henderson, D.A. (1999). Risk of a deliberate release of smallpox virus: Its impact on virus destruction. Johns Hopkins University Center for Civilian Biodefense Studies. Available: *http://www.hopkins-biodefense.org/pages/agents/risk.html*. Accessed on March 15, 2004.

Horsburgh, C.R. (1998). Editorial: What it takes to control tuberculosis. *American Journal of Public Health, 88*(7), 1015–1016.

Institute of Medicine. (2000). *Calling the shots: Immunization finance policies and practices*. Washington, DC: National Academy of Sciences.

Ku, L., St. Louis, M., Farshy, C., Arai, S., Turner, C.F., Lindberg, L.D., et al. (2002). Risk behaviors, medical care, and chlamydial infection among young men in the United States. *American Journal of Public Health, 92*(7), 1140–1143.

Lauer, G., & Walker, B.D. (2001) Hepatitis C virus infection. *New England Journal of Medicine, 345*(1), 41–53.

Leslie, M., et al. Update: Hanta virus pulmonary syndrome—United States, 1999. (1999). *Morbidity and Mortality Weekly Report, 48*(24), 521–525.

Mackenzie, E.R. (1998). *Healing the social body: A holistic approach to public health policy*. New York: Garland Publishing.

Malhotra, A., & Krilov, L. (2000). Influenza and respiratory syncytial virus. *Pediatric Clinics of North America, 47*(2), 353–372.

McCullough, D. (2001). *John Adams*. New York: Touchstone.

Mee, C. (2001). Hepatitis C: Speaking out about the silent epidemic. *Nursing, 31*(3), 36–42.

Mertz, K.J., Ransom, R.L., St. Louis, M.E., Groseclose, S.K.,

Hadgu, A., Levine, W.C., et al. (2001). Prevalence of genital chlamydial infection in young women entering a national job training program, 1990–1997. *American Journal of Public Health, 91*(8), 1287–1290.

Mullins, M.E. (2002, September 24). West Nile's spread exposes health agency's weakness. *USA Today,* 11A.

Nass, M. (2002). The anthrax vaccine program: An analysis of the CDC's recommendations for vaccine use. *American Journal of Public Health, 95*(5), 715–721.

National Institutes of Health Office of AIDS Research (OAR). (2001). *National Institutes of Health: HIV/AIDS research programs.* Bethesda, MD: Author.

Neumann, D.A. (2002). Letter from the NPI director. *NPI Bulletin, 2*(2), 2.

NIAID. (2002). *Tuberculosis.* Bethesda, MD: National Institute of Allergy and Infectious Diseases, National Institutes of Health.

Olsen, J.M. (2002, June 22). Europe decreed free of polio. *The Fresno Bee,* p. A12.

Polio at all-time low, but WHO warns not to let efforts slide. (2002, June/July). *The Nation's Health,* p. 10.

Prisco, M.K. (2002). Update your understanding of influenza. *The Nurse Practitioner, 27*(6), 32–39.

Quander, L. (2001, Spring). HIV/AIDS prevention programs: What's working with our youth? In *HIV Impact, A Closing the Gap Newsletter of the Office of Minority Health* (pp. 1–2, 4). Washington, DC: U. S. Department of Health & Human Services, Office of Minority Health.

Reichman, L.B., & Andriote, J. (2002). *Guidelines for the diagnosis of latent tuberculosis infection for the 21st century.* Newark, NJ: New Jersey Medical School National Tuberculosis Center.

Saraiya, M., Cookson, S.T., Tribble, P., Silk, B., Cass, R., Poonja, S., et al. (2002). Tuberculosis screening among foreign-born persons applying for permanent US residence. *American Journal of Public Health, 92*(5), 826–829.

Sarbah, S.A., & Younossi, Z. (2000). Hepatitis C: An update on the silent epidemic. *Journal of Clinical Gastroenterology, 30*(2), 1–26.

Satcher, D. (1996). CDC's first 50 years: Lessons learned and relearned. *American Journal of Public Health, 86*(12), 1705–1708.

Schultz, T.R. (2002). Straight talk about community-acquired pneumonia. *Nursing 32*(1), 46–49.

Scutchfield, F.D., & Keck, C.W. (2001). *Principles of public health practice.* Albany, NY: Delmar.

Sibley, C.L. (2002). Smallpox vaccination revisited. *American Journal of Nursing, 102*(9), 26–32.

Spake, A. (2002). Small defense. *U.S. News & World Report, 133* (13), 64.

United States Agency for International Development. (2001a). *Effective prevention strategies in low HIV prevalence settings.* Washington, DC: Family Health International.

United States Agency for International Development. (2001b). *USAID child survival and disease programs fund progress report.* Washington, DC: Author.

United States Department of Health and Human Services. (1991). *Healthy people 2000: National health promotion and disease prevention objectives* S/N 017-001-00474-0). Washington, DC: U. S. Government Printing Office.

United States Department of Health and Human Services. (2000). *Healthy people 2010* (Conference ed., Vols. 1 & 2). Washington, DC: U. S. Government Printing Office.

Veenema, T.G. (2002). The smallpox vaccine debate. *American Journal of Nursing, 102*(9), 33–38.

WHO. (2004). Communicable disease surveillance and response (CSR), SARS. Available at: *http://www.who.int/entity/CSR/SARS/country/2003_06_04/en.* Accessed on March 15, 2004.

WHO reviews, approves acceptable HIV/AIDS drugs. (2002, May). *The Nation's Health,* p. 14.

World Health Organization. (1998). *Report of the director-general.* Geneva: Author.

Wright, C. (2002, November). CDC issues guidelines for state, local smallpox response. *The Nation's Health,* pp. 1, 25.

SELECTED READINGS

Berkman, A. (2001). Confronting global AIDS: Prevention and treatment. *American Journal of Public Health, 91*(9), 1348–1349.

Brown-Peterside, P., Rivera, E., Lucy, D., Slaughter, I., Ren, L., Chiasson, M.A., et al. (2001). Retaining hard-to-reach women in HIV prevention and vaccine trials: Project ACHIEVE. *American Journal of Public Health, 91*(9), 1377–1379.

Centers for Disease Control and Prevention. (2002d). Trends in sexual risk behaviors among high school students—United States, 1991–2002. *Morbidity and Mortality Weekly Report, 51*(38), 856–859.

Dicker, L.W., Mosure, D.J., Levine, W.C., et al. (2000). Impact of switching laboratory tests on reported trends in *Chlamydia trachomatis* infections. *American Journal of Epidemiology, 51,* 430–435.

Essex, M., Mboup, S., Kanki, L., Marlink, R.G., & Tiou, S.D. (2002). *AIDS in Africa* (2nd ed.). Norwell, MA: Kluwer Plenum.

Karon, J.M., Fleming, P.L., Steketee, R.W., & DeCock, K.M. (2001). HIV in the United States at the turn of the century: An epidemic in transition. *American Journal of Public Health, 91*(7), 1060–1068.

Kolata, G. (1999). *Flu: The story of the great influenza pandemic of 1918 and the search for the virus that caused it.* New York: Farrar Straus & Giroux.

Lansky, A., Lehman, J.S., Gatwood, J., Hecht, F.M., & Fleming, P.L. (2002). Changes in HIV testing after implementation of name-based HIV case surveillance in New Mexico. *American Journal of Public Health, 92*(11), 1757.

Lee, K. (2000, Spring). The toll of HIV/AIDS on minority women. *HIV Impact, A Closing the Gap Newsletter of the Office of Minority Health* (pp. 1–2). Washington, DC: U. S. Department of Health and Human Services, Office of Minority Health.

Lifson, A.R., Halcon, L.L., Hannan, P., St. Louis, M.E., & Hayman, C.R. (2001). Screening for sexually transmitted infections among economically disadvantaged youth in a national job training program. *Journal of Adolescent Health, 28,* 190–196.

Meadows, M. (2001). *Understanding vaccine safety* [Reprint from FDA Consumer Magazine]. Publication No. (FDA) 01-9001. Rockville, MD: U. S. Food and Drug Administration.

Murrill, C.S., Weeks, H., Castrucci, B.C., Weinstock, H.S., Bell, B.P., Spruill, C., et al. (2002). Age-specific seroprevalence of HIV, hepatitis B virus, and hepatitis C virus infection among injection drug users admitted to drug treatment in six U.S. cities. *American Journal of Public Health, 92*(3), 385–387.

Nossal, G. (2002). Protecting our progeny: The future of vaccines. *Perspectives in Health, 7*(2), 8–13.

O'Leary, A. (2002). *Beyond condoms: Alternative approaches to HIV prevention.* Norwell, MA: Kluwer Plenum.

Peterson, J.L., & DiClemente, R.J. (2000). *Handbook of HIV prevention.* Norwell, MA: Kluwer Plenum.

St. Lawrence, J.S., Montano, D.E., Kasprzyk, D., Phillips, W.R., Armstrong, K., & Leichliter, J.S. (2002). STD screening, testing, case reporting, and clinical and partner notification practices: A national survey of U.S. physicians. *American Journal of Public Health, 92*(11), 1784–1788.

Susser, I., & Stein, Z. (2000). Culture, sexuality, and women's agency in the prevention of HIV/AIDS in southern Africa. *American Journal of Public Health, 90*(7), 1042–1048.

Swartz, A. (2002, September/October). Breaking the silence: The black church addresses HIV. *HIV Impact, A Closing the Gap Newsletter of the Office of Minority Health* (pp. 1–2). Washington, DC: U. S. Department of Health and Human Services, Office of Minority Health.

Thomas, J.C. & Weber, D.J. (2001). *Epidemiologic Methods for the Study of Infectious Diseases.* Oxford: Oxford University Press.

Turner, C.F., Rogers, S.M., Miller, H.G., Miller, W.C., Gribble, J.N., Chromy, J., et al. (2002) Untreated gonococcal and chlamydial infection in a probability sample of adults. *Journal of the American Medical Association. 287,* 726–733.

Urgvarski, P.J. (2001). The past 20 years of AIDS. *American Journal of Nursing, 101*(6), 26–29.

Weinstock, H., Dale, M., Linley, L., & Gwinn, M. (2002). Unrecognized HIV infections among patients attending sexually transmitted disease clinics. *American Journal of Public Health, 92*(2), 280–283.

Word, B.M. (2002). Barriers to adolescent vaccination: Adolescents, the orphans of immunization practices. *NPI Bulletin, 2*(2), 3,5.

Zabos, G.P., & Trinh, C. (2001). Bringing the mountain to Mohammed: A mobile dental team serves a community-based program for people with HIV/AIDS. *American Journal of Public Health, 91*(8), 1187–1189.

Internet Resources

American Public Health Association: *http://www.apha.org/*

Center for International Health Information: *http://www.cihi.com*

Centers for Disease Control and Prevention: *http://www.cdc.gov*

CDC National Prevention Information Network: *http://www.cdcnpin.org*

HCV Advocate: *http://www.hcvadvocate.org*

Hepatitis Foundation International: *http://www.hepfi.org*

Immunization Action Coalition immunization Web sites: *http://www.immunize.org/* *http://www.immunizationinfo.org/* *http://www.harlemtbcenter.org/*

National Immunization Program (NIP): *http://www.cdc.gov/nip*

National Institute of Allergy and Infectious Diseases: *http://www.niaid.nih.gov*

National Institutes of Health: *http://www.nih.gov*

WHO Network for Global Influenza Surveillance: *http://www.who.int/csr/disease/influenza/surveillance/en/*

10

Environmental Health and Safety

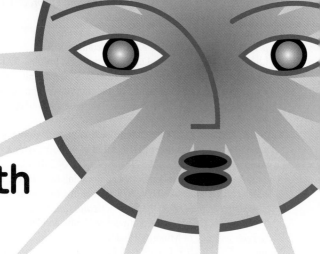

Learning Objectives

Upon mastery of this chapter, you should be able to:

- Discuss the importance of applying an ecologic perspective to any investigation of human-environment relationships.

- Explain the concepts of prevention and long-range environmental impact and their importance for environmental health.

- Discuss at least five global environmental concerns and describe hazards associated with each area.

- Relate the effect of the described hazards on people's health.

- Discuss appropriate interventions for addressing these health problems, including community health nursing's role.

- Describe how national health objectives for the year 2010 target environmental health.

- Describe strategies for nursing collaboration and participation in efforts to promote and protect environmental health.

In 2002, Dixon reported in *Family and Community Health* that children are being affected by air pollution in many ways, including "reduced lung function, increased morbidity, increased use of health care services, and infant mortality" (2002, p. 9). Brown, Gardner, Sargent, et al. (2001) studied the relation of housing policies to risk of lead exposure at addresses where lead-poisoned children lived. They found that the risk of identifying children with high blood levels for lead was 4 times higher at addresses with limited enforcement. In 2000, the World Health Organization reported that 16,000 people worldwide die from injuries every day. "For every person who dies of injuries, several thousand injured persons survive, but many of them are left with permanent disabling sequelae" (Krug, Sharma, & Lozano, 2000, p. 523).

Our environment—the conditions within which we live and work, including the quality of our air, water, food, and working conditions—strongly influences our health status. Consequently, the study of environmental health has tremendous meaning for community health nurses. Broadly defined, **environmental health** is concerned with assessing, controlling, and improving the impact people make on their environment and the impact of the environment on them. The field of environmental health is concerned with all those elements of the environment that influence people's health and well-being. The conditions of workplaces, homes, or communities, including the many forces—chemical, physical, and psychological—present in the environment that affect human health, are important considerations.

Different environments pose different health problems and benefits. Consider the effects of acid rain, soil erosion, and insect invasions on a rural community or the effects of industrial toxic wastes, auto emissions, and airport noise on urban residents. The health effects of a hot, dry climate are different from those of an arctic area, and the environmental conditions of an industrialized nation are dramatically different from those of a developing country.

This chapter describes conceptual and theoretic approaches to environmental health and examines historical perspectives, global environmental health issues, and the primary environmental areas of concern to community health nurses. The primary environmental areas include air pollution, water pollution, unhealthy and contaminated food, waste disposal, insect and rodent control, and safety in the home, worksite, and community.

CONCEPTS AND THEORIES CENTRAL TO ENVIRONMENTAL HEALTH

Assessing environmental health means more than looking for illness or disease-causing agents; it also means examining the quality of the environment. Do the conditions of both the manmade and the natural environment combine to provide a health-enhancing milieu? Are people's surroundings safe and life-sustaining? Are they clean and aesthetically enriching? Is the environment not only physically but also psychologically health-enhancing? To answer these questions and gain greater understanding, the nurse needs to consider the conceptual and theoretic approaches that are essential to assessing and controlling environmental health.

Preventive Approach

The study of environmental health has become increasingly complex as people's influence on the environment has increased. With the unprecedented advances in science and technology that have taken place in the past few decades, society's ability to affect the environment has expanded and the implications are not fully comprehended. New forms of energy, new synthetic chemical substances, and genetic engineering research bombard us with such rapidity that it is almost impossible to anticipate all the potential side effects on the environment and, in turn, on people's health. For each advance and "improvement," the toll to be paid is frequently unknown. In addition, new environmental threats emerge in light of real and potential terrorist attacks that include the use of chemicals, biological agents, radiation, and the destruction of the environment by force.

For these reasons, the concept of prevention is vital to environmental health. Scientists must use foresight as they design innovations; government agencies, business organizations, and citizens must play watchdog; and those concerned with human and environmental health must monitor new developments and intervene to prevent problems from occurring. Health practitioners need to determine causal links between people and their environment, with an eye to improving the health and well-being of both. Nurses, in particular, must be aware of environmental factors that have the potential to either promote or adversely affect the health of communities. All three levels of prevention (primary, secondary, and tertiary) must be employed, but most important is primary prevention. Prevention of a disease or *hazard* (a source of danger and risk particularly affecting human health) from occurring at all has the greatest benefit to the community.

Although small-scale preventive and health-promoting measures, such as safety education in the home or workplace, are important, it is the larger environmental problems that ultimately place many, if not all, members of a given community at risk. Community health nurses can develop an understanding of these environmental threats as well as the collaborative skills needed to work with other members of the public health team to prevent or alleviate them.

Ecologic Perspective

It is important to consider issues of environmental health from an **ecologic perspective**, keeping in mind the total relationship or pattern of relationships among people and their environment. Even when environmental health efforts focus on a specific health hazard or single environmental factor that poses a health threat, a broad view of human/environment relationships must be maintained. In most cases, a single causal factor cannot be isolated, because there may be many causal relationships. An outbreak of food poisoning, for example, may be attributed to the *Salmonella* organism. However, it is most likely also associated with improper food handling and restaurant standards, which, in turn, may be affected by inadequate inspections and monitoring (Cruz, Katz, & Suarez, 2001). The multiple relationships present in any environmental situation have been referred to as a *web* and the multiple causes of a problem as a *web of causation* (see Chapter 8).

An **ecosystem** is a community of living organisms and their interrelated physical and chemical environment; no one factor, whether organism or substance, can be viewed in isolation from the rest of its environment. Within an ecosystem, any manipulation of one element or organism may have hazardous effects on the rest of the system. Therefore, no one factor, whether organism or substance, can be viewed in isolation. For example, in produce processing, there are several points at which contamination can occur: at production and harvest (growing, picking, and bundling); during initial processing (washing, waxing, sorting, and boxing); during distribution (trucking); and during final processing (slicing, squeezing, shredding, and peeling). Several different pathogens are associated with a variety of foodborne diseases from produce and animals grown and raised in the United States, Mexico, and Central America (U. S. Department of Agriculture [USDA], 2000) (Table 10–1). Pathogens may have been introduced in the irrigation water, with the manure, or from lack of field sanitation during production and harvest; from contaminated wash water and handling at initial processing; from contaminated ice and dirty trucks during distribution; or in the final processing from dirty wash water, improper handling, or cross-contamination. Raw meat, poultry, seafood, and eggs are not sterile. Plastic-wrapped boneless chicken breasts and ground meat, for example, were once part of live chickens or cattle. By taking an ecologic approach to the study of environmental health, the community health nurse acknowledges that people can affect their environment and the environment can affect them. Preventive and health promotive measures may be applied to all aspects of the environment as well as to the people in it. Humans share this planet with millions of other living creatures and must consider the ecologic balance and anticipate the far-reaching consequences of their actions before introducing environmental change with contaminants or toxic agents. A **contaminant** is organic or inorganic matter that enters a medium, such as water or food, and renders it impure. A **toxic agent** is a poisonous substance in the environment that produces harmful effects on the health of humans, animals, or plants.

Using a model similar to the epidemiologic triad introduced in Chapter 8, a triangle of human disease ecology is created. This model stresses the links between habitat, population, and behavior (Fig. 10–1). *Habitat* includes aspects of the environment in which people live, including housing, workplaces, communication systems, flora, fauna, climate, topography, services, and economic and political structures of societies and local communities. *Population* factors include the characteristics of the population (age, gender, and genetic predisposition), which help to determine health status and disease susceptibility. *Behavioral* factors include health-related beliefs and behaviors, which are shaped by a range of social and economic factors. The triangular relationship among these factors suggests that there are no real boundaries between them and that the health of populations is a result of the interaction of all factors. It also indicates that action on one part of the system in isolation is unlikely to be effective without complementary action on other relevant factors.

Environmental justice is a movement that has sought to ensure that no particular part of the population is disproportionately burdened by the negative effects of pollution (American Public Health Association [APHA], 1999). Industrial plants, waste facilities, and other potential polluters are more likely to be situated in poorer communities, and pollutants from these facilities can make the people who live there ill. In one slum neighborhood in Bhopal, India, in 1984, one of the world's worst industrial cataclysms occurred. At least 3800 people died and 200,000 were injured (171,382 with temporary injuries and 18,922 permanent injuries) when methylisocyanate was uncontrollably released from a Union Carbide Plant (Yassi, Kjellstrom, de Kok, & Guidotti, 2001). It is very possible that, as poor countries industrialize and embrace Western development and consumerism, there will be more disasters. However, action can be taken in advance to prevent such incidents. Environmental legislation, preventive maintenance strategies, worker-training programs, environmental education programs, research on product safety, development of systematic hazard-evaluation models, emergency planning, and disaster preparedness are all examples of possible preventive activities.

In the United States, it is not unusual to identify communities that are exposed to higher levels of pollutants than others. Members of these communities are not well equipped to deal with pollution problems because of their limited involvement in the political process. In addition, they may not be aware of their exposure to pollutants and may be more vulnerable to health problems because of poor nutrition and inadequate health care.

Aesthetics is the appreciation of beauty that is culturally pleasing to the person observing the person, place, or thing. Even accounting for cultural differences, there are some things, such as a woodland path, a rocky beach, or a colorful sunset, that most people would find aesthetically pleasing. How does the aesthetics or beauty of our environment affect us? People themselves are the best sources for ideas regarding those things that they cherish as being beautiful. However, an environment that is free of waste material, clutter, and foul smells and that includes well-landscaped surroundings can contribute to the inhabitants' well-being.

The benefits of aesthetically pleasing surroundings are difficult to measure. Nevertheless, we know how good it

TABLE 10-1

Bacteria That Cause Foodborne Illness

Bacteria	Found	Transmission	Symptoms
Campylobacter jejuni	Intestinal tracts of animals and birds, raw milk, untreated water, and sewage sludge.	Contaminated water, raw milk, and raw or undercooked meat, poultry, or shellfish.	Fever, headache, and muscle pain followed by diarrhea (sometimes bloody), abdominal pain, and nausea that appear 2 to 5 days after eating; may last 7 to 10 days.
Clostridium botulinum	Widely distributed in nature, soil, water, on plants, and intestinal tracts of animals and fish. Grows only in little or no oxygen.	Bacteria produce a toxin that causes illness. Improperly canned foods, garlic in oil, vacuum-packaged and tightly-wrapped food.	Toxin affects the nervous system. Symptoms usually appear 18 to 36 hours, but can sometimes appear as few as 4 hours or as many as 8 days after eating; double vision, droopy eyelids, trouble speaking and swallowing, and difficulty breathing. Fatal in 3 to 10 days if not treated.
Clostridium perfringens	Soil, dust, sewage, and intestinal tracts of animals and humans. Grows only in little or no oxygen.	Called "the cafeteria germ" because many outbreaks result from food left for long periods in steam tables or at room temperature. Bacteria destroyed by cooking, but some toxin-producing spores may survive.	Diarrhea and gas pains may appear 8 to 24 hours after eating; usually last about 1 day, but less severe symptoms may persist for 1 to 2 weeks.
Escherichia coli O157:H7	Intestinal tracts of some mammals, raw milk, unchlorinated water; one of the several strains of *E. coli* that can cause human illness.	Contaminated water, raw milk, raw or rare ground beef, unpasteurized apple juice or cider, uncooked fruits and vegetables; person-to-person.	Diarrhea or bloody diarrhea, abdominal cramps, nausea, and malaise; can begin 2 to 5 days after food is eaten, lasting about 8 days. Some, especially the very young, have developed hemolytic-uremic syndrome (HUS) that causes acute kidney failure. A similar illness, thrombotic thrombocytopenic purpura (TTP), may occur in adults.
Listeria monocytogenes	Intestinal tracts of humans and animals, milk, soil, leaf vegetables; can grow slowly at refrigerator temperatures.	Ready-to-eat foods such as hot dogs, luncheon meats, cold cuts, fermented or dry sausage, and other deli-style meat and poultry, soft cheeses and unpasteurized milk.	Fever, chills, headache, backache, sometimes upset stomach, abdominal pain and diarrhea; may take up to 3 weeks to become ill; may later develop more serious illness in at-risk patients (pregnant women and newborns, older adults, and people with weakened immune systems).
Salmonella (over 2300 types)	Intestinal tracts and feces of animals; *Salmonella enteritidis* in eggs.	Raw or undercooked eggs, poultry and meat, raw milk and dairy products, seafood, and food handlers.	Stomach pain, diarrhea, nausea, chills, fever, and headache usually appear 8 to 72 hours after eating; may last 1 to 2 days.
Shigella (over 30 types)	Human intestinal tract; rarely found in other animals.	Person-to-person by fecal-oral route; fecal contamination of food and water. Most outbreaks result from food, especially salads, prepared and handled by workers with poor personal hygiene.	Disease referred to as "shigellosis" or bacillary dysentery. Diarrhea containing blood and mucus, fever, abdominal cramps, chills, and vomiting; 12 to 50 hours from ingestion of bacteria; can last a few days to 2 weeks.
Staphylococcus aureus	On humans (skin, infected cuts, pimples, noses, and throats).	Person-to-person through food from improper food handling. Multiply rapidly at room temperature to produce a toxin that can cause illness.	Severe nausea, abdominal cramps, vomiting, and diarrhea occur 1 to 6 hours after eating; recovery within 2 to 3 days—longer if severe dehydration occurs.

Food Safety and Inspection Service, United States Department of Agriculture; Center for Food Safety and Applied Nutrition, United States Food and Drug Administration.

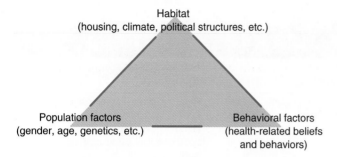

FIGURE 10–1. The triangle of human disease ecology. (Adapted from Curtis, S., & Taket, A. [1996]. *Health and societies: Changing perspectives.* London: Arnold.)

makes us feel when we experience it, that we would like to linger there longer, and that we would like to not let it disappear. If people were able to feel this way about their home, their neighborhood, and their community, the world would be a more harmonious and healthier place.

Long-Range Environmental Impact

When studying environmental health, it is important to consider the effect of positive or negative changes on the environment and on the people, animals, and plants living in it. This **environmental impact** must be viewed not only in terms of its consequences for people living now but also in terms of its long-range impact on the human species. One must consider the health of future generations as well as present ones. Considerations should include food and fuel limitations of the natural environment, attendance to conservation through balancing of present and future needs, and prevention of the consequences of environmental abuse. This last point broadens the focus even more. Certainly, one should determine how current practices and toxins are hurting humans, but it is also imperative to discover what threats they pose to the biosphere and thus to future generations— their long-range environmental impact. For example, carbon monoxide gas given off by factories and automobiles is toxic and can be lethal, causing dizziness, headaches, and lung diseases in humans who inhale it at certain concentrations. It has also been found to reduce the atmosphere's ozone layer, which protects us against ultraviolet irradiation. Therefore, it poses a serious ecologic threat for the future. A study by the Institute of Medicine (1999) calls for more research to help policy makers weigh the possible environmental risks of any new industrial or business facility against the potential job and tax benefits for local citizens.

EVOLUTION OF ENVIRONMENTAL HEALTH

Environmental influences on health have been present throughout human history. Interactions with the environment, and the conditions of that environment, have shaped

humans' mental, emotional, and physical health since the beginning of time. From ancient tribal practices of burial of excreta to modern-day sewage treatment, humans have been concerned with how the environment would provide for their needs and affect their well-being.

Global Perspective

In an effort to promote human health, people have taken steps to control, alter, and adapt to their environment. Demonstrations of this concern go back to Biblical times, when the Israelites observed strict rules governing food preparation, practiced sanitation, and quarantined people with infectious diseases (eg, leprosy).

As populations became more settled and urbanized, many different environmental health concerns developed. Community actions to deal with these developments have been recorded as far back as 2500 BC. Archaeologists have discovered remnants of sophisticated water and waste systems in ancient cities of northern India and in the Middle Kingdom of Egypt. Early Roman engineers built aqueducts for supplying fresh water, and they developed management operations for overseeing water and sewage systems (McGrew, 1985).

A major environmental issue in the medieval world was the spread of infectious diseases brought about by the growth of cities, increased trade, and wars. Plague, spread by rodents, appeared in the writings of Dionysius in the 3rd century AD. The most severe infectious diseases were outbreaks of leprosy and bubonic plague during the 13th and 14th centuries (McGrew, 1985). As leprosy spread and peaked in Europe in the early 13th century, people recognized a connection between the environment and spread of the disease. They instituted epidemic control by isolating people with signs of the disease and checking newcomers to the community. Therefore, long before science had discovered the true causes of these diseases, people were instinctively changing or avoiding harmful environmental circumstances in an effort to promote health. Simple city ordinances restricted locals from washing their clothes or tanners from cleaning their skins in rivers that supplied drinking water. A law passed in London in 1309 governed the disposal of wastes into the Thames River. Similarly, people passed rules governing the sale of old or spoiled meat to local residents, and "in Basel, leftover fish were displayed at a special inferior food stall and sold only to strangers" (McGrew, 1985, p. 139). This early concern for sanitary conditions became a major focus in public health, reaching its peak between 1840 and 1880.

The social hygiene movement called for societal transformation to create a truly healthful environment (McGrew, 1985). During the middle to late 1800s, Florence Nightingale in England and Dr. Ignace Semmelweiss in Vienna pioneered the promotion of clean hospital and surgical conditions to prevent illness. Oliver Wendell Holmes made the connection between exposure to sepsis and maternal infection in Boston in 1843. John Snow first documented environmental spread of disease in London in 1850 when he linked the spread of cholera with contaminated drinking water (Kerns, 2001). The work of Pasteur and Koch demonstrated the role of bacteria in disease. All of these, in addition to greater use of the microscope, shed further light on the relationship of the environment to health.

Awareness of the environmental impact on health was first documented in a "Report on an Inquiry into the Sanitary Conditions of the Labouring Population of Great Britain" by Edwin Chadwick in 1842 (Turnock, 1997). This document addressed the necessity for a healthy environment. About the same time, a similar report in the United States, called "Report of the Sanitary Commission of Massachusetts," by Lemuel Shattuck, provided original insights into environmental health issues, including smoke prevention, pest control, sanitation programs, and food regulations (Teutsch & Churchill, 2000). These documents marked the first organized concern for public health and environmental health controls. Since that time, the focus has gradually expanded from sanitation to the problems generated by advances in technology, chemical production, and pollution, which are discussed in this chapter.

An important international agency, the World Health Organization (WHO), was created in 1948 and has helped to identify and address world health problems, including issues of environmental concern. Because many modern technological discoveries cause far-reaching health hazards that affect the environment and the health of the entire global population, this organization and others like it will play increasingly important roles in the future.

National Perspective

In the United States, all levels of government have worked diligently to assess, prevent, and correct environmental health hazards. The major environmental health efforts of the federal government have come primarily since the early 1970s. Local governments assume responsibility for proper waste disposal, pure water supply, and efficient sanitary and safety conditions within the community. State governments, represented by different agencies, handle broader issues that deal with the creation of state regulations, policies, and supervision of local health efforts (Williams & Torrens, 1999). The federal government is charged with establishing and enforcing health standards and regulations. During the past 20 years, the public concern for people's health in relation to the environment, as well as concern for the environment itself, has stimulated increased government actions. The Environmental Protection Agency (EPA) was established in 1971 and was given extensive authority over all environmental concerns and protection of public health. The Food and Drug Administration (FDA) was established within the Public Health Service in 1968; the Occupational Safety and Health Administration (OSHA), for regulation, and the National Institute for Occupational Safety and Health (NIOSH), for research, were both established in 1970. The Public Health Service, under the U. S. Department of Health and Human Services (USDHHS), has helped to focus environmental control efforts through development of objectives published in 1979 and again in 1991. Its 1991 document, *Healthy People 2000,* listed objectives in major target areas. In the 2000 follow-up document, *Healthy People 2010,* objectives for improvement in environmental health parameters continue (Display 10–1).

Private business has become more conscious of health and safety issues as those issues have been enhanced by legislation such as the Products Liability Law and monitored by the Products Safety Commission. Private business and industry have often been accused of having total disregard for the health of the environment and its effect on human health, but this image seems to be changing slowly. Many companies, confronted by concerned environmentalists or consumer protection groups that have formed in recent years, have been forced to change their practices. Boycotts of products, listings of environmentally conscientious firms, and general public outrage have put a stop to many harmful practices. A number of companies have been concerned for some time with the environmental impact of their business operations; they have sought not only reduction of health hazards but also ways to promote environmental and public health. Timber companies, for example, have actively engaged in reforestation projects. Private business has been a major contributor to many nonprofit, environmentally concerned projects and agencies, such as the Sierra Club.

Maintaining a healthy environment and balanced ecology and promoting the health of those living in it remain challenging. Past efforts to accomplish these goals have been only partially successful. However, increased public awareness and concern for future generations have exerted tremendous pressure to create new and more effective legislative acts and activities (Display 10–2).

MAJOR GLOBAL ENVIRONMENTAL CONCERNS

The global perspective, and specifically the national perspective, of environmental health provides us with a picture of humankind's attempts to protect populations. However, for much of our world's history, protecting people, other living beings, or the earth itself has not been a priority or even a concern. Because of this history, there are major global environmental concerns now facing the world, including overpopulation, ozone depletion and global warming, deforestation, wetlands destruction, desertification, energy depletion, inadequate housing, aesthetics, and environmental justice issues.

Overpopulation

Human population took hundreds of thousands of years to grow to 2.5 billion in 1950; since then, in less than 50 years, it has more than doubled to 5.9 billion (Population Action International, 1998). Many believe that this exponential popu-

D I S P L A Y   1 0 – 1

Healthy People 2010 Objectives Related to Environmental Health

In 1998, it was reported by the U.S. Department of Health and Human Services, in the *Healthy People 2010 Objectives for Public Comment*, using midpoint data, that progress (or lack of it) was made in the following areas:

1. Reduce asthma morbidity, measured by reduced asthma hospitalizations, to no greater than 43 per 10,000 population. Special target populations: Blacks, nonwhites, and children.
   1999: 94 per 10,000
2. Reduce prevalence of serious mental retardation among school-aged children to no more than 124 per 10,000 children.
   1995: 1991–1994 prevalence was 131 per 10,000.
3. Reduce outbreaks of waterborne disease from infectious agents and chemical poisoning to no more than 2 per year. Special target populations: People served by public or investor-owned water systems.
   1987–1996 average: 6 outbreaks per year.
4. Reduce the prevalence of blood lead levels among children to zero. Target: total elimination. Special target population: Inner-city, low-income, black children.
   1991–1994: 4.4% of children aged 1 to 5 years had blood lead levels exceeding 10 µg/dL.
5. Reduce the proportion of people exposed to air that does not meet the Environmental Protection Agency (EPA) health-based standards for harmful air pollutants. Target air pollutants include ozone, carbon monoxide, nitrogen dioxide, sulfur dioxide, particulates, and lead.
   1997: ozone, 43%; particulate matter, 12%; carbon monoxide, 19%; nitrogen dioxide, 5%; sulfur dioxide, 2%; lead, <1%. 2010 target: 0%.
6. Increase to at least 20% the proportion of homes in which homeowners/occupants have tested for radon concentrations and concentrations have been found to pose minimal risk or have been modified to reduce risk to health, as a means to reduce the incidence of lung cancer.
   1998: An estimated 17% of the nation's homes had been tested for radon concentrations.
7. Reduce air toxic emissions to decrease the risk of adverse health effects caused by airborne toxins.
   Baseline 1993: 8.1 million tons of toxins were released into the air. Target: 2.0 tons—a 75% improvement.
8. Increase recycling of municipal solid waste.
   1996 baseline: 27% of total municipal solid waste generated was recycled. Target: 38% of municipal solid waste generated recycled.

9. Increase the proportion of people to at least 95% who receive safe drinking water supplies that meet the regulations of the Safe Drinking Water act.
   1995: 73% of community water systems met safe drinking water standards, which is the same as the baseline year of 1998; however, the EPA continues to issue additional safe standard levels.
10. Reduce potential risks to human health from surface water. This will be measured by a decrease in the proportion of surface waters (lakes, streams, and so forth) that do not support beneficial uses, such as fishing and swimming.
   This is a developmental objective with no percentages set; however, in 1994 40% of the nation's surface waters were too polluted for fishing or swimming.
11. Provide testing for lead-based paint in at least 50% of homes built before 1950.
   1998: 16% of people living in homes built before 1950 reported that the house paint had been analyzed for lead content.
12. Increase the number of new homes constructed to be radon resistant.
   1997: 1.4 million new homes. Target: 2.1 million additional new homes.
13. Eliminate significant health risks from hazardous waste sites on the EPA's National Priority List. This will be measured by performing site cleanups sufficient to eliminate specified health threats. The year 2010 target is 98%.
   1995: 90% of the recommendations were followed among the 1232 hazardous waste sites.
14. Increase or maintain the number of territories, tribes, states, and the District of Columbia that monitor environmental diseases. (These diseases include lead poisoning, other heavy metal poisoning, pesticide poisoning, carbon monoxide poisoning, heatstroke, hypothermia, acute chemical poisoning, methemoglobinemia, and respiratory diseases due to environmental factors.)
   1999 baseline: 4–41 jurisdictions. Target: 2010: 10–51 jurisdictions.
15. Reduce the proportion of children aged 6 and younger who are regularly exposed to tobacco smoke at home.
   1994: 27% of household with children under age 6 expose their children to tobacco smoke at least 4 days per week. Target: 10%.

(U.S. Department of Health and Human Services [2000]. *Healthy people 2010* [Conference ed., Vols. I & II]. Washington, DC: Government Printing Office.)

DISPLAY 10-2

Selected Environmental Health Acts/Agencies/Activities Influencing Health in the United States

Date	Act/Agency/Activity
1850	The Shattuck Report
1872	The American Public Health Association was founded
1872	The American Forestry Association was established
1890	Yosemite National Park in California became the first national park in the United States
1936	The National Wildlife Federation was founded
1970	The Environmental Protection Agency was formed
1970	The Clean Air Act
1970	Poison Prevention Packaging Act
1970	Occupational Health and Safety Act (OSHA)
1970	National Institute of Occupational Safety and Health (NIOSH) formed
1970	Hazardous Materials Transportation Control
1970	National Environmental Policy Act
1970	First annual Earth Day was held
1971	Lead-Based Paint Poisoning Prevention Act
1972	Federal Water Pollution Control Act Amendments
1972	Noise Control Act
1974	Safe Drinking Water Act (amended in 1996)
1976	Resource Conservation and Recovery Act
1976	Toxic Substances Control Act
1977	Clean Water Act
1979	U.S. Department of Health and Human Services helped to focus environmental control efforts
1980	Low Level Radiation Waste Policy Act
1980	Comprehensive Environmental Response, Compensation, and Liability Act (Superfund)
1991	*Healthy People 2000* set environmental health objectives as a priority
1992	The United States, the European community, and 153 other nations signed the United Nations Framework Convention on Climate Change (UNFCCC), an agreement pledging to reduce greenhouse gases to the 1990 level by the year 2000
1995	*Healthy People 2000: Midcourse Review and 1995 Revisions* gave update on environmental health progress
1996	The Food Quality Protection Act
1996	The World Health Organization, scientists, and United Nations officials called for stronger efforts to combat global warming
2000	*Healthy People 2010* used the 1995 review and revisions and input from professionals from around the country to establish 2010 environmental health goals

lation growth will level off if actions are taken now, or, if no actions are taken, there will be a dramatic reduction because of environmental disaster (Ford, 2000). Uncontrolled population growth is indisputably a public health issue.

The world's population is still increasing by more than 80 million people per year. This rate is expected to continue until 2010, at which point, it will gradually decline to about 40 million a year by 2050 (Population Action International, 1998; WHO, 2000). However, even with a worldwide trend toward smaller families, we will continue to add at least another 2 billion people to our small planet in the next 50 years.

The burden of the population growth is being carried by the poorest developing countries, such as in Africa and India, where 90% of the growth is occurring. More than 95% of future population growth is also expected to occur in these regions. Between one third and one half of the population in most developing countries is younger than 15 years of age, in part because advances in public health have lowered mortality among all age groups, but especially among infants and children.

In some nations, the population is projected to shrink. If low fertility rates continue in Germany, Italy, Russia, and Spain, their populations will decrease by 5% to 15% by the year 2025. In contrast, countries such as Nigeria, Zaire, and Jordan have high fertility rates, and it is likely that their populations will more than double over the same period.

What do these statistics and trends mean for the health of populations and the ecosystem? When a population exceeds the ability of its ecosystem to either support it or acquire the support needed, or when it exceeds its ability to migrate to other ecosystems in a manner that preserves its standard of living, the population is said to be experiencing **demographic entrapment**. Such a population faces the four tragedies of entrapment. Depending on cultural, political, and ecologic factors, it can starve, die from disease, slaughter itself or others, or be supported indefinitely by aid from others.

Government's Role

The government has a responsibility to prevent a population from exceeding the limits of the nation's resources and boundaries. The possible methods of preventing overpopulation, or solutions to it, are controversial, depending on one's culture, religious beliefs, and personal values and convictions. Ideally, the political system governing a country has a responsibility to provide a well-formed infrastructure of health and safety services for its population; economic development that provides employment, housing, and services; and political strength to provide stability to the nation. Many countries with unstable political systems are unable to deal effectively with overpopulation issues.

Nurse's Role

Public health professionals, including community health nurses, have a responsibility in the area of overpopulation, both globally and locally. Productive interventions include the following: (1) teaching families that birth spacing improves child and maternal survival and that a planned family is the best environment for a child's development; (2) preventing high-risk pregnancies such as those among teens and adult women who are infected with the human immunodeficiency virus (HIV) or have the acquired immunodeficiency syndrome (AIDS) (National Instiiutes of Health, 2001); (3) preventing the growing epidemic of HIV/AIDS; (4) providing family planning education to prevent worldwide deaths from unsafe abortions; and (5) providing prenatal care—because healthy mothers equal healthy children. These are key areas in which public health efforts can reap major rewards for families.

Air Pollution

For many centuries, people have known that air quality affects human health. In Europe and America in the 1800s and early to middle 1900s, documented episodes of concentrated air pollution due to thermal atmospheric inversion caused many reported deaths. **Pollution** refers to the act of contaminating or defiling the environment to the extent that it negatively affects people's health. Air pollution is now recognized as one of the most hazardous sources of chemical contamination. It is especially prevalent in highly industrialized and urbanized areas where concentrations of motor vehicles and industry produce large volumes of gaseous pollutants.

Air pollution is a global problem. Decades of environmentally insensitive industrial development in eastern Europe and the Soviet Union, as it was then known, has caused serious life- and health-threatening air pollution. In the Czech Republic, one of the most heavily polluted countries, air pollution may be responsible for up to 3% of all deaths. There is evidence that tens of thousands of people in these countries have developed respiratory and cardiovascular problems from airborne contaminants, and 75% of the children in many industrial areas of these countries have respiratory disease. A study of low-level air pollution in Helsinki, Finland, demonstrated that symptoms of ischemic cardiac and cerebrovascular diseases may be provoked by pollutants in concentrations lower than those given as guidelines in many countries and lower than previously shown. Air quality guidelines for Europe are recommended by the WHO, and guidelines that the United States follows are developed by the Environmental Protection Agency (Yassi et al., 2001). In the United States from 1970 to 1997, overall emissions of the six major pollutants the federal government measures (carbon monoxide, nitrogen oxides, hydrocarbons, particulate matter, sulfur dioxide, and lead) decreased by 31%. However, in 2000, the EPA reported that approximately 101 million people in the United States lived in 114 areas designated as nonattainment areas for at least one of the critera pollutants (Dixon, 2002).

Airborne pollutants have adverse effects on many areas of human life; costs to property, productivity, quality of life, and especially human health are enormous. The list of diseases and symptoms of ill health associated with specific air pollutants is lengthy, ranging from minor nose and throat irritations, respiratory infections, and bronchial asthma to emphysema, cardiovascular disease, lung cancer, and genetic mutations (Fig. 10–2).

As with other toxic chemicals, it is often difficult to establish a cause-and-effect relationship between air pollution and illness. A relatively short, high level of exposure is normally easier to identify. There have been a number of poignant examples. One acute episode in Donora, Pennsylvania, in 1948 caused 20 deaths, and 1190 people were sickened (almost 43% of the area's population). Another occurred in London in 1952, when an atmospheric inversion trapped coal-burning smoke and fog over the city for almost a week. Between 4000 and 8000 people, mostly the elderly and those who were vulnerable because of respiratory and cardiac diseases, died as a result (Yassi et al., 2001). Although these disasters and others like them are dramatic and frightening, the effects of long-term exposure to low levels of pollution, such as passive smoking exposure in the home, are perhaps even more threatening (Gaffney, 2001). They are definitely more difficult to record, measure, understand, define, correlate, and control. It may be impossible to ever document their total effects.

Certain geographic areas are more susceptible to the ill effects of air pollution because of weather conditions or physical terrain. The episode in London occurred when a lack of wind combined with low temperatures to create a temperature inversion—a phenomenon in which air that normally rises is trapped under a layer of warm air, allowing air contaminants to build up to intolerable levels. Los Angeles, another city troubled by air pollution, is surrounded by mountains that prevent winds from clearing away smoke and fumes. A further condition occurs in urban areas: city buildings create a "heat island effect" in which warm air traps pollution in the atmosphere around the city. In examining the effects of air pollution, it is necessary to take into account the climate conditions and topography of an area.

The EPA has developed a tool to provide the public with timely and easy-to-understand information on local air quality and whether air pollution levels pose a health concern. The Air Quality Index (AQI) lets the public know how clean the air is and whether they should be concerned for their health. The AQI is focused on health effects that can happen within a few hours or days after breathing polluted air (Table 10–2). Depending on the topography and general air flow patterns of the area, some communities use the index to inform the public as to when use of wood-burning fireplaces or burning of trash piles or leaves is inadvised or illegal.

Dusts, Gases, and Naturally Occurring Elements

Dusts can contain numerous types of chemical irritants and poisons. Many hazardous dusts are associated with the workplace; for example, coal miners have developed black lung

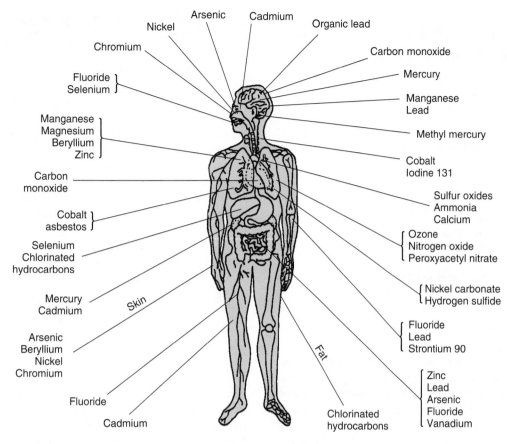

FIGURE 10-2. Body system targets of major air pollutants.

disease from inhaling coal dust, and a respiratory disease called silicosis is caused by exposure to silica dust (common in mining, sandblasting, and tunnel work). Dusts are also associated with farming and grain elevator work, as well as highway construction. Asbestos fibers, which are found in insulation and fireproofing materials, textiles, and many other products, have been associated with lung cancer. Although people who smoke are at 30 times greater risk of developing lung cancer than those who do not smoke, passive smoking is estimated to cause approximately 3000 lung cancer deaths in nonsmokers each year, and 150,000 to 300,000 infants and children younger than 18 months of age experience lower respiratory tract infections. In addition, asthma and other respiratory conditions are triggered or worsened by tobacco smoke (USDHHS, 2000).

Although much air pollution results from some type of human activity, naturally occurring elements, such as pollen from plants and flowers, ash from volcanic eruptions, and airborne microorganisms, can also have ill effects on health. A long list of gaseous pollutants, including sulfur oxides and nitrogen oxides produced by industrial emissions, pose additional problems for community health. Such gases cause respiratory disease, asphyxiation, and other problems in humans and can harm plant and animal life as well. Other gases, in-

cluding chlorine, ozone, sulfur dioxide, and carbon monoxide, are all harmful to individual health as well as to the broader environment and the ecosystem.

Another gas that has been a topic of concern in recent years is radon. This colorless, odorless, radioactive gas is formed by the breakdown of uranium in rock, groundwater, and soil in some geographic areas (Yassi et al., 2001). It is associated with increased lung cancers in the United States, especially in miners. However, it can seep into basements of houses and enter buildings through cracks in basement walls or through sewer openings, exposing people who inhabit, attend school, or work in the affected buildings. Furnaces and exhaust fans can help pull radon into a house, although the highest levels tend to be found in basements where the gas enters. Home testing for radon was recommended by the EPA and the U. S. Public Health Service starting in 1988. Sealing the cracks in basement walls and covering dirt floors can substantially reduce radon levels.

Healthy People 2010 (USDHHS, 2000) has two objectives focused on radon concerns. One goal is to increase the proportion of persons who live in homes tested for radon concentrations from 17% to 20%, and the other is to increase the number of new homes constructed to be radon resistant from 1.4 million (in 1997) to 2.1 additional new homes by 2010.

TABLE 10-2

The Air Quality Index (AQI)

AQI Values	Levels of Health Concern	Colors
When the AQI is in this range...	...air quality conditions are...	...as symbolized by this color.
0–50	Good	Green
51–100	Moderate	Yellow
101–150	Unhealthy for Sensitive Groups	Orange
151–200	Unhealthy	Red
201–300	Very Unhealthy	Purple
301–500	Hazardous	Maroon

Agency for Toxic Substances and Disease Registry (ATSDR) (2001). *Air pamphlet.* Washington, DC: ATSDR.

WHAT DO YOU THINK?

Ticks of the Ixodidae family have a wide geographic distribution, including parts of the subarctic regions. They are vectors for several diseases, such as Lyme disease and tick-borne encephalitis (TBE). Hosts for the tick include several animals: birds, rodents, and deer. If infected with the pathogen, a vector tick can pass it on to humans through its blood-sucking capacity. Ticks as well as their host animals and habitat are all dependent on changes in local weather patterns. Future climatic change, brought about by global warming, would affect the complicated ecologic interactions associated with the transmission of tickborne diseases. As a result, tickborne diseases may spread into new areas that are located at higher northern latitudes and altitudes than present endemic regions.

E. Lindgren of Sweden (Yassi et al., 2001)

Acid Precipitation (Acid Rain)

The emission of hazardous chemicals into the earth's atmosphere has a serious effect on the environment. Air pollutants such as sulfur dioxide from power plant emissions or nitrogen oxides from motor vehicle exhaust combine with rainwater, snow, and other forms of precipitation to produce sulfuric and nitric acid, commonly called "acid rain." The problem has been most severe and most heavily documented in Canada (from emissions from the U. S. Midwest) and Scandinavia (from emissions arising in Germany and Britain). Similar situations occur in Russia and Eastern Europe and probably in China, India, and Central Asia, and can extensively change the biology of small bodies of water (Yassi et al., 2001). Although acid rain does not seem to pose any direct danger to humans, it kills small forms of life and endangers the forest and freshwater ecologies. An increased accumulation of carbon dioxide in the atmosphere from fuel combustion is altering the climate and contributing to a condition called the "greenhouse effect" (see What Do You Think?)

Ozone Depletion and Global Warming

Two new and very threatening environmental hazards, stratospheric ozone layer depletion and global warming, are closely related. **Global warming** is the trapping of heat radiation from the earth's surface that increases the overall temperature of the world, causing a greenhouse effect (Yassi et al., 2001). This warming is caused by carbon dioxide and other gases that enter the atmosphere through a depleted ozone layer and become trapped. The direct health effects of ozone depletion include increased risks for skin cancer and cataracts. Greater indirect effects could result from the global warming through damage to the food chain, an increase in the global population exposed to vector-borne diseases, raised ocean levels, and a variety of effects on crop production (Agency for Toxic Substances and Disease Registry, 2001;

Yassi et al., 2001). For example, scientific studies based on mathematical models indicate that a global mean temperature increase of 1°C to 2°C would enable mosquitos to extend their range to new geographic areas, leading to 45% to 60% increases in cases of malaria by 2050. In addition, there are already at least 25 million people, sometimes called environmental refugees, who can no longer support their families in their homelands because of drought, soil erosion, desertification, deforestation, and other environmental problems (WHO, 2000) (see Research: Bridge to Practice).

In the past, changes in the earth's climate resulted from natural causes and enabled the evolution of species over hundreds of thousands of years. The accumulation of stratospheric ozone shields the earth from damaging ultraviolet light, filtering and reducing the extent of radiation that reaches the earth. Today, human activities are affecting our climate in serious and immediate ways. It is being destroyed as a result of chemical interactions among air pollutants, primarily chlorofluorocarbons (CFCs). Most of the ozone-destroying chemicals and greenhouse gases are produced in the wealthier countries.

Government's Role

Government regulation of air pollution has been relatively slow. In 1963, the federal government passed the first series of Clean Air Acts. These set standards for air quality and industrial emissions and delegated funds to assist in pollution control programs. Although progress has been made, further public health efforts are needed to help identify pollution sources and related health hazards (see Display 10–2).

Even if the air is cleaner than it was 30 years ago, there is work yet to be done. The EPA has instituted rules to force

RESEARCH: BRIDGE TO PRACTICE

Patz, J.A., McGeehin, M.A., Bernard, S.M., et al., (2001, September). The potential health impacts of climate variability and change for the United States: Executive summary of the report of the health sector of the U. S. National Assessment. *Environmental Health, 64,* 20–28.

In 1997, the U. S. National Assessment of the Potential Consequences of Climate Variability and Change was established as part of the U. S. Global Change Research Program, which began in 1990. The work involved an assessment of the potential impacts of climate change over two time frames—from the present to 2030 and from 2030 to 2100—for geographic regions of the United States.

Outcomes from the assessment determined that U. S. climate will be characterized by increased temperatures, altered hydrologic cycle, and increased variability. There are two fluctuations climatologists are concerned about: the short- to medium-term fluctuations that are measured within a 30-year period, such as El Niño or La Niña, and climate change, which refers to a fundamental shift in the mean state of the climate over a longer period.

Projections are partially based on historical data and indirect measurements found in ice cores, tree rings, and other paleodata. In the past 100 years, the global surface temperature has warmed by 0.7°F to 1.4° F. In the contiguous United States, temperatures have increased by 1° F, and precipitation has been increasing. Certain populations within the United States, such as the poor, the elderly, children, and immunocompromised individuals, may become more vulnerable to many of the health risks that are exacerbated by climate change. For example, the urban poor are less likely to have air conditioning, which is an adaptive response strategy to reduce illnesses and deaths during heat waves. In another example the United States is an aging society—the U.S. population grew 45% from 1960 to 1994, while the number of those older than 65 years of age increased by 274%. As a result, we have large numbers of people with increased vulnerability to infectious disease or external environ-

mental stresses such as extreme heat—and poverty, which increases with age, adds to their vulnerability.

The potential health impacts of climate variability and change can be listed, but with layers of uncertainty. First, methods that project changes in climate over time will continue to improve, but existing climate models are unable to accurately project regional-scale impacts. Next, because basic scientific information on the sensitivity of human health to aspects of weather and climate is limited, we are unsure of the effects of climate changes on humans. Third, the adaptability and vulnerability of people based on population density, level of economic and technological development, local environmental conditons, preexisting health status, quality and availability of health care, and the public health infrastructure factor into their wellness level. People of color who live in poverty in inner-city areas are at risk for multiple health problems, not the least of which are environmentally induced diseases and injuries. These people then become at greater risk with the advent of global climatic changes, according to the U.S. National Assessment findings. The potential impacts of projected climate change on health include temperature-related illnesses and deaths from prolonged heat waves; health effects related to increasing storms, tornadoes, hurricanes, and precipitation extremes; air pollution-related health effects from a warming global temperature, waterborne and foodborne disease that may increase due to changes in precipitation, temperature, humidity, salinity, and wind; and increasing vector-borne and rodent-borne diseases that are altered with the weather patterns

Although it is fairly comprehensive, the U.S. National Assessment did not address the impact that changes in the hydrologic cycle might have on crop production and food storage in the United States or the long-term effects of stratospheric oxone depletion. However, it did find that most of the U.S. population is presently protected against adverse health outcomes associated with weather or climate, although certain demographic and geographic populations are at increased risk.

---

reductions in nitrogen oxide emissions by 2003, at a cost of $1.7 billion for the power industry. The automobile is a continued target as a source of pollutants, and new steps will include reducing sulfur in gasoline, tightening emission standards, and removing a loophole that allows sports utility vehicles to defy emission standards.

In 1997, the EPA identified 10 ways in which people can help stop global warming. These remain useful suggestions that the community health nurse can use and pass along to clients:

1. Reduce home energy usage (eg, keep heat lower in the winter and air conditioning higher in the summer, shut off lights in rooms not occupied, unplug appliances when not in use).
2. If considering buying or building a new house, make sure it is energy-efficient.
3. Buy products that feature reusable, recyclable, or reduced packaging to save the energy required to manufacture new containers.
4. When buying a car, consider a fuel-smart car, one

that gets more miles to the gallon than your current vehicle.

5. Consider transportation alternatives such as mass transit, car pooling, bicycling, and telecommuting. When you do drive, keep your car tuned up and its tires properly inflated to save on fuel costs.

6. Insulate your home to save money and energy, caulk windows and doors, and tune up your furnace and air conditioner.

7. Encourage your utility company to do its part by offering energy from clean sources (landfill gas recovery, high-efficiency natural gas-fired power plants, or renewable sources such as solar and wind).

8. Get involved at work by ensuring that your company has joined EPA programs such as Green Lights, ENERGY STAR Buildings, and Waste Wi$e recycling programs, and by buying office equipment with an ENERGY STAR label (indicating high efficiency, which saves energy and money, results in better performance, and helps prevent air pollution).

9. Plant trees. Trees absorb carbon dioxide, a greenhouse gas, from the air. Join family members, neighbors, or community service groups in planting trees in your yard, along roadways, and in parks.

10. Educate others. Let friends, family, and clients know about these practical, energy-saving steps they can take to save money while protecting the environment.

Nurse's Role

Community health nurses can influence air quality through detection, community education, and lobbying for appropriate legislation. People are exposed to numerous impurities in the air in their homes and workplaces. Nurses can promote health by helping to detect indoor pollutants and informing people of existing or potential dangers. Many household products and building materials emit vapors that can cause problems. Cigarette smoke and cigar smoke are common indoor pollutants that can have ill effects on nonsmokers as well as smokers. Infants and other vulnerable persons are at risk from such exposure (Dixon, 2002; Gaffney, 2001). Carbon monoxide poisoning may result from stove and furnace emissions or from car exhaust accumulating in a garage. Radon gas trapped in basements or tightly insulated homes is also a major concern. Nurses can assist with prevention or elimination of these health hazards by ensuring that the indoor environment is well ventilated (oxygenated) and heating equipment properly maintained and by looking for possible sources of pollution.

Water Pollution

Water is such an essential element to human survival that the available quantity and quality of water within a community has become a prime environmental health issue. Water has many uses other than consumption by humans. It serves as a means of transportation. It cleans and cools the body or other

objects. It is the basis for many forms of recreation and sports, such as swimming and boating, and it provides a vehicle for disposing of human and industrial wastes and controlling fires. Apart from serving human needs, water also acts as a medium for sustaining other living organisms, as a home to plant and animal life, and as a means of carrying and distributing necessary nutrients in the environment. Although nursing's environmental health role concerns the safe consumption of water by humans, it is important, taking an ecologic perspective, to keep in mind water's other uses and users.

Drinking water comes from two main sources: surface water (such as lakes and streams) and underground sources (called groundwater), which collects in areas known as aquifers and comes to the surface through wells and springs. In general, underground sources are thought to be less subject to contamination than surface sources, which are open to runoff from agricultural pesticides or industrial wastes. However, groundwater too may be contaminated if seepage occurs. In the Middle Ages, disease epidemics spread as people drank water contaminated by human waste; this is still a problem today in developing countries and, at times, in other countries if flooding occurs. Well water may contain fecal contaminants from improper septic tank drainage. Toxic agents that may affect groundwater include buried hazardous wastes, nitrate contamination of wells in rural areas, and arsenic in drinking water, which is linked to bladder and lung cancer (APHA, 2001; Rose, 2002).

In most industrialized nations, lack of sufficient water for drinking has not been a serious issue. Areas with limited water supplies have devised facilities to store water during high-flow periods so it is available to satisfy the year-round needs of a given community. Adequate water supply to meet agricultural demands still has not been achieved, however.

The major concern with regard to water is its purity. In March 2002, EPA Administrator Christie Whitman called water quantity and quality "the biggest environmental issue that we face in the 21st century" (Lavelle & Kurlantzick, 2002). Water can be contaminated and made unsafe for drinking in many different ways. Three are discussed here.

1. Water may be infected with bacteria or parasites that cause disease. *Giardia lamblia* is a parasite that enters the water supply through contamination from human or wild animal feces. It can cause giardiasis, a gastrointestinal disease that results in diarrhea and malabsorption of nutrients. For example, beavers in the northern Cascade Mountains often contaminate water. Humans using the area for recreation must treat the water with iodine before drinking it. Water may also be contaminated with bacteria such as *Vibrio cholerae*, resulting in cholera, or with viruses leading to hepatitis A (Yassi et al., 2001).

2. Toxic substances such as pesticides are introduced by humans into water systems and constitute another form of water pollution. These substances may contaminate streams, lakes, and wells. Industrial pollutants may also enter drinking water through oil spills, careless dumping, or buried hazardous wastes that seep into underground

water sources. Such wastes not only harm the quality of the water but also have been implicated in diseases such as leukemia. They can contaminate local fish and shellfish, making them unfit for consumption. Mercury poisoning from contaminated seafood on the Atlantic coast is a case in point: by 1988, one third of the nation's shellfish beds had been closed because of pollution. In 2002, six drinking water wells in Bourne, Massachusetts, had to be closed because it was discovered that they were contaminated with perchlorate, a rocket fuel component that had leaked from a nearby military reservation. And in Chesapeake, Virginia, almost 200 women sued their water system, claiming that miscarriages they suffered in the 1980s and 1990s were traceable to trihalomethanes, chemicals produced when chlorine reacted with their region's murky river water (Lavelle & Kurlantzick, 2002).

3. Pollutants may upset the ecosystem, affecting natural organisms that help purify water systems. Power plants or other industries dissipate excess heat into lakes and streams and cause water temperatures to rise. This thermal pollution kills off beneficial organisms in the water.

In response to the various potential water pollutants, most cities and local communities with public or semipublic water systems in operation have set up water testing and treatment purification centers to ensure safe drinking water. Unfortunately, testing for bacteria and toxins often does not occur until after illness has been reported. Another major problem arises in rural areas, where most water supplies are private and therefore not subject to systematic testing and treatment. Testing of water for coliforms as indicator organisms has proved useful. Water frequently is treated with chlorine to disinfect it, but this has led to risk of chloroform exposure.

Recreational uses of water, such as public swimming, have health implications. Lakes, oceans, rivers, and even hot tubs often carry infectious agents and result in a number of health problems, including swimmers' itch, diarrheal diseases, and granulomatous pneumonitis (Rose et al., 1998). Many disease outbreaks have been caused by polluted water systems serving campgrounds, parks, and other public areas.

The marine ecosystem can be altered by any changes that affect the oceans, such as water temperatures at the surface, nutrient levels, winds, currents, and precipitation patterns. This can lead to possible increases in diseases transmitted from fish and shellfish, toxic "red tides," and a dormant form of cholera that develops when pH, temperature, salinity, and nutrient levels are insufficient (Patz et al., 2001). In addition, research has shown that coming in contact with marine waters that are contaminated with domestic sewage can cause nonenteric illnesses, including febrile respiratory illness from fecal streptococci and ear ailments from fecal coliform exposure among swimmers.

Government's Role

Most of the responsibility for maintaining water quality rests with state and local governments. The federal government took a needed step in 1974 by passing the Safe Drinking Wa-

ter Act, which gave the EPA authority to establish water standards and to ensure that these standards were upheld. The federal government also provided funds to assist state and local governments in this effort. However, policies related to groundwater quality protection need continued monitoring. In 1998, the EPA developed a Right-to-Know report, which tells consumers about contaminants in their drinking water. These long-awaited rules set the minimum requirements for healthy drinking water and helped to ensure the safety of drinking water supplies (EPA, 2002; Lavelle & Kurlantzick, 2002; Yassi et al., 2001). Saltwater intrusion caused by changes in sea level is threatening drinking water supplies in many communities along the East Coast. The state of Florida has resorted to building desalinization plants.

Globally, because of the enormous health problems in developing nations caused by unclean water, WHO declared the 1980s as the International Clean Water Decade and established a goal to have safe drinking water for all by the year 1990. This goal was not met; only 50% of the world's population had a safe water supply in 1980, 55% in 1985, and 66% in 1990 (WHO, 2000). Efforts to address water purity globally continue to assume high priority; however, the focus is shifting from drinking water quality alone toward overall improvement of the environment.

Nurse's Role

What role can community health nurses play in the effort to keep water safe? As nurses work in a community, they can help by examining household or city drinking water. Is there a strange odor or discoloration? Are particles or sediment visible in the water? Being aware of drinking water quality and possible contaminants in a given locality alerts the nurse to consider possible causal relationships if a problem exists. Asking clients to observe and report changes in water quality further assists the nurse in the monitoring process. If such changes occur, the proper authorities, such as health department officials, should be notified and water samples tested. Community health nurses can also be alert to increased incidence of illnesses that might be water related. For example, if several children exhibit similar symptoms, the nurse might inquire as to whether all have been swimming in the same pool or drinking from the same water fountain. Although water quality monitoring is ultimately the responsibility of environmental health authorities, it behooves the nurse, as a collaborating member of the health team, to observe and report any information that would further the goal of safe and healthy water for communities.

Deforestation, Wetlands Destruction, and Desertification

Deforestation is the clearing of tropical and temperate forests for cropland, cattle grazing, or urbanization. Elimination of these natural habitats is dooming some species of insects and animals to **extinction**, the loss of a species from the earth forever. **Wetlands** are natural inland bodies of shallow water, such as marshes, ponds, river bottoms, and flood plains, that filter contaminated surface waters and support wildlife reproduction and growth. They can be as small as a neighborhood seasonal stream bed or as large as the Everglades in Florida. At one time, the Everglades covered the lower 20% of the state, but the U. S. Army Corps of Engineers converted thousands of acres into housing developments 60 years ago. The destruction of this major U. S. wetland has caused numerous species of wildlife to disappear from the area or become extinct. There is discussion to reclaim some of the land and convert it back to much-needed wetlands. **Desertification** refers to the conversion of fertile land into desert, which is unable to support crop growth or wildlife.

Any natural or manmade process that changes life-supporting regions into land for other use or into barren wastelands upsets the ecosystem of the area. The destruction of forests and the upturning of earth for urban sprawl uncovers organisms hidden for eons, to which humans and animals are then exposed. In addition, gases that were once absorbed by these lost trees remain in the atmosphere and contribute to ozone depletion, which increases global warming. Deforestation, in turn, contributes to desertification, because forests provide protection for the surrounding topsoil by way of their roots, fallen leaves, and undergrowth. When this protection is lost, landslides and other geographic changes occur. Global temperature increases cause the drying up of riverbeds and create desert areas that are unable to support the people who once inhabited them. Drought, famine, and starvation often follow in such areas. The loss of forests and wetlands along with increasing desertification affects millions of people each year, with a potential for catastrophic environmental damage in the future.

Government's Role

Our government has the power to make decisions that save the wetlands and forests in the United States. The decision to save these lands is made when constituents express their concern loudly enough for their congressperson or senator to hear and respond positively. Often, developers of housing and industrial facilities are more influential, and their interests prevail. If the importance of the wetlands and forests is not recognized where decisions are made, then they will be lost.

Nurse's Role

Community health nurses can make a difference in this area. Perhaps no other person knows a community more intimately than the community health nurse. This role gives a valid voice of concern at the local level. By using leadership and collaborative skills, the nurse can initiate grassroots efforts to save wetlands and forests in the community. Chapters 13 and 16 provide information for bringing about change, beginning at the local level.

Energy Depletion

Most of the energy sources we use today are not renewable. Wood has been used for thousands of years and was our first fuel. It is still a primary source of home heating for most of the world's population (with resultant deforestation and air pollution). Natural gas for heat and fuel can be a highly efficient energy source, but pipelines must be built for hundreds or thousands of miles in some cases—a luxury that smaller and poorer countries cannot afford. Coal takes thousands of years to create, and worldwide sources will soon be depleted. Some countries do not have coal as a natural resource and have similar problems with natural gas.

Nuclear energy has been used for at least 35 years. This source of energy has been controversial since its first use yet it has proved to be an effective power product. Nevertheless, there have been some near-disasters and real disasters caused by human error. In 1979, a nuclear power plant on Three Mile Island near Harrisburg, Pennsylvania, had a near-disaster in one of its cooling towers; fortunately, the nuclear core was never exposed. This scare caused many people in the United States to lobby against nuclear power plants in their communities. The largest radiation disaster occurred in April, 1986, at the Chernobyl nuclear power plant in Ukraine. Five million people in Ukraine, Belarus, and the Russian Federation were exposed to ionizing radiation. Twenty-eight of the 444 people at the plant who were directly exposed died within 3 months, and 300 were hospitalized. Psychological effects among people living in the surrounding areas resulted from the lack of information immediately after the accident, the stress and trauma of compulsory relocation, a break in social ties, and fear that radiation exposure could cause health damage in the future. There has been an increase in the incidence of childhood thyroid cancer, particularly in Belarus. Ultimately, it is estimated that the aftereffects of this nuclear disaster will cause 6600 more deaths from cancer and leukemia (Yassi et al., 2001). The area remains unsafe to enter today.

Government's Role

Other renewable sources of energy need to be discovered, rediscovered, or tapped. Newer and more "environmentally friendly" energy sources are used experimentally in limited areas. They include landfill gas recovery, solar power, and wind power. Here are a few examples in the United States of how these sources can make a difference:

- A National Wind Coordinating Committee, established by utility companies, consumers groups, state and federal regulators, and the U. S. Department of Energy, has instituted experimental projects in six northeastern, midwestern, and southeastern sites. The resulting savings in energy costs were expected to reach $484 million.
- The U. S. Department of Energy is working closely with industry to develop photovoltaic systems for harnessing the rays of the sun to generate power. During the 1996 Olympics in Atlanta, the swimming competitions took place under lights powered by photovoltaics.
- The U. S. Department of Energy is working to address the need for growing and harvesting crops that can be turned into biomass fuels and to reclaim waste products from agricultural crops and forestlands for generating electricity. Two demonstration projects are in progress—the Vermont Gasifier Project and the Hawaii Biomass Gasifier Facility.

- The U. S. Department of Energy also is involved in geothermal projects. One includes the development of a pipeline that involves geysers in California. Another is from a consortium of more than 70 utility companies, promoting the use of geothermal heat pumps.

It will take both a global effort to increase awareness and an accompanying technology to use these energy sources in enough areas to make an environmental difference.

Nurse's Role

A community health nurse may not have a direct role in the creation of new energy sources or the use of a particular source. However, the nurse can educate people about energy conservation, discuss alternative energy sources presently available in the community, and encourage people to become interested in and knowledgeable about the importance of the potential for energy depletion in the future.

Conservative use of existing energy sources can be a part of the community health nurses's teaching with families in the community. In addition to saving precious energy resources, measures taken to cut energy use can save the family money spent on monthly utility bills. Conservation methods include ensuring that a home or apartment is well insulated and free from drafts: broken windows and improperly fitted windows or doors are kept repaired, caulking and weatherstripping is used where needed, and heating and cooling of the home are modified by setting the thermostat at 68 degees in the winter and no lower than 76 degrees in the summer. Families should be encouraged to wear warmer clothing or layers of clothing indoors in the winter and to dress in cool garments made of cotton in the summer. In the summer, using indoor freestanding fans or ceiling fans and closing the blinds on the sides of the home where the afternoon sun comes in help to keep a home cooler and allow the inhabitants to keep the thermostat higher while remaining comfortable.

In many communities, the utility company provides home energy inspections free of charge to help families recognize areas in their home where they are losing energy. Often these programs provide funding to make the needed changes, especially among families with low income.

Inadequate Housing

Housing is of central importance to quality of life. Ideally, it minimizes disease and injury and contributes much to physical, mental, and social well-being. Perhaps we cannot appreciate the kind of housing that people in most of the world call home. Because of lack of exposure to developing countries and poor countries, most Americans think of poor housing as being a house that is smaller than desirable, lacks a fresh coat of paint, needs some repairs, and has an unkempt yard; or an apartment in a poor neighborhood with graffitied walls, unpredictable plumbing, and unsafe elevators. This is unfortunate enough in a country such as the United States, but it is far above the substandard living conditions that obtain in most of the world.

At least 600 million urban-dwelling people in Africa, Asia, and Latin America live in life- and health-threatening homes and neighborhoods. Most live in overcrowded dwellings, with four or more persons to a room in tenements, cheap boarding houses, or shelters built on illegally occupied or subdivided land. In Chile, just 30 minutes outside of Santiago, there are shantytowns in fields that resemble piles of trash at a dump. These "homes" have no water or electricity. Tens of millions are homeless and sleep in public or semipublic places—including pavement dwellers and those who sleep in bus shelters, train stations, or parks (WHO, 2000).

Government's Role

The WHO (2000) has identified nine features of the housing environment that have important direct or indirect effects on the health of their occupants. WHO considers the home and its surrounding environment as being "the health burden of poor housing":

1. The structure of the shelter: Does it protect the occupants from extremes of heat or cold and insulate against noise and invasion by dust, rain, insects, and rodents?
2. The extent to which the provision for water supplies is adequate—from both a qualitative and a quantitative point of view
3. The effectiveness of provision for the disposal (and subsequent management) of excreta and liquid and solid wastes
4. The quality of the housing site, including the extent to which it is structurally safe for housing and the provisions made to protect it from contamination (provision for drainage being among the most important)
5. Overcrowding, which can lead to household accidents and increased transmission of airborne infections such as acute respiratory infectious diseases, pneumonia, and tuberculosis
6. The presence of indoor air pollution associated with fuels used for cooking or heating
7. Food safety standards, including the extent to which the shelter has adequate provision for storing food to protect it against spoilage and contamination
8. Vectors and hosts of disease associated with the domestic and peridomestic environment
9. The home as a workplace—where the use and storage of toxic or hazardous chemicals and unsafe equipment may present health hazards

Nurse's Role

In this area of environmental health and safety, the community health nurse has great influence. Much of the nurse's commitment to the community focuses on assessment, planning, intervention, and evaluation of a client's home and surrounding environment. The role may call for client education about home improvements, advocacy for routine maintenance of rental housing conditions, or assistance to clients who live on the streets or in shelters so that they can locate and secure more permanent and adequate safe housing (see Using the Nursing Process).

USING THE NURSING PROCESS

A Family Living in Substandard Housing

BACKGROUND

Ethel and Harvey Wolder live with their three children in a two-bedroom trailer in a small trailer park with minimal amenities which is increasingly occupied by very poor families and drug users. They own their old trailer, which is very small, but pay $260 a month for rental of the space. Other housing costs include propane (for heat, hot water, and cooking) and electricity, which runs about $150 a month for the poorly insulated trailer. The park is on the outskirts of town, and Harvey takes their car to drive into town for work, leaving Ethel and the children without transportation. They are unhappy where they live and have an opportunity to sell their trailer but don't know where they could afford to live that would be better. They think they will be able to afford an apartment at up to $600 per month, and their monthly take-home income is $1400. The family would like you to help them.

ASSESSMENT

You ask the family to
1. Describe what they are looking for in future housing (size, location, amenities, cost)
2. Prepare a copy of their monthly budget.
3. Share their goals for next year and the next 5 years.

After an assessment you discover that Harvey is a veteran, Ethel is able to work part-time, the family would like to own their own home, $600 a month rent might be difficult based on their budget and increasing needs of growing children, they can sell their trailer with $3000 left over, and they would like to live in the city nearer Harvey's work but would temporarily live in an apartment.

NURSING DIAGNOSIS

A highly motivated, close, and functional family with interest and assets that would allow them to live in a larger apartment or small home.

PLAN/IMPLEMENTATION

You work with the family to
1. Locate an adequate apartment or small home for purchase.
2. Work within their budget while locating adequate housing.
3. Locate housing options that are "children-friendly."
4. Explore the possibility of eligibility for a Veterans Administration (VA) home loan, a Housing and Urban Development (HUD) home purchase, a Habitat for Humanity home, or a subsidized apartment based on their income.

EVALUATION

1. Harvey and Ethel sold their trailer and moved to a three-bedroom apartment, where they pay only $400 a month in exchange for helping to maintain the small complex of 16 apartments.
2. They have a 1-year plan to purchase a home and are using Harvey's days off to look at homes for sale.
3. They applied to the VA for the paperwork to be eligible for a VA loan.
4. They are exploring local availability of HUD homes and Habitat for Humanity homes with your help, because they were unfamiliar with these opportunities.

SUMMARY

The clients are content with their apartment, are able to manage the maintence responsibilities at the apartment complex, are saving $100 per month, and are excited about their future plans as homeowners.

Unhealthy or Contaminated Food

This section describes how the supply of food, particularly the quality of that food, is affected by the environment, and what health hazards are associated with food. The community health nurse needs to ask: "How does the environment influence the safety of food for human consumption?" Three types of hazardous foods must be considered when examining food as a possible health problem: inherently harmful foods, contaminated foods, and foods with toxic additives.

Inherently Harmful Foods

Poisonous foods, such as certain types of mushrooms or inedible berries, do not pose a serious threat to most people. The general public can identify and avoid harmful plants and substances, so poisonings are rare. There are, however, numerous household plants and outdoor flowers, shrubs, and trees that are poisonous if consumed. Children are at risk because some of these plants bear berries or colorful flowers that can capture a child's interest, including the following:

Asparagus fern	Mountain-ash
Azalea	Oak
Begonia	Oleander
Chrysanthemum	Philodendron
Holly	Poinsettia
Honeysuckle	Poison ivy
Jade plant	Rhododendron
Jerusalem cherry	Rubber plant
Medicine aloe	Schefflera
Mistletoe	Spider plant

Contaminated Foods

Contaminated foods pose a more serious health problem. The Centers for Disease Control and Prevention (CDC) estimates that 76 million people in the United States experience foodborne illnesses each year, accounting for 325,000 hospitalizations and more than 5000 deaths—an average of almost 100 deaths per week (National Institute of Allergy and Infectious Diseases [NIAID], 2002). Food may contain harmful bacteria that cause outbreaks of disease, such as *Salmonella enteritidis, Campylobacter jejuni, Clostridium botulinum, Shigella sonnei,* or *Escherichia coli* O157:H7. These are the most common or serious of the more than 250 different known foodborne diseases (Chin, 1999; NIAID, 2002). Of these, salmonellosis is the most common.

An estimated 5 million *Salmonella* infections occur annually in the United States (Chin, 1999); they account for $1 billion yearly in direct and indirect medical costs (NIAID, 2002). Salmonellosis is characterized by sudden onset of headache, abdominal pain, diarrhea, nausea, vomiting, fever, and dehydration. The acute enterocolitis may develop into septicemia or a severe focal infection, such as endocarditis, meningitis, pneumonia, or pyelonephritis. Infants, the elderly, and debilitated persons are at greatest risk for death. It is conservatively estimated that 33% of poultry, 15% of pork, and 10% of beef products nationwide are contaminated with *Salmonella* because of inadequate processing and shipping methods. Cooking destroys the organism, but problems may be caused by eating undercooked foods (eg, rare roast beef) or handling raw meats.

There are several types of *Campylobacter* bacteria, but most cases of campylobacteriosis are casued by *C. jejuni.* It is the leading cause of bacterial diarrheal illness in the United States, affecting an estimated 2.4 million people every year. It causes between 5% and 14% of all diarrheal illness worldwide and primarily affects children younger than 5 years of age and young adults (15 to 29 years). In the United States, few people die from *Campylobacter* infection. Humans get infected from handling raw poultry, eating undercooked poultry, drinking nonchlorinated water or raw milk, or handling infected animal or human feces. Most frequently, poultry and cattle waste are the sources of the bacteria, but feces from puppies, kittens, and birds also may be contaminated.

Symptoms of the disease include diarrhea that is often bloody, abdominal cramping and pain, nausea and vomiting, fever, and fatigue. Symptoms usually lasts for 2 to 5 days,

and the diagnosis is made by laboratory testing to identify the organism in the stool of an infected person. Most people get better with no special treatment.

Botulism is a rare but serious illness caused by botulinum toxin produced by *C. botulinum* bacteria. The toxin affects the nerves and, if untreated, can cause paralysis and respiratory failure. An average of 110 cases of food, infant, and wound botulism are reported to the CDC each year, and 10 to 30 foodborne botulism outbreaks are reported every year. Although this illness does not occur frequently, it can be fatal if not treated quickly and properly. *C. botulinum* is anaerobic, which means that it can survive and grow with little or no oxygen; therefore, it can be found in low-acid foods in sealed containers. Outbreaks of the infection come from home-canned foods with low acid content, such as asparagus, green beans, beets, and corn, in addition to more unusual sources such as chili peppers, tomatoes, and improperly handled baked potatoes wrapped in aluminum foil. Syptoms of foodborne botulism include double vision, drooping eyelids, slurred speech, dry mouth, difficulty swallowing, and weak muscles. Symptoms begin within 18 to 36 hours after eating contaminated food. A health care provider can use laboratory tests to identify the toxin in the blood or stool of an infected person. If diagnosed early, botulism can be treated successfully with an antitoxin that blocks the action of the bacterial toxin circulating in the blood, but recovery takes many weeks. People who develop severe botulism experience breathing failure and paralysis and need to be put on ventilators. Ways to prevent foodborne botulism include following strict hygienic steps when home canning, refrigerating oils that contain garlic or herbs, keeping baked potatoes wrapped in aluminum foil hot until served (or refrigerating them), and considering boiling of home-canned foods before eating them, to kill any bacteria that might be in the food. *C. botulinum* was approved by the FDA in 1989 as a treatment for two eye muscle disorders and in 2000 for cervical dystonia. In April 2002, the FDA approved this toxin for temporary improvement in the appearance of moderate to severe frown lines between the eyebrows; it is marketed under the name Botox.

S. sonnei infection, also called bacillary dysentery, is an infectious disease caused by *Shigella* bacteria that is transmitted by the fecal-oral route. The CDC estimates that more than 400,000 cases occur every year in the United States, with about 18,000 cases reported to the CDC. People can be infected by eating food or drinking beverages contaminated by infected food handlers who did not wash their hands properly after using the bathroom, eating vegetables grown in fields containing sewage, eating food contaminated by flies that were bred in infected feces, or drinking or swimming in contaminated water. Outbreaks of shigellosis frequently occur in tropical or temperate climates, especially in areas with severe crowding or poor hygiene, and sometimes in day care and institutional settings. Symptoms include fever, tiredness, watery or bloody diarrhea, nausea and vomiting, and abdominal pain.

The last infectious foodborne disease discussed here is caused by one serotype of the *E. coli* bacterium. *E. coli*

O157:H7 is a particularly harmful type of *E. coli*. The designation O157:H7 refers to the chemical compounds found on the bacterium's surface. This type produces one or more related, powerful toxins that can severely damage the lining of the intestines. *E. coli* and its toxins have been found in undercooked or raw hamburgers, salami, alfalfa sprouts, lettuce, unpasteurized milk, apple juice and apple cider, and contaminated well water. Unsuspecting swimmers have been infected by accidentally swallowing unchlorinated or underchlorinated water in swimming pools contaminated by human feces. Symptoms of *E. coli* O157:H7 include nausea (and occasionally vomiting), severe abdominal cramps, watery or very bloody diarrhea, and tiredness that begins from 2 to 5 days after eating contaminated food. Most people recover from the infection without treatment. However hemolytic-uremic syndrome (HUS), a serious complication, can lead to kidney failure. In North America, HUS is the most common cause of acute kidney failure in children, who are particularly prone to this complication. Prevention of *E. coli* infection can be enhanced by eating only thoroughly cooked beef and beef products, cooking ground beef patties to an internal temperature of 160°F, avoiding unpasteurized juices, drinking only pasteurized milk, and washing fresh fruits and vegetables thoroughly before eating them raw or cooking them.

There are other causes of foodborne illnesses. Parasitic transmission usually takes the form of trichinosis, which is caused by ingestion of *Trichinella spiralis* in undercooked pork and is rarely seen in the United States. Various types of worm infestations have created serious health problems, particularly in developing countries. Viral food transmission is rare. Different types of chemical food contamination result from improper food handling or processing (eg, dirty machines used in food processing factories), from use of pesticides and herbicides by farmers, and from polluted water (eg, mercury in fish) (WHO, 2000).

International trade and travel, together with changes in demographics, consumer lifestyles, food production, and microbial adaptation, have led to the emergence of new foodborne diseases. Globalization of the food supply means that people are exposed, through foods purchased locally, to pathogens native to remote parts of the world. As a result of international travel, people who are exposed to foodborne hazards in a foreign country may bring the disease into their own country when they return, possibly exposing others in a location thousands of miles from the original source of the infection (Yassi et al., 2001).

Foods With Toxic Additives

A third health hazard from food comes from the intentional introduction of additives to food products. Because present-day consumers demand convenience foods and time-saving devices—and businesses want to produce food items with long shelf-lives, enhanced flavor, and lasting, vibrant colors—many foreign chemicals and synthetic products have been added to foods. Animals that are raised for food, such as chickens, pigs, and beef cattle, are often fed or injected with substances to speed their growth. As consumers shift toward healthier eating, they do not know and are only starting to question the effects these additives may have over time. For example, red dye no. 2 once was added to improve the color of certain food products but has since been identified as carcinogenic. Preservatives and chemical flavorings such as saccharin have also proved hazardous in large doses. It is still questionable what small doses may do with prolonged use. More recently, questions have been raised about potential long-range effects of NutraSweet, a sugar substitute. Furthermore, such natural flavor enhancers as salt and processed sugars appear in excessive quantities in some canned and packaged foods and are linked to unhealthy dietary consequences such as hypertension or obesity. In small doses these additives may not be harmful, but when additives are consumed in combination and over prolonged periods, they may create serious health consequences.

A more recent concern is the intentional contamination of food or water supplies with toxic substances or bacteria by foreign or domestic terrorist groups or by countries who consider us their enemy. Such potential terrorist activities could disable large portions of the population while striking fear among the rest. Homeland security efforts, begun in 2002, are addressing the primary and secondary prevention practices needed to protect against such possibilities. Homeland security in regard to environmental health and safety is discussed later in this chapter and in Chapter 6.

Food Irradiation

One promising tool for global food safety not yet mentioned is food irradiation. It is a process of imparting ionizing energy to food to kill microorganisms. Sometimes it is referred to as "electronic pasteurization." Just as with traditional heat pasteurization of milk, food irradiation can enhance the safety of foods such as meat, chicken, seafood, and spices, which cannot be pasteurized by heat without changing their nature to a cooked rather than a raw form. Irradiation is not a substitute for safe food handling and good manufacturing practices by processors, retailers, and consumers, but it is a method of promoting food safety that has been approved by some 50 countries worldwide. It has been applied comercially in the United States, Japan, and several European countries such as Belgium, France, and the Netherlands for many years, in some for longer than two decades.

Only certain ionizing energy sources can be used for food irradiation. Permitted gamma sources are the isotopes cobalt 60 and cesium 137. More recently, electron beams (e-beams) have become available as a source of ionizing energy in the United States and other countries. All of the previously mentioned organisms that cause foodborne diseases can be eradicated with the use of food irradiation. Although many questions have been raised about its safety and efficacy, food irradiation, according to the WHO, "is a thoroughly tested process and when established guidelines and procedures are followed, it can help ensure a safer and more plentiful food supply" (International Food Information Council [IFIC], 2002, p. 8).

Government's Role

It is the legal responsibility of food producers, processors, and manufacturers to guarantee the quality and safety of food products. However, conflicting motives, such as concern over loss of profit, often lead to careless or inadequate monitoring. Governmental regulatory agencies exist on the local, state, and federal levels to set standards and control the quality of food sold to the public. Such public health authorities as the FDA, the U. S. Department of Agriculture, and the USDHHS are all necessary to help ensure the purity of commercial food products. Included in their jurisdiction is supervision of the food service industry. Licensing requirements, sanitation standards, and inspections serve as control measures.

Governmental agencies cannot cover all the bases, however. For example, inadequate inspection of the quality of commercial fish sold for food has led to numerous outbreaks of hepatitis A and other illnesses. With the wide variety of possible contaminants and potential dangers, consumers' best protection lies in supervising their own food quality (see Important Telephone Numbers and Internet Resources at the end of this chapter).

The national budget in 2003 included an additional $4.3 billion for homeland security, to be used primarily by the National Institutes of Health, CDC, and FDA (APHA, 2002). In addition to vaccines, increased security, and upgrading of laboratories, there would be increased spending for food safety activities at FDA, including inspection of imported food. The Institute of Medicine, in their executive summary (Manning & Goldfrank, 2002), indicated that biologic agents with adverse effects on human health include viruses, bacteria, fungi, and toxins, some of which can be introduced into the food supply.

The distinguishing feature of biological agents other than toxins is their ability to propagate— exposure to an extremely small amount can lead to an overwhelming infection and in some cases the victim may even become a source of infection for additional victims. This propagation within the exposed person takes time, however, so the effects of viruses, bacteria, and fungi may not become apparent until days or weeks after the initial exposure. Diagnosis of infection in individual patients will also be rendered more difficult because most of the agents considered to be likely threats are very rarely seen in U. S. cities and the initial syptoms that they produce (fever, headache, general malaise) are also characteristic of those produced by many common diseases" (Manning & Goldfrank, 2002, p. 4).

Nurse's Role

Community health nurses can have a significant impact through health education. Most bacterial and viral foodborne diseases can be prevented if people know and practice proper cooking and storage of food as well as proper personal hygiene (Display 10–3).

DISPLAY 10–3

Ten Golden Rules for Safe Food Preparation

To prevent and control foodborne disease, the World Health Organization has developed the following rules:
1. Choose food processed for safety.
2. Cook food thoroughly.
3. Eat cooked food immediately.
4. Store cooked food carefully.
5. Reheat cooked foods thoroughly.
6. Avoid contact between raw foods and cooked foods.
7. Wash hands repeatedly.
8. Keep all kitchen surfaces meticulously clean.
9. Protect foods from insects, rodents, and other animals.
10. Use pure water.

(Chin, J. [Ed.]. [1999]. *Control of communicable diseases manual* [17th ed.]. Washington, DC: American Public Health Association.)

Nurses can teach the basics of keeping perishable products sufficiently refrigerated, discarding foods that may be old or spoiled, cooking foods thoroughly, and bringing water to a full boil when appropriate to be certain of eliminating microbes. Reheating leftovers in slow cookers, steam tables, or chafing dishes is not recommended because foods may stay for too long in the "danger zone," between 40°F and 140°F (USDA, 2000). Bacteria multiply rapidly at these temperatures.

A consumer education program that is sponsored by the Partnership for Food Safety Education is called Fight BAC! This is a public-private partnership of industry, government, and consumer groups created to educate the public about safe food handling to help reduce foodborne illness. Educational material are available for use by teachers, health educators, and community health nurses when working with groups in the community (USDA, 2000).

Nurses can emphasize washing and cleaning of produce and tools used in food processing, including the preparer's own hands. Finally, nurses can educate people to watch for signs of contamination. A dented can, for example, may signal the presence of living bacteria that are using the oxygen within the container and contaminating its contents. Nurses can raise public awareness regarding the conditions of supermarkets, restaurants, and other food handlers. They can also help promote community standards, enabling legislation, and policies for safer food supplies.

Waste Disposal

The United States generates more solid and hazardous waste per capita than any other industrialized nation. In 1990, each person in the United States produced, on average, 4.3 lb of combustible or landfill-maintained waste per day. In 1995, this figure was 4.4 lb, equivalent to 1600 lb of municipal solid waste each year (Fig. 10–3). More frightening is the fact that U. S. industry produces the equivalent of more than 1 ton of *hazardous* waste per person each year. In addition, some 8.1 million tons of toxins were released into the air in 1993. The year 2010 target is 2.0 tons (USDHHS, 2000).

With the vast amounts of waste produced in the form of household garbage, human excreta, and agricultural and industrial byproducts, including hazardous chemical and radioactive substances, it is no wonder that waste management and disposal has become an important and pressing topic in recent decades. New technology has effectively addressed some of the problems, but there is still much need for improvement. Solid and hazardous wastes pose a wide range of public health concerns. Therefore, it is imperative that health officials, including community health nurses, become aware of the possible health hazards that these wastes present to individuals and to communities.

Disposal of Human Waste

One of the oldest environmental health hazards comes from improper disposal of human excreta. Although industrialized nations have successfully addressed the problem, it continues to be widespread in developing nations and in rural, poverty-stricken communities. Human wastes, particularly feces, provide a perfect environment in which bacteria and disease-causing parasites can live and reproduce. Therefore, contaminated drinking water, food grown in contaminated soil, and, of course, direct contact with the contaminated water or soil can cause infections. For example, hookworm, a problem in the United States in the early part of the 20th century, usually enters the body through the skin of bare feet (Yassi et al., 2001).

Disposal of Garbage

Dumping, burning, and burying are the most common solid-waste disposal methods. Dumping is problematic, because garbage dumps provide perfect conditions for the breeding of rats, flies, and other disease-carrying organisms and may potentially be a source of water contamination from runoff. Dumps also are eyesores that take up valuable land resources. Burning, although it reduces the volume of garbage, produces noxious odors and pollutes the air.

In 2002, much of the air over the city of Fresno, California, was polluted for longer than 3 weeks when a 5-acre private garbage dump, some three stories high, caught fire. It continued to burn and smolder despite the best efforts of several fire-fighting companies using water and eventually foam. Because the dump was piled so high, the interior of the pile could not be reached in a timely manner. Hundreds of citizens living up to a mile from the dump site suffered upper respiratory tract symptoms, and a haze was created over the city. Asthmatic children and adults suffered greater symptoms. Nearby schools cancelled outdoor activities (eg, recess in elementary schools) and after-school sports for weeks. By the time the fire was almost extinguished, several public and private health care providers (hospitals and clinics) collaborated and offered a free screening service, held at a local school, for those who were worried that their health may have been affected negatively by the fire. This was an important service that demonstrated a coordinated volunteer effort, because those affected were mostly low-income families living in the economically depressed section of the city nearest the dump, people who were most likely to be without health insurance.

Sanitary landfills have generally replaced dumps as a more effective way to dispose of refuse by burying it. With proper handling, including covering and daily sealing (to prevent insect and rodent breeding), this method has proved satisfactory for solid waste and eliminates such problems as occurred in California.

Disposal of Hazardous Waste

Disposal of toxic chemical and radioactive wastes produced by industry is another grave concern. The threat is serious, because one cannot be certain of all of the effects of these wastes or whether present methods of disposal are foolproof. Furthermore, many of these wastes escape containment or accidentally leak into water systems and into the soil to contaminate drinking water and food.

Primary methods of hazardous waste disposal include burial in double-lined cells in landfills, surface impoundments for special treatment and storage, waste-injected underground steel- and concrete-lined wells, solid waste piles, and land treatment facilities. Some hazardous wastes are incinerated before disposal. With the disposal of hazardous

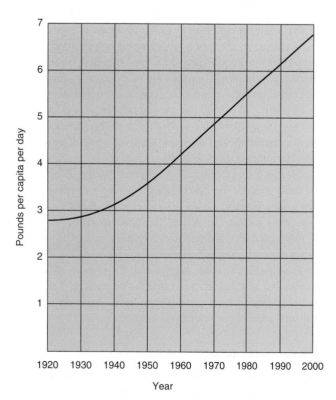

FIGURE 10–3. United States trend in per capita refuse production.

waste, it is always a concern that storage containers may not be leakproof, and interference with dump sites or storage facilities may expose the environment to these toxic substances. Examples of chemical contamination have been discovered in communities such as Elizabeth, New Jersey; Times Beach, Michigan; and Love Canal, New York, where residents developed cancer and other health problems because of exposures to toxic chemicals. There is also the continuing problem of securing disposal sites for the increasing volume of hazardous wastes. Communities seek the advantages of new technology but do not wish to bury the resulting wastes in their backyards. In many instances, legislators and public officials have faced serious conflict in their efforts to locate acceptable toxic waste dump sites.

With burgeoning industry and new technology in the world today, society has developed more sophisticated means of energy production, more labor-saving devices, and more practical and innovative products. This massive new product development has created a problem for the environment—how to handle the vast amount of waste created from discardable goods, byproducts of production, and the "throwaway" mentality. For example, more than 18 billion disposable diapers, which alone are estimated to account for 2% of municipal wastes, are used each year in the United States. Until the late 1990s, the diapers were made of durable plastics and were estimated to resist deterioration for up to 500 years after burial in a landfill. They are now made of treated paper with an absorbent gel within the diaper, and about 40% of the diaper product in most brands is biodegradable. One mom-entrepreneur in Sweden created a 70% biodegradable diaper called Nature Boy & Girl that sells in the United States (Stanley, 2002). It is possible to create an environmentally friendly product. However, when questioned, 99% of disposable diaper users say they discard them directly into the trash instead of flushing fecal material down the toilet. Consequently, a large amount of raw, untreated sewage is ending up in landfills, with the potential for serious problems in the future. Not only does the development of such products take an enormous toll on natural resources, but the quantity and nature of the resulting wastes also pose serious health hazards and environmental problems. Improper disposal of domestic products, such as toxic insect sprays, some household cleaners, partially used paint cans, used auto oil, and termite fumigation chemicals, causes health dangers (Calvert et al., 1998).

Government's Role

The government's role is to establish standards for safe waste disposal and to monitor and enforce compliance. In most modernized urban areas, the public sewage system handles waste by treating raw sewage and disposing it into a body of water. In most instances in the United States, state health departments oversee proper waste treatment and disposal. In rural areas where people usually have private septic systems, the supervision of proper waste handling is difficult and not as consistent. Health workers in rural settings should be alert to the potential dangers posed by inconsistent monitoring.

More research is needed to determine the effects of various disposal methods and to improve disposal practices. It is imperative that people not only learn how to dispose of wastes safely—to protect humans, the environment, and future generations—but that they also look seriously at other options. More emphasis must be placed on transforming waste into usable products, increasing the amounts and kinds of recycling done, and reducing the amount of refuse produced in the first place.

Nurse's Role

Community health nurses can encourage the positive actions described by educating the public and lobbying for enabling legislation. Nurses can promote greater sensitivity among citizens to the problems of accumulating waste with its potential health hazards, encourage clients to buy products that can be recycled, and discourage use of aerosol spray containers, plastics, and other nonrecyclable items. Such information sharing occurs during home visits when conducting family and home assessments; during group educational opportunities that arise in apartment complexes or neighborhoods where several families are being served; with school children when the community health nurse is invited into the classroom by the teacher; or in conjunction with environmental health services when a community is blighted by waste management problems and the nurse speaks to groups of parents, teens, or children. The possibilities are limited only by the nurse's imagination, priorities, community connections, and time constraints.

Insect and Rodent Control

All human communities are affected by the insects and rodents living in their environment. On the least dangerous level, they can cause irritation (eg, mosquito or flea bites) and discomfort (eg, infestations of bedbugs or lice). They can also pose a direct threat to health through such things as attacks by diseased rats or squirrels. Insects and rodents can consume and, in turn, contaminate food. However, by far the most serious health hazard they impose is through their role as *vectors,* nonhuman carriers of disease organisms that can transmit these organisms directly to humans.

The most common vectors are mosquitos, flies, ticks, roaches, fleas, rats, mice, and ground squirrels. All of these vectors can serve as reservoirs for germs that they then transmit through physical contact with humans or by contaminating human foodstuffs or water. Table 10–3 summarizes some of the diseases spread by vectors. Cases of vector-spread diseases range from the 14th-century bubonic plague epidemic spread by rat fleas, which killed a quarter of the European population, to the mosquito-spread outbreaks of West Nile virus that began in New York in 1999.

Government's Role

Vector surveys, research, and control are usually left to local and state health departments. These agencies have also im-

TABLE 10-3

Diseases Transmitted By Various Insect Vectors

Vector	Disease	Pathogen
Mosquitoes		
Anopheles sp	Malaria	*Plasmodium* sp (protozoa)
Culex sp	Filariasis	*Wuchereria bancrofti* and *malayi* (nematodes)
Culex sp	Encephalitis	Arbovirus
Aedes aegypti	Yellow fever	Arbovirus
Aedes aegypti	Dengue	Arbovirus
Biting Flies		
Deerfly	Filariasis	*Loa loa* (nematode)
Black fly	River blindness	*Onchocerca volvulus* (nematode)
Tsetse fly	Sleeping sickness	*Trypanosoma gambiense* and *rhodesiense* (protozoa)
Sand fly	Kala-azar	*Leishmania donovani*
	Tropical ulcer	*Leishmania tropica*
	Cutaneous leishmaniasis	*Leishmania mexicana*
	Espundia	*Leishmania braziliensis* (protozoa)
	Phlebotomus fever	Arbovirus
Other Insects		
Gnats	Filariasis	*Mansonella ozzardi* (nematode)
Rat flea	Plague	*Yersinia pestis* (bacteria)
	Murine typhus	*Rickettsia mooseri*
Body louse	Epidemic typhus	*Rickettsia prowazekii*
	Trench fever	*Rickettsia quintana*
Tick	Rocky Mountain spotted fever	*Rickettsia rickettsii*
Tick	Colorado tick fever	Arbovirus
Mite	Riskettsialpox	*Rickettsia akari*

(Blumenthal, D., & Ruttenber, J. [1994]. *Introduction to environmental health* [2nd ed.]. New York: Springer.)

plemented community awareness and pest control programs. Once vectors have been found, health workers can attempt to control them through many methods. Approaches used in the past included trapping of rodents, poisoning, spraying with pesticides, and eliminating areas where vectors breed (eg, draining or filling marshes to control mosquito populations). It is essential in planning any approach to consider the possible health hazards to humans or other living organisms and the effect the method will have on the ecosystem—how it may upset the ecologic balance. In 1986, WHO advocated that the most basic, yet effective, approach is to improve sanitary conditions and practices to the extent that the condition encouraging the multiplication of insects and rodents no longer exists (WHO, 1986).

Nurse's Role

The community health nurse can contribute through awareness of the presence and possible health threat of rodents and insects. By remaining alert to the presence of rodents and insects in homes, schools, and communities, nurses can take measures to educate affected persons and notify proper au-

thorities when corrective action is needed. They can assist this effort by surveying homes and neighborhoods for exposed rubbish or conditions that might attract insects and rodents. They can also promote preventive efforts through education and influencing policy makers.

Some of the simple changes families can make that will help to eliminate rodents and insects include the following:

- Ensure that screens exist on all open windows, and use screen doors.
- Wash dishes, pots, and pans after meals, and clean counter surfaces.
- Keep pet food off the floor; fill the pet dish when the pet eats, and do not leave it on the floor for extended periods.
- Keep foodstuffs that insects may infest, such as cereals, corn meal, and flour, in closed plastic containers.
- Ensure that doors and windows fit properly; use calking if the outside can be seen through gaps in doors or windows.
- Keep floors swept and vacuumed in rooms where people eat, to eliminate food supply for rodents and insects; preferably, eat only in the kitchen or dining room.
- Remove trash bags that include food scraps and food

packaging from the home daily and place in garbage containers that are kept outside and have tight-fitting lids.

Safety in the Home, Worksite, and Community

As we have seen, the environment of the home, the workplace, and the community at large significantly affects people's health. This section addresses six additional problems that affect people's safety: exposure to toxic chemicals, radiation exposure, injury hazards, noise pollution, psychological hazards, and facing terrorist dangers.

Exposure to Toxic Chemicals

The number of natural and synthetic chemicals in the environment and the threats they pose to human and environmental health are overwhelming. Approximately 10 million chemical compounds were synthesized in laboratories in the 20th century (Yassi et al., 2001). Most chemicals are intermediates in the manufacture of end products for human use. All chemicals are toxic to some degree, with the health risk being primarily a function of the severity of the toxicity and the extent of exposure. About 1500 toxins constitute the greatest threat of hazardous exposures, but only some 450 have established threshold limit values and adequate toxicity testing. Several hundred new chemicals come into use each year that are basically untested (Schecter, 1998). This section presents a general overview of the different categories of environmental chemicals, where they are found, the dangers they impose, and community health nurse's role in forestalling or detecting those dangers.

Toxic chemicals include those that do not contain carbon, are not derived from living matter, are usually of mineral composition, and have an inherent capacity to cause injury to a living organism (Yassi et al., 2001). Inorganic toxic chemicals include halogens, corrosive materials, and metals. Substances such as zinc, cadmium, lead, iron, calcium, sodium, potassium, magnesium, and copper often play an important and healthful role in human physiology, but they become toxic if a person is exposed to large quantities. A toddler's accidental ingestion of several chewable vitamins with iron can cause mild gastrointestinal distress or—if many are ingested—devastating physiologic damage.

Lead is a toxic agent that is frequently found in occupational or industrial settings. Workers must be careful to avoid inhaling lead fumes or exposing their families to lead dust on their clothing. Lead was once widely used in paint and can still be found in leaded gasoline and batteries. It is the top environmental health hazard for children, with 890,000 young children in the United States affected annually (Cohen, 2001; Markowitz & Rosner, 2000). According to the Agency for Toxic Substances and Disease Registry (ATSDR), lead is ranked first among the top 10 hazardous substances in people of all ages. It is especially dangerous in children, whose high metabolic activity makes them more susceptible (Brown et al., 2001). In utero lead exposure is another concern. Even low-level exposure to lead has a dangerous cumulative effect leading to nerve damage, neurobehavioral problems, learning disabilities, and mental retardation (Yassi et al., 2001). This has been observed, for example, in children who play outside and are exposed to the lead in ambient air or play near roadways where dirt has absorbed lead from gasoline. Low levels of lead have been detected in household dust, in drinking water, and in foods and beverages.

In occupational settings, workers have been exposed to lead since long before the Industrial Revolution, because lead was used for making pipes, pigments, and bullets. Workers in some occupations such as smelters have been exposed to high levels of lead, as have those exposed to leaded gasoline and lead-containing paints. Fortunately, now we are aware of the dangers of lead exposure, and it can be avoided or the worker protected. However, if lead is present in the environment, children can be accidentally exposed.

Community health nurses need to check with clients for possible exposure and examine client homes for lead-based paint. Lead-based paint is now restricted in residential use, but any painted building that is more than 35 years old may still have lead paint. In particular, nurses can warn parents to keep their young children from eating paint chips from windowsills, walls, or furniture painted with lead-based paint; to keep them away from lead-infused dirt near roads; and to avoid dust and debris when older buildings are being torn down or renovated.

Mercury is also highly toxic. It is used in many scientific instruments, electronic equipment, crop fungicides, and the processing of dental fillings. Historically, mercury was used in goldsmithing, mirror-making, explosive detonators, and as an antiseptic and antifungal agent. Inorganic mercury can be changed through bacterial action in industrial processes to more toxic organic compounds, as in the bleach used for paper manufacturing. Toxic mercurials then escape into the environment and contaminate the food chain. In 1953, at Minanata Bay on the island of Kyushu, Japan, many persons died and more were disabled with permanent neurologic impairment from eating mercury-contaminated seafood. In Iraq in 1972, hundreds of fatalities occurred among people who used treated seed to make bread (Yassi et al., 2001).

Other harmful metals include aluminum, which recently was associated with certain mental disorders and has been found in high levels in the brain tissues of patients with Alzheimer's disease (Schecter, 1998). Chromium, nickel, and arsenic are other toxic compounds.

Many toxic chemicals are byproducts of the petroleum industry, including many alcohols, ethers, hydrocarbons (eg, benzene), medicines, and plastics that contain carbon. Ingestion or exposure can cause cancer, liver and kidney disease, birth defects, and many other health problems. Pesticides for household and crop use, particularly dichlorodiphenyltrichloroethane (DDT), have created major health hazards. DDT, a very dangerous chemical used for pest control, was banned in 1972 in the United States because of environmental and health concerns. However, it is still present in the environment and continues to be used illicitly, posing a danger to farmers and migrant farmworkers in particular. It has also been used legally in certain countries to control malaria.

Exposure to toxic chemicals can have far-reaching effects on humans. People may come in contact with them in their homes through building materials, cleaning products, or airborne dust. Another source is the workplace, where many different compounds are created and used each day. Toxic substances also may be transferred home from the workplace in motor vehicles and on clothing or shoes. In the greater community, pollutants in the air and food chain create further hazards. Toxic chemicals can cause illness when they are inhaled, come into contact with the skin (as in industrial accidents where chemicals are spilled), or are ingested (as when a child drinks from a liquid cleaning solvent bottle). Table 10–4 lists some common workplace carcinogens.

Exposure to Radiation

Radiation is technically defined as a process by which energy is propagated through space or matter. Natural radiation from the sun, soil, and minerals can be found in virtually all areas of the earth's environment. The largest natural source of radiation exposure is airborne radon. Some radioactive substances produce particles, and others produce rays (Fell-Carslon, 2003). Radiation in its manmade form has numerous beneficial uses in science and industry for lasers, radiographs that help in the diagnosis of disease, and production of nuclear energy. It is found in many home electronic devices, such as television sets, smoke detectors, and microwave ovens (see Levels of Prevention Matrix). Other manmade forms of radiation can be produced for negative purposes, such as conventional bombs laced with radioactive material, called "dirty bombs" (see later discussion).

Regardless of its source, radiation is a threat to human health in the workplace and in the general environment. The extent of danger depends on the dose and type of radiation. For example, casualties among miners can be attributed to their prolonged and intense exposure to radioactive minerals such as uranium. Prolonged exposure can cause skin ulcers, damage to cells, cancer, premature aging, kidney dysfunction, and genetic disorders in the children of those whose cells have been damaged. Naturally occurring radioactive materials are present in tobacco and further threaten the health of smokers. A two-pack-a-day cigarette smoker receives more than 10 times the long-term dose-rate limit for radiation exposure.

T A B L E   10–4

Occupational Carcinogens

Carcinogen	Cancer Site	Examples of Exposed Occupations
4-Aminodiphenyl Auramine β-Naphthylamine Magenta Benzidine	Bladder	Dye manufacturing, rubber manufacturing
Arsenic	Skin, lung, liver	Metal smelting, arsenic pesticide production, metal alloy workers
Asbestos	Lung, mesothelium, gastrointestinal tract	Asbestos miners, insulators, shipyard workers
Benzene	Leukemia (blood-forming organs)	Petrochemical workers, chemists
Bischloromethyl ether (BCME)	Lung	Organic chemical synthesizers
Cadmium	Prostate	Cadmium alloy workers, welders
Chromium/chromates	Lung, nasal sinuses	Chromate producers, metal workers
Coke oven emissions	Lung, kidney	Coke oven workers
Foundry emissions	Lung	Foundry workers
Leather dust	Nasal cavity, nasal sinuses, bladder	Shoe manufacturing
Nickel	Lung, nasal passages	Nickel smelting, metal workers
Radiation (x-rays)	Leukemia (blood-forming organs), skin, breast, thyroid, bone	Radiologists, industrial radiographers, atomic energy workers
Radon gas	Lung	Uranium and feldspar miners
Soots, tars, and oil Petroleum (aromatic hydrocarbons)	Skin, lung, bladder, scrotum	Roofers, chimney sweepers, shale oil workers
Ultraviolet light	Skin	Outdoor workers
Vinyl chloride	Liver, brain, lung	Polyvinyl chloride synthesizers, rubber workers
Welding fumes	Lung	Welders
Wood dust	Nasal passages	Hardwood workers, furniture makers

(Blumenthal, D., & Ruttenber, J. [1994]. *Introduction to environmental health* [2nd ed]. New York: Springer.)

LEVELS OF PREVENTION MATRIX

SITUATION: Increase to at least 20% the proportion of homes in which homeowners/occupants have tested for radon concentrations (baseline: 11% in 1994). (From *Healthy People 2010* [USDHHS, 2000].)

GOAL: Using the three levels of prevention, negative health conditions are avoided, or are promptly diagnosed and treated, and the fullest possible potential is restored.

PRIMARY PREVENTION		SECONDARY PREVENTION		TERTIARY PREVENTION		
Health Promotion and Education	*Health Protection*	*Early Diagnosis*	*Prompt Treatment*	*Rehabilitation*	*Primary Prevention*	
					Health Promotion and Education	*Health Protection*
Conduct community education regarding the nature and dangers of inhaling radon gas	Require sealed basement construction to avoid release of radon into building from underlying soil	Periodic testing of radon levels	Circulate air with fans in homes with low concentrations Use fan and positive-ion generator to decrease inhaled concentrations	Seal cracks in basement floors and walls Install subslab exhaust system below basement floors	Educate the surrounding community members regarding their risk	Require building modifications where radon concentrations are high

A certain amount of natural radiation exposure from the sun is important for the absorption of vitamin D. However, intentional exposure by sunbathing, still a popular activity in many areas, must be tempered with the use of lotions with sunscreen. The highest screening protection factor (SPF) considered effective is a factor of 30. This should be used by people of all ages when exposed to the sun for more than 10 to 15 minutes in winter or summer. Sunscreen is more important at higher elevations and when participating in outdoor snow activities, such as skiing, because the snow reflects the sun's rays (Display 10–4).

A major area of concern centers on the problems associated with nuclear energy and nuclear weapons. The production of radioactive wastes, the threat of accidental exposure from unsafe reactors, and possible fallout from weapons testing generate real fears. These fears were confirmed by the nuclear reactor accidents at Three Mile Island and Chernobyl, which allowed radioactive ions to escape into the atmosphere. Accidents of this type are uncommon, however, and the safe operation of nuclear power plants exposes communities to much less radiation than other sources, such as medical or natural radiation. The risk of radiation exposure as a weapon of war or terrorist activity is discussed later.

Injury Hazards

An environmental characteristic that must be considered in assessing health risks is a community's level of physical safety.

How likely is it that injuries will occur? This is a very important question when one considers that in the United States unintentional injuries kill more people during the first three decades of life than any other cause of death (National Center for Injury Prevention and Control [NCIPC], 2001). In 1997, a total of 95,644 Americans died from unintentional injuries (USDHHS, 2000). Groups at highest risk are the young, the elderly, the poor, minorities, and rural residents (Table 10–5).

Not surprisingly, motor vehicle crashes cause more than 42,000 deaths and 3 million injuries per year (NCIPC, 2001). The second-ranked cause of injury death is falls, followed by poisoning, drowning, and residential fires. Alcohol plays a major role in many of these injuries and subsequent deaths, particularly with motor vehicle crashes and drownings (USDHHS, 2000). Additionally, many unintentional injuries occur in the home (see Chapter 30 for home-safety assessment).

Another area of safety concern is violence. Individuals, families, schools, and communities are frequently at risk for violent acts stemming from domestic quarrels and abuse, dysfunctional behavior, and crime. Violence and the injuries and deaths it causes are becoming one of the most urgent health problems in the United States. About 35% of injury-related deaths are intentional, primarily homicides and suicides. Use of handguns and domestic abuse make women, children, and the elderly particularly at risk for injury and death (NCIPC, 2001).

Community health nurses have a responsibility to assess situations for the threat of potential physical harm and to

T A B L E 1 0 – 5

Ten Leading Causes of Deaths by Age Group, 1998 (With Injuries/Homicide/Suicide Highlighted)

Age Groups

Rank	<1	1–4	5–9	10–14	15–24	25–34	35–44	45–54	55–64	65+	Total
1	Congenital Anomalies 6,212	Unintentional Injuries 1,935	Unintentional Injuries 1,544	Unintentional Injuries 1,710	Unintentional Injuries 13,349	Unintentional Injuries 12,045	Malignant Neoplasms 17,022	Malignant Neoplasms 45,747	Malignant Neoplasms 87,024	Heart Disease 605,673	Heart Disease 724,859
2	Short Gestation 4,101	Congenital Anomalies 564	Malignant Neoplasms 487	Malignant Neoplasms 526	Homicide 5,506	Suicide 5,365	Unintentional Injuries 15,127	Heart Disease 35,056	Heart Disease 65,068	Malignant Neoplasms 384,186	Malignant Neoplasms 541,532
3	SIDS 2,822	Homicide 399	Congenital Anomalies 198	Suicide 317	Suicide 4,135	Homicide 4,565	Heart Disease 13,593	Unintentional Injuries 10,946	Bronchitis Emphysema Asthma 10,162	Cerebro-vascular 139,144	Cerebro-vascular 158,448
4	Maternal Complications 1,343	Malignant Neoplasms 365	Homicide 170	Homicide 290	Malignant Neoplasms 1,699	Malignant Neoplasms 4,385	Suicide 6,837	Liver Disease 5,744	Cerebro-vascular 9,653	Bronchitis Emphysema Asthma 97,896	Bronchitis Emphysema Asthma 112,584
5	Respiratory Distress Synd. 1,295	Heart Disease 214	Heart Disease 156	Congenital Anomalies 173	Heart Disease 1,057	Heart Disease 3,207	HIV 5,746	Cerebro-vascular 5,709	Diabetes 8,705	Pneumonia & Influenza 82,989	Unintentional Injuries 97,835
6	Placenta Cord Membranes 961	Pneumonia & Influenza 146	Pneumonia & Influenza 70	Heart Disease 170	Congenital Anomalies 450	HIV 2,912	Homicide 3,567	Suicide 5,131	Unintentional Injuries 7,340	Diabetes 48,974	Pneumonia & Influenza 91,871
7	Perinatal Infections 815	Septicemia 89	Bronchitis Emphysema Asthma 54	Bronchitis Emphysema Asthma 98	Bronchitis Emphysema Asthma 239	Cerebro-vascular 670	Liver Disease 3,370	Diabetes 4,386	Liver Disease 5,279	Unintentional Injuries 32,975	Diabetes 64,751
8	Unintentional Injuries 754	Perinatal Period 75	Benign Neoplasms 52	Pneumonia & Influenza 51	Pneumonia & Influenza 215	Diabetes 636	Cerebro-vascular 2,650	HIV 3,120	Pneumonia & Influenza 3,856	Nephritis 22,640	Suicide 30,575
9	Intrauterine Hypoxia 461	Cerebro-vascular 57	Cerebro-vascular 35	Cerebro-vascular 47	HIV 194	Pneumonia & Influenza 531	Diabetes 1,885	Bronchitis Emphysema Asthma 2,828	Suicide 2,963	Alzheimer's Disease 22,416	Nephritis 26,182
10	Pneumonia & Influenza 441	Benign Neoplasms 53	HIV 29	Benign Neoplasms 32	Cerebro-vascular 178	Liver Disease 506	Pneumonia & Influenza 1,400	Pneumonia & Influenza 2,167	Septicemia 2,093	Septicemia 19,012	Liver Disease 25,192

Source: National Center for Health Statistics, 2000.

Chart developed by the National Center for Injury Prevention and Control, CDC.

DISPLAY 10-4

The TAN Commandments

1. Don't sunbathe.
2. Wear protective clothing and a wide-brimmed hat when in the sun for more than 15 minutes.
3. Don't spend time in the sun without a sun-screening lotion.
4. Use a sun-screening lotion with the highest SPF available (SPF 30).
5. Reapply sun-screening lotion periodically, especially after swimming or perspiring.
6. Stay out of the sun when the sun's rays are the most direct, usually between 10 AM and 2 PM.
7. Remember that even on cloudy days you can burn—use sun-screening lotion and/or protective clothing.
8. Be aware that sun exposure can be dangerous in any season. Wear sun-screening lotion and/or protective clothing when gardening in the spring, swimming in the summer, hiking in the fall, or skiing in the winter.
9. Although people of all ages and races can be affected by the sun's rays, infants and children are especially vulnerable because their skin is more sensitive and the sun's effects are cumulative. Be especially vigilant in protecting children with hats, clothing, and sun-screening lotion.
10. Take additional precautions if living or vacationing at higher altitudes, where the effects of sun exposure are greater.

work with other professionals to design preventive measures. Safety education and primary prevention is a major role of the community health nurse. This teaching can begin one-on-one or in groups of pregnant women attending clinics or Women, Infants, and Children (WIC) appointments. The topics to be discussed are many but usually include anticipatory guidance to enhance infant safety, creating a child-proof home, and acquiring a car seat and using it properly. Topics and clients will change as the nurse branches out to preschools, schools, youth clubs, parent-teacher organizations, and other groups. The nurse may become a resource for others who do the teaching, and knowing where to find safety information, brochures, and other "handouts" is important in information dissemination. The subjects of levels of prevention with personal and stranger (individual or group) violence is discussed further in Chapters 25 and 36.

Exposure to Noise Pollution

People in the United States are bombarded by noise from many sources. Noise has two definitions. One, related to its physical properties, defines noise as *a sound, generally random in nature, the spectrum of which does not exhibit clearly defined frequency components.* A simpler and more subjec-

tive definition is *any unwanted sound* (Behar, Chasin, & Cheesman, 2000). Household appliances, traffic, radios, machinery, and voices are typical noise sources. However, a teen's loud music choice may be a source of noise. Noise is measured three ways. First, noise is measured by the magnitude of the noise, or *decibels*. A whisper may measure 10 to 20 decibels, and a fire engine siren may measure 80 to 100 decibels. Another way to measure is by the high and low tones of the noise, referred to as *frequency*. A male voice usually has a lower frequency than a female voice does, and a drum is lower than a flute. A third factor is the *time history,* or the length of time one has been exposed to the noise.

Noise has been cited as a major environmental health problem. Prolonged exposure (months to years) to extremely loud noises, such as pneumatic drills or rock music, can cause temporary or permanent hearing loss (Behar, Chasin, & Chessman, 2000). Other noises, perhaps occasional machinery noises at the workplace or residential exposure to airport traffic, can lead to general annoyance; headaches; sleep, speech, and task interference; alterations in emotions; stress; lowered body resistance to disease; ulcers; and aggravation of existing physical disorders. The effects vary in severity depending on the intensity and duration of the noises and the disposition of the people concerned.

There are four methods of control. First, the source of the noise can be relocated (eg, having the teen band practice in the garage instead of the family room) or replaced (eg, fixing or replacing a broken toy or appliance). Another method is to do something about the path of the noise. A barrier, enclosure, or muffler may be effective. This is often seen along highways where 8- to 10-foot walls have been built between the highway traffic noises and housing developments. An automobile muffler serves a similar purpose of "muffling" the engine's sound. A third method of control is to relocate the receiver. For instance, if parents are annoyed by the loudness and music choice of their teenager, they may want to go to another room in the house. Finally, the receiver can use hearing protectors such as ear plugs. For example, airline ground-crew members wear highly sophisticated hearing protectors.

Community responses to noise pollution take many forms. There are usually community standards for noise abatement after 10 PM and before 8 AM. Police will respond if a neighbor complains about a loud neighborhood party. As highways creep into suburban neighborhoods, barriers are erected in the form of walls or noise-absorbing trees and shrubbery. Standards for the decibel levels of appliances and tools are set by manufacturers, following OSHA standards. Packaging instructions indicate whether hearing protectors should be used when the tool or piece of equipment is in use.

Community health nurses can inform families of the damage or annoyance noises can inflict and help people quiet their environment. If community-generated noise comes from industry, the nurse can collaborate with health team members of the offending company and work to bring about positive changes that improve the relationship between the company and the community. In one low-income community during the 1950s, an aluminum factory created a loud, repetitive booming noise all day long that made it impossible for people in nearby housing to speak to each other within their homes without raising their voices or shouting. It was impossible to sit on a porch and hear someone nearby speak. OSHA did not exist at the time, and community attempts at changing the situation did not make an impact. It was not until the company's manufacturing processes changed years later that the community felt relief. In the meantime, many families left the neighborhood as soon as they were able, leaving the housing choices near the factory for the uniformed.

Exposure to Biologic Pollutants

Biologic pollutants or hazards include all of the forms of life, as well as the nonliving products they produce, that can cause adverse health effects (Yassi et al., 2001). Some common indoor biologic pollutants include animal dander (minute scales from hair, feathers, or skin), dust mite and cockroach parts, fungi, molds, infectious agents (bacteria and viruses), plants, pollen, and a wide variety of toxins and allergens. The recently discovered type of biologic hazard called the *prion* (disease-producing protein particle) has been related to a number of diseases, including Creutzfeldt-Jacob ("mad cow") disease (Yassi et al., 2001).

Breathing indoor air contaminated with biologic pollutants can cause health problems or make existing health problems worse, especially among infants, young children, the elderly, and those with chronic illnesses. The effects range from allergic symptoms (conjunctival inflammation, rhinitis, sneezing, nasal congestion, itching, dyspnea, coughing, wheezing, chest tightness, headache, and malaise) to infections and toxicity (Last, 1998).

Home conditions that promote this type of pollution include damp areas, which encourage the growth and buildup of biologic pollutants. It is estimated that 30% to 50% of all structures, mostly in warm, moist climates, have damp conditions. In addition, there are particular items and areas in homes and personal environments where biologic pollutants are commonly found and where proper cleaning or care is especially important. These include

- Humidifiers and dehumidifiers
- Bathrooms without vents or windows
- Kitchens without vents or windows
- Refrigerator drip pans
- Laundry rooms with an unvented dryer
- Unventilated attics
- Damp basement floors with carpeting
- Bedding
- Closets on outside walls
- Heating/air conditioning systems
- Bookshelves, curio cabinets, and other areas that accumulate dust
- Dog and cat bedding, litter boxes, bird cages, fish tanks, and so forth
- Areas with water damage (around windows, the roof, or the basement)

- In automobile ventilation systems where moisture pools after use of the air conditioner

The most important role of the community health nurse is to assess clients' homes for possible biologic pollutants and then to provide them with the information they need to correct or improve the situation. If clients are renting a house or apartment and the dampness is caused by structural conditions or owner negligence, the nurse may act as an advocate for the clients to remedy the potentially hazardous situation. Display 10–5 includes a list of assessment questions the nurse should apply during home visits when clients may have been exposed to biologic pollutants.

DISPLAY 10–5

Assessment Questions to Detect Biologic Pollutants in Homes

- ❑ Does anyone in the family have frequent headaches, fevers, itchy watery eyes, a stuffy nose, dry throat or a cough?
- ❑ Does anyone complain of feeling tired or dizzy all the time?
- ❑ Is anyone wheezing or having difficulties breathing on a regular basis?
- ❑ Did these symptoms appear after you moved to this home/apartment?
- ❑ Do the symptoms disappear when you go to school or work or go away on a trip, and return when you come back home?
- ❑ Have you (or your landlord or apartment manager) recently remodeled your home or done any energy conservation work, such as installing insulation, storm windows, or weather stripping?
- ❑ Does your home feel humid?
- ❑ Can you see moisture on the windows or on other surfaces, such as walls and ceilings?
- ❑ What is the usual temperature in your home? Is it very hot or cold?
- ❑ Have you recently had water damage?
- ❑ Do you have a basement? Is it wet or damp?
- ❑ Is there any obvious mold or mildew in the basement, closets, bathrooms?
- ❑ Does any part of your home have a musty or moldy odor?
- ❑ Is the air stale?
- ❑ Do you have pets? (Consider all—including fish, turtles, snakes.)
- ❑ Do you have house plants? Do they show signs of mold?
- ❑ Do you have air conditioners or humidifiers that have not been properly cared for or cleaned?
- ❑ Does your home have cockroaches or rodents?

(Adapted form U.S. Consumer Product Safety Commission, 1996.)

Psychological Hazards

A discussion of environmental health and safety would not be complete if it overlooked the psychological hazards that people must face in their environments. Environment plays a significant role in the mental health of a community. The psychological variables that affect people often lead to physiologic illnesses. Such elements as noise, overcrowding, traffic, lack of privacy, unavailability of work, lack of natural beauty, and boredom can be detrimental to peoples' well-being.

Another psychological hazard is urban crowding. Early studies on crowding done by J. B. Calhoun demonstrated serious effects on behavior. When healthy, naturally clean laboratory mice were forced to live in overcrowded conditions, they experienced dramatic behavior changes. Gross insanitary conditions led to aggressive behavior, attacks by strong mice on the weak, symptoms of regression and mental disturbance, mating decline, and neglect or cannibalization of weaker offspring. Although this is an extreme example, it perhaps provides some insight into the conditions of urban areas and the psychological stress that urban conditions can create (Nakamura, 1999).

The daily psychological stresses of the modern world are innumerable. Excessive stimulation comes from rapid societal changes created by new technology, an accelerated pace of living, increased work production demands, and other causes. All can create potential health hazards.

Facing Terrorist Dangers

An unfortunate addition to the list of environmental hazards is the fear of, preparation for, or reponse to a terrorist attack. All of us are affected directly or indirectly by our environment. Therefore, an actual attack on our environment, no matter how large or small, affects everyone. Perhaps you do not know anyone who was injured or killed during the terrorist attacks of September 11, 2001, that shook the United States and other nations, but the disaster came into your home day after day on your television screen. Remarkable video footage showed the events and their aftermath in graphic detail and was repeatedly aired after the attacks. Thus, even people who were nowhere near the locations of the attacks experienced substantial stress responses.

The RAND Corporation researched the effects on people through a telephone survey of a nationally representative sample of U. S. households 3 to 5 days after the attacks. When adults were asked whether they became upset when something reminded them of what happened, 30% stated that they exprienced substantial stress; 16% related having subtantial stress from repeated disturbing memories, thoughts, or dreams about what happened; 14% had difficulty concentrating; 11% had trouble falling or staying asleep; and 9% felt irritable or had angry outbursts. Of all people questioned around the country 44% had at least one of the above symptoms. Children, when questioned, reported similar complaints; 35% had at least one of the same symptoms, and 47% worried about their safety or the safety of a loved one (Schuster et al., 2001). In additon, the researchers asked how people coped. Almost all talked about their thoughts and feelings with friends and family, more than 90% prayed, about 60% participated in a public activity, 40% avoided watching television and other reminders, and about 37% donated blood, money, or gifts.

The fear of terrorist attacks is real. What about the prevention of future attacks? Are the country's preparations going to be enough? Are the preparations planned being accepted by the public? Are people still fearful, or have they been lulled into complacency? Is the government doing what it can with the development of the Department of Homeland Security, alerting the public of the threat level for impending terrorist activities, and mobilizing a system to provide smallpox vaccines or potassium iodide (KI) doses to the people?

All of these occurences are making people feel more secure or more fearful, depending on who you talk to. Community health nurses are in the middle of many of these decisions and have their own thoughts. In 2003 nurses were some of the health care responders to receive smallpox immunizations. They are in the homes in communities where questions are asked or opinions sought. What can community health nurses say or do to help the community approach decision-making with assurance and to help reduce or prevent fears when the nurses may have their own doubts and fears? These are challenging questions with many possible answers.

As with other community health concerns, nurses can provide the best services by being honest, staying current, and providing correct information and education, being supportive, and giving a listening ear. When individuals or groups participate in plans to promote their own safety, it provides an outlet for their fears and gives them something constructive to focus on. The nurse might suggest that people volunteer, serve on community safety committees, or contact legislative representatives if they have strong feelings about proposed bills. When people feel in control of their situation, fears are reduced.

It is important for community health nurses to stay informed regarding governmental guidelines that involve smallpox immunizations and the availability and benefits of KI. In addition, they can educate people about remaining safe in their communities and where and when to report any suspicious behavior or activities they observe. They can also educate clients about what the various terrorist threat levels mean as they go about their day-to-day activities. They can allow clients to ventilate their fears and concerns and can provide the support clients need. Most importantly, community health nurses should encourage people to cope with their fears in constructive ways and to go about their lives positively, not letting unwarranted fears control them and alter their life plans.

Community health nurses can reassure the public about the actions being taken by the federal, state, and local governments to provide protection. Homeland security involves state and local needs assessments so that changes can be made, state and regional response plans so that all of the people can be protected, Emergency Response Decision Support Systems (ERDSS) to provide critical surveillance data, and education and training tools for first responders and medical staff for personnel involved in prevention, management, and post-event response. Much has been planned and developed to secure our country since September of 2001. Most lay people are aware only of the changes at airports, but this is just one segment of national homeland security measures.

Government's Role

The government plays an active role in promoting public safety. Standards and regulations have been set at the federal level regarding toxic chemicals, radiation exposure, occupational safety practices, noise abatement, biologic hazards, terrorist threats, and other safety issues. State and local governments seek to enforce business, industry, and community compliance with these standards. Health departments and other government agencies assist with monitoring of chemical use and production as well as promotion of public education programs to alert people to the presence and potential dangers of toxic chemicals and exposure to radiation in the environment. Researchers are examining the biologic effects of chemicals and radiation. Those in medical and dental fields have developed simple safety procedures, such as having patients wear lead aprons during radiographs and having technicians stand behind leaded walls. The U. S. Public Health Service holds responsibility for monitoring nuclear plants and other possible sources of radiation to protect the public.

Because the government holds companies liable for the safety of their products, industry now invests considerable resources into researching and designing safe goods. Many products have been modified to make them more safe, such as childproof caps on medication bottles, flame-retardant children's clothing, and seat belts and airbags in automobiles. Industries must also warn consumers if one of their products is inherently dangerous (eg, toys with sharp edges or parts small enough to be ingested by toddlers). Bright-orange, frowning faces on bottles that contain harmful substances have helped to warn consumers and reduce the number of poisonings. Children learn to avoid poisonous plants and other potential hazards through school and community education efforts.

Community safety organizations, government agencies, and public health officials all play their part in assessing community safety and taking measures to prevent accidents. Organizations such as the Consumer Protection Agency and Health Care Without Harm, as well as consumer advocates such as Ralph Nader, continue to serve as watchdogs for environmental safety. Federal and state legislation to enforce speed limits has helped to reduce the number of automobile crashes, and supervision of recreational and occupational areas has led to discovery of health hazards and promoted the development of safety programs. State-established boating safety regulations and the assigning of adequate lifeguards to monitor busy swimming beaches are measures that help to reduce the number of recreational accidents. Community surveys of intersections where multiple traffic crashes have occurred have led to installation of traffic signals and a reduction of crashes.

The role of government in reduction or control of violence and psychological hazards has been less effective. Certain federal-level agencies, such as the National Institute for Mental Health; NIOSH; the U. S. Departments of Labor, Commerce, and Transportation; and the Department of Homeland Security influence standards and regulations affecting psychological well-being. Legislation regarding firearm use and penalties associated with domestic abuse and physical violence have become more stringent. Nonetheless, both violence and psychological hazards continue to be serious public health problems that are preventable and deserve greater attention.

Nurse's Role

It is difficult to monitor all the possible contacts a person or community may be experiencing with toxic chemicals, biologic agents, or radiation, but such monitoring is necessary in order to estimate health risks and establish correlations. Multiple exposures in small doses from many different sources may add up. Are clients' homes well ventilated? Is the burning of fossil fuels polluting the air with sulfur oxides? Does home, school, or worksite insulation contain asbestos? Are all household chemical agents stored in a childproof place? Is the home free of molds and other biologic hazards? Monitoring difficulties arise from the many opportunities for exposure to toxic chemicals, biologicals, or radiation; cumulative exposure over time; and the fact that disease symptoms may not appear until years after exposure, when the agent may no longer be in the immediate environment. The best protection is to promote and monitor the safe use and disposal of chemical hazards, seek out and treat or remove biologic contaminants, and limit radiation exposure to prevent health problems from occurring.

Community health nurses can promote environmental safety and prevent injuries in many ways. Six target area settings in which to concentrate preventive measures are highways, homes, worksites, schools, farms, and recreational sites. Working with the police, fire personnel, social services, schools, drug rehabilitation counselors, and many other community groups, the nurse can help to develop programs targeted at preventing drunk driving, firearm misuse, failed smoke detectors, unsafe playground equipment, and much more. In homes, nurses can encourage safe storage of toxic materials and removal of biologic hazards. Railings can be installed on stairways and in bathrooms used by elderly individuals. Gates at the tops of stairways and window guards can prevent falls by small children. Nonskid decals can be used in bathtubs to prevent slipping.

Safety education offers one of the most vital preventive measures. When people are made aware of possible dangers and unsafe areas, they can avoid injuring themselves. Local community programs to educate people on the dangers of driving while intoxicated, to instruct them on the proper handling of home machinery such as chainsaws, or to encourage safe use of fireworks during holiday celebrations can also help to reduce injuries. In the event that an injury does occur, public education about appropriate responsive actions can help to reduce the potential impact. Promotion of first aid and cardiopulmonary resuscitation (CPR) classes can be beneficial.

Community health nurses need to be aware of the effects noise can have on hearing health and overall well-being. This knowledge will help the nurse identify specific health problems caused by increased noise. Teaching employers, employees, teachers, and children about the potential harm of repeated loud noises in their environment, even the noise from a headset that is turned to a high decibel level, is essential.

Education as a preventive measure against injuries applies particularly in the case of natural disasters. Although a tornado or earthquake cannot be prevented, people can be prepared in the event that one does occur. By running fire drills in schools and workplaces and by informing people of the location of safe and unsafe places to take shelter during an electrical storm or hurricane, or what to do in an earthquake or flood, nurses can help to forestall or minimize tragic events (see Chapter 20).

It is necessary for community health nurses to be aware of psychological hazards in the environment, to recognize the potential they have for affecting both psychological and physiologic health, and to encourage stress reduction wherever possible. Some specific ways in which community health nurses can promote a psychologically healthy environment include active lobbying for control and prevention of domestic abuse and violence, neighborhood crime prevention, reduction of workplace stressors, and the development of educational and support programs to reduce lifestyle stressors.

Finally, the fear of terrorist activities creates psychological damage and increases stress, whether or not an actual event occurs. People need to have useful information so that they can make informed decisions while participating in constructive outlets for their fears. The community health nurse has many roles to play with clients while promoting homeland security.

STRATEGIES FOR NURSING ACTION IN ENVIRONMENTAL HEALTH

Each of the preceding sections has discussed actions and given examples of ways in which the community health nurse can be involved in environmental health. To summarize, the nurse has a two-part challenge: (1) to help protect the public's health from potential threats in the environment and (2) to help protect and promote the health of the environment itself, so that it can be life- and health-enhancing for its human inhabitants. The following strategies for collaboration and participation provide a summary of the nurse's role and can assist the nurse in addressing this two-part goal:

1. Learn about possible environmental health threats. The nurse has a responsibility to keep abreast of current environmental issues and to know the proper authorities to whom problems should be reported.
2. Assess clients' environment and detect health hazards. Careful observation and an environmental checklist can assist in this assessment.
3. Plan collaboratively with citizens and other professionals to devise protective and preventive strategies. Remember that environmental health work is generally a team effort.
4. Assist with the implementation of programs to prevent health threats to clients and the environment.
5. Take action to correct situations in which health hazards exist. Nurses can use direct intervention (eg, in an unsafe home situation), notify proper authorities, or publicly protest if corrective measures are beyond their sphere.
6. Educate consumers and assist them to practice preventive measures. Examples of preventive measures include radon testing in homes and well-water testing in rural communities.
7. Take action to promote the development of policies and legislation that enhance consumer protection and promote a healthier environment.
8. Assist with and promote program evaluation to determine the effectiveness of environmental health efforts.
9. Apply environmentally related research findings and participate in nursing research.

SUMMARY

Environmental health is a discipline encompassing all of the elements of the environment that influence the health and well-being of its inhabitants. Public health workers, including community health nurses, need to monitor and determine causal links between people and their environment with a concern as to how they may promote the health and well-being of both.

An ecologic perspective of environmental health is important to understand the human-environment relationship and how the health of one affects the health of the other. Prevention and strategic or long-range concerns are also important in considering environmental health, because what is done today may affect the health of many generations in the future.

There are major global environmental concerns such as overpopulation, ozone depletion and global warming, defor-

CLINICAL CORNER

OCCUPATIONAL ENVIRONMENTAL HEALTH AND THE NURSE'S ROLE

Scenario

Metropolis Tool Company is a manufacturing plant that employs 1200 workers. Most of the employees work in assembly or data entry jobs. Recently, there have been increasing complaints of work-related stress, with employees citing pressure to perform and produce at higher levels as the root of the stress. You are an occupational health nurse working for the company.

It has come to your attention that there has been a significant increase in insurance claims for the following conditions:

- Stress-related migraine headaches
- Early pregnancy leave for women experiencing low maternal weight gain

Metropolis Tool Company has been in business for more than 29 years. Recently, competition in the manufacturing industry has increased, and the company's executives are looking for ways to cut expenses. Insurance premiums cost the company a considerable amount, and rates will increase if the number of claims continues to rise. Your employer recently became aware of the problems leading to increased utilization of disability benefits. He approached you and asked you to "fix" these problems in an expeditious manner.

Available assessment data that may be related to the problems include the following:

- The plant recently moved to rotating shifts and is now operating around the clock
- Staff layoffs are predicted within 6 months
- Increasing corporate competition has led to higher productivity standards and expectations

Questions

1. Discuss additional assessment data needed and how you will go about gathering these data.
2. Describe your role related to the issue of environmental health and safety.
3. Discuss interventions that your program may perform at the following levels of prevention:
   - Primary
   - Secondary
   - Tertiary
4. Your supervisor in your role of occupational health nurse is a company vice president. He is very knowledgeable about business but knows little about health issues. Where will you turn to obtain information to assist you in addressing the problems identified in this scenario?
5. How will you evaluate the effects of your interventions?
6. What issues does this scenario elicit regarding:
   Fears and anxiety in this role
   Lack of immediate resources (supervisor)
   Social justice
   Building partnerships within your communities
   Globalization of public health

---

estation, desertification and wetlands destruction, energy depletion, air pollution, water pollution, unhealthy or contaminated food, waste disposal, insect and rodent control, biologic pollutants, safety (in the home, worksite, and community), and protection from terrorist activity. Each has its own set of problems, concerns, and solutions.

Both public and private sectors are involved in regulating, monitoring, and preventing environmental health problems and have accomplished much during the past 35 years. Much, however, is still left to be done, and new problems continue to develop. The community health nurse is an important member of the team of health professionals who promote and protect the reciprocal relationship between the environment and the public's health. The nurse can follow several important strategies to accomplish the two-part goal of protecting the public's health from environmental threats and promoting a healthy and health-enhancing environment.

ACTIVITIES TO PROMOTE CRITICAL THINKING

1. You are planning a visit to a young family who live in an older home. You know that older homes may have radon, lead pipes and lead-based paint, asbestos insulation, and other safety, fire, and health threats, such as those from biologic pollutants. Using the nursing process, design a plan for (a) determining whether any of these threats are present, (b) deciding what actions should be taken if the dangers exist, (c) assisting the family in taking corrective action, and (d) evaluating successful removal of existing threats.

2. Data from the local health department show that, in the past year, five people from the same rural portion of the county died of cancer. What collaborative actions would be appropriate for you to take to determine whether there is an environmental relationship? What other members of the health team should be involved in the investigation? Write a letter to the mayor and the county commissioners to justify why nurses should be involved in this study.

3. Select an article from the mass media (eg, newspaper, weekly news magazine) that deals with an "environmental health" problem. Analyze and critique the article by answering the following questions: What are the characteristics of the community involved? What appear to be the sources of the problem? What evidence is provided in the article to substantiate the cause? Does the news coverage describe health effects? What population is at risk? Does the coverage provide adequate information for consumers to understand the problem and seek any needed assistance? What suggestions do you have for improving the article?

4. Design a list of items to include in a checklist for assessing clients' home, school, or worksite environments. Consider each of the environmental areas of concern described in this chapter and what potential health threats might be present in each area. Review this list with an environmental health expert for accuracy and completeness. Use the list as a teaching tool with two different sets of clients, and evaluate its effectiveness for assessment and diagnosis of environmentally related health hazards.

5. Identify an environmental health problem in your community or state. Become informed about this problem by talking with experts in the area, reading recent literature and research reports, and searching the Internet for information about the problem. Meet with a senator or congressperson who has been involved in legislation related to the problem, and learn what he or she plans to do about it. Summarize what you have learned, and present it in writing as a letter to the editor of your city newspaper (see Clinical Corner.)

6. Assess what your community is doing to protect itself from terrorist activities by contacting the health department nursing and environmental health services, hospitals, police, and emergency medical services in your community. Use the information to enhance services you provide in the community.

REFERENCES

Agency for Toxic Substances and Disease Registry (ATSDR). (2001). *Air pamphlet*. Washington, DC: ATSDR.

American Public Health Association. (1999). More research needed to guide policy on environmental justice. *Nation's Health, 29*(3), 4.

American Public Health Association. (2001). Arsenic in drinking water linked to bladder, lung cancer. *Nation's Health, 11*, 5.

American Public Health Association. (2002, March). Bioterrorism preparedness key in 2003 budget proposal. *The Nation's Health, 1*, 11.

Behar, A., Chasin, M., & Cheesman, M. (2000). *Noise control: A primer*. San Diego, CA: Singular.

Blumenthal, D., & Ruttenber, J. (1994). *Introduction to environmental health* (2nd ed.). New York: Springer.

Brown, M.J., Gardner, J., Sargent, J.D., Swartz, K., Hu, H., & Timperi, R. (2001). The effectiveness of housing policies in reducing children's lead exposure. *American Journal of Public Health, 91*(4), 621–624.

Calvert, G.M., Mueller, C.A., Fajen, J.M., Chrislip, D.W., Russo, J., Briggle, T., et al. (1998). Health effects associated with sulfuryl fluoride and methyl bromide exposure among structural fumigation workers. *American Journal of Public Health, 88*(12), 1774–1780.

Chin, J. (Ed.). (1999). *Control of communicable diseases manual* (17th ed.). Washington, DC: American Public Health Association.

Cohen, S.M. (2001). Lead poisoning: A summary of treatment and prevention. *Pediatric Nursing, 27*(2), 124–130.

Cruz, M.A., Katz, D.J., & Suarez, J.A. (2001). An assessment of the ability of routine restaurant inspections to predict food-borne outbreaks in Miami-Dade County, Florida. *American Journal of Public Health, 91*(5), 821–823.

Curtis, S., & Taket, A. (1996). *Health and societies: Changing perspectives*. London: Arnold.

Dixon, J.K. (2002). Kids need clean air: Air pollution and children's health. *Family and Community Health, 24*(4), 9–26.

Environmental Protection Agency. (2001). *Protecting your drinking water*. Washington, DC: Office of Ground Water and Drinking Water.

Environmental Protection Agency. (1997). *Climate change and public health*. Washington, DC: Office of Policy, Planning, and Evaluation.

Fell-Carlson, D. (2003). Terrorist danger. *Nurseweek, 16*(3), 21–23.

Ford, B.J. (2000). *The future of food*. New York: Thames & Hudson.

Gaffney, K.F. (2001). Infant exposure to environmental tobacco smoke. *Journal of Nursing Scholarship, 33*(4), 343–347.

Institute of Medicine. (1999). *Toward environmental justice: Research, education and health policy needs*. Washington, DC: National Academy Press.

International Food Information Council (IFIC). (2002). *Food irradiation: A global food safety tool*. Zagreb, Croatia: Rudjer Bokovic Institute.

Kerns, T. (2001). *Environmentally induced illnesses: Ethics, risk assessment, and human rights*. Jefferson, NC: McFarland & Company.

Krug, E.G., Sharma, G.K., & Lozano, R. (2000). The global burden of injuries. *American Journal of Public Health, 90*(4), 523–526.

Last, J.M. (1998). Housing and health. In R.B. Wallace (Ed.), *Maxcy-Rosenau-Last public health and preventive medicine* (14th ed.). Stamford, CT: Appleton & Lange.

Lavelle, M., & Kurlantzick, J. (2002, August 12). The coming water crisis. *U. S. News & World Report, 133*, 22–30.

Manning, F.J., & Goldfrank, L. (Eds.). (2002). *Preparing for terrorism: IOM executive summary*. Washington, DC: National Academy Press.

Markowitz, G., & Rosner, D. (2000). "Cater to the children": The role of the lead industry in a public health tragedy, 1900–1955. *American Journal of Public Health, 90*(1), 36–46.

McGrew, R. (1985). *Encyclopedia of medical history* (pp. 137–141). New York: McGraw-Hill.

Nakamura, R.M. (1999). *Health in America: A multicultural perspective*. Boston: Allyn and Bacon.

National Center for Injury Prevention and Control. (2001). *Injury Fact Book 2001–2002*. Atlanta, GA: Centers for Disease Control and Prevention.

National Institute of Allergy and Infectious Diseases. (2002). *Foodborne diseases*. Bethesda, MD: National Institutes of Health.

National Institutes of Health. (2001). *HIV/AIDS-related research activities: Women and girls and HIV/AIDS*. Bethesda, MD: Author.

Patz, J.A., McGeehin, M.A., Bernard, S.M., et al. (2001, September). The potential health impacts of climate variability and change for the United States: Executive summary of the report of the health sector of the U. S. National Assessment. *Environmental Health, 64*, 20–28.

Population Action International. (1998). *Fact sheet. What birth dearth? Why world population is still growing*. Washington, DC: Author.

Rose, C.S., Martyny, J.W., Newman, L.S., Milton, D.K., King, T.E., Jr., Beebe, J.L., et al. (1998). "Lifeguard lung": Endemic granulomatous pneumonitis in an indoor swimming pool. *American Journal of Public Health, 88*(12), 1795–1800.

Rose, J.B. (2002, August 30). A world of water hazards. *The Baltimore Sun*. Accessed February 15, 2004, from *http://www.waterandhealth.org/drinkingwater/hazards.html*

Schecter, A.J. (Ed.). (1998). Environmental health. In R.B. Wallace (Ed.), *Maxcy-Rosenau-Last public health and preventive medicine* (14th ed.). Stamford, CT: Appleton & Lange.

Schuster, M.A., Stein, B.D., Jaycox, L.H., Collins, R.L., Marshall, G.N., Elliott, M.N., et al. (2001). A national survey of stress reactions after the September 11, 2001, terrorist attacks. *New England Journal of Medicine, 345*, 1507–1512.

Stanley, B. (2002, July 3). Mother nature. *The Fresno Bee*, C1, C6.

Teutsch, S.M., & Churchill, R.E. (2000). *Principles and practice of public health surveillance*. Oxford: Oxford University Press.

Turnock, B.K. (1997). *Public health: What it is and how it works*. Gaithersburg, MD: Aspen.

United States Consumer Product Safety Commission. (1996). *Biological pollutants in your home*. Washington, DC: U.S. Government Printing Office.

United States Department of Agriculture. (2000). *Foodborne illness: What consumers need to know*. Washington, DC: Author.

United States Department of Health and Human Services. (1991). *Healthy people 2000: National health promotion and disease prevention objectives* (Publication no. S/N 017-001-00474-0). Washington, DC: U. S. Government Printing Office.

United States Department of Health and Human Services. (2000). *Healthy people 2010* (Conference ed., Vols. I & II). Washington, DC: U. S. Government Printing Office.

Venes, D., & Thomas, C. (Eds.). (2001). *Taber's cyclopedic medical dictionary* (19th ed.). Philadelphia: F. A. Davis.

Williams, S.J., & Torrens, P.R. (1999). *Introduction to health services* (5th ed.). Albany, NY: Delmar.

World Health Organization. (1986). *Health and the environment* (WHO Regional Publications, European Series, no. 19) (pp. 12–16). Vienna: Author.

World Health Organization. (2000). *The world health report 2000*. Geneva, Switzerland: Author.

Yassi, A., Kjellstrom, T., de Kok, T., & Guidotti, T.L. (2001). *Basic environmental health*. Oxford: Oxford University Press.

SELECTED READINGS

Baffigo, V., Albinagorta, J., Nauca, L., Rojas, P., Alegre, R., Hubbard, B., et al. (2001). Community environmental health assessment in Peru's desert hills and rainforest. *American Journal of Public Health, 91*(10), 1580–1585.

Barnett, M. (2002, August 5). Making a stink: Neighbors say sewage sludge fertilizer makes them ill. *U. S. News & World Report*, 48–50.

Butterfield, P. (2000). Recovering a lost legacy: Nurses' leadership in environmental health. *Journal of Nursing Education, 39*(9), 385–386.

Cohn, L.D., Hernandez, D., Byrd, T., & Cortes, M. (2002). A program to increase seat belt use along the Texas-Mexico border. *American Journal of Public Health, 92*(12), 1918–1920.

Cohen, R.E. (2000). *Mental health services in disasters: Manual for humanitarian workers.* Washington, DC: Pan American Health Organization.

Eckel, W.P., Rabinowitz, M.B., & Foster, G.D. (2001). Discovering unrecognized lead-smelting sites by historical methods. *American Journal of Public Health, 91*(4), 625–627.

Fitzpatrick, K., & LaGory, M. (2000). *Unhealthy places: The ecology of risk in the urban landscape.* New York: Routledge.

Geiger, H.J. (2001). Terrorism, biological weapons, and bonanzas: Assessing the real threat to public health. *American Journal of Public Health, 91*(5), 708–709.

Guidry, M., Vischi, T., Han, R., & Passons, O. (2001). *Healthy people in healthy communities.* Washington, DC: Department of Health and Human Services.

Kerr, M.J., Brosseau, L., & Johnson, C.S. (2002). Noise levels of selected construction tasks. *AIHA Journal, 63,* 334–339.

Larsson, L.S., & Butterfield, P. (2002). Mapping the future of environmental health and nursing: Strategies for integrating national competencies into nursing practice. *Public Health Nursing, 19*(4), 301–308.

Lawson, A.B., & Williams, F.L.R. (2001). *An introductory guide to disease mapping.* Chichester, UK: John Wiley & Sons.

Maliha-Nebus, J. (2002). Industrial pollution: A nurse fights back. *Reflections on Nursing Leadership/Sigma Theta Tau International, 28*(4), 25–26, 37.

Olden, K., Guthrie, J., & Newton, S. (2001). A bold new direction for environmental health research. *American Journal of Public Health, 91*(12), 1964–1967.

Patterson, J., Brody, C., Pierce, A., & Vivio, D. (2001). *Green birthdays.* Washington, DC: Health Care Without Harm and American College of Nurse-Midwives.

Retting, R.A., Persaud, B.N., Garder, P.E., & Lord, D. (2001). Crash and injury reduction following installation of roundabouts in the United States. *American Journal of Public Health, 91*(4), 628–631.

Ruvinsky, R. (2002, September 9). A long, slow autumn: An army of imported pests is devouring the nation's trees. *U. S. News & World Report,* 66–68.

Speer, S.A., Semenza, J.C., Jurosaki, T., & Anton-Culver, H. (2002). Risk factors for acute myeloid leukemia and multiple myeloma: A combination of GIS and case-control studies. *Journal of Environmental Health, 64,* 9–16.

Waller, P.F. (2001). Public health's contribution to motor vehicle injury prevention. *American Journal of Preventive Medicine, 21*(Suppl. 4), 3–4.

Wright, C. (2002, November). CDC issues guidelines for state, local smallpox response. *The Nation's Health, 1,* 25.

U. S. Agency for International Development. (2001). *Child survival and disease programs fund progress report, fiscal year 2001.* Washington, DC: Author.

Important Telephone Numbers

Consumer Product Safety Commission: 1-800-638-CPSC

Food Information and Seafood Hotline (U. S. Food and Drug Administration): 1-800-FDA-4010

Indoor Air Quality Information Clearinghouse (U. S. Environmental Protection Agency): 1-800-438-4318

Local American Lung Association: 1-800-LUNG-USA

Meat and Poultry Hotline (U. S. Department of Agriculture): 1-800-535-4555

National Institute of Occupational Safety and Health: 1-800-35-NIOSH

National Lead Information Center: 1-800-LEAD-FYI

National Pesticides Telecommunications Network: 1-800-858-PEST

Nuclear Regulatory Commission Radiation Protection and Emergency Response Program: (301) 415-8200

Ozone Hotline (U. S. Environmental Protection Agency): 1-800-296-1996

Radiation Emergency Assistance Center/Training Site (REAC/TS): (865) 576-3131

Internet Resources

Agency for Toxic Substances and Disease Registry (ATSDR): *www.atsdr.cdc.gov*

American Nurses Association. (1997). *Position statements: Lead poisoning and screening.* Available: *http://www.nursingworld. org/readroom/position/social/sclead.htm*

Fight BAC!: *http://www.fightbac.org*

Health Care Without Harm: *http://www.noharm.org*

National Food Safety Initiative: *http://www.foodsafety.com*

Partnership for Food Safety Education: *http://www.fightbac.org*

Population Action International: *http://www.populationaction.org*

U. S. Environmental Protection Agency: *http://www.epa.gov/globalwarming*

U. S. Food and Drug Administration: *http://www.fda.gov/*

U. S. Food and Drug Administration, Office of Health Affairs: *http://www.fda.gov/oc/oha*

U. S. National Response Team: *http://www.nrt.org*

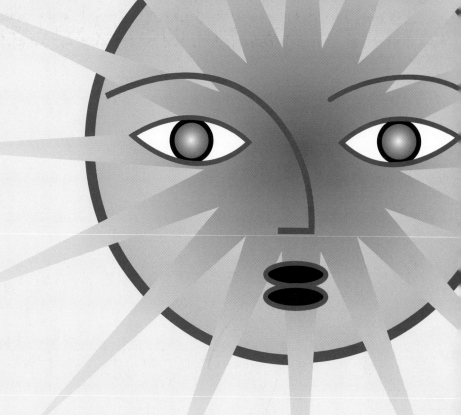

Tools of Community Health Nursing

11

Communication, Collaboration, and Contracting

Key Terms

- Active listening
- Brainstorming
- Channel
- Collaboration
- Communication
- Contracting
- Critical pathway
- Decoding
- Delphi technique
- Electronic meetings
- Empathy
- Encoding
- Feedback loop
- Formal contracting
- Informal contracting
- Message
- Nominal group technique
- Nonverbal messages
- Nursing informatics
- Paraphrasing
- Receiver
- Sender
- Verbal messages

Learning Objectives

Upon mastery of this chapter, you should be able to:

- Identify the seven basic parts of the communication process.
- Describe four barriers to effective communication in community health nursing and how to deal with them.
- Explain three sets of skills necessary for effective communication in community health nursing.
- Discuss four techniques for enhancing group decision-making.
- Describe five characteristics of collaboration in community health.
- Compare the three phases common to the collaboration process.
- Identify four features of contracting in community health nursing.
- Discuss the value of contracting to both clients and community health nurses.
- Design an aggregate-level contract useful in community health nursing.

C ommunication, collaboration, and contracting are primary tools for community health nurses. They form the basis for effective relationships that contribute both to the prevention of illness and to the protection and promotion of aggregate health. To use them skillfully in community health practice, it is important to understand the meaning and value of these concepts. For the nurse accustomed to communicating one-on-one with clients, communication with aggregates and a host of professionals requires new skills. The computer, with its Internet and e-mail capabilities, adds another dimension to communication and brings the world into the home and work settings. Unlike ordinary social relationships, collaborative relationships are based on a team approach with shared responsibilities and mutual participation in establishing and carrying out goals. Clients and health care professionals enter into a working agreement, or contract, tailored to address specific client needs. The concept of contracting can further assist the collaborative process. This chapter examines these tools and discusses their integration into community health nursing practice.

COMMUNICATION IN COMMUNITY HEALTH NURSING

Groups cannot exist without communication, nor can nurses practice without communication. These facts often are taken for granted, since most people spend almost 70% of their waking hours communicating: speaking, listening, reading, or writing. Yet the quality of people's communication has far-reaching effects. Lack of effective communication can lead to misunderstanding, poor performance, interpersonal conflict, ineffective programs, weak public policy, and many other undesirable outcomes (Marshall & Houseman, 1999; Tan, 2001). To communicate, people must have, construct, or create shared realities and meanings. In other words, they must engage in an exchange that is both understood and meaningful. **Communication** means transfering meaning and enhancing understanding.

Communication is the lifeblood of effective community health nursing practice. It provides a two-way flow of information that nourishes professional-client and professional-professional relationships. It also establishes the base of information on which health planning decisions are made and programs developed. For communication to take place, clients and professionals need to send and receive messages. As participants in the communication process, community health nurses play both roles: sender and receiver. The nurse working with a group of abused women must learn to "read" the messages these women send. Similarly, as a member of a health planning team, the nurse must be able to elicit ideas as well as contribute to the planning process by speaking and acting in ways that communicate effectively.

Communication serves several functions in community health nursing. It provides information for decision-making at all levels of community health. From the choice of goals for a small group to health policy affecting a population at risk, decisions are enhanced through effective communication. It functions as a motivator by clarifying information so that consensus is reached and the people involved can move forward with commitment to shared goals. Effective communication facilitates expression of feelings and promotes closer working relationships. It also controls behavior by providing clear expectations and boundaries for group-member actions.

The Communication Process

Communication occurs as a sequence of events or a process. The process is made up of seven basic parts that work together to result in the transference and understanding of meaning. These parts are (1) the message, (2) a sender, (3) a receiver, (4) encoding, (5) a channel, (6) decoding, and (7) a feedback loop.

The first part of the communication process is a **message**, which is an expression of the purpose of communication. Without the message, there can be no communication. The next two parts are a sender and a receiver. The **sender** is the person (or persons) conveying a message, and the **receiver** is the person (or persons) to whom the message is directed and who is its actual recipient. The fourth step is the act of **encoding**, which refers to the sender's conversion of the message into symbolic form. This involves how the sender translates the message to the receiver. It can be accomplished through verbal or nonverbal means. For example, a nurse teaching breathing techniques to a prenatal class may explain verbally while also demonstrating the correct procedures. The degree of the sender's success in encoding is influenced by the sender's communication skills, knowledge about the topic of the message, attitudes related to the message and the receiver, and the beliefs and values held by the sender. The fifth part involves a **channel,** or the medium through which the sender conveys the message. The channel may be a written, spoken, or nonverbal expression. Examples include an e-mail stating a request, a report providing information, a written health plan, a verbal request for clarification, or a facial expression indicating confusion. Communication channels may be formal, such as a written grant proposal, or informal, such as a face-to-face verbal statement or an e-mail message.

Once the sender has conveyed a message through a channel, the receiver must translate the message into an understandable form, called **decoding**, which is the sixth part of the communication process. The receiver's ability to decode the message is influenced by knowledge of the topic, skills in reading and listening, attitudes, and sociocultural values. The seventh and final part is a **feedback loop**, which refers to the receiver's indication that the message has been understood (decoded) in the way that the sender intended (encoded). It requires feedback from the receiver to the sender, serving as a check on the success of the transference of meaning (Tan, 2001). Figure 11–1 portrays the seven steps of the communication process.

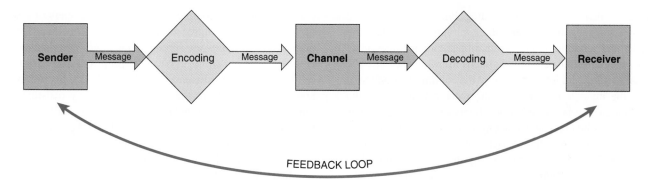

FIGURE 11–1. The communication process (feedback loop).

Communication Barriers

Community health nurses should be aware of the barriers that block effective communication. This section discusses four barriers that pose particular problems: selective perception, language barriers, filtering, and emotions (Robbins, 2003).

Selective Perception

Receivers in the communication process interpret a message through their own perceptions, which are influenced by their own experience, interests, values, motivations, and expectations. They project this perceptual screen onto the communication process as they decode a message. They might distort or misinterpret meaning from the sender's original intent. For example, the nurse may propose a class session on nutrition to a group of elderly persons, and the clients may translate that message to mean a focus on dieting, which is not the intended meaning. Nurses can overcome this barrier by using the feedback loop to ask clients or others involved to restate their understanding of the message. In this case, the nurse could ask the elderly clients what the term *nutrition* means to them. This provides an opportunity for clarification and correction of misunderstandings, which is an essential step in the communication process.

Language Barriers

People interpret the meaning of words differently, depending on many variables such as age, education, cultural background, and primary spoken language. An adolescent understands the terms "cool," "tight," and "dude" to mean that something is fashionable or desirable, whereas an 80-year-old woman might not understand the current slang terms. In community health, nurses work with a wide range of clients and professionals whose disparate ages, education levels, and cultural backgrounds lead to different speech patterns (Sharpe, 2001). The use of scientific terminology or jargon by some health professionals can be confusing, as in the case of the Hmong refugee woman who was asked whether her son had experienced enuresis. Using unfamiliar terms can become barriers to communication. Client differences must be taken into consideration during the communication process.

Filtering Information

A third barrier to communication is filtering, which means manipulation of information by the sender to influence the receiver's response. To gain favor with receivers, senders sometimes say what they believe receivers want to hear rather than the whole truth (Robbins, 2003). Clients sometimes use filtering during a needs assessment process, giving only partial or distorted information because they think this is what health professionals want to hear. Another intent of filtering is to slant information. Prepared minutes from a meeting or a department's quarterly report can emphasize some points and omit or deemphasize others, giving (sometimes unintentionally) false impressions that influence decision-making.

Emotional Influence

How a person feels at the time a message is sent or received influences its meaning. Senders can distort messages and receivers can interpret messages incorrectly when emotions cloud their perception. Emotions can interfere with rational and objective reasoning, thus blocking communication. Nurses need to be aware of their own emotions as they send messages. They also need to ascertain the emotional status of clients or health professionals with whom they are communicating to avoid misunderstandings. As an example, parents may be upset about the health status of a child injured at school; messages from the school nurse can result in vague, conflicting, and muddled exchage of information if the nurse is not aware of the parents emotional state (Sharpe, 2001).

Core Communication Skills

Overcoming the barriers to effective communication just described requires the development of sound communication skills. Community health nurses need to cultivate three sets of communication skills: sending skills, receiving skills, and interpersonal skills.

Sending Skills

Sending skills enable nurses to transmit messages effectively. Through these skills, nurses convey information to clients and other persons. Two important considerations influence clarity and effectiveness of message sending. First, the extent of the nurse's self-awareness affects the communication. Does the nurse feel anxious, angry, tired, impatient, or concerned? Does the nurse find certain individuals irritating or offensive? What motives and interests prompt the communication? Second, the nurse's awareness of the receivers influences the sending of messages. What do clients or the professionals with whom the nurse is interacting want or need? Is the message suited to their cultural background and level of understanding? Does the message have significance for them? How are receivers responding as the nurse sends the message?

Two main channels are used to send messages: nonverbal and verbal. **Nonverbal messages**, those conveyed without words, constitute almost two thirds of the messages transmitted in normal communication. People send messages nonverbally in many ways. Personal appearance, dress, posture, facial expression, and physical distance between sender and receiver all communicate messages. These nonverbal statements may enhance or discredit what someone says verbally (Robbins, 2003). Body language often speaks louder than words. Facial expressions convey acceptance or rejection, interest or boredom, anger or patience, fear or confidence. Gestures and bodily movements such as clenched hands, crossed arms, tapping fingers, hands on hips, or a turned shoulder all communicate messages. Eye contact or lack of it carries additional meaning. Tone of voice and use of silence also send nonverbal messages. Accepting food in certain situations may communicate acceptance and the desire to be friendly. Nonverbal messages may have different cultural meanings or social interpretations (Spector, 2000). Nurse self-awareness and validation of meaning can save considerable misunderstanding.

Verbal messages are communicated ideas, attitudes, and feelings transmitted by speaking or writing. Nurses cannot assume that the intent of their words always is understood by clients or other professionals. Effective sending skills depend on asking for feedback to make certain that receivers have understood the verbal message's intent. Communication is more effective if speakers avoid using jargon that is unfamiliar to clients. Like all occupations, nursing has its own vocabulary or jargon that may not be understood by clients, perhaps making them feel ignorant or inferior. For example, the terms "critical pathways" or "case-management approach" might have little meaning to a community group. Nurses must make a special effort to avoid using jargon that is part of nursing's everyday speech. The basic rules for effective sending can be summarized in this manner:

1. Keep the message honest and uncomplicated.
2. Use as few words as possible to state it.
3. Ask for reactions (feedback) to make certain that it is understood.

Receiving Skills

Receiving skills are as important to communication as sending skills. They involve not only listening to what people say but also observing their behavior. They enable nurses to receive accurate and complete messages. If members of a seniors' exercise class agree to certain exercises but do not participate in them, they are sending a message. What message is their behavior sending? Were the proposed exercises too difficult? Did they misunderstand the nurse's instructions about how to perform the exercise? Are they resisting in other areas of the program? Effective receiving skills require attention to nonverbal as well as verbal messages and seeking feedback to understand their meaning.

An essential skill needed for receiving messages is **active listening** or reflective listening, which is the skill of assuming responsibility for and understanding the feelings and thoughts in a sender's message. Instead of expecting clients or others to help the nurse understand, the nurse should actively work to discover what clients mean. Understanding the message from the sender's perspective demands careful attention. It arises from a genuine interest in what the speaker has to say. Active listeners demonstrate their interest, perhaps by sitting forward, sustaining eye contact, nodding the head, and asking occasional questions for clarification (Kar, Arcalay, & Alex, 2001). At times, **paraphrasing**, or stating back to the sender what was heard by the receiver, is helpful in clarifying the sender's meaning. This helps the nurse to avoid daydreaming or pretending to be listening, both of which block communication. Also, the content and feeling of the sender's message is overwhelming at times, and the nurse becomes preoccupied with formulating a response rather than actively listening. In these situations, paraphrasing can help the nurse to stay focused. An example of the skill of paraphrasing is as follows:

> Client: *"I don't think I can manage my elderly mother at home any longer. I know she never wanted to go to a nursing home, but with my job and the kids, caring for her is becoming impossible. My husband is so helpful, I feel guilty burdening him. But I'll be going against my mother's wishes if I place her somewhere."*
>
> Nurse: *"You feel frustrated caring for your mother and your family while maintaining a job, and you're not sure what is the best action to take?"*

Nurses also can listen actively by asking reflective questions that restate what clients or others have said to clarify the received meaning. Reflective questions have a twofold purpose: to show a sincere attempt to understand the senders' messages, and to make clear that the messages and the people who send them are important to the nurse. An example of a reflective question follows:

> Class members state, *"Quitting smoking is impossible."*
>
> The nurse asks, *"Do you feel you can't quit smoking?"*

Active listening helps to communicate acceptance and increase trust, especially when the listener refrains from making any negative judgments of the message or the way it is delivered. A critical response to the message by the listener cuts off communication. Active listening enables nurses to encourage clients to deliberate carefully and to exercise problem-solving skills; it avoids the pitfall of telling receivers what to do. By asking reflective questions, the nurse continues to clarify the messages clients send.

Interpersonal Skills

Effective communication in community health nursing also requires interpersonal skills. Three types of interpersonal skills build on sending and receiving skills but go beyond the mere exchange of messages. They are showing respect, empathizing, and developing trust.

Showing Respect

Showing respect means conveying the attitude that clients and others have importance, dignity, and worth. Community health nurses can express respect by treating ideas and comments as valuable and worthy of attention. Nurses can demonstrate an interest in wanting to understand the situation from the other person's point of view. Nurses show respect by the manner in which they address people—for instance, by using the courtesy titles of "Mr." or "Mrs." until it is determined how the client wants to be addressed. On a more subtle level, the tone of voice the nurse uses can either show respect or make people feel inferior and insignificant. Clients, community members, and other professionals need to feel respected if they are to enter fully into the mutual exchange necessary for effective communication (Display 11–1).

Empathizing

Empathizing is another important interpersonal skill. **Empathy** is the ability to communicate understanding and to vicariously experience the feelings and thoughts of others (Balzer-Riley, 2000). Nurses show empathy by reflecting another person's feelings and expressing that message in the receiver's language. The nurse should use the same terms and, if possible, the same tone of voice as the other person did. For example, the nurse should assume a serious manner if the speaker seems serious. Empathy conveys the message, "This is the way it seems to me. Is that correct?" The nurse should keep validating the speaker's true feelings to be certain that the message is being interpreted correctly. Empathy focuses attention on receivers and their feelings and reduces clients' anxiety and defensiveness. It shows that the nurse shares their concerns and makes them feel that their contributions are valued (Balzer-Riley, 2000).

Developing Trust

Developing trust is necessary for effective communication. Clients and others will not express their true feelings if they do not fully trust the nurse. Many times, clients say what they think the nurse wants to hear. They may agree to a plan of action simply because they do not want to displease the nurse, or they may hide their true feelings be-

DISPLAY 11-1

Health Communication—One Disparity: Low-Literacy Clients

Most poorly educated populations, those with the lowest literacy levels, have the highest mortality and morbidity. Changing demographics suggest that low literacy is an increasing problem among certain racial and ethnic groups, non–English-speaking populations, and persons older than 65 years of age, although the majority of people with low literacy are white native-born Americans (U. S. Department of Health and Human Services, 2000). Yet it has been well documented that most health information pamphlets, brochures, and other materials cannot be read or comprehended by low-literacy adults. Communication with these high-risk groups should be simplified and should include easy-to-read materials. At the same time, there is the danger of making the communication so simple that the reader feels insulted. Low literacy does not necessarily mean low intelligence. How does the nurse find the right balance?

The goal of communication is to achieve understanding. If clients are to understand health communication—whether the messages are spoken or written—they must be given ample opportunity to provide feedback. Pamphlets and other written health information should be reviewed by their intended audiences before final printing and distribution. Proposed users should comment on the readability and acceptability of both text and graphics. With spoken communication, nurses should regularly solicit feedback to make certain that messages are understood.

cause they think that the nurse is eager for a decision. Agreeing with others, especially with people who are in powerful positions and from different cultures, is the polite and respectful thing to do in some cultures (Spector, 2000). The nurse who is unaware of this fact may interpret the client's agreement as understanding, and a "teachable moment" is lost.

Nurses develop trust in the communication process by showing that they truly accept others, that they believe in them as people. Trust generates trust; as the nurse shows confidence in clients and the other professionals with whom the nurse is communicating, they will respond in kind. Treating people as fully participating partners in the communication process means demonstrating that they are trustworthy and responsible. Trust also is developed through an open, honest, and patient approach with others. Candid discussion in a flexible time frame encourages people to share their real feelings and to move at their own pace. As trust develops, communication becomes more free-flowing and productive.

Factors Influencing Communication

Effective communication, both sending and receiving, is strongly influenced by three factors: previous experiences, culture, and relationships.

Previous experiences of both sender and receiver influence their perceptions and the meanings they attach to messages. For example, adolescents who are having difficulty with parents' authority may hear the nurse's suggestion to "learn more about sexually transmitted diseases" as a command or effort to exert control. Requests for clarification help to verify that messages are being received as intended.

The respective cultures of sender and receiver influence understanding and acceptance of messages. A nervous laugh, appropriate as an outlet in one culture, may appear rude and disrespectful to someone from another culture. Silence, which in Native American cultures indicates patience and thoughtfulness, may be interpreted as weakness or indifference to someone not familiar with their cultural practices. With many clients, the nurse must communicate cross-culturally, which requires patience and constant effort to ensure accurate and inoffensive messages (Kar, Alcalay, & Alex, 2001; Spector, 2000).

Because much of community health nursing involves groups, the relationships among group members can significantly influence communication effectiveness. When many people are involved, group communication patterns can be complex, and interaction requires skill on the nurse's part to elicit feedback from all members and to generate a common understanding among the group's members.

Group Decision-Making

An important aspect of communicating with groups in community health is group decision-making. Community health nurses are regularly involved in this activity. Nurses working in the community face different decision-making challenges from those encountered by their hospital colleagues. Nurses need to understand how groups function as they make decisions, and they need to learn techniques for facilitating group decision-making.

Group Functions in Decision-Making

Groups, regardless of size, perform many functions. Four functions are of particular relevance to group decision-making:

1. Group members share information. In community health nursing, groups often include clients, health professionals, and community members who share their experience and expertise to arrive at solutions and decisions.
2. Groups present diverse views, which enriches the number and types of alternatives in the problem-solving process.
3. Groups influence their members' thinking by broadening their perspectives and presenting new ways of thinking about the issues. This influencing function can improve the quality of group decision-making.

4. Groups progress toward consensus or resolution by discussing a set of alternatives and arriving at solutions. Time pressures and the desire for completion help to move this process along.

Techniques for Enhancing Group Decision-Making

As a member of many decision-making groups in the community, the community health nurse can facilitate the process through certain techniques. Robbins (2003) describes four useful strategies: brainstorming, nominal group technique, Delphi technique, and electronic meetings.

Brainstorming

Brainstorming is an idea-generating process that encourages group members to freely offer suggestions. When brainstorming, members sit around a table (if group size permits) and take turns presenting ideas. They are encouraged to be creative and unusual; no idea is too bizarre. Furthermore, no criticism or discussion is allowed until all ideas have been exhausted and recorded. This technique is helpful for generating creative possibilities and is most useful in the early stages of decision-making.

Nominal Group Technique

Nominal group technique is a group decision-making method in which ideas are pooled and discussed face-to-face after members initially think and write down their ideas independently. In this approach, members meet together but spend time silently writing down their ideas first. Afterward, members take turns presenting one idea at a time to the group without discussion until all ideas have been recorded. Discussion then follows for clarifying and judging. Next, members independently and silently rank-order the ideas and read these rankings to the group. This allows the decisions to be narrowed down to the one with the highest aggregate ranking.

Delphi Technique

Delphi technique is a method of arriving at group consensus through a systematic pooling of individuals' judgments by using a written questionnaire and suggestions. Members do not need to be physically present to participate. It follows a series of steps:

1. Identify problem or topic and design questionnaire to elicit responses from members.
2. Members respond independently and anonymously and return the questionnaire.
3. Compile responses centrally, then send results and a new questionnaire to members.
4. Members offer new responses or solutions, based on earlier results, and return these.
5. Repeat steps 3 and 4 as needed until consensus is reached.

This process is useful for polling experts who may be geographically distant from one another. It also provides a way to reach a decision without group members unduly influencing each other. Its disadvantages are that it is time-consuming and can be expensive.

Electronic Meetings

Electronic meetings provide a fourth group decision-making method. This method, currently used more in business settings, applies nominal group technique combined with computer technology. Group members sit around a table, and each is furnished with a computer—tabletop, laptop, or hand-held personal digital assistant (PDAs) (Enger & Segal-Isaacson, 2001). As issues are presented, members use their computers to key in their responses, which are anonymously displayed on a large projection screen. Group decisions also are displayed for group viewing. This method promotes greater honesty and speed; in fact, experts claim that electronic meetings are significantly faster than face-to-face meetings (Robbins, 2003).

In community health, the availability of such technology may be limited in many settings. Nonetheless, computer-assisted decision-making is becoming increasingly useful and available. Computers are used in conjunction with other group decision-making techniques for recording ideas and research findings, tabulating rankings, and conducting simulations.

Nursing Informatics

Nursing informatics is a term for the collective technologic sciences currently available to nurses in the health care delivery system for the delivery of nursing care. One of the most useful definitions of nursing informatics that remains current comes from Graves and Corcoran (1989, p. 227):

A combination of computer science, information science, and nursing science designed to assist in the management and processing of nursing data, information, and knowledge to support the practice of nursing and the delivery of nursing care.

Nursing informatics as a nursing specialty was approved in 1992 by the American Nurses Association. It encompasses computer science, information science, and nursing science (Saba, 2001). The computer is changing all aspects of health care. Educational efforts include online journals, workshops, courses, and conferences for professionals and instructional video disks for clients. The documentation process increasingly uses the computer, with paperless charting not far off. This technology is no longer used exclusively in acute care settings but in the community at clinics, with home health nurses, with advanced practice nurses, and in public health nursing settings. Various practitioners use the computer to research diseases, treatment methodologies, and educational resources for clients. Consultation regarding complex client health problems is enhanced by computers with two-way visual capabilities. Gebbie (1999), in an editorial in the *American Journal of Public Health,* suggested a core curriculum for all employed public health professionals to include nine topics, with informatics being one of them. Informatics can provide a framework for interdisciplinary study and research, thus enhancing individual and group decision-making.

In many community health settings, the computer has been used to compile client health records; for Medicare, Medicaid, and other insurance billing; and for community health nursing assignments. More and more, community health nurses access computerized nursing information systems that assist with quality measurement and improvement (see Chapter 15), home visiting documentation according to protocol computer tools, documentation of all client contacts, time management, and work schedules. The technique of documenting everything on paper in handwriting is being replaced. Client "charts" are becoming client disks, which are accessed by passwords with laptop computer technology that can be brought into the home. For all students early in the educational process, required courses include typing and computer technology, so that students can efficiently use the "writing and documenting" format of the 21st century.

Computerized geographic information systems (GSIs) allow community health and safety organizations to use three-dimensional graphics to locate and track diseases, toxic waste sites, groundwater sources, vehicle crashes on roads in a region, county, or census tract, and so on. With such information, community health and safety can be enhanced. Traffic patterns can be altered to make roads safer; health care personnel resources can be redistributed based on disease distribution; and dumps and waste sites can be relocated to protect valuable ground water sources—three examples of the usefulness of GSIs.

COLLABORATION AND PARTNERSHIPS IN COMMUNITY HEALTH NURSING

Collaboration, for community health nurses, means a purposeful interaction between nurses, clients, other professionals, and community members based on shared values, mutual participation, and joint effort. It involves building trust and confidence and "is like a marriage in which a partner can speak for you even though you are not at the meeting" (Corrigan, 2000, p. 177). These thoughts highlight two basic features of collaboration: it has a goal, and it involves several parties assisting one another to achieve that goal. The overriding purpose or goal of collaboration in community health practice is to benefit the public's health. To that end, many players must work together. There are key strategies for establishing partnerships and collaboration with interprofessional team members (Allender et al, 1997):

- Think "outside the box" when looking for partners or collaborators.
- The partners must be part of the planning.
- Plans are *guides* toward a goal—stay flexible.
- When adding new partners, be prepared to re-plan.
- Maintain different levels of collaboration (different team members have more resources, come in later to the project, or leave the project earlier).

DISPLAY 11-2

Cross-Cultural Collaboration Guidelines

1. Practice—we get better at cross-cultural collaboration when we practice it.
2. Do not use generalizations about other cultures to stereotype or oversimplify your ideas about another person or group.
3. Do not assume that there is only one right way (yours) to communicate. Keep questioning your assumptions about the "right way" to communicate.
4. Do not assume that breakdowns in communication occur because other people are on the wrong track. Search for ways to make communication work, rather than searching for who should receive the blame.
5. Listen actively and empathetically. Try to put yourself in the other person's shoes, especially when another person's ideas or perceptions are different from your own. Be willing to step outside your comfort zone.
6. Respect other opinions.
7. Stop, suspend judgement, and try to look at the situation as an outsider.
8. Be aware of power imbalances and the effects on communication.
9. Remember that cultural norms may not apply to the behavior of any particular individual. Start from where they are. Check your interpretations and ask for clarification.

- Use consensus-building techniques that are creative and visual.
- Establish a shared vision, then share the plans and the leadership.

Addressing the needs of aggregates requires a variety of team players. Community health nursing practice draws on the expertise and assistance of numerous individuals. The list includes health planners and policy makers, epidemiologists, biostatisticans, community citizens, demographers, environmentalists, educators, politicians, housing experts, safety professionals, and industrial hygienists in addition to physicians, social workers, psychologists, physical therapists, and most of the other professionals involved in health services. Depending on the need to be addressed, community health nurses may work with many of these people on a single project. Furthermore, perhaps the most important team players are community clients—those populations and groups who are the targets of community health services. Clients' cultural background, experience in collaboration and partnership building, perspectives, and expressions of need provide important information for the planning and delivery of services (Display 11–2). Their participation, either collectively or through representatives, ensures more comprehensive and accurate information as well as commitment to fully using the health programs designed for their benefit.

Characteristics of Collaboration and Partnerships

To explore the meaning of collaboration in the context of community health nursing, this section examines five characteristics that distinguish collaboration from other types of interaction: shared goals, mutual participation, maximized resources, clear responsibilities, and set boundaries.

Shared Goals

First, collaboration in community health nursing is goal directed. The nurse, clients, and others involved in the collaborative effort or partnership recognize specific reasons for entering into the relationship. For example, a lumber company with 150 employees seeks to develop a wellness program. The community health nurse, company employee representatives, a safety expert, an industrial hygienist, a health educator, an exercise therapist, a nutritionist, and a psychologist might work together to develop specific physical and mental health goals. The team enters into the collaborative relationship with broad needs or purposes to be met and specific objectives to accomplish.

Mutual Participation

Second, in community health nursing, collaboration involves mutual participation; all team members contribute and are mutually benefitted (Green, Daniel, & Novick, 2001). Collaboration involves a reciprocal exchange in which individual team players discuss their intended involvement and contribution. The lumber company representatives may outline assessed areas of need, such as back strengthening exercises to facilitate lifting and reduce strain. The professionals, including the nurse involved in the collaboration, will offer their own specific ideas and expertise to design the wellness program.

Maximized Use of Resources

A third characteristic of collaboration is that it maximizes the use of community resources. That is, the collaborative partnership is designed to draw on the expertise of those who are most knowledgeable and in the best positions to influence a favorable outcome. If the lumber company team has identified a need for health education materials, the nurse and other members of the collaborating team may explore health education resources through the local health department and within their own professions.

Clear Responsibilities

Fourth, the collaborating team members work in partnership and assume clearly defined responsibilities. As in a football team, each member in the partnership plays a specific role with related tasks. The nurse may play a case-management or group leadership role, whereas others assume roles appropriate to their areas of expertise. Effective collaboration clearly designates what each member will do to accomplish the identified goals. The nurse, for example, might coordinate the planning effort for the lumber company wellness program and work with the health educator to develop classes on various topics. The psychologist might advise on a chemical dependency program, and the industrial hygienist would provide assistance with safety measures. Each member of the team develops an understanding of individual responsibilities based on realistic and honest expectations. This understanding comes through effective communication. The collaborating partners explore necessary resources, assesses their capabilities, and determines their willingness to assume tasks.

Set Boundaries

Fifth, collaboration in community health practice has set boundaries, with a beginning and an end that fall within the goals of the communication. An important part of defining collaboration is determining the conditions under which it occurs and when it will be terminated. The temporal boundaries sometimes are determined by progress toward the goal, sometimes by the number of team member contacts, and often by setting a time limit. The collaborating group might target 6 months as a completion date for the lumber company wellness program and establish a time line with designated activities to reach the goal. Once the purpose for the collaboration has been accomplished, the group as a formal entity can be terminated.

In some settings, the partnership may desire to continue to work on other, mutually agreed upon activities. If so, the process begins again with different goals. Some partnerships are ongoing. For example, a university with a department of nursing might use a neighborhood community center for clinical experiences for the students. The community center has needs that may include health assessments and in-home health teaching among community members, flu shots given at the center for elders without transportation, or health education classes for the adults in an English as a Second Language (ESL) class or for preschoolers in a Head Start program. The center and the university work in partnership so that, each semester, ongoing services are provided by the nursing students and coordinated by a faculty member or graduate nursing student in collaboration with the community center staff. Each partner wins. The students receive a rich educational experience, and the neighborhood center gets services they would otherwise do without. Within such a model, there are opportunities for students and volunteers. Students from other educational disciplines—social work, theater arts, physical therapy, early elementary education, and other areas—can be integrated into a center that serves people of all ages. Professionals (eg, dentist, pediatrician) who are willing to volunteer (eg, one-half or one day per week) enhance the services provided, as can lay volunteers, who can read to the children, answer the telephone, or participate in fund-raising. Any number of possibilities exist when people collaborate and work in partnership together.

Fostering Client Participation

This chapter has stressed that communication and collaboration are based on mutual participation. The extent of clients' involvement in that participation varies, however, depending on their readiness and ability to participate (Chatterjee & Leonard, 2001). The client's level of wellness at the time of the initial professional-client encounter directly influences participation. Some people are not physically or emotionally well enough to assume an active role in the relationship. Women recently discharged from the hospital after a mastectomy, for example, have many physical and emotional adjustments with which to cope. Their families, too, must expend additional energies to provide needed support and to cope with the temporary loss of the woman's usual role in the family. They may find it difficult to engage actively in identifying their needs and goals at the start of the collaborative process. The nurse may have to take a stronger initial leadership role; however, the goals of collaboration are not abandoned. Gradually, as the client's wellness level improves, the nurse can encourage more active participation.

Sometimes a client's previous experiences with health personnel limit participation in collaboration. Clients from poverty-stricken areas, those from different cultural backgrounds, or those with little education may need extensive encouragement to participate actively. Also, clients who were not previously encouraged to participate in decision-making by physicians, nurses, or other professionals may follow the pattern of a passive role and not truly collaborate. Unless the nurse persists in efforts to reduce the dependence of clients, the relationship can fall short of the therapeutic goals.

The nurse's own view of collaboration also influences the degree of client participation. Nurses who are accustomed to relating to clients in an adult-to-child manner restrict client involvement. If nurses see their position as more informed and the client's position as one of complete ignorance and need, a paternalistic relationship may develop. All clients have resources on which to build, and the community health nurse helps clients to discover these resources and use them to enhance collaboration and attain health goals.

Clients who initiate or seek service frequently are best able to assume an active participant role; examples include abused women seeking protection and elderly widowed persons seeking support. These clients have already demonstrated a sense of responsibility for their health by identifying a need and asking for assistance. They also are experts regarding their situation. This intimate knowledge of the problem makes the client an expert partner and a colleague in problem-solving. The nurse still must work carefully to build mutual participation and respond with concern and caring to foster continued interest and participation by clients.

Structure of Collaborative Relationships

Effective collaboration occurs within a particular structure and sequence. During this process, the work of identifying and meeting the client's needs takes place. Because most collaborative and partner relationships are bound by time, the structure involves several phases: (1) a beginning phase when the team relationship is just being established; (2) a middle, working phase; and (3) a termination phase when the relationship ends.

The first phase is a period of establishing and defining the team relationship. All of the team members, including clients, are getting to know each other; they seek to establish communication patterns and develop trust. From these bases, they identify the clients' needs and determine the goals toward which they will work.

The middle phase occurs when team members start working together to accomplish desired goals. Their work may include assessment and planning as well as implementation and evaluation. The cycle of the nursing process is repeated as needed during this working phase until goals are satisfactorily accomplished.

The termination phase occurs when the need for team members to work together has ended. When team members have grown close in the relationship, termination can be difficult. Termination should never occur abruptly or without participation. It often requires careful advance preparation to make certain that all parties understand when and why it is taking place. Termination helps to ensure a clearcut end to the collaborative relationship. For example, a nurse, physician, social worker, psychologist, and nutritionist collaborated with a refugee group for almost 1 year. As the group's multiple needs declined, the professionals began to taper off their assistance. Two months before the relationship was ended, termination of the group was discussed. At first, client group members were frightened at the loss of group support, but slowly they took ownership and control, and with their newly acquired skills they assumed more responsibility for their health needs.

CONTRACTING IN COMMUNITY HEALTH NURSING

Contracting means negotiating a working agreement between two or more parties in which they come to a shared understanding and mutually consent to the purposes and terms of the transaction. Some kinds of contracts are familiar, such as when a buyer signs a contract agreeing to pay a certain amount over a certain period of time to purchase an automobile. Paying tuition for an education involves a form of contracting: although no formal document is signed, students agree with an educational institution on a purpose (to obtain a degree), with the terms of the contract being regular tuition payments and regular learning opportunities over a specified period of time. For students in individual university courses,

their syllabus is a contract. It spells out what is offered, what is expected, and what the ouctcomes may include.

In contrast to legal contracts, which are written and legally binding, contracts in a collaborative relationship or a nurse-client alliance are flexible and changing and are based on mutual understanding and trust. They are working agreements that may be renegotiated continuously between clients and health professionals. The flexibility built into nurse-client contracting makes it a valuable tool for community health nurses.

The same format is followed with clients who are receiving home health care services. The contract that develops from the partnership between client and home health care nurse often is referred to as a **critical pathway**. It consists of the written plans for client care with a timetable. This represents a more formal type of contracting: it is typically a fiscally driven and agency-required tool designed to document standards and quality of care while reducing costs (see Chapters 15 and 37).

Characteristics of Contracting

The concept of contracting, as used in the collaborative relationship, incorporates four distinctive characteristics: partnership and mutuality, commitment, format, and negotiation.

Partnership and Mutuality

All aspects of contracting involve shared participation and agreement between team members; they become partners in the relationship. There is also a mutuality to the nurse-client relationship: if we were to document nurse-client collaboration on a continuum, paternalism would be at one extreme and autonomy at the other. Mutuality becomes the midpoint, balance, or ideal of these two extreme positions. For example, a parenting group of 15 couples requested community health nursing involvement. The group entered into a mutual partnership with the nurse and came to an agreement on what they needed and what the nurse could provide. Together they developed goals, outlined methods to meet those goals, explored resources to help achieve them, defined the time limits for the contract, and outlined their separate responsibilities. The contract involved reciprocal negotiation and shared evaluation. A partnership with mutuality means that all parties are responsible for setting up and carrying out the terms of the agreement within a dynamic balance. Display 11–3 shows an individual service plan, which includes a contract, that is used by one community health nursing program in a California county health department with clients in their Perinatal Outreach Education program.

Commitment

Second, every contract implies a commitment. The involved parties make a decision that binds them to fulfilling the purpose of the contract. In community health collaboration, contracting does not mean making a binding agreement in the legal sense; rather, it is a pledge of trust and dedication. Accompanying that sense of dedication is a strong motivation to see the contract through to completion. All parties feel

DISPLAY 11-3

Client Service Plan with Contract

Madera County Public Health Department
Public Health Nursing: Client Individual Service Plan

Client Name: _Angelica Luz-Smith_   Client Signature: _Angelica Luz-Smith_

Case Manager: _J. Allender, RN, PHN_   Start Date: _6-02-04_

Date: 6-02-04	Client Goal:	Case Manager: Teaching/Counseling/Referral	Follow-up/Reassessment Date: 6-30-04	Follow-up/Reassessment Date: _____
Strengths Identified: Desires to have a healthy baby	1. Eat 5 fruits + vegetables daily	−value of fruits + vegs	Outcome/Evaluation	Outcome/Evaluation
	A. Start with 1–2 fruits + 1–2 vegetables/day	−nutrients not available in any "vitamin"	−Client eating 4 vegs/day on 24 hr dietary recall	
Problems/Risks/Concerns Identified:		−reviewed vegs–client likes corn, canned green beans, V-8 juice	−Client eating 1 fruit/day (banana)	
Doesn't like vegetables	B. Try new ones (use list provided) at least 1/week	−reviewed fruits–client likes apples, bananas + strawberries	Teaching– −reviewed fruits in season	
Doesn't like many fruits	(May use cheese and/or ranch dressing)	−Cl will try peas + carrots + pears	−client will try a fresh peach or grapes each day	
Date: _____	Client Goal:	Case Manager: Teaching/Counseling/Referral	Follow-up/Reassessment Date: _____	Follow-up/Reassessment Date: _____
Strengths Identified:			Outcome/Evaluation	Outcome/Evaluation
Problems/Risks/Concerns Identified:				

responsible for keeping promises; all want to achieve the intended outcomes. When the nurse and the parenting group identified their separate tasks, they committed themselves: "Yes, we will do thus and so."

Format

Format, the third distinctive feature of contracting, involves outlining the specific terms of the relationship. Clients and professionals gain a clear idea of the purpose of the relationship, their respective responsibilities, and the specific limits within which they will work. The format of contracting provides the framework for collaboration. Once the terms of the contract have been spelled out, there is no question about what has to be done, who is to do it, or within what time frame it is to be accomplished. This format helps to avoid the difficulty of terminating long-term relationships and shifts health care responsibilities from the professionals to the individual or group. At times, having something in writing helps the client "legitimize" the nurse-client interaction. The goals and specific objectives are visualized and can be referred to and followed by all parties, as seen in Display 11–3.

Negotiation

Finally, contracting always involves negotiation. The nurse and other team members propose to accept certain responsibilities and then ask whether the clients agree. The nurse might ask, "What do you feel you can do to achieve this goal?" A period of give-and-take then occurs in which ideas are discussed and conclusions and consensus are reached. Team members may find over time that terms or goals on which they had agreed need modification. Perhaps clients have assumed more responsibility than they can realistically handle at this time and need to redefine their specific responsibilities. Perhaps the nurse feels a need to involve another professional in the collaborative process. The importance of effective interpersonal communication between clients and professionals to keep contracts updated is emphasized. Negotiation during contracting allows for changes that facilitate the ultimate achievement of goals. It provides built-in flexibility and encourages ongoing communication among all team members. Negotiation gives contracting a dynamic quality.

Value of Contracting

The value of contracting has been demonstrated in many settings and disciplines. Contracts have been used for many years in psychiatric and other nursing settings to promote client self-respect, problem-solving skills, autonomy, and motivation. Other disciplines, such as social work, have long used contracting as a tool in the helping relationship to enhance realistic planning and emphasize partnership (Sauer, 1973). Educational contracts between students and instructors have proved valuable for facilitating learning. In the Levels of Prevention Matrix, the three levels of prevention are used to provide a framework of care for elderly clients in a contract format.

Community health nursing also has used the concept of contracting for many years. Without always labeling it as contracting, community health nurses have used these techniques with clients who, for example, want to lose weight. In this case, the contract involves mutual agreement on certain exercise and eating patterns for clients and teaching and

---

LEVELS OF PREVENTION MATRIX

SITUATION: A population of elderly individuals, interacting with a community health nurse on a monthly basis at a senior center health clinic, will experience healthful living to the fullest extent of their ability.

GOAL: Using the three levels of prevention, negative health conditions are avoided, or promptly diagnosed and treated, and the fullest possible potential is restored.

PRIMARY PREVENTION		SECONDARY PREVENTION		TERTIARY PREVENTION			
Health Promotion and Education	*Health Protection*	*Early Diagnosis*	*Prompt Treatment*	*Rehabilitation*	*Primary Prevention*		
					Health Promotion and Education	*Health Protection*	
Assess health status Identify specific activities that will improve current health status and functional ability. Provide homework for elders to work on between meetings with the community health nurse.	Provide needed immunizations, (eg, flu, pneumonia, tetanus/diphtheria).	Identify factors contributing to existing health limitations and functional status. Refer to appropriate professionals as needed for diagnosis	In collaboration with elders, select appropriate activities to achieve individual and group goals designed to resolve health limitations and functional status. Encourage client follow-up of treatment regimen designed by community health nurse or other health care practitioner.	In collaboration with elders, select appropriate activities to prevent recurrence of health problems or to restore a healthful level of functioning within their limitations.	Promote healthful lifestyle with adequate diet, rest/sleep, and exercise.	Maintain appropriate immunization schedule.	

support responsibilities for the nurse. Often, it has set a time limit, such as 6 months, within which to achieve the intended weight loss. In each case, a partnership is developed, with agreement about the purpose of the relationship and the conditions under which it will be carried out. Nurses and clients are, in effect, contracting.

As more nurses seek to promote client autonomy and self-care, the wide applicability of contracting to nursing practice is being increasingly recognized (Balzer-Riley, 2000). Community health nurses have provided care for infants receiving total parenteral nutrition, worked with outpatients receiving chemotherapy, and collaborated with prenatal groups, postpartum mothers, and home health clients using various forms of contracting with the clients.

The advantages of contracting in community health nursing are summarized as follows:

1. It involves clients in promoting their own health.
2. It motivates clients to perform necessary tasks.
3. It focuses on clients' unique needs, regardless of aggregate size.
4. It increases the possibility of achieving health goals identified by collaborating team members.
5. It enhances all team members' problem-solving skills.
6. It fosters client participation in the decision-making process.
7. It promotes clients' autonomy and self-esteem as they learn self-care.
8. It makes nursing service more efficient and cost-effective.

Potential Problems with Contracting

Emphasis on contracting as a method rather than a concept can create problems. If a client has experienced contracts only in a business setting, it is possible to carry the stereotype of a cold, formal arrangement into the nursing practice setting. Some nurses fear that asking clients to negotiate a contract will place clients under stress, impede the development of trust, and negatively influence the relationship. Others have found that some clients prefer to have the nurse make decisions for them and are not ready to enter into any kind of negotiation. These problems in contracting can be overcome by understanding the true concept of contracting.

Process of Contracting

Contracting applies basic principles of adult education: self-direction, mutual negotiation, and mutual evaluation (Gustafson, 1977; Hanson, 2001). It need not be a formal, written, or complex negotiation. Contracting can be formal or informal, written or verbal, simple or detailed, and signed or unsigned by client and nurse. It should be adapted to the particular client's abilities to assess, plan, implement, and evaluate, which may vary greatly from situation to situation. The tool shown in Display 11–3 seeks input from the client. The client's goals are mutually set, and the goals are spelled out. Initial interventions are dated, as are follow-up and reassessment visits. In addition,

there is a place for a continuing assessment of outcomes and for evaluation on future dates. Like all nursing tools, contracting enhances client health only if it is adapted to each particular set of client needs and abilities.

Contracting follows a sequence of steps. As a working agreement, it depends on knowing what clients want, agreeing on goals, identifying methods to achieve these goals, knowing the resources that collaborating members bring to the relationship, using appropriate outside resources, setting limits, deciding on responsibilities, and providing for periodic reviews. Each of these tasks requires discussion among members of the contractual group. The tasks are incorporated into the contracting process and can be described in eight phases that follow the nursing process:

Assessment

1. *Explore needs:* Assess clients' health and needs: done by clients, nurse, and other relevant persons

Nursing Diagnosis/Goal Setting

2. *Establish goals:* Discussion followed by agreement among contracting members on goals and objectives

Plan/Intervention

3. *Explore resources:* Define what each member has to offer and can expect from the others; identify appropriate resources and agencies
4. *Develop a plan:* Identify methods, activities, and a time line for achieving the stated goals
5. *Divide responsibilities:* Negotiate the activities for which each member will be responsible
6. *Agree on time frame:* Setting limits for the contract in terms of length of time or number of meetings

Evaluation

7. *Evaluation:* Formative and summative assessments of progress toward goals occur at agreed-on intervals
8. *Renegotiation or termination:* Agree to modify, renegotiate, or terminate the contract

As community health nurses use this process to negotiate a contract, they must adapt it to each situation. The sequence of phases may change, and some steps may overlap. Nevertheless, the basic elements remain important considerations for successful contracting (Fig. 11–2).

Levels of Contracting

Community health nurses use contracts at levels ranging from formal to informal. The degree of formality depends on the demands of the situation. To fund a community health program for preventing child abuse, for example, a formal contract in the form of a written grant proposal may be needed; or, to conduct a wide-scale needs assessment of a homeless population, the services of an epidemiologist and statistician may require a formal contract to clarify roles and expectations. **Formal contracting** involves all parties' negotiating a written contract by mutual agreement, signing the agreement, and sometimes having it witnessed or notarized. This level of contract has been used with mental health or substance-abusing clients,

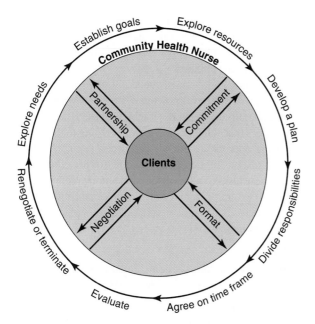

FIGURE 11-2. The concept and process of contracting. Contracting is based on four distinctive features shown here as spokes that support a wheel. These features form the basis for a reciprocal relationship between clients, nurse, and other persons. This relationship is not static; it is a dynamic process that moves through phases, represented here as the outer rim of the wheel. The process moves forward, focused on meeting clients' needs, and enables the collaborating group to facilitate ultimate achievement of clients' goals.

where the seriousness of the working agreement and the need to actively involve the client are important aspects of therapy.

Some situations best lend themselves to a modified and less formal use of contracting, in which the nursing plan becomes the written contract. For example, a school nurse forms a support group for pregnant adolescents. The nurse uses modified contracting by discussing with the girls the purpose of the group and the number of sessions needed and obtaining their agreement to attend all sessions.

Informal contracting involves some form of verbal agreement about relatively clearcut purposes and tasks. A client group may agree to prioritize their list of needs, the nurse may agree to conduct health teaching sessions, the social worker may agree to obtain informational materials, and so on. Sometimes, nurses use contracting informally without realizing it. They conclude a session with clients by agreeing with them about the purpose and time of the next meeting. Conscious use of contracting, however, is a more effective way to provide structure for the relationship and foster client involvement, regardless of the level at which it is applied.

The level of contracting also may change during the development of communication and collaboration. Clients often need education about their options. Initially, they may have difficulty in identifying needs and making choices. The professional team can work to promote clients' self-confidence and help them to assume increasing responsibility for their own health (see The Global Community). Through these efforts,

THE GLOBAL COMMUNITY

INTERNATIONAL COLLABORATION TO PREVENT HIV/AIDS IN LOW PREVALENCE SETTINGS

The diversity of human immunodeficiency virus (HIV) infection throughout populations in the world is striking. Sixteen countries (all in sub-Sarahan Africa) report an overall adult HIV prevalence greater than 10%. Twenty-eight countries report a 1% to 5% prevalence rate. The remaining 119 countries in the world have a less than 1% prevalence rate among adults. The low prevalence rates can lull countries into a false security that they do not have a problem, and consequently they may not have systems in place to prevent HIV infection and the acquired immunodeficiency syndrome (AIDS). This translates into impediments at all levels, from policy formulation to prevention planning and implementation strategies, and ultimately in individual behavior change. Countries with low prevalence often think that low prevalence means low priority, have no desire or ability to prioritize the response to HIV, and think that "we have no problem here."

Countries and their populations have additional barriers that make prevention difficult. Legal, social, and economic conditions affect the whole society and how resources are spent. Education, religious barriers, gender roles, and social pressures impact prevention activities in different ways in the 119 countries.

Many international agencies (UNICEF, UNESCO, WHO, PAHO, World Bank, USAID, the Joint United Nations Programme on HIV/AIDs [UNAIDS], the Asia Pacific InterCountry Team, and Family Health International) have worked together to create recommended prevention strategies that will reach countries as diverse as China, India, Indonesia, and Bangladesh. International collaboration as an overall strategy is helping countries overcome the problem areas that hinder an effective prevention response. Teams from these agencies who know the target communities, cultures, and populations use their skills to help a country develop infrastructures and policy, provide education, and encourage use of prophylactics using strategies that fit with the uniqueness of the population.

The collective experiences from more than 20 years of dealing with this disease can help the low-prevalence countries keep their prevalence rates low, and make them lower, as they deal with their barriers.

(From UNAIDS. [2001]. *Effective prevention strategies in low HIV prevalence settings.* Washington, DC: Family Health International.)

contracting becomes a consciously recognized part of the relationship, and clients become fully participating partners.

SUMMARY

Communication and collaboration are important tools for community health nurses to promote aggregate health. Communication involves the transfer and understanding of meaning between individuals. The communication process comprises seven parts: a message, a sender, a receiver, encoding, a channel, decoding, and a feedback loop. Barriers to effective communication include selective perception, language barriers, clients filtering out parts of the message, and emotional influence. Core skills essential to effective communication in community health nursing include sending skills, which allow the nurse to transmit messages effectively; receiving skills, which allow the nurse to receive accurate and complete messages; and interpersonal skills, which allow the nurse to interact and respond to the messages from clients. These skills include special techniques of active listening, the ability to show respect regardless of the message (whether positive or negative), the ability to empathize with clients' thoughts and feelings, and the ability to develop trust. Many factors can influence the quality of communication, such as negative previous experience, cultural influence, and relationships among the people involved. The community health nurse must consider all of these factors when trying to foster good communication.

In community health, nurses frequently need to promote communication in groups and in group decision-making. Decisions made by groups have many advantages, including sharing of members' experience and expertise, diversity of opinions, potential for broadening members' perspectives, and a focus on arriving at consensus solutions. There are several methods of enhancing group decision-making, including brainstorming, nominal group technique, Delphi technique, and electronic meetings. Nursing informatics, encompassing all of the computer-generated tools created to enhance communication, is changing the form of communicating in community health nursing, as it has in the acute care setting.

Collaboration and partnership building is a purposeful interaction among the nurse, clients, community members, and other professionals based on mutual participation and joint effort. It is characterized by shared goals, mutual participation, maximized use of resources, clear responsibilities, and set boundaries. Clients play an important role in the collaborative relationship.

Contracting also is a helpful tool in promoting clients' participation, independence, and motivation. It is used at all levels in community health nursing to promote partnership in the collaborative process, to encourage commitment to health goals, and to ensure a format and a means for negotiation among the collaborating group. Contracts can be formal or informal, written or verbal, simple or complex. The nurse must know the needs and abilities of clients and must tailor the type of contracting to best suit the client's particular situation.

ACTIVITIES TO PROMOTE CRITICAL THINKING

1. Discuss how you would handle the communication barrier of selective perception with a group of clients.
2. Practice active listening with a colleague and analyze the factors that interfered with your total concentration. Identify three actions to take to improve your active listening and apply them during the next week, keeping a log of your progress.
3. Use nominal group technique with a group of classmates to arrive at a rank-ordering of barriers to cross-cultural communication. What did you learn about arriving at a quality decision in the process?
4. Organize a group of classmates to represent a group of clients, professionals, and community members who are collaborating to address the needs of an inner-city homeless population. Analyze how well you integrated the five characteristics of collaboration into your activity.
5. Explain the concept of contracting as it applies to aggregates. Discuss its four distinctive characteristics and the advantages that contracting offers to the community health nurse.
6. Develop a hypothetical contract with a group of elderly widows who need support and outlets for their loneliness. What other community members and professionals might be helpful as part of a collaborative team to address the widows' needs?
7. Become a good listener. This exercise asks you to list your closest friends, relatives, school peers, and work associates. Rank them on a scale of 1 to 10, with 1 meaning always fascinating and 10 meaning boring. If you find that you've labeled most as boring, you probably have one of two problems: you are either socializing and working with the wrong people, or you are a poor listener. The likelihood is the latter. To improve listening skills, compliment people and encourage them; this increases the chance that they will continue conversing with you and is a valuable skill in both your personal and professional life.
8. Experiment in communication. This can be used with your peers or as part of a group teaching project on communication with elementary or high school students:

Purpose

To demonstrate the differences between one-way and two-way communication and to demonstrate the advantages of the latter.

Setting

Can be conducted in the classroom with any size group. Each person will need paper and pencil.

Procedure

Have the group members select one person whom everyone believes can communicate clearly and effectively to be the "sender." Place this person so that he or she is out of sight but can be clearly heard by the rest of the group ("receivers"). The sender is to describe a diagram, and the receivers are to draw it.

Using Diagram 1, the sender explains the diagram so that the receivers are able to recreate it exactly, following the sender's directions without any further communication with the sender or with other group members. Time the exercise. When the receivers are finished, rank the accuracy of their drawings by placing them on a Likert scale (a 10-point scale, from 1 as Least accurate to 10 as Most accurate). Ask receivers how they felt and how the sender probably felt. Ask the sender how she or he felt.

Next, begin the two-way communication demonstration by allowing the sender to remain in sight of the group as he or she explains Diagram 2 and the receivers draw it. Allow the receivers to ask questions. The sender may reply but may not use gestures. Record the time required, and rank the drawings for accuracy. Discuss how the receivers felt and how the sender probably felt. Ask the sender how she or he felt this time.

Analysis

Compare your findings with the following statements:
A. Two-way communication takes longer.
B. Two-way communication results in greater accuracy among the drawings.
C. In one-way communication, the sender often feels relatively confident; the receiver, uncertain or frustrated.
D. In two-way communication, the sender may feel frustrated or angry; the receiver relatively confident.

REFERENCES

Allender, J.A., Carey, K.T., Castanon, J.G., Garcia, B., Gonzalez, B., Hedge, G., et al. (1997, April). *Interprofessional training project: California State University, Fresno. Serving children and families*. Monmouth, OR: Teaching Research Division.

Balzer-Riley, J. (2000). *Communications in nursing: Communicating assertively and responsibly in nursing. A guidebook* (4th ed.). St. Louis: Mosby.

Chatterjee, N., & Leonard, L. (2001). Partners-in-health: A new front line for disease prevention and health promotion in the community. *American Journal of Health Education, 32*(1), 52–55.

Corrigan, D. (2000). The changing role of schools and higher education institutions with respect to community-based interagency collaboration and interprofessional partnerships. *Peabody Journal of Education, 75*(3), 176–195.

Enger, J.C., & Segal-Isaacson, A.E. (2001). The ABCs of PDAs. *Nursing Management, 32*(12), 60–62.

Gebbie, K.M. (1999). The public health workforce: Key to public health infrastructure. *American Journal of Public Health, 89*(5), 660–661.

Graves, J., & Corcoran, D. (1989). The study of nursing informatics. *Image: Journal of Nursing Scholarship, 21*(3), 227–231.

Green, L., Daniel, M., & Novick, L. (2001). Partnerships and coalitions for community-based research. *Public Health Reports, 116*(Suppl. 1), 20–31.

Gustafson, M.B. (1977). Let's broaden our horizons about the use of contracts. *International Nursing Review, 24*(1), 18–19.

Hanson, G.F. (2001). Refocusing the nursing skills laboratory. In A.H. Lowenstein & M.J. Bradshaw (Eds.), *Fuszard's innovative teaching strategies in nursing* (3rd ed., pp. 269–277). Gaithersburg, MD: Aspen.

Kar, S.B., Arcalay, R., & Alex, S. (2001). *Health communication: A multicultural perspective*. Thousand Oaks, CA: Sage.

Marshall, S.G., & Houseman, C.A. (1999). *Communicating in nursing*. Philadelphia: Lippincott Williams & Wilkins.

Robbins, S.P. (2003). *Essentials of organizational behavior* (7th ed.). Upper Saddle River, NJ: Prentice-Hall.

Saba, V.K. (2001). Nursing informatics: Yesterday, today and tomorrow. *International Nursing Review, 48*, 177–187.

Sauer, J.K. (1973, summer). The process of contracting in the helping relationship. *Minnesota Welfare*, 12–14, 23.

Diagram 1

Diagram 2

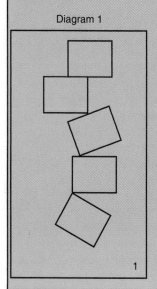

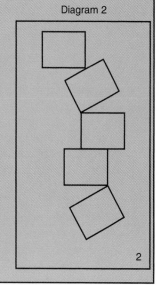

Sharpe, C.C. (2001). *Telenursing: Nursing practice in cyberspace.* Westport, CT: Auburn House.

Spector, R.E. (2000). *Cultural diversity in health and illness* (5th ed.). Upper Saddle River, NJ: Prentice-Hall Health.

Tan, J.K.H. (2001). *Health management information systems: Methods and practical applications* (2nd ed.). Gaithersburg, MD: Aspen.

United Nations Programme on HIV/AIDS (UNAIDS). (2001). *Effective prevention strategies in low HIV prevalence settings.* Washington, DC: Family Health International.

United States Department of Health and Human Services. (2000). *Healthy people 2010* (Conference ed., Vols. I & II). Washington, DC: U.S. Government Printing Office.

SELECTED READINGS

Alexander, C., & McKenna, S. (2001). A sound partnership for end-of-life care. *American Journal of Nursing, 101*(12), 75–77.

Arons, R.R. (2001). Using technology to advance the public's health. *American Journal of Public Health, 91*(8), 1178–1179.

Berkowitz, B., & Wolff, T. (2000). *The spirit of the coalition.* Washington, DC: American Public Health Association.

Brown, S.G., & Davis, S. (2000). Putting a new face on self-sufficiency programs. *American Journal of Public Health, 90*(9), 1383–1384.

Guttman, N. (2000). *Public health communication interventions: Values and ethical dilemmas.* Thousands Oaks, CA: Sage.

Hardin, S., & Langford, D. (2001). Telehealth's impact on nursing and the development of the interstate compact. *Journal of Professional Nursing, 17*(5), 243–247.

Heinemann, G.D., & Zeiss, A.M. (2002). *Team performance in health care assessment and development.* Norwell, MA: Kluwer Plenum.

Hojat, M., Nasca, T.J., Cohen, M.J.M., Fields, S.K., Rattner, S.L., Griffiths, M., et al. (2001). Attitudes toward physician-nurse collaboration: A cross-cultural study of male and female physicians and nurses in the United States and Mexico. *Nursing Research, 50*(2), 123–128.

Jenkins, R.L., & White, P. (2001). Telehealth advancing nursing practice. *Nursing Outlook, 49*(2), 100–105.

Jones, J., & Moore, S.M. (2001). Telehealth: Can nursing values be preserved? In H. R. Feldman, *Nursing leaders speak out: Issues and opinions* (pp. 55–61). New York: Springer.

Kim, J.J., Cho, H., Cheon-Klessig, Y.S., Gerace, L.M., & Camilleri, D.D. (2002). Primary health care for Korean immigrants: Sustaining a culturally sensitive model. *Public Health Nursing 19*(3), 191–200.

Malone, G., & Morath, J. (2001). Pro-patient partnerships. *Nursing Management, 32*(7), 46–47.

Maurana, C.A., & Rodney, M.M. (2000). Strategies for developing a successful community health advocate program. *Family and Community Health, 23*(1), 40–49.

Pan American Health Organization. (2001). *Building standard-based nursing information systems.* Washington, DC: Author.

Rice, R.E., & Katz, J.E. (2001). *The internet and health communication: Experiences and expectations.* Thousand Oaks, CA: Sage.

Riegelman, R., & Persily, N.A. (2001). Health information systems and health communications: Narrowband and broadband technologies as core public health competencies. *American Journal of Public Health, 91*(8), 1179–1183.

Saba, V.K., & McCormick, K.A., (Eds.). (2001). *Essentials of computers for nurses: Informatics in the next millennium.* New York: McGraw-Hill.

Scholes, M., et al. (2000). *International nursing informatics: A history of the first forty years, 1960–2000.* London: British Computer Society.

Strader, T.N., Collins, D.A., & Noe, T.D. (2000). *Building healthy individuals, families, and communities: Creating lasting connections.* Norwell, MA: Kluwer Plenum.

Sullivan, M., & Kelly, J.G. (2001). *Collaborative research: University and community partnership.* Washington, DC: American Public Health Association.

Young, K.M. (2000). *Informatics for healthcare professionals.* Philadelphia: F.A. Davis.

Internet Resources

American Medical Informatics Association (AMIA): *http://www.amia.org*

British Computer Society Nursing Specialist Group: *http://www.man.ac.uk/bcsnsg*

Canada's Health Informatics Association: *http://www.coachorg.com*

Cumulative Index to Nursing and Allied Health Literature (CINAHL): *http://www.cinahl.com*

International Medical Informatics Association (IMIA): *http://www.amia.org*

Midwest Alliance for Nursing Informatics: *http://www.maninet.org*

Health Informatics Society of Australia (Vic.), Inc.: *http://www.hisavic.aus.net*

National Institute for Dispute Resolution: *http://www.nidr.org*

North Carolina Nurses Association Council on Nursing Informatics: *http://www.unc.edu/dbailel/CONI/*

Whole Nurse Informatics Page: *http://www.wholenurse.com/informatics.htm*

12

Health Promotion Through Education: Theories, Models, and Tools

Key Terms

- Accommodation (Piaget)
- Adaptation (Piaget)
- Affective domain
- Anticipatory guidance
- Assimilation (Piaget)
- Cognitive domain
- Gestalt-field
- Learning
- Operationalize
- Psychomotor domain
- Teaching

Learning Objectives

Upon mastery of this chapter, you should be able to:

- Identify how the nurse collaborates with other professionals using *Healthy People 2010* as a guide for educational and community-based programs.

- Describe the community health nurse's role as educator in promoting health and preventing or postponing morbidity.

- Identify educational activities for the nurse to use that are appropriate for each of the three domains of learning.

- Select learning theories that are applicable to an individual, family, or aggregate client.

- Identify health teaching models for use when planning health education activities.

- Select teaching methods and materials that facilitate learning for clients at different developmental levels.

- Develop teaching plans focusing on primary, secondary, and tertiary levels of prevention for clients of all ages.

- Identify teaching strategies for the community health nurse to use when encountering clients with special learning needs.

- Locate appropriate multimedia resources to enhance client learning.

T hink of a time when you were so influenced by a teacher that you stopped an unhealthy habit, altered a long-held belief, or embarked on a new endeavor. What precisely was it that motivated the change? Was it simply the content of the teaching, or was it how the teacher presented the content? What is good teaching, and why is it important to community health nursing?

Teaching has been a critical part of the community health nurse's role since the origins of the profession, and it frequently is the primary role or function. Community health nurses develop partnerships with clients to achieve behavior changes that promote, maintain, or restore health. This partnership focuses on self-care—the ability to effectively advocate and manage a person's own health. The rationale for health teaching is to equip people with the knowledge, attitudes, and practices that will allow them to live the fullest possible life for the greatest length of time. The goals of *Healthy People 2010* emphasize not only health status and longevity but also the quality of our lives; they state that even the later years should be full of vigor (U. S. Department of Health and Human Services [USDHHS], 2000). Table 12–1

provides a list of *Healthy People 2010* objectives for educational, community-based programs.

When the community health nurse identifies a need that is best met through health education, the nurse is faced with a series of questions: How can I teach effectively? What content should I cover? What method of presentation will communicate most effectively? What resources can I use as teaching tools? How do I know when the client has grasped the information or mastered the skills? How do I help clients with special learning needs? The nurse must understand what makes teaching effective, how teaching skills are acquired, and how mastery is measured. This chapter addresses these questions and discusses teaching as a basic intervention tool in community health nursing practice.

Teaching is a specialized communication process in which desired behavior changes are achieved. The goal of all teaching is learning. Learning is thought to mean gaining knowledge, comprehension, or mastery. These are nebulous terms, and a more acceptable definition suggests that **learning** is a process of assimilating new information that promotes a permanent change in behavior. All people have been

TABLE 12–1

Healthy People 2010 Objectives for Educational and Community-Based Programs

Objective	2010 Goals	Baseline
High school completion	Increase the high school completion rate to at least 90%.	85%
School health education	Increase to at least 70% the proportion of middle/junior high and senior high schools that require 1 school year of health education.	28%
Undergraduate health risk behavior information	Increase to at least 25% the proportion of undergraduate students attending postsecondary institutions who receive information from their college or university on all six priority health risk behavior areas—behaviors that cause unintentional and intentional injuries, tobacco use, alcohol and other drug use, sexual behavior, dietary patterns that cause disease, and inadequate physical activity.	6%
School nurse-to-student ratio	Increase to at least 50% the proportion of the middle/junior and senior high schools that have a nurse-to-student ratio of at least 1:750.	28%
Work site health-promotion programs	Increase to 100% the proportion of work sites (with more than 50% employees) that offer a comprehensive health-promotion program to their employees.	95%
Participation in employer-sponsored health-promotion activities	Increase to at least 50% the proportion of all employees (over age 18) who participate in employer-sponsored health-promotion activities.	28%
Patient satisfaction with health care provider communication	This objective is developmental: increase the proportion of patients who report that they are satisfied with the patient education they receive from their health care organization.	—
Community-based health promotion	This objective is developmental: increase the proportion of tribal and local health service areas or jurisdictions that have established a community health promotion program that addresses multiple *Healthy People 2010* focus areas.	—
Culturally appropriate community health-promotion programs	Increase the proportion of local health departments to at least 50% that have established culturally appropriate and linguistically competent community health-promotion and disease-prevention programs for racial and ethnic minority populations.	13–27%
Elderly participation in community health promotion	Increase to at least 90% the proportion of people age 65 and older who have participated during the preceding year in at least one organized health-promotion program.	12%

(U.S. Department of Health and Human Services. [2000, January]. *Healthy people 2010* [Conference ed., Vols. I & II]. Washington, DC: Author.)

presented with information that was not interesting, relevant to their needs, or comprehensible. In such situations, learning was difficult, if not impossible. The nurse as a teacher seeks to transmit information in such a way that the client demonstrates a relatively permanent change in behavior. After learning, clients are capable of doing something that they could not do before learning took place. Effective teaching is a cause; learning becomes the effect. To teach effectively, especially in the community where teaching is the focus of care, nurses need to understand the various domains of learning and related learning theories.

DOMAINS OF LEARNING

Learning occurs in several realms or domains: cognitive, affective, and psychomotor. Understanding of the differences among the domains and of the related roles of the nurse provides the background necessary to teach effectively.

Cognitive Domain

The **cognitive domain** of learning involves the mind and thinking processes. When the meaning and relationship of a series of facts is grasped, cognitive learning is experienced. The cognitive domain deals with the recall or recognition of knowledge and the development of intellectual abilities and skills (Bloom, 1956). There are six major levels in the cognitive domain (Gronlund, 1970): knowledge, comprehension, application, analysis, synthesis, and evaluation. To **operationalize** these levels (ie, put these ideas or concepts into words that can be used), verbs are used. As the goal of the learning or behavioral objective changes, so do the verbs, indicating the learning to be accomplished within that particular level of the cognitive domain. Notice that the objectives at the beginning of each chapter in this text follow this format, using a variety of verbs to indicate the expected level of learning. A representative sample of behavioral objectives focusing on nutrition and appropriate cognitive-level verbs is included in the discussion of each level.

Knowledge

Knowledge, the lowest level of learning according to Bloom's taxonomy (1956), involves recall. If students remember material previously learned, they have acquired knowledge. This level may be used with clients who are unable to understand underlying reasons or rationales, such as young children or people who have had strokes. Stroke clients may need to remember that medication should be taken daily, that regular exercise restores function, and that drinking alcohol should be avoided, although they may not grasp the reasons behind these measures. Five-year-olds may need to identify healthful foods rather than understand why they are nutritious.

A knowledge-level behavioral objective might be, "The client can *recall* the names of six fruits to eat as nutritious

snacks." Other knowledge-level verbs include *define, repeat, list,* and *name.*

Comprehension

The second level of cognitive learning, comprehension, combines remembering with understanding. Teaching aims at instilling at least a minimal understanding. Nurses want clients to grasp the meaning and to recognize the importance of suggested health behaviors.

An example of a comprehension-level behavioral objective might be, "The pregnant client will *describe* a well-balanced diet during pregnancy." Other appropriate verbs at the comprehension level include *discuss, explain, identify, tell,* and *report.*

Application

Application is the third level of cognitive learning, in which the learner is able not only to understand material but also to apply it to new situations. Application approaches the possibility of self-care when clients use their knowledge for improvement of their own health. The test of application is a transfer of understanding into practice. Therefore, to encourage application, the nurse can design teaching plans that provide clients with knowledge that can be put into practice. For example, a program used this approach to increase knowledge and change attitudes and beliefs regarding breast cancer. Awareness and mammography participation increased significantly among Latina women who participated in a multimedia breast cancer education intervention (Valdez, Banerjee, Ackerson, & Fernandez, 2002). In the home setting, a nurse may suggest that a diabetic client write down glucometer readings to show the nurse at the next visit. A school nurse could ask adolescents in a weight-loss group to keep a diet record for a week, draw up a diet plan, and share this plan with the group at the next meeting. In contrast, the construction worker who understands on-the-job hazards but seldom wears a protective hat in the work area has yet to transfer knowledge and comprehension into practice or application.

An example of an application-level behavioral objective might be, "The client will *practice* eating well-balanced meals at least two times a day." Other verbs at this level include *apply, use, demonstrate,* and *illustrate.*

Analysis

The fourth level of cognitive learning is analysis; at this level, the learner breaks down material into parts, distinguishes between elements, and understands the relationships among the parts. This level of learning becomes a preliminary step toward problem-solving. The learner carefully scrutinizes all of the variables or elements and their relationships to each other to explain the situation. A family that studies its own communication patterns to identify sources of conflict is using analysis. A mother analyzes when she seeks to determine the cause of an infant's crying. After viewing the total situation, she breaks it down into variables such as hunger, pain, overstimulation, loneliness, type of crying, and intensity of crying. She examines these parts and draws conclusions about their relationships. In health teaching, community health nurses foster clients' analytic skills by (1) demonstrating how to isolate the parts in a situation, and (2) encouraging the clients to consider the relationships among the parts and to draw conclusions from their thinking.

An analysis-level behavioral objective for senior citizens trying to learn more about low-fat foods might be, "The seniors should be able to *compare* the fat content in a variety of packaged foods." Other verbs at the analysis level include *differentiate, contrast, debate, question,* and *examine.*

Synthesis

Synthesis, the fifth level of cognitive learning, is the ability not only to break down and understand the elements of a situation, but also to form elements into a new whole. Synthesis combines all of the earlier levels of cognitive learning to culminate in the production of a unique plan or solution. Clients who achieve learning at this level not only analyze their problems but also find solutions for them. For example, a nurse may assist mental health clients in a therapy group to examine their frequent depression and then to generate their own plan for alleviating it. A young couple who want to toilet train their 2-year-old child may learn the physiologic and psychological dimensions of toilet training, analyze their own situation, and then develop strategies (their own plan) for training the child. Nurses facilitate synthesis by assisting and encouraging clients to develop their own solutions with specific plans. After a problem is identified, the client should be asked, "What are some possible causes? Do you see anything that has been overlooked about the problem?" If the client asks for a solution, the nurse should encourage synthesis by asking, "What are some possible solutions to this problem that you might carry out?"

An example of a synthesis-level behavioral objective for a client on a sodium-restricted diet might be, "The client will be able to *prepare* an enjoyable meal using low-sodium foods." Other verbs at this level include *compose, design, formulate, create,* and *organize.*

Evaluation

The highest level of cognitive learning is evaluation: at this level, the learner judges the usefulness of new material compared with a stated purpose or specific criteria (Gronlund, 1970). Clients can learn to judge their own health behavior by comparing it with standards established by others—such as complete abstinence from smoking, maintenance of normal weight, or exercising three times a week. Alternatively, clients may establish their own criteria. For example, a parent support group might design activities to enhance parent-child communication, then judge their performance by using their desired outcomes as evaluation criteria. When nurses aim for this level of client learning, they have made self-care a concrete objective. Evaluation, because it goes beyond attempts at problem-solving, enables the client to judge the adequacy of solutions, to critique lifestyle and health-related behaviors, and to anticipate needed improvements.

An example of a behavioral objective at the evaluation level might be, "The clients in a nutrition class will be able to *measure* the cholesterol content in one portion of the low-cholesterol dish they brought to share." Other verbs at this level include *judge, rate, choose,* and *estimate.*

How to Measure Cognitive Learning

Cognitive learning at any of the levels described can be measured easily in terms of learner behaviors. Nurses know, for instance, that clients have achieved teaching objectives for the application of knowledge if their behavior demonstrates actual use of the information taught. Client roles in cognitive learning range from relatively passive (at the knowledge level) to active (at the evaluation level). Conversely, as clients become more active, the nurse's role becomes less directive. Notice that not all clients need to be brought through all levels of cognitive learning, nor does every client need to reach the evaluation level for each aspect of care. For some clients and situations, comprehension is an adequate and effective level; for others, the nurse should focus on the application level as the level of achievement. Table 12–2 illustrates client and nurse behaviors for each cognitive level.

TABLE 12–2

Cognitive Learning: Case Study in Controlling Diabetes

Level	Illustrative Client Behavior	Illustrative Nurse Behavior
Knowledge (recalls, knows)	States that insulin, if taken, will control own diabetes	Provides information
Comprehension (understands)	Describes insulin action and purpose	Explains information
Application (uses learning)	Adjusts insulin dosage daily to maintain proper blood sugar level	Suggests how to use learning
Analysis (examines, explains)	Discusses relationships between insulin, diet, activity, and diabetic control	Demonstrates and encourages analysis
Synthesis (integrates with other learning, generates new ideas)	Develops a plan, incorporating above learning, for controlling own diabetes	Promotes client formulation of own plan
Evaluation (judges according to a standard)	Compares degree of diabetic control (outcomes) with desired control (objectives)	Facilitates evaluation

Affective Domain

The **affective domain** in which learning occurs involves emotion, feeling, or affect. This kind of learning deals with changes in interest, attitudes, and values (Bloom, 1956). Here, nurses face the task of trying to influence what clients value and feel. Nurses want clients to develop an ability to accept ideas that promote healthier behavior patterns even if those ideas conflict with the clients' own values.

Attitudes and values are learned (Bigge, 1992). They develop gradually, as the way an individual feels and responds is molded by family, peers, experiences, and societal influences. These feelings and responses are the result of imitation and conditioning. In this way, clients acquire their health-related beliefs and practices. Because attitudes and values become part of the person, they are difficult to change unless the nurse is aware of how they develop.

Affective learning occurs on several levels as learners respond with varying degrees of involvement and commitment. At the first level, learners are simply receptive; they are willing to listen, to show awareness, and to be attentive. The nurse aims at acquiring and focusing learners' attention (Gronlund, 1970). This limited goal may be all that clients are ready for at the early stages of the nurse-client relationship.

At the second level, learners become active participants by responding to the information in some way. Examples are a willingness to read educational material, to participate in discussions, to complete assignments (eg, keeping a diet record), or to voluntarily seek out more information.

At the third level, learners attach value to the information. Valuing ranges from simple acceptance through appreciation to commitment. For example, a nurse taught members of a therapy group several principles concerning group effectiveness. An explanation of the importance of a democratic group process and ways to improve group skills was given. Members showed acceptance when they acknowledged the importance of these ideas. They showed appreciation of the ideas by starting to practice them. Commitment came when they assumed responsibility for having their group function well.

The final level of affective learning occurs when learners internalize an idea or value. The value system now controls learner behavior. Consistent practice is a crucial test at this level. Clients who know and respect the value of exercise but only occasionally play tennis or go for a walk have not internalized the value. Even several weeks of enthusiastic jogging is not evidence of an internalized value. If the jogging continues for 6 months, 12 months, or longer, learning may have been internalized.

Affective learning often is difficult to measure. This elusiveness may influence community health nurses to concentrate their efforts on cognitive learning goals instead. Yet client attitudes and values have a major effect on the outcome of cognitive learning—desired behavioral changes. Therefore, both cognitive and affective domains must remain linked in teaching; otherwise, results quickly fade.

Attitudes and values can change in the same way that they were first learned, that is, through imitation and conditioning (Redman, 2001). Role models, particularly individuals from the client's peer group who practice the desired health behaviors, can be a strong influence. Support groups such as mastectomy clubs or chemical dependency support groups can have a powerful role-model effect. Frequently, the nurse is viewed as a role model by clients; for this reason, nurses should be careful to demonstrate healthy behaviors.

Attitudes often change when the nurse provides clients with a satisfying experience during the learning process. The nurse who recognizes clients' participation in a group, praises them for completing assignments, or commends them for sticking to diet plans will have more success than the nurse who only criticizes failures. Another point to remember is that clients can develop a close relationship with the nurse during the teaching-learning process. When this occurs, some limited sharing of the nurse's experiences in managing personal health issues may be appropriate to let clients know that the nurse, too, is human. This can be an effective addition to teaching strategies if it feels comfortable and is used wisely. Table 12–3 shows client and nurse behaviors for each level of affective learning.

To influence affective learning requires patience. Values and attitudes seldom change overnight. Remember that other forces continue to reinforce former values. For example, a middle-aged housewife may want to pursue a career for self-fulfillment, but she might not do so because she has children in high school and feels that their needs come first. A young man who can verbalize to the nurse the importance of safe sex

T A B L E   1 2 – 3

Affective Learning: Case Study in Family Planning

Level	Illustrative Client Behavior	Illustrative Nurse Behavior
Receptive (listens, pays attention)	Attentive to family planning instruction	Directs client's attention
Responsive (participates, reacts)	Discusses pros and cons of various methods	Encourages client involvement
Valuing (accepts, appreciates, commits)	Selects a method for use	Respects client's right to decide
Internal consistency (organizes values to fit together)	Understands and accepts responsibility for planning for desired number of children	Brings client into contact with role models
Adoption (incorporates new values into lifestyle)	Consistently practices birth control	Positively reinforces healthy behaviors

may be uncomfortable discussing the subject with his partner, jeopardizing his compliance with the nurse's instruction.

Psychomotor Domain

The **psychomotor domain** includes visible, demonstrable performance skills that require some kind of neuromuscular coordination. Clients in the community need to learn skills such as infant bathing, temperature taking, breast or testicular self-examination, prenatal breathing exercises, range-of-motion exercises, catheter irrigation, walking with crutches, and how to change dressings.

For psychomotor learning to take place, three conditions must be met: (1) learners must be capable of the skill, (2) learners must have a sensory image of how to perform the skill, and (3) learners must practice the skill.

The nurse must be certain that the client is physically, intellectually, and emotionally capable of performing the skill. An elderly diabetic man with tremulous hands and fading vision should not be expected to give his own insulin injections; it could frustrate and harm him. An accessible person who is more physically capable should be enlisted and taught the skill. Clients' intellectual and emotional capabilities also influence their capacity to learn motor skills. It may be inappropriate to expect persons of limited intelligence to learn complex skills. The degree of complexity should match the learners' level of functioning. However, educational level should not be equated with intelligence. Many clients have had limited formal schooling but are able to learn complex skills for themselves or as caregivers after thorough instruction. Developmental stage is another point to consider in determining whether it is appropriate to teach a particular skill. For example, most children can put on some article of clothing at 2 years of age but are not ready to learn to fasten buttons until well past their third birthday.

Learners also must have a sensory image of how to perform the skill through sight, hearing, touch, and sometimes taste or smell. This sensory image is gained by demonstration. To teach clients motor skills effectively, the nurse has to provide them with an adequate sensory image. The nurse must demonstrate and explain slowly, one point at a time, and sometimes repeatedly, until clients understand the proper sequence or combination of actions necessary to carry out the skill.

The third necessary condition for psychomotor learning is practice. After acquiring a sensory image, clients can start to perform the skill. Mastery comes over time as clients repeat the task until it is smooth, coordinated, and unhesitating. During this process, the nurse should be available to provide guidance and encouragement. In the early stages of practice, the nurse may need to use hands-on guidance to give clients a sense of how the performance should feel. When clients give return demonstrations, the nurse can make suggestions, give encouragement, and thereby maximize the learning. For example, a nurse demonstrates passive range-of-motion exercises on a client's wife to show her how the exercises should feel (giving her a sensory image). The wife then learns to perform the exercises on her husband. During practice, feedback from the nurse enables the wife to know whether the skill is being performed correctly.

The psychomotor domain, like the cognitive and affective domains, ranges from simple to complex levels of functioning. It is necessary to exercise judgment in assessing clients' ability to perform a skill. Even clients with limited ability often can move to higher levels once they have mastered simple skills. Nurse behaviors that influence psychomotor learning are shown in Table 12–4.

LEARNING THEORIES

A *learning theory* is a systematic and integrated look into the nature of the process whereby people relate to their surroundings in such ways as to enhance their ability to use both themselves and their surroundings more effectively. Nurses have and use a particular theory of learning, whether consciously or unconsciously, and that theory, in turn, dictates their way of teaching. It is useful to discover what that learning theory is and how it affects the nurse's role as health educator.

Some of the learning theories developed by educational psychologists in the 20th century remain influential. They are grouped into four categories: behavioral, cognitive, social, and humanistic. Recently, the adult learning theory of Malcolm Knowles (1980, 1984, 1989) has influenced client teaching. A brief examination of these categories and the specific theories of each follows.

Behavioral Learning Theories

Behavioral theory (also known as stimulus-response or conditioning theory) approaches the study of learning by focusing on behaviors that can be observed, measured, and

T A B L E   1 2 – 4

Nurse Behaviors in Psychomotor Learning		
The Nurse	**Provides Sensory Image**	**Encourages Practice**
Determines capability: Assesses client's physical, intellectual, and emotional ability	Demonstrates and explains	Uses guidance and positive reinforcement

changed. Developed early in the 20th century, behavioral theory work primarily is associated with three famous names: Ivan Pavlov (1957), Edward Thorndike (1932, 1969), and B. F. Skinner (1974, 1987). To a behavioralist, learning is a behavioral change—a response to certain stimuli. Therefore, the behaviorialistic teacher seeks to significantly change learners' behaviors through a series of selected stimuli.

The stimulus-response "bond" theory proposes that, with conditioning, certain causes (stimuli) evoke certain effects (responses). The teacher promotes acquisition of the desired stimulus-response connections so that transfer of learning can occur in another situation having the same stimulus-response elements. Pavlov's early work with stimulus-response and involuntary reflex actions is the best-known application of this theory. Pavlov conditioned a dog to anticipate food by ringing a bell at feeding time. Initially, the dog would salivate as the food was brought to the cage. However, after time, the dog would salivate at hearing the bell, before seeing or smelling the food.

Two other behavioral theories are conditioning with no reinforcement (Thorndike) and conditioning through reinforcement (Skinner). No-reinforcement theorists focus on the learner's innate reflexive drives to accomplish the desired response after conditioning, such as when the nurse repeatedly emphasizes to a group of pregnant women that their prenatal classes promote a positive delivery experience and healthy newborns. In contrast, the reinforcement theorists use successive, systematic changes in the learner's environment to enhance the probability of desired responses. For example, a school nurse might give rewards (balloons, coloring books, crayons) to children who attend each class on safety.

Cognitive Learning Theories

Jean Piaget is the most widely known cognitive theorist. His theory of cognitive development contributed to the theories of Kohlberg (moral development) and Fowler (development of faith). Piaget (1966, 1970) believed that cognitive development is an orderly, sequential, and interactive process in which a variety of new experiences must exist before intellectual abilities can develop. His work with children led him to develop five phases of cognitive development, from birth to 15 years of age (Table 12–5).

Each stage signifies a transformation from the previous one, and a child must move through each stage sequentially. The three abilities of **assimilation** (reacting to new situations by using skills already possessed), **accommodation** (being sufficiently mature so that previously unsolved problems can now be solved), and **adaptation** (the ability to cope with the demands of the environment) are used to make the transformation. Nurses must understand their audience's learning stage to ascertain how to approach teaching for that developmental stage. The nurse can see how the use of puppets with 3-year-olds may be a beneficial addition to a presentation on safety, whereas a group of young teens with diabetes may respond to information on the consequences of taking or not taking their insulin.

The **Gestalt-field** family of cognitive theories assumes that people are neither good nor bad—they simply interact with their environment, and their learning is related to perception (Wertheimer, 1945/1959, 1980). This theory defines learning as a reorganization of the learner's perceptual or psychological world (Bigge, 1992).

The first Gestalt-field theory, called *insight theory*, regards learning as a process in which the learner develops new insights or changes old ones. Learners sense their way intuitively and intelligently through problems. However, the "insight" is useful only if the learner understands its significance. For example, Lana dropped out of high school after the birth of her daughter; after attending a career planning class offered by a community health nurse, she realizes that she has limited job skills and that if she knew how to use a computer she could get a better job. This learner understood the significance of her insight. The second theory, *goal-insight*, is similar to the insight theory but goes beyond intuitive hunches to tested insights. Teachers subscribing to this theory promote insightful learning but assist learners in developing higher-quality insights. For example, Lana takes a beginning and then an advanced computer class and is offered a higher-paying job. The community health nurse discusses Lana's successes with her, asks Lana whether she ever thought about going to college, and mentions the added benefits of college-level course work. Lana reflects on this for a while and begins to think about completing the requirements to go to junior college, because if she had an associate degree she could be promoted to supervisor. In the third theory, *cognitive-field theory*, the learner is seen as pur-

T A B L E   1 2 – 5

Piaget's Five Phases of Cognitive Development		
Age	**Stage**	**Behavior**
Birth to 2 yr	Sensorimotor stage	The child moves focus from self to the environment (rituals are important).
2–4 yr	Preconceptual stage	Language development is rapid and everything is related to "me."
4–7 yr	Intuitive thought stage	Egocentric thinking diminishes, and words are used to express thoughts.
7–11 yr	Concrete operations stage	Child can solve concrete problems and recognize others' viewpoints.
11–15 yr	Formal operations stage	Child uses rational thinking and can develop ideas from general principles (deductive reasoning) and apply them to future situations.

posive and problem-centered. Teachers seek to help learners gain new insights and restructure their lives accordingly. For example, Lana confers with the community health nurse about her choices and has changed her thinking about herself so much that she is planning to get an apartment in a neighborhood that is better for her child and may continue taking classes "for the fun of it" after she completes her degree in a few months.

Social Learning Theories

The aim of social learning theory is to explain behavior and facilitate learning. An important social theorist, Bandura (1977, 1986), pointed out that apparent but not real relationships often are dysfunctional, producing undesirable or inappropriate behavior. He described three ways that dysfunctional beliefs develop:

1. In coincidental association, outcomes typically are preceded by numerous events, and the client selects the wrong events as predictors of an outcome. For example, Juanita had a negative experience with a man who wore a hearing aid. Afterward, all of her experiences with men who wore hearing aids were negative. She reached the conclusion that all men who wear hearing aids were undesirable. This client's beliefs became a self-fulfilling prophecy.
2. In inappropriate generalization, one negative experience provokes negative feelings for future experiences. For example, Shauna had a purse snatched by a teenager and generalized that all teenagers are bad. Three-year-old Ryan accidentally drank some spoiled milk. He generalized that milk tastes bad and now refuses to drink it.
3. In perceived self-inefficacy, "Persons who judge themselves as lacking coping capabilities, whether the self-appraisal is objectively warranted or not, will perceive all kinds of dangers in situations and exaggerate their potential harmfulness" (Bandura, 1986, p. 220). For example, an older client, William, tells the community health nurse about two missing social security checks, but he refuses to take a bus to the post office. He states that he does not know what to say to the postal clerk and has read about senior citizens getting mugged on buses. He refused to follow up on his lost income.

Social learning theory focuses on the learners. They are benefitted by role models, building self-confidence, persuasion, and personal mastery. Self-efficacy can lead to the desired behaviors and outcomes. Juanita may begin to separate her negative experiences with men from their hearing disabilities after attending a class on building self-esteem suggested by the nurse. Through some positive experiences with teenagers organized by the nurse, Shauna may learn that not all teenagers are bad. The nurse can suggest to Ryan's mother that he may be persuaded to drink chocolate milk. She then can slowly reintroduce plain milk. William might find the courage and self-confidence to solve future problems after the nurse introduces him to another gentleman in the apartment complex who feels confident in the neighborhood.

Humanistic Learning Theories

Humanistic theories assume that there is a natural tendency for people to learn and that learning flourishes in an encouraging environment. Two of the best-known humanists are Abraham Maslow and Carl Rogers. Abraham Maslow developed the classic hierarchy of human needs in the 1940s. It suggests that a person's first needs are physiologic (eg, air, food, water). Once these needs are met, people work to fulfill safety and security needs. Third is the need for love and a sense of belonging; then come self-esteem needs (positive feelings of self-worth). Only after these needs are met do people work toward self-actualization or "becoming all that we can be" (Maslow, 1970).

In community health nursing, the clients' needs must be considered when planning health education programs. For example, it would be difficult for a group of young mothers to concentrate on learning about proper infant nutrition if they are worried about their babies crying in the next room or about an abusive partner who doesn't want them out of the house. Their need to care for their children (need of love and belonging) or for their personal well-being (security and safety) would be greater than the need to learn about future health considerations (self-esteem, self-actualization). Likewise, it is impossible for learning to take place if a room is so warm that the participants are falling asleep (ie, physiologic needs are not being met).

Carl Rogers developed the client-centered counseling approach that has long been important in psychotherapy. He believed the role of the therapist should be nondirective and accepting and proposed approaching clients in a warm, positive, and empathetic manner to get in touch with their feelings and thoughts. Rogers soon applied his beliefs to education, suggesting that the learning environment be learner centered (1969, 1989). The outcome of a learner-centered educational environment is that the students become more self-directed and guide their own learning. Rogers believed that the learner is the person most capable of deciding how to find the solutions to problems. The client identifies the problem and, given time and space, can find a way through the problem to a solution. The nurse acts as a facilitator in this learning process. As an example, a 55-year-old man wants to quit smoking after a prolonged upper respiratory tract infection, aggravated by his habit, and comes to a stop-smoking class conducted by a nurse in the county health department.

Knowles' Adult Learning Theory

In the last 20 to 30 years, a variety of techniques have been developed to help adults learn. One of the main discoveries is that adults as learners are different from children. They do not learn differently, but are a different kind of learners. Knowles (1984) suggested that there are four characteristics of adult learners, and these characteristics have implications for adult learning. Adults are self-directed in their learning; they have a lifetime of experience to draw on when learning; their readiness to learn is focused on requirements for their personal and occupational roles; and adults have a problem-centered time perspective in that the learners have a need to learn so that it can be applied and tried out quickly. Display 12–1 describes the characteristics of adult learners and implications for nurses working with adults in more detail.

HEALTH TEACHING MODELS

Theories on learning provide a general understanding of how people learn. In addition, various health teaching models specifically focus on explaining individual health experiences, behaviors, and actions. These models fit with the

DISPLAY 12–1

Characteristics and Implications for Knowles' Adult Learning Theory

Characteristics	Learning Implications
Self-concept Adult learners are self-directed.	Openness and respect between teacher and learner. The learner plans and carries out own learning activities. Learner evaluates own progress toward self-chosen goals.
Experience Adults have a lifetime of experience and define self in terms of this experience.	Teaching methods focus on experiential activities. Discovering how to learn from experience is key to self-actualization. Mistakes are opportunities for learning.
Readiness to learn Learning is focused on social and occupational roles.	Experiential learning opportunities focus on requirements for occupational and social roles. Learning peaks when there is a need to know. Adults can best assess own readiness to learn and teachable moments.
Need to learn Adults have a problem-centered time perspective.	Teaching needs to be problem-centered rather than theoretically oriented. Teacher needs to teach what the learners need to learn. Learners need to apply and try out learning quickly.

learning theories to give nurses a more accurate picture of the client and the clients' learning needs. Five useful ones are described here: the Cloutterbuck Minimum Data Matrix (CMDM), the Health Belief Model (HBM), Pender's Health Promotion Model (revised) (HPM), and the PRECEDE and PROCEED models.

The Cloutterbuck Minimum Data Matrix

The CMDM generates a comprehensive base of client information. This information is prerequisite to the in-depth level of critical analysis and synthesis needed to produce quality health care outcomes in the 21st century. It assumes an interdisciplinary perspective and educates the nurse to recognize and incorporate client diversity into care. In teaching, it assists the nurse in conceptualizing clients beyond the institutional, individual, and biomedical perspectives (Cloutterbuck & Cherry, 1998). The model helps the nurse to discern the life circumstances or chain of events that have jeopardized a client's health (Fig. 12–1).

The model comprises a set of empiric variables that are "known to influence consumer health status, behavior, and outcomes" (Cloutterbuck & Cherry, 1998, p. 386). For example, in the personal variables dimension, there are items such as age, ethnicity, level of education, and self-care practices. These variables are distributed across three dimensions: personal, situational, and structural. Information generated by the CMDM creates a more comprehensive profile than information gathered in the traditional biomedical health care system. This information, such as client health beliefs and practices and a broad range of personal factors, can be instrumental in helping the nurse design and implement health education programs to promote positive changes in clients' health. Although community health nurses have a long tradition of considering the client holistically, this matrix helps the nurse visualize the complexity of factors influencing clients' health. It helps to identify and challenge assumptions, recognize the importance of context, imagine and explore alternatives, and use reflective skepticism. When the nurse approaches individuals, families, and groups prepared with complete information, all of the caregiving—especially the appropriateness and effectiveness of the teaching—is enhanced.

The Health Belief Model

This section and the next describe two closely associated health models. The HBM, which was developed by social psychologists and brought to the attention of health care professionals by Rosenstock (1966), has undergone much empiric testing. The HBM is useful for explaining the behaviors and actions taken by people to prevent illness and injury. It postulates that readiness to act on behalf of a person's own health is predicated on the following (Strecher & Rosenstock, 1997):

Perceived susceptibility to the condition in question

Perceived seriousness of the condition in question

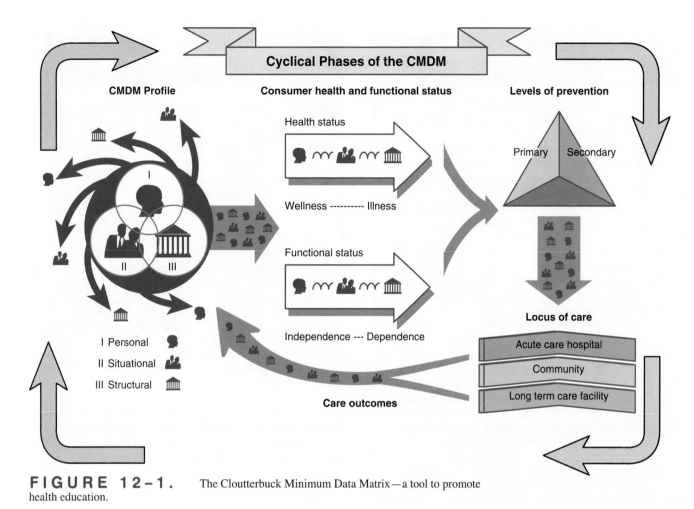

FIGURE 12-1.   The Clootterbuck Minimum Data Matrix—a tool to promote health education.

Perceived benefits to taking action

Barriers to taking action

Cues to action, such as knowledge that someone else has the condition or attention from the media

Self-efficacy—the ability to take action to achieve the desired outcome

For example, using concepts from this model, researchers looked at beliefs about the ability to control diabetes and beliefs about the degreee to which family members supported a targeted Mexican-American population in following their diabetes treatment regimen (Brown, Becker, Garcia, et al., 2002). Unable to find many tools to measure diabetes-related health beliefs the researchers took ideas from some older tools and designed a culturally-sensitive education and group support intervention (Brown & Hanis, 1999). They realized how influential health beliefs are in managing one's health, whether in promoting or improving health or in trying to control a disease.

Pender's Health Promotion Model

The revised HPM (Pender, Murdaugh, & Parsons, 2001) modifies the HBM and focuses on predicting behaviors that influence health promotion. In addition, the HPM includes the variable of interpersonal influence of others, including family and health professionals. Being able to predict health promotion behaviors enhances the community health nurse's ability to work with clients. Awareness of their characteristics, experiences, comprehension of their health-related issues, perceived barriers, self-efficacy, support (or lack of it) from significant others, and commitment provides the nurse with a picture that paints the client-nurse role and gives direction for action-taking. "The HPM is a competence- or approach-oriented model [and] does not include 'fear' or 'threat' as a source of motivation for health behavior" (Pender, et al., 2001, p. 61). The HPM is based on the theoretical propositions found in Display 12–2.

Using these propositions, researchers explored clients' health behaviors in many studies conducted in the 1980s, 1990s, and into the 21st century. They looked at health-promoting behavior among workers, ambulatory cancer patients, older adults, incarcerated men, rural older women, university students, men in cardiac rehabilitation programs, adolescent girls, human immunodeficiency virus (HIV)-seropositive men, and married and unmarried mothers, to name a few of the populations that have been studied by nurse researchers and others.

The revised HPM contains significant changes from the original model and is outlined to provide clarity in Display 12–3.

DISPLAY 12-2

Theoretical Propositions of the Health Promotion Model

1. Inherited and acquired characteristics along with prior behavior influence beliefs, affect, and health-promoting behavior.
2. People engage in behaviors from which they anticipate deriving personally valued benefits.
3. Perceived barriers can constrain action to change behavior and the behavior itself.
4. Perceived self-efficacy to embrace a given behavior increases the likelihood to commit to action and implementing the behavior.
5. Greater perceived self-efficacy results in fewer perceived barriers.
6. Positive affect toward a behavior results in greater perceived self-efficacy, which can result in increased positive affect.
7. When positive affect is associated with a behavior, commitment and action are increased.
8. People are more likely to commit to and participate in health-promoting behaviors when significant others model the behavior, expect it, and provide assistance and support for the behavior.
9. Others—family members, peers, and health care providers—are important sources of influence that can positively or negatively influence commitment to and implementation of health-promoting behavior.
10. Situational influences can positively or negatively influence commitment to and implementation of health-promoting behavior.
11. The greater the commitment to a behavior change, the more likely the change will be maintained over time.
12. Distracting demands over which the person has little control may affect commitment to a behavior change.
13. Commitment to a behavior change is less likely to be maintained when other actions are more attractive and preferred.
14. People can modify the interpersonal and physical environments to create incentives for behavior changes.

(Adapted from Pender, N.J., Murdaugh, C.L., & Parsons, M.A. [2001]. *Health promotion in nursing practice* [4th ed.]. Upper Saddle River, NJ: Prentice-Hall.)

DISPLAY 12-3

Components of the Revised Health Promotion Model

Personal Characteristics and Experiences
  Past related behavior
  Biopsychosocial factors
Cognitive and Affective Behaviors
  Perceived benefits
  Perceived self-efficacy
  Action-related affect
  Influence of others and their role in support and as models
  Situational influence
Outcome Behavior
  Competition—demands and preferences
  Commitment to the plan
  Health promotion behavior

(Adapted from Pender, N.J., Murdaugh, C.L., & Parsons, M.A. [2001]. *Health promotion in nursing practice* [4th ed.]. Upper Saddle River, NJ: Prentice-Hall.)

The community health nurse's role of teacher focuses heavily on assessment and identification of strengths and weaknesses at each level. From the information gathered, the nurse can develop a diagnostic statement describing the learning needs of clients.

The PROCEED model had been associated with the PRECEDE model as the community health nurse proceeds to plan, implement, and evaluate health education programs. This acronym stands for Policy, Regulatory, and Organizational Constructs for Educational and Environmental Development. The four steps in this model include implementation, process, impact, and outcome evaluation of the teaching process (Richards, 1997). The nurse builds on the assessment and diagnosis formulated from the PRECEDE model. The steps are similar to the nursing process and, because of this familiarity, have become useful tools for nurses teaching in the community.

TEACHING AT THREE LEVELS OF PREVENTION

Nurses should develop teaching programs that coincide with the level of prevention needed by the client. The three levels (defined in Chapter 1) of primary, secondary, and tertiary prevention are demonstrated in the Levels of Prevention Matrix for nurses who teach clients, families, aggregates, or populations.

Ideally, the nurse focuses teaching at the primary level. If nurses were able to reach more people at this level, it would help to diminish the years of morbidity and limit subsequent infirmity. Many people experience disabilities that might have been prevented if primary prevention behaviors had been incorporated into their daily activities.

The PRECEDE and PROCEED Models

First publicized by Green and Kreuter (1991), the PRECEDE model was developed for educational diagnosis. The acronym PRECEDE stands for Predisposing, Reinforcing, and Enabling Causes in Educational Diagnosis and Evaluation. It includes seven levels in formulating educational diagnoses (Table 12–6).

T A B L E   1 2 – 6

Seven Phases of the PRECEDE Model

Role of community health nurse as teacher: assessment, identification of strengths and weaknesses, and formulation of diagnoses.

Level (Phases)	Description (Questions)
Phase I Social diagnosis	Assessing the learner's quality of life. What are the group's general concerns?
Phase II Epidemiologic diagnosis	Identifying health problems. What are the specific problems related to the social diagnosis?
Phase III Behavioral and environmental diagnosis	Identifying risk factors. What are the health related behaviors?
Phase IV Educational diagnosis	Identifying predisposing, reinforcing, and enabling factors at each level. What are the predisposing, enabling, and reinforcing factors?
Phase V Analysis of educational diagnosis	Which of the priority factors will be focused on during the educational plan?
Phase VI Administrative and policy-making diagnosis	Assessing administrative and organizational resources. What specific objectives and resources are needed for the health education plan?
Phase VII Evaluation	What are the results of the educational plan?

Because the primary level of prevention is not possible in all cases, a significant share of the nurse's time is spent teaching at the secondary or tertiary level. An example is an 88-year-old woman with a fractured hip who has returned home after 3 weeks of physical therapy at a skilled nursing facility. The nurse assesses the client's environment, gait, functional limitations, safety, and adherence to medication and initiates needed referrals. The teaching focuses on rehabilitation and prevention of a secondary problem that may affect the healing process and the client's health and safety in general.

EFFECTIVE TEACHING

Teaching is an art. It was described in the classic book, *The Educational Imagination* by E.W. Eisner (1985). Teaching can be performed with such skill and grace that the client becomes part of a well-orchestrated event with learning as the natural outcome. Instead of relying on prescribed teaching methods, the skillful nurse can make judgments based largely on client qualities, situations, and needs that guide the experience to fruition. The desired changes emerge in the course of the interaction rather than at a level conceived before the teaching. Before the community health nurse can reach this level of artistry, there is much to learn about being an effective teacher.

Teaching-Learning Principles

Teaching lies at one end of a continuum. At the other end is learning. Without learning, teaching becomes useless in the same way that communication does not occur unless a message is both sent and received (Lorig, 2000). Both the teacher and the learner have responsibilities on that continuum. Learners must take responsibility for their own learning (Bastable, 2003). Teachers obstruct that process if they assume complete responsibility for bringing about changed behavior. Clients can be directed toward health knowledge, but they will not learn unless they have the desire to learn. Teaching, then, becomes a matter of facilitating both the desire and the best conditions for satisfying it. Teaching in community health nursing means to influence, motivate, and act as a catalyst in the learning process. Nurses bring information and learners together and stimulate a reaction that leads to a change (Rankin & Stallings, 2001). Nurses facilitate learning when they make it as easy as possible for clients to change. To do this, the nurse needs to understand the basic principles underlying the art and science of the teaching-learning process and the use of appropriate materials to influence learning (Table 12–7).

Client Readiness

Clients' readiness to learn influences teaching effectiveness (Rankin & Stallings, 2001). Two facets of client readiness have been identified. Both emotional readiness, a state of receptivity to learning, and experimental readiness, the learner's knowledge and understanding, must be assessed by the nurse. For instance, one community health nurse found that a young primipara was not ready for prenatal teaching on fetal growth and development. She had strong fears, the nurse discovered, that "losing her figure" would make her sexually unattractive to her husband. Until these anxieties

LEVELS OF PREVENTION MATRIX

SITUATION: Several examples of teaching at three levels of prevention

GOAL: Using the three levels of prevention, negative health conditions are avoided, or promptly diagnosed and treated, and the fullest possible potential is restored.

PRIMARY PREVENTION		SECONDARY PREVENTION		TERTIARY PREVENTION		
Health Promotion and Education	*Health Protection*	*Early Diagnosis*	*Prompt Treatment*	*Rehabilitation*	*Primary Prevention*	
					Health Promotion and Education	*Health Protection*
Health education: a nurse teaches a class on sensible weight control for teenagers	Immunizations: a nurse teaches the importance of pneumonia and flu vaccines for seniors, followed by an immunization clinic	Screening and case-finding: a nurse takes blood pressure measurements from all family members at each home visit and teaches them the importance of maintaining a healthy blood pressure reading	Treatment: a nurse teaches clients how to navigate through the complexities of the health care delivery system to receive prompt treatment	Restore function: a nurse teaches a stroke survivor about home safety, alternative housing options, physical therapy, and retraining opportunities	Health teaching: a nurse teaches about the importance of diet, rest, and exercise to prevent a secondary health problem	Maintenance: a nurse observes clients with tuberculosis where they live while taking their oral medication on a daily basis (DOT therapy)

T A B L E   1 2 – 7

Seven Principles for Maximizing the Teaching-Learning Process

Teaching Principles	Learning Principles
1. Adapt teaching to clients' level of readiness.	1. The learning process makes use of clients' experience and is geared to their level of understanding.
2. Determine clients' perceptions about the subject matter before and during teaching.	2. Clients are given the opportunity to provide frequent feedback on their understanding of the material taught.
3. Create an environment that is conducive to learning.	3. The environment for learning is physically comfortable; offers an atmosphere of mutual helpfulness, trust, respect, and acceptance; and allows for free expression of ideas.
4. Involve clients throughout the learning process.	4. Clients actively participate. They assess needs, establish goals, and evaluate their learning progress.
5. Make subject matter relevant to clients' interest and use.	5. Clients feel motivated to interest and learn.
6. Ensure client satisfaction during the teaching-learning process.	6. Clients sense progress toward their goals.
7. Provide opportunities for clients to apply material taught.	7. Clients integrate the learning through application.

(Adapted from Knowles, M. [1980]. *The modern practice of adult education: Androgogy versus pedagogy* [2nd ed.]. Chicago: Follett.)

had subsided, the teaching would remain ineffective. Clients' needs, interests, motivation, stress, and concerns determine their readiness for learning.

Another factor that influences readiness is educational background. If a group of women who never completed grade school meet to learn how to care for a sick person in the home, material should be presented simply, factually, and in terms that they understand. To discuss complex concepts of health, illness, and scientific research would be above their level of readiness. However, increasingly complex concepts can be introduced as the nurse works with the women and assesses their readiness to assimilate advanced concepts.

Maturational level also affects readiness. An adolescent mother who still is working on normal developmental tasks of her age group, such as seeking independence or selecting a career path, may not be ready to learn parenting skills. Readiness of the client determines the amount of material presented in each teaching session. The pace or speed with which information is presented must be manageable. A moderate amount of anxiety often increases client receptivity to learning; however, high or low levels of anxiety can have the opposite effect.

Client Perceptions

Clients' perceptions also affect their learning, serving as a screening device through which all new information must pass (Rankin & Stallings, 2001). Individual perceptions help people interpret and attach meaning to things. A wide range of variables affects human perception. These variables include values, past experiences, culture, religion, personality, developmental stage, educational and economic level, surrounding social forces, and the physical environment. One client may view the experience of parenting as a positive, growth-producing relationship; another may see it as a conflict-ridden, unhappy experience to avoid. Each kind of perception has a different consequence for teaching and learning. In another example, the nurse working with adolescents to educate them about the dangers of substance abuse should understand that adolescents seeking independence need to feel that they have options and choices and do not want to be told what to do.

Frequently, clients use selective perception. They screen out some statements and pay attention to those that fit their values or personal desires. For example, a nurse is teaching a client the various risk factors in coronary disease; the individual screens out the need to quit smoking and lose weight, paying attention only to factors that would not require a drastic change in lifestyle. Nurses must know their clients, understand their backgrounds and values, and learn about their perceptions before health teaching can influence their behavior.

Educational Environment

The setting in which the educational endeavor takes place has a significant impact on learning (Breckon, Lancaster, & Harvey, 1998). Students probably have had the experience of sitting in a cold room and trying to concentrate during a lecture or of being distracted by noise, heat, or uncomfortable seating. Physical conditions such as ventilation, lighting, decor, room temperature, view of the speaker, and whispering need to be controlled to provide the environment most conducive to learning.

Equally important for learning is an atmosphere of mutual respect and trust. The nurse needs to convey this attitude both verbally and nonverbally. The way the nurse addresses clients, shows courtesies, and gives recognition makes a considerable difference in establishing clients' respect and trust. Both nurse and clients need to be mutually helpful and considerate of one another's needs and interests. All participants in the educational experience should feel free to express ideas, should know that their views will be heard, and should feel accepted despite differences of opinion and perspective. According to Knowles, this requires that the nurse refrain from seeming judgmental or inducing competitiveness among learners. Knowles adds that the teachers should share their own feelings and knowledge "as a colearner in the spirit of inquiry" (1980, p. 58) (see Research: Bridge to Practice).

Client Participation

The degree of participation in the educational process directly influences the amount of learning (Bastable, 2003). One nurse discovered this principle while working with a group of clients who were nearing retirement. After talking to them about the changes they would face and receiving little response, the nurse shifted to a different method of teaching. Pamphlets on social security benefits were distributed, and everyone was asked to read them during the week and come the next week with questions generated by the pamphlets. This strategy prompted the group to slowly begin to participate in their own learning.

When the nurse works with clients in a learning context, one of the first questions to discuss is, What does the client want to learn? As Carl Rogers (1969, p. 159) stated:

> Learning is facilitated when the student participates responsibly in the learning process. When he chooses his own directions, helps to discover his own learning resources, formulates his own problems, decides his own course of action, lives with consequences of each of these choices, then significant learning is maximized.

The amount of learning is directly proportional to the learners' involvement. In another example, a group of senior citizens attended a class on nutrition and aging, yet made few changes in eating patterns. It was not until the members became actively involved in the class, encouraged by the nurse to present problems and solutions for food purchasing and preparation on limited budgets, that any significant behavioral changes occurred.

RESEARCH: BRIDGE TO PRACTICE

Valdez, A., Banerjee, K., Ackerson, L., & Fernandez, M. (2002). A multimedia breast cancer education intervention for low-income Latinas. *Journal of Community Health, 27*(1), 33–51.

In this study, researchers field-tested a multimedia health education intervention designed to provide breast cancer education for low-income Latinas, using Bandura's social learning theory (SLT). Breast cancer screening rates among Latinas have yet to reach the recommended levels established by the *Healthy People 2010* initiative (USDHHS, 2000), even with the availability of subsidized mammograms for low-income women since 1991. Almost 1200 foreign-born Latina women with less than 8 years of education, low income, and age younger than 65 years participated in the study.

The women were randomly assigned to a control or intervention group. The multimedia intervention (video, animation, stills, music, and narrative) was specifically designed to document knowledge, attitudes, and intentions toward mammography screening. All intervention techniques used were developed for low-education, low-income, and low-literacy Latina populations.

The intervention was evaluated in two stages—at the field study stage for knowledge, attitudes, and intentions toward breast cancer screening and a follow-up stage 4 months later for actual mammography behavior. According to SLT, a message's effectiveness and credibility depend on the characteristics of the presenter. A presenter who appears to share the values and beliefs of the audience is perceived as more credible and authentic. Therefore, in this study, Latina social models were used to represent women's experiences with breast cancer in realistic settings. The breast cancer modules were developed using input from experts, health care workers, and low-education, low-income Latinas similar to those targeted in this intervention.

The results for the intervention group included significantly higher correct answer responses on all knowledge items except one on insurance. Mean breast cancer knowledge scores were significantly different from those in the control group. Attitude and belief differences were not significant except for one item: that breast cancer could be cured if detected early. For likelihood of screening intentions, there was significance in only one respect: to ask a doctor about getting a mammogram.

Overall results showed that multimedia technologies can be used to effectively provide health information to low-education, minority women. The entire breast cancer program came in a kiosk that could be used by a variety of educators in different settings, such as clinic waiting rooms or a client's home. In addition, the kiosk could be programmed to offer information on a range of topics.

Contracting, in which the client participates in the process as a partner to determine goals, content, and time for learning, can contribute to client learning. Contracting in the context of teaching can develop a sense of accountability in clients for their own learning. Contracting is discussed in Chapter 11.

Subject Relevance

Subject matter that is relevant to the client is learned more readily and retained longer than information that is not meaningful (Lorig, 2000). Learners gain the most from subject matter that is immediately useful to their own purposes. This is particularly true of adult learners, who have more life experiences that can be related to learning and who tend to see the immediate relevance of the material taught (Knowles, 1980).

Consider two middle-management men taking a physical fitness course offered by their employer. One, the father of a Boy Scout, has agreed to co-lead his son's troop on a 2-week backpacking trip in the mountains. He wants to get in shape. The second man is taking the course because it is required by the company. Its only relevance to his own purposes is that it prevents incurring the disfavor of his boss. There is little question about which man will learn and retain the most. The course has considerable relevance and meaning to the first man and little to the second.

Relevance also influences the speed of learning. Diabetics who must give themselves daily injections of insulin to live learn that skill quickly. When clients see considerable relevance in the learning, they accomplish it with speed. According to Rogers (1969), 65% to 85% of the time allotted for learning various subjects could be deleted if learners perceived the material to be related to their own purposes. This is seen in the short period of time that it takes for families to learn the skills needed to provide home care for a family member in need (Baltazar, Ibe, & Allender, 1999).

When the subject matter is relevant to the learner, there also is greater retention of knowledge. On seeing the usefulness of the material, the learner develops a strong motivation to acquire it and use it and is less likely to forget it. Even in instances when a previously learned motor skill has not been used for years, it often is quickly recaptured when it is needed.

Client Satisfaction

Clients must derive satisfaction from learning to maintain motivation and increase self-direction (Lorig, 2000). Learners need to feel a sense of steady progress in the learning process. Obstacles, frustrations, and failures along the way discourage and impede learning. Many stroke clients with potential for rehabilitation give up trying to regain speech or move paralyzed limbs because they become too frustrated, discouraged, and dissatisfied. On the other hand, clients who experience satisfaction and progress in their speech and muscle retraining maintain their motivation and work on exercises without prompting (Diamantopulos, 1999). Nurses can promote client satisfaction through support and encouragement.

Realistic goals contribute to learner satisfaction. Objectives should be set within the learner's ability, thereby avoiding the frustration resulting from a task that is too difficult and the loss of interest resulting from one that is too easy. Setting objectives requires agreement on goals, periodic reviews, and revision of goals if they become too easy or too difficult. Nurses further promote clients' learning satisfaction by designing tasks with rewards. One school nurse led a class for obese adolescents, and together they set the goal of a weekly 2-lb weight loss. The nurse helped the group to design a plan that included counting calories, reducing fat in their diets, increasing physical activity, and a buddy system to bring about behavior change. As members in the group achieved monthly goals, they were encouraged to reward themselves with a pair of earrings, new nail polish, or a special outing as a group. These students found this learning experience satisfying because goals were attainable and their progress was rewarded. Instead of competing with one another, the group set out to help each member achieve the goal. As a result, most kept the weight off after the class had finished.

Client Application

Learning is reinforced through application (Lorig, 2000). Learners need as many opportunities as possible to apply the learning in daily life. If such opportunities arise during the teaching-learning process, clients can try out new knowledge and skills under supervision. Learners are given an opportunity to begin integrating the learning into their daily lives at a time when the teacher is there to help reinforce that pattern. Take a prenatal class as an example. The learning only begins with explanations of proper diet, exercise, breathing techniques, hygiene, and avoidance of alcohol and tobacco. More learning occurs as the group members discuss these issues and apply them intellectually, exploring ways to practice them at home. Additional reinforcement comes by demonstrating how to do these activities. Sample diets, demonstrations of exercises, posters, pamphlets, or models may be used. The group can begin application in the classroom by making diet plans, exercising, role-playing parenting behavior, or engaging in group problem-solving. The members then can be encouraged to apply these activities on a daily basis at home and to share their results at future sessions.

Frequent use of newly acquired information fosters transfer of learning to other situations. The major goal of prevention and health promotion depends on such a transfer. For instance, mothers who learn and practice a well-balanced diet that is free of non-nutritious snacks can be encouraged to of-

fer more nourishing foods to other family members. A family that practices asepsis and good handwashing techniques when caring for a postsurgical wound can learn to transfer this same principle to prevention of infection in daily living.

Teaching Process

The process of teaching in community health nursing follows steps similar to those of the nursing process:

1. *Interaction:* Establish basic communication patterns between clients and nurse.
2. *Assessment and diagnosis:* Determine clients' present status and identify clients' need for teaching (keeping in mind that clients should determine their own needs).
3. *Setting goals and objectives:* Analyze needed changes and prepare objectives that describe the desired learning outcomes.
4. *Planning:* Design a plan for the learning experience that meets the mutually developed objectives; include content to be covered, sequence of topics, best conditions for learning (place, type of environment), methods, and materials (eg, visual aids, exercises). A written plan is best; it may be part of the written nursing care plan.
5. *Teaching:* Implement the learning experience by carrying out the planned activities.
6. *Evaluation:* Determine whether learning objectives were met and if not, why not. Evaluation measures progress toward goals, effectiveness of chosen teaching methods, or future learning needs.

Interaction

Reciprocal communication must take place between nurse and client. It is essential in the helping relationship and requisite to effective use of the nursing process. Community health nurses need to develop good questioning techniques and listening skills to determine clients' learning needs and levels of readiness (see Chapter 11).

Assessment and Diagnosis

Identifying clients' learning needs presents a challenge to the nurse. Too often, teaching occurs based on the nurse's assumption of what the learner needs to know. In client education, nurses have a responsibility to tailor their teaching to clients' real and perceived needs. Knowles (1980, 1984, 1989) described educational needs as gaps between what people know and what they need to know to function effectively. He related that the potential learners, the sponsoring organization, and the community all help to determine the needs to be addressed in the teaching-learning situation.

Assessing educational needs may be accomplished in several ways. The nurse can use surveys, interviews, open forums, or task forces that include representative clients as members. The principle to remember is that clients should be involved in identifying what they want to learn. When a "need" to learn something, such as the importance of immunizing children, is identified by the nurse rather than by clients, the nurse may need to "sell" clients on the importance of the topic. Nurses need to use approaches that assist clients toward their own awareness of the need.

Setting Goals and Objectives

Once a need has been clearly identified, the nurse and clients can establish mutually agreed-on goals and objectives. Goals are broad statements of intent, and objectives are more specific descriptions of intended outcome (Mager, 1975). Sometimes, in a teaching situation, an objective may be broken down into short-term and long-term goals. For example, the nurse may have identified a group's desire to stop smoking. The need and teaching goals might be stated as follows:

Need: A group of smokers wish to stop their addiction to nicotine.

Short-term goal: All members of the group will stop smoking within 1 month.

Long-term goal: Ninety percent of group members will remain tobacco-free for 6 months.

Objectives should be stated in measurable behavioral terms, using a grammatical structure that contains a subject, verb, condition/criterion, and time frame. That is, each objective should include a single idea that describes an outcome that can be measured within a certain time frame. To accomplish the short- and long-term goals of smoking cessation, educational objectives are developed from the levels of cognitive learning covered earlier in this chapter. Each behavioral objective is stated in measurable terms and includes a verb that coincides with one of the six levels within the cognitive domain (Display 12–4). Objectives might appear as follows:

At the end of the program all clients should be able to:
1. *List* three reasons why smoking is unhealthy.
2. *Identify* at least two factors that influenced their smoking habit.
3. *Apply* a series of action steps leading to smoking cessation within 1 month.
4. *Examine* the steps as they contribute to living tobacco-free in the first 3 months.
5. *Design* a way to live a fulfilled, tobacco-free life.
6. *Evaluate* successful strategies to remain tobacco-free for 6 months.

Each of these objectives (1) refers to a subject; (2) can be readily measured—because each describes a specific outcome, condition, criterion, or expected behavior; (3) uses a verb for stating cognitive outcomes; and (4) includes a specific time frame. Well-written objectives meet these four criteria and enhance evaluation of the success of the educational effort.

Planning

Teaching preparation and the planning of it are all-important (Lowenstein, 2001). Although nurses teach individuals and families informally, it is generally best to have a written plan when teaching. The formalization of creating a written plan provides a framework within which the nurse can function securely, knowing that the topic is well thought out and presented and individualized for a specific client group. This plan should include the following: (1) subject; (2) intended audience; (3) dates, times, and places; (4) short- and long-term goal statements; (5) teaching-learning methods; (6) ac-

D I S P L A Y   1 2 – 4

Sample Verbs for Stating Cognitive Outcomes

Knowledge	Comprehension	Application	Analysis	Synthesis	Evaluation
Define	Translate	Interpret	Analyze	Compose	Judge
Repeat	Restate	Apply	Distinguish	Plan	Appraise
Record	Describe	Employ	Appraise	Propose	Evaluate
List	Discuss	Use	Calculate	Design	Rate
Recall	Recognize	Practice	Experiment	Formulate	Value
Name	Explain	Operate	Differentiate	Arrange	Revise
Relate	Express	Schedule	Test	Assemble	Score
Underline	Identify	Sketch	Compare	Collect	Select
	Locate	Shop	Contrast	Construct	Choose
	Report	Practice	Criticize	Create	Assess
	Review	Demonstrate	Diagram	Set up	Estimate
	Tell		Inspect	Organize	Measure
			Debate	Manage	
			Inventory	Prepare	
			Question		
			Relate		
			Categorize		
			Examine		

tivies and assignments; (7) course outline of topics; and (8) evaluation method and criteria.

Teaching

The class, seminar, workshop, or small-group teaching should be conducted according to the plan described earlier. Even with one-on-one teaching, these eight steps should be planned in advance, because each client has a different cultural background, education, intellectual level, and learning need. Use of a variety of teaching methods addresses the unique needs of learners and makes the teaching interesting. Include and combine such methods as lectures, discussions, role-playing, demonstrations, and videos (see Teaching Methods and Materials).

If necessary, assignments can be made, such as readings, presentations, keeping journals, practice experiences, or return demonstrations designed to reinforce and synthesize the learning. The teaching methods used and activities selected are important parts of the teaching plan. The teacher will find that a well-designed plan enhances the smoothness and effectiveness of the teaching situation; problems in teaching often can be related to a poorly developed plan.

Evaluation

The final step of evaluation is a critical one in the teaching-learning process. According to Tyler (1949, p. 106), "evaluation is the process for determining the degree to which changes in behavior are actually taking place." At this point, the nurse determines whether the goals and objectives for the educational experience have been met and if not, why not. Clear, measurable objectives facilitate evaluation. For example, to measure the third objective in the stop-smoking program previously noted, "Apply a series of action steps that will lead to smoking cessation within 1 month," the nurse may ask group members to share the steps that they will use and then have a group discussion about the ideas shared. To measure the sixth objective, "Evaluate successful strategies to remain tobacco-free for 6 months" would require follow-up contacts and relying on self-reporting. Adatsi (1999) reported that 195 clients were monitored for 1 year after participation in a smoking-cessation program in Duluth, Minnesota, and 49% remained tobacco free. The American Lung Association estimates that only 20% to 30% of smokers typically remain abstinent for 1 year after quitting. The authors attributed the success of the Minnesota program to gearing intervention to the client's stage of readiness to quit, based on a model that describes four stages through which smokers move as they attempt to change their smoking habit. In addition, the participants got the support of planned and periodic contact from program staff over the 12 months follow-up period, which included evaluation of strategies that worked or did not work for the participant's individual stage.

If objectives have not been met or have been met only partially, this too requires attention. The nurse should explore this outcome with the clients to determine what factors hindered their success and what actions might be helpful. Partially met objectives give the nurse a place to begin with the group at follow-up sessions and should not be considered a failure.

Teaching Methods and Materials

Teaching occurs on many levels and incorporates various types of activities. It can be formal or informal, planned or unplanned. Formal presentations, such as lectures with groups, usually are planned and fairly structured. Some teaching is less formal but still planned and relatively structured, as in group discussions in which questions stimulate exploration of ideas and guide thinking. Informal levels of teaching, such as counseling or **anticipatory guidance** (in which the client is assisted in preparing for a future role or developmental stage), require the teacher to be prepared, but there is no defined plan of presentation. Perhaps the nurse uses a pamphlet or agency protocol steps as a guide. All nurses use one or a combination of methods and a variety of materials to facilitate the teaching-learning process. However, nurses need to expand their repertoire of teaching methods and to avoid relying on one or two methods. Generating a variety of teaching methods stimulates creative thinking. Nurses use knowledge from physiology, pathology, sociology, and psychology in their practice, and, when teaching, nurses can benefit from using concepts, principles, and teaching methods derived from education, especially adult education. This chapter closes by discussing four commonly used teaching methods (lecture, discussion, demonstration, and role playing), teaching materials for enhanced learning, and how to effectively teach the client with special learning needs (Fig. 12–2).

Lecture

The community health nurse sometimes presents information to a large group, such as a local parent-teacher association, a women's club, or a county board of commissioners. Under such circumstances, the lecture method, a formal kind of presentation, may be the most efficient way to communicate general health information. However, lecturers tend to create a passive learning environment for the audience unless strategies are devised to involve the learners. Many individuals are visual rather than auditory learners. To capture their attention, slides, overhead projections, computer-generated slide presentations, or videotapes can supplement the lecture. Allowing time for questions and discussion after a lecture also actively involves the learners. This method is best used with adults, but even they have a limited attention span, and a break at least midway through a presentation of 1 hour or longer will be appreciated. Distributing printed material that highlights and summarizes the content shared, or supplements it, also reinforces important points.

Discussion

Two-way communication is an important feature of the learning process. Learners need an opportunity to raise questions, make comments, reason out loud, and receive feedback

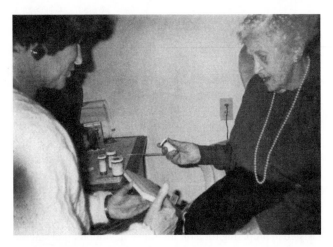

FIGURE 12–2.   Teaching methods and tools vary with clients' learning needs. On this home visit, the nurse uses a weekly medication container to help an elderly woman with limited vision devise a plan for taking her medications.

to develop understanding. When discussion is used in conjunction with other teaching methods such as demonstration, lecture, and role playing, it improves their effectiveness. In group teaching, discussion enables clients to learn from one another as well as from the nurse. The nurse must exercise leadership in controlling and guiding the discussion so that learning opportunities are maximized and objectives are met. Discussions that are organized around specific questions or topics are more fruitful.

Demonstration

The demonstration method often is used for teaching psychomotor skills and is best accompanied by explanation and discussion, with time set aside for return demonstration by the client or caregiver. It gives clients a clear sensory image of how to perform the skill. Because a demonstration should be within easy visual and auditory range of learners, it is best to demonstrate in front of small groups or a single client. Use the same kind of equipment that clients will use, show exactly how the skill should be performed, and provide learners with ample opportunity to practice until the skill is perfected.

This is an ideal method to use in a client's home as well as in groups. The materials and supplies that the client will use when unaided by the nurse should be used in the demonstration. This might be the time when the nurse uses improvising skills. Helping families figure out ways to accomplish goals with materials found at home often becomes the hallmark of an experienced community health nurse. The new mother learns how to bathe her baby safely in the kitchen sink. The nurse assists several low-income parents in using household items to make inexpensive toys (eg, mobiles from plastic coat hangers, string, and pictures from a magazine; bean bags using dry beans and scraps of fabric). The husband learns how to change dressings over his wife's central line site using sterile technique while conserving supplies purchased on their

fixed income. Each activity takes a different type of psychomotor skill and ingenuity on the part of the nurse.

Role-Playing

At times, having clients assume and act out roles maximizes learning. A parenting group, for example, found it helpful to place themselves in the role of their children; their feelings about various ways to respond became more apparent. Reversing roles can effectively teach spouses in conflict about better ways to communicate. To prevent role-playing from becoming a game with little learning, plan the proposed drama with clear objectives in mind. What behavioral outcomes should be achieved? Define the context (the "stage") clearly so that everyone shares in the situation. Then define each role ahead of time, making sure that participants understand their performance roles. Emphasize that no wrong or right performance exists, and that participants should behave the way people behave in everyday life. Avoid having people play themselves, because it can embarrass them and make it difficult for them to achieve objectivity. After the drama has concluded, elicit discussion with carefully prepared questions. This technique can be used with staff, coworkers, young children, teenagers, and adults. However, it can be a risk-taking experience for some people, and they may be reluctant to participate. The nurse should use judgment, begin with volunteers, and avoid pushing this technique on unwilling or nonreceptive people. Build up to full participation.

Teaching Materials

Many different kinds of teaching materials are available to the nurse. They often are used in combination and are useful during the teaching process. Visual images—such as PowerPoint presentations, pictures, slides, posters, chalkboards, flannel boards, videotapes, CDs, bulletin boards, flash cards, pamphlets, flyers, charts, and gestures—can enhance most learning. Americans readily learn from television; it appeals to sight and sound and grabs attention. Learning of both positive and negative health behaviors through television can be more effective and efficient than traditional teaching methods. As an example, researchers found that situation comedy television shows (sitcoms) during Black prime time programs on national television stations had more commercials for candy, chocolate, and soda than did general prime time shows (Tirodkar & Jain, 2003). However, there are many programs on educational, public television channels and network channels that can be recommended by the nurse. Other tools, such as anatomic models and improvised or purchased equipment, provide clients with both visual and tactile learning experienes. Still others, such as interactive computer games or instruction, actively involve the learners.

The choice of teaching materials varies with the clients' interests and abilities and the resources available. Teaching often occurs in casual conversations, spontaneously in situations in which clients raise unexpected questions, or when a crisis arises. In these instances, nurses draw on their background of knowledge and exercise professional judgment in their selection of content, methods, and materials.

Several different types of printed educational support materials are available, such as pamphlets, brochures, booklets, flyers, and informational sheets. Each should be evaluated for its appropriateness and effectiveness with particular individuals, families, or groups. Many come from state and local official sources. Nurses can create their own handouts by using the Internet and a computer, customizing them to the needs of individual clients. The Internet has vast health resources that can be combined with the desktop publishing capabilities of the nurse's computer to create one-of-a-kind materials for clients. The nurse can get educational information from state, federal, and international health agencies such as state health departments, the Food and Drug Administration (FDA), the Centers for Disease Control and Prevention (CDC), the National Institues of Health (NIH), and the World Health Organization (WHO). Other materials come from nonprofit national agencies such as the American Diabetes Association (ADA), the March of Dimes, the American Association for Retired Persons (AARP), and the American Heart Association (AHA). Materials from these sources can be acquired in mass quantity for free or at a nominal cost to the nurse or agency. Major manufacturers of infant formulas, foods, diapers, and toys are good sources for literature on growth and development, safety, and caring for infants and children. Pharmaceutical companies develop educational material for the public, as do the manufacturers of in-home supplies and equipment. Usually, these are excellent sources of information for families or groups; however, the nurse needs to assess the material for appropriateness. Also, beware that the commercial message in the literature does not outweigh the educational impact, making it misleading or confusing to the client.

Factors to be considered with all educational literature include the material's content, complexity, and reading level. There are several ways to assess the readability of the printed word. One that is easy to use is the Fog Index. It is a rough way of determining the years of schooling needed to understand printed material. It works by analyzing words and sentence length. The higher the Fog Index, the more difficult the reading level. A Fog Index of 6 is a sixth-grade reading level, and 11 is the junior year in high school. The steps include the following:

1. Take a sample of approximately 100 words. Count the number of sentences. If semicolons and commas are used instead of periods, count each clause as a separate sentence.
2. Divide the number of sentences into the exact number of words, which gives the number of words per sentence.
3. Count the words with three or more syllables, excluding those that became three syllables because of "es" or "ed" at the end. Also, do not count names.
4. Add the number of words with three or more syllables to the average number of words per sentence.
5. Multiply the total by 0.4.
6. Use the resulting whole number (without rounding) as the Fog Index. It represents the number of years of schooling needed to understand the writing sample.

Culturally appropriate health education materials must be acquired or developed for the predominant cultural and linguistic minority populations taught by the nurse. Developing printed materials is an important first step, but the development of video, audio, and public service announcements in community-appropriate languages is also necessary.

Finally, nurses teach by example. Actions speak louder than words. If a nurse teaches the importance of washing hands to reduce disease transmission and then begins a newborn assessment without hand washing, the message of observed actions carries more impact than the words. Nurses who exhibit healthy practices use themselves as tools and serve as role models as well as health teachers.

Clients With Special Learning Needs

At times, the nurse experiences a challenging teaching situation with an individual, family, or group. These challenges may involve clients who have cultural or language differences, hearing impairments, developmental delays, memory losses, visual perception distortions, problems with fine or gross motor skills, distracting personality characteristics, or demonstrations of stress or emotions. Regardless of the situation, the nurse will feel most comfortable and confident if she or he is prepared to deal with these situations before they are experienced (see What Do You Think?).

Before beginning to teach a client, family, or aggregate, thorough preparation is important for successful learning to occur. This includes finding out whether it is possible to teach in English or whether other modifications are needed as the teaching plan is being developed. Nurses should never assume anything, including the primary language spoken by clients, their visual or hearing ability, or their capacity to understand. When teaching unfamiliar groups, the nurse can obtain from a center manager, caretaker, or program director information regarding the interests and abilities of the members. These human resources are invaluable in planning any teaching when English may be a second language or when other barriers exist that may impede success if they are not known by the nurse. The phases of the nursing process continue to guide the nurse as a teacher.

WHAT DO YOU THINK?

More than 90 million Americans have limited literacy skills. Almost 2 million U. S. residents cannot speak English, and millions more speak it poorly. How effective is your teaching when populations are not English speaking or have limited English skills?

Another difficulty that can arise is unexpected behavior from a client who disrupts the group process. The client may monopolize the discussion, answer questions asked of others, burst out with personal experiences that have no relevance to the topic, become irate at the comments of others, or sit silently and never speak. This can be unnerving to even the most experienced nurse. Any behavior that has the potential to distract the other learners needs to be diffused by the nurse. This is accomplished by caringly giving the recognition sought by the person while also setting limits. More information on client behavior and appropriate communication techniques can be found in Chapters 11 and 23.

SUMMARY

Much of community health nursing practice involves teaching. More than simply giving health information to clients, the purpose of teaching is to change client behavior to healthier practices. If these practices are internalized and implemented regularly, years of morbidity and premature mortality can be avoided, contributing to the quality and length of the human life span. *Healthy People 2010* focuses on teaching to improve the quality of life.

Understanding the nature of learning contributes to the effectiveness of teaching in community health. Learning occurs in three domains: cognitive, affective, and psychomotor. The cognitive domain refers to learning that takes place intellectually. It ranges in levels of learner functioning from simple recall to complex evaluation. As learners move up the scale of cognitive learning, they become more self-directed; the nurse then assumes a more facilitative role.

Affective learning involves the changing of attitudes and values. Learners may experience several levels of affective involvement, from simple listening to adopting the new value. Again, as the client increases involvement, the nurse becomes less directive.

Psychomotor learning involves the acquisition of motor skills. Clients who learn psychomotor skills must meet three conditions: they must be capable of the skill; they must develop a sensory image of the skill; and they must practice the skill.

Learning theories can be grouped into four broad categories: (1) behaviorist theories, which view learning as a behavioral change accomplished through stimulus-response or conditioning; (2) cognitive learning theories, which seek to influence learners' understanding of problems and situations through promoting their insights; (3) social learning theories, which explain dysfunctional behavior and facilitate learning; and (4) humanistic theories, which assume that people have a natural tendency to learn and that learning flourishes in an encouraging environment. Knowles' adult learning theory provides a framework to understand adult characteristics and appropriate teaching interventions.

Health teaching models work together with the learning theories to give nurses a more accurate picture of the client and the client's learning needs. Five models were explored in this chapter. The CMDM is designed as a teaching mechanism to create a comprehensive base of client information that enhances all care, including client teaching. The HBM is useful in explaining the behaviors that are triggered by people with an interest in preventing diseases, and the revised HPM modifies the HBM and focuses on predicting behaviors that influence health promotion. The PRECEDE model, an acronym standing for Predisposing, Reinforcing, and Enabling Causes in Educational Diagnosis and Evaluation, is designed to address educational diagnosis, focusing heavily on assessment and identification of strengths and weaknesses. The fifth model, PROCEED, is an acronym for Policy, Regulatory, and Organizational Constructs for Educational and Environmental Development. The steps in this model include implementation, process, and impact and outcome evaluation of the teaching process, building on the assessment and diagnosis formulated from the PRECEDE model.

Teaching in community health nursing is the facilitation of learning that leads to behavioral change in the client. Ideally, this is done at the primary level of prevention. However, much of the nurse's work is done at the secondary and tertiary levels. The nurse uses several teaching-learning principles to facilitate the learning process, such as clients' readiness for learning, clients' perceptions, learners' physical and emotional comfort within an educational setting, degree of client participation, relevant subject matter, allowing clients to derive satisfaction from learning, and reinforcing learning through application.

The teaching process in community health nursing is similar to the nursing process, including steps of interaction, assessment and diagnosis, goal setting, planning, teaching, and evaluation. The teaching may be formal or informal, planned or unplanned, and methods may range from structured lecture presentations and discussions to demonstration and role-playing. Selection of teaching materials depends on how well they suit learners and help to meet the desired objectives. Sources of teaching materials that are free or inexpensive can enhance the nurses' teaching but need to be evaluated for effectiveness. The nurse needs to know how to help learners with special needs, those with physical or mental disabilities, those who are from a different culture or who speak a different language, and those who monopolize the discussion, become emotional, or are hostile. The nurse must be prepared for each situation to effectively teach the individual, family, or group.

ACTIVITIES TO PROMOTE CRITICAL THINKING

1. What learning theories discussed in this chapter most closely reflect your own position? How can they be applied in your practice?

2. A child day care center is in your service area. What populations in this setting are potential recipients of health teaching? How would you assess each group's learning needs?

3. Your city governmental officials often make decisions that appear to reflect a lack of knowledge regarding health and health care. How might you "educate" them using the concepts and principles described in this chapter?

4. Discuss the differences between cognitive, affective, and psychomotor learning. Why do cognitive and affective learning need to be linked in health teaching?

5. Develop a flyer or program for an educational presentation for clients using behavioral objectives that match the learning level desired.

6. Select one of the health teaching models. Use the model to plan an educational program for a group of teenagers. How did the use of the model enhance your teaching?

7. Explore the possible use of role models as teaching tools for community health nursing practice. What examples exist in your community? What new ones might you develop?

8. You are teaching an aggregate of middle-aged women about menopause. One woman monopolizes the class by telling stories and talking negatively about her husband. The other women are getting upset with her. How do you resolve the situation?

9. Using the Internet, locate Web sites of companies, public service agencies, and voluntary health agencies that offer free or low-cost educational material. Either request useful material to be used with clients now or bookmark a selection of sites to refer to later as needed, developing a resource file.

REFERENCES

Adatsi, G. (1999). Health going up in smoke: How can you prevent it? *American Journal of Nursing, 99*(3), 63–67.

Baltazar, V., Ibe, O.B., & Allender, J.A. (1999). Maintaining optimum nutrition among elderly clients at home. In S. Zang & J.A. Allender (Eds.), *Home care of the elderly* (pp. 98–121). Philadelphia: Lippincott Williams & Wilkins.

Bandura, A. (1977). *Social learning theory.* Englewood Cliffs, NJ: Prentice-Hall.

Bandura, A. (1986). *Social foundations of thought and action: A social cognitive theory.* Englewood Cliffs, NJ: Prentice-Hall.

Bastable, S.B. (2003). *Nurse as educator: Principles of teaching and learning for nursing practice* (2nd ed.). Boston: Jones & Bartlett.

Bigge, M.L. (1992). *Learning theories for teachers* (5th ed.). New York: Harper Collins.

Bloom, B. (Ed.). (1956). *Taxonomy of educational objectives: The classification of educational goals. Handbook I: Cognitive domain.* New York: Longman.

Breckon, D.J., Lancaster, B., & Harvey, J.S. (1998). *Community health education: Settings, roles, and skills for the 21st century* (4th ed.). Gaithersburg, MD: Aspen.

Brown, S.A., Becker, H.A., Garcia, A.A., Barton, S.A., & Hanis, C.L. (2002). Measuring health beliefs in Spanish-speaking Mexican Americans with type 2 diabetes: Adapting an existing instrument. *Research in Nursing and Health, 25,* 145–158.

Brown, S.A., & Hanis, C.L. (1999). Designing a culturally-referenced intervention for Mexican Americans with type 2 diabetes: The Starr County diabetes education study. *The Diabetes Educator, 25,* 226–236.

Cloutterbuck, J.C., & Cherry, B.S. (1998). The Cloutterbuck Minimum Data Matrix: A teaching mechanism for the new millenium. *Journal of Nursing Education, 37*(9), 385–393.

Diamantopulos, D. (1999). Caring for the elderly client with neurological deficits. In S. Zang & J.A. Allender (Eds.), *Home care of the elderly* (pp. 388–411). Philadelphia: Lippincott Williams & Wilkins.

Eisner, E.W. (1985). *The educational imagination* (2nd ed.). New York: Macmillan.

Green, L.W., & Kreuter, M.W. (1991). *Health promotion planning: An educational and environmental approach* (2nd ed.). Mountain View, CA: Mayfield.

Gronlund, N.E. (1970). *Stating behavioral objectives for classroom instruction.* New York: Macmillan.

Knowles, M. (1980). *The modern practice of adult education: Androgogy versus pedagogy* (2nd ed.). Chicago: Follett.

Knowles, M. (1984). *The adult learner: A neglected species* (3rd ed.). Houston: Gulf.

Knowles, M. (1989). *The making of an adult educator: An autobiographical journey.* San Francisco: Jossey-Bass.

Lowenstein, A.J. (2001). Strategies for innovation. In A.J. Lowenstein & M.J. Bradshaw (Eds.), *Fuszard's innovative teaching strategies in nursing* (3rd ed., pp. 18–28). Gaithersburg, MD: Aspen.

Lorig, K. (2000). *Patient education: A practical approach* (3rd ed.). Thousand Oaks, CA: Sage.

Mager, R.F. (1975). *Preparing instructional objectives* (2nd ed.). Belmont, CA: Pitman Learning.

Maslow, A.H. (1970). *Motivation and personality* (2nd ed.). New York: Harper and Row.

Pavlov, I.P. (1957). *Experimental psychology and other essays.* New York: Philosophical Library.

Pender, N.J., Murdaugh, C.L., & Parsons, M.A. (2001). *Health promotion in nursing practice* (4th ed.). Upper Saddle River, NJ: Prentice-Hall.

Piaget, J. (1966). *The origin of intelligence in children*. New York: Norton.

Piaget, J. (1970). Piaget's theory. In P.H. Mussen (Ed.), *Charmichael's manual of child psychology* (Vol. 1). New York: Wiley.

Rankin, S.H., & Stallings, K.D. (2001). *Patient education: Principles and guidelines* (4th ed.). Philadelphia: Lippincott Williams & Wilkins.

Redman, B.K. (2001). *The practice of patient education* (9th ed.). St. Louis: Mosby.

Richards, E. (1997). Motivation, compliance, and health behaviors of the learner. In S.B. Bastable (Ed.), *Nurse as educator: Principles of teaching and learning* (pp. 124–144). Boston: Jones & Bartlett.

Rogers, C. (1969). *Freedom to learn*. Columbus, OH: Merrill.

Rogers, C. (1989). *Freedom to learn for the eighties*. Columbus, OH: Merrill.

Rosenstock, I.M. (1966). Why people use health services. *Milbank Memorial Fund Quarterly, 44*, 94–127.

Skinner, B.F. (1974). *About behaviorism*. New York: Knopf.

Skinner, B.F. (1987). *Upon further reflection*. Englewood Cliffs, NJ: Prentice-Hall.

Strecher, U.J., & Rosenstock, I.M. (1997). The health belief model. In K. Glanz, F.M. Lewis, & B.K. Rimer (Eds.), *Health behavior and health education: Theory, research and practice* (2nd ed., pp. 41–59). San Francisco: Jossey-Bass.

Thorndike, E.L. (1932). *The fundamentals of learning*. New York: Teachers College Press.

Thorndike, E.L. (1969). *Educational psychology*. New York: Arno Press.

Tirodkar, M.A., & Jain, A. (2003). Food messages on African-American television shows. *American Journal of Public Health, 93*(3), 439–441.

Tyler, R.W. (1949). *Basic principles of curriculum and instruction*. Chicago: University of Chicago Press.

U. S. Department of Health and Human Services. (2000). *Healthy people 2010* (Conference ed., Vols. I & II). Washington, DC: Author.

Valdez, A., Banerjee, K., Ackerson, L., & Fernandez, M. (2002). A multimedia breast cancer education intervention for low-income Latinas. *Journal of Community Health, 27*(1), 33–51.

Wertheimer, M. (Ed.). (1945/1959). *Productive thinking*. New York: Harper & Row.

Wertheimer, M. (1980). Gestalt theory of learning. In G.M. Gazda & R.H. Corsini (Eds.), *Theories of learning: A comparative approach*. Ithasca, IL: Peacock.

SELECTED READINGS

Anderson, S., & Keller, C. (2002). Examination of the transtheoretical model in current smokers. *Western Journal of Nursing Research, 24*(3), 282–294.

Banks-Wallace, J., Enyart, J., Lewis, L., Lewis, S., Mitchell, S., Parks, L., et al. (2002). Development of scholars interested in community-based health promotion research. *Western Journal of Nursing Research, 24*(4), 326–344.

Conobbio, M.M. (2000). *Mosby's handbook of patient teaching* (2nd ed.). St. Louis: Mosby.

Dreger, V., & Tremback, T. (2002). Optimize patient health by treating literacy and language barriers. *AORN Journal, 75*(2), 280–293.

Halforn, N., & Hochstein, M. (2002). Life course health development: An integrated framework for developing health, policy, and research. *The Milbank Quarterly, 80*(3), 433–472.

Health Resources and Services Administration. (2002). *Web teaching materials: Compendium to how to start a youth web advisory program*. Washington, DC: Department of Health and Human Services.

Gingiss, P. (2000). *Building a future without HIV/AIDS: What do educators have to do with it?* Washington, DC: American Association of Colleges for Teacher Education.

Kerr, M.J., Lusk, S.L., & Ronis, D.L. (2002). Explaining Mexican American workers' hearing protection use with the health promotion model. *Nursing Research, 51*(2), 100–109.

Knowles, M. (1975). *Self-directed learning: A guide for learners and teachers*. New York: Associated Press.

Lee, J.W., Jones, P.S., Mineyama, Y., & Zhang, X.E. (2002). Cultural differences in responses to a Likert scale. *Research in Nursing & Health, 25*, 295–306.

Lewin, K. (1951). *Field theory in social science*. New York: Harper.

Long, M. (2000). *The psychology of education*. London: Routledge.

McNicholas, S.L. (2002). Social support and positive health practices. *Western Journal of Nursing Research, 24*(5), 772–787.

Morrell, R.W. (Ed.). (2002). *Older adults, health information, and the world wide web*. Mahwah, NJ: Lawrence Erlbaum Associates.

Murray, R.B., & Zenter, J.P. (2001). *Health promotion strategies through the life span* (7th ed.). Upper Saddle River, N.J.: Prentice-Hall.

Nelson, D.E., Brownson, R.C., Remington, P.L., & Parvanta, C. (Eds.). (2002). *Communicating public health information effectively: A guide for practitioners*. Washington, DC: American Public Health Association.

Norman, L.D., McArthur, D., & Miles, P. (2001). Partnership model for teaching population health care improvement. *Nursing Administration Quarterly, 26*(1), 7–13.

Parsons, R., Hinson, S., & Sardo-Brown, D. (2001). *Educational psychology: A practitioner–researcher model of teaching*. London: Wadsworth.

Poland, B.D., Green, L.W., & Rootman, I. (Eds.). (2000). *Settings for health promotion: Linking theory and practice*. Thousand Oaks, CA: Sage.

Rafiroiu, A.C., Sargent, R.G., Parra-Medina, D., Drane, W.J., & Valois, R.F. (2003). Covariations of adolescent weight-control, health-risk and health-promoting behaviors. *American Journal of Health Behavior, 27*(1), 3–14.

Redman, B.K. (2003). *Patient self-management of chronic disease: The health care provider's challenge*. St. Louis: Mosby.

Williamson, D.L., & Drummond, J. (2000). Enhancing low-income parents' capacities to promote their children's health: Education is not enough. *Public Health Nursing, 17*(2), 121–131.

Valente, T.W. (2002). *Evaluating health promotion programs*. New York: Oxford University.

Winslow, E.H. (2001). Patient education materials: Can patients read them, or are they ending up in the trash? *American Journal of Nursing, 101*(10), 33–38.

13

The Community Health Nurse as Leader, Change Agent, and Case Manager

Key Terms

- Autocratic leadership style
- Autonomous leadership style
- Case management
- Change
- Empiric-rational change strategy
- Empowerment
- Evolutionary change
- Force field analysis
- Leadership
- Normative-reeducative change strategy
- Participative leadership style
- Planned change
- Power
- Power bases
- Power-coercive change strategy
- Power sources
- Revolutionary change
- Stages of change
- Transactional leadership
- Transformational leadership

Learning Objectives

Upon mastery of this chapter, you should be able to:

- Describe three characteristics of leadership.
- Summarize five leadership theories.
- Compare and contrast five leadership styles.
- Describe five leadership functions.
- Differentiate between four power bases and four power sources.
- Discuss the concept of empowerment and its significance for community health nursing.
- Explain the three stages of change.
- Discuss the eight steps in planned change.
- Identify three planned change strategies.
- Summarize six principles for effecting change in community health.
- Describe the case-management role of the community health nurse.

Influencing people to change to healthier beliefs and practices lies at the heart of all community health nursing. With clients at every level, from families and groups to large aggregates, the ability to influence change requires knowledge and skill in the practice of leadership, the acquisition and use of power, the management of change, and skillful case management.

How do nurses carry out their roles as both leaders and change agents at the aggregate level? Many examples can be cited. A community health nurse becomes a member of the Governor's Commission on Children with Developmental Disorders. In addition to recognizing the entire state as a community and those with developmental disorders as a special population, the nurse assists the commission to formulate new policies for meeting the needs of this group of people. Another nurse, as a member of a metropolitan health planning board, works to improve health care for a group of Hmong immigrants from Southeast Asia. In a rural community of farms and small towns, the county health department nurse organizes a grassroots task force concerned about the increasing number of injuries from farm machinery. The task force decides to survey farm families to determine the causes and develop preventive measures. All three of these nurses are involved in leadership and change at the aggregate level. They are working to change people's beliefs regarding health and healthful activities and to involve them in creating organized responses to community problems.

Community health nurses also lead people to change at the organizational level. For example, a staff nurse in a public-health nursing agency who feels overburdened by paperwork, is burned out, and lacks clear goals for daily tasks observes that other staff members seem to be feeling the same. At a staff meeting, the nurse brings up the problem of job stress and suggests that everyone read an article on the subject to discuss at the next staff meeting. The first discussion is successful, and a regular staff-development meeting evolves with rotating leadership. Over a few months' time, the staff begins to feel more focused in their work and more capable of coping with job stress. Consequently, their morale improves. This is one example of how a nurse can lead informally to bring about organizational change. At another agency, several of the nurses had young families and felt the stress of being away from their families on a daily basis while working full-time. A group of the nurses worked out a plan whereby they could job-share and extend their hours in the department on fewer days per week. This plan seemed to meet their needs, and when it was presented to nursing administration it was well received, because it also solved a larger organizational problem of needing to see some families very early in the morning or in the early evening and enabled the immunization clinic to have an earlier starting time. The results of both agency's plans not only left individuals feeling better able to cope with their jobs but also improved the health of the organizations and the quality of their services.

Many nurses do not see themselves as leaders, nor do they wish to become leaders. These nurses often assume that leadership entails a formal position with heavy administrative responsibilities. Although this sometimes is the case, leadership also takes place informally in nursing practice. Being an expert practitioner, case manager, role model, and mentor for peers are important leadership roles (Kelly, 2000). In other words, nurses can be leaders in the profession and within their organization by the nature of their nursing skills and should remember that professional accountability includes these leadership roles.

Many nurse theorists advocate that all nurses should exercise leadership and accept responsibility for continually revitalizing professional nursing practice, broadening nursing's sphere of influence, and improving health services (Swansburg & Swansburg, 2002). Habel (1999) declared, "The world is in the midst of a major transformation as civilization moves from the industrial era into the communication age and beyond. The changes affecting the world and the healthcare industry will provide unique opportunities for nurses who develop their leadership potential" (p. 10). For community health nurses, the opportunities for leadership are staggering. Among them are the need to influence health reform, promote healthy public policies, and design more effective health services. Other authors stress that nurses must prepare themselves to move into clinical and administrative leadership positions (Cherry & Jacob, 2002; Marquis & Huston, 2000).

Becoming an effective leader, change agent, and case manager requires specialized knowledge and skills. This chapter examines the theoretic and applied aspects of leadership, power, and change. It describes how leadership, empowerment, and effecting change are inextricably linked and how community health nurses incorporate them into practice.

WHAT IS LEADERSHIP?

Leadership has been studied for decades, and many theorists in the social sciences and business domains have contributed to its definition. Noteworthy definitions of leadership constructed by nurses always identiy **leadership** as an interpersonal process. In this process, one person influences the activities and decisions of another person or group of persons toward the accomplishment of a desired goal (Cherry & Jacob, 2002; Huber, 2000). Therefore, leadership simply is the use of personal characteristics or qualities to influence others (Bleich, 1999). Leadership involves creating a vision and guiding and directing people's beliefs and behavior toward fulfilling that vision. It accomplishes goals with and through people. To lead requires interacting with other people to influence them to achieve a goal.

Three major characteristics of leadership are implied in these descriptions: it involves a purpose or goal, it is interactive with people, and it influences people.

Leadership Is Purposeful

Leadership always has a goal (Bleich, 1999). No act of leadership exists without a reason. A mayor seeks low-cost housing for the poor; a community health nurse wants to see teenaged parents develop parenting skills; a minister desires transportation that is accessible to physically challenged parishioners. In each instance, the leader has a purpose and involves others in accomplishing that purpose. A leader works to achieve goals by making them clear, attainable, specific, and agreeable to the follower constituency.

Leadership Is Interpersonal

Leadership always involves a social exchange, a relationship between the two parties of leader and followers (Cherry & Jacob, 2002). These parties mutually agree on roles and share information in a variety of patterns: a community agency's director of nursing sets policy and standards for client services; a nurse chairing a community task force makes informal suggestions to members. In both cases, the leader and followers must maintain a relationship that fosters ongoing communication and facilitates the movement-toward-a-goal process.

Leadership Is Influential

Leadership is influential, that is, it motivates others to change their behaviors and achieve a goal (Shinitzky & Kub, 2001). Leaders are creative problem-solvers who use their imagination to visualize new connections between ordinary events; they continually analyze the efficiency of the status quo and ask "what if" questions. For example, in a suburb of a large city, a nurse received reports that several children had encountered rats while playing, and two children had been bitten. A casual survey revealed alleys with piles of garbage and trash that attracted rats. The nurse, as a leader, wanted to influence or motivate members of the community to eliminate this public health problem. To achieve this goal, the nurse needed to influence local citizens. The nurse began by inviting the parents of children who had encountered rats to call their neighbors together. At that meeting, the nurse facilitated the discussion and offered suggestions; the group decided to form a task force and hold a cleanup day with proper disposal of refuse and adequate containers. As a leader, this nurse offered guidance and direction, thus influencing the ideas and activities of this group of followers. In this situation, the nurse analyzed the efficiency of the status quo and asked the "what if" questions. In summary, then, leadership in community health means to influence people toward development of an optimally healthy lifestyle and environment. Any purposeful effort to influence behavior is an example of leadership; therefore, every community health nurse can act as a leader.

LEADERSHIP THEORIES

Some nurses effectively influence change in community health, and others do not. What explains the difference? What accounts for effective leadership? Six theoretic approaches provide insight into the nature of leadership: trait theory, behavioral theory, contingency theory, leadership style theories, transformational theory, and charismatic theory.

Trait Theory

"The 'great man,' or 'trait' theory, was derived from the Greek philosopher Aristotle's belief that only a few people are born with the traits necessary to be great leaders" (Habel, 1999, p. 11). During the Industrial Revolution, researchers theorized that certain individuals exhibited specific personality qualities—or traits—that made them leaders, including intelligence, enthusiasm, self-confidence, charisma, and decisiveness (Table 13–1). They concluded at first that leaders were born with these characteristics but later determined that, for some, these traits were acquired. However, trait theorists were unable to identify specific qualities possessed by *all* leaders. For example, in 1967, Geier reviewed 20 different research investigations that had isolated 80 different traits of leaders but found only 5 traits to be common to four or more of the studies. Vance and Larson (2002) looked at leadership research in business and health care and cited the "complex evolutionary nature of leadership research" (p. 165) that has spanned the past 50 years. They found that trait theory research was the most common topic studied in business research literature; it was the focus of 31.1% of 1911 citations from 1986 to 1999. Most research has identified six traits that distinguish leaders from nonleaders:

1. Desire to lead
2. Ambition and energy
3. Intelligence
4. Self-confidence
5. Honesty and integrity
6. Job-relevant knowledge

The trait theory has had only limited success in enlarging our understanding of leadership. Its flaws include a failure to examine the needs of followers and different work settings and situations. Furthermore, today's focus in organizations is on patient outcomes, and most trait theory research does not make

T A B L E 13–1

Leadership Qualities Enhancing Effectiveness

Intelligence	Personality	Abilities
Knowledge	Adaptability	Social participation
Decisiveness	Creativity	Interpersonal skills
Speaks fluently	Cooperativeness	Ability to enlist
Judgment ability	Self-confidence	cooperation
	Emotional stability	Tact and diplomacy
	Independent thinking	Popularity and prestige
	Personal integrity	

(Adapted from Bass & Stogdill, 1990; Gibson et al., 1999; and Swansburg, 1996.)

a connection between a specific leadership trait and an identified patient outcome. Additionally, the theory does not clarify the relative importance of various traits, because different traits take on greater or lesser importance depending on the leadership situation. Finally, it does not reveal whether traits are already present or are acquired as a result of leadership.

Behavioral Theory

Dissatisfied with the limitations of the trait approach, researchers began in the 1940s to focus on the behavior of leaders during interaction with followers. Behavioral theory proposes that leaders' behaviors, rather than their personality traits, are the chief determinants of who will become leaders and how effective they will be. This approach holds out the hope that leadership ability can be developed.

As stated earlier, leadership involves accomplishing goals with and through people. Consequently, behavioral theorists determined that leaders must be concerned with production to achieve goals and with relationships to show concern for people. These two dimensions, concern for people and concern for productivity or tasks, became the focus of many studies in nursing and business (Huber, 2000; Stordeur, Vandenberghe, & D'hoore, 2000; Vance & Larson, 2002). Research shows that leaders who exhibit high concern for tasks while neglecting concern for people tend to be less effective (Fig. 13–1). Similarly, leaders demonstrating high concern for people with little emphasis on tasks do not yield desired results. Leaders who show high concern for people and a high concern for production (see Fig. 13–1, upper right quadrant) are the most effective. These behavioral research findings, however, could not demonstrate a leadership style that was effective in all situations.

Contingency Theory

Contingency theory describes leadership in terms of the leader's ability to adapt to the situation. It became the focus of research starting about the mid-1960s, when researchers recognized that predicting leadership success is more complex than had been envisioned previously. The type of leadership used in one organization is not always successful in another. Leadership success is contingent on the situation that dictates which style of leadership should be used.

As researchers began to examine the situational factors that influence leadership effectiveness, several contingency models emerged. The classic Fiedler's Leadership Contingency Model indicates three measures of the kind of power and influence that the group gives to its leader: the relationship between the leader and the group members, the group's task structure, and the positional power of the leader (Fiedler, 1967). Because every situation is unique, leadership is a dynamic process of adapting the leader's style to the demands of the situation. Hersey, Blanchard, and Johnson (1996) refer to this process as "adaptive leader behavior" and say that leadership style should be adapted to the followers' level of maturity, immaturity, or ability and willingness to assume responsibility. Its implications for community health nursing are summarized as follows: the more nurses adapt their style of leadership behavior to meet the particular situation and the needs of clients or followers, the more effective they will be in reaching health-related goals (Fiedler, 1969; Swansburg & Swansburg, 2002).

Attribution Theory

Attribution theory says that leadership is made up of a set of characteristics ascribed or attributed to leaders by other people. For example, Mother Theresa was considered exceptionally inspiring and humane, characteristics that were attributed to her because of people's perceptions of her style and accomplishments. People also judge whether the leader's behavior is a personal attribute (internally caused) or is dictated by the situation (externally caused). This theoretic approach combines aspects of trait, behavioral, and contingency theories to explain leadership style and effectiveness.

Charismatic Theory

Charismatic theory says that leadership occurs because of a magnetic and inspirational personality and behavior. The charismatic leader inspires others by getting an emotional commitment from them and arousing strong feelings of loyalty and enthusiasm (Habel, 1999). Charismatic theory is similar to attribution theory in that followers attribute extraordinary leadership ability to someone who exhibits exceptional appeal and persuasive ability. Examples include Martin Luther King, Jr., Fidel Castro, and William Jefferson

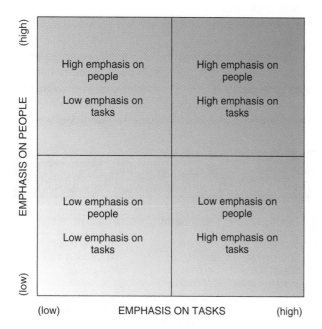

FIGURE 13–1. Leadership behavior grid. (Hersey, P., Blanchard, K., & Johnson, D.E. [1996]. *Management of organizational behavior* [7th ed.]. Upper Saddle River, NJ: Prentice-Hall.)

(Bill) Clinton. Being a charismatic leader does not always produce, nor does it guarantee, a positive situation for followers. Habel (1999) and Swansburg & Swansburg (2002) describes charismatic leaders as follows:

1. Emerge during a crisis or in troubled times
2. Advocate a vision that differs from the status quo
3. Accurately assess the situation
4. Communicate self-confidence
5. Use personal power
6. Make self-sacrifices
7. Are magnetic, persuasive, and spellbinding
8. Use unconventional strategies
9. Can be good or evil

Followers of charismatic leaders, for their part:

1. Trust in the leader's beliefs
2. Have similar beliefs
3. Exhibit affection for, obedience to, and unquestioning acceptance of the leader
4. Believe that they can contribute to the mission advocated by the leader

Research shows a high correlation between charismatic leadership and followers' high performance and satisfaction. Furthermore, individuals can learn "charismatic" behaviors. Therefore, this type of leadership is not limited solely to those who are born with these qualities. Finally, charismatic leadership is a powerful style and because of that power there is greater responsibility on the part of the leader to lead followers in positive ways. As an example, a community health nursing agency has a charasmatic nursing leader. This leader has a vision for the agency, and she assesses clearly the needs in the community and the talents of agency staff nurses. She is unafraid to take risks and is fair and generous with work assignments, rewards, and positive feedback to staff nurses. The staff enjoy working with her so much that some have given up better-paying jobs to stay in this setting with this leader. Someone who is such a charismatic leader could make decisions that were less than beneficial for the community. It would take awhile for the followers to realize that they were following someone who was not looking out for the best interests of the community, the agency, or the employees.

LEADERSHIP STYLES

Early research by Kurt Lewin, in the 1930s, examined three general styles of leadership related to forces within the leader, within the group members, and within the situation: (1) autocratic, (2) participative (democratic), and (3) autonomous (formerly called laissez-faire) (Swansburg & Swansburg, 2002). Recently, theorists have distinguished between a transactional style of leadership and a transformational style.

Autocratic Leadership Style

Autocratic leadership style is an authoritarian style in which leaders use their power (usually the power of their po-

sition) to influence their followers. The autocratic leader makes decisions alone and gives orders, expecting others to obey without question. This style generally is evident in the military. Suggestions from followers are not, as a rule, invited or accepted. The leader is dominant, and followers have little power or freedom of choice. This type of leader is more interested in task accomplishment than in concern for followers. In an extreme crisis, an autocratic style can enhance results and even survival. Sometimes, a nurse finds that members of a group expect to be led in an autocratic style. They may see the nurse as the qualified expert among them. However, autocratic leadership has a tendency to promote hostility, aggression, dependency on the leader, or apathy, which decreases initiative. It may stifle creativity and innovation. Autocratic leadership must be used with caution, and many current organizational structures do not lend themselves to its practice (Huber, 2000; Swansburg & Swansburg, 2002).

Participative Leadership Style

Participative leadership style is a democratic style in which leaders involve followers in the decision-making process (Swansburg & Swansburg, 2002). These leaders are people who are oriented to and focus on relationships and teamwork. This form of leadership has become increasingly popular, because it promotes followers' self-esteem and increases motivation and productivity. Leaders using this style encourage all members of the group to have a voice and to participate in consensus decision-making. Some participative leaders encourage followers to exercise more freedom and power than others do. Generally, however, this leadership style allows followers considerable freedom to make choices.

Autonomous Leadership Style

Autonomous leadership style is facilitative and encourages group members to select and carry out their own activities and to function independently. The leader's role is to set general parameters and to facilitate followers' progress. This style is used in certain industries in which creative design of new products (eg, computer applications, medical technologies) is being encouraged. It is effective in a group whose members have both the motivation and the competence to achieve the goals. Although someone is formally the leader, this style uses little or no direct influence; rather, the leader exercises indirect influence by establishing an overall purpose and encouraging follower creativity and innovation. In some situations, where more guidance and direction is needed, this laissez-faire approach results in low productivity and follower frustration (Swansburg & Swansburg, 2002).

Building on these leadership styles, Hersey, Blanchard, & Johnson (1996) developed a continuum of leadership behavior (Fig. 13–2) that describes style in relation to concern for people versus concern for production. Research shows

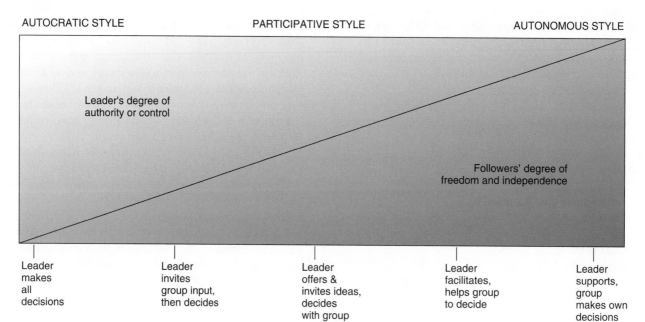

AUTOCRATIC STYLE   PARTICIPATIVE STYLE   AUTONOMOUS STYLE

Leader's degree of
authority or control

Followers' degree of
freedom and independence

| Leader makes all decisions | Leader invites group input, then decides | Leader offers & invites ideas, decides with group | Leader facilitates, helps group to decide | Leader supports, group makes own decisions |

FIGURE 13–2.   Leadership styles continuum. (Adapted from Hersey, P., Blanchard, K., & Johnson, D.E. [1996]. *Management of organizational behavior* [7th ed.]. Upper Saddle River, NJ: Prentice-Hall.)

that autocratic leaders are concerned about goals and are more task oriented, whereas participative leaders are more concerned about people and emphasize relationships.

Transformational Versus Transactional Leadership Styles

In **transactional leadership**, leader and followers engage in a reciprocal transaction. During this transaction, the roles and tasks of the followers are clarified and assigned as the group works to accomplish the goal. Most of the early leadership theories describe transactional leadership.

In the last decade or so, the literature has increasingly emphasized a type of leadership that is more charismatic (Bass, 1998; Vance & Larson, 2002). **Transformational leadership** is a new leadership paradigm that encompasses the intuitive and emotional nature of people and inspires followers to high levels of commitment and effort to achieve group goals while emphasizing interpersonal relationships (Ward, 2002). Transformational leaders gain the respect and trust of their followers; instill in them a sense of pride and mission; communicate high expectations; promote intelligent, rational problem-solving; and give followers individualized consideration (Bass, 1998). It is leadership that creates purposes for institutions.

Transformational leaders are reflective leaders with attributes of self-knowledge, authenticity, expertise, vision, flexibility, and shared leadership who effectively use the following strategies (Cherry & Jacob, 2002; Huber, 2000; Ward, 2002):
1. Use charisma.
2. Get to know the followers.
3. Help the followers to learn and develop via intellectual stimulation.

4. Provide individualized consideration.
5. Give generous feedback.
6. Give responsibility and status.
7. Give rewards to the followers.
8. Communicate information.
9. Produce greater effort, effectiveness, and satisfaction in followers.

Community health nurses are being challenged to engage in transformational leadership; however, nurses need to determine the most appropriate leadership style by assessing the unique qualities of each situation, their followers' needs and degree of independence, and their own personalities and abilities.

LEADERSHIP FUNCTIONS

What are the functions of leadership in community health nursing? Community health nursing leaders are professionals who embrace challenges; synthesize, process and promote healing; analyze and cure. Leaders challenge the process and inspire shared visions, enabling others to perform to their ultimate ability. Leaders know how to ask the right questions, how to develop problem-solving networks to find solutions to these questions, and how to marshal human energy and commitment to create the solutions. Specifically, five essential functions are required for effective leadership at any level:
1. The creative function
2. The initiating function
3. The risk-taking function
4. The integrative function
5. The instrumental function

These functions do not occur in any particular order; rather, they operate simultaneously throughout the leadership process.

Creative Function

Leaders must be creative and must envision new and better ways to solve problems. This first step involves creative thinking about problems, which includes developing methods and activities for carrying out their solutions. This function requires knowledge to stimulate sensory perceptions, curiosity, openness, sensitivity to problems, and flexibility. For instance, a group of nursing students participated in a community leadership experience in an alternative high school for adolescent parents and children. After a community assessment, the students planned a health fair focusing on issues identified as needed by the mothers and their children. But after they began working on their health fair plan, their creativity sparked dozens of new ideas, and the services at the health fair expanded from providing screening and health information to formalizing a baseline of health data on all of the teenagers. In order to not lose a valuable community contact and the assessment information gathered, the students shared their actions with nursing students entering the leadership course the next semester, encouraging them to continue to build on their successful efforts. This fostered continuity of services to the school population and provided a valuable leadership experience for new students. It was a win-win situation for the community and nursing students.

The creative leadership function includes generating ideas and developing designs for action. It also involves risk-taking and inventive problem-solving when buffering resisting forces. Finally, it includes empowering others to use their own creativity to accomplish goals.

Initiating Function

A leader introduces change and sets its process in motion. For a nurse, the initiating function includes convincing clients or followers of the need for change, starting the problem-solving process, and launching the activities needed to carry out the plan. Like all of the other leadership functions, it requires decision-making skills. For example, after seeing an increased number of adolescent pregnancies in the high school, a school nurse convinces the board of education of the need for a sex education program initiated at the junior high school level. The nurse also works to establish a prenatal counseling group and initiates a series of parenting seminars tailored to the teenaged parents in the high school. The initiating function begins the process toward goal accomplishment. It is the stimulus that starts clients or followers on their way to meet personal or agency goals.

Risk-Taking Function

Every leader is faced with uncertainty, and to proceed under uncertain conditions is to be a risk-taker. Leaders cannot guarantee outcomes. Most nurses working with families or groups in the community frequently encounter unpredictable variables. Examples include uncertainty about whether new government policies will alter programs and funding or whether a proposed program will be well received by clients and will bring about the needed change. The leadership process requires careful planning based on all available data and the creation of scenarios to predict all possible obstacles and outcomes. It requires preparation of alternative courses of action, should earlier plans fail. Nevertheless, some variables cannot be predicted beyond a certain point, and leaders must be willing to take risks and expose themselves to possible failure and embarrassment. Taking risks also means that they may expose clients or followers to potential negative outcomes. Effective leaders, however, take calculated risks; they weigh the potential consequences, pro and con, of each action before proceeding. Their concern is to minimize perceived barriers and harmful consequences and maximize positive outcomes for followers (see Bridging Financial Gaps).

Integrative Function

The integrative aspect of the leadership role focuses on strengthening collective ties and uniting clients or followers through a strong sense of purpose. The leader reminds the followers of their goals, encourages pride in their group identity, stabilizes intragroup relations, and mediates interpersonal conflict (Kouzes & Posner, 2003). Community health nurses working with families, groups, and aggregates frequently find members at odds or at cross-purposes with one another. Individuals in any group setting tend to have their own hidden agendas and separate needs. One job of the nurse leader is to keep the client group on target by clarifying and reinforcing the goals that they have mutually identified. The integrative function requires good interpersonal skills for establishing positive relationships with, as well as between, followers. This function supports the aim of promoting member commitment and cooperation.

Instrumental Function

Leaders also must keep followers moving in the right direction; this is the purpose of the instrumental or facilitative function. Inspired by vision and goals, the leader serves as an enabler to move followers to act (Kouzes & Posner, 2003; Sullivan, Decker & Jamerson, 2001). For nurse leaders, this function involves good communication. They must keep in constant touch with clients or followers to make certain that goals and activities are understood and agreed on, and to encourage both negative and positive feedback. Leaders further stimulate followers to progress toward achievement of goals by reinforcing desired behaviors and by setting the pace themselves. The latter is particularly important for gaining followers' respect and sustained commitment. To set the pace means that nurse leaders must demonstrate competence, practice what they preach, and demonstrate their belief in the followers and in what the followers are being asked to accomplish.

BRIDGING FINANCIAL GAPS

Koniak-Griffin, D., Anderson, N.L.R., Verzemnieks, I, & Brecht, M. (2000). A public health nursing early intervention program for adolescent mothers: Outcomes from pregnancy through 6 weeks postpartum. *Nursing Research, 49*(3), 130–138.

It is generally recognized that teen pregnancy and parenting continue to be a major public health problem. The social and economic well-being of the nation is affected by maternal-child health. It is imperative that adolescent mothers have the support to become self-sufficient. In addition, federal welfare reform legislation demands a plan for economic independence. This includes employment after 2 years of welfare enrollment and a lifetime limit of 5 years of welfare enrollment. This is a short span of time for pregnant teens who have not completed their education.

This study was conducted in Southern California with a randomized selection of underserved minority teens. The study was designed to evaluate the effects of an early intervention program (EIP) that used a public health nursing model. The EIP was designed to look at health and social outcomes of teen mothers and infants and at the quality of mother-child interaction, compared with similar teen parents experiencing traditional public health nursing. The EIP consisted of 17 home visits by public health nurses that were conducted from the middle of the pregnancy through the first year of motherhood on approximately a monthly basis. During the home visits, the public health nurses applied a variety of interventions in five areas: health, sexuality and family planning, maternal role, life skills, and social support. Counseling was provided in relation to maternal role issues, education, and mental health issues. The experimental group also participated in preparation-for-motherhood classes. Postpartum visits included information on family planning, infant care, and well-baby health care. Furthermore, the test group experi-enced examination of educational and vocational goals and options, completion of problem-solving worksheets, letter-writing, and individualized videotape parenting instruction and feedback. Referrals were initiated as needed for mental health counseling, family planning, and child care.

The adolescents receiving traditional public health nursing care received one or two prenatal home visits and one visit after delivery. Assessment, counseling, self-care, preparation for childbirth, educational plans, postpartum recovery, nutrition, home safety, family planning, and well-baby care were topics discussed in these few visits. Both groups received regular telephone calls by the nurses to prevent attrition and to arrange and confirm home visits.

The conclusions of the study indicate that both groups benefitted from the traditional and the EIP nursing care in terms of prenatal and perinatal outcomes. However, the EIP group outcomes were associated with decreased infant morbidity during the first 6 weeks of life and decreased maternal school dropout, with a greater likelihood of the teens' attending high school or junior college or graduating from high school. Each of these two positive outcome areas, in addition to creating better outcomes for the participants, contributed in the long run to decreased client and state or federal program costs. Health care provider, medication, and hospital costs were reduced with the lower infant morbidity, and with decreased maternal school dropout there was a greater opportunity for future financial achievement, self-sufficiency, and freedom from relying on welfare.

Suggestions for the future include replicating this study in other communities, broadening the study in the agency where it took place, and encouraging researchers to continue to get information about innovative programs into the nursing literature, so that others may learn from successful programs and initiate them across the country.

POWER AND LEADERSHIP

Power is the ability to influence or control other people's behavior to accomplish a specific purpose. Leadership and power are closely related, because leaders use power in the process of achieving goals. The concept of power has both positive and negative connotations. Positive synonyms for power are strength, energy, force, and might. Although the power to influence people for good is a goal in community health, power also may be abused. Authority, control, domination, coercion, and manipulation are negative terms often associated with power.

Although power often is viewed as being exercised by the leader, many see power as a social relationship of mutual dependency that can create different scenarios to address different work situations (Brown, 2002). A leader has only as much power over the followers as the followers grant to the leader. The leader is dependent on the followers. At the same time, the greater the followers' dependency on the leader, the greater is the power that the leader has over the followers.

If a college student is financially dependent on her parents, the parents have a certain economic power over the student. But the amount of power held by the parents also depends on how much the student earns independently and spends. People make choices. Followers can choose how dependent on the leader they wish to be, as well as the amount of power that they wish to exercise for themselves. Leaders also can choose the amount of power that they exert and the degree of their dependency on their followers. Therefore, the amount of power a person has over others is determined by two things: (1) the amount that a person chooses to take, and (2) the amount that others are willing to give.

Power Bases and Power Sources

Where does power originate? What gives people the ability to influence others? In 1959, French and Raven identified five bases of power: (1) coercive power, which uses force to gain compliance; (2) reward power, which provides something of value in exchange for compliance; (3) expert power, which exerts influence by using special knowledge or skills; (4) legitimate power, which is derived from the person's position or title; and (5) referent power, which comes from other people's admiration and emulation of the power holder. These five categories proved useful but did not clearly distinguish between bases of power and sources of power (Sullivan, Decker, & Jamerson, 2001).

Power Bases

Power bases refer to knowledge or skills possessed by the power holder that enable the power holder to exert influence over others. As a power holder, a person's power bases are the things controlled by the person. Power bases come from four types of power: information power, persuasive power, reward power, and coercive power.

Information Power

Information power refers to a person's access to or possession of valued information. It often has been said that knowledge is power. When individuals control unique information needed for such things as decision-making, they are in positions of power. The Internet gives information power, which is an empowering experience. Being knowledgeable about computers and how to retrieve global data can empower nurses and clients alike.

Persuasive Power

Persuasive power is the ability to influence people to adopt changed beliefs and actions through convincing discussion. The discussion may take such forms as argumentation, entreaty, or expostulation. A political leader who arouses a crowd to rally around a certain cause and a clergyman passionately raising money for the poor are both using persuasive power.

Reward Power

Reward power is the ability to influence people by granting rewards that they view as valuable. People comply with a request if they believe that a positive benefit will result from their compliance. They are thus voluntarily granting power to the person giving the reward. When a child is offered candy for good behavior or an employee a raise in salary if performance improves, the individuals offering the benefits have reward power.

Coercive Power

Coercive power refers to forced compliance based on fear. People comply with orders if they believe that not doing so would result in penalty, pain, or death. A mother threatening her children with loss of their allowance to get them to complete their homework has coercive power. A robber holding a gun to the head of a jewelry store owner has coercive power.

Power Sources

Power sources refer to qualities or situations from which the power holder gains a power base (Swansburg & Swansburg, 2002). Although individuals may hold one or more of the types of power just described in their power base, the question still remains: "Where does that power originate?" There are generally considered to be four sources of power: a person's position, personal qualities, expertise, and opportunities.

Position or Legitimate Power

Position or legitimate power means the ability to influence or control people as a result of a formal position. A formal position of authority, such as chief executive officer, classroom teacher, or nursing department head, gives the person power over those who are lower in the structural hierarchy. Position power enables a person to use various power bases. For example, a college professor exercises persuasive and reward power, a police officer uses coercive power, and a secretary applies information power.

Personal or Referent Power

Personal or referent power is the ability to influence others because of the person's personality. Trait theory and charismatic theory demonstrate that personal characteristics or personality style is a source of power. An individual who is charming, articulate, or physically dominating usually influences others through personal power.

Expert Power

Expert power refers to the ability to influence people based on specialized knowledge or skills. Expertise in some specialized area enables the leader to use one or more of the power bases. For example, a computer expert's knowledge is the source for information power as well as persuasive power when making computer-related decisions. Nurses, physicians, environmentalists, epidemiologists, and tax accountants have expert power.

Opportunity Power

Opportunity power is the ability to influence people by taking advantage of a special or timely situation. Rosa Parks seized an opportune moment in history to create awareness and change concerning civil rights. (Although her significant contributions to civil rights bravely began 50 years ago, when she refused to give up her seat on a bus in 1955 to a white passenger, she received the nation's highest civilian honor, a Congressional Gold Medal, in 1999 for her subsequent civil rights work.) In a crisis (eg, at the scene of a car accident), someone who does not necessarily have a position of power often emerges to take charge and tell people what to do. That person is using opportunity power. Being in the right place at the right time and using that opportunity to influence people is drawing on opportunity power.

Empowerment for Change in Community Health

Community health nurses need to develop their sources of power. Nurses can move into positions of influence in the health system as professional practitioners, managers, teachers, researchers, and consultants. They can use these positions to exercise information power, persuasion power, reward power, or coercive power to effect change. Nurses also can capitalize on their personal characteristics as a power source. Self-knowledge becomes critical in cultivating this power source. Nurses need to know their own strengths, limitations, and proclivities to find and sharpen the traits that will enhance their ability to influence people. Developing expertise is another source of nurse empowerment. In community health, nurses who expand their knowledge and competence in such areas as group dynamics, health policy and politics, computer technology, epidemiologic research, occupational health, school health, environmental health, health planning, or community assessment can use this expertise to build their power base of knowledge, persuasion, reward, and coercion. Nurses also need to take better advantage of opportunities in their personal and professional lives—instances in which they can influence decisions because of their rich power bases. Sometimes, nurses shy away from chances to serve on influential committees in the community, testify before the legislature on important health issues, attend community meetings where issues are being aired, or provide input for planning decisions. These are only a few of the opportunities through which community health nurses can gain power and influence change. Nursing's input into discussions of health reform or Medicare coverage for elders' perscriptions are prime examples of gaining nursing power and influence.

Empowerment is a process of developing knowledge and skills that increase a person's mastery over life-changing decisions. To empower means to enable. As community health nurses learn to empower themselves, they can then empower others. Empowerment is therapeutic physically, mentally, and spiritually for the nurse, the agency, and the community (Huber, 2000; Kuokkanen & Leino-Kilpi, 2000). To empower people in the community requires helping them to develop competence to take charge of their lives and find ways to meet their own needs. It means helping them to develop knowledge and skills so that they can participate in their social and political worlds. Nurses can assist community clients to develop the four power sources for themselves: using their position, capitalizing on personal characteristics, developing expertise, and taking advantage of opportunities.

The elderly population, for example, could be encouraged to take advantage of a local election (opportunity power) to lobby for crime prevention. Older urban women could participate in a community breast cancer education program along with social support to gain knowledge (expert power) about breast health and breast cancer early detection. Such programs have proved effective in detecting cancer early and promoting longevity (Skinner, Arfken, & Waterman, 2000).

Vulnerable groups in the community, such as the homeless or abused women and children, often perceive themselves to be powerless. To promote client choice and self-determination requires empowering strategies that foster clients' self-esteem. To promote clients' self-esteem, nurses can provide consistent affirmations, set clear expectations, encourage increasing responsibility, model empowering behavior, facilitate client choices, and promote a sense of meaning and hope (Koniak-Griffin, et al., 2000). When people are unable to act in a positively autonomous manner (eg, abusive parents, the mentally ill), the nurse may need to use persuasive or coercive power bases to protect them and the people affected by their actions.

Empowerment of self and others is therapeutic and spiritual (Swansburg & Swansburg, 2002). It is germane to effective leadership for all nurses and community health nurses especially. The use of power can and should be a positive force for protecting and promoting individual, organizational, and aggregate health.

THE NATURE OF CHANGE

To be a leader is to effect change in people's behaviors. When nurses suggest that families adopt healthier communication patterns, they are asking them to change. Teaching parenting skills to teenagers is introducing a change. Promoting a community's self-determination in choosing a safer environment requires that the individuals involved must change. Because community health nursing's responsibility is to accomplish health goals and thus promote change, nurses cannot lead without introducing change into people's lives. Therefore, it becomes imperative for community health nurses to understand the nature of change, how people respond to it, and how to effect change for improved community health.

Definitions and Types of Change

Change is "any planned or unplanned alteration of the status quo in an organism, situation, or process" (Lippitt, 1973, p. 37). This classic definition explains that change may occur either by design or by default. Over the years, various theorists have contributed to understanding the nature of change. From a systems perspective, change means that things are out of balance or the system's equilibrium is upset (Marriner-Tomey, 2002; Swansburg & Swansburg, 2002). For instance, when a community is devastated by a flood, its normal functioning is thrown off balance. Adjustments are required; new patterns of behavior become necessary. Other classic theorists explain change as the process of adopting an innovation (Spradley & McCurdy, 1994). Something different, such as an organization-wide smoke-free policy, is introduced; change occurs when the innovation is accepted, tried, and integrated into daily practice. Some have explained change in terms of its effect on behavior—change requires adjustment in thinking and behavior, and people's responses to change vary according to their perceptions of it. Change threatens the security that people feel when following established and familiar patterns (Cherry & Jacob, 2002). It generally requires adopting new roles. Change is disruptive.

The way people respond to change depends partly on the type of change. The change process can be described as sudden or drastic (revolutionary) or gradual over time (evolutionary).

Evolutionary change is change that is gradual and requires adjustment on an incremental basis. It modifies rather than replaces a current way of operating. Some examples of evolutionary change include becoming parents, gradually cutting back on the number of cigarettes smoked each day, and losing weight by eliminating desserts and snacks. Because it is

gradual, this kind of change does not require radical shifts in goals or values. For the most part, people resist discarding their own ideas. Accepting another's idea can reduce their self-esteem and is resisted. Gradual change may "ease the pain" that change brings to some individuals. This type of change sometimes may be viewed as reform (see The Global Community).

Revolutionary change, in contrast, is a more rapid, drastic, and threatening type of change that may completely upset the balance of a system. It involves different goals and perhaps radically new patterns of behavior. Sudden unemployment, stopping smoking overnight, losing the town's football team in a plane accident, suddenly removing children from abusive parents, or suddenly replacing human workers with computers are examples of revolutionary changes. In each instance, the people affected have little or no advance warning and little or no time to prepare. High levels of emotional, mental, and sometimes physical energy and rapid behavior change are required to adapt to revolutionary change. If the demands are too great, some may experience defense mechanisms such as incapacitation, resistance, or denial of the new situation. (See Chapter 20 for a detailed discussion of coping with stress and defense mechanisms.)

THE GLOBAL COMMUNITY

Jones, P.S., O'Toole, M.T., Hoa, N., Chau, T.T., & Muc, P.D. (2000). Empowerment of nursing as a socially significant profession in Vietnam. *Journal of Nursing Scholarship, 32*(3), 317–321.

The nursing profession and the leadership among nurses in Vietnam are poised for empowerment as a socially significant profession. Historically, nursing in Vietnam has reflected a crisis orientation. Throughout years of war, nursing care was carried out by people trained in basic first aid. This practice, forged out of necessity, created a legacy of ambiguity concerning the role of nurse and who is qualified to practice nursing.

In addition, it has been difficult to establish professional nursing education programs in Vietnam. Physicians dominate as nursing faculty members by 10 to 1. They teach medical management and following physicians' orders, thus perpetuating physician control of the fledgling profession of nursing.

This sounds bleak for the health of the nation and is reminiscent of our own nursing history. Nevertheless, the nurses persevere. The Vietnamese Nursing Association (VNA) was established in 1990. In 1992, a nursing office was established in the cabinet of the Ministry of Health. Each of Vietnam's 61 provinces has a chief nurse in the provincial health service department; there are 539 district health centers and 9941 communal

health stations. The leadership among Vietnamese nurses recognizes the job that lies ahead for the nursing profession in this country. The following goals and expectations are seen as essential by the VNA to promote the leadership of nursing in Vietnam:

1. Strengthen nursing organization and management in acute care facilities and in the community.
2. Strengthen the VNA as the professional organization to represent Vietnamese nurses.
3. Improve the nation's quality of health.
4. Improve the implementation of comprehensive care.
5. Create postgraduate and retraining courses and programs.
6. Establish a national policy for nursing education.
7. Revise the curriculum for all levels of nurses in the country.
8. Create university programs to educate nursing faculty at the baccalaureate and master's degree levels.
9. Develop standards and regulations for nursing practice.
10. Develop a national mechanism to administer licensing examinations.

Vietnamese nurses have a monumental challenge ahead, but they are becoming empowered to make needed changes. They have the creativity and energy to enhance the leadership of the nursing profession in Vietnam.

The impact of a proposed change on a system clearly depends on the degree of the change's evolutionary or revolutionary qualities, a factor to be considered in planning for change. Some situations lend themselves better to one kind of change than the other. A community in need of improved facilities for the handicapped (eg, ramps, wider doors) can introduce this change on an evolutionary, incremental basis, whereas a community that is involved in an unsafe, intolerable, or life-threatening situation, such as a flood or serious influenza epidemic, may require revolutionary change.

Stages of Change

The phrase **stages of change** refers to the three sequential steps leading to change: unfreezing (when desire for change develops), changing (when new ideas are accepted and tried out), and refreezing (when the change is integrated and stabilized in practice). These stages were first described by Kurt Lewin in the 1940s and early 1950s and have become a cornerstone for understanding the change process in more recent years (Huber, 2000; Lewin, 1947, 1951; Lippitt, Watson, & Westley, 1958; Noone, 1987).

Unfreezing

The first stage, unfreezing, occurs when a developing need for change causes disequilibrium in the system. A system in disequilibrium is more vulnerable to change. People are motivated to change either intrinsically or by some external force. People have a sense of dissatisfaction; they feel a void that they would like to fill. The unfreezing stage involves initiating the change.

Unfreezing may occur spontaneously. A family requests help in solving a problem with alcoholism; a group seeks assistance in adjusting to retirement; a community desires a solution to noise pollution. However, the nurse as change agent may need to initiate the unfreezing stage by attempting to motivate clients, through education or other strategies, to see the need for change.

Changing/Moving

The second stage of the change process, changing or moving, occurs when people examine, accept, and try the innovation. For instance, this is the period when participants in a prenatal class are learning exercises or when elderly clients in a senior citizens' center are discussing and trying ways to make their apartments safe from accidents. During the changing stage, people experience a series of attitude transformations, ranging from early questioning of the innovation's worth, to full acceptance and commitment, to accomplishing the change. The change agent's role during this moving stage is to help clients see the value of the change, encourage them to try it out, and assist them in adopting it (Huber, 2000).

Refreezing

The third and final stage in the change process, refreezing, occurs when change is established as an accepted and permanent part of the system. The rest of the system has adapted to it. Because it is no longer viewed as disruptive, threatening, or new, people no longer feel resistant to it. As the change is integrated, the system becomes refrozen and stabilized. It is evident that refreezing has occurred when weight loss clients, for example, are routinely following their diets and losing weight, or when senior citizens are using grab bars in their bathrooms and have removed scatter rugs from their homes, or when a community has erected stop signs and established crosswalks at dangerous intersections.

Refreezing involves integrating or internalizing the change into the system and then maintaining it. Because a change has been accepted and tried does not guarantee that it will last. Often, there is a tendency for old patterns and habits to return; consequently, the change agent must take special measures to ensure maintenance of the new behavior. A later section discusses ways to stabilize change.

PLANNED/MANAGED CHANGE

Leaders in community health nursing have been change agents for decades. They have planned and managed change in a variety of systems. **Planned change** is a purposeful, designed effort to effect improvement in a system with the assistance of a change agent (Spradley, 1980). Planned change, also known as managed change (Swansburg & Swansburg, 2002), is crucial to the development of successful community health nursing programs. The following characteristics of planned change are key to its success:

The change is purposeful and intentional: There are specific reasons or goals prompting the change. These goals give the change effort a unifying focus and a specific target. Unplanned change occurs haphazardly, and its outcomes are unpredictable.

The change is by design, not by default: Thorough, systematic planning provides structure for the change process and a map to follow toward a planned destination.

Planned change in community health aims at improvement: That is, it seeks to better the current situation, to promote a higher level of efficiency, safety, or health enhancement. Planned change aims to facilitate growth and positive improvements. Plans to provide shelter and health care for a homeless population, for example, are designed to improve this group's well-being.

Planned change is accomplished through an influencing agent: The change agent is a catalyst in developing and carrying out the design; the change agent's role is a leadership role.

Planned Change Process

The planned change process involves a systematic sequence of activities that follows the nursing process. Following its eight basic steps leads to the successful management of change: (1) recognize symptoms, (2) diagnose need, (3) analyze alternative solutions, (4) select a change, (5) plan the change, (6) implement the change, (7) evaluate the change, and (8) stabilize the change (Spradley, 1980). Figure 13–3

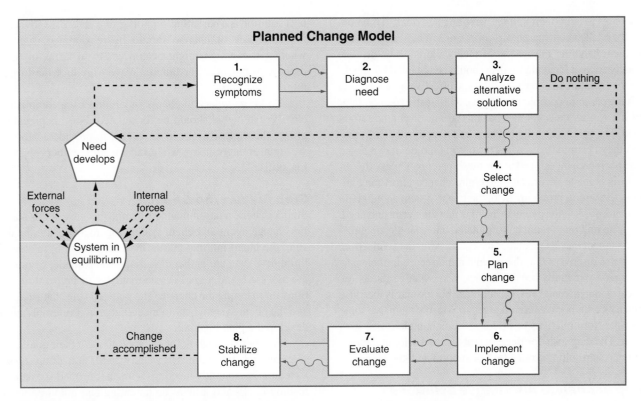

FIGURE 13–3. Planned change model. The planned change process begins when one recognizes a need. When the change agent fails to respond to a need for change, the need continues and may escalate. Client system (those involved and affected by the change) and change agent must work together throughout the entire planned change process. Their respective roles vary depending on the situation and the player's abilities, but no planned change is truly effective without utilization of this collaborative relationship. The client system (*wavy arrow*), which may be an entire community, will fluctuate in its involvement with the change process. The change agent (*straight arrow*), as a good leader, analyzes the situation thoroughly, plans carefully, and sets a steady course for effecting the change.

shows how forces acting on a system create a need for change using the planned change model.

Step 1: Recognize (Assess) Symptoms

The first step in managing change is to recognize and assess the symptoms that indicate a need for change. In this step, it is necessary to gather and examine the presenting evidence, not diagnose or jump ahead to treatment. For instance, assume that a group of clients shows interest in receiving help with parenting skills. The nurse cannot assume that these clients feel inadequate in the parent role, nor can the nurse assume that they lack information about parenting or are having difficulty with their children. The nurse must assess the specific needs to discover that some of the parents have trouble talking to their teenagers, others wonder whether their children's behavior is normal, a few question how strictly they should set limits, and still others are not certain about how to handle punishment. These symptoms are pieces of evidence that will assist diagnosis in the next step. This first step is an assessment phase. Before moving on, however, change agents need to ask themselves what their motives are for pursuing this change. Inappropriate motives of the change agent, such as wanting to feel needed, can cloud judgment and interfere with effective management of change.

Step 2: Diagnose Need

Diagnosis means to analyze the symptoms and reach a conclusion about what needs changing. First, describe the situation as it is now (the real) and compare it with the way it should be (the ideal). For example, loud arguing and conflict may be normal and functional behavior for an adolescent support group. There is no discrepancy between the real and the ideal and, therefore, no need for change within the group. If, however, there is a discrepancy between the real and the ideal, then a need exists and a change effort is justified (Hersey, Blanchard, & Johnson, 1996). For example, the community health nurse, in talking with a group of parents, hears the following comment: "I'm not sure how much freedom to allow Karen. She came in late twice last week and I'm not sure how to punish her." Clearly, the nurse notices a discrepancy between this family's present and ideal situations; hence, there is a need.

The next step is to determine the nature and cause of the need. Gathering data by questioning clients, checking the literature, or seeking consultation is important for making a more accurate diagnosis. The parents should be questioned in more detail about the difficulties that they are having with their children. Ask questions such as the following: How do they feel about being parents? What are the most difficult aspects of parenting for them? Have they read any books or used any other resources to help them in their parenting activities? To whom do they talk about parenting problems? When they have a problem handling the raising of their children, how do they usually solve it? Secondary data should be obtained by checking the literature to determine the most effective approaches to solving parenting problems or by consulting an expert on family life to get ideas about what this group of parents might need. The parents also should be asked directly what information they desire or need. Conclusions should be drawn about the specific changes needed for these parents. Unless the diagnosis is made accurately, the entire change effort may address the wrong problem. Also, the client system should help to diagnose. Ask the parents what it is that they want and need.

The findings should be formulated into a single, diagnostic statement that also includes the cause. After data collection, the nurse discovers that the parents are insecure in their parenting roles, partially because of lack of knowledge about how to carry out parental responsibilities, but primarily because they lack a supportive reference group. Most of them live some distance from relatives or no longer maintain close ties with them. The diagnosis for these parents is insecurity in the parenting role resulting from a lack of support and knowledge.

Step 3: Analyze Alternative Solutions

Once the diagnosis and its cause are determined, it is time to identify solutions or alternative directions to follow. Brainstorming is helpful here, and the client system should be involved as much as possible in the process. Reviewing the literature is helpful at this point to suggest solutions tried by others. Make a list of all reasonable, broad alternatives and then analyze them thoroughly to determine the advantages, disadvantages, possible consequences, and risks involved in each. For the parents, general alternatives might be considered, such as family counseling, a support group, or education in family life. Each of these alternatives has some advantages and disadvantages toward meeting the parents' need for confidence in their roles.

Next, each alternative should be analyzed. For example, the counseling solution could provide insight and awareness into family behavior. It would give family members opportunities to express feelings and gain understanding of how other members feel. However, it would not provide a frame of reference that the clients could use to compare their own parenting behaviors with other acceptable ones, nor would it provide adult peer support for the parents. The consequences of this alternative most likely would be to promote parents' self-understanding and better family communication. Risks would include the possibility that children, especially teenagers, might not be willing to participate and that parents might not gain self-confidence in their roles. Each alternative should be examined to determine its usefulness and feasibility, again using literature and other resources (eg, consultants) to learn the best ways to meet the parents' need for change.

Step 4: Select a Change

After all alternatives have been carefully analyzed, the best solution must be selected. The parents favor the idea that the best solution is a parenting support group. The risks involved in the choice of change should be reexamined, such as whether this action might be too costly in terms of time, money, or potential for failure. Ways to reduce these risks might be explored.

To know what the change is aiming to accomplish, a clearly stated goal should be formulated. For this parenting group, the mutually agreed-on goal is to provide a supportive, reinforcing climate while increasing members' parenting skills.

Step 5: Plan the Change

Step 5 is at the heart of planned change, because at this stage, the change agent and client system together prepare the design, the blueprint, that guides the change action. In steps 1 through 4, data are gathered, a diagnosis is made, resources are assessed, and a goal is established—all preparatory actions for planning the change. The plan tells the change agent and the client system how to meet that goal. Preferably, they develop the plan together.

Talk with the parents about ways to meet their goal, considering such possibilities as weekly discussion groups on selected topics, monthly meetings with an informed speaker, or reading books and articles on parenting and holding regular sessions to discuss their application. After analysis and discussion, the group decides to meet one evening a month, rotating the location among members' homes. Group sessions will include a variety of approaches: a speaker will be invited every 4 months, a book or article discussion will be held quarterly, and the remaining meetings will be spent on topics of the group's choice. All sessions will provide opportunities for parents to discuss their concerns or problems. The nurse and the group design this plan around a set of objectives.

The most important activity in planning is to have clear, specific objectives. These should be measurable and, preferably, stated as outcomes. For example, the following objective is measurable and describes an outcome: "By the end of the second session, each parent in the group will have participated in the discussion at least once." It is helpful to prepare a list of activities to help accomplish each objective and to develop a time plan. It also is important to assess the potential costs in terms of time, money, materials, and the number of people needed and to determine the resources available. Design the evaluation plan and start a list of ways to stabilize (refreeze) the change.

During planning, it is useful to perform a **force field analysis** (Hersey, Blanchard, & Johnson, 1996), a technique developed by Kurt Lewin for examining all positive (driving) and negative (restraining) forces that are influencing a change situation. Force field theory says that there are driving forces, which favor change, and restraining forces, which decrease or discourage change. Examples of driving forces include clients' desire to be healthier, to be more productive, or to have a safe environment. Examples of restraining forces include apathy, habits, fear of something new, perceived loss of power, low self-esteem, insecurity, and hostility (Swansburg & Swansburg, 2002). When the strength of the driving forces is equal to the strength of the restraining forces, equilibrium exists. To introduce a change and move the client system to a higher level of health, that balance must be altered. The change agent either increases the driving forces, decreases the restraining forces, or both. The change agent uses force field analysis to study both sets of forces and to develop strategies to influence the forces in favor of the change (Fig. 13–4).

The procedure for conducting a force field analysis follows a few simple steps. The change agent may perform the analysis alone but preferably consults with clients and a change-planning resource group such as community health colleagues. The steps for conducting force field analysis are as follows:

1. Brainstorm to produce a list of all driving and restraining forces. (For the parenting group, one driving force is the parents' desire to be more successful parents; a restraining force might be lack of group agreement on discussion topics.)
2. Estimate the strength of each force.
3. Plot the forces on a chart such as the one shown in Figure 13–4.
4. Note the most important forces, then research and analyze them.
5. List and document possible responses or actions that might strengthen each important driving force or weaken each important restraining force.

Finally, as a consideration in planning the change and in analyzing the driving and restraining forces, the change agent studies the social network and interactions within the system involved in the change. The change agent needs to be aware of formal and informal leaders, cliques within larger groups, influential persons, and all other social network influences on the change process. For instance, one nurse attempting to improve the infant-feeding practices among a group of young southeast Asian mothers failed to consider the strong cultural influence of the infants' grandmothers living nearby. The older women had strong opinions based on long-held cultural traditions about what infants were to eat and how they were to be fed. To ignore their influence could cause the proposed change to fail; involving the grandmothers could be a way of turning their influence into a driving force for the change.

Step 6: Implement the Change

The implementation step involves enacting the change plan. Because the objectives and activities have been clearly defined in previous steps, the change agent and client system know what needs to be done and how to begin the process. For example, the parenting group and their nurse/change agent begin group discussions meeting every Tuesday evening at a local school.

At the start of implementation, be certain that all persons concerned clearly understand and are prepared for the change. When working with an aggregate, for example, the nurse may do most of the planning with a few key members. The nurse must be sure that each member who will be affected by the proposed change understands (1) what to expect, (2) the meaning of the change, and (3) what will be required of them in adapting to it. An unprepared client system, especially in a large group or organization, may bring disaster (Tiffany & Lutjens, 1998). No matter how well a change effort is planned, people who are unprepared for it may resist it strongly and render it useless.

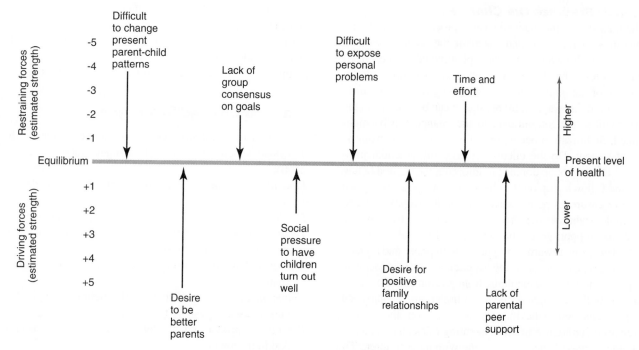

FIGURE 13–4.   Analysis of restraining and driving forces.

When implementing change that will affect a large group of people, such as introduction of a mass screening or immunization program, it is helpful to do a pilot study. The pilot study is done to test the change on a small scale, iron out problems, and revise the change before implementing it in the larger system. One advantage of a pilot study is that it demonstrates the change to the client system on a small scale, which is less threatening, so that clients are more receptive. It gives people time to adjust their thinking and to discover that the change will not disrupt their lives too much or require drastic adaptations.

Step 7: Evaluate the Change

The success of step 7 depends on how well the change is planned. Well-written objectives with specific criteria for their measurement make the evaluation step simpler. However, evaluation does not end with saying whether the objectives were met. Each objective requires analysis: (1) Was it met? (2) What evidence (documentation) shows that it was met? (3) Was it accomplished using the best means possible, or would another method have been better? The objective for the parenting group stated that each member should enter into the discussion by the end of the second session. Although this objective could easily be evaluated by the nurse leader, the objective could have been improved by a more specific description of how this participation would occur. A better method to achieve this objective would have been to suggest that more active group members could solicit ideas from those who did not have an opportunity to speak. This would facilitate more group participation, rather than having the nurse leader calling on nontalkers to speak. Finally, considering the evaluation, the change agent makes needed modifications in the change before stabilization.

Step 8: Stabilize the Change

The final step in the planned change process requires taking measures to reinforce and maintain the change (see Fig. 13–3). A well-developed change plan includes a design for stabilization. The change agent actively encourages continued use of the innovation by establishing two-way communication; in this way, future resistance can be overcome, and the client's full commitment to the change can be maintained. Stabilization occurs by soliciting reactions from the client system. Do the clients perceive any potential problems? Do they have doubts? Reinforcing the desired behavior and following up on the change as long as necessary will help to ensure its permanence. Alcoholics Anonymous, for example, stabilizes the change to nondrinking by providing a regular support group that reinforces the nondrinking pattern. The group rewards compliance with praise and replaces drinking with other satisfying experiences, such as social acceptance, to keep the alcoholic from returning to the old behavior. In the example of the parenting group, the nurse stabilizes changed behaviors by focusing on the group's increased confidence in their parenting roles and emphasizing the increased success in coping with their children. The

group decides to reward successes by giving a "Parent of the Month" plaque to the member who demonstrates the most growth in parenting skills and agrees to nominate one member as "Parent of the Year" in the community newspaper contest. After stabilization occurs and the system achieves a new equilibrium (see Fig. 13–4), the change agent-client system relationship can be terminated for this specific change effort.

Applying Planned Change to Larger Aggregates

We have viewed the planned change process primarily in the context of introducing change to smaller aggregates. Community health nurses also use these eight steps when managing change at organization, population group, community, and larger aggregate levels. For example, a nurse may suspect that there is a widespread lack of confidence among young parents. This hypothesis could be tested through a survey using a mailed questionnaire to determine parenting needs among the entire community's population of young parents. If symptoms are present (step 1), the nurse, in collaboration with health department personnel or other appropriate professionals, could analyze the symptoms and reach a diagnosis (step 2), perhaps that many young parents in the community are lacking in confidence and knowledge of parenting skills. Several approaches to meeting this need could be considered, such as instituting a parenting center in the community with satellite clinics, organizing churches or clubs to sponsor parenting support groups, or working through the community college system to hold workshops and classes on parenting skills (step 3). The most feasible and useful alternative could be selected (step 4), and a parenting program for the community planned (step 5) and implemented (step 6). The nurse, with parents and other professionals involved, then would evaluate the outcomes (step 7) and make necessary adjustments in the parenting program before finally stabilizing it (step 8), making certain that this change, undertaken to meet a population group need, remains an established and effectively functioning service.

Planned Change Strategies

Several change strategies have been published. One author described seven categories of change strategies (Huber, 2000):

Educational: help adopters to see problems and develop skills

Facilitative: provide resources to ease implementation

Technostructural: alter the interaction among technology, structure, and physical space

Data-based: use the collection and use of data to make social change

Communication-related: spread information through channels in a social system

Persuasive: produce change by means of urging, reasoning, and inducement

Coercive: control rewards and punishments to threaten and produce change

Here we focus on the three major change strategies: (1) empiric-rational (similar to technostructural, data-based, and communication-related strategies), (2) normative-reeducative (similar to educational, facilitative, and persuasive strategies), and (3) power-coercive (similar to coercive strategy). In a given situation, the change agent may use one or a combination of these strategies to effect a change.

Empiric-Rational Change Strategies

Empiric-rational change strategies are strategies used to effect change based on the assumption that people are rational and, when presented with empiric information, will adopt new practices that appear to be in their best interest. To use this approach, which is common in community health, new information is offered to people. For instance, most family planning programs use empiric-rational strategies. Clients are given basic information (communication-related strategy) on reproductive anatomy and physiology, and they are told about the benefits of contraception with an explanation of a variety of family planning methods. Health workers hope that once clients have this information, they will adopt some method of family planning. Some clients respond well to this approach, and others do not. The difference lies in client ability and interest in self-help. The nurse/change agent uses empiric-rational strategies with clients who can assume a relatively high degree of responsibility for their own health. In some respects, this set of strategies parallels the participative leadership style (see Fig. 13–2), which fosters maximum client autonomy and may use technostructural or data-based strategies.

Normative-Reeducative Change Strategies

Normative-reeducative change strategies are strategies used to influence change that not only present new information but directly influence people's attitudes and behaviors through persuasion. It is a sociocultural reeducation. This approach assumes that people's attitudes and practices are determined by sociocultural norms and that they need more than presentation of information to change behavior. This approach strengthens client self-understanding, self-control, and commitment to new patterns through direct urging and influence. For example, a health education program that aims to increase safety practices in an industrial setting not only provides safety information such as posters and warning signs but also uses persuasive tactics such as individual rewards for safe practices, division recognition for minimum number of accidents, or discipline for noncompliance. Nurses use normative-reeducative strategies with clients who have a measure of self-care skill but at the same time need external assistance to effect lasting behavioral change. This type of client is found in teaching, counseling, and therapy situations.

Power-Coercive Change Strategies

Power-coercive change strategies use coercion based on fear to effect change. Change agents may derive power from the law (eg, health regulations, administrative policies), from position (political, social, or managerial), from a group (social, work, or professional), or from personal power (eg, personal charisma, competence, respect of followers). They use this power to coerce change; the result is forced compliance on the part of the client system. Some situations, particularly those that are life-threatening, may require power-coercive strategies. In community health practice, power-coercive strategies may be used with people who cannot help themselves or in situations that threaten individuals' safety or the public's health. An example is the stringent enforcement of infection control policies regarding the treatment of contaminated objects such as used needles and the safe disposal of infectious wastes. In another example, if officials find a restaurant to be in violation of health codes, they will either force compliance with the code or close the restaurant. Occasionally, clients cannot exercise responsibility because of temporary or permanent physical or psychological incapacitation; examples may include mentally ill individuals, abusive parents, or developmentally disabled persons. In such cases, the nurse may need to use the power of the law to effect changes that are in clients' best interests. Although power-coercive strategies are appropriate in some situations, they should be used with caution because they can rob people of opportunities to grow in autonomy and capacity for self-care.

Planned change strategies may be combined; for instance, a normative-reeducative approach might have a power-coercive backup. This combination is evident in programs that educate and persuade groups of people to be immunized against an impending epidemic or to keep their garbage contained to avoid insect and rodent infestation. Behind this normative-reeducative strategy is an implied coercive threat of official disapproval, or worse, if the clients are noncompliant.

The effectiveness of a change strategy, then, varies with each situation and particularly with the degree of client capacity for self-care. As in the approach to leadership styles and use of power discussed earlier in this chapter, the nurse/change agent adapts strategies to fit each change situation. It is important to remember that "strategies need to be chosen carefully to match the change process and to enhance effectiveness. Strategies need to be congruent and not cancel each other out" (Huber, 2000, pp. 305–306).

Principles for Effecting Positive Change

Community health nurses introduce change every day that they practice. Every effort to solve a problem, prevent another problem from occurring, meet a potential community need, or promote people's optimal health requires changes. For these changes to be truly successful, so that desired outcomes are reached, they must be managed well. The following six principles provide guidelines for effecting positive change: (1) principle of participation, (2) principle of resistance to change, (3) principle of proper timing, (4) principle of interdependence, (5) principle of flexibility, and (6) principle of self-understanding.

Principle of Participation

Persons affected by a proposed change should participate as much as possible in every step of the planned change process (Marriner-Tomey, 2002). This involvement is important for several reasons. Collaboration with those who have a vested interest in the change can produce a wealth of ideas and insights that can greatly improve the change plan. Furthermore, such participation can help remove obstacles and reduce resistance. Participation ensures a greater likelihood that the change will be accepted and maintained. One nurse, for instance, when planning with a school's parent-teacher association for a drug education program, involved students as well as teachers and parents. As a result, she secured all their support and cooperation, gained many helpful suggestions that she had not considered, and discovered that students were more responsive to the program because the change plan was specifically tailored to their needs.

Principle of Resistance to Change

Because all systems instinctively preserve the status quo, the change agent can expect people to resist change (Swansburg & Swansburg, 2002). The homeostatic mechanism operating in any system seeks to maintain equilibrium; change poses a threat to that stability and security. Furthermore, all systems experience inertia; that is, they resist beginning movement. People do not undertake a change until they are convinced of its worth. Resistance may also come from a conflict over goals and methods or from misunderstanding about what the change will mean and require. Involving people in the planned change process, as discussed in the previous section, is one way to overcome resistance. Another way is establishing and maintaining open lines of communication in order to make ideas clearly understood and to resolve disagreements quickly. Prepare clients thoroughly for the change, provide support and patience during the change process, and encourage response and expression of feelings (Tiffany & Lutjens, 1998).

Principle of Proper Timing

Sometimes a change, even a well-designed and much needed one, should be postponed because the present is not the right time to introduce it. For example, perhaps the client system is experiencing too many other changes to handle the stress of this one. Other projects or activities in which the client system is currently engaged may compete for energy and other resources, depleting the energy and resources needed to make the proposed change successful. For example, in November, some middle-aged women, eager to start a book club that focused on discussion of preparing for midlife changes

(including menopause, "empty-nest" syndrome, and planning for retirement), had to postpone the project because the holidays were approaching. Shopping, entertaining, and vacations made it impossible to give the kind of time and energy needed to make the book club effective.

Proper timing is as important to a planned change as well-timed seed planting is to a good harvest. The change idea must be appropriate, the change recipient prepared, the climate right, and the resources available before the change can be fostered to grow into full maturity and usefulness.

Principle of Interdependence

Every system has many subsystems that are intricately related to and interdependent on one another. A change in one part of a system affects its other parts, and a change in one system may affect other systems. For example, a county community nursing agency made a change in its use of home health aides. Because many homebound clients needed more care than the agency staff could provide, the agency contracted with a private home-care service for extra home health aides. These paraprofessionals worked in the homes of agency clients, supplementing the care given by agency staff. The private company preferred to supervise its own aides, whereas the county agency had a policy of using community health nurses to supervise aides. The county agency was legally responsible and professionally accountable for the quality of care given to clients. The private company wanted to retain control of its workers. The matter was resolved by contracting with a different private service that would accept the county agency's supervision. The change, however, had affected the roles of nurses and aides within the system as well as the relationships between the two systems.

This principle of interdependence reminds the nurse that change does not take place in a vacuum. When workers learn new health and safety practices associated with their jobs, their relationships with one another, and their bosses, their overall productivity in the organization may easily be affected. One must anticipate and prepare for the impact of the proposed change on the clients involved, other persons, departments, organizations, or even geographic areas.

Principle of Flexibility

Unexpected events can occur in every situation. This fifth principle emphasizes two points. First, the nurse needs to be able to adapt to unexpected events and make the most of them. Perseverance and flexibility are the marks of a creative change manager (Clampitt & DeKoch, 2001; Swansburg & Swansburg, 2002). One community health nurse had tried unsuccessfully to contact a young mother who was reportedly abusing her 2-year-old son. After several phone calls and visits to an empty house, she finally found the mother and son at home with a neighbor who insisted on staying for the entire visit. At first the nurse was irritated by the neighbor's presence and viewed it as interfering with her goal of getting to know the mother and child. Then she realized that her presence offered an opportunity to learn more about the situation through the neighbor's input and viewed it as an opportunity to influence another client as well. She asked whether the neighbor had children and began to include both women in the discussion, explaining what she had to offer in terms of health teaching and support. This nurse was flexible in her approach to this situation.

The second point to remember about flexibility is that a good change planner anticipates possible blocks or problems by preparing strategies and alternative plans. During step 3 of the planned change process, it is helpful to rank the alternative solutions considered. Then, if the first choice does not work out for some reason, an alternative is ready to be put into action. Flexibility involves a willingness to consider a variety of options and suggestions from many sources (Clampitt & DeKoch, 2001).

Principle of Self-Understanding

Self-understanding is essential for an effective change agent (Hersey, Blanchard, & Johnson, 1996). A leader and change agent should be able to clearly define his or her role and learn how others define it. It is important to understand one's values and motives in relation to each change that one might ask people to make. Nurses also should understand their personality traits and typical leadership styles so that they can capitalize on or alter them in order to be more effective leaders and change agents. Understanding oneself is crucial to learning to make use of one's best qualities and skills to effect change.

CASE MANAGEMENT IN COMMUNITY HEALTH NURSING

One of the most important leadership roles of a community health nurse is that of case manager. **Case management** is a strategy to coordinate care through a process of managing quality, access, and cost to manage the risks with vulnerable groups (Yoder-Wise, 1999). It involves face-to-face relationships across a variety of health care agencies and services and their representatives. For community health nurses, this has been the method of caregiving for more than 100 years. However, it was introduced in the acute care setting, with enthusiasm, in the 1990s as a "delivery innovation" and a panacea for harnessing escalating costs and insurance premium increases (Powell, 2000).

Regardless of the setting or wellness level of the client population, case management takes interdisciplinary collaboration, the working together of professionals across health, education, and welfare domains, moving clients toward specific, measurable outcomes. The nurse works with clients using all available agencies and services to reach predetermined goals.

The settings in which community health nurses work frequently incorporate the case-management role as part of third-party reimbursement partnerships. For instance, a school nurse may conduct annual physical examinations, in-

cluding hearing and vision screening, height and weight measurements, and a head-to-toe assessment, for high-risk students receiving Medicaid or for those in the Children's Health Insurance Program (CHIP).

The nurse plans follow-up when assessment data determine that there is a potential or existing health problem. This may take the form of nutrition classes for a group of children and their parents or referring a child to an ophthalmologist for strabismus. Additionally, the nurse collaborates with others working in the best interest of the child, such as the school dietitian, physical education and classroom teachers, family physician, or other helping professionals already working with the families of children with nutrition problems. For the child with strabismus, the nurse coordinates follow-up with the classroom teacher, medical specialist, family, and hospital staff if correction of the problem entails surgery.

Populations at risk in the community benefit from the intensive relationship that promotes coordination of care through the case-management delivery system. The most effective case manager benefits from using leadership skills (including creativity and flexibility), developing her or his power base, tapping the appropriate power sources, and participating as an effective change agent. High-risk populations depend on the case-management skills of the nurse.

LEADERSHIP ROLES OF COMMUNITY HEALTH NURSES

Community health nurses exercise the functions of leadership in ever-widening spheres of influence, as shown in Figure 13–5. The central aim of this leadership role is to positively influence community health. The first area of focus is

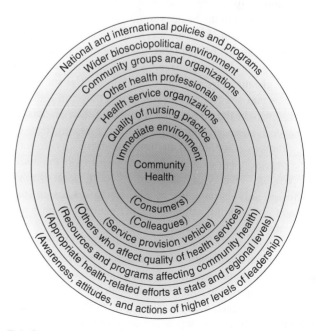

FIGURE 13–5. Areas of potential leadership influence within community health nursing practice.

to improve the immediate environment, which includes physical, psychological, social, and spiritual factors, by influencing consumer health-related behavior. Community health nurses exercise leadership when they influence the quality of nursing practice of their coworkers through, for instance, providing opportunities for professional growth and development and peer review and consultation. They may also influence the service provision vehicle, the agency or organization through which care is offered, by accepting a formal leadership position or by serving on committees and taking an active part in quality management and improvement. For example, here are some areas of influence associated with various positions in a large community health nursing agency:

Director: Influences organizational policy and decision-making

Associate director: Influences management of specific aspects of the organization

Supervisor: Influences structure and process of providing services

Case manager: Influences coordination of assessment and referral activities

Team leader: Influences day-to-day quality of nursing practice

Staff nurse: Influences client health, behavior, and environment

In other settings for community health nursing practice, such as rural or occupational environments, there may be only one nurse present to provide leadership that encompasses many, if not all, of these activities. Beyond the agency itself, the leadership role of each nurse extends to influencing those community attitudes, programs, and environmental factors that affect community health. Each nurse must assess the situation and determine the kind and extent of leadership needed.

Community health nurses may influence other professionals involved in the health system through ongoing communication to promote awareness of health needs and facilitate development of appropriate services. Nurses may influence groups and organizations, such as clubs, churches, or the legislature, by keeping them informed about health problems and suggesting ways in which they can improve health levels in the community. Extending their leadership influence even wider, community health nurses may focus on the wider biosociopolitical environment of the city, county, state, or region. For example, a nurse may support antismoking programs or may campaign for proper disposal of toxic wastes. Finally, community health nursing leadership may extend to influencing national and international policies and programs that affect health, such as those of the World Health Organization. Participating in citizens' lobbies, serving on national committees, or contacting senators and representatives at the national and international levels are some of the many possible actions nurses could take. The number of spheres in which the community health nurse exercises a leadership role varies, depending on health needs, the work situation, the nurse's abilities, and available time.

Conditions for Effective Nursing Leadership

The ultimate test of nurse leadership is in the outcomes. Are goals met? What did the leader accomplish? Reaching a successful outcome involves certain factors. Adherence to these factors contributes to positive results, but violation of one or more of them creates negative results. They form the conditions necessary for leadership to be effective.

1. Team members, followers, or clients must have the background knowledge of what is being suggested, advised, or directed in order to make compliance possible.
2. Team members, followers, or clients must be able to carry out the suggestion. They must have access to the needed resources or have their abilities developed as needed.
3. The required action must be consistent with the personal values and interests of team members, followers, or clients.
4. The required action must be consistent with the collective purposes, values, and norms of the team members, followers, or clients—that is, be in tune with group or agency goals.

Central and most important to effective leadership is a relationship of trust, respect, and mutual exchange between leader and followers. It is through this transformational relationship that community health nurses can satisfy the conditions for effective leadership and accomplish positive health outcomes.

Effectiveness of Followers

A great deal of attention has been focused on leadership. Yet for every leader there must be followers. There is evidence that the success of leadership depends on the effectiveness of followers (Yoder-Wise, 1999). Simple observation demonstrates that some followers do a good job of supporting leader goals, whereas others may be indifferent or incompetent. What role do followers play in successful leadership outcomes? It is becoming evident that ineffective followers may be more of a handicap to accomplishing goals than ineffective leaders.

Four qualities are characteristic of effective followers (Yoder-Wise, 1999):

1. *Commitment:* They are committed to the vision, goals, and purpose of the leadership effort, in addition to concern for their own goals. They are physically and psychologically dedicated to their work.
2. *Self-management:* Effective followers manage their own lives well, working independently and not needing close supervision. They are disciplined and can think and solve problems for themselves.
3. *Integrity:* Effective followers are honest and trustworthy. Their ideas, judgment, and ability to follow through can be trusted. They have high moral and ethical standards, acknowledge their mistakes, and give credit where it is appropriate.

4. *Competence:* Effective followers learn to master the skills necessary for accomplishing leadership goals. They seek to expand their competence and have higher standards for their own performance than the job requires.

In addition, these traits are observed in effective followers (Yoder-Wise, 1999):

1. They perceive the needs of both the leader and other staff.
2. They demonstrate cooperative and collaborative behaviors.
3. They exert the power to communicate through various channels.
4. They remain fully accountable for actions while relinquishing some autonomy and conceding certain authority to the leader.
5. They exhibit willingness to both lead and follow peers, as the situation warrants, allowing for competency-based leadership.
6. They assume responsibility to understand what risks are acceptable for the organization and what risks are unacceptable.

As a community health nurse, you can seek to enhance these qualities in yourself when you perform a follower role as well as encourage these qualities and traits in clients.

SUMMARY

Community health nurses, at every level of practice, must be leaders and change agents in order to influence people to adopt healthier behaviors. Formally or informally, they act as leaders to change people's health beliefs and practices and promote organized responses to community health problems. For example, they may provide leadership in initiating programs to meet the needs of at-risk populations such as the homeless, or they may lead groups such as the elderly toward self-empowerment.

Leadership includes three important characteristics: it is purposeful, it is interpersonal—involving interaction with others—and it is influential in that the change agent influences others toward accomplishing a goal. Several theories assist in understanding leadership. Their differing emphases include personality traits, leader behaviors, adapting leadership to the situation, differing leadership styles, attributed qualities, and charisma. Leadership styles may be autocratic, participative, or autonomous. In additon, some leadership is transactional, focused more on roles, tasks, and accomplishing goals, whereas other leadership is transformational, emphasizing inspiring motivation and commitment in followers.

Leadership influence depends on the use of power. This power is based on the ability to use information, be persua-sive, grant rewards, and enforce compliance. The sources of these abilities or power bases come from the leader's position of authority or influence, the leader's personality, the leader's expertise, and effective use of opportunities. Nurses need to empower themselves and others to effect change in community health.

The purpose of leadership is to effect change, which alters the equilibrium in a system; it may occur gradually, with time for people involved to adjust, or it may occur in a drastic fashion, such as in a crisis or natural disaster. Change occurs in three stages: unfreezing when the system is ready for change, changing when the innovation is implemented, and refreezing when the change is stabilized.

Planned or managed change is a purposeful, designed effort to effect improvement in a system with the help of a change agent. It involves a process of eight steps, similar to the nursing process, which nurses can use to create change. These steps include the following: assessing symptoms, diagnosing need, analyzing alternative solutions, selecting a change, planning the change, implementing the change, evaluating the change, and stabilizing the change. During planned change, the nurse can use one or a combination of several change strategies. However, the three major change strategies—a rational approach of providing information to influence people to change, an educative approach of combining new information with persuasion to effect change, and a coercive approach of enforcing compliance—are encompassing strategies. Several important principles serve as guidelines for community health nurses to effect change. They include involving all persons affected by the change, introducing change in a timely fashion, considering the impact of the change on other systems, being flexible, and understanding oneself and one's own qualities, which can be groomed to provide the most effective leadership.

Case management is an important leadership function in an agency employing community health nurses. In this role, the nurse coordinates client care, collaborating with other professionals to meet client needs. Although this role is familiar to the public health sector, it is an innovative caregiving method in other health care settings.

Finally, effective leadership incorporates the functions of creative problem-solving, initiating ideas and events, taking risks, uniting people around a purpose, and facilitating movement toward the goal. Community health nurses use these leadership functions in the context of ever-widening spheres of potential influence. They inspire and motivate people to believe in themselves, develop high self-esteem, and empower themselves to solve problems and effect change.

ACTIVITIES TO PROMOTE CRITICAL THINKING

1. As a staff community health nurse with case-management responsibilities, you have been asked to chair an ad hoc committee in your health department made up of interdisciplinary colleagues and community members. The committee's task is to plan a health fair for the local community.

   a. As chairperson of the committee, discuss how you would exercise each of the five leadership functions as you chair the planning committee.

   b. Identify and analyze your own sources of power and bases of power. Which of these power bases and sources would you use to influence committee members and community citizens?

   c. Describe your leadership style and determine whether it is appropriate for this situation and group.

   d. Outline the specific planned change steps that your committee needs to ensure a successful health fair with outcomes that promote improved levels of community health.

   e. Select one specific objective of your health fair (eg, cholesterol screening of an at-risk aggregate with reduced cholesterol levels in a year). Does the proposed objective require an evolutionary or revolutionary change in citizens' health-related behaviors? Justify your choice of the type of change.

   f. Explain the strategies that you would use to effect the change.

   g. Six principles for effecting positive change are presented in this chapter. Briefly discuss how you would use each one as you and your committee develop the health fair.

   h. How would your role of case manager in this agency assist you in your work on this committee?

   i. As the committee leader, you suggest that someone use the Internet to search for resources to help the committee enhance the materials available at the health fair. What appropriate health fair materials can you find on the Internet?

2. Characteristics of leadership exercise: The purpose of this exercise is to identify the characteristics of an effective leader. This exercise has six steps, which can be done with a large group of peers or with students in grades 7 to 12 as part of a teaching project.

   a. Give each group member 10 minutes to individually list the characteristics of an effective leader, stated in single words, phrases, or short sentences. Identify the most important characteristic by making a check next to it.

   b. Divide the group into equal subgroups of 8 to 10 members, each of which is to select two observers from among its members.

   c. Instruct the observers separately to look for persons who exhibit some of the leadership characteristics that are being identified in their groups.

   d. Instruct each group to share among themselves within a 20-minute period the lists of characteristics previously prepared by individual members and to collectively agree on the priority order of the characteristics.

   e. For the next 10 minutes, have each group discuss the process by which they worked, with contributions by the observers. Were there effective leaders in the subgroups? What characteristics did they display?

   f. During a final 10-minute period, discuss with the whole group the styles of behavior that seemed particularly helpful in sharing views on leadership characteristics. Discuss learning outcomes of the exercise.

REFERENCES

Bass, B.M. (1998). *Transformational leadership: Industrial, military, and educational impact*. Mahwah, NJ: Lawrence Erlbaum Associates.

Bass, B.M., & Stogdill, R.M. (1990). *Bass and Stogdill's handbook of leadership: Theory, research, and managerial applications* (3rd ed.). New York: Free Press.

Bleich, M.R. (1999). Managing and leading. In P. Yoder-Wise (Ed.), *Learning and managing in nursing* (2nd ed., pp. 3–20). St. Louis: Mosby.

Brown, C.L. (2002). A theory of the process of creating power in relationships. *Nursing Administration Quarterly, 26*(2), 15–33.

Cherry, B., & Jacob, S.R. (2002). *Contemporary nursing: Issues, trends, & management*. St. Louis: Mosby.

Clampitt, P.G., & DeKoch, R.J. (2001). *Embracing uncertainty: The essence of leadership*. Armonk, NY: M.E. Sharpe.

Fiedler, F.E. (1967). *A theory of leadership effectiveness.* New York: McGraw-Hill.

French, J., Jr., & Raven, B. (1959). The bases of social power. In D. Cartwright (Ed.), *Studies in social power.* Ann Arbor: University of Michigan, Institute for Social Research.

Geier, J.G. (1967). A trait approach to the study of leadership in small groups. *Journal of Communication, 4,* 316–323.

Gibson, J., Ivancevich, J., & Donnelly, J. (1999). *Organizations: Behavior, structure, processes* (10th ed.). Hightstown, NJ: McGraw-Hill.

Habel, M. (1999). Wanted: Nurse leaders for the new millennium. *NurseWeek, 12*(9), 10–11.

Hersey, P., Blanchard, K., & Johnson, D.E. (1996). *Management of organizational behavior* (7th ed.). Upper Saddle River, NJ: Prentice-Hall.

Huber, D. (2000). *Leadership and nursing care management* (2nd ed.). Philadelphia: W.B. Saunders.

Jones, P.S., O'Toole, M.T., Hoa, N., Chau, T.T., & Muc, P.D. (2000). Empowerment of nursing as a socially significant profession in Vietnam. *Journal of Nursing Scholarship, 32*(3), 317–321.

Kelly, L.S. (2000). Where leaders are born: Living the mentoring continuum. *Reflections in Nursing Leadership, 26*(3), 8–9.

Koniak-Griffin, D., Anderson, N.L.R., Verzemnieks, I., & Brecht, M. (2000). A public health nursing early intervention program for adolescent mothers: Outcomes from pregnancy through 6 weeks postpartum. *Nursing Research, 49*(3), 130–138.

Kouzes, J.M., & Posner, B.Z. (2003). *The leadership challenge: How to get extraordinary things done in organizations* (3rd ed.). San Francisco: Jossey-Bass.

Kuokkanen, L., & Leino-Kilpi, H. (2000) Power and empowerment in nursing: Three theoretical approaches. *Journal of Advanced Nursing, 31(1),* 235–241.

Lewin, K. (1947). Frontiers in group dynamics: Concept, method, and reality in social science; social equilibria and social change. *Human Relations, 1*(1), 5–41.

Lewin, K. (1951). *Field theory in social science: Seleted theoretical papers.* New York: Harper & Row.

Lippitt, G.L. (1973). *Visualizing change: Model building and the change process.* La Jolla, CA: University Associates.

Lippitt, R., Watson, J., & Westley, B. (1958). *The dynamics of planned change.* New York: Harcourt.

Marquis, B.L., & Huston, C. J. (2000). *Leadership roles and management functions in nursing* (3rd ed.). Philadelphia: Lippincott Williams & Wilkins.

Marriner-Tomey, A. (2002). *Guide to nursing management and leadership* (6th ed.). St. Louis: Mosby.

Noone, J. (1987). Planned change: Putting theory into practice—utilizing Lippitt's theory. *Clinical Nurse Specialist 1*(1), 25–29.

Powell, S.K. (2000). *Case management: A practical guide to success in managed care* (2nd ed.). Philadelphia: Lippincott Williams & Wilkins.

Shinitzky, H.E., & Kub, J. (2001). The art of motivating behavior change: The use of motivational interviewing to promote health. *Public Health Nursing 18*(3), 178–185.

Skinner, C.S., Arfken, L., & Waterman, B. (2000). Outcomes of the Learn, Share, and Live breast cancer education program for older urban women. *American Journal of Public Health, 90*(8), 1229–1234.

Spradley, B.W. (1980). Managing change creatively. *Journal of Nursing Administration, 10*(5), 32–37.

Spradley, J., & McCurdy, D. (1994). *Conformity and conflict: Readings in cultural anthropology* (8th ed.). New York: Harper Collins.

Stordeur, C., Vandenberghe, C., & D'hoore, W. (2000). Leadership styles across hierarchical levels in nursing departments. *Nursing Research, 49*(1), 37–41.

Sullivan, E.J., Decker, P.J., & Jamerson, P. (2001). *Effective leadership and management in nursing* (5th ed.). Upper Saddle River, NJ: Prentice-Hall.

Swansburg, R.C. (1996). *Management and leadership for nurse managers* (2nd ed.). Sudbury, MA: Jones & Bartlett.

Swansburg, R.C., & Swansburg, R.J. (2002). *Introductory management and leadership for nurses* (3rd ed.). Sudbury, MA: Jones & Bartlett.

Tiffany, C.R., & Lutjens, L.R.J. (1998). *Planned change theories for nursing: Review, analysis, and implications.* Thousand Oaks, CA: Sage.

Vance, C., & Larson, E. (2002). Leadership research in business and health care. *Journal of Nursing Scholarship, 34*(2), 165–171.

Ward, K. (2002). A vision for tomorrow: Transformational nursing leaders. *Nursing Outlook, 50*(3), 121–126.

Yoder-Wise, P.S. (1999). *Leading and managing in nursing* (2nd ed.). St. Louis: Mosby.

SELECTED READINGS

American Nurses Association. (1996). *Scope and standards for nurse administrators.* Washington, DC: American Nurses Publishing.

Boykin, A., & Schoenhofer, S. (2001). The role of nursing leadership in creating caring environments in health care delivery systems. *Nursing Administration Quarterly, 25*(3), 1–7.

Chinn, P.L. (2001). *Peace and power: Building communities for the future* (5th ed.). Boston: Jones & Bartlett.

Fast, B., & Chapin, R. (2000). *Strengths-based care management for older adults.* Baltimore, MD: Health Professions Press.

Feldman, H.R. (2001). *Strategies for nursing leadership.* New York: Springer.

Gebbie, K.M., & Hwang, I. (2000). Preparing currently employed public health nurses for changes in the health system. *American Journal of Public Health, 90*(5), 716–721.

Grohar-Murry, M.E., & DiCroce, H.R. (2003). *Leadership and management in nursing* (3rd ed.). Upper Saddle River, NJ: Prentice-Hall.

Kunstler, B. (2001). Building a creative hothouse: Strategies of history's most creative groups. *The Futurist, 35*(1), 22–29.

Lamond, D., & Thompson, C. (2000). Intuition and analysis in decision making and choices. *Journal of Nursing Scholarship, 32*(4), 311–314.

Laschinger, H.K.S., Finegan, J., & Shamian, J. (2001). Promoting nurses' health: Effect of empowerment on job strain and work satisfaction. *Nursing Economics, 19*(2), 42–52.

Longest, B.B., Rakich, J.S., & Darr, K. (2000). *Managing health services, organizations, and systems* (4th ed.). Baltimore: Health Professions Press.

Novick, L.F., & Mays, G.P. (2000). *Public health administration: Principles for population-based management*. Gaithersbug, MD: Aspen.

Perra, B.M. (2000). Leadership: The key to quality outcomes. *Nursing Administration Quarterly, 24,* 56–61.

Powell, S.K. (2000). *Advanced case management: Outcomes and beyond*. Philadelphia: Lippincott Williams & Wilkins.

Simms, L., Price, S., & Ervin, N. (2000). *Professional practice of nursing administration* (3rd ed.). Albany, NY: Delmar.

Snow, J.L. (2001). Looking beyond nursing for clues to effective leadership. *Journal of Nursing Administration, 31*(9), 440–443.

Yukl, G.A. (2002). *Leadership in organizations* (5th ed.). Upper Saddle River, NJ: Prentice-Hall.

14

Research in Community Health Nursing

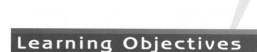

Learning Objectives

Upon mastery of this chapter, you should be able to:

- Explain the difference between quantitative research and qualitative research.
- Describe the eight steps of the research process.
- Differentiate between experimental and nonexperimental research design.
- Analyze the potential impact of research on community health nursing practice.
- Evaluate the application of a community-based research study.
- Identify the community health nurse's role in conducting research and using research findings.

S tudents new to community health nursing often ask, "Can anything I do really make a difference in the lives of my clients?" They are often shocked and discouraged by the crushing poverty they see, the overwhelming sense of helplessness experienced by many of their clients, and the continual recurrence of substance abuse, domestic violence, job failure, and criminal activity. They may ask, "Why should I bother to make home visits to pregnant teens? Why should I offer smoking cessation classes at the local homeless shelter? Why should I teach clients about the importance of taking their antituberculosis medications? Will it really matter?"

Recent community health nursing research validates that nursing care *does* matter and that you really *can* make a difference. For example, David Olds and his colleagues (Kitzman et al., 2000) examined the enduring effects of a nurse home visitation program on a group of primarily Black urban women and found that 3 years after visits ended, when compared with the women in the control group, the participants had:

- Fewer subsequent pregnancies
- Longer intervals between the births of their first and second children
- Fewer closely spaced subsequent pregnancies, and
- Fewer months of using welfare (Aid to Families with Dependent Children) and food stamps.

Women in the home visitation program had an average of only seven visits during their pregnancies and approximately one visit per month during the first 2 years of their children's' lives—a relatively small investment of time and resources with potentially priceless returns.

Olds later joined with Eckenrode and colleagues (2001) to study child maltreatment and the early onset of problem behaviors. They concluded that a 2-year program of nurse home visitation did moderate the risk of child maltreatment after the group of low-income, unmarried women and their first-born children were reexamined as the children were turning 15 years old.

An earlier longitudinal study by Olds and colleagues (1997), conducted with a primarily White sample in a semirural setting for a 15-year period, found that regular visits by public health nurses to poor, unmarried women and their first-born children resulted in dramatic differences when compared with similar mothers and children in a control group. Many of the women in the study were younger than 19 years of age, and nurses made an average of 9 prenatal visits and 23 child-related visits (up to age 2 years). There were statistically significant differences in the following outcomes:

- Fewer subsequent pregnancies and live births
- Longer intervals between first and second births
- Fewer incidences of reported child abuse and neglect
- Fewer months on public assistance and food stamps
- Fewer arrests and convictions
- Less reported impairment by alcohol or other drug use

The effects of the intervention continued for up to 15 years after the birth of the first child. This is powerful evidence for the effectiveness of regular public health nursing visits to this vulnerable client group. The minor costs of public health nurse visits are more than offset by the large savings in both dollars and human suffering. This evidence of the effectiveness of public health nursing visits can be gleaned only through conducting formal nursing research.

Research is the systematic collection and analysis of data related to a particular problem or phenomenon. Research that is properly conducted and analyzed has the potential to yield valuable information that can affect the health of large groups of people. Indeed, it often serves as the basis for changes in health care policies and programs. In the current national atmosphere of managed care and obstinately rising health care costs, the importance of valid research on how health care dollars can be spent to benefit the greatest number of people cannot be overemphasized.

This chapter examines research as it relates to community health nursing. It discusses the differences between quantitative and qualitative research and then describes the eight steps in the research process. A community-based research study is analyzed, and the nurse's role with respect to research in community health is discussed.

QUANTITATIVE AND QUALITATIVE RESEARCH

Scientific inquiry through research is generally pursued by means of two different approaches: quantitative research and qualitative research. **Quantitative research** concerns data that can be quantified or measured objectively. This could be as simple as counting the number of children receiving vaccination for varicella in immunization clinics during the past month and noting the number of reported cases of postvaccination complications. One example of a rather simple quantitative study involved counting the number of times that medications were discussed on an Internet listserv for school nurses. Reutzel and Patel (2001) wanted to know more about medication management problems reported by school nurses, so for 5 months they monitored discussion threads (or postings on a single subject) dealing with medications. They counted the number of times school nurses mentioned particular drugs or medication-related problems and found that prescription drugs, namely Ritalin, generated queries most often. School nurses had questions about administration, therapeutic appropriateness, storage, and documentation of medications. They mentioned pharmacists or pharmacies in only 14% of the postings. The researchers concluded that school nurses could benefit from greater collaboration with pharmacists, more explicit policies and guidelines, and further research in this area.

More variables can be added to quantitative studies. An example is a study examining the effects of alcohol-free instant hand sanitizers and a placebo product on school absences (White, Shinder, Shinder, et al., 2001). In addition to their regular hand-washing activities at school, 729 kindergarten through sixth grade students were assigned to one of two groups. The students in one group were given a spritz bottle containing alcohol-free instant hand sanitizer, and the others were given spritz bottles with a placebo substance. Absences were monitored for 5 weeks, and the group using the hand sanitizer had 31.1% fewer absences than the group using the placebo.

Quantitative research is helpful in identifying a problem or a relationship between two or more variables, such as type of treatment (eg, hand sanitizer versus placebo) and an outcome (decreased absenteeism). In so doing, quantitative studies tend to examine isolated parts of problems or phenomena and do not generally pay attention to the larger context or overall health of individuals. Quantitative research involves a reductionistic tendency (focusing on the parts rather than the whole) and, if used exclusively, can limit nursing knowledge because many of the important aspects of client services (eg, quality of life, grieving, spirituality) cannot be measured objectively.

A more subjective or qualitative approach is needed to study those areas that need a broader focus or that do not lend themselves to objective measurement. **Qualitative research** emphasizes subjectivity and the meaning of experiences to individuals. An example of this type of research is a study conducted by a group of nurses who looked at factors affecting the use of health and social services by elderly Russian immigrants (Aroian, Khatutshy, Tran, et al., 2001). A combination of semistructured individual interviews and focus groups was used to gather qualitative data from 17 elderly Russian immigrants, 8 adult children caregivers, and 15 health care providers serving this population. Many previous anecdotal reports from health professionals had indicated an overuse of health and social services by this population. However, a few prior research studies had contradicted this idea.

The nurse researchers analyzed the content of their interview transcripts and found that all three groups of respondents agreed unanimously that the Russian immigrants in this study heavily relied on primary health care services and homemaker services. Instead of simply "counting" the number of times elderly immigrants used services, the researchers were able to get a sense of why they did so. All three groups agreed that loneliness and depression related to immigration in later life promoted the elders' preoccupation with their health. The elders viewed good health as important and necessary so that they would not become burdens to their caregiving children. This helped explain their frequent doctor visits. They also had very high expectations for medical services in the United States, expecting cures for all of their ailments. They wanted as many free services as they could obtain—revealing another cultural factor in the overuse of services. An additional facilitating factor was the large number of Russian-speaking health care providers in the area, which made it easy for them to communicate and to navigate the health care system. This qualitative approach resulted in a much more fine-grained analysis of the problems facing elderly Russian immigrants.

It is not uncommon to find research studies in which both quantitative and qualitative approaches are used. A study on cigar and marijuana use in adolescents (Stoltz & Sanders, 2000) employed both quantitative methods (ie, self-report

questionnaires) and a qualitative approach (ie, focus groups). Questionnaire results revealed a statistically significant relationship between cigar and marijuana use ($P < .005$). Another finding revealed the positive relationship between the number of cigars smoked and the number of close friends smoking cigars. In the focus groups, the nurse researcher asked questions to discern the decision-making process of teens and why they chose to smoke. Respondents reported that both cigar and marijuana use were more often group activities "associated with luxurious relaxation" (p. 34)—a different experience from that reported by cigarette smokers, who generally smoked alone to relieve tension (see The Global Community).

Another method of analyzing research in community health uses a statistical procedure known as **meta-analysis** to evaluate the results of many similar quantitative research studies in an attempt to integrate the findings. By combining results of many similar studies, meta-analysis affords greater statistical power and can give the researcher a more complete overall perspective, especially when research on a certain issue may seem inconclusive (Gordis, 1996). An example of this type of research is a meta-analysis of epidemiologic studies on malignant melanoma (Huncharek & Kupelnick, 2002). The researchers were puzzled because the majority of studies indicated that sunscreen use was a risk factor for development of malignant melanoma. This seemed to go against common sense. By pooling the data of 11 case-control studies and employing various statistical analyses, they were able to determine that there was a wide variation in outcome for most studies. This was probably related to problems with selection of subjects, which caused confounding variables to be introduced and a subsequent inaccurate result. Using the techniques of meta-analysis, they found no statistically significant association between sunscreen use and malignant melanoma.

Another study, an integrative review of the literature on infant exposure to environmental tobacco smoke, included no meta-analysis of statistical findings (Gaffney, 2001). However, the nurse researcher examined the results of 10 international research studies with more than 20,000 subjects, looking for common themes in the findings. She found that infant colic, sudden infant death syndrome, lower respiratory tract infections, gastroesophageal reflux, and recurrent otitis media were positively associated with environmental tobacco smoke. Maternal smoking was a very significant predictor of babies' health outcomes. Many of the studies examined relied on self-report, which can be problematic because some respondents want to give socially desirable responses and may underreport their cigarette use. Public health nurses working with infants and mothers who smoke can use this type of research to assist them with promoting smoking cessation.

STEPS IN THE RESEARCH PROCESS

All effective research follows a series of predetermined, highly specific steps. Each step builds on the previous one

THE GLOBAL COMMUNITY

Smoking is a worldwide concern. Research is still needed to determine rates or patterns of smoking in the United States and many other countries. The World Health Organization has been monitoring cigarette smoking across the globe (Molarius et al., 2001). Scientists in Australia (Hill, White & Effendi, 2002), Russia (Kemppainen, Tossavainen, Vartianinen, et al., 2002), Argentina (Morello, Duggan, Adger, et al., 2001), China (Hesketh, Jian Ding, & Tomkins, 2001), as well as the United States (Vlahov, Galea, Resnick, et al., 2002; Delnevo, Pevzner, Steinberg, et al., 2002; Morabia, Costanza, Bernstein et al., 2002; Perez-Stable, Ramirez, Villareal, et al., 2001) have studied cigarette smoking among various populations. Although California and many other states have passed laws to decrease smoking in public places (Magzamen & Glantz, 2001) and added new cigarette taxes to discourage smoking (Bartosch & Pope, 2002), smoking in other countries around the world is increasing. East Asian countries account for 38% of the world's smokers (Jha, Ranson, Nguyen, et al., 2002). Approximately 80% of the world's smokers live in low- or middle-income countries.

Beyond just counting the number of new smokers, it is important to know what methods of smoking prevention and cessation are effective and what further harmful effects of smoking are being uncovered. A study by Wakschlag and colleagues (2002) analyzed a number of current research studies about the in utero effects of maternal smoking and subsequent antisocial behavior of offspring. They used a causal framework to determine that there is consistent support for (although not absolute proof of) an etiologic role of prenatal maternal smoking in the onset of antisocial behavior. The odds for development of antisocial behavior in children of mothers who smoked were 1.5 to 4 times greater than in children not exposed to cigarette smoke. This is certainly another important reason to educate pregnant mothers about the

benefits of not smoking. Horta and associates (2001), American researchers, studied breast-feeding women and found that those mothers who smoked were almost twice as likely to wean their babies from breast feeding earlier than those who did not smoke.

A Finnish study found that smoking during pregnancy was very common among young women—especially those living in the northern and eastern parts of the country and those with less education. Jaakkola and associates (2001) noted that despite educational campaigns and increased professional knowledge about the adverse effects of smoking, young women were continuing to smoke. They suggested that public health officials target rural areas and young, less educated, unmarried women in their smoking education and prevention efforts.

This information from U. S. and foreign researchers can provide nurses in the community with valuable information. Imagine that you are a public health nurse in a poor, rural county. You have noticed that the rates of cigarette smoking have increased among high school girls. Your state is interested in reducing the rates of smoking overall, and particularly among pregnant women.

1. What information could you gather to research the adverse effects of smoking on children of pregnant women?
2. What types of local data could you collect about smoking and adverse effects and how would you analyze the data?
3. How can studies like the one from Finland be useful to community health nurses in the United States? Why is a global perspective helpful?
4. Think of several questions that you could pose regarding cigarette smoking and smoking cessation. What type of research design would be most appropriate to each question? How would you collect and analyze data? Think of methods you could employ to share the results of your research.

---

and provides the foundation for the eventual discussion of findings. Alone or in collaboration with others, community health nurses use the following eight steps to complete a research project:

1. Identify an area of interest.
2. Formulate a research question or statement.
3. Review the literature.
4. Select a conceptual model.
5. Choose a research design.
6. Obtain Institutional Review Board or Human Subjects Committee approval
7. Collect and analyze data.

8. Interpret results.
9. Communicate findings.

Identify an Area of Interest

Identifying the problem or area of interest is frequently one of the most difficult tasks in the research process. It is important that the problem or interest is not too broad, that the resources and opportunity to study it are available, and that it has relevance to community health nursing practice.

The problem needs *specificity* (ie, it must be specific enough to direct the formulation of a research question). For example, concern about child safety is too broad a problem; instead, the focus could be on a narrower subject, such as use of child restraints and car seat availability and use in the community.

The problem must also be *feasible*. Feasibility concerns whether the area of interest can be examined given available resources. For example, a statewide study of the needs of pregnant adolescents might not be practical if time or funding is limited, but a study of the same group in a given school district could be more easily accomplished.

The *meaning* of the project and its *relevance* to nursing must also be considered, such as exploring the implications for nursing practice in the study of pregnant adolescents. Areas for study often evolve from personal interests, clinical experience, or philosophical beliefs. The nurse's specialty influences the selection of a problem for study and also the particular perspective or approaches used. The community health nurse functions within a context that emphasizes disease prevention, wellness, and the active involvement of clients in the services they receive. Clients' physical and social environments, as well as their biopsychosocial and spiritual domains, are of major concern. Community health nurses think in terms of the broader community; their research efforts are developed with the needs of the community or specific populations in mind.

Problems recently identified and studied within community health nursing include the following:

- The effects of maternal employment and prematurity on child outcomes in single-parent families (Youngblut, Brooten, Singer, et al., 2001)
- The effects of nurse home visitation on maternal life course (Kitzman, Olds, Sidora, et al., 2000)
- The limiting effects of domestic violence on a nurse home visitation program to prevent child abuse and neglect (Eckenrode, Ganzel, Henderson, et al., 2000)
- Protective and risk behaviors of rural minority adolescent women (Champion & Kelly, 2002)
- Health perceptions of Mexican-American women (Mendelson, 2002)
- Effects of two frequencies of walking on cardiovascular risk-factor reduction in Mexican-American women (Keller & Trevino, 2001)
- Health risk behaviors among adolescents attending rural, suburban, and urban schools (Atav & Spencer, 2002)
- Infection control among professional tattooists in Minneapolis and St. Paul, Minnesota (Raymond, Pirie, & Halcon, 2001).

Each of these problem areas provides direction for the formulation of related research questions.

Formulate a Research Question or Statement

The research question or statement reflects the kind of information desired and provides a foundation for the remainder of the project. The manner in which the question or statement is phrased suggests the research design for the project. For example, the question, "What are nurses' attitudes toward pregnant women who use crack cocaine?" determines that the design will be simple, nonexperimental, and exploratory (see later discussion). In contrast, the question, "What is the effect of an educational program on nurses' attitudes toward drug-abusing pregnant women?" suggests an experiment that will evaluate changes in nurses' attitudes toward pregnant women who use crack cocaine after receiving an educational intervention. The first research question suggests a broad, open-ended conversation with participants (nurses), asking them to discuss their attitudes toward pregnant women who use crack cocaine. From the data obtained, general themes and patterns will emerge, leading the researcher to some overall conclusions. The second question examines the effects that an educational program may have on nurses' attitudes about pregnant women who use crack cocaine. This is most likely a quantitative, evaluative study that may involve pretesting to determine the nurses' attitudes, conducting one or more classes, and then posttesting to determine whether there was any change in attitude.

Well-formulated research questions identify (1) the population of interest, (2) the variable or variables to be measured, and (3) the interventions (if any). It is very important when formulating research questions that specific terms be used to clearly represent the variables being studied. For example, if "stress" is identified as the variable measured in the research question, then it is important to note how "stress" is being defined. For instance, the researcher who wants to measure stress experienced by clients waiting for human immunodeficiency virus (HIV) test results must be careful not to measure other related variables, such as trait anxiety or depression. Consistency of terms used is crucial to the success of a project, so investigators must formulate the research question carefully. One needs to be clear about the variable and what is being measured to ensure validity of the results.

Good examples of research questions addressed recently by community health nurses include the following:

- How are social support, self-esteem, and hope [*variables*] associated with positive health practices [*variables*] among urban minority adolescents [*population of interest*] (Mahat, Scoloveno, & Whalen, 2002)?
- What are the barriers and solutions [*variables*] to implementing school-based hepatitis B immunization programs identified by school nurses [*population of interest*]? (Guajardo, Middleman, & Sansaricq, 2002)?
- What is the role of school nurses in China (Yu, 2002)?
- How does acculturation status [*variable*] affect birth outcomes and family planning compliance [*variables*] among Hispanic teens [*population of interest*] (Jones, Kubelka, & Bond, 2001)?
- Is there a relationship between adolescent parenting [*population of interest*] and school attendance and achievement [*variables*] (Casserly, Carpenter, & Halcon, 2001)?
- What are adolescents' [*population of interest*] knowledge, behavior, influences, risk, and perceptions of HIV [*variables*] (Facente, 2001)?

- What are the risk factors for breast cancer [*variables*] in Jordanian women [*population of interest*] (Petro-Nustas, Norton, & Al-Masarweh, 2002)?
- What factors are associated with recovery [*variables*] in a sample of urban residential fire survivors [*population of interest*] (Keane, Houldin, Allison, et al., 2002)?

Review the Literature

There are two phases in a review of the literature. The first phase consists of a cursory examination of available publications related to the area of interest. Although several nursing research journals publish studies reflecting all areas of nursing practice, most specialty areas have journals dedicated to specific interests. *Public Health Nursing, Family and Community Health, Journal of Community Health Nursing, American Journal of Public Health, Journal of School Health,* and *Journal of School Nursing* are some of the journals that publish the research results of interest to community health nurses. In this phase, the investigator develops knowledge about the area of interest that is somewhat superficial but sufficient to make a decision about the value of pursuing a given topic. If considerable research has already been conducted in the area, the investigator may decide to ask a different question or to pursue another area of interest.

The second phase of the literature review involves an in-depth, critically evaluated search of all publications relevant to the topic of interest. The goal of this phase is to narrow the focus and increase depth of knowledge. Journal articles describing research conducted on the topic of interest provide the most important kind of information, followed by clinical opinion articles (information on the topic described by experts in the field) and books. Journal articles provide more up-to-date information than books do, and systematic investigations provide a foundation for other studies. Prior research that has already been done on the topic of interest provides a solid foundation for later replication studies.

Criteria for compiling a good review of the literature include (1) using articles that closely relate to the topic of interest (relevancy); (2) using current articles that provide up-to-date and recent information—usually within the past 5 years (earlier articles may be included based on their importance to the area of interest); and (3) including primary and secondary sources. A *primary source* is a publication that appears in its original form. A *secondary source* is an article in which one author writes about another author's work. Primary sources are preferred over secondary sources because the information can be reviewed in its original form; this affords the investigator a more accurate and firsthand account of the study, from which personal conclusions can be drawn. For example, Horowitz and colleagues (2001) described the results of their experimental study using an interactive coaching intervention to promote responsiveness between depressed mothers and their infants. In their literature review, they cite many other studies using various interventions, including one by Armstrong and associates (1999),

which concluded that home visiting programs to vulnerable families promoted more secure mother-infant attachment and decreased depressive symptoms in mothers. The Armstrong article was important and useful for understanding interventions that may promote bonding and decrease maternal depression, but it became a secondary source for the later study dealing with a specific type of coaching intervention. Direct reading of the Armstrong article would provide a primary source for information gained specifically from that research, which undoubtedly led the more current researchers toward their choice of intervention.

A major component of a review of literature is the investigator's critical evaluation of information collected. The conceptual base and research methods of studies must be critically assessed regarding the appropriateness of the methods used and the conclusions drawn, as well as how carefully the research was conducted. Examination of the primary literature source assists this process. For nurses unskilled in this type of assessment, consultation with an experienced researcher can be helpful.

After a careful and comprehensive review of the literature, the investigator writes a clear description of the information related to the area of interest. Conflicting findings are included, and each study or article is referenced. This review provides the basis for the proposed study. The conclusions from the literature review become the basis for the new study's assumptions and methodology. The hypothesis must be built up by basing the assumptions on previous research studies, rather than making a "leap of knowledge."

Select a Conceptual Model

In relation to research, a **conceptual model** is a framework of ideas for explaining and studying a phenomenon of interest. A conceptual model conveys a particular perception of the world; it organizes the researcher's thinking and provides structure and direction for research activities. Models are like a hanger or framework on which to "hang" concepts or variables, and they should be used to guide the design and methods for collecting research data.

All fields of study, whether nursing, psychology, sociology, or physics, specify the major concerns and boundaries for their activities. Nursing is concerned with the interaction between humans and the environment in relation to health (Burns & Groves, 1999). Widely used classic nursing conceptual models such as Orem's (1985) self-care model or King's (1989) open systems model reflect the boundaries and major concerns of nursing as a profession. Although nurse investigators frequently and successfully use conceptual models developed within other fields, the advantage of using nursing models is that they provide an understanding of the world in terms of nursing's major concerns.

The investigator can become familiar with various conceptual models by reviewing the literature in the area of interest and by reading any of the many texts available on conceptual models. A thorough understanding of the major concepts of a potential model and their relationships is necessary before one attempts to use a model as a framework for a study.

For example, Benda (2001) drew from several conceptual models of risk-taking behavior in choosing the particular constructs that represent assets and deficits in a theoretical model predicting adolescent unlawful behavior by gender and region (urban or rural settings). Benda cited several studies in a review of the literature (Beman, 1995; Hawkins, Catalano, & Miller, 1992; Newcomb, 1997) but noted that the Multiple Problem Behavior Index used by Jessor and colleagues (1995) contained the strongest set of predictors of problem behavior while examining interactions between protective and risk factors. Benda wanted to extend the line of research based on this model and chose to strengthen it by incorporating additional elements found in more current literature. Benda's further goal was to note whether there were differences in unlawful behavior between males and females and between rural and urban adolescents. Jessor's model consisted of protective factors (or assets) and risk factors (or deficits). The protective factors included positive orientation toward school and health, attitudinal intolerance of deviance, positive relations with adults and perceived regulatory controls, the use of friends as models for conventional behavior, and involvement in prosocial activities. Risk factors were low self-esteem, low expectations for success, hopelessness, and low parent-friend agreement. Friends serving as models for problem behavior and low grade point average were also noted risk factors. Problem behaviors such as sexual intercourse, problem drinking, marijuana use, and delinquency were predicted based on knowledge of the protective and risk factors delineated in this model.

The results of Benda's study showed that there were some differences between male and female subjects, as well as urban and rural subjects. Being abused as a child and caregiver substance abuse had positive relationships to unlawful behavior for both males and females and for adolescents in both rural and urban settings. However, caregiver attachment was only inversely related to unlawful behavior for females. Association with delinquent peers and use of excuses were positively related to unlawful behavior for males, and parental monitoring had a larger inverse relationship to unlawfulness for males than for females. Religiosity for rural youth demonstrated a much larger inverse relationship to unlawful behavior than for urban youth. The use of Jessor's model provided clues to Benda's further development of a more sophisticated theoretical model of assets and deficits leading to unlawful behavior.

The results of Benda's research provide important information for community health nurses and others working with at-risk youth.

Choose a Research Design

The design of a research project represents the overall plan for carrying out the study. This overall plan guides the conduct of the study and, depending on its effectiveness, can influence investigators' confidence in their results. A major consideration in selecting a particular design is to try to control as much as possible those factors that are not included in the study but can influence the results. For example, Douglas and coworkers (1999) wanted to discover the percentage of homes with functioning smoke alarms. They initially conducted a telephone survey, a commonly used method of survey research in community health, and found that 71% of households reported functioning smoke alarms. Concerned that this might be an inflated number, they conducted an on-site survey to confirm the results. After face-to-face interviews, they found that only 66% of householders reported having functioning alarms. However, when researchers actually tested the smoke alarms in those homes, only 49% were fully functioning. By having researchers actually test the smoke alarms, this design controlled for inflated results of the more convenient and economic telephone survey. The community health nurse needs to determine the most efficient methods of obtaining necessary data.

In another example, researchers themselves controlled the variables to ensure true results. Kerr and colleagues (2001) knew from their review of the literature that posters encouraging exercise at the point of choice between stairs and escalators in public shopping areas could be effective in promoting greater use of stairs. They incorporated this fact into the design of their study. They used a control site and a study site (both shopping malls) and collected baseline data and a first observation 2 weeks after placing posters. Then, they followed up with stair-riser banners containing multiple messages placed on alternate stairs. Both sites were equal at baseline and the first observation; however, at the second observation time (at 4 weeks), there was a 6.7% increase in use of the stairs at the site with stair-riser banners. This simple yet novel approach motivated more people to use the stairs.

Complete descriptions of various research designs and specific methodologies are available in basic nursing research texts. For the purposes of this chapter, a few important considerations underlying design selection are described. First, quantitative approaches use two major categories of research design: experimental and nonexperimental (or descriptive).

Experimental design requires that the investigators institute an intervention and then measure its consequences. Investigators hypothesize that a change will occur as a result of their intervention, and then they attempt to test whether their hypothesis was accurate.

Experimental design requires investigators to randomly assign subjects to an **experimental group** (those receiving the intervention) and a **control group** (those not receiving the intervention). This process, called **randomization**, is the systematic selection of research subjects so that each one has an equal probability of selection. For example, Dahlquist and colleagues (2002) evaluated a distraction intervention for preschool children who had to undergo repeated chemotherapy injections. Twenty-nine children age 2 to 5 years were randomly assigned to one of two groups: (1) distraction by a developmentally appropriate electronic toy or (b) wait-list control. Children in both groups were videotaped at three sessions without distraction. Children in the intervention group were videotaped on three additional occasions during either intramuscular or surgically placed subcutaneous intravenous access port chemotherapy treatment. Distress was measured by coded observation (videotape), parent rating of child distress, and nurse rating of child distress. The results indicated that those in the distraction group had significantly improved anticipatory distress (74% saw improvement), procedural distress (59%), and recovery distress (62%). The novel distraction continued to be effective over the several weeks of the study. If the children had not been randomly assigned to the groups, there would be a greater likelihood that the results could be questioned (ie, more pain-sensitive children or more older children might have been in one group).

Another important distinction made within the experimental category of research is between true experiments and quasi-experiments. **True experiments** are characterized by instituting an intervention or change, assigning subjects to groups in a specific manner (randomization), and comparing the group of subjects who experience the manipulation with the control group. **Quasi-experiments** lack one of these elements, such as the randomization of subjects. Community health nurses conduct quasi-experiments more often than true experiments because it is often difficult (sometimes impossible) to use randomization.

A quasi-experimental study was conducted by Resnicow and coworkers (2001), who wanted to know if the addition of a motivational interviewing intervention would result in significantly increased fruit and vegetable intake among Black churchgoers. They assigned subjects from 14 churches to one of three treatment conditions: (1) a comparison group, who received nutrition education materials only; (2) a self-help intervention group, who received a video, a cookbook, and other materials along with one telephone cue call; and (3) a self-help intervention group, who received the same materials, one telephone cue call, and three telephone counseling calls (including motivational interviewing) at 3, 6, and 10 months after study initiation. Subjects in the third group, who received motivational interviewing counseling calls, reported increasing their intake of fruits and vegetables by 1.1 servings per day. Serum carotenoid levels supported their self-reports.

Nonexperimental designs (also called *descriptive designs*) are used in research to describe and explain phenomena or examine relationships among phenomena. Examples of this approach include examining the relationship between sex and smoking behaviors among adolescents, describing the emotional needs of families of clients with Alzheimer's disease, and determining the attitudes of parents in a given community toward sex education in the schools. In each of these instances, the focus of the research is on the relationships observed or the description of what exists. Greendale and associates (2002) conducted a pilot study to evaluate the effectiveness of yoga for women with hyperkyphosis (dowager's hump). Participants were assigned to 12 weeks of twice-weekly 1-hour yoga classes. Improvement in some timed physical performance measures was noted, as were perceived improvements and positive comments from participants' diaries.

Another example of a nonexperimental design is the study by McDonnell and coworkers (2001), who wanted to know what factors were associated with successful adherence to tuberculosis medication regimens. In a convenience sample of 62 adults, they determined a self-reported adherence score of 92.6% and noted that higher levels of adherence were associated with higher income (more than $11,000 per year), education beyond high school, perceived support for taking medications and absence of barriers, no current alcohol use, strong intentions to adhere to medication regimens, and a high capacity for self-care. Belief in the usefulness and benefit of medications was found to strongly correlate with intentions to adhere. From the results of this study, a community health nurse could deduce the importance of regularly teaching patients about the benefits of adhering to their antituberculosis medication regimens.

Such nonexperimental designs are often the precursors of experiments. For example, DeSantis and colleagues (1999) examined attitudes and values regarding sexuality in a small group of Haitian immigrant parents and their adolescent children. Interviews with the subjects revealed that there were considerable differences between parents and adolescents regarding the topics of sex education, contraception, and expectations about premarital sexual intercourse. Both adolescents and parents lacked accurate information about contraception, yet both believed that the main responsibility for education about sexuality and contraception remained with parents. The researchers determined that there was a need for culturally appropriate sexuality and reproductive health education. Once such an intervention is developed, further research can evaluate its appropriateness and, ultimately, its effectiveness. Other lines of clinically based research can also be designed. The choice of research design influences the ability to generalize the results, and the attention given to the details of the study affects the value of the knowledge derived. Research done with larger numbers of participants drawn from a geographically diverse area is more complete than small scale, exploratory studies done in an isolated area. Valid tools or instruments and appropriately applied statistical methods lead to greater confidence in the results of the study.

Obtain Institutional Review Board or Human Subjects Committee Approval

Whenever research is to be conducted that involves human subjects, prior approval must be gained from either an Institutional Review Board or a Human Subjects Committee. The reason for this approval is to safeguard the rights of prospective study participants. Each health department should have a committee or a gatekeeper, such as the Health Officer, who understands the federal guidelines for protecting subjects involved in research studies.

One of the most egregious examples of exploitation of human subjects was a study carried out by the U. S. Public Health Service. The Tuskegee study, begun in 1932 and ended in 1972, sought to learn more about syphilis and to justify treatment services for Blacks in Alabama (Centers for Disease Control and Prevention, 2003). The 399 men with syphilis in the study had agreed to be examined and treated. However, they were misled about the exact purpose of the study and were not given all of the facts; therefore, they were unable to give truly informed consent. Even after penicillin became the drug of choice for treatment of syphilis, in 1947, the researchers failed to offer this treatment to the infected participants. Because of this experiment and earlier Nazi atrocities, the Nuremberg Code and the Declaration of Helsinki were adopted by the world scientific community and then revised in 1975.

The following ethical principles are widely viewed as basic protections for research participants. Freedom from harm or exploitation encompasses several aspects. First, no research can be done that may inflict permanent or serious harm. Second, the research study must be stopped if it becomes evident that harm may come to participants. Debriefing, or allowing participants to ask questions of the researcher at the conclusion of the study, as a means of protecting from any unseen psychological harm, is also a component. There should be some identified benefits from participation in the research study, and any costs or risks should be clearly enumerated so that participants can more easily determine the cost/benefit ratio. Subjects should also be told that they can withdraw from the study at any time without prejudice or penalty (known as self-determination). Consent forms should include full disclosure of the nature of the study, the time and commitment required of subjects, the researcher's contact information and a pledge of confidentiality (assurance of privacy).

Vulnerable subjects, determined by the federal guidelines, include children, mentally or emotionally disabled people, physically disabled people, institutionalized people, pregnant women, and the terminally ill. Special care must be taken to ensure protection of vulnerable subjects. Once approval has been obtained from the proper entities, data collection can begin.

Collect and Analyze Data

The value of the data collected in any research project largely depends on the care taken when measuring the concepts of concern or variables. The specific tool used to measure the variables in a study, often a questionnaire or interview guide, is called an **instrument.** The accuracy of the instrument used and the appropriateness of the choice of instruments can clearly influence the results. For instance, Spielberger's State-Trait Anxiety Inventory is a well-researched question-

naire used in studying anxiety levels in adults. It has been shown to accurately measure state anxiety and the more stable tendency toward anxious personality–trait anxiety. One could infer that more accurate measurements of anxiety could be found using this instrument than a researcher-developed questionnaire that has never been tested for validity and reliability.

Validity and Reliability

Two tests are used to evaluate instrument accuracy: validity and reliability. **Validity** is the assurance that an instrument measures the variables it is supposed to measure. If a written questionnaire is being used in the study, the questions included would be evaluated to make certain that they are appropriate to the subject (content validity) and that the variable of interest is actually being measured (construct validity).

For example, Fry and Duffy (2001) described the conceptual development and psychometric evaluation of their Ethical Issues Scale. They developed this scale in response to the increasing number of ethical dilemmas facing nurses. After an extensive search of the literature and focus group research, they modeled their questionnaire after a previously developed 32-item scale used in a study of Maryland nurses. New items were added and content validity was examined by a panel of bioethics expert nurses. Finally, a sample of 2090 New England nurses completed the scale. Random sample cross-validation was done by splitting the sample into two subsamples, one used for calibration and the other for validation of the instrument. Item analysis, confirmatory principal components analysis, and internal consistency reliability analysis were performed. On statistical analysis, three factors were verified: (1) end-of-life treatment decisions (eg, withdrawing or withholding life-sustaining treatments), (2) patient care issues (eg, allocation and use of expensive resources or procedures), and (3) human rights issues (eg, patient privacy and confidentiality).

Reliability refers to how consistently an instrument measures a given research variable within a particular population. Test-retest reliability ensures that similar results are obtained by the same instrument in the same population on two separate testings. If similar results are obtained on two separate occasions, the test can be considered reliable. Fry and Duffy (2001) could conduct test-retest reliability studies by administering their questionnaire twice (with an interval between testings) to the same group of subjects. If their responses were similar enough each time to indicate a high stability of the questionnaire, then test-retest reliabililty would be established.

Statistical tests and measurements are often used to analyze subjects' responses to questionnaires to evaluate internal consistency. A questionnaire is internally consistent to the extent that all of its subparts measure the same characteristic. Cronbach's alpha is often cited as a measure of internal consistency. The end-of-life treatment issues subscale was reported by Fry and Duffy (2001) to have a Cronbach's alpha of .86 in the calibration sample and .85 in the validation sample. Measures for the patient care issues were reported as .84 and .82, and the human rights issues subscale had a Cronbach's alpha of .74 for both samples. Cronbach's alpha is reported as a correlation coefficient, so the closer the value is to +1.0, the greater the degree of internal consistency. Results higher than .7 are generally regarded as desirable.

Within the area of community health nursing research, instruments appropriate to the measurement of nursing concepts (eg, caring) are often not available. Researchers may use questionnaires that have been designed and tested by other investigators, or they may begin the tedious task of developing their own. Both approaches to measuring the variables of interest are acceptable; however, using available instruments of known reliability and validity saves considerable time.

Methods of Collecting Data

A variety of methods can be used to collect data, including self-report (subjects report their own experience verbally or in written form), observation (investigators observe subjects and document their observations), physiologic assessment (investigators use measures of physical evidence such as blood pressure or impaired mobility), and document analysis (investigators review and analyze written materials such as health records). For example, using these four methods, investigators examining the stress level of the caregiver when a family member chooses to die at home might do the following:

1. Design or use an existing written questionnaire or interview schedule (self-report)
2. Outline a schema, such as a list of potential stress-induced behaviors, for observing caregivers as they function in the home (observation)
3. Measure various physiologic indicators of stress, such as hypertension, insomnia, or poor diet (physiologic assessment)
4. Ask caregivers to keep a diary of their activities and feelings for 2 weeks, then analyze the diaries for evidence of stress (document analysis).

In most instances, the nature of the data to be collected dictates the best method of collection. One or more methods may be appropriate, given the topic of concern. In the example mentioned, a combination of the first three methods would probably be appropriate, or the diary could be substituted for the questionnaire (see Voices from the Community).

Methods of Analyzing Data

Once collected, data must be analyzed so that a meaningful interpretation can be made. Statistical procedures reduce great amounts of information to smaller chunks that can be easily interpreted. When deciding on an appropriate statistical procedure, it is helpful to consider the two major categories of statistical analysis: descriptive and inferential statistics.

Descriptive statistics portray in quantitative or mathematical terms the data collected. Commonly used descriptive statistical methods include calculating the average number or

VOICES FROM THE COMMUNITY

Back pain is a very common complaint, but it is often difficult to determine its causes. Here is the introduction to an article by a very young author in the *American Journal of Public Health,* who was interested to know whether other students had back or shoulder pain from carrying their heavy backpacks.

"The tale of student and public health researcher Shruti Iyer may turn out to be a reprise of 'The Emperor's New Clothes,' in which the child sees what all the townspeople cannot.

"Shruti was just a sixth grader in Houston, Texas, when her own back began yowling in pain. She considered the possibility that the cumbersome backpack she lugged to school might be the culprit. She interviewed other students in her immediate school and discovered that more than half of them also had back and shoulder pains that they attributed to their backpacks, sports bags, musical instruments, and other 'carry-on' items.

"Shruti turned her investigation into a science fair project and subsequently expanded the study, making it quantitative and international. She then went beyond science fairs, presenting her findings at professional society meetings and in publications, and she initiated a wide-ranging public health campaign. All this in less than 5 years: Shruti entered 10th grade in the fall of 2000."

Guyer, R. L. (2001). Backpack = back pain. *American Journal of Public Health, 91*(1), 16–19.

mean of a particular set of occurrences and calculating standard deviations (how much each score on the average deviates from the mean) and percentages. For example, an investigator analyzing data collected from 50 clients with chronic pain might find their mean pain score to be 4.96 (on a scale from 0 [no pain] to 10 [worst pain]), with a standard deviation of 0.83. These descriptive statistics suggest that clients are grouped around the middle of the pain scale and differ very little in the amount of pain they experience. The investigator may also report that more than 95% of the female clients experience pain rated between 4 and 6 on the 10-point pain scale. These descriptive statistics can be reported graphically (using graphs or charts) or in written form as shown in Table 14–1.

Inferential statistics involve making assumptions about features of a population based on observations of a sample. For example, the Gallup Poll, which surveys a sample of the population to determine what opinion they hold on a particular topic (eg, favorite presidential candidate), uses

T A B L E   1 4 – 1

Pain Ratings		
Value	Frequency	Percent (%)
3.00	1	2.0
4.00	11	22.0
5.00	30	60.0
6.00	6	12.0
7.00	1	2.0
8.00	1	2.0
MEAN 4.96	STANDARD DEVIATION 0.83	

inferential statistics to estimate the proportion of the total population that favors that candidate (Jaeger, 1990). The potential for **generalizability**, the ability to apply the research results to other similar populations, has great value to health professionals. It allows researchers to test their hypotheses on smaller groups before instituting widespread changes in methods, programs, and even national health policies.

Inferential statistics are also used to test hypotheses in research; they provide information about the likelihood that an observed difference between two or more groups could have happened just by chance or might be the result of some intervention or manipulation. These statistical procedures provide a determination of the extent to which changes or differences between sets of data are attributable to chance fluctuations and estimate the confidence with which one can make generalizations about the data. For example, in the previously cited study by Dahlquist and coworkers (2002), in which preschool children receiving chemotherapy injections were assigned to an intervention group (distraction by an electronic toy) or a control group (no distraction), the differences between the two groups in the number of subjects who showed improvement in levels of distress could be tested with the use of inferential statistics. The results would give researchers a better sense of whether the differences between those numbers were caused by their intervention or by experimental error or chance. There are many inferential statistical techniques, and they vary considerably in their complexity; however, the goal of each technique is the same: to determine the true relationship or differences between the variables under investigation.

It is appropriate to use both descriptive and inferential statistics to analyze the data from a study. For example, in a study designed to examine the effects of prenatal education on the health status of pregnant women, investigators might use inferential statistics to find a significant difference in health status between the group who experienced the educational program (experimental group) and the group who did not (control group). The investigators might also use descriptive statistics to report the percentage of women from the experimental group who attended all classes and the means and standard deviations for the women's health status scores.

Interpret Results

The explanation of the findings of a study flows from the previously formulated research plan. The findings need to be a logical conclusion, based on the building blocks of the literature review, conceptual framework, research question, and methodology. You can't jump to a conclusion for which you have not laid a foundation. Findings need to make sense, to be sensible and logical. When findings support the directions developed in the research plan, their interpretation is relatively straightforward. For example, a group of community health nurse investigators might design a study to determine the effect of parenting classes on the self-esteem of single welfare mothers between 21 and 35 years of age. They could use Coopersmith's (1967) ideas on self-esteem as their conceptual model, hypothesize that self-esteem will improve as a result of the classes, and design an experiment to test their idea. If self-esteem does, in fact, increase, their finding flows logically from their framework.

If the findings do not support the hypothesis of the study, investigators question various aspects of the research to develop an explanation. In this instance, a number of questions could be posed. Coopersmith posited that self-esteem would relate to feelings of success in a given endeavor. Can that position be inaccurate? Could the parenting classes have been ineffective? Perhaps they did not enhance feelings of success. Were there problems with the methodology used: were there too few subjects or intervening occurrences that affected the results? All of these questions and more could be considered in an attempt to explain the results.

If the study is descriptive in nature (ie, one that was designed to describe particular characteristics of a population), the direction of the findings is not a concern. A detailed, accurate report of the results and their implications alone is appropriate. Given either an experimental or a descriptive design, the importance of accuracy cannot be overemphasized. Leaps of faith when reporting the results of a study are not appropriate unless labeled as such. For example, one could not conclude from the study on parenting classes that these classes develop expert parenting skills, given that parenting skills were not assessed.

A valuable contribution can be made to the advancement of nursing knowledge when investigators use their results to make suggestions for future research. The investigators' knowledge of a particular area and their experience in conducting a specific study give them an excellent background for identifying future research possibilities.

Communicate Findings

The findings of nursing research projects need to be shared with other nurses regardless of the studies' outcomes. Findings contrary to the researcher's expectation are a valuable contribution to other researchers and consumers of research. Negative as well as positive findings can make a valuable contribution to nursing knowledge and influence nursing practice. Whether or not the hypothesis was verified is not the most important part of research; it is equally important to know about results that are inconclusive or not statistically significant, because this information is also necessary to build the science of nursing. For instance, in a study by Eckenrode and colleagues (2000), researchers found that participants who received nurse home visitation during pregnancy and through the child's second birthday had significantly fewer child maltreatment reports with the mother as perpetrator or the study child as subject than did participants not receiving nurse home visitation. However, for mothers reporting more than 28 incidents of domestic violence, no significant reductions were noted. This is important information, because domestic violence may limit the effectiveness of these types of programs. In the future, researchers may want to include questions about domestic violence when trying to evaluate the effectiveness of this type of intervention.

The research report should include the key elements of the research process. The research problem, methodology used, results of the study, and the investigators' conclusions and recommendations are presented. Whether investigators are presenting their findings verbally or writing for publication, they need to discuss the implications of their findings for nursing practice.

IMPACT OF RESEARCH ON COMMUNITY HEALTH AND NURSING PRACTICE

Research has the potential to have a significant impact on community health nursing in three ways, by affecting (1) public policy and the community's health, (2) the effectiveness of community health nursing practice, and (3) the status and influence of nursing as a profession. Community health nurses have been involved in research addressing all three of these dimensions.

Public Policy and Community Health

Research with policy implications for addressing the health needs of aggregates has been conducted on numerous topics. Many studies done by nurses and others have examined issues related to prevention, lifestyle change, quality of life, and health needs of specific at-risk populations (see Selected Readings).

Often both quantitative and qualitative methods are useful when conducting **health policy evaluation** studies to determine whether existing health services are appropriate and accessible, as well as effective. Remler and Glied (2003) wanted a better understanding of why many Americans who qualify for health insurance programs do not participate in them. They examined more than 100 articles about health insurance and other health policy–driven programs and found similar patterns and themes across all areas. The most consistent predictor of client participation was the size of the

benefit measured over time, and they suggested that longer periods of coverage might promote greater participation. They noted that Medicare, Part A, had the highest percentage of participation (99%), whereas participation in Medicaid for eligible uninsured children ranged between 50% and 70%.

The results of health policy studies can influence public policy, the quality of services, and, in turn, the public's health. In California, health policy promotes smoke-free restaurants and public places. Recently, this ban on tobacco has been extended to bars (Magazmen & Glantz, 2001).

An example of a study that could lead to health policy changes was done by Keller and Trevino (2001). They studied the effects of walking (either 3 or 5 days per week) on reduction of cardiovascular risk factors in Mexican-American women. All participants were instructed to walk at 50% of their target heart rate for 30 minutes per day (same intensity and duration). Researchers made weekly telephone calls to participants to give support and reinforce the protocols. Body composition and blood lipid measures were taken as a baseline and at 12 and 24 weeks. While control group subjects gained weight and had increased blood lipids at the end of the study, those in the 3-day-a-week group had improvements in all areas. Those in the 5-day-a-week group showed improvements at the 12-week mark but had weight gains and increased blood lipid levels at the end of the study. Researchers noticed that participants in the 5-day-a-week group became increasingly nonadherent to their protocol and actually spent less time per week walking than women in the 3-day-a-week group. The lower frequency of walking was shown to have the greatest benefit for this group of previously sedentary Mexican-American women because they were able to sustain their protocol and integrate it into their daily routines.

Clearly, this study has implications for public health and nursing practice. The Hispanic population is increasing in the United States. Because the number and proportion of overweight adults in this country have continued to increase, the significance, both in terms of quality of life for those at risk of coronary heart disease and cost savings to the health care system, cannot be overemphasized. Actions to be taken based on the study's findings should include regular counseling on low-intensity, low-frequency exercise for high-risk populations.

Another example of research useful for changing public policies is a study done by Stone and associates (2000). They determined the incidence of falls from windows in Hamilton County, Ohio. Over a 7-year period, they examined cases listed in the trauma registry of a children's hospital. Children most at risk for morbidity or mortality from falls from windows included children younger than 5 years of age, Black children, and male children. All deaths in the study occurred within the city limits of Cincinnati, where more multiple-level buildings are located. The researchers reviewed the literature and found that 90% of falls from windows can be prevented by the use of window guards. They cited as an exemplary case New York City, where the health department started a campaign to decrease deaths due to falls from windows. They implemented reporting guidelines, community education, and free installation of window guards. After 2 years, deaths fell by 50%, and legislation was passed mandating window guards. Ten years later, falls from windows had decreased by 96%. The authors stated that "lack of epidemiologic data and lobbying efforts by property owners" (p. 32) had thwarted previous attempts at policy change and legislation in Ohio. This study provided some significant empiric evidence for necessary legislation.

Community Health Nursing Practice

A primary purpose for conducting community health research is to gain new knowledge that will improve health services and promote the public's health. Consequently, most nursing research has implications for nursing practice. Many studies focus on a specific health need or at-risk population and then suggest nursing actions to be taken based on study findings. An example is an outcomes evaluation study done by Bensussen-Walls and Saewyc (2001) examining the effectiveness of teen-focused care for high-risk pregnant adolescents. In this retrospective study, outcomes for participants in a teen-centered prenatal care clinic were compared with matched cases receiving traditional adult-centered obstetric services at either a university medical center or a health maintenance organization (HMO). Results revealed that teen clinic participants missed fewer appointments, had more vaginal deliveries and higher birth weights, and were more likely to be enrolled in supplemental Medicaid programs. They also were more likely to attend 2-week and 6-week postpartum visits. Although postpartum comparison data were missing, the contraception rates for clients of the teen clinic were high (87.5%), as were the rates of breast feeding (62%) and postpartum return to school (63%). The results from this study provided useful information for nurses in targeting the unmet needs of this population.

Some nursing research specifically addresses nursing practice. For example, Sadler and colleagues (2001) examined the knowledge, attitudes, and behaviors of 194 American–Asian Indian women toward early detection of breast cancer. They found that adherence to monthly breast self examination (BSE) was low (only 40.7%), but that between 61.3% and 70% of the women reported having had a mammogram within the previous year (a relatively high rate). Breast cancer knowledge was reported as inadequate, but interest in sharing information with others was high. The authors noted practice implications for public health nurses in teaching Asian Indian women and recruiting them to teach other women about early detection of breast cancer. For example, emphasis on public health nurses teaching BSE to Asian Indian women might be changed to teaching key leaders in this community about breast cancer facts and prevention methods—information to share with small groups of women in their homes. Public health nurses might emphasize how to get low-cost mammograms, because this is something these clients are more likely to practice than BSE.

It is important for public health nurses to have a sound knowledge base to effectively teach their clients in the community. Broderick and colleagues (2002) examined the baseline knowledge of public health nurses before presenting a "train the trainer" program on iron poisoning. Pretest scores averaged 56%, and they found that 71% of public health nurses did not identify iron as a leading household poison. At posttest, public health nurses averaged a score of 96%, and, in a follow up survey, 87% of them stated that they had used the program information to educate their clients about iron poisoning.

Nursing's Professional Status and Influence

The third way in which research has a significant impact on community health nursing is in its potential to enhance nursing's status and influence. As community health nursing research sheds light on critical health needs of at-risk populations, exposes deficiencies in the health care system, demonstrates more efficient and cost-effective methods for delivering services, and documents the effectiveness of nursing interventions, the profession will gain a stronger voice and have a greater impact on health policy and programs.

An example of community-oriented research was conducted by Rothman and associates (2002). Community-developed strategies were used in a program to reduce lead poisoning in a poor area of Philadelphia. Four census tracts were selected for intervention on the basis of pre-1950 built housing, poverty level, and percentage of Black citizens. Matching control census tracts were also studied. Adult block parties (using educational and motivational strategies) and interactive educational sessions for children (eg, puppet shows) were used over the 3 years of study. Approximately 1200 children and 900 adults participated. Initially, overall lead poisoning awareness was low. Testing of homes revealed that more than 90% were positive for lead. After the first intervention year, there was a 27% increase in the number of children tested for lead in the intervention census tracts, and only a 10% increase in the control census tracts. There was an 11% reduction in the percentage of children with excess blood lead levels in the intervention group, and only a 3% reduction in the control group. Participants readily accepted this community-developed and community-based intervention by nurses and a physician from Temple University. This research enhanced nursing's role in the community by engaging with community members on their turf and demonstrating nurses' roles in research (see What Do You Think?).

In many poor communities, most of the population can be on some type of public assistance. Welfare reform is a concern to many professionals, not just community health nurses. Youngblut and colleagues (2001) examined the effects of maternal employment and infant prematurity on later child outcomes. They chose low-income single-parent families, the majority of whom (more than 66%) were African-American. A total of 60 preterm and 61 full-term preschool children were

WHAT DO YOU THINK?

Much of the research in community health is published by physicians, university researchers, and government-sponsored scientists. Public health nurses
contribute to this research by conducting their own
studies and also by partnering with other established
researchers. What would happen to the practice and
credibility of community health nursing if nurses
ceased to conduct and publish research?

assessed for cognitive functioning and child behavioral performance. Mother-child relationship was also determined, as
were current employment, employment patterns, and desire to
be employed. Regardless of gestational status, children of employed mothers scored significantly higher on achievement
than those of unemployed mothers. More hours of employment was also related to better cognition and achievement
outcomes. The researchers theorized that this may be the result of better financial resources and mothers' increased feelings of self-worth. Those mothers whose actual and desired
employment status did not match were thought to be more
likely to be depressed, explaining their reports of having
fewer positive interactions with their children. Researchers
concluded that the current welfare reform legislation might
have a potential for positive effects on child development.

There is strong documentation for the effectiveness of
community health nursing interventions. Nurses in the community setting must provide empiric proof of their worth as
professionals as well as the needs of their clients. This kind
of information must be made visible and used to influence
legislators, planners, administrators, and other decision-
makers in health care. As this occurs, nursing's status and influence will increase.

THE COMMUNITY HEALTH NURSE'S ROLE IN RESEARCH

The advantages of community health nursing include a focus
on health promotion and disease prevention; provision of services across the lifespan where people live, work, and learn;
development of community capacity building for health; and
working with partnerships, coalitions, and policy makers to
promote a healthier environment. Community health nurses
have two important responsibilities with respect to research in
community health: (1) to apply research findings and (2) to
conduct nursing research. First, because research results provide essential information for improving health policy and the
delivery of health services, community health nurses need to
be knowledgeable consumers of research. That is, they need
to be able to critically examine research reports and apply
study findings to improve the public's health.

Many research textbooks describe the steps one can take
to thoroughly assess a research study. Begin by looking carefully at the title and the journal in which the article is found.
Abstracts afford an opportunity to quickly preview the article. The quality of the journal (based on its history, circulation, and caliber of editorial board, among other factors) is
another consideration. Authors' educational and affiliative
credentials give clues to their credibility and could reveal any
financial interest they might have in relation to their research
outcomes. For instance, authors whose research studies are
funded by drug companies could have a conflict of interest,
and the results of those studies could be questioned. Examine the currentness of references and the extensiveness of the
authors' literature review. When reading the article, keep in
mind the steps in the research process and note how carefully
the authors followed each one. Ask the following questions:

*   Was the research question clearly stated?
*   Was the literature review complete and current?
*   Was there an appropriate conceptual framework?
*   How was the sample selected?
*   Did the methodology follow logically from the research
    question and the conceptual framework?
*   Were the instruments used valid and reliable and de-
    scribed in sufficient detail?
*   Were the methods of data collection and data analysis
    clearly identified?
*   Did the authors give ideas for future nursing research
    based on this study?

Carefully review the findings and discussion sections of the
research article to determine what implications this study
might have for nursing practice. Talk with colleagues and
peers about the implications of the study and ways in which
it might be replicated or its line of research extended.

Community health nurses have many opportunities to
apply the results of other investigators' research, but a necessary prerequisite is to be informed about research findings.
As an essential part of their role, community health nurses
must read the journals in public health and community health
nursing. Subscribing to some of these journals enables nurses
to make regular review of research an ongoing part of their
professional practice. Nursing agencies and employment
sites in community health can encourage nurses to become
more knowledgeable about research findings by subscribing
to journals and circulating them among staff, by holding
seminars to discuss recent research results, and by promoting
nurses' application of research findings in their practice.

Second, although the amount and quality of community
health nursing research are expanding, many more community health nurses need to conduct research themselves. An
increasing number of nurses have developed skill in research
through advanced preparation and conduct investigations related to aggregate health needs. Other community health
nurses work collaboratively with trained investigators on a
variety of research projects affecting community health.
Whether initiated by the nurse or involving the nurse as a
team member, these projects are an opportunity to influence

the types of research questions that are addressed and the ways in which the research is carried out, ultimately affecting the community's health.

SUMMARY

Involvement in community health nursing research can be an exciting opportunity to contribute to the body of nursing knowledge and influence changes in nursing practice and in community health programs and policies. Research findings also enable community health nurses to promote health and prevent illness among at-risk populations and to design and evaluate community-based interventions.

Research is defined as the systematic collection and analysis of data related to a particular problem or phenomenon. *Quantitative research* concerns data that can be measured objectively. It is helpful in identifying a problem or a relationship between two or more variables; however, because it requires the researcher to focus on a part instead of the whole, if used exclusively it can limit nursing knowledge. *Qualitative research* emphasizes subjectivity and the meaning of experiences to individuals.

The research process includes eight steps:
1. Identify an area of interest.
2. Specify a research question or statement.
3. Review the literature.
4. Select a conceptual model.
5. Choose a research design.
6. Collect and analyze data.
7. Interpret the results.
8. Communicate the findings.

Although the process is the same regardless of nursing specialty, community health nurses have a unique opportunity to expand nursing knowledge in relation to community health issues and the health needs of aggregates and families.

Research has a significant impact on community health and nursing practice in three ways. It provides new knowledge that helps to shape health policy, improve service delivery, and promote the public's health. It contributes to nursing knowledge and the improvement of nursing practice. And it offers the potential to enhance nursing's status and influence through documentation of the effectiveness of nursing interventions and broader recognition of nursing's contributions to health services.

Nurses must become responsible users of research, keeping abreast of new knowledge and applying it in practice. Nurses must learn to evaluate nursing research articles critically, assessing their validity and applicability to their own practice. Nurses should subscribe to and read nursing research journals and discuss research studies with colleagues and supervisors. More community health nurses must also conduct research studies of their own or in collaboration with other community health professionals. A commitment to the use and conduct of research will move the nursing profession forward and enhance its influence on the health of at-risk populations.

ACTIVITIES TO PROMOTE CRITICAL THINKING

1. As a community health nurse working in a large city, you notice a group of small children playing in a vacant, unfenced lot bordered by a busy street. List three research questions you might consider using to study the situation.
2. You want to determine whether a group of sexually active teenagers who are at risk for acquired immunodeficiency syndrome (AIDS) would be receptive to an educational program on HIV/AIDS. Formulate a research question, describe a conceptual framework you might use in your study, and defend your choice.
3. Select a community health nursing research article from the references and readings listed in this chapter (or choose one of your own) and analyze its potential impact on health policy and on community health nursing practice.
4. You have just completed a study on the effectiveness of a series of birth control classes in three high schools, and the results show a reduction in the number of pregnancies over the last year. Describe three ways in which you could disseminate this information to your nursing colleagues and other community health professionals.
5. You are alarmed to note that the new area to which you have been assigned has high rates of tuberculosis. Using the Internet and your college library databases to research this topic, determine the most effective forms of treatment and discuss the feasibility of implementing some new approaches with your specific target population.

REFERENCES

Armstrong, K.L., Fraser, J.A., Dadds, M.R., & Morris, J. (1999). A randomized, controlled trial of home visiting to vulnerable families with newborns. *Journal of Paediatric Child Health, 35*, 237–247.

Aroian, K., Khatutsky, G., Tran, T., & Balsam, A. (2001). Health and social service utilization among elderly immigrants from the former Soviet Union. *Journal of Nursing Scholarship, 33*(3), 253–258.

Atav, S., & Spencer, G.A. (2002). Health risk behaviors among adolescents attending rural, suburban, and urban schools: A comparative study. *Family & Community Health, 25*(2), 53–64.

Bartosch, W., & Pope, G. (2002). Local enactment of tobacco control policies in Massachusetts. *American Journal of Public Health, 92*(6), 941–943.

Beman, D.S. (1995). Risk factors leading to adolescent substance abuse. *Adolescence, 30*, 201–208.

Benda, B.B. (2001). Conceptual model of assets and risks: Unlawful behavior among adolescents. *Adolescent and Family Health, 2*(3), 123–131.

Bensussen-Walls, W., & Saewyc, E. (2001). Teen-focused care versus adult-focused care for the high-risk pregnant adolescent: An outcomes evaluation. *Public Health Nursing, 18*(6), 424–435.

Broderick, M., Dodd-Butera, T., & Wahl, P. (2002). A program to prevent iron poisoning using public health nurses in a county health department. *Public Health Nursing, 19*(3), 179–183.

Burns, N., & Groves, S.K. (1999). *Understanding nursing research* (2nd ed.). Philadelphia: WB Saunders.

Casserly, K., Carpenter, A., & Halcon, L. (2001). Adolescent parenting: Relationship to school attendance and achievement. *Journal of School Nursing, 17*(6), 329–335.

Centers for Disease Control and Prevention (CDC). (2003). *The Tuskegee syphilis study: A hard lesson learned.* Retrieved on November 24, 2003, from *http://www.cdc.gov/nchstp/ od/tuskgee/time.htm*

Champion, J.D., & Kelly, P. (2002). Protective and risk behaviors of rural minority adolescent women. *Issues in Mental Health Nursing, 23*, 191–207.

Coopersmith, S. (1967). *The antecedents of self-esteem.* San Francisco, CA: Freeman & Company.

Dahlquist, L., Pendley, J.S., Landthrip, D., Jones, C., & Steuber, P. (2002). Distraction intervention for preschoolers undergoing intramuscular injections and subcutaneous port access. *Health Psychology, 21*(1), 94–99.

Delnevo, C., Pevzner, E., Steinberg, M., Warren, C., & Slade, J. (2002). Cigar use in New Jersey among adolescents and adults. *American Journal of Public Health, 92*(6), 943–945.

DeSantis, L., Thomas, J.T., & Sinnett, K. (1999). Intergenerational concepts of adolescent sexuality: Implications for community-based reproductive health care with Haitian immigrants. *Public Health Nursing, 16*(2), 102–113.

Douglas, M.R., Mallonee, S., & Istre, G.R. (1999). Estimating the proportion of homes with functioning smoke alarms: A comparison of telephone survey and household survey results. *American Journal of Public Health, 89*(7), 1112–1114.

Eckenrode, J., Ganzel, B., Henderson, C., Smith, E., Olds, D.L., Powers, J., et al. (2000). Preventing child abuse and neglect with a program of nurse home visitation: The limiting effects of domestic violence. *JAMA, 284*(11), 1385–1391.

Eckenrode, J., Zielinski, D., Smith, E., Marcynyszyn, L., Henderson, C., Kitzman, H., et al. (2001). Child maltreatment and the early onset of problem behaviors: Can a program of nurse home visitation break the link? *Developmental Psychopathology, 13*(4), 873–890.

Facente, A. (2001). Adolescents and HIV: Knowledge, behaviors, influences, and risk perceptions. *Journal of School Nursing, 17*(4), 198–203.

Fry, S.T. & Duffy, M.E. (2001). The development and psychiatric evaluation of the Ethical Issues Scale. *Journal of Nursing Scholarship, 33*(3), 273–277.

Gaffney, K. (2001). Infant exposure to environmental tobacco smoke. *Journal of Nursing Scholarship, 33*(4), 343–347.

Gordis, L. (1996). *Epidemiology.* Philadelphia, PA: WB Saunders Co.

Greendale, G., McDivit, A., Carpenter, A., Seeger, L., & Huang, M.H. (2002). Yoga for women with hyperkyphosis: Results of a pilot study. *American Journal of Public Health, 92*(10), 1611–1614.

Guajardo, A., Middleman, A., & Sansaricq, K. (2002). School nurses identify barriers and solutions to implementing a school–based Hepatitis B immunization program. *Journal of School Health, 72*(3), 128–130.

Hawkins, J.D., Catalano, R.F., & Miller, J.U. (1992). Risk and protective factors for alcohol and other drug problems in adolescence and early adulthood: Implications for substance use prevention. *Psychological Bulletin, 112*, 64–105.

Hesketh, T., Jian Ding, Q., & Tomkins, A. (2001). Smoking among youths in China. *American Journal of Public Health, 91*(10), 1653–1655.

Hill, D., White, V., & Effendi, Y. (2002). Changes in the use of tobacco among Australian secondary students: Results of the 1999 prevalence study and comparisons with earlier years. *Australian-New Zealand Journal of Public Health, 26*(2), 156–163.

Horowitz, J.A., Bell, M., Trybulski, J., Munro, B.H., Moser, D., Hartz, S., et al. (2001). Promoting responsiveness between mothers with depressive symptoms and their infants. *Journal of Nursing Scholarship, 33*(4), 323–329.

Horta, B., Kramer, M., & Platt, R. (2001). Maternal smoking and the risk of early weaning: A meta-analysis. *American Journal of Public Health, 91*(2), 304–307.

Huncharek, M., & Kupelnick, B. (2002). Use of topical sunscreens and the risk of malignant melanoma: A meta-analysis of 9,067 patients from 11 case-control studies. *American Journal of Public Health, 92*(7), 1173–1177.

Jaakkola, N., Jaakkola, M.S., Gissler, M., & Jaakkola, J.K. (2001). Smoking during pregnancy in Finland: Determinants and trends. *American Journal of Public Health, 91*(2), 284–286.

Jaeger, R.M. (1990). *Statistics: A spectator sport* (2nd ed.). Newbury Park, CA: Sage.

Jessor, R., Van Den Bos, J., Vanderryn, J., Costa, F., & Turbin, M. (1995). Protective factors in adolescent problem behavior: Moderator effects and developmental change. *Developmental Psychology, 31*, 923–933.

Jha, P., Ranson, M., Nguyen, S.N., & Yach, D. (2002). Estimates of global and regional smoking prevalence in 1995, by age and sex. *American Journal of Public Health, 92*(6), 1002–1006.

Jones, M., Kubelka, S., & Bond, M. (2001). Acculturation status, birth outcomes and family planning compliance among Hispanic teens. *Journal of School Nursing, 17*(2), 83–89.

Keane, A., Houldin, A., Allison, P., Jepson, C., Shults, J., Nuamah, I., et al. (2002). Factors associated with distress in urban residential fire survivors. *Journal of Nursing Scholarship, 34*(1), 11–17.

Keller, C., & Trevino, R.P. (2001). Effects of two frequencies of walking on cardiovascular risk factor reduction in Mexican American women. *Research in Nursing and Health, 24*, 390–401.

Kemppainen, U., Tossavainen, K., Vartiainen, E., Pantelejev, V., & Puska, P. (2002). Smoking patterns among ninth-grade adolescents in the Pitkaranta district (Russia) and in eastern Finland. *Public Health Nursing, 19*(1), 30–39.

Kerr, J., Eves, F., & Carroll, D. (2001). Encouraging stair use:

Stair-riser banners are better than posters. *American Journal of Public Health, 91*(8), 1192–1193.

Kitzman, H., Olds, D., Sidora, K., Henderson, C., Hanks, C., Cole, R., et al. (2000). Enduring effects of nurse home visitation on maternal life course: A 3-year follow-up of a randomized trial. *Journal of the American Medical Association, 283*(15), 1983–1989.

Magazmen, S., & Glantz, S.A. (2001). The new battleground: California's experience with smoke-free bars. *American Journal of Public Health, 91*(2), 245–252.

Mahat, G., Scoloveno, M., & Whalen, C. (2002). Positive health practices of urban minority adolescents. *Journal of School Nursing, 18*(3), 163–169.

McDonnell, M., Turner, J., & Weaver, M.T. (2001). Antecedents of adherence to antituberculosis therapy. *Public Health Nursing, 18*(6), 392–400.

Mendelson, C. (2002). Health perceptions of Mexican American women. *Journal of Transcultural Nursing, 13*(3), 210–217.

Molarius, A., Parsons, R., Dobson, A., Evans, A., Fortmann, S., Jamrozik, K., et al. (2001). Trends in cigarette smoking in 36 populations from the early 1980s to the mid-1990s: Findings from the WHO MONICA project. *American Journal of Public Health, 91*(2), 206–212.

Morabia, A., Costanza, M., Bernstein, M., & Rielle, J. (2002). Age at initiation of cigarette smoking and quit attempts among women: A generation effect. *American Journal of Public Health, 92*(1), 71–74.

Morello, P., Dugan, A., Adger, H., Anthony, J., & Joffe, A. (2001). Tobacco use among high school students in Buenos Aires, Argentina. *American Journal of Public Health, 91*(2), 219–224.

Newcomb, M.D. (1997). General deviance and psychological distress: Impact of family support/bonding over 12 years from adolescence to adulthood. *Criminal Behavior and Mental Health, 7*, 368–400.

Olds, D., Eckenrode, J., Henderson, Cl., Kitzman, H., Powers, J., Cole, R., et al. (1997). Long-term effects of home visitation on maternal life course and child abuse and neglect: Fifteen-year follow-up of a randomized trial. *Journal of the American Medical Association, 278*(8), 637–643.

Perez-Stable, E., Ramirez, A., Villareal, R., Talavera, G., Trapido, E., Suarez, L., et al. (2001). Cigarette smoking behavior among US Latino men and women from different countries of origin. *American Journal of Public Health, 91*(9), 1424–1430.

Petro-Nustas, W., Norton, M., & Al-Masarweh, I. (2002). Risk factors for breast cancer in Jordanian women. *Journal of Nursing Scholarship, 34*(1), 19–25.

Raymond, M.J., Pirie, P.L., & Halcon, L.L. (2001). Infection control among professional tattooists in Minneapolis and St. Paul, MN. *Public Health Reports, 116*, 249–257.

Remler, D., & Glied, S. (2003). What other programs can teach us: Increasing participation in health insurance programs. *American Journal of Public Health, 93*(1), 67–74.

Resnicow, K., Jackson, A., Wang, T., De, A.K., McCarty, F., Dudley, W., et al. (2001). A motivational interviewing intervention to increase fruit and vegetable intake through Black churches: Results of the Eat for Life trial. *American Journal of Public Health, 91*(1), 1686–1693.

Reutzel, T.J., & Patel, R. (2001). Medication management problems reported by subscribers to a school nurse listserv. *Journal of School Nursing, 17*(3), 131–139.

Rothman, N., Lourie, R., & Gaughan, J. (2002). Lead awareness: North Philly style. *American Journal of Public Health, 92*(5), 739–741.

Sadler, G.R., Dhanjal, S., Shah, N.B., Shah, R.B., Ko, C., Anghel, M., et al. (2001). Asian Indian women: Knowledge, attitudes, and behaviors toward breast cancer early detection. *Public Health Nursing, 18*(5), 357–363.

Stoltz, A., & Sanders, B. (2000). Cigar and marijuana use: Their relationship in teens. *Journal of School Nursing, 16*(4), 28–35.

Stone, K., Lanphear, B., Pomerantz, W., & Khoury, J. (2000). Childhood injuries and deaths due to falls from windows. *Journal of Urban Health, 77*(1), 26–33.

Vlahov, D., Galea, S., Resnick, H., Ahern, J., Boscarino, J., Bucuvalas, M., et al. (2002). Increased use of cigarettes, alcohol, and marijuana among Manhattan, New York, residents after the September 11th terrorist attacks. *American Journal of Epidemiology, 155*(11), 988–996.

Wakschlag, L., Pickett, K., Cook, E., Benowitz, N., & Leventhal, B. (2002). Maternal smoking during pregnancy and severe antisocial behavior in offspring: A review. *American Journal of Public Health, 92*(6), 966–974.

White, C., Shinder, F., Shinder, A., & Dyer, D. (2001). Reduction of illness absenteeism in elementary schools using an alcohol-free instant hand sanitizer. *Journal of School Nursing, 17*(5), 258–265.

Youngblut, J.M., Brooten, D., Singer, L., Standing, T., Lee, H., & Rodgers, W.L. (2001). Effects of maternal employment and prematurity on child outcomes in single parent families. *Nursing Research, 50*(6), 346–355.

Yu, X. (2002). The role of school nurses in Beijing, China. *Journal of School Health, 72*(4), 168–170.

SELECTED READINGS

Atav, S., & Spencer, G. (2002). Health risk behaviors among adolescents attending rural, suburban, and urban schools: A comparative study. *Family and Community Health, 25*(2), 53–64.

Barner-Boyd, C., Fordham N.K., & Nacion, K.W. (2001). Promoting infant health through home visiting by a nurse-managed community worker team. *Public Health Nursing, 18*(4), 225–235.

Barr, R.G., Diez-Roux, A., Knirsch, C., & Pablos-Mendez, A. (2001). Neighborhood poverty and the resurgence of tuberculosis in New York City, 1984–1992. *American Journal of Public Health, 12*(9), 1487–1493.

Brady, G., Case, A., Himmelstein, D., & Woolhandler, S. (2002). No care for the caregivers: Declining health insurance coverage for health care personnel and their children, 1988–1998. *American Journal of Public Health, 92*(3), 404–408.

Choudhry, U.K., Jandu, S., Mahal, J., Singh, R., Sohi-Pabla, H., & Mutta, B. (2002). Health promotion and participatory action research with South Asian women. *Journal of Nursing Scholarship, 34*(1), 75–81.

Cohen, L. (2002). Reducing infant immunization distress through distraction. *Health Psychology, 21*(2), 207–211.

Cornelius, L., Smith, P., & Simpson, G. (2002). What factors hinder women of color from obtaining preventive health care? *American Journal of Public Health, 92*(4), 535–539.

Cullen, K., Ash, D., Warneke, C., & deMoor, C. (2002). Intake of soft drinks, fruit-flavored beverages, and fruits and vegetables by children in grades 4 through 6. *American Journal of Public Health, 92*(9), 1475–1478.

DeBaryshe, B., Yuen, S., & Rodriguez-Stern, I. (2001). Psychosocial adjustment in Asian American/Pacific Islander youth: The role of coping strategies, parenting practices, and community social support. *Adolescent and Family Health, 2*(2), 63–71.

Dilorio, C., Hartwell, T., & Hansen, N. (2002). Childhood sexual abuse and risk behaviors among men at high risk for HIV infection. *American Journal of Public Health, 92*(4), 214–219.

Falck, R., Wang, J., Carlson, R., & Siegal, H. (2002). Variability in drug use prevalence across school districts in the same locale in Ohio. *Journal of School Health, 72*(7), 288–293.

Fishbein, M., Hall-Jamieson, K., Zimmer, E., von Haaften, I., & Nabi, R. (2002). Avoiding the boomerang: Testing the relative effectiveness of antidrug public service announcements before a national campaign. *American Journal of Public Health, 92*(2), 238–245.

Fisher, J., Fisher, W., Bryan, A., & Misovich, S. (2002). Information-motivation-behavioral skills model-based HIV risk behavior change intervention for inner-city high school youth. *Health Psychology, 21*(2), 177–186.

French, S., Jeffrey, R., Story, M., Breitlow, K., Baxter, J., Hannan, P., et al. (2001). Pricing and promotion effects on low-fat vending snack purchases: The CHIPS study. *American Journal of Public Health, 91*(1), 112–117.

Halpern, C., Oslak, S., Young, M., Martin, S., & Kupper, L. (2001). Partner violence among adolescents in opposite-sex romantic relationships: Findings from the National Longitudinal Study of Adolescent Health. *American Journal of Public Health, 91*(10), 1679–1685.

Hamel, C., Guse, L., Hawranik, P., & Bond, J. (2002). Advance directives and community-dwelling older adults. *Western Journal of Nursing Research, 24*(2), 143–158.

Hennrikus, D., Jeffrey, R., Lando, H., Murray, D., Brelje, K., Davidann, B., et al. (2002). The SUCCESS project: The effect of program format and incentives on participation and cessation in worksite smoking cessation programs. *American Journal of Public Health, 92*(2), 274–279.

Huebner, C.E. (2002). Evaluation of a clinic-based patient education program to reduce the risk of infant and toddler maltreatment. *Public Health Nursing, 19*(5), 377–379.

Ibald-Mulli, A., Stieber, J., Wichmann, H.E., Koenig, W., & Peters, A. (2001). Effects of air pollution on blood pressure: A population-based approach. *American Journal of Public Health, 91*(4), 571–577.

Krieger, N. (2002). Is breast cancer a disease of affluence, poverty, or both? The case of African American women. *American Journal of Public Health, 92*(4), 611-613.

Lazovich, D., Parker, D., Brosseau, L., Milton, F., Dugan, S., Pan, W., et al. (2002). Effectiveness of a worksite intervention to reduce an occupational exposure: The Minnesota wood dust study. *American Journal of Public Health, 92*(9), 1498–1505.

Lee, R., & Cubbin, C. (2002). Neighborhood context and youth cardiovascular health behaviors. *American Journal of Public Health, 92*(3), 428–436.

Manfredi, C., Crittenden, K., Cho, Y., Engler, J., & Warnecke, R. (2002). Maintenance of a smoking cessation program in public health clinics beyond the experimental evaluation period. *Public Health Reports, 116*, 120–135.

McCaffery, J., Pogue-Geile, M., Muldoon, M., Debski, T., Wing, R., & Manuck, S. (2001). The nature of the association between diet and serum lipids in the community: A twin study. *Health Psychology, 20*(5), 341–350.

O'Connor, M., Maddocks, B., Modie, C., & Pierce, H. (2001). The effect of different definitions of a patient on immunization assessment. *American Journal of Public Health, 91*(8), 1273–1275.

Phipps, M., & Sowers, M. (2002). Defining early adolescent childbearing. *American Journal of Public Health, 92*(1), 125–128.

Prigerson, H., Maciejewski, P., & Rosenheck, R. (2002). Population attributable fractions of psychiatric disorders and behavioral outcomes associated with combat exposure among U.S. men. *American Journal of Public Health, 92*(1), 59–63.

Richardus, J., & Kunst, A. (2001). Black-White differences in infectious disease mortality in the United States. *American Journal of Public Health, 91*(8), 1251–1253.

Spicer, R., Cazier, C., Keller, P., & Miller, T. (2002). Evaluation of the Utah student injury reporting system. *Journal of School Health, 72*(2), 47–50.

Thomas, K., Rubino, L., O'Connor, A., & Nachman, S. (2002). How common is choosing to discontinue treatment for HIV? *American Journal of Public Health, 92*(3), 364.

Wang, P., Demler, O., & Kessler, R. (2002). Adequacy of treatment for serious mental illness in the United States. *American Journal of Public Health, 92*(1), 92–98.

Wynd, C. (2002). Testicular self-examination in young adult men. *Journal of Nursing Scholarship, 34*(3), 251–255.

Young, L., & Nestle, M. (2002). The contribution of expanding portion sizes to the U.S. obesity epidemic. *American Journal of Public Health, 92*(2), 246–249.

Young, T., D'Angelo, S., & Davis, J. (2001). Impact of a school-based health center on emergency department use by elementary school students. *Journal of School Health, 71*(5), 196–198.

Internet Resources

American Nurses Foundation: *http://www.nursingworld.org/anf/*
National Institute of Nursing Research: *http://www.nih.gov/ninr*
Sigma Theta Tau International Registry of Nursing Research: *http://www.stti.iupui.edu/VirginiaHendersonLibrary/Registryof NursingResearch.aspx*
Midwest Nursing Research Society: *http://www.mnrs.org*
Southern Nursing Research Society: *http://www.snrs.org*
Eastern Nursing Research Society: *http://www.enrs.org*
Western Institute of Nursing: *http://www.ohsu.edu.son-win/*
International Council of Nurses: *http://www.icn.org*
Triservice Nursing Research Program/Military Nursing: *http://www.usuhs.mil/tsnrp*
Current Clinical Trials: *http://www.clinicaltrials.gov*
Irish Nursing Research site: *http://www.nurse2nurse.ie*

15

Quality Measurement and Improvement in Community Health Nursing

Key Terms

- Audit
- Benchmarking
- Concurrent review
- Evidence-based nursing
- Peer review
- Quality assurance
- Quality care
- Quality circles
- Quality improvement
- Quality indicators
- Quality measurement
- Retrospective review
- Risk assessment
- Standards of care
- Total quality management

Learning Objectives

Upon mastery of this chapter, you should be able to:

- Develop a working knowledge of quality improvement and management terms.

- Discuss five factors affecting quality measurement and improvement in community health nursing.

- Compare and contrast six models for measuring and improving the quality of care and their usefulness in community health nursing.

- Identify six techniques used in quality measurement and improvement in community health programs.

- Discuss the role of the nurse within quality measurement and improvement programs in community health nursing agencies.

T hink about your most recent experience at your health care provider's office, clinic, or hospital. What were your expectations for the care you would receive and the manner in which that care would be provided? Were these expectations met? Why or why not? How would you approach the task of measuring and improving the quality of the care that you received? Indeed, what is quality care?

Quality is a relative term that describes something with high merit or excellence as compared to an accepted standard or norm. In industry, for example, products are typically measured against a predetermined standard of quality established by field testing. Quality experts test sample products for durability, consistency of performance, and other characteristics and then recommend improvements in the products to meet consumer expectations. Most companies constantly monitor and control their purchase of supplies, their methods of production, their products' packaging, and their distribution networks to ensure that standards are met and that customers are satisfied. In health care, the wide variety of situations, roles, settings, and services makes identification and adoption of quality standards somewhat more challenging. But during the past 50 years, serious efforts have been made to set standards for measurement and improvement of health care services. **Quality care** means that the services provided match the needs of the population, are technically correct, and achieve beneficial results.

The escalating costs of health care in recent years have caused consumers and third-party payers to demand quality care at a more reasonable cost. Efforts to control costs have led to changes in the health care delivery system, most notably the emergence of managed care. Health care costs are largely beyond a community health nurse's direct control, but nurses do have control over the delivery of quality care, and they can evaluate the quality of their own nursing care and the outcomes of that care. They can use these evaluations to determine whether clients are receiving the best service possible and how to use limited resources to support the most critical improvements and programs.

This chapter discusses how quality services in the community are measured and improved and the pivotal role of the community health nurse in achieving quality care.

TERMINOLOGY OF QUALITY IMPROVEMENT AND MANAGEMENT

This chapter contains many new terms that are specific to the focus of quality improvement and management. The terms presented in this section are used more generally in quality measurement and improvement literature and provide a foundation for understanding the concepts in this chapter. In addition, some terms are no longer in general use and are described as part of historical development of quality management.

Formal quality management in the health care field began in earnest in the early 1970s. Nursing's efforts were in **quality assurance**, an approach that was developed and used during the 1950s and 1960s, predating its use in other health care fields. Quality assurance efforts included initial setting of standards, formal auditing, and **peer review,** in which peer professionals use an organized system to assess the quality of care being delivered (Phaneuf, 1976). It includes methods of ensuring that quality care is being delivered through the use of the following three-phase process: (1) comparing a health care situation with preestablished criteria believed to represent quality care; (2) identifying care strengths, deficiencies, and opportunities for improvement; and (3) introducing changes in the health care system. (The term *quality assurance* can be misleading and is no longer used. It assumes that if the three-phase process is carried out, quality care can be assured. Although identifying areas that need to be modified or enhanced certainly may improve care, *assuring* quality is a more ambitious outcome than the behaviors in the process can accurately deliver.)

Faced with limited available resources and escalating costs of care, health care agencies began in the 1980s to engage in **quality measurement**; the goal was to be able to identify services and programs that best serve the needs of the community. Studying the impact of intervention and instituting tighter controls on the delivery of specific community health nursing services may not automatically result in satisfied clients or healthier clients; however, such methods can contribute to **quality improvement** of the care delivered by the health care organization.

Quality indicators, or quality-focused objectives, are used to determine whether a goal has been achieved and to measure client outcomes or process outcomes. For example, one measurable outcome might be, "All clients will receive a home visit within 24 hours after the agency receives the referral." Quality indicators ensure that quality issues are dealt with routinely within all organizational program evaluations.

Total quality management (TQM) is a comprehensive term referring to the systems and activities used to achieve all aspects of quality care within a given agency. Quality indicators are a part of this broader concept.

FACTORS AFFECTING QUALITY MEASUREMENT AND IMPROVEMENT

A variety of factors promote quality measurement and improvement. These include (1) professional self-regulation of clinical competence, (2) certification and accreditation, (3) legislation and regulation, (4) reimbursement, and (5) consumer demands.

Nursing's Self-Regulation

In the mid-1800s, nurses began to assume responsibility for maintaining standards in the services they provided by requiring minimum levels of education. Nursing education began with a few intuitive, service-minded people who applied practical knowledge in the care of the ill. By the late 1800s, nursing education had become formalized, with many hospitals providing 1- to 3-year training programs for nurses. By the 1920s, the education of nurses began to be standardized, with mandatory licensure nationwide. Educational opportunities, including programs developed in colleges and universities, improved options. Today, nursing education includes standardized basic and advanced clinical preparation with many options, including advanced practitioner and doctoral preparation in nursing.

Various accrediting organizations were established in the early 1900s to oversee and stimulate nursing schools to keep up with changes in health care. Two of the most influential organizations are the American Nurses Association (ANA), which began in the 1890s, and the National League for Nursing (NLN), which was formed in 1952 from seven organizations established in the early 1900s (see Chapter 2).

The ANA first developed functions, standards, and qualification committees in 1952. In 1973, ANA's Congress for Nursing Practice published a generic set of standards of nursing practice based on the work of these committees, laying the foundation for professional nursing practice (ANA, 1998). This generic standard has served as the root of today's current standards of practice in 22 nursing specialties. Nine scope and standards for specialty areas are included for nurses who provide care in the community: addictions nursing, college health nursing, nursing in correctional facilities, specialized nursing in developmental disabilities and/or mental retardation, forensic nursing, home health nursing, parish nursing, psychiatric-mental health nursing, and public health nursing. The newest sets of standards, for public health nursing (Display 15–1) and home health nursing (see Chapter 37), were developed in 1999 (ANA, 1999b, 1999c). In 1983, the ANA developed **standards of care,** which are desired goals that can be used to help plan and evaluate school nursing practice. (See Chapter 28 for more information on the role of the school nurse.)

The NLN (and subsequently the National League for Nursing Accreditation Center, or NLNAC) was the voluntary and specialized accrediting body for nursing programs until 1999. In 2000, the Commission for Collegiate Nursing Education (CCNE) was established as an autonomous arm of the American Association of Colleges of Nursing (AACN) and approved by the U. S. Department of Education as an official accrediting agency for baccalaureate and graduate nursing education programs, thereby offering a choice of accrediting agencies for those programs. Either agency works closely with a nursing program to maintain educational standards.

In the 1980s and 1990s, the ANA focused quality issues on nurses and their responsibility and accountability for the quality of care their clients receive. Each nurse is responsible for interpreting and implementing the standards of nursing practice and must participate with other nurses in the decision-making process for auditing, peer review, and assessing and evaluating the quality of nursing care being delivered.

DISPLAY 15–1

American Nurses Association Scope and Standards for Public Health Nursing

The public health nurse:
1. Assesses the health status of populations using data, community resources identification, input from the population, and professional judgment.
2. Analyzes collected assessment data and partners with the people to attach meaning to those data and determine opportunities and needs.
3. Participates with other community partners to identify expected outcomes in the populations and their health status.
4. Promotes and supports the development of programs, policies, and services that provide interventions that improve the health status of populations.
5. Assures access to and availability of programs, policies, resources, and services to the population.
6. Evaluates the health status of the population.
7. Systematically evaluates the availability, accessibility, acceptability, quality, and effectiveness of nursing practice for the population.
8. Evaluates his or her own nursing practice in relation to professional practice standards and relevant statutes and regulations.
9. Acquires and maintains current knowledge and competency in public health nursing practice.
10. Establishes collegial partnerships while interacting with health care practitioners and others, and contributes to the professional development of peers, colleagues, and others.
11. Applies ethical standards in advocating for health and social policy and delivery of public health programs to promote and preserve the health of the population.
12. Collaborates with the representatives of the population and other health and human service professionals and organizations in providing for and promoting the health of the population.
13. Uses research findings in practice.
14. Considers safety, effectiveness, and cost in the planning and delivery of public health services when using available resources, to ensure the maximum possible health benefit to the population.

(From American Nurses Association [1999]. *Scope and standards of public health nursing practice.* Washington, DC: Author.)

Peer review is an ongoing process of assessing performance against the standards and criteria that indicate quality care in a specific agency. It involves periodic review of caregiving practices by staff nurses, who may make shared home visits with their peers or observe peers teaching groups of clients or implementing the services of programs or projects.

Over the past 35 years, nursing has developed increasingly more formalized nursing care review models and implemented them throughout the profession. The ANA has contributed to formal quality improvement evaluative processes through the development of models, quality of care and peer review guidelines, and nursing care standards, including those for community health nursing and home health nursing. In addition, nursing case management and managed care concepts have been incorporated in publications produced by the ANA since 1982. More recently, ANA publications have addressed current trends that include nursing quality indicators. These measurements provide critical evidence-based information and insights into nursing's contribution to client outcomes (ANA, 1999a, 2000a). In addition, there is a trend in nursing practice for nurses to practice **evidence-based nursing**, which involves the process of making clinical decisions using the best available research evidence, clinical expertise, and client preferences, in the context of available resources (Amarsi, 2002). Patient or client outcomes as indicators of quality of care received are measurable and become indicators of the care given, including client teaching. Nursing has adapted and applied these models, guidelines, standards, and concepts in many inpatient, ambulatory care, and community nursing settings.

The American Nurses Credentialing Center (ANCC) was established in 1989 and assumed responsibility for the ANA certification programs. Professional certification is a confirmation of knowledge and expertise within a defined area of nursing. It assures the public that the credentialed nurse is competent at an advanced level and has had this competency confirmed through examination and years of practice. Continuation of the credential is maintained by further examination, practice, or other actions deemed examples of expertise in the area. ANCC (2003) provides an opportunity for clinical certification of nurses who have achieved the baccalaureate (BSN) and have had several years of clinical practice in more than 25 clinical specialties. The most common ANCC certifications that community health nurses may find helpful to hold include the following:

Nurse Generalists
 College health nurse
 Community health nurse
 Home health nurse
 School nurse
 Women's health
Nurse Practitioner (NP)
 Ambulatory nurse practitioner (ANP)
 Family nurse practitioner (FNP)
 Geriatric nurse practitioner (GNP)
 Pediatric nurse practitioner (PNP)
 School nurse practitioner (SNP)
Clinical Nurse Specialist (CNS)
 CNS in community health nursing
 CNS in home health nursing
Nurse Administrator
 Nursing administration
 Nursing administration advanced

Certification examinations and ongoing continuing education units (CEUs) provide additional means for achieving and maintaining a high level of nursing skills. In addition, associations of nurses in specific disciplines influence the standards of care provided by supporting their own certification programs. They also establish forums of support for nurses through regularly scheduled meetings and periodic conferences that focus on advances in the specific disciplines.

By 1952, all states, the District of Columbia, and all U. S. territories had enacted nurse practice acts to ensure that minimum standards of education, practice, and expertise are maintained. In addition to graduating from a state-approved school of nursing and passing a state-recognized examination, nurses are required to accrue an annual or biannual number of CEUs as part of their qualifications for nursing license renewal (Cherry & Jacob, 2002).

Certification and Accreditation of Health Care Organizations

The many responsibilities that hospitals and other health care organizations have to their clients, staffs, boards of directors, and funders complicate their functioning and have the potential to compromise care. As these organizations have developed and diversified, many methods for managing their large staffs, multiple departments, and missions have emerged. Institutional attention to quality-of-care issues first appeared in the 1940s and 1950s. At that time, it became clear that organizations delivering health care services needed to monitor those services to meet the goals of the organization and its consumers and to survive in a competitive environment. External certification and accreditation processes began at about the same time (Catalano, 2003). These processes verify an organization's ability to provide adequate service. Voluntary accreditation boards, such as the Joint Commission on Accreditation of Healthcare Organizations (JCAHO), examine all types of health care organizations—inpatient and outpatient care facilities, health care networks, and health plans—and help them attend to all facets of their operations, thus establishing appropriate priorities. For example, they certify all organizations that receive Medicare or Medicaid dollars. In reviewing an organization for accreditation, they consider how quality is affected by such factors as staff recruitment, organizational structure, management effectiveness, billing practices, and planning. They also require, in all agencies that they certify, evidence of effective quality measurement and improvement programs that use an interdisciplinary team approach (Lewis & Latney, 2002).

Through the 1970s, accrediting bodies focused most of their attention on hospitals. In the 1980s, the attention shifted to include ambulatory or outpatient care, long-term care, and home health care. That shift occurred for many reasons, but the high costs of care and competition for health care dollars were the leading reasons why such agencies sought accreditation (Ellis & Hartley, 2001). Since 1965, the Community

Health Accreditation Program, Inc. (CHAP) has existed as a joint venture between the American Public Health Association (APHA) and the NLN. It was the first accrediting body for community-based health organizations in the United States, and it has set a standard of excellence through its accreditation services and publications geared to home health care, hospice care, and community health care organizations. As an independent evaluating body based on a voluntary commitment to excellence by home and community health care organizations, CHAP is attempting to determine levels of excellence (quality) in home care services.

Legislation and Regulation

Legislation and regulation of health care services are the functions of individual states. Agencies must be licensed by the state, staffed by trained and licensed people, and prepared to provide the services offered. State licensure or accreditation standards are monitored by regular state inspections and annual surveys. If an agency provides a variety of technically sophisticated services, such as mammography or ultrasonography, additional state inspections may occur.

Most often, health care organizations apply for and receive federal or state grants to support specific programs or services. These grants are often a major part of the agency budget, and if the services do not maintain a specified standard of quality, funding will be discontinued. The withdrawal of financial support may cause other services to be discontinued as well, leaving clients with fragmented or discontinuous care.

Financial Reimbursement

As mentioned earlier, financial reimbursement is often linked to the state through grants that provide funding for immunization programs, maternal and infant services, and other specific programs. Without this important source of financial support, many agencies would have to limit services. Other sources of funding include Medicare, Medicaid, and private insurers. These federal, state, and privately financed programs for large populations in the United States have rigid rules and regulations regarding standards of care provided to beneficiaries.

Monitoring of specific aspects of care is often done in response to funders' requirements for periodic progress reports rather than as part of a program of quality management. If monitoring is done only for reimbursement purposes, the total quality of the program is not the agency goal, as it should be. Health care agencies cannot survive without relying on reimbursement sources, but quality management should be a mission of the agency regardless of the source of funding.

Consumer Demands

Which health care provider or health care agency consumers choose to use is often based on presumed or assumed caregiving services and the quality of those services. Health care consumers are provided with many choices when selecting health care services. This competition in the health care marketplace is beneficial to consumers. When consumers are knowledgeable receivers of health care services, they can demand quality care as they define it. They make decisions regarding health care services based on quality domains, such as

Proficiency—capability, expertise, or knowledge of the staff and the manner in which services are provided

Judgment—consistency, objectivity, and reasonable interpretation of regulations

Responsiveness—timeliness, assistance, and guidance

Communication—clarity of verbal and written expression

Accommodation—the behavior or interpersonal skills of staff

Relevance—significance and pertinence of the encounter with staff

The decisions regarding these domains are based on consumers' perception of the care received. This perception is an important piece of the quality measurement and improvement program within an organization.

MODELS FOR QUALITY MANAGEMENT AND IMPROVEMENT

Models of client caregiving are based on structure, process, and outcome: ideally, they provide *structure* to guide nurses through the *nursing process* to reach desired *client outcomes*. Each of the following models has all three components, some working more effectively than others, depending on the agency and its philosophy. Six quality management models are presented in this section: the Donabedian model, the Quality Health Outcomes model, the ANA model, the upwardly spiraling feedback loop model, the Omaha classification system, and the Quality Practice Settings Attribute model.

Donabedian Model

Donabedian (1966, 1969, 1981, 1985, 2002), the country's premier researcher on health care quality, proposed a model for the structure, process, and outcome of quality that has been widely used over the past 35 years as the framework for more elaborate models. The care environment structure—from philosophy, to facility resources, to personnel—is the first component. Next are the processes responsible for improving or stabilizing the client's health status, such as standards, attitudes, and effectiveness of tools used in caregiving (eg, nursing care plans). Finally, the resultant outcomes are causally linked indicators of quality, such as client health care goals and effectiveness of service.

The Donabedian model is recognized as a simplistic and basic method of measuring quality. It lends itself to rehabilitation and is the model used in several settings. It has been part of federally supported research conducted at Duke University in Durham, North Carolina (Hoenig et al., 1999).

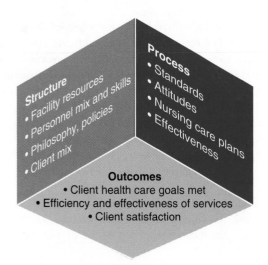

FIGURE 15–1. Structure, process, and outcome of quality model.

Structure, process, and outcome can be depicted in a box-shaped model (Fig. 15-1).

Quality Health Outcomes Model

Mitchell and colleagues (1998) took the time-tested Donabedian model a step further. The Quality Health Outcomes model includes the client in the model and proposes a two-dimensional relationship among components. Interventions always act through the system and the client, creating a dynamic model. The uniqueness of this model is the postulate that there are "dynamic relationships with indicators that not only act upon, but reciprocally affect the various components" (Mitchell, Ferketich & Jennings, 1998, p. 43). A major criticism of other models is that they do not lend themselves to the population focus of community health nursing. However, this model includes community as a client. Figure 15–2 depicts the Quality Health Outcomes model.

American Nurses Association Model

The ANA provides a quality improvement model based on standards of care and quality indicators within the Donabedian framework of structure, process, and outcome. Adopted by the ANA in 1975, the model was developed by Lang to

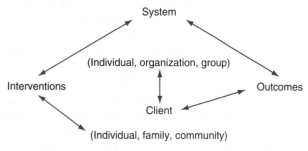

FIGURE 15–2. Quality health outcomes model.

depict the multiple components of evaluation of client care (ANA, 1975). The ANA model has changed as more information has been gathered through research and as the profession of nursing has grown; however, it has proved beneficial over time (Bull, 1996). This circular and continuous model suggests ongoing evaluation. Its core includes the agency's philosophy or mission statement, which identifies the values of the agency and reflects its views of clients, nursing, the community, and health. Defining the beliefs of the agency is the first step in improving quality. The three components of structure, process, and outcome are depicted as pie-shaped wedges located around this central core. Specific nursing actions are added to more closely interrelate each section and make the transition to the next section smoother (Fig. 15–3).

Although each component is important, agencies rely on positive client outcomes as key indicators of success. Successful outcomes are the purpose of the agency's existence and the key to positive evaluation by accrediting bodies. Moreover, continued reimbursement by third-party payers, such as private insurance companies, Medicare, and Medicaid, depends on successful outcomes.

Upwardly Spiraling Feedback Loop Model

This model takes the ANA model one step further. It adds a feedback loop that makes the process dynamic and subject to change in response to ongoing feedback, which is used to assess and then implement revisions in care or plans. Figure 15–4 illustrates this idea. The right pole of the model represents the continuum of a client's health needs and personal health behaviors, from the client's current status to optimal

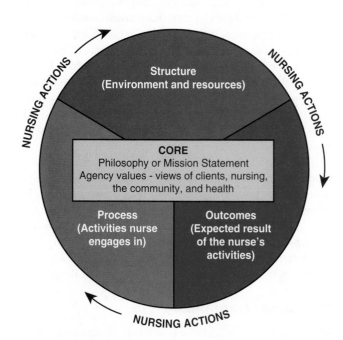

FIGURE 15–3. The ANA quality assurance model.

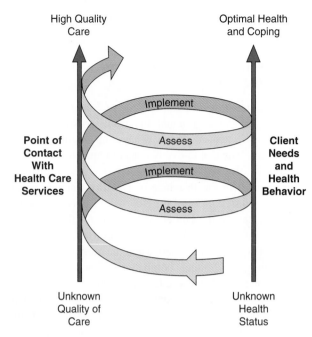

FIGURE 15–4.   Upwardly spiraling quality assurance feedback loop.

health and coping. The left pole depicts the contacts between the client and the health care system. The spiral's movement from pole to pole demonstrates the quality assessment activities that nurses use to assess their clients, revise nursing care or plans, and implement changes. Any changes are assessed again at a future date as part of the ongoing review process.

This ongoing and repetitive process should result in improvements in the quality of care and the client's health. The model makes two basic assumptions: first, that specific nursing activities are known to maintain and promote health; second, that positive results are brought about by positive interventions.

This model shows the distance between the two poles of client needs and behaviors and contacts with the health care delivery system. It demonstrates that nurses should step back from the everyday demands of direct client care and assess that care and the desired outcomes. More specifically, stepping back from the process prompts nurses to do the following:

1. Identify and prioritize the health problems and needs of the populations served.
2. Determine the systems, nursing actions, or outcomes in terms of client behaviors that are facilitated by the nurse.
3. Examine the success or failure of nursing efforts with a specific group.
4. Adjust nursing care, systems, or client goals as needed.
5. Plan for future quality assessments.

Omaha System

This model was developed and refined during four research projects conducted between 1975 and 1992 in the Omaha

Visiting Nursing Association. It was designed to increase the effectiveness and efficiency of nursing practice in the agency (Bowles & Naylor, 1996; Martin, Leak & Aden, 1997). It is a comprehensive model and includes the following components:

Patient classification scheme—offers nurses a holistic, standardized method for client assessment and nursing diagnosis and problem identification

Intervention scheme—provides a framework for documenting plans and interventions in the client record in the areas of health teaching, guidance, and counseling; treatments and procedures; case management; and surveillance

Supervisory shared visit tool—a supervisor's evaluation instrument used for formative and cumulative evaluation of community health nurses within the agency

Problem rating scale for outcomes—consists of a Likert-type scale that is a systematic and recurring method used to document the progress of clients in the record and in case conferences during their time of service in the agency. It is used in conjunction with any problem in the Problem Classification Scheme (a list of problems, modifiers, and signs/symptoms provided in the Omaha System).

The Omaha system has measurement approaches that make it a useful model for determining the quality of nursing care provided to individuals and families. Evaluation focuses on process indicators, client outcome measures, and satisfaction with care (Bowles & Naylor, 1996; Martin, Leak & Aden, 1997). With the use of this multifocal approach, measurement of nursing practice becomes comprehensive (Table 15–1). However, this model was designed to evaluate care to individuals and families. Evaluation of care to populations needs a different set of indicators; they must include, for instance, health trend data, morbidity and mortality statistics, and community system comparisons.

The Omaha System was used with an aggregate when a group of county health department community health nurses conducted an assessment of a community's need for a satellite health clinic in a rural part of the county. The nurses gathered data on population needs, age, health status, and accessibility to health care by surveying clients who lived in rural zip code areas and used the main health department. They also conducted a survey by mail of additional residents who were not presently using the health department clinic system for immunizations, screening for tuberculosis or sexually transmitted diseases, or well-baby visits, to see whether these people had unmet needs. After carefully analyzing the data, they began three operating 4-hour clinics during the first week of each month in an empty storeroom of the community pharmacy.

After funding the clinics for 6 months, the health department evaluated the effectiveness of this nursing service. The number of emergency-room visits for infants in the area was compared with the number of visits during a similar period before the satellite clinic was established, as was the number of cases of influenza and pneumonia

TABLE   15-1

Components of the Omaha System Model

I Domains

4 Environmental choices
12 Psychosocial choices
15 Physiologic choices
9 Health-related behavior choices
(A place for "other" in each of the above domain choices)

II Client data

Brief subjective/objective data

III Problems and signs/symptoms

From a list of 35 problems and modifiers

IV Ratings

Knowledge, behavior, status of client—on a scale of 1 to 5

V Interventions

One (or more) of four intervention areas and target areas:
　Health teaching, guidance, and counseling
　Treatments and procedures
　Case management
　Surveillance
These data sets are used as outline information to provide consistent, yet individualized care to clients when nurses involved in the care change over time. Because the information comes from predetermined sets of data, care can be easily assessed for audit and quality improvement in an agency. Gaps and overlapping services become apparent, and interventions can be modified as needed.

among residents older than 65 years of age. Finally, clients were surveyed in regard to their satisfaction with nursing care and services and were asked if there were any additional services they needed. Survey outcomes were supportive of continuing the clinics and adding an additional well-baby clinic, a dental clinic, and a prenatal clinic. Clients liked the convenience: older residents did not have to drive the 35 miles to the main clinic; parents were able to keep more closely to the recommended schedule for their children's immunizations, and they liked the shorter wait. Follow-up after human immunodeficiency virus (HIV) screening included the formation of an HIV/AIDS support group for clients and families in the rural area, meeting a need that no one had previously identified. The nurses combined clinic responsibilities with home visits in the area on clinic days and were able to do case finding, improving the overall health of this rural area.

The nurses were evaluated and their charts were audited with the use of traditional tools, and clients received the same periodic surveys. Case conferences continued to be held among the nurses serving the rural area, and, at times, cases were presented among the larger group of nurses. By modifying the comprehensive Omaha Visiting Nursing Associa-

tion measurement approaches, they met the quality measurement needs of a population.

The Quality Practice Setting Attributes Model

This model, developed by the College of Nurses of Ontario in Canada, provides the foundational framework for a unique quality improvement approach to creating quality practice environments. The College of Nurses of Ontario is the regulatory body for 138,000 registered nurses and registered practical nurses in the Province of Ontario, Canada; it has functions similar to those of the Boards of Registered Nursing in each state in the United States. The Quality Practice Setting Attributes Model is used as a tool to assist in ensuring the quality of nursing practice and the nursing profession by promoting continuing competence among nurses in Canada (College of Nurses of Ontario, 2002).

This nurse-centered model of quality improvement is designed to contribute to the best possible health outcome for the client, regardless of health care setting. The components of this quality assurance program include reflective nursing practice, practice review, and practice setting consultation. The first two components focus on nurses' individual responsibility for maintaining competence throughout their careers; the practice setting consultation focuses on the practice environment in which nursing care is delivered.

The governing body for nurses in Ontario, Canada, has relied on the Quality Practice Setting Attributes Model to improve nursing care quality in their province. The model identifies seven key systems attributes in the work enviornment that create a quality practice setting. Figure 15–5 portrays this model and its components.

QUALITY MEASUREMENT AND IMPROVEMENT TECHNIQUES

Quality should not be an event. It should be how business is conducted and a way of life. Quality means always seeking ways to improve what is being done and what client outcomes are achieved. Quality management programs should consider quality to be an ongoing process and a standard rather than an afterthought of a specific event. The many terms used for describing various aspects of quality management may seem confusing, if not overwhelming. To evaluate a quality business, which any health care agency can and should be, several techniques may be used. In addition, nursing is seeking to improve its practice through the use of tools that assist in identifying and continually updating nursing diagnoses, nursing intervention classifications, and nursing outcome classifications (see later discussion).

Assessing Risk

Risk assessment is a process of identifying factors that lead to negative events. It can be a formal process that uses a tool,

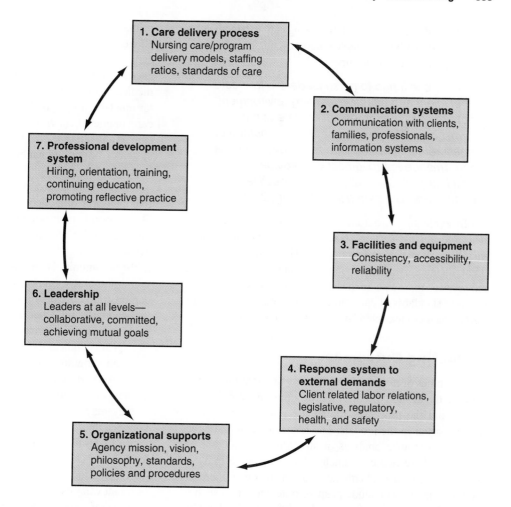

FIGURE 15-5.
The quality practice setting attributes model.

such as a questionnaire or a checklist called a *risk assessment inventory* (RAI). It can also proceed informally (eg, a nurse with knowledge about primary health promotion is aware that children are at higher risk for preventable diseases if they are not immunized and that pregnant women who gain more than 50 lb during pregnancy are at an increased risk for complications).

An RAI is designed to inventory specific factors that put people at a higher risk for certain events. For example, falls among older adults are often viewed as single events. However, their occurrences have been associated with a number of intrinsic (client or host) and extrinsic (environmental) factors. Intrinsic factors include aspects of the older person's physical and mental health, such as dizziness, weakness, difficulty ambulating, poor vision, confusion, and impaired memory or judgment. Use of medications, including sedatives or psychotropic drugs, is another intrinsic factor. Extrinsic factors are associated with the environment. They include proper footwear, lighting, glare, slippery and wet surfaces, and obstacles. Just one of these factors could cause a fall, but most often falls are "multifactorial" (Tideiksaar, 2002).

Knowing a population's risk factors for certain events helps with planning prevention strategies. Once the potential for risks is determined and assessed, plans can begin

with designing goals and objectives for the intervention strategy.

Setting Measurable Goals and Objectives

Planned programs should have specific goals to help identify who the program is supposed to serve, what services are provided, the length of time during the services are to be provided, and the resources that are needed. Then, measurable objectives are developed that describe the expected outcomes. Use of selected verbs indicates the expected level of achievement, such as "Clients will be able to demonstrate safe administration of insulin after three home visits" or "Parents will have their infants' recommended immunizations up to date by 24 months of age." Goal setting is done when developing an educational program (see Chapter 12) or an entire health program or service. These statements of measurable goals are then examined during the program evaluation. Without such statements, accurate evaluations cannot be conducted.

Outcome measurement requries nursing to shift to outcome-based practice based on research that leads to evidence-based practice (DePalma, 2002; Hill, 1999). Each is intertwined with the other. For nursing care to become outcome focused with measurable outcomes, nurses must leave behind a task-based environment.

The key challenge to nurse leaders is to create an efficient and effective learning environment that provides outcomes-based care at the lowest cost. This environment where outcomes measurement and management drive continual performance improvement will provide a healthier profession and a more effective professional practice (Hill, 1999, pp. 2–3).

In evaluating programs and care, outcomes must be measured against certain standards. Standards are generic guidelines of expected functioning. They can focus on the client, the caregiver, or the organization (finances). All care and services must also be measured against these guidelines. The core standards of care, practice, and finance must be integrated and compatible if they are to ensure quality care.

Evaluating Outcomes

The outcomes or results of care (having the right things happen) are the desired effect of the structure (having the right things) and the processes (doing the right things), as described earlier in the models. The focus on client outcomes demands continued analysis of structure and process, because it is these two components that produce desirable or undesirable outcomes. With the focus on outcomes, there has been an impetus to include positive outcome terms such as improved health status, functional ability, perceived quality of life, and client satisfaction. Client satisfaction is measured by how closely a client's expectations of nursing care match the perception of the nursing care actually received (Gordon, 2003). Client satisfaction, as one outcome measurement, can be determined by a telephone survey or a mailed questionnaire (Donabedian, 1969).

If the responses indicate that a program is meeting its goals, maintaining set standards, and having positive client outcomes and satisfied clients, the program is providing quality care. However, the accuracy of using outcomes as a primary measure of quality care is limited, because some clients have unsatisfactory outcomes despite receiving good care. Factors other than specific health interventions influence outcomes. These factors include a client's adherence to medically prescribed treatments; the progress of chronic or terminal disease beyond the capabilities of medicine, nursing care, or client behaviors; and the client's ability to respond to care as a result of such situations as a compromised immune system. Community health nurses need to keep such factors in mind when evaluating care.

Quality indicators of client outcomes are the quantitative measures of a client's response to care (Gordon, 2003). Defining and quantifying client outcomes from these indicators are worthwhile processes that enable the nursing staff to evaluate the results of the care they provide. The goal of care in the community is successful client outcomes. By starting with measurable indicators, successful outcomes can be demonstrated in quantifiable terms. When client care meets the standards set, client satisfaction—another quality outcome indicator—is greater.

Quality indicators are part of the broader quality management program and are used to determine goal achievement. A chart audit is a useful method to measure the frequency of quality indicator occurrence. For example, an agency may have a quality indicator such as, "All infants younger than 6 months of age are weighed on each home visit." Every fifth chart of infants visited in March, June, September, and December during a designated year is audited for documentation of the number of home visits and the number of infant weights recorded. A sampling of charts is sufficient to measure goal achievement and specific quality indicators. It is generally accepted that a sample of 20 randomly selected cases will provide useful information. If the population to be sampled numbers more than 200, some sources recommend that the sample include more than 20 cases.

Quantifying the indicators also can be accomplished through a rate or ratio of events for a defined population and time frame. Such indicators can be tailored to express almost any patient outcome (Williams, 1991). For example, in Display 15–2, the nursing staff sets a standard for the number of urinary tract infections (UTIs) the agency will tolerate in

DISPLAY 15-2

Quantifying Outcome Indicators

$$\text{Outcome indicators} = \frac{\text{Number of patient care events}}{\text{Total number of clients or total number of times at risk for event during a given period}}$$

Example:

$$\text{Occurrence of urinary tract infections in clients with indwelling urinary catheters} = \frac{\text{Number of clients experiencing urinary tract infections related to long-term use of indwelling urinary catheters from January 1 to March 1, 2005}}{\text{Number of clients with long-term indwelling urinary catheters from January 1 to March 1, 2005}}$$

clients with indwelling urinary catheters (perhaps 5% to 7%, depending on client age, diagnosis, family support, and home environment). In another situation, a public health nursing service has a standard to make home visits to first-time mothers and babies born at one hospital, within 5 days of delivery, 95% of the time. To evaluate this goal, the dates of initial home visits to first-time mothers and the birth dates of the infants are measured from a sample of client records during several measurement periods. These are both examples of assessing quality outcome indicators.

It is necessary to have indicators when setting standards in order to measure the success and quality of programs at home or in the community. The same types of indicators are used in acute care settings, with the focus appropriate to that population. If the standards are being met but client outcomes are unacceptable, the process indicators are explored for possible areas of weakness. Such areas may need further study to identify the cause of the poor client outcomes. For example, a process indicator such as the catheter care protocol used by an agency or the communication system between hospital and health department nurses may be examined to determine, respectively, the cause of infections or the reason why initial home visits are delayed. In addition, Medicaid and Medicare regulations in some states mandate that a percentage of records be audited each year.

While striving for excellence and best practices, agencies are using the benchmarking process. **Benchmarking** uses continuous, collaborative, and systematic processes for measuring and examining internal programs' strengths and weaknesses and includes studying another's processes in order to improve one's own (Lewis & Latney, 2002). Internal benchmarking occurs within the organization, between departments or programs. External benchmarking occurs between similar agencies providing like services. For example, a home care agency may have developed a clinical pathway that has proved useful with clients with congestive heart failure (CHF); another agency could benefit by using the same clinical pathway. In another example, an agency may use clinical practice guidelines obtained from a specialty organization along with information from a national database; another agency could benefit from this knowledge. This is a way for an agency to identify what is achievable while comparing and contrasting how others provide quality services.

Contributions of NANDA, NIC and NOC, and OASIS

The North American Nursing Diagnosis Association (NANDA) system of nursing diagnoses was designed for the acute care setting. This system of diagnoses stays current through the addition of new diagnoses and modification of older ones as medical care progresses. They are used with modifications and community-appropriate, family-centered diagnoses in the Omaha System and in home care through the Home Health Care Classification system. Another system that is specific to home health care is used when clients are admitted to care, when they have episodes of hospitalization, when they are recertified for home care, and when they are discharged from care. This system is the Outcomes and Assessment Informaton Set (OASIS). It is a Medicare requirement that data must be gathered using a standardized patient assessment technique. Data are shared with the federal agency, Health Care Financing Administration (HCFA), at the specific times mentioned. In this way, a national databank is developed that includes quality and client satisfaction with care received (see Chapter 37). These are useful tools; some identify client problems, teaching needs, and strengths, and others evaluate quality and client satisfaction.

The addition of such tools to the caregiving responsibilities of nurses is a result of continued research in the area of quality improvement and management. Change is the "norm" for health care practitioners, and the increased documentation responsibilities should be viewed as useful tools designed to enhance client care.

NANDA diagnoses are foundational to forming nursing intervention classifications (NIC) and nursing outcome classifications (NOC). Nursing interventions have been largely invisible due to inability to articulate the contributions of nurses to the care of clients. A classification system helps nurses document their actions. In the early 1960s, Aylelotte was a pioneer in measuring client outcomes. She suggested documenting changes in characteristics of clients to evaluate nursing care delivery. Most outcomes work from that time through the 1980s focused on clients' self-care skills (Gordon, 2003). In the 1990s, work on nursing interventions and outcomes provided nurses in many settings with a formalized classification system that is useful in delivering care. Nursing outcomes, especially useful in the community, are different from medical outcomes and include client knowledge and behaviors, safety, use of resources, home maintenance, and caregiver status.

Employing Quality Circles

Nursing staff in the community can use quality circles to improve the quality of care provided to clients. **Quality circles** are a participative management approach in which employees and managers share the responsibility for decision-making and problem-solving in client care. The concept of quality circles is based on several well-established motivational and management theories (Herzberg, Mauser & Snyderman, 1968; Maslow, 1954). The quality circles approach has been used in Japan since it was introduced after World War II by Dr. W. Edwards Deming (Swansburg & Swansburg, 2002). Ishikawa (1985) is recognized as a motivator for the movement in Japan. More recently, quality circles have been used in American industry as a participative management tool based on W. G. Ouchi's Theory Z (Ouchi, 1981). Quality circles are being used as effective tools in the health care arena (Swansburg & Swansburg, 2002). Although this management technique was first only used in the acute-care setting, it is now being identified as an excellent tool for those providing care in the home and community. The use of quality circles promotes shared decision-making and helps health care agencies achieve program goals and enhance multidisciplinary and interdisciplinary collaboration (Hibbard, 2003).

For a quality circle to be an effective problem-solving group, it must incorporate the following aspects (Hibbard, 2003; Swansburg & Swansburg, 2002):

• Problems are identified and solved by using the energies of nurses working in groups.
• Contributions made by individuals and groups are recognized.
• Continuous mechanisms are in place for further learning, decision-making, and nursing research.
• Processes are instituted for advocacy and negotiation, power from knowledge, networking through consultation, communication, collaboration, and coordination.

Central to achieving these purposes is the expectation that the formation of a quality circle ensures unity and a common sense of purpose. Employees are more satisfied in environments that are open and supportive of opportunities for self-determination and creative expression and in which their ideas are valued (Swansburg & Swansburg, 2002). The quality circle approach promotes such environments. Staff members share their expertise, experiences, and ideas, and they critique the handling of past situations. This profoundly useful quality improvement tool uses sharing and quality practices to go beyond routine auditing of key nursing activities. The emphasis on group processes facilitates increased understanding among a staff who must consider the quality of care delivered by the department or agency and must work together across a range of skills, management levels, and job assignments to solve problems related to the nursing goals.

Measuring Client Satisfaction

The health care practices that consumers value have been receiving more attention in recent years. The client's perception of quality care has become very important, as health care agencies or programs compete for clients. However, client satisfaction is difficult to define. Many studies using reliable and valid measurement tools indicate that clients identify quality care by such attributes as kindness, pleasantness, the ability to listen and care, flexibility, and proficiency. In addition, the quality of the nurse–client interaction in providing holistic care is frequently mentioned when clients are asked about the quality of care received (Hibbard, 2003; Moore & Coddington, 2002).

The final step of the nursing process—the evaluation—is often the weakest, yet it is one of the most crucial components. Failure to thoroughly evaluate services and care can result in delivery of mediocre nursing care. If the delivery and outcome of care are not evaluated, then care may continue at an unsafe or below-minimum standard. No longer will consumers tolerate mediocre care, nor can agencies afford to provide such care. Today's health care consumer demands a high level of quality care from beginning to end.

This may begin by the pleasantness and timeliness of the first telephone call and continue with the proficiency and flexibility of services, to efficiency of the follow-up survey 2 weeks after the termination of service. Questionnaires or telephone surveys can be used to collect feedback from clients. If clients are not satisfied, they may select a different agency, or they may be unreceptive to delivered services and refuse to come to the door, which often occurs in public agencies. Lack of follow-up and noncompliance with mutually set goals can often be traced to dissatisfaction with certain aspects of the care received.

In public agencies, many clients do not solicit the services they receive. As a result, adherence to instructions or goals, as in teaching parenting skills to substance abusers, educating pregnant teens, or instructing older adults about their medication, becomes an even more important and challenging issue. Issues of adherence also make it difficult to use questionnaires or surveys to gather information on client satisfaction. However, satisfaction may be determined through qualitative measures, such as statements from clients and family members. Quantitative measures include such indicators as the number of times clients make themselves available for visits or adhere to caregiving measures. Another factor affecting clients' perceptions of the care they receive is the nurse-to-client ratio. In many public programs, because one-on-one nursing care is not cost-effective, more care is delivered to the aggregate. Use of such aggregate approaches as group classes may affect the client's perception of quality service. In addition, only the most motivated and receptive clients may attend group sessions, which means that reticent or disinterested clients do not contribute to the evaluation process.

Auditing

Auditing is another technique for improving quality. An **audit** is an organized effort whereby practicing professionals monitor, assess, and make judgments about the quality and appropriateness of nursing care provided by peers as measured against professional standards of practice. A variety of audit tools can help achieve the best and most comprehensive data. These tools include record reviews, checklists, questionnaires, and surveys. They provide the audit committee with quantitative data with which to make decisions about future care as it relates to the agreed standards. Collaboration with the entire staff in the process is essential to increasing incentives for adhering to the standards (Norman, McArthur, & Miles, 2001). The information gathered can also support plans for revising the standards as client needs change. In some instances, the audit committee is empowered to implement those changes. Otherwise, the committee should receive follow-up reports on their recommendations from those who have taken the actions. In either case, the results of recommended actions should be reevaluated at a specified future date by the same group (ANA, 2000b; JCAHO, 2003).

Retrospective Review System

The most commonly known audit process is the **retrospective review** of client charts. This review is a quality assessment process that examines patterns of care over a specified period of time and includes closed-record audits and a statistical review of trends in services provided. Specific components of a home visit or care provided are reviewed, such as documented teaching, an infant's height and weight, the nurse's signature, or dates of care. However, the assumption that there is a relationship between the quality of documentation and the quality of nursing care is questionable. This type of audit should be viewed as a continuous process of reflective exploration rather than an attempt to determine the quality of care. There is a need for exploratory tools as well as evaluative tools. One tool does not give an agency a holistic picture of care provided. An agency that relies on only one tool can get a distorted and incomplete view of the care delivered.

Concurrent Review System

A **concurrent review** system is done on clients who are presently being visited or who are receiving care and uses the chart audit, clients' opinions, and observations of the health center environment. This approach combines a retrospective review with assessment of current clients' opinions and observations, while the care is still occurring. Combined data are tabulated and consolidated and can be used to improve care after being shared with the staff. To understand such an audit system, staff members must be oriented during work sessions in which they review a client record using the combined monitoring tools. In this way, staff members gain insight and become invested in the system. All changes or new systems used to improve quality of care, such as charting methods or audit systems, must be shared with staff from the beginning to enhance "buy-in" and ownership, which will promote adaptation to the new system.

QUALITY MEASUREMENT AND IMPROVEMENT IN COMMUNITY HEALTH NURSING

Do the people in health care fields know what their customers want, need, and like? Can satisfied consumers of health care services be identified? Often, the answers to these questions are no, leaving health care agencies with little knowledge about how to target their services.

The unique population-focused role of community health carries with it the challenge of sorting out top-priority health care needs from the many competing client needs. There are many areas of community health in which the current system of services does not meet the needs of large segments of the population. Frequently seen are preventable injuries, illnesses, and deaths caused by accidents, chemical abuse, sexually transmitted diseases, domestic violence, violent deaths, and suicide. Deficiencies in health services are also evident in the ways that care is delivered to those with existing problems, such as adolescent parents, disabled children, frail elderly, and people entrenched in cycles of poverty and illness.

New and innovative public health programs arise from the realization by public health practitioners that time-honored methods have become ineffective in addressing the problems of those at risk. New strategies need to be found. Such realizations come from scrutinizing public health services. This careful examination requires objective data on services and self-reflection about the health care delivered. The process of continually improving and ensuring quality provides a framework for collecting and evaluating these data on an ongoing basis (Swansburg & Swansburg, 2002) (see The Global Community).

Characteristics of Quality Health Care

An agency operates from an agreed-upon definition of quality. That definition is incorporated into the agency's mission statement or philosophy and is the basis on which a quality health care program can be built. In other words, a quality health care program is built on the concepts that the agency and its staff value. Such a program must consider everything that has an impact on the agency and the clients it serves. The following six characteristics are considered essential in a quality community health program:

1. It is comprehensive and addresses the interrelated health needs of the entire person or community.
2. It demonstrates organizational competency and operates from within an expertly managed and financially sound organizational system.
3. It demonstrates professional competency and a commitment to an environment that encourages personal excellence among a competent staff.
4. It is accessible and demonstrates that its services are readily available to its clients in a timely manner, despite the financial, cultural, emotional, or geographic barriers that may exist.
5. It is efficient and demonstrates that it consistently makes the best use of available and, at times, limited resources.
6. It is effective and demonstrates its consideration of client priorities and concern with the positive effects of the health status of clients as measured by client outcomes, client satisfaction ratings, and the client's ability to return to the same program when needed.

These six characteristics provide a framework for evaluating the quality of community health care delivery. Consider how these six characteristics might be used to assess a program or services for adolescent mothers. (1) Are we looking at all the health care needs of our typical teen mothers? (2, 3) Is the care being provided and delivered by competent staff who provide excellent care, from an agency that is well managed? (4) Are these young mothers actually functioning at a higher level as a result of our care, and do we connect

THE GLOBAL COMMUNITY

Amarsi, Y. (2002). Evidence-based nursing: Perspective from Pakistan. *Reflections on Nursing Leadership,* *28*(2), 28–29, 45–46.

In this article the author explores some of the constraints of evidence-based nursing (EBN) practice in developing countries. Although it is difficult, there are reasons why nurses should pursue EBN which include legitimizing and seeking greater professionalism in nursing practice in terms of enhanced authority and autonomy; helping nurses build their academic careers; following the wake of EBM; and improving nursing practice and raising standards of care.

Ideally, EBN focuses on what is important to nursing without care being sacrificed to scientific evidence. This is difficult in areas where resources are rich. Implementation of EBN in the countries of Southeast Asia such as Pakistan, Bangladesh, and Sri Lanka and in those of East Africa such as in Kenya, Uganda, and Tanzania faces overwhelming constraints.

First, in most of these countries health is a government responsibility, and not a high one, with most health care in the public sector. Health services are underfunded, resources are maldistributed, and basic resources such as clean water and antiseptics are a struggle to obtain. In this environment, it is unreasonable to expect computers and the needed software for EBN.

Second, nursing is not a recognized profession, and nursing education is hospital based. Only a handful of nurses have a baccalaureate education, and even fewer have graduate degrees. Under such circumstances, it is difficult to make research available to nurses. Their skills must be developed in information technology, problem solving, and critical thinking—all essential to implementing EBN.

A third constraint is the limited resources in these countries in relation to the contextual relevance of the evidence obtained by research studies. In addition, the research-based findings may not be culturally or socially acceptable to the client and family, because the studies come from outside of these countries.

Fourth, there are limited resources for research. The basics of food, shelter, security, and transportation come first, and much-needed resources are used in those areas.

Finally, nurses in developing countries are overworked and undertrained, without the time available for adequate preparation toward EBN. Nurses in the 21st century in all countries must use appropriate evidence to improve nursing practice and consequently the health of the people for whom they care. It is much more difficult for these nurses, and they must do it without outside help. They must develop their own expertise by obtaining higher education, strive to build institutional commitment and develop the work environment and culture toward EBN, obtain funding to facilitate technologic advancement, develop innovative strategies to conduct and disseminate research, and build collaboration in the international nursing community in the areas of research, practice, and education.

These nurses have major challenges to overcome, but with the support of the international health care community they may be able to improve health in their countries.

---

with these women during their first trimester and find ways to effectively interact with them to meet their needs throughout their pregnancy and postpartum period? (5) Are the services provided consistent with the mother's specific needs, or are they too generalized to make efficient use of available funds? (6) Are the women satisfied with their care and do they return to our agency for continued services after this pregnancy?

Such questions provide the basis for studying each dimension of quality. Each question refers to one of the key dimensions within the agency's mission statement or philosophy (Fig. 15–6).

Outcomes Check Points for Quality

A program of quality can have specific check points and outcomes that are determined by the agency's mission statement

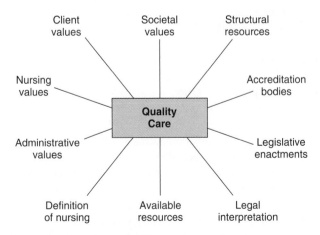

F I G U R E   1 5 – 6 .   Factors affecting quality nursing care.

and are measurable. In an attempt to strengthen the home care industry, 11 check points for quality can be measured. These check points are divided into three categories:

1. Client/family outcomes
   a. Client/family empowerment
   b. Caregiver relationship
   c. Knowledge and information needs
   d. Family support
   e. Client/family expectations
2. Clinical outcomes
   a. Functional ability
   b. Physiologic functioning
3. Organizational outcomes
   a. Team building
   b. Commitment to quality
   c. Coordination of care
   d. Financial viability

Ideally, a comprehensive community health nursing program addresses in some fashion all of the agency services, the processes and resources used to accomplish the services, and client expectations and outcomes. This is done to improve quality and efficiency and is part of an organized assessment process.

Role of the Nurse in Quality Measurement and Improvement

Although nurses who deliver care directly to clients are not managers as such, improving quality is a "management" activity, not only of administration personnel but of the practicing nurses as members of the team. Community health nurses may not be responsible for a staff or agency budget and functioning, but they are responsible for managing a caseload of clients with needs of varying degrees of urgency. With judicious use of the resources available, they must provide priority services that promote the highest possible level of personal and group functioning and health. Any activities the community health nurse engages in to realize these goals contribute to the quality management program.

Some quality improvement activities for community health nurses include daily prioritizing of care needs for a caseload of clients, seeking supervision or skills development for a difficult case, systematizing charting so that needed documentation is efficiently completed (eg, using flow sheets to chart maternal–child health visits), proposing better ways to organize care of chronically ill clients, and establishing new agency procedures. All of these actions demonstrate that nurses are evaluating their work and looking for ways to improve care. Staff meetings, quality circle meetings, peer review, and case conferences are common settings for nurses to bring the lessons of their practices to the larger group for examination and potential adoption.

It is the role of nursing administration to develop a formalized quality management program that includes a three-pronged focus, based on a classic approach to quality man-

agement: (1) review organizational structure, personnel, and environment; (2) focus on standards of nursing care and methods of delivering nursing care (process); and (3) focus on the outcomes of that care (Donabedian, 1985). These formal evaluations include peer review audits (documented care delivered by peers), client satisfaction assessments, review of agency policies and procedures, analysis of demographic information, and the like (Ellis & Hartley, 2001).

Nurses who are new to formal quality improvement activities in the work setting need to recognize the value of these efforts and their part in ensuring that quality care is being delivered. Direct service providers are the best judges of care problems and their potential solutions. For this reason, it is critical that quality assurance reviews and other quality improvement activities focus on issues relevant to staff and client concerns and be structured so they can be accomplished quickly and with minimal effort. When these activities are clear, concise, and well integrated into daily routines, they become less time-consuming, and staff members can see the positive client outcomes as rewards for their contributions to the process. Moreover, when health care providers have the opportunity to systematically examine the care they provide, they can generate useful ideas for improving that care and can identify care issues sooner.

Whether small or large, health care agencies are complex organizations with interrelated components. The nursing staff has input into or some control over the quality of care delivered to clients who use the services of the agency. The following paragraphs review the nurse's role in each of the three areas of structure, process, and outcomes.

Structure

The organizational structure and financial stability of the agency should allow the mission statement or philosophy to be realized. The agency should be client focused, with sufficient resources to maintain present services and introduce additional services as needed. Public agencies need to operate within budget and also have a well-developed system of acquiring additional funding for new services through grants and contract expansion. Private agencies should operate efficiently enough to realize a profit that encourages the owners and boards of directors to continue to support the services. They should look for additional ways to solicit clients in addition to employing highly motivated and qualified staff.

Process

The agency should maintain standards set by the professional staff that comply with or surpass those recommended by the accrediting bodies mentioned earlier. The staff is encouraged to contribute to evaluation of the standards and revise them as needed. Staff members need to keep themselves current by attending in-service training sessions and acquiring additional education appropriate to their job requirements. The staff members work collaboratively with others across disciplines to improve the quality of care given in the community by using a variety of participative management tools (eg, audit instruments, quality circles). The agency is supportive of its staff and the needs of individuals. Staff turnover is minimal because employee values are compatible with the goals of the agency. Administration and staff have a compatible working relationship. A system of quality review is in place, and each staff member contributes to this process as a member of a peer review committee or quality improvement or assurance committee. Staff members also listen to clients and provide an outlet to evaluate the care received (eg, questionnaires, surveys, interviews), and the agency acts on client suggestions and comments.

Outcomes

Standards of care are met or surpassed. Client outcomes are consistent with agency goals and quality care. They are measured against set standards. Client satisfaction is monitored, and a system of improving client satisfaction is part of the agency's agenda.

All services an agency provides should be reviewed periodically to determine whether standards are meeting the present needs of the population and whether the nursing staff are implementing these standards. The nursing services used most frequently, such as well-child care, self-care education with chronically ill adults, and various screening programs, are excellent places to begin the review. Usually, these services involve the entire nursing staff and consume a significant amount of nursing care time.

The focus on commonly served high-risk groups presents an opportunity to optimize care delivery as well as to benefit high-risk clients. Children living in neighborhoods that are known to have high lead toxicity rates from leaded paint in older homes stand to benefit tremendously from a consistently implemented lead screening, treatment, and advocacy program. Without review, such a program may not achieve its goals of decreasing toxic levels of lead in area children.

Incidents of poor client outcome are important areas for further study. Through clinic or home visit records, community nurses can routinely review documentation of deceased or hospitalized clients to assess whether any aspect of the clinic's care or home visit activities might have prevented these occurrences. For instance, the case of a child with repeated high serum lead levels who requires hospitalization for chelation might stimulate a clinic's examination of the adequacy of parent education regarding environmental sources of lead. The clinic could also explore the effectiveness of its advocacy with the area's lead-abatement staff to ensure needed repairs in leaded homes and the removal of families to safe housing while repairs are being made.

As another example, a review of the charts of hospitalized clients who take multiple medications can be conducted to ascertain whether teaching or compliance issues regarding medication contributed to each client's hospitalization. The results may prompt a change in home-visit teaching techniques, an increase in the frequency of visits, or a change in

vital-sign parameters for notifying a physician. Persistence of problems and deficiencies could be a clue that the community health nurse needs additional education in this area or that the nurse's caseload is too heavy and therefore exceeds the ability of the nurse to provide minimally expected care. Once the cause is determined, implementation of appropriate changes can commence, after allowing adequate time for the staff to address critical issues. Should additional education be needed, it is the responsibility of the coordinating, in-service, or staff education nurse to provide or arrange for the needed education.

Given adequate resources, including sufficient time, information, and support, good care is the norm. Occasionally, quality-of-care problems result from an individual provider's performance. Recommendations are made for counseling or another type of intervention by that person's supervisor, and appropriate corrective action should be taken to resolve the problem and preserve the employee's potential contributions as a successful team member.

Future Trends

Major changes in quality measurement and improvement have been occurring in recent years. At present, there are several activities and initiatives that will affect the quality of health care services, including public health, in the future.

Public health officials representing the Centers for Disease Control and Prevention (CDC), the American Public Health Association (APHA), and state and territorial health offices have formed a coalition to develop performance standards for state and local public health systems nationwide ("Coalition unveils," 1999). These "partners" believe that performance standards will have a profound impact on the quality of public health delivery systems. The standards will act as critical tools for measuring and refining public health practice, documenting accountability, benchmarking quality improvement in performance, and justifying investment in public health infrastructure. " What gets measured, gets done," stated the coalition members ("Coalition unveils," 1999).

Another major effort began in 1999 when a White House planning committee was convened to design and initiate actions to establish a National Forum for Health Care Quality Measurement and Reporting (NQF). The planning committee also recommended that a Strategic Framework Board (SFB) be established. This group began to develop a conceptual framework to define the scope of a new national system that would move the nation toward a coordinated health care system (McGlynn, 2003). The long-awaited national accreditation process is being developed by the National Committee for Quality Assurance (NCQA) and JCAHO through the recently formed National Quality Measurement and Reporting System (NQMRS). As reported by McGlynn (2003, p. I-3), "The purpose of the NQMRS is to:

- Evaluate the degree to which the U. S. health care system is providing safe, effective, timely, and patient-centered care.

- Assess whether the delivery of high-quality care is efficient and equitable.
- Enable substantial progress to be made toward achieving established national goals.
- Provide easily accessible information on quality to a variety of audiences, including consumers, purchasers, and providers, to facilitate individual and collective decision-making.
- Provide information that regulators, purchasers, and providers can use to support continued improvement and achievement of goals."

NQMRS reviewed the priorities established in *Healthy People 2010* (U. S. Department of Health and Human Services, 2000), used literature reviews conducted by The Rand Corporation, based its foundation on evidence, and wrote goal statements that were designed to be compelling to consumers and clinicians as a driver for change (McGlynn, 2003). Out of this research, a conceptual framework for the NQMRS was created (Fig. 15–7).

The ANA is testing quality indicators for the acute-care setting. In addition, an advisory committee on community-based non–acute-care quality indicators has been established. The group is defining and testing the feasibility of an initial set of indicators across health care settings that are nursing sensitive (ie, the ability to exceed, meet, or fall below expected quality indicators is reflected in the nurse's actions with clients). The group has identified the following areas where there is adequate research regarding a link to quality care: symptom severity, therapeutic alliance, client satisfaction, protective factors, level of function, risk reduction, and utilization of services.

OASIS, mentioned earlier in this chapter, is a fairly new tool. This tool is designed to enhance the measurement of quality services to the nation's elders in long-term care and creates the ability to benchmark with comparable agencies. Similar changes initiated by JCAHO are occurring in home care.

What benefits and costs will potentially be associated with these changes for clients, community health nurses,

community health care organizations, third-party payers, and indeed, the national health care delivery system? Time will tell what positive, or possibly negative, effects these changes may have. These represent some of the quality measurement and improvement activities at the national, state, and local levels of health care delivery in the community. The community health nurse must stay informed about legislative changes that affect how care and services are measured, as well as professional organization standards and agency policies.

SUMMARY

Quality measurement and quality improvement for community health nursing are vital. Quality measurement and improvement programs seek to ensure that sufficient health care services are provided in a timely manner and that the services being provided are very likely to produce positive effects on the health and perception of health of those being served. Factors affecting the outcome of quality include nursing's self-regulation, certification and accreditation, legislation and regulation, reimbursement, and consumer demands.

The multiple models or frameworks on which quality management systems are based include a classic way of looking at programs through organizational structure, process, and outcomes, along with the interrelatedness of each component. The six models presented in this chapter are structured in unique ways that enable them to meet the differing needs of community agencies.

Over time, quality management techniques have changed, becoming more inclusive and using participative management systems. Current techniques include risk assessment, the setting of measurable goals and objectives, evaluating outcomes, employing quality circles, measuring client satisfaction, and using retrospective and concurrent review of documentation during the audit process. The current

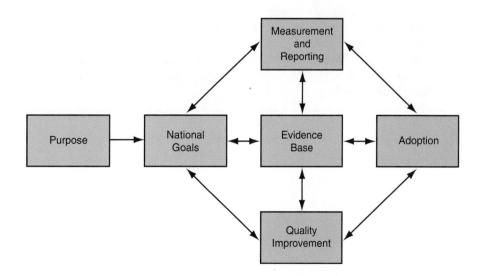

FIGURE 15–7.
NQMRS conceptual framework.

techniques provide new ways to involve staff in participative management opportunities. All services an agency provides should be reviewed periodically to determine whether the current standards are being met. Increasing focus has been placed on quality care indicators such as client outcomes and client satisfaction because of the increasing competition among health care providers.

Identification of quality health care characteristics and "checkpoints" for quality helps the community health care practitioner recognize the quality indicators of best practice. These also give community health nurses direction for their role in quality measurement and improvement. This role is grounded in the structure, process, and outcomes of caregiving and services provided.

Quality measurement and improvement initiatives are a fairly new addition to the health care delivery system, having taken hold in the 1970s with nursing in a leadership position. Whether quality measurement and improvement techniques are formally or informally practiced, whenever nurses monitor, assess, and judge the quality and appropriateness of care as measured against professional standards the interests of clients are being served.

Local agencies, professional organizations, and official agencies at the state and national levels are developing standards, techniques, and tools designed to improve quality, measure care and services, and determine client outcomes. This development is likely to continue into the 21st century, with a constant view toward positive client outcomes.

CLINICAL CORNER

QUALITY ASSURANCE

As a school nurse in a large urban high school, your duties have ranged from violence prevention program coordinator and clinic specialist to parent group liaison. The high school is located in the inner city of an East Coast metropolitan area. The demographics of the student population reflect the diversity of the city: 30% of the students are white, 25% are Hispanic, 20% are black, 10% are Southeast Asian, and the remaining 15% represent a wide range of other cultures and ethnicities. There are approximately 3000 students enrolled in the school.

Until recently, the school's family planning program services have been contracted out to a community-based family planning clinic. The clinic was paid $60,000 per year to provide students with family planning services. Recently, there has been a significant increase in the number of unplanned pregnancies among students at the school. This problem, combined with anticipated budget cutbacks, led the school board to sever its ties with the contracted clinic. With supreme confidence in your abilities, your supervisor has volunteered you for the job of starting up a school-based family planning/STD prevention clinic.

Quality management issues in the past have included
• School staff does not refer students to the clinic. Rationale is unknown.

• Although the predetermined agreement of $60,000/year is to include all students who may remain anonymous when presenting for care, utilization is reportedly low.
• STD and pregnancy rates have continued to rise in the past 3 years.
• Clients complain of language barriers and culturally insensitive staff members.

QUESTIONS

1. What additional information do you need to improve the quality of care given?
2. How will you go about obtaining necessary information?
3. The current budget is $60,000 per year to the contracted agency. The school board has allotted $56,000 for the upcoming fiscal year. Can you provide higher-quality care at a lower cost? Brainstorm about your plan; include a budget along with anticipated outcomes.
4. What issues does this scenario elicit regarding
   Fears and anxiety in this role
   Lack of immediate resources (eg, supervisor)
   Social justice
   Building partnerships within your communities
   Globalization of public health

ACTIVITIES TO PROMOTE CRITICAL THINKING

1. Refer to an existing community health nursing program (home health agency, public health nursing service, or adult health clinic) in your community and evaluate its quality based on the characteristics of a quality community health program.

2. Using one of the six models for quality management discussed in this chapter, create a quality management program in a community family planning agency. Select another model and create a quality management program in a prenatal clinic. How do the different models serve the agencies selected?

3. Select a community program with which you are familiar. Identify one topic for study, and develop one or more standards and criteria you can use to measure the actual service provided.

4. Using the organizational tools (philosophy, mission, procedures, and protocols) of a community agency, participate in a quality circle with peers to improve an identified area of care an agency provides.

5. Using the Internet and selecting various portals, locate recent nursing journal articles that focus on quality measurement and improvement. Are some of the models described in this chapter being used? Are there new models in the literature? If so, how different are they from the ones presented here? Would they be more useful in the community? Why or why not? (See Clinical Corner.)

REFERENCES

Amarsi, Y. (2002). Evidence-based nursing: Perspective from Pakistan. *Reflections on Nursing Leadership, 28*(2), 28–29, 45–46.

American Nurses Association. (1975). *A plan for implementation of the standards of nursing practice.* Kansas City, MO: Author.

American Nurses Association. (1983). *Standards of school nursing practice.* Kansas City, MO: Author.

American Nurses Association. (1998). *Standards of clinical nursing practice.* Washington, DC: Author.

American Nurses Association. (1999a). *Nursing quality indicators: Guide for implementation* (2nd ed.). Washington, DC: Author.

American Nurses Association. (1999b). *Scope and standards of home health nursing practice.* Washington, DC: Author.

American Nurses Association. (1999c). *Scope and standards of public health nursing practice.* Washington, DC: Author.

American Nurses Association. (2000a). *Nursing quality indicators beyond acute care: Literature review.* Washington, DC: Author.

American Nurses Association. (2000b). *Nursing quality indicators beyond acute care: Measurement instruments.* Washington, DC: Author.

American Nurses Credentialing Center. (2003). *Advanced practice certification catalog.* Washington, DC: Author.

Bowles, K.H., & Naylor, M.D. (1996). Nursing intervention classification systems. *Image. Journal of Nursing Scholarship, 28*(4), 303–308.

Bull, M.J. (1996). Past and present perspectives on quality of care in the United States. In J. A. Schmele (Ed.), *Quality management in nursing and health care* (pp. 141–157). Albany, NY: Delmar.

Catalano, J.T. (2003). *Nursing now! Today's issues, tomorrow's trends* (3rd ed.). Philadelphia: FA Davis.

Cherry, B. & Jacob, S.R. (2002). *Contemporary nursing: Issues, trends, and management* (2nd ed.). St. Louis: Mosby.

Coalition unveils standards for public health practice. (July 1999, Part I). *The Nation's Health.* Washington, DC: American Public Health Association.

College of Nurses of Ontario, Quality Assurance Program. *http://www.cno.org/frame_quality.html.* Accessed on February 5, 2002.

DePalma, J.A. (2002). Proposing an evidence-based policy process. *Nursing Administration Quarterly, 26*(4), 55–61.

Donabedian, A. (1966). Evaluating the quality of medical care. *Milbank Memorial Fund Quarterly, 44,* 166–206.

Donabedian, A. (1969). Medical care appraisal: Quality and utilization. In *Guide to medical care administration.* New York: American Public Health Association.

Donabedian, A. (1981). *The criteria and standards of quality.* Ann Arbor, MI: Health Administration Press.

Donabedian, A. (1985). *Explorations in quality assessment and monitoring* (Vol. 3). Ann Arbor, MI: Health Administration Press.

Donabedian, A. (2002). *An introduction to quality assurance in health care.* New York: Oxford University Press.

Ellis, J.R., & Hartley, C.L. (2001). *Nursing in today's world: Challenges, issues, and trends* (7th ed.). Philadelphia: Lippincott Williams & Wilkins.

Gordon, M. (1998, September 30). Nursing nomenclature and classification system development. *Online Journal of Issues in Nursing.* Retrieved November 11, 2003, from *http://www.nursingworld.org/ojin/tpc7/tpc7_1.htm.*

Herzberg, F., Mauser, B., & Snyderman, B. (1968). *The motivation to work.* New York: John Wiley.

Hibbard, J.H. (2003). Engaging health care consumers to improve the quality of care. *Medical Care, 41*(Suppl. 1), I61–I71.

Hill, M. (1999). Outcomes measurement requires nursing to shift to outcome-based practice. *Nursing Administraion Quarterly, 24*(1), 1–16.

Hoenig, H., Horner, R.D., Duncan, P.W., Clipp, E., & Hamilton, B. (1999). New horizons in stroke rehabilitation research [Review]. *Journal of Rehabilitation Research and Development, 36*(1), 19–31.

Ishikawa, K. (1985). *What is total quality control?* Englewood Cliffs, NJ: Prentice-Hall.

Lewis, P.S., & Latney, C. (2002). Achieve best practice with an evidence-based approach. *Nursing Management, 33*(12), 24, 26–29.

Martin, K., Leak, G., & Aden, C. (1997). The Omaha system: A research-based model for decision making. In B.W. Spradley & J.A. Allender (Eds.), *Readings in community health nursing* (5th ed., pp. 316–324). Philadelphia: Lippincott-Raven.

Maslow, A. (1954). *Motivation and personality.* New York: Harper & Row.

McGlynn, E.A. (2003). Introduction and overview of the conceptual framework for a national quality measurement and reporting system. *Medical Care 41*(Suppl. 1), I1–I7.

Mitchell, P.H., Ferketich, S., & Jennings, B.M. (1998). Quality health care outcomes model. *Image: Journal of Nursing Scholarship, 30*(1), 43–46.

Norman, L.D., McArthur, D., & Miles, P. (2001). Partnership model for teaching population health care improvement. *Nursing Administration Quarterly, 26*(1), 7–13.

Ouchi, W.G. (1981). *Theory Z.* Reading, MA: Addison Wesley.

Phaneuf, M.C. (1976). *The nursing audit and self-regulation in nursing practice.* New York: Appleton Century Crofts.

Swansburg, R. & Swansburg, R.C. (2002). *Management and leadership for nurse managers* (3rd ed.). Boston: Jones and Bartlett.

Tideiksaar, R. (2002). *Falls in Older People: Prevention & Management (3rd ed.),* Baltimore, MD: Health Professions Press.

U. S. Department of Health and Human Services. (2000). *Healthy people 2010* (Conference ed., Vols. 1 & 2). Washington, DC: Author.

Williams, A.D. (1991). Development and application of clinical indicators for nursing. *Journal of Nursing Care Quality, 6*(1), 1–5.

SELECTED READINGS

Bradley, M., & Thompson, N.R. (2000). *Quality management integration in long-term care: Guidelines for excellence.* Baltimore, MD: Health Professions Press.

Brown, S.J. (2001). Managing the complexity of best practice health care. *Journal of Nurisng Care Quality, 15*(2), 1–8.

Chambers, N., & Jolly, A. (2002). Essence of care: Making a difference. *Nursing Standard, 17*(11), 40–44.

Grembowski, D. (2001). *The Practice of Health Program Evaluation.* Thousand Oaks, CA: Sage.

Hibbard, J.H. (2002). Engaging health care consumers to improve the quality of care. *Medical Care, 41*(Suppl. 1), I48–I80.

Institute of Medicine. (2001). Crossing the quality chasm: A new health system for the 21st century. Report by the Committee on Quality Health Care in America. Washington, DC: National Academy Press.

Morse, J.M., Penrod, J., & Hupcey, J.E. (2000). Qualitative outcome analysis: Evaluating nursing interventions for complex clinical phenomena. *Journal of Nursing Scholarship, 32*(2), 125–130.

Nolan, M.T. & Mock, V. (2000). *Measuring Patient Outcomes.* Thousand Oaks, CA: Sage.

Pan American Heath Organization. (2001) *Health Systems Performance Assessment and Improvement in the Region of the Americas.* Geneva: World Health Organization.

Pearson, M.L., Lee, J.L., Chang, B.L., Elliott, M., Kahn, K.L., & Rubenstein, L.V. (2000). Structured implicit review: A new method for monitoring nursing care quality. *Medical Care, 38*(11), 1074–1091.

Perra, B.M. (2001). Leadership: The key to quality outcomes. *Journal of Nursing Care Quality, 15*(2), 68–73.

Ryan, P. & Lauver, D.R. (2002). The efficacy of tailored interventions. *Journal of Nursing Scholarship, 34*(4), 331–337.

Sabin, J.E., O'Brien, M.F., & Daniels, N. (2001). Strengthening the consumer voice in managed care: II. Moving NCQA standards from rights to empowerment. *Psychiatric Services, 52*(10), 1303–1305.

Schalock, R.L. (2001). *Outcome-based evaluation* (2nd ed.). Norwell, MA: Kluwer Plenum.

Suri, S. (2002). Using medical and information techonology for improving quality of care. *Journal of Ambulatory Care Management, 25*(1), 33–39.

Valente, T.W. (2002). *Evaluating health promotion programs.* New York: Oxford University Press.

Wesorick, G. (2002). 21st century leadership challenge: Creating and sustaining healthy, healing work cultures and integrated service at the point of care. *Nursing Administration Quarterly, 26*(5), 18–32.

Zander, K. (2002). Nursing case management in the 21st century: Intervening where margin meets mission. *Nursing Administration Quarterly, 26*(5), 58–67.

Zerwekh, J., Thibodeaux, R., & Plesko, R. (2000). Chart it once: Innovation in public health documentation. *Journal of Community Health Nursing, 17*(2), 75–83.

Internet Resources

American Nurses Association: *http://www.ana.org*
American Nurses Informatics Association: *http://www.ania.org*
Case Management Society of America: *http://www.cmsa.org*
Community Health Accreditation Program, Inc. (CHAP): *http://www.chapinc.org/*
Interagency Collaborative on Nursing Statistics (ICONS): *http://www.iconsdata.org*
Joint Commission on Accreditation of Healthcare Organizations (JCAHO): *http://www.jcaho.org*
Nursing Standard Online: *http://www.nursing-standard.co.uk*

16

Policy Making and Community Health Advocacy

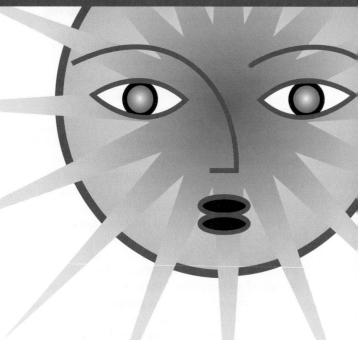

Learning Objectives

Upon mastery of this chapter, you should be able to:

- Define health policy and explain how it is established.
- Analyze the influence of health policy on community health and nursing practice.
- Explain the role of special interest groups in health care reform and policy making.
- Define political empowerment and describe ways in which community health nurses can become politically empowered.
- Identify the four stages in the policy process and briefly explain what each entails.
- Explain the role of community health nurses in determining a community's health policy needs.
- Identify the 10 steps in mobilizing a community for political action.
- Describe the steps involved in how a bill becomes law.
- Explain several methods of communicating with legislators on policy issues.
- List at least four political strategies for community health nursing.

A s a nursing student, you probably have a vision of health care that is more accessible, equitable, cost-effective, and quality-oriented than the present system. Unfortunately, as you enter the current health care system, you will soon recognize that vision alone is not enough. For a myriad of reasons, nurses have had a difficult time just making policy makers aware of the value of their input, not to mention the vital role that nurses play in providing essential health care services. Although most nurses recognize the importance of their role as providers of health care, many do not recognize the importance of their role in influencing or making legislation in relation to their practice or to community health.

Behind all legislation and health care regulation, there are power struggles. Only the naive think that others will be persuaded by facts alone. There are social and political factions at work; special interest groups, business, and industry each bring their power into play. Because the outcomes of these struggles determine the availability and quality of all health and social services, nurses need to develop an operational knowledge of health policy and political process in order to protect individuals, families, communities, and their nursing practice.

Fortunately, nursing's interest and representation in public affairs are growing. Nurses are competing successfully for fellowships in public policy, such as the Robert Wood Johnson Health Policy Fellows Program and the Kellogg National Fellowship Program. In 1992, Eddie Bernie Johnson, RN (D., Texas), became the first nurse to be elected to the U.S. House of Representatives. She was one of nine nurses who ran for the 103rd Congress (Mason, Leavitt & Chaffee, 2002). More recently, several nurses have served as elected officials at the state and national levels. In addition, nurses are influential representatives in support of policies, bills, or laws that reflect issues affecting the population's health and well-being (Wakefield, 2002).

This chapter examines health policy, the political process involved in determining health policy, and the role of community health nursing in the process. The underlying bias is that community health nurses should not only provide input to policy circles through advocacy but should be leaders who sit at the decision-making tables. The purpose is to emphasize the need for community health nurses to understand their role and power in providing an essential influence and unique perspective in health care.

POLICY MAKING

Policy is an authoritatively stated course of action that guides decision-making. It is how an institution, organization, agency, or government exercises its authority; it is based on that group's goals and exists to provide guidelines for operation. Policy can (and should) be written formally, but many policies are unwritten, unclear, or "hidden" to prevent public or legal review. Government policy that makes decisions af-

fecting the public—whether the government is local, state, or federal—is called **public policy**.

Policies attempt to express the collective interests and beliefs of the social system or institution that generates them. Changes in public policy usually come about because policy makers perceive that something is not functioning as it should or because the political pressure is so great that a change is mandated. A policy is made because the perceived benefits outweigh the perceived costs, at least to the decision makers. The "something" that needs changing can be as large and complex as the health care system or as small and simple as a local agency's name. The latter will not be perceived as small and simple by those with a vested interest in the name. As an example, during the development of the National Institute of Nursing Research (NINR) from the National Center of Nursing Research (NCNR) in 1993, those involved struggled long and hard to secure a name for this institute that accurately reflected its mission.

Policies are enforced by the agency or organization for whom they were created. For example, noncompliance with employment policies in a health care agency, such as not following protocol designed to ensure client safety or ignoring a specific dress code that identifies employees to clients and portrays professionalism, may result in termination of services. Violation of a government policy, such as illegally selling drugs, may result in a fine or imprisonment. Public policy is usually backed by laws or regulations.

All public policy is inextricably linked to economics. The growth of the health care system is driven by economic conditions and profit motives as well as competition promoted by the political climate (Harrington & Estes, 2001). Policy problems come about because policies, to a great extent, determine who gets what in a society or institution. In other words, policy problems occur because resources are being redistributed, with the result that some receive a greater share and others receive less.

Health Policy

Health policy is any policy that constitutes the governing framework (structure, process, and outcomes) for providing health services on a local, state, national, or even international level. *Structure* is the number and types of agencies, programs, and services, as well as providers and targeted clients. *Process* is the manner in which the agencies, programs, and services are going to be provided, managed, and funded, as well as how clients are to receive services. *Health policy outcomes* are the actual consequences of health policy implementation and are described in terms of effectiveness, efficiency, equity, innovativeness, and empowerment. Figure 16–1 outlines health policy from this perspective.

The passage of health care legislation at the federal and state levels ultimately leads to the implementation of health policy at a local level. For example, the Omnibus Budget Reconciliation Act (OBRA) of 1993 recognized the Vaccines for Children (VFC) program as a critical need. As a re-

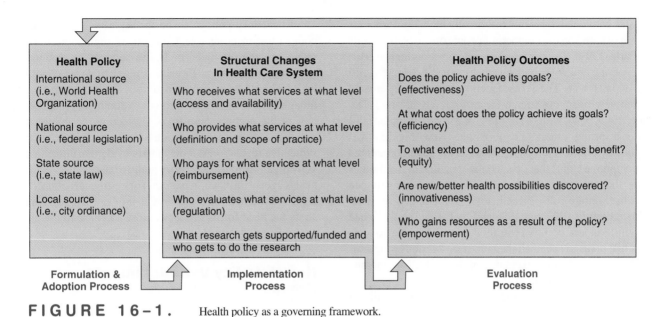

Health Policy	Structural Changes In Health Care System	Health Policy Outcomes
International source (i.e., World Health Organization)	Who receives what services at what level (access and availability)	Does the policy achieve its goals? (effectiveness)
National source (i.e., federal legislation)	Who provides what services at what level (definition and scope of practice)	At what cost does the policy achieve its goals? (efficiency)
State source (i.e., state law)	Who pays for what services at what level (reimbursement)	To what extent do all people/communities benefit? (equity)
Local source (i.e., city ordinance)	Who evaluates what services at what level (regulation)	Are new/better health possibilities discovered? (innovativeness)
	What research gets supported/funded and who gets to do the research	Who gains resources as a result of the policy? (empowerment)

Formulation & Adoption Process   Implementation Process   Evaluation Process

F I G U R E   1 6 – 1 .   Health policy as a governing framework.

sult, the President's Childhood Immunization Initiative (CII), a nationwide effort to vaccinate all children in the United States, was implemented in October 1994. This federal health policy provides guidelines and resources by combining the efforts of both public and private health care providers at the local level to vaccinate children, regardless of ability to pay.

Similarly, in response to the assessed need for a more secure homeland after the terrorist attack on September 11, 2001, the federal government proposed creating a new Department of Homeland Security, with plans coming to the decision level in 2002 and the appointment of a head of this new department in 2003. Under this new department, the nation's security, protection, and emergency response activities are rolled into a single federal department. Included in the mix are some of the activities of the U. S. Department of Health and Human Services (USDHHS), with transfer of responsibilities from agencies such as the Centers for Disease Control and Prevention (CDC) and Health Resources and Services Asdministration (HRSA). Some public health experts and legislators were worried the plan would fragment the nation's broad-based public health system and hinder overall responsiveness, thus negatively affecting people at the local level. Representative Henry Waxman, a Democrat from California, stated, "If our public health system is structured and viewed exclusively through the lens of fighting terrorism, it may seriously weaken our ability to respond to other threats to the health of the American people" (Late, 2002). Such conflicts in health policy at the federal level have "trickle-down" effects at the local level that can cause gaps in services and overlap of responsibilities. Ideally, such issues should be resolved before decisions are finalized—although this is not always the case.

Ultimately, health policy is about health care choices and should reflect a community's values (Mason, Leavitt & Chaf-

fee, 2002). However, the power to make policy decisions for any community is spread among a number of stakeholders (ie, anyone with a vested interest), who may not live in the community. Because there are so many people with vested interests in the health care system, it is unlikely that anyone can know the real and full impact of a health policy on a given community until after the policy has been implemented.

Theoretically, health policy should empower the community for which it is intended, but conflicts can arise if one community's empowerment threatens the values of another. For example, there has been much conflict and argument over the controversial policies regarding government funding of abortions for low-income women. Some community groups oppose this policy, arguing that it violates the greater policy of preserving life, whereas other groups support it, saying that it protects and promotes the overall health of the community. Such conflict dilutes the empowering ability of a given health policy.

Health policy also empowers the health care provider by deeming the provider's services to be essential, subsidizing the provider's education, and directly reimbursing the provider. Because health policies affect a community's health status and determines who will be reimbursed for what by whom, political considerations are involved at every step of their development, implementation, and evaluation. If health policy fails to provide a workable framework at the community level, the health care needs of communities are not met in a cost-effective manner.

For example, in 1996, Congress passed and President Clinton signed the watershed welfare reform bill, which was predicated on a centuries-old notion of "forcing" the poor out of poverty. This law, after being in effect for several years, dramatically rendered millions of people ineligible to receive federal assistance. However, it increased the amount spent on the remaining families and left billions of dollars unspent as states continued to receive historically high fixed amounts of money based on the numbers of people on old welfare rolls (DeParle, 1999). The percentage unspent was as high as 91% in Wyoming and 76% in Idaho and as low as 6% in Missouri and 4% in Hawaii. The excess federal welfare money created a "rich new financing stream for anti-poverty efforts" (DeParle, 1999, p. 1), which, for a few years baffled some states while inspiring others. For example, New Mexico was plagued by political infighting between the governor and the state Supreme Court that delayed the spending of the monies while thousands of jobless New Mexicans were dropped from the welfare rolls. Nonetheless, New Mexico received $751 million in 1997 and 1998 and by the end of 1998 had $242 million left, or 32% of its total grant. The state government had plans to spend all the money on "various programs for the poor, such as expanding child-care for low-income workers" (DeParle, 1999, p. 20).

These diverse examples are a reminder that the intent of a policy may not be its outcome. The policy intent reflected by this bill was to reduce an expensive government program, but it continued to cost the federal government the same amount of money while denying access to critical safety net programs, thereby undermining the health of millions of families in some states. A few years after the passage of this legislation, the national leadership changed. The federal government became aware of the overage at the same time that the federal feduciary stream began to slow in response to the country's economic downturn. As a result, the excess funds have been all but eliminated, again without benefit to those in need.

Health policies can be distributive or regulatory. **Distributive health policy** promotes nongovernmental activities that are thought to be beneficial to society as a whole. An example of a distributive policy is the Nurse Training Act, Title VIII of the Public Health Service Act, which was established in 1965 and provided federal subsidies for nursing education in an effort to address the need for more nurses. *Redistributive health policy* changes the allocation of resources from one group to another, usually to a broader or different group. Medicare is an example of redistributive policy in that provisions under Medicare were expanded to provide a broader range of benefits and coverage to needy groups, such as those older than 65 years of age and the permanently disabled of any age.

Regulatory health policy is policy that attempts to control the allocation of resources by directing those agencies or persons who offer resources or provide public services. For example, there are government regulations that set standards for licensure of health care organizations (eg, hospitals) and health care providers (eg, nurses). Regulatory public health policy is often used to protect the health of the community (Kovner & Jonas, 2002). An example in the United States is the mandatory reporting of certain communicable diseases. On the international level, regulatory health policy has a broad scope, including areas such as international communicable disease control, trade, human rights, armed conflict and arms control, and the environment (Fidler, 1999).

Regulatory policy can be further categorized as either competitive or protective. Competitive regulation limits, or structures, the provision of health services by designating who can deliver them. Protective regulations set conditions under which various private activities can be undertaken. Although professional licensure is most commonly identified as having the primary purpose of protecting the public, such policy is competitive regulation in terms of its social impact. Protective regulation is more clearly evident in utilization review organizations (regulatory bodies that critically examine health agency utilization patterns) or certificates of need (the legal requirement that a potential provider agency demonstrate the need for its services before a license to practice is granted; see Chapter 15).

Health Policy Debate and Interest Groups

Health policy debate centers on issues such as the overall cost of health care reform, the amount of control the federal government will exercise over the entire health care system, and the extent to which various individuals and groups, including nurses, will be harmed (or perceive they will be harmed) by a proposed reform. Any policy involving redistribution of income will be opposed most vigorously by those affected most negatively. For example, early in the nurse practitioner movement, physicians were threatened by the advanced practice status of nurses and how it might influence their client base and income. The effective lobbying and influence of the American Medical Association (AMA), a powerful interest group, contributed to the state by state limitations placed on the practice of nurse practitioners. However, eleven states now grant nurse practitioners direct third-party reimbursement for their services without a physician as the primary care provider (Catalano, 2003).

The most significant obstacles to the passage of effective health care legislation today are special interest groups and partisan politics. A **special interest group** is a group of people who share a common goal and are politically active in attempting to influence policy makers to support that goal. Policy solutions are, more often than not, eliminated by the outcry of politically motivated special interest groups. These interest groups come in many forms, such as business groups, labor groups, neighborhood groups, minority groups, religious groups, environmental groups, and even nursing specialty groups. The AMA, the tobacco industry, and the National Rifle Association (NRA) constitute three of the most powerful special interest forces in the United States today. The AMA has a significant influence on delivery of health services; the tobacco industry continues to promote smoking and tobacco use; and the NRA fights against restrictions on ownership of guns, which contribute to high death and injury statistics. The impact these groups have on public policy decisions is immeasurable. Interest groups employ many tactics to influence policy decisions, including public hearings, campaigns, litigation, protest, public relations, and, especially, lobbying.

Similarly, there are agencies designed to promote the health of the American public. The American Public Health Association (APHA) guides public health advocacy. "APHA leaders, representatives and staff rely on APHA policies when they advocate on Capitol Hill, communicate with federal leaders, endorse legislation, form partnerships and promote research," ("APHA policies," 2002a). **Lobbying** is the process by which an individual or group acts on the behalf of others to influence specific decisions of policy makers, such as legislators. Many special interest groups and organizations employ one or more full-time lobbyists to represent their interests. In addition to attending hearings and giving public testimony, these individuals work behind the scenes to influence policy makers through informal sessions and written communications.

The four most powerful special interest groups in health care have been physicians, hospitals, insurance companies, and the drug industry (Lee & Estes, 2003). Physicians recognized the implications and consequences of health policy in relation to their profession decades ago and have become increasingly empowered through most of this century. Medicine's strong social and political influence is the result of many factors, among them a strong professional organization (the AMA), active political lobbying for their interests, and formation of strategic coalitions with respected individuals and scientific groups.

Hospitals have lost some of the power they had earlier in the 20th century as insurance companies have increased in power and influence as a special interest group. At the same time, increasing numbers of physicians have become associated with health maintenance organizations (HMOs), decreasing their direct influence in hospitals. The most significant impact on the influence of hospitals occurred with the implementation of the prospective payment system in the mid-1980s. Under this system, hospitals no longer were reimbursed for each day a client was hospitalized; instead, they were paid based on a client profile schedule. This gave hospitals an incentive to discharge clients quickly. This trend continues today, with clients recuperating at home, not in the hospital.

The influence of insurance companies rose steadily as the influence of the hospital declined, and it remains a formidable force today. Insurance companies direct the quality and quantity of client care in most instances. If Medicare and Medicaid are included in the "pool" of insurance companies, the influence is overwhelming.

The drug industry is a fourth special interest group. Billions of dollars are spent annually by drug companies to develop, test, and market new medications. The only way they can recover development costs and make a profit is to ensure that their products are sold to millions of clients. Therefore, they must convince primary care providers to prescribe new medications and must charge high prices for them. This cycle of development, marketing, and more development continues in a highly competitive marketplace, and the consumer is an unwitting victim. Elderly clients are most vulnerable to the spiraling costs of drugs, because many of them have fixed incomes and live with chronic illnesses that require long-term polypharmacy. Many elderly individuals take four, five, or six different medications, and some spend more than $1000 per month for their medications.

Policy, Politics, and Community Health Nursing

Health policy provides the conditions for empowering or disempowering certain groups in a variety of ways. Community health nurses must understand that power is an essential and primary concept inherent to all political and policy systems. A power base can be created through collaboration, cooperation, and communication (Catalano, 2003). To be politically effective, nurses must negotiate and compromise with other interest groups. By forming strong health care coalitions, nurses gain a stronger voice in policy decisions affecting them and their clients (see The Global Community).

Politics is inherent in any system in which resources are absolutely or relatively scarce and there are competing interests for those resources. **Politics** is an interactive process of influencing others to make decisions that favor (or at least do not threaten) a person's or group's chosen position and that allocate scarce resources to support that position (Mason, Leavitt & Chaffee, 2002). An example of nursing's increasing influence on federal research development and funding policies was the initial provision of $63,531,000 in funds for the NINR in 1994, compared with $3,467,000 for Allied Health.

The health care system is governed through complex interactions among various government representatives, health professionals, consumers, third-party payers, and employers who may not agree on one another's roles and jurisdictions in health care. These groups use politics to survive, as well as to pursue their respective health care interests and goals. There is no single source of governance or health policy, nor do the groups share a single set of values or goals. The health care system is a large bureaucracy with many different agendas. Politics in the government is demonstrated by the fact that literally thousands of legislative bills are drafted each year, yet only a few are ever signed into law and go on to influence citizens. Although the political system within a local community may be less formalized, it has a profound influence on the collective health and well-being of its residents.

In the past, public policy has restricted nurses primarily in three related ways—scope of practice limitations, exclusionary definitions, and limits on eligibility for reimbursement. Although most community health nursing services constitute primary care (first contact, continuous, comprehensive, and coordinated), most health policy definitions of primary care exclude community health nurses as providers of primary care. As a result, community health nurses are not paid directly for their services, may require physician supervision, and have client responsibilities that continually test their practice limits.

It is a major problem when health policy does not recognize nurses as providing reimbursable health care services or primary care services in any community context. The

THE GLOBAL COMMUNITY

Wakefield, M. (2002). What would Florence do? *Reflections on Nursing Leadership, 28*(4), 12–16, 37.

In this article, Dr. Mary Wakefield, a nurse and director of the Center for Rural Health, University of North Dakota, Grand Forks, and appointed to the Institute of Medicine's Committee on Quality of Health Care in America in 1999, discusses our present health care system. She mentions how clients benefit from the expertise of highly educated nurses, state-of-the-art technology, new and beneficial pharmaceuticals, and evidence-based practice. With Internet information reaching the most rural citizens in the country, consumers have access to telehealth technology that allows them to direct their own health. Yet there are vulnerabilities in the system, with compromised quality of care, decreasing access to care, especially among the chronically ill and the unemployed and underemployed, and difficulty in financing health care. Our advanced technology comes with a hefty price tag—increasing health care costs by 50%. Consumer health insurance premiums are rising and out-of-pocket health care expenses are increasing while more than 40 million Americans remain uninsured.

Nurses, the essential caregivers, are victims of poorly targeted cost-saving efforts that lead to burnout and compromised patient care. Practicing nurses are getting older and fewer are coming into the profession to replace those retiring. Schools of nursing are expensive for universities to fund, nursing faculty are greying, conse-

quently smaller numbers of students are coming into nursing. Legislation in 2002 increased funding for nursing education, but this effort alone is not going to make the changes needed. What can nurses do to change our expensive, yet at times inaccessible system when our own ranks are stretched to the maximum?

First, we must think creatively about using the visibility and public recognition of the nursing shortage to our advantage. We are being asked for our opinions and to speak on actions that need to be taken. We need to work across disciplines and initiate discussions with stakeholders to inform and chart a new course out of this current crisis of complex issues. Sigma Theta Tau International, as our nursing honor society, is an example of an ideal organization through which nurses can "cast a wide net of influence." We need to communicate with policy makers, using language that they can relate to, both individually and collectively. We need to engage our elected officials at local, state, and national levels and do what we do best—educate them. We need to be at the table with policy makers. If that isn't possible, we must write letters (to legislators and newspapers), support those legislators who deserve our support, invite policy makers to speak at nurse-based functions, and educate fellow nurses and other health care providers.

The crisis in our health care delivery system and the critical long-term shortage of nurses cannot be ignored. The status quo is unacceptable. It is not a condition Florence Nightingale would ignore—and we cannot afford to either.

---

exclusion of nurses, other than nurse practitioners, in primary care legislation and health policy statements practically eliminates the possibility of community health nurses receiving direct fees for services or even practicing without the supervision of a physician. Community health nurses should be one of the major sources of political influence (Gebbie, Wakefield, & Kerfoot, 2000), although many strong and well-organized forces resist nursing's direct involvement in the politics and policy making of health care.

In spite of health policy restrictions on reimbursement and scope of practice, the demand for community health nursing services is stronger than ever. Community health nursing has grown in part because many areas were abandoned or delegated by physicians, such as home- and community-based ambulatory care and primary care. In addition, the country's focus on homeland safety and preparation against terrorist activities has placed public health and the role of its nurses and other public health specialists in the forefront, such as with the administration of smallpox vaccinations and community bioterrorism plans in 2003. Finally, the importance and im-

pact of quality community health care is receiving the national and political focus it deserves. Competencies for health care practitioners were identified by the Pew Foundation more than a decade ago and included caring for the community's health, emphasizing primary care, expanding access to effective care, practicing prevention, involving clients and families in the decision-making process, promoting healthy lifestyles, understanding the role of the physical environment, accommodating expanded accountability, and participating in a racially and culturally diverse society. Clearly, these are competencies that have long been expected of—and practiced by—community health nurses.

Changes currently being considered in federal health policy may present an opportunity to revisit the issue of giving community health nurses authority consistent with their actual practice. One commonly stated goal of health care reform is to provide more services to more people at a lower cost. Community health nurses are well positioned to do just that.

At the global level, nurses from many different cultures and countries, who speak many different languages, are working in their respective communities to promote the public's health. Protocols developed by the World Health Organization (WHO) are used by health, social, and environmental team members who are working together. Politics is encountered on the international and regional levels, as well as within the WHO (see Chapter 21).

No practicing nurse can escape politics, whether it be in the workplace or in the context of local, state, or federal government. However, there are still many social and professional barriers that hinder nurses from becoming a unified, powerful political force. Fragmented communication patterns isolate individual nurses and prevent them from interacting on issues of health policy beyond their immediate work environment. Also, tight resources limit opportunities and strain nurse relationships in the workplace. In addition, prevailing methods of evaluation and reward in the workplace often undermine attempts to create an environment that is more conducive to political involvement of nurses beyond work issues. Finally, passivity and apathy are still problems within the profession. We *are* a profession and are responsible for ourselves and our practice. The nursing profession has gained a much stronger political voice in recent years, and nurses are learning to build strategic alliances and power bases. It is each nurse's responsibility to continue to value, support, and foster political thinking and behavior that enhances the profession and its future.

Community health nurses need to learn to manage their immediate work environment effectively and be able to participate in the context of a larger political system to support quality health care (Gebbie, Wakefield, Kerfoot, 2000). They must work to create a supportive health care culture that encourages frequent interaction among the various constituencies. Political involvement is an important means to achieve this goal. Community health nurses, like all people, may hold significantly different or conflicting opinions about theory, methods, and the direction of health care. These differences should be aired and debated to promote dialogue and creative solutions to health care problems. Community health nurses face an unparalleled opportunity to influence health policy through political involvement (Catalano, 2003).

Health Care Reform: Implications for Community Health

Although the U. S. health care system has made remarkable advances in practice, education, technology, and facilities over the past 50 years, these have come at a very high cost. Inflation, running to double digits in some years, has compounded the problem. The United States has been spending an extraordinary and disproportionate amount of its national income on health care. In 2002, 14% of the gross national product (GNP) was spent on health care (CT Coalition for Universal Health Care, 2003).

The most troubling issues about the health care delivery system are the growing aggregate cost and the seemingly disproportionate fraction of income that citizens pay for care, compared with those in other nations (Kovner & Jonas,

2002). According to virtually all measures, health care spending in the United States is the highest in the world. Annual health care expenses are greater than $1 trillion, and the President's proposed budget for 2003 called for $489 billion to fund the USDHHS (mainly Medicare, Medicaid, and the Children's Health Insurance Program [CHIP]), with $4.3 billion earmarked for bioterrorism spending ("Bioterrorism preparedness," 2002b).

Four major factors influence rising health care costs: general nationwide inflation, additional inflation specific to the health care industry, population growth, and changes in the nature and intensity of health care service delivery (Kovner & Jonas, 2002). Furthermore, the American public has expectations of the health care delivery system, nurtured by physicians over the years, that are unrealistic. When resources are finite in a health care system that focuses on secondary and tertiary prevention, the health of everyone cannot be optimized. However, community health's focus on primary prevention allows the limited resources to be available to those who need them.

There are also problems with accessibility of health care for certain segments of the population. Despite the enormous cost, approximately 44.3 million people lacked health insurance in 1998 (USDHHS, 2000). "Substantial disparities remain in health insurance coverage for certain populations. Among the non-elderly population, approximately 31% of Hispanic persons lacked coverage in 1997, a rate that is double the national average" (USDHHS, 2000, p. 1–9). One in four pregnant women receives no prenatal care, and only 45% and 53% of African-American and Hispanic elders, respectively, received influenza vaccinations (USDHHS, 2000). These figures suggest why the United States ranks among the highest in the industrialized world in infant mortality and 19th in the world in life expectancy for women (25th for men) (USDHHS, 2000). These statistics indicate that we are spending more money but getting less for the dollars spent.

President Clinton reenergized the health care debate by making health care reform a major theme of his 1992 presidential campaign and a primary goal of his first term in office. The proposed Clinton plan (the Health Security Act of 1993) was supposed to provide quality health care to everyone, regardless of ability to pay, while curbing the rise of medical costs. This legislation stirred national debate and controversy and ultimately was defeated in 1994. Between 2001 and 2003, President Bush considered proposals to add a drug benefit package to Medicare coverage, but partisan issues stalled its passage for years. However, in 2003 a compromise bill passed, and Medicare was reorganized to phase in a drug benefit between 2004 and 2006 that offsets medication costs for the neediest elders. These defeats and compromises demonstrate the complexities of health care reform at the federal level and the influence of partisan politics and special interests, including business, labor, the insurance industry, government, education, health care providers, and consumers. The failure of the 103rd Congress to pass the Health Security Act of 1993 and the stalling of pharmacy coverage for Medicare recipients sent signals to the health care industry that attempts to shape the health care system were not likely to come easily from the federal government. In his classic work, Starr (1982, p. 411) stated that health care reform will remain elusive "as long as opposing interests remain sufficiently strong to block almost any coherent course of action, conservative or progressive." Indeed, the fiscal need for health care reform may be the only force that can overcome such widespread resistance. The managed care movement that took the United States by storm in the 1990s and has continued into the new millennium has made profound changes in health care choices and accessibility for much of the population. These changes are not necessarily perceived as positive by the public. Although managed care attempts to contain costs while ensuring quality of care, it has not solved all of the problems. The health care system continues to cost too much and serve too few (see Voices from the Community).

One group with an enormous stake in health care reform is the disabled community. People with disabilities have significant health care needs, yet they are often uninsured or underinsured. This population includes people of all ages, with the greatest percentage being older than 65 years of age. In the current U. S. health system, enormous sums are spent— mostly out of pocket—on nursing homes and hospitals and much less on outpatient, home health, preventive care, or personal assistance services. It is the latter services that are most needed by the disabled community (see Chapter 34).

The challenge for U. S. health care reform in this new century is to reduce costs and increase accessibility. What is needed is a change from the present uncoordinated system to a consolidated health services delivery system that is accountable for costs, quality, and outcomes. Strategically, enhancing quality health care and reducing health care costs are the primary yardsticks for any health policy. Community health professionals must work to convince the political players that the health of the community is directly tied to quality health services, accessibility, and reasonable costs. As the need to restrain health care spending continues and health care dollars remain tight, beginning community health nurses (and others) must learn to integrate more fully the principles of community-based comprehensive care into the delivery of a more population-based approach to health care. Convincing policy makers to support these priorities is key to successful health care reform.

Political Empowerment and Professional Organizations

Politics is an inherent part of any professional organization's operations. It is through participation in organizations that many nurses develop and refine their political skills. A strong professional organization offers a more collective diversity and realistic forum for political issues and debate and for enhancing a nurse's visibility. Leaders of professional organizations sit on decision-making boards, influence public policy, and define priorities for their communities. Professional organizations become seats of political empowerment. **Political empowerment** is a conscious state in which an individual, group, or organization becomes recognizably influential in determining policy. The nurse who is visible and influential in professional organizations can raise community awareness and mobilize community support.

Professional organizations sometimes come under fire from people outside their membership. Some believe professional organizations are nothing more than efforts to carve out turf or claim dominion at the expense of others. Regardless of criticisms, professional organizations provide an essential mechanism for nurses to be collectively empowered. One nurse's opinions may not be recognized, nor would one nurse have the resources to promote a cause, but several thousand nurses together can do so. Effective nursing organizations monitor governmental regulations and lobby public officials on a regular basis. They also work together with other organizations to influence how the public views nursing, to set standards for nursing practice, and to participate in interdisciplinary efforts to shape public policy. An example is the document *Nursing's Agenda for Health Care Reform* (American Nurses Association [ANA], 1994), which was endorsed by more than 60 professional nursing organizations (Display 16–1). This proposal for reforms in the U. S. health care system, which was presented to legislators and many others, raised national consciousness and gave nurses a strong voice in shaping health reform. It became the policy statement of the nursing profession.

Personal politics, as much as any other factor, sharpens conflict among individual nurses and makes communication difficult. The pursuit of personal agendas over the common good results in a piecemeal approach to problems and promotes polarization. **Polarization** is the process by which a group is severely split into two or more factions over a political issue. Polarization can be so intense that people perceive one another as good or wicked depending on their ideological opinions. One of the primary goals of a professional nursing

VOICES FROM THE COMMUNITY

"The goal of managed care is to prevent and cure disease among members of the managed care plan. However, although the primary duty of managed care organizations is to their members, the organizations function within a larger community, and their operations must be consistent with public health goals. On the other hand, the goal of public health is to ensure the health of the community at large, and public health officials see their duty as promulgating this approach among all health care providers in the community."

(From Levi, J. [2000]. Managed care and public health. *American Journal of Public Health, 90*[12], 1823).

DISPLAY 16-1

Nursing's Agenda for Health Care Reform

This radical proposal called for "a new paradigm in U.S. health care delivery based upon a community and health model, a patient-focused system of care, patient self-determination with informed consent, a balance of health and illness services, a value on care and caring, and an expanded health care work force with direct consumer accessibility to professional nurses" (Betts, 1996, p. 4). In addition it called for "a federal standard of a uniform basic benefits package for all U.S. citizens and residents, financed through a public–private partnership, delivering a continuum of services, in convenient, accessible sites by a variety of qualified providers whose activities would balance services for health and illness while improving quality of care, which would be measured and openly reported" (Betts, 1996, p. 4).

association is to build a collective voice for nurses. A strong professional association limits polarization by developing the political skills of its members and ensuring that its structure and processes equitably meet the needs of its constituencies. This is the essence of politics: people must listen to one another, learn from others' viewpoints, and compromise to ensure the most positive outcomes from their endeavors.

Policy Systems and Policy Analysis

A **policy system** is an entity that receives input from external sources and has legal authority to generate or revise policies that govern or manage the constituents the system represents. Policy systems (eg, city and county governments) are interrelated, complex, and highly political and receive input from many sources (eg, voters, lobbyists, special interest groups, the media). Policy systems produce an output by generating policy, which in turn determines feedback for subsequent policy decisions. Their boundaries are defined by their legal authority to make only certain types of policy decisions at a particular level. Ideally, policy systems revise or make policy (output) based on comprehensive, accurate information (input) from a variety of sources, including feedback from all constituencies that are affected by the policy.

Policy analysis is the systematic identification of causes or consequences of policy and the factors that influence it (Kovner & Jonas, 2002). Often, nurses confuse policy advocacy with policy analysis. This mistake can be detrimental in community health nursing. Policy advocacy is subjective, whereas policy analysis should be objective. More importantly, policy analysis should come before policy advocacy.

Community health nurses need a simple policy analysis framework to be effective in any practice arena. Nurses use the framework to determine the intentions and possible ca-

pacity of policy systems governing their practice, as well as their community. This framework allows nurses to protect themselves and, more importantly, to protect clients, whether families or groups.

Nurses can take several approaches when analyzing a policy that affects the health of a community or target population. They can look at the reasons for policy formulation, the groups of people affected by the policy, or the policy's possible long-range consequences. When analyzing policy, nurses need to answer two general questions: (1) who benefits from this policy? and (2) who loses from this policy? Whether the policy should be advocated by the community as a whole depends on the degree to which the policy benefits the community without being detrimental to individuals or the country.

Figure 16–2 provides a simple model for studying health policy. If nurses know something about the forces shaping health policy and the policy process, they are in a better position to influence policy outcomes. The model identifies four major stages in the policy process: formulation, adoption, implementation, and evaluation. Policy formulation involves identifying goals, problems, and potential solutions. Policy adoption involves the authorized selection and specification of means to achieve goals, resolve problems, or both. Implementation follows adoption and occurs when the policy is put to use. Policy evaluation means comparing policy outcomes or effects with the intended or desired effects.

Stages 1 and 2: Policy Formulation and Adoption

Health policy formulation is the stage at which a policy is conceptualized and ultimately defined. It is approached in at least two ways. Most commonly, a health problem is identified, such as the increased infant mortality rate associated with teenage pregnancy, and health policy is developed to correct that particular problem. Another approach to policy formulation emphasizes health planning more than corrective actions, at least initially (Longest, 2002). This is a goal-oriented approach. Health goals and strategies for achieving the goals are identified. In this more proactive approach, resources may be created as well as allocated for health services. Although either approach to policy formulation may lead to the solution of a health problem, the goal-oriented approach is less reactive in that it does not require problem identification before the making of health policy.

The social and political conditions that affect policy formulation are limitless, but public need and public demand *should* be the strongest influences (Kovner & Jonas, 2002). Health care providers can stimulate a community to identify its health needs and demand health policies to fulfill its needs. During this process, the community health nurse should recognize that each community is unique, with its own mix of health services and public expectations.

Stage 3: Policy Implementation

Implementation of health policy occurs when an individual, group, or community puts the policy into use. It involves

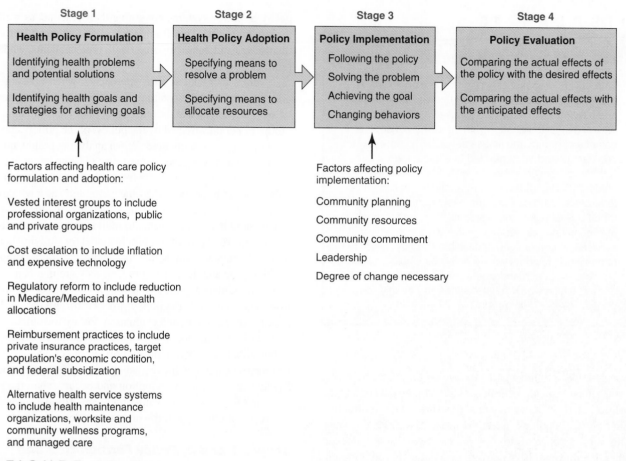

Stage 1	Stage 2	Stage 3	Stage 4
Health Policy Formulation Identifying health problems and potential solutions Identifying health goals and strategies for achieving goals	**Health Policy Adoption** Specifying means to resolve a problem Specifying means to allocate resources	**Policy Implementation** Following the policy Solving the problem Achieving the goal Changing behaviors	**Policy Evaluation** Comparing the actual effects of the policy with the desired effects Comparing the actual effects with the anticipated effects

Factors affecting health care policy formulation and adoption:

Vested interest groups to include professional organizations, public and private groups

Cost escalation to include inflation and expensive technology

Regulatory reform to include reduction in Medicare/Medicaid and health allocations

Reimbursement practices to include private insurance practices, target population's economic condition, and federal subsidization

Alternative health service systems to include health maintenance organizations, worksite and community wellness programs, and managed care

Factors affecting policy implementation:

Community planning

Community resources

Community commitment

Leadership

Degree of change necessary

FIGURE 16–2.   Policy analysis model. Policy analysis examines the entire process to determine (1) who benefits from the policy and (2) who loses from the policy.

overt behavior changes as the policy is put into nursing practice. The extent of compliance with a policy is the most direct measure of the policy's implementation (Harrington & Estes, 2001). *Noncompliance* refers to conscious or unconscious refusal to follow the policy directives. Community health nurses have always been health policy implementers and, recently, evaluators, regardless of whether these roles were consciously chosen.

Implementation of health policy is an essential part of effective, comprehensive client care for many documentable reasons. It should now be apparent that policies come in many forms and can have statutory or nonstatutory origins. Nurses are most cognizant of the latter in the form of procedure manuals and institutional guidelines. Communities are most aware of policies that limit or restructure their activities and growth, such as curfews and zoning regulations.

Once a health policy is written and adopted, its successful implementation depends heavily on the manipulation of many variables. For example, the implementation of day care standards depends, in part, on how they are interpreted and what resources are available to enforce them. The community health nurse as an implementer assesses the capacity of the community to formulate and define strategies that will enhance the community's compliance with the policy. This phase of policy analysis does not focus on the merits or short-

comings of the policy, in contrast to policy formulation, adoption, and evaluation.

Stage 4: Policy Evaluation

Comparing what a policy does with what it is supposed to do is *evaluation*. Evaluation of a policy should result in continuation of the policy in its original form, revision or modification of the policy, or termination of the policy. Laws and policies are created to express the collective and powerful interests of the political system that generated them (Kovner & Jonas, 2002; Longest, 2002). The need for a particular health policy may be temporary, but a policy is difficult to change once it is adopted and implemented. Once a policy system is in operation, vested interests evolve as a result and become political influences. These vested interests, under the guise of jobs, positions, titles, and wealth, are perceptibly jeopardized by any change in the health policy that helped create them. Hence, tradition in the form of old policies tends to prevail.

One form of policy evaluation examines the health outcomes that are believed to be attributable to the health policy. Indicators such as mortality and morbidity statistics are used. However, the manner in which the outcomes are defined and measured is highly political and is more subjective than many recognize. For example, mortality statistics are often treated as objective data, yet the way in which the data are collected and the formulas used can often render them more subjective. For example, if data regarding driving under the influence of alcohol or drugs are not included in data on deaths from motor vehicle crashes, or if smoking data are left out of data on deaths from lung cancers, policy decisions based on such data may be seriously misdirected.

Perhaps the major premise that should underlie policy evaluation is that the goal of health policy is to design a system wherein health services are equitably distributed and appropriate care is given to the right people at a reasonable cost. This premise leads to the following basic criteria for evaluation:

1. Are the health services appropriate and acceptable to the population?
2. Are the health services accessible (physically and financially)?
3. Are the health services comprehensive?
4. Is there continuity of care?
5. Is the quality of the services adequate?
6. Is the efficiency of the services adequate?
7. Is there an ongoing (formative) evaluation of the services?
8. Is there a final (summative) evaluation of the services?
9. Is appropriate action taken based on the findings of the evaluations?

Regardless of the factors that affect policy evaluation, continual comparison is necessary between what a community believes and wants in health care and what it is getting. Nurses have a responsibility to increase community awareness of health issues. They help the community make sure that its health needs are met through productive, desirable health policies.

COMMUNITY HEALTH ADVOCACY

The health of a nation stems from the health of its communities, and nurses have a solid tradition in serving the community's needs (Mason, Leavitt, & Chaffee, 2002). Nurses improve the quality of health services through community health advocacy. *Advocacy,* as defined in Chapter 3, refers to the community health nurse's role of pleading the cause or working on behalf of others. **Community health advocacy** refers to efforts aimed at creating awareness of and generating support for meeting the community's health needs. Both nurses and communities have a common goal—the best possible health services for all. The community health nurse helps communities achieve this goal by being politically active, as well as providing effective health programs. As an advocate, the nurse works directly with community constituencies to support vulnerable groups such as low-income families, children, and the elderly. For example, community health advocacy might mean creating public awareness of the needs of battered women and exerting pressure on policy makers to provide protective legislation, or it might mean demonstrating the effectiveness of early intervention. There is a need for nurses to have good data because they base their practice on evidence derived from well-conducted research.

This recognition of a community's rights in determining its health policies inherently involves conflict. Nurses as community advocates are under pressure to help the population define specific goals, to delegate or implement actions to achieve these goals, and to establish controls to see that a community moves toward these goals. Sometimes, specific health goals prove elusive or they have no validity save that they are agreed upon. One thing is certain—the goals, constraints, and consequences of actions are seldom known precisely at a community level.

Community health advocacy causes change to occur at the community level. The change can be through legislation at the local level (eg, traffic laws), the state level (eg, revision of a nurse practice act), or the federal level (eg, expansion of Medicaid coverage for a target population). The change can also be regulatory (eg, higher reimbursement for home health care services) or budgetary (eg, federal financing of training for nursing students). To be effective, community health nurses must serve as an impetus for change at the community level by increasing the community's awareness and supporting the community's decisions regarding health policies.

Determining a Community's Health Policy Needs

Data about a community's problems and needs are often incomplete. This results in ineffective policy decisions and usually occurs because people within a community allow others to determine policy for them instead of with them. If consultation with important policy implementers such as community leaders or community health nurses is not considered, ineffective health policy is likely to be enacted. Notable efforts to prevent these types of omissions in relation to health care policy have occurred in the formulation of the original *Healthy People* document, *Healthy People 2000: National Health Promotion and Disease Prevention Objectives* and in the current *Healthy People 2010* (U.S. Department of Health and Human Services, 1991, 2000). These documents were developed with input from numerous groups and individuals, among whom nurses were well represented. They propose a national strategy for improving the health of the United States over the decade of the 1990s and, in the newer document, the first decade in the new millennium.

It is essential that the community health nurse take an active role in identifying a community's health policy needs. The nurse serves as a facilitator in assessing the community's unique health care needs in relation to its existing health care policies. Legislation and policy must be reviewed from the community's viewpoint, as opposed to an individual's viewpoint. Both public health efforts and community health systems are confronted with conflicting interests when individual rights interfere with aggregate rights. However, the community health nurse's primary mission is to promote and preserve the health of populations or aggregates for the benefit of the entire community (see Research: Bridge to Practice).

To identify the health policy needs of a community requires an ongoing, comprehensive assessment of the com-

RESEARCH: BRIDGE TO PRACTICE

Raube, K. & Merrell, K. (1999). Maternal minimum-stay legislation: Cost and policy implications. *American Journal of Public Health, 89*(6), 922–923.

In the fall of 1996, President Clinton signed the Newborns' and Mothers' Health Protection Act, which requires insurers to cover hospitalization for a minimum period for mothers and newborns after delivery, namely 48 hours after normal vaginal deliveries and 96 hours after cesarean deliveries. Some attribute the swift adoption of federal and state minimum-stay laws, in part, to the absence of compelling data from researchers on the outcome of shorter stays. In the research literature, there is disagreement about the appropriate length of stay for healthy newborns and cost-effectiveness of longer stays.

In this light, the hospital discharge records for more than 167,000 women who gave birth in Illinois during a 12-month period before the new law was enacted were analyzed for client (maternal and infant) outcomes. Readmissions for women who gave birth and received a routine discharge were 1.1%; 2.1% of the newborns were readmitted during the first 2 weeks of life. Jaundice was the most common cause of newborn readmissions, accounting for more than one third. Using the data from this analysis to determine the percentage of total spending on maternal and infant admissions and readmissions, the net effect of the law ranges from a savings of just 0.1% to a significant cost savings of 20.2%.

Is this policy decision accomplishing what it intended to do—improve client outcomes and save money? The analysis has some important limitations in seeking answers to this question. This study gives no evidence of improved maternal and infant outcomes related to longer hospital care. There is no discussion on promising alternatives such as postdischarge home nursing visits. Public health nursing visits can be made to selected high-risk families on the day of or after discharge for infant and maternal assessment and teaching. Home health care visits can be made to monitor in-home phototherapy to treat newborn physiologic jaundice, once diagnosed by a primary health care provider in an outpatient setting, perhaps eliminating most of the infant readmissions related to jaundice.

This study may highlight that the rush to implement minimum-stay legislation is not accomplishing what it intended to do and is an expensive reaction to outcomes that were not well documented before more cost-effective models of care were tried.

munity, or what some policy analysts call a "community diagnosis." Chapter 18 identifies the dimensions or variables of a community that are important in making a community assessment. Research studies sometimes provide data for policy formulation. A study by Sargent and associates (1999) examined the association between state housing policy and lead poisoning in children in two census tracts in different states. They found that the percentage of children with lead poisoning was three times higher in Providence County, Rhode Island, than in Worcester County, Massachusetts. Although both counties had similar percentages of pre-1950s housing, the researchers concluded that Massachusetts policy, which requires lead paint abatement of children's homes and places liability for lead paint poisoning on property owners, contributed to substantially reduced childhood lead poisoning in that state. Such data can be used to influence policy formation in other parts of the country.

Community Organization for Political Action

Political action refers to actions taken by an individual or group to influence the political decisions of others toward issues or policies beneficial to the welfare of the individual or group. Organizing a particular community for political action involves taking the following steps:

1. In your role as the community health nurse, identify yourself as a potential community organizer. In this beginning step, nurses must perform a self-assessment in terms of what they have to offer the community.
2. Identify problems, concerns, and issues. This information should come from the community's perspective, not merely that of individuals. Such information may be obtained directly by conducting a survey in the community and indirectly by looking at vital statistics, voting practices, and the lifestyle of the community.
3. Assess the physical community. Physical environment can have a significant influence on a community. Characteristics of the location in which a population lives set the stage for particular health problems and practices. Information about the physical environment can be obtained from a variety of sources, such as a windshield survey (see Chapters 10 and 18).
4. Assess community strengths, resources, and interests. This information is an important indicator of the community's health potential and ability to organize for political action. In this step, the nurse identifies community skills and assesses community strengths and limitations.
5. Assess political influences in the community. Each community has its own power base and political structure. Gaining knowledge of community political systems enables the nurse to identify key people and operations that

are essential to the successful implementation of health goals. The community health perspective has a political advantage in terms of votes if the community is clearly defined and can be unified on a particular health issue.

6. Evaluate alternative courses of action. Community decision-making is facilitated when the community is well informed. The nurse can play an important role in the decision-making process by helping to identify possible outcomes and alternative courses of action to meet health goals. Each community, as well as each individual, has a different perspective, knowledge level, and ability to make changes. Decision-making is influenced by the impact the decision can have on the social systems of the community.

7. Redefine objectives, priorities, and the community health nurse's goals. After a careful assessment of the community's needs, the community health nurse must compare the existing programs and policies to the defined needs and goals. If an incongruent relationship does exist, plans must be made to redefine and reshape existing and future policy directions.

8. Develop a plan of action. Planning for an entire community requires the nurse to collaborate with other professionals and representatives of the community's social systems. Each member of the planning team is considered an equal resource, and each member's input is vital to the successful implementation of the plan. Target audiences include federal policy officials, state and local policy officials, community groups, the business community, professional groups, major institutions such as hospitals or universities, research organizations, advocacy groups, and the general public.

9. Implement the plan. Implementation first and foremost requires effective communication of the plan to those who have a vested interest in such a way that they will support it or at least not block it. One must figure out a way of reconciling differences that exist among those who (1) favor taking major action, but in different ways; (2) favor taking action, but in incremental steps; or (3) only see the necessity of correcting certain problem areas, such as allowing workers to transfer the same health insurance coverage when they change jobs. Implementation of a plan requires several important considerations: involvement by representatives of the population to be affected, proper timing, and preparedness. When implementing a community action plan, it is critical that the nurse is prepared and understands the common ground that racial and ethnic groups share without losing sight of their differences (Wolff, Young, & Maurana, 2001). Understanding the community's cultural values and media behavior is the first step to bridging cultural gaps. The second step is to choose the right messages. When the CDC tested public service announcements about AIDS through focus groups, it found that single-race panels and multicultural panels reacted quite differently. In other words, a multicultural panel's perspective is not complete in itself.

10. Evaluate the outcome of the planned action. Evaluation of a plan or program requires analysis of the observed outcomes based on the specific goals, objectives, and criteria that were adopted. Evaluation should be a continuous process that guides decision-making for the future.

THE LEGISLATIVE PROCESS AND INFLUENCING LEGISLATION

Theoretically, at the local level, health policies are guidelines for the implementation of health laws. A community's policy system exerts its control in distributing its health resources through its health policies. Sometimes, nurses and clients come to think of policies as statutes and therefore as difficult to change as law. In reality, community health policies are often an interpretation of health laws and, at best, serve as a strategy for implementing health laws, whether they be state or federal.

The nurse's role as an indirect care provider includes active involvement in the community's political arena (Des Jardin, 2001; Ray & Roberts, 2002). Nurses particularly have a responsibility to generate new ways of providing health care and to modify or improve existing health care. To influence and initiate changes in the health care system, the nurse needs to know about the legislative process and be directly involved in setting the health policy agenda for a community. The nurse also needs to know how to influence the passage of legislation or modify existing legislation, ideas promoted more than 20 years ago by Williams (1983). These skills are essential for all professional nurses because they are major ways that nurses can provide leadership in the improvement of health care.

How a Bill Becomes Law

All state governments and the three branches of the federal government make decisions that affect health care. All nurses have opportunities to provide input on the initiation, formulation, and revision of legislation at the local, state, and federal levels. Proposed drafts of bills originate from many places, because the sources of legislative ideas are relatively unlimited. An idea may be forwarded to a legislator by individuals, groups, government agencies, or other interested parties. The process can be initiated when a concerned citizen or group writes or talks to a legislator.

The legislative process is well defined and is guided by rules at all levels of government (U.S. House of Representatives, 1981). The process is similar at the state and federal levels, with the exception of some minor peculiarities. Public libraries have copies of a state's legislative process, or information may be obtained from the state's printing office.

There is a requirement that certain types of federal bills be initially considered in the House of Representatives, as opposed to the Senate. This may not be true at the state level, depending on the particular state's constitution. Once a senator or representative is found who is willing to author a bill, discussion takes place about what current law needs changing or what needs to be added to existing laws. When authoring a bill, a senator or representative consults with a legislative council. This council consists of legal specialists who assist legislators with the drafting of bills. The drafted bill is returned to its originator in the form of an "author copy." Content is carefully reviewed to ascertain that the bill does, in fact, state what it was intended to state.

A bill can be introduced at any time while the House is in session as long as the sponsoring representative has endorsed the bill and placed the proposal in the House's hopper. The procedure is more formal for the Senate, and any senator can postpone a bill by raising objections to it. All sponsored bills are assigned a legislative number and referred to committee. There are 16 standing committees of the Senate, 22 standing committees of the House of Representatives, and 5 joint committees. Most standing committees have two or more subcommittees.

Formal statements and details pertaining to each bill are published in the *Congressional Record* and printed for distribution. At the federal level, a bill may be considered at any time during the 2-year life of the Congress during which it was introduced.

The chairperson of the committee to which a bill has been referred must submit the bill to the appropriate subcommittee assigned to work on it within a specified time period, usually 2 weeks. The exception occurs when the majority of the committee members of the majority party vote to have the bill considered by full committee. Traditionally, many committees and subcommittees have had a policy that any member who insists on a committee hearing on a particular bill should have it. Standing committees must have regular meetings at least once per month while in session, and the chairperson may call additional meetings.

The legislators appointed to a committee conduct the hearing on a bill. At the federal level, a bill may have no hearings or several hearings at one time in different committees. At the federal level, the author of a bill is seldom a member of the committee hearing the bill, whereas at the state level, the bill's author may have connections not available to other legislators or the audience.

The committee chairperson selects individuals to present the first testimony at hearings. Individuals or representatives of groups who have requested to speak about the bill may or may not be called for testimony. Testimony can always be submitted in writing (Display 16–2). It is a frustrating political reality that one may go to committee hearings planning to speak or expecting to hear witnesses, only to find that the voting action was determined before the meeting. Astute individuals and groups not only monitor legislation but also tactfully lobby legislators before committee and subcommittee hearings.

After a bill has been studied and testimony heard, there are three types of recommendations the committee can make:

DISPLAY 16–2

How to Prepare for Public Testimony

If you provide testimony, it will be under the scrutiny of a House or Senate panel. Use this information to help present your testimony:

Be prepared!

Dress professionally.

Be familiar with your prepared remarks.

Have remarks printed in large, bold font.

Practice your remarks enough to be comfortably familiar with them.

Have copies of your remarks for others as needed.

Identify some questions that you may be asked, and think through your responses.

Prepare appropriate responses for when you do not know the answer to some questions.

Keep testimony brief, concise, and succinct. (Ray & Roberts, 2002)

(From Ray, M.M., & Roberts, S.C. [2002]. Nurses as lobbyists: Individual and collective strategies for influencing others. *AWHONN Lifelines, 6*[5], 438–442.)

---

(1) the committee approves the bill and is ready to forward it (due pass); (2) the committee revises the bill (due pass with amendments); (3) the committee refers the bill to another committee. If the bill is set aside by any committee, it will eventually die; in this way, committees can actually veto bills. Bills are usually revised and then forwarded or set aside. If a committee votes to pass a bill, a committee report is written that includes the bill's purpose, its scope, and the reasons for the committee's approval. Containing a section-by-section analysis of the bill, the committee's report is one of the most valuable sources of information regarding policy formulation and adoption.

Amendments to state bills and federal bills are handled differently. At the state level, the original bill retains its assigned number throughout the legislative process, regardless of amendments. At the federal level, amending occurs in "markup" sessions. A new bill is printed and reintroduced with a new number after each markup session. Obviously, it is more difficult to follow a bill through the federal process. Also, it should be noted that thousands of bills and joint resolutions are introduced each year, yet fewer than 10% are enacted as laws.

After committee action, the bill goes on the calendar and awaits a reading before the originating house. The house considers the bill, and, at this point, its author states reasons why the bill is needed and responds to questions. Only legislators of the house may speak at the floor vote. The house may pass the bill or defeat the bill at this third reading. If the author knows in advance that there are not enough votes for the bill's passage, he or she may take action to delay the vote. At this point, considerable compromises, negotiations, tradeoffs, and other strategies come into play. Success greatly depends on the author's power base and political maneuvering ability.

If a bill passes the first house, it is forwarded to the second house. For example, if a bill passes the Senate, it then goes to the House of Representatives. It enters as a new bill with an introduction and first reading. In the second house, the bill is again assigned to committee. The committee recommends due pass, due pass as amended, or amend and rerefer. After this committee's actions, the bill has a second reading on the floor of the second house. The third reading results in a floor vote. If any changes have been made to the bill by the second house, it is returned to the originating house for concurrence. If significant differences prevent concurrence, the bill is referred to a conference committee consisting of members from both houses.

The conference committee action is a very important step to which the public has no access. This committee determines which version of the bill, or compromise from both versions, will go forward in the conference report. At this point a great deal of political trading goes on, and major deals

are cut. After adoption by both houses, the bill is enrolled and goes to the President.

The President has three options: to sign, to hold, or to veto the bill. Signing the bill causes it to become law. Holding the bill without signing it may be done for timing or political reasons, but even without signing the bill becomes law after a delay of 10 days if Congress is still in session. Vetoing the bill sends it back to Congress with the President's objections attached. Congress can override this veto by a two-thirds majority vote in both houses; if the veto is overridden, the bill becomes law despite the President's objections.

Figure 16–3 outlines the process by which a bill becomes law. The fact remains that statutory law is only the beginning. The legislature enacts statutory law, which enables a government agency to administer the law by means of regulation. Law is measured only in court. There are few laws other than criminal law by which one may be cited for noncompliance without going through a report mechanism. The executive branch, as represented by a government agency, administers the law through regulation. In the case of registered nurses, it is the Board of Registered Nursing that ad-

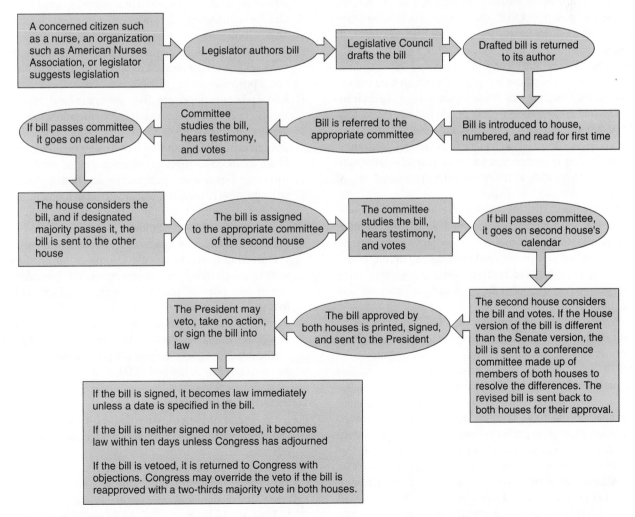

FIGURE 16–3.   This flow chart diagrams the legislative process through which a bill becomes a federal law.

ministers laws related to nursing education, licensure, and practice (most often called Nurse Practice Acts). This group is also accountable for disciplining registered nurses who do not meet the requirements of the law.

A Political Strategy for Nursing

Community health nursing must be clearly defined as having a necessary and integral role with clearcut responsibilities in the health care system. The role must be understood and appreciated by the public and legislators. The "selling" or marketing of the role can begin at the community or grassroots level but must also occur at the state and national levels. Ideas of opposition groups or interest groups with conflicting goals must be met with constructive criticism and compromise. During this process of defining and marketing nursing, nurses should present a positive and unified image to the public, legislators, and opposition groups (Mason, Leavitt & Chaffee, 2002).

Nursing, like all other professions, has internal struggles and disagreements, but these internal disagreements need to be downplayed in the political arena. Nursing needs to present a unified, professional influence. Nursing holds a great deal of power, but that power remains unexerted when various internal interests are polarized (Swansburg & Swansburg, 2002). A change in image is overdue. Nurses outnumber all other health care providers and are as well educated as most. They have enhanced the health care system throughout all its struggles. Nurses need to improve their individual and collective self-concept and learn to be personally and politically assertive (Mason, Leavitt & Chaffee, 2002). They must assist each other in achieving the highest possible levels of maturity, education, public service, and professionalism with a focus on growth (Swansburg & Swansburg, 2002).

Nurses must give one another credit for their accomplishments and learn to support and assist one another. Community health as a movement was created by nurses, yet many other groups are ready to take the credit. Many leaders in nursing have received little recognition from their peers. Nurses need their colleagues' respect and recognition.

A greater financial base for promoting nursing must be established. As with any investment, nurses must first invest money in their professional organizations, in supporting the work of nurse lobbyists, and in promoting research and dissemination of information about nursing's contributions, before expecting any returns. Also, it must be recognized there is an inherent risk to be taken by being politically involved before any short-term gains or, more importantly, long-term gains can be expected. Gains for clients and for the profession as a whole have been minimized because, until now, nurses have not taken an active enough role in policy decision-making and have not been unified in their political voice. Once the profession as a whole becomes empowered and assumes authority, autonomy, and recognition, individ-

ual nurses will be individually empowered to achieve their personal goals.

Individual Guidelines for Political Involvement

Community health nurses need to develop skill and experience to function effectively in the policy/political arena. Three major goals should be accomplished by the nurse as an individual in the political arena: generating support, creating legitimacy, and resolving conflicts. These goals are fulfilled when the community health nurse follows certain guidelines.

Generating Support

1. Present yourself well by promoting a positive and professional image. Dress and act accordingly.
2. Communicate your ideas effectively. Be knowledgeable and prepared, and state your position well. Use clear, concise, and understandable terms.
3. Learn the importance of socialization skills. Legislators attend local social and community functions for constituents. Invite a legislator to attend a social event at which a concern or issue can be discussed in a relaxed manner.
4. Get yourself known. Network both inside and outside the profession.
5. Recognize your skills to initiate, organize, and participate and use the nursing process. Apply these skills to the political process.
6. Know who your representatives are at the local, state, and federal levels and other groups and organizations that share the same legislative goals. Get in touch with them and keep them informed of health issues and their potential impact.
7. Make a concerted effort to influence a legislator to take a particular position on prospective legislation. Offer to write position papers. Become involved in lobbying, writing, and presenting testimony when legislators hold hearings on prospective legislation.
8. Support a candidate's campaign by donating money or by volunteering time and energy. Campaign for candidates who support nursing and community health, provided the rest of their political platform is agreeable. Get involved in campaigns early.
9. Join a **political action committee (PAC)**, which is formed by a group or organization to endorse and financially back its candidates and support the group's position on issues (Des Jardin, 2001; Ray & Roberts, 2002; Wakefield, 2002).

Creating Legitimacy

1. Keep abreast of current issues in health care and nursing and share information with your colleagues and elected officials.
2. Register to vote and encourage other nurses to do so. Hold a voter registration drive. Be sure to vote and communicate with legislators when a health issue surfaces.
3. Belong to and become involved in professional nursing organizations, such as the ANA and the National League

for Nursing, and outside professional organizations, such as the American Public Health Association and the American Hospital Association.

4. Become involved on committees and boards within your agency and community, such as boards of directors, state boards of registered nursing, health planning boards and committees, city planning boards, and the League of Women Voters.

5. Run for office. Start by running for an office at the local level, or, if you are known in your community, consider state or national office. Nurses need representation from nurses in the governmental system at all levels.

6. Become knowledgeable about the political process. Become familiar with the committees that handle health care legislation.

Resolving Conflict

1. Plan your strategies well. Be able and willing to negotiate and compromise with conflicting views or interest groups. However, always keep the goals of nursing as your primary concern over those of other professions.

2. Be proactive rather than reactive on health issues whenever possible. Anticipate health concerns and issues and accumulate resources to be better prepared to negotiate rather than simply react to poor policies.

3. Communicate with tact and respect. Each person has a right to his or her own beliefs. Avoid insults and overly aggressive behavior. Balance cooperation, collaboration, strength, and assertiveness. Be positive.

4. Have an open mind in considering issues. Every political position has both pros and cons and should be weighed carefully to avoid a narrow viewpoint. Know opposing viewpoints well and be prepared to provide accurate rebuttal information.

Communicating With Public Officials

One form of political participation is communication with legislators. The purpose of this contact is to sway the public official's view toward or against a specific bill or political position. The nurse can influence a legislator's opinion by means of oral and written communication through telephone calls, personal visits, telegrams, mailgrams, and letters. To be effective as a private citizen or as a member of a group, the nurse needs to know the process and appropriateness of each type of communication.

Written Communication

Legislators and government officials are more likely to be influenced by letters that express personal opinion and provide useful data than by form letters or mass telegrams. Form communications are tallied by an administrative assistant, but personal communication often reaches legislators directly. E-mail may be a legislator's or government official's preferred method of communication. A considerable amount of data convincingly presented is necessary to change a legislator's opinion (Display 16–3).

Personal Visits

An amazing number of bills are enacted with no input from constituents. Lobbyists exert great influence, as do other legislative colleagues and persons who use their physical proximity to a legislator or the persuasive tactic of trading favors to sway legislators' decisions.

Personal visits by nurses to their legislators can have a profound impact. Many legislators welcome additional expert information and respect the professional commitment involved in making the visit. Because legislators are very busy, with as little as 3 to 5 minutes for an interview, a visit will be more profitable if the nurse sends a one-page briefing sheet or letter before the meeting. Discussion with a legislator's staff members can also be worthwhile and may be the only route open. These individuals do the legislator's background research and help to develop the positions and language contained in the bills. Staff members are the gatekeepers and are often more knowledgeable than the legislator about the issues and have more time to discuss them.

Community health nurses, as advocates for a health issue, must know the opposition's arguments and be prepared to counter them. The prepared nurse is able to communicate far more effectively with the legislator and staff.

Attending Hearings and Providing Testimony

Community health nurses attending a legislative hearing can have considerable impact on a pending bill or proposed regulation. Singly or as an organized group, the nurses' physical presence communicates to legislators that they are concerned, informed, and ready to take action. Again, nurses need to be prepared in advance of the hearing. Resources such as a government relations committee or the state nurses' association can provide useful information on the issues surrounding the bill. Other existing communication networks, such as nurses involved in political action committees, can provide additional information.

After becoming versed in the particular topic of a bill, the community health nurse may want to provide testimony (see Display 16–2). Testimony may be given verbally at the time of a hearing, or it may be written in advance. The content differs little from what should be included in a letter, with the exception of supportive materials, such as actual research or survey data, and the style of presentation.

Party politics has a significant impact on the conduct of legislative business. At times, votes reflect party allegiance and platforms rather than individual legislators' responses to the information provided at the hearing or through constituents' letters. For this reason, the numbers of any given party in each house can make a considerable difference in passing bills. Organized lobbying groups can exert more pressure on legislators to override party decisions.

DISPLAY 16–3

Effective Communication With Legislators and Government Officials

Effective communication persuades with facts, logic, and brevity. It requires the nurse to be well prepared. In writing a public official, the following points should be considered:

1. A neat, clear, handwritten letter is acceptable, although a typewritten/computer-generated letter is preferable. Always address the letter appropriately with name and address on the letter and envelope and use appropriate salutations.

U.S. President

Name	The President
Address	The White House
	Washington, DC 20500
Salutation	Dear Mr. or Mrs. President:
Closing	Sincerely,

U.S. Senator

Name	The Honorable Jane Doe
Address	United States Senate
	Washington, DC 20510
Salutation	Dear Mr. or Ms. Doe:
Closing	Sincerely,

U. S. Congressperson

Name	The Honorable John Doe
Address	U.S. House of Representatives
	Washington, DC 20515
Salutation	Dear Representative/Congressperson Doe:
Closing	Sincerely,

U.S. Secretary of Health and Human Services

Name	The Honorable Jane Doe
Address	200 Independence Ave, SW
	Washington, DC 20201
Salutation	Dear Ms. Jane Doe:
Closing	Sincerely,

Governor

Name	The Governor
Address	State Capitol
	City, State, ZIP
Salutation	Dear Governor Doe:
Closing	Sincerely,

Mayor or City Council Member

Name	Mayor (or) Council Member
Address	City Hall
	City, State, ZIP
Salutation	Dear Mayor or Council Member:
Closing	Sincerely,

2. When a bill is in committee, correspond with all members of the committee. The content of the letter may be the same, but each letter should be individually typed or handwritten.
3. Plan the wording of your letter to make points concisely and succinctly. Letters are scanned before they are read. The following is a content outline of what is appropriate to include in the correspondence:
   a. One sentence that clearly states the issue
   b. One sentence that clearly states your individual or group position
   c. A statement that delineates the status of the proposed legislation (eg, where it is in the legislative process and what appears to be its disposition)
   d. A list of the reasons to support or oppose the pending legislation
      (1) Financial
      (2) Groups adversely affected
      (3) Weaknesses of opposing view
      (4) Specific benefits that override weaknesses of your view, benefits of the opposing view, or both
   e. Specific data that support these reasons
      (1) Dollar amounts
      (2) Number of groups affected and their names
      (3) Numbers within those groups
      (4) Delineation of processes, systems, equipment, and loopholes that have adverse or positive effects
   f. A clear, concise statement of the action that you want the legislator to take on the piece of legislation such as to vote for or against the legislation; meet with you or your organization; ask for additional information; convey contents of letter to interested, influential persons; provide you with those persons' names and titles so you can contact them; or other similar action.

Community health nurses who support a bill and wish to testify should contact the author of the bill; if opposed, they should notify the bill's author and the chairperson of the committee in which the bill is being heard. They must be sure they are working from or responding to the latest version of a bill (with amendments). Organized groups with registered lobbyists are most familiar with the process and may provide the best entree to committee hearings as a participant. It should be remembered that votes are counted by the bill's au-

thor before the committee meets, and, if the number is not sufficient for a due pass, there are many ways to postpone an official vote.

Running for Public Office or Seeking an Appointment

Perhaps running for public office or seeking an appointment is the best way for the community health nurse to express his or her convictions and effect change. The steps mentioned in the discussion of the three goals—generating support, creating legitimacy, and resolving conflict—can be used to place the nurse in the best position to be successful as a candidate for political office or appointment.

The local level is an appropriate beginning for most people just entering the political arena. The nurse should become aware of positions coming open and know where his or her expertise and interest can best be used. Most political positions have terms of office or term limits, after which the incumbent must run for the office again or step down. Good beginning positions might be in local educational systems as president of a parent-teachers association or as a member of a school board. There are positions on advisory boards, governing boards, and boards of directors for nonprofit organizations, such as the Epilepsy Foundation or the American Cancer Society. Those whose interests are with specific aggregates, health departments, acute-care facilities, or other health- and service-related organizations and who have strong connections in these settings should consider a board member position for an aggregate living center. After becoming well known for work at the local level, the nurse might consider other political offices, such as member of the board of education, county board of supervisors, city council member, or mayor. The election strategy needs to be well planned, the necessary funding organized, and the necessary paperwork filed. Of course, basic eligibility requirements of age, residency, and citizenship must be met. Major political parties provide training for potential candidates.

Once the nurse becomes known in the community, a state or national political office or appointment can be considered (ANA, 1993). Nurses and the community as a whole benefit by representation from nurses in all levels of the government. For community health nurses, the basic skills needed for aggregate nursing can carry over into the political arena. These skills include the ability to assess aggregate health needs, to communicate and collaborate effectively with others, to educate people regarding health promotion and disease prevention, to conduct and be a consumer of health research, to lead others and effect positive change, and to gain power and wield it effectively. Nurses can speak on issues with a strong voice and influence health and public policy. To do this, they must be prepared to meet the challenge of public service. Again, participation in the steps to meet the three goals mentioned earlier give nurses that preparation.

The need for nurses who are prepared to influence the system is even more urgent today, as health care policy reaches a crisis in terms of continued rising costs, personnel shortages, and limited access to services—problems not resolved by the managed care movement. The knowledge and experience gained in the political arena build confidence and skill for community health nurses to influence health policy and, ultimately, the public's health.

Nurses must depend on professional and political organizations and current literature for guidance in studying policy and becoming politically active. Many organizations are politically significant to community health nurses; a listing of some national level websites can be found at the end of this chapter. The chief objective is to provide directions in which political contacts and knowledge can be developed by the community health nurse.

SUMMARY

The need for health care reform has become critical as the costs of health care continue to rise. The United States spends a disproportionate percentage of the national budget on health care, yet there are still major segments of the population that do not have adequate access to quality health services. Because of these economic concerns, health care reform and policy making have become politically charged issues involving many groups and factions, including not only health care providers and health care professionals but also government, third-party payers, insurance companies, and others with vested interests.

Many people are just beginning to realize that health care is a business. It has always been a business—we are just more aware of it now because of scarcity of resources. Many believe that business interests and efforts to curb rising costs may divert public services away from community health issues such as preventive and primary care. Because community health nurses know community needs and the value of such services, they need to be a major force in the political arena where health policy decisions are being made. Community health nurses need to become politically aware and active to ensure quality health services—working as community health advocates. They must collaborate with community constituents and with nurses and other professionals to ensure the safety and well-being of groups and populations at risk.

Although nurses' influence has been limited in the past, they must learn how to empower their own profession, themselves, and the communities they work with by becoming politically active and aware. If they are to fulfill their mission of promoting, protecting, and preserving the health of aggregates, they must become policy makers as well as policy implementers. They must learn to use policy systems and the political process so that their voice is heard and they have influence in policy decision-making. They must learn to formulate, implement, and evaluate health policies. They must understand the legislative process and how to influence that process. The politically involved nurse should aim to accomplish three primary goals: (1) generating support for his or her views, by communicating ideas effectively and getting to know and influence representatives at local, state, and national levels; (2) creating professional legitimacy, by keeping abreast of current issues in health care and nursing and becoming involved in professional nursing organizations, community boards or committees, or political office at the local, state or national level; and (3) resolving conflict and being able to effectively negotiate and compromise.

Many resources and opportunities exist to help community health nurses study policy issues and make political contacts. Community health nurses must recognize societal changes and their potential impact on community health. They must also be able to analyze policy and become active in the political process to influence policy decisions that are in the community's best interests.

ACTIVITIES TO PROMOTE CRITICAL THINKING

1. Investigate a major health policy system in your community or state; discover how it works, and determine whether community health nurses are represented in this system. Areas to investigate include the boundaries of the system, the authority by which the system generates health policy, how the system receives input (formally and informally), resources the policy system uses and allocates to others, and the system's output over the past few years.

2. Describe a legislative bill related to community health at either the state or federal level and the issues involved in it. Identify who is sponsoring the bill, who is opposing it, and why. Determine who will be affected by the bill if it passes and in what ways they will be affected. Discuss what you, as a community health nurse, could do to be involved in this bill, and then develop a political action plan to support or oppose the bill. Write a letter to your legislator regarding your position.

3. Carefully review your own health care plan and determine whether you believe it is an adequate and equitable plan. Describe the plan and the issues involved in it. Include what health services are covered and who is authorized to provide services and receive direct reimbursement. Also determine who qualifies for the plan, who

is excluded, and what conditions can disqualify a person or a family once they have been covered by the plan. Compare the cost of this plan to one other plan.

4. Attend a meeting of a professional organization, board of directors, government agency, or council when a health policy or health care issue is on the agenda. Analyze the positions of the major interest groups involved and describe to what extent economics comes into the discussion. Describe who controls the discussion and how this is done.

5. Interview a health care administrator in your local area and determine this person's position on health care reform and the rationale for the position. Determine at what levels this administrator is politically active and involved in influencing policy.

6. Several Web sites for government agencies and organizations are shared in this chapter. Contact two or three of them. What resources can you get from these sites? How can you use the information as a community health nurse? Did these sites lead you to other sites? If they did, contact these additional sites and write down the additional Web site addresses in the margin of the chapter for future reference.

REFERENCES

American Nurses Association. (1993). *Positioned for power: Obtaining government appointments for nurses.* Washington, DC: Author.

American Nurses Association. (1994). *Nursing's agenda for health care reform.* Washington, DC: Author.

APHA policies can guide public health advocacy. (2002). *The Nation's Health, 5.*

Betts, V.T. (1996). Nursing's agenda for health care reform: Policy, politics, and power through professional leadership. (Politics, power, and practice). *Nursing Administration Quarterly, 20,* 1–9.

Bioterrorism preparedness key in 2003 budget proposal. (2002). *The Nation's Health, 1,* 11.

Catalano, J.T. (2003). *Nursing now: Today's issues, tomorrow's trends* (3rd ed.). Philadelphia: F.A. Davis.

CT Coalition for Universal Health Care. Available at: *http://cthealth.server101.com.* Accessed on March 17, 2004.

DeParle, J. (1999, August 29). Leftover money for welfare baffles or inspires states. *The New York Times,* pp. 1, 20–21.

Des Jardin, K. (2001). Political involvement in nursing: Politics, ethics, and strategic action. *AORN Journal, 74*(5), 614–627.

Fidler, D.P. (1999). *International law and infectious diseases.* Oxford: Clarendon Press.

Gebbie, K.M., Wakefield, M., & Korfoot, K. (2000). Nursing and health policy. *Journal of Nursing Scholarship, 32*(3), 307–315.

Harrington, C., & Estes, C.L. (2001). *Health policy: Crisis and reform in the U. S. health care delivery system* (3rd ed.). Boston: Jones & Bartlett.

Kovner, A. R., & Jonas, S. (2002). *Jonas and Kovner's health care delivery in the United States* (7th ed.). New York: Springer.

Late, M. (2002, August). Homeland department plan may undermine public health. *The Nation's Health*. Washington, DC: American Public Health Association.

Lee, P.R., & Estes, C.L. (Eds.). (2003). *The nation's health* (7th ed.). Boston: Jones & Bartlett.

Levi, J. (2000). Managed care and public health. *American Journal of Public Health, 90*(12), 1823–1824.

Longest, B.B. (2002). *Health policymaking in the United States* (3rd ed.). Chicago: Health Administration Press.

Mason, D.J., Leavitt, J.K., & Chaffee, M.W. (Eds.). (2002). *Policy and politics in nursing and health care* (4th ed.). Philadelphia: W.B. Saunders.

Raube, K., & Merrell, K. (1999). Maternal minimum-stay legislation: Cost and policy implications. *American Journal of Public Health, 89*(6), 922–923.

Ray, M.M., & Roberts, S.C. (2002). Nurses as lobbyists: Individual and collective strategies for influencing others. *AWHONN Lifelines, 6*(5), 438–442.

Sargent, J.D., Dalton, M., Demidenko, E., Simon, P., & Klein, R.Z. (1999). The association between state housing policy and lead poisoning in children. *American Journal of Public Health, 89*(11), 1690–1695.

Starr, P. (1982). *The social transformation of American medicine.* New York: Basic Books.

Swansburg, R., & Swansburg, R.C. (2002). *Management and leadership for nurse managers* (3rd ed.). Boston: Jones & Bartlett.

U. S. Department of Health and Human Services. (1991). *Healthy people 2000: National health promotion and disease prevention objectives* (S/N 017–001–00474–0). Washington, DC: U. S. Government Printing Office.

U. S. Department of Health and Human Services. (2000). *Healthy people 2010* (Conference ed., Vols. 1 & 2). Washington, DC: U.S. Government Printing Office.

U. S. House of Representatives. (1981). *Our American government: What is it? How does it function? 150 questions and answers.* (House Document No. 96–351). Washington, DC: U.S. Government Printing Office.

Wakefield, M. (2002). What would Florence do? *Reflections on Nursing Leadership, 28*(4), 12–16, 37.

Williams, C.A. (1983). Making things happen: Community health nursing and the policy arena. *Nursing Outlook, 31,* 225–228.

Wolff, M., Young, S., & Maurana, C.A. (2001). Community advocates in public housing. *American Journal of Public Health, 91*(12), 1972–1973.

SELECTED READINGS

Anderson, G., & Hussey, P.S. (2001). Comparing health system performance in OECD countries. *Health Affairs, 20,* 219–232.

American Public Health Association. (2000). *APHA advocates' handbook: A guide for effective public health advocacy.* Washington, DC: Author.

Artz, M. (2002). Log on to mobilize political power. *The American Journal of Nursing, 102*(9), 24.

Betts, V.T., & Cherry, B. (2002). Health policy and politics. In B. Cherry & S.R. Jacob (Eds.), *Contemporary nursing: Issues, trends, and management* (pp. 219–237). St. Louis: Mosby.

Gabel, S. (2001). *Leaders and healthcare organizational change: Art, politics and process.* Norwell, MA: Kluwer Plenum.

Hoffman, B. (2003). Health care reform and social movements in the United States. *American Journal of Public Health, 93*(1), 75–85.

Hooker, T., & Speisseger, L. (2002). *Public health: A legislator's guide.* Washington, DC: USDHHS Health Resources and Services Administration.

Institute for the Future. (2000). *Health and health care 2010: The forecast, the challenge.* San Francisco: Jossey-Bass.

Kealy, M., Kendig, S., Ray, M., Nolan, L., Percy-McDaniel, H., & Roberts, S. (2000). *AWHONN legislative handbook: How to get started.* Washington, DC: Association of Women's Health, Obstetric and Neonatal Nurses.

Maurana, C.A., & Rodney, M.M. (2000). Strategies for developing a successful community health advocate program. *Family Community Health, 23,* 40–49.

O'Rourke, T. (2002). Health care reform: Insights for health educators. *American Journal of Health Education, 33*(5), 297–300.

Sarikonda-Woitas, C., & Robinson, J.H. (2002). Ethical health care policy: Nursing's voice in allocation. *Nursing Administration Quarterly, 26*(4), 72–80.

Wallace, D.C. (2001). Health policy and planning. In J.L. Creasia & B. Parker, *The Bridge to Professional Nursing Practice* (3rd ed., pp. 203–227). St. Louis: Mosby.

Internet Resources

Agency for Health Care Research and Quality (AHCRQ): *http://www.ahcrq.gov/*

American Public Health Association (APHA): *http://www.apha.org*

The Association of Women's Health, Obstetric and Neonatal Nurses (AWHONN): *http://www.awhonn.org*

Thomas (U.S. Government Legislative Information): *http://www.thomas.loc.gov*

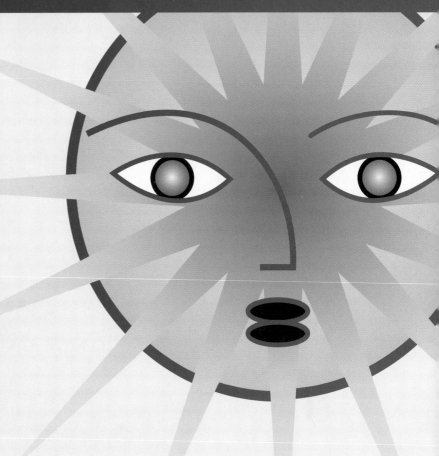

Community as Client

17

Theoretical Basis of Community Health Nursing

Key Terms

- Bioterrorism
- Community-oriented, population-focused care
- Genetic engineering
- Global economy
- Migration
- Model
- Relationship-based care
- Technology
- Tenet
- Theory

Learning Objectives

Upon mastery of this chapter, you should be able to:

- Discuss two essential characteristics of nursing service when a community is the client: community-oriented, population-focused care, and relationship-based care.

- Describe the contributions of at least five models of nursing practice to community health.

- Explain the benefits of applying eight tenets of public health nursing to community health nursing.

- Identify at least five social issues that influence contemporary community health nursing care.

When you open the door of a senior center where you will be promoting cardiovascular fitness, advocating for exercise equipment, and suggesting changes in the on-site meal program, how might theories of community health nursing contribute to your success? When you approach your city council about the need to increase staffing of public health services, what models of community health nursing practice might support your argument? What is meant by *theories, models,* and *tenets,* and what is their relevance to day-to-day community health nursing practice? These are the key issues explored in this chapter. First, however, we revisit some of the fundamental characteristics of community health nursing that we began to explore in Chapter 1.

WHEN THE CLIENT IS A COMMUNITY: CHARACTERISTICS OF COMMUNITY HEALTH NURSING PRACTICE

Nursing exists to address people's health care needs, and nurses fulfill this purpose through their work in various specialty areas. Specialties are characterized by the unit of care for which the specialty is responsible and by the goal of the specialty. Each specialty requires a particular area of knowledge and a set of skills for excellence in practice.

Community health nursing is a specialty in which the unit of care is a specific community or aggregate and the nurse has responsibility to promote group health. The goal of this specialty is health improvement of the community. The skills required for excellence in community health nursing practice include epidemiology, research, teaching, community organizing, and interpersonal relational care, as well as many others (see The Global Community).

In summary community health nursing is characterized by community-oriented, population-focused care and is based on interpersonal relationships. In the following sections, each of these characteristics is examined in more depth.

Community-Oriented, Population-Focused Care

As was discussed in Chapter 1, a *community* is a group of people who have some characteristics in common, are bounded by time, interact with one another, and feel a connection to one another. For example, members of an Internet-based support group for people with colitis are a community. They share similar experiences and concerns, and they often influence one another's behavior. For instance, they may recommend food choices or complementary therapies to one another. Members of a class of community health nursing students are also a community. Because they begin and end their studies in a particular month and year, they are bonded by time, and they certainly share certain values and feel a sense of connection to one another.

THE GLOBAL COMMUNITY

Nurses from Aga Khan University provided prenatal and postnatal checkups for women in urban slums in Karachi, Pakistan. After an analysis of the clinic's records, the nurses validated consistently high rates of anemia among these women. The nurses used this information to help develop and promote a program to reduce anemia that included screening all pregnant women and new mothers both at the clinic and in the community, providing iron prescriptions and pills at low cost, and teaching the women about the importance of iron intake, sources of iron-rich foods, how and when to take the pills, and normal side effects of iron supplementation. This program was successfully implemented and reduced anemia among pregnant women and new mothers so significantly that it became part of primary health care programs in other urban slum areas in Pakistan.

(Z. Ladhani, personal communication, July 20, 1999)

Community orientation is a process that is actively shaped by the unique experiences, knowledge, concerns, values, beliefs, and culture of a given community. For example, when an outbreak of hepatitis occurs, the community health nurse does more than simply treat infection in individuals. The nurse also

- Uses disease-investigation skills to locate possible sources of infection
- Determines how the community's knowledge, values, beliefs, and prior experiences with infectious disease may influence its interpretation of the disease, response to the outbreak, and treatment preferences
- Uses knowledge and suggestions gathered from the community to develop, in collaboration with other health professionals, a community-specific program to prevent future outbreaks

A community-oriented nurse who provides education about sexually transmitted diseases to a group of students at a Catholic college includes consideration of community values regarding sexual behavior. Similarly, a community-oriented nurse who provides nutritional counseling to a community of Hispanic seniors considers the meaning of food in this culture, the types of food most commonly consumed, and the cooking methods most commonly used.

A *population* is any group of people who share at least one characteristic, such as age, gender, race, a particular risk factor, or disease. Smokers and breast cancer survivors are two populations. The concept of population may also include delineation by time (eg, all children born in the year 2004). The nurse's place of employment commonly limits the population that the nurse serves. For example, a nurse who works for a county health department is limited professionally to caring for the population of that county.

A *population focus* implies that a nurse uses population-based skills such as epidemiology, research in community assessment, and community organizing as the basis for interventions. For example, a population-focused nurse employed by an autoworkers' union may study all cases of repetitive-use injury occurring in the auto industry in the United States in the past 5 years, develop a program for reducing repetitive-use injury, and lobby industry executives for adoption of the program.

Community-oriented, population-focused care employs population-based skills and is shaped by the characteristics and needs of a given community. Community health nurses provide community-oriented, population-focused care when they count and interview homeless people sleeping in a park and, based on these data, help develop a program to provide food, clothing, shelter, health care, and job training for this population.

Relationship-Based Care

Relationship-based care incorporates the value of establishing and maintaining a reciprocal, caring relationship with the community. It is a necessary and feasible aspect of community health nursing practice and is foundational to caring effectively for the community's health. A reciprocal, caring relationship with the community involves listening, participatory dialogue, and critical reflection, and it may also involve sociopolitical elements of practice such as advocacy, community empowerment, and movement to action (Shields & Lindsey, 1998).

Community health nurses provide relationship-based care when they meet regularly with groups of female inmates to learn about their physical and psychosocial health care needs and the needs of their families and then use the information gathered to advocate for this population with prison officials and other professionals in the community. A nurse also provides relationship-based care when working with parents of children with cancer, a psychologist, and a hospital chaplain to determine the needs of each family and to facilitate formation of a self-help group. In both these examples, community health nurses are working to establish and maintain ongoing relationships with other professionals in the community and with their communities of clients.

THEORIES AND MODELS FOR COMMUNITY HEALTH NURSING PRACTICE

A **theory** is a set of systematically interrelated concepts or hypotheses that seek to explain or predict phenomena. For example, the "big bang theory" seeks to explain the series of events that occurred during the earliest moments in the history of our universe. In contrast, a **model** is a description or analogy used as a pattern to enhance our understanding of something that is known. For example, the fluid mosaic model of the eucaryotic cell membrane is a verbal and visual description that enhances understanding of cell-membrane structure and function. Both theories and models have been developed to describe, clarify, and guide nursing practice. Three theories and seven models that have particular relevance to the practice of community health nursing are described here.

Nightingale's Theory of Environment

Florence Nightingale's environmental theory has great significance to nursing in general and to community health nursing specifically, because it focuses on preventive care for populations. While organizing and supervising a nursing service for soldiers in the Crimean War, Nightingale kept meticulous records. Her observations suggested that disease was more prevalent in poor environments and that health could be promoted by providing adequate ventilation, pure water, quiet, warmth, light, and cleanliness. The crux of her theory was that poor environmental conditions are bad for health and that good environmental conditions reduce disease (Nightingale, 1992).

There is no consensus of opinion on specific conditions that ensure people's health. Some people believe that, in addition to a clean environment, social services such as public transportation, education, and health care are necessary. In thinking about services that promote the health of communities, it is useful to consider

- Why these services were created
- Who benefits from the services
- Who pays for the services
- The cost to the people using the services
- The public's perception of the services

For example, if ventilation in a city's homeless shelter is inadequate, the community health nurse who plans to advocate for capital improvements to the shelter needs to consider who pays for the shelter as well as the public's perception of the shelter.

Orem's Self-Care Model

Dorothy Orem, a nurse administrator and educator, focused on the concept of *self-care*—learned, goal-oriented actions to preserve and promote life, health, and well-being. She described people who need nursing care as those who lack ability in self-care (Orem, 2001). If a demand for self-care exceeds the client's ability, the client experiences a self-care deficit and nursing intervention becomes appropriate. The goal of nursing action is to help people recognize their self-care demands and limitations and increase their self-care ability. Nursing care also functions to meet clients' self-care needs until they are able to care for themselves.

Orem further described three types of requirements that influence people's self-care abilities:

- Universal requirements, common to all human beings, are self-care activities essential to meet physiologic and psychosocial needs.
- Developmental requirements are activities necessary to help people progress developmentally.
- Health-deviation requirements are activities needed to help people deal with a diminished level of wellness.

Although Orem's theory focused primarily on individuals, it can be applied to community health nursing. Populations and communities can be considered to have a collective set of self-care actions and requirements that affect the well-being of the total group. If an aggregate's demands for self-care exceed its ability, the aggregate experiences a self-care deficit and community health nursing intervention is indicated. According to this theory, the goal of community health nursing is to promote a community's collective independence and self-care ability.

For example, a riverside community that ingests large quantities of fish contaminated with heavy metals might have self-care deficits related to the lack of awareness that eating local fish is dangerous and that some subpopulations such as pregnant women and young children are especially vulnerable. The community health nurse should help the community become aware of the risk and identify other food sources. The nurse should also help the community lobby government and industry to reduce pollution and clean up the river.

Neuman's Health Care Systems Model

Betty Neuman, a leader in mental health nursing and nursing education, proposed a systems model (Neuman, 1982; Neuman & Fawcett, 2002) that can be adapted to view clients as aggregates. In this model, people are seen as open systems that constantly and reciprocally interact with their environments. Each system is greater than the sum of its parts, and wellness exists when the parts of the system interact in harmony with each other and with the system's environment. Four sets of variables, or influences, make up each system's "whole." These are physiologic, psychological, sociocultural, and developmental variables. Given these variables, each system has a unique response to stressors and to those tension-producing stimuli that may cause disequilibrium or illness.

A system's response to stressors may be envisioned as a series of concentric circles (Fig. 17–1). In the center is a core of basic survival abilities, such as a community's ability to make the best use of its natural resources. Surrounding this core are three boundaries. The innermost boundary is a flexible line of resistance that encompasses internal defenses, such as a community's collective sense of responsibility for raising healthy children. The second boundary is the system's normal line of defense, such as a community's police force or voluntary fire brigade. The third boundary is a dynamic, flexible line of defense, a buffer that prevents stressors from invading the system's normal line of defense. An example is regular maintenance of a community's roads and bridges.

In Neuman's model, stressors can originate from the internal environment or the external environment. Examples of internal stressors include a high proportion of low-income residents or an inadequate system of water purification. External stressors might include natural disasters, war, or a downturn in the global economy. The role of community health nursing, then, is to assist communities in remaining stable within their environments.

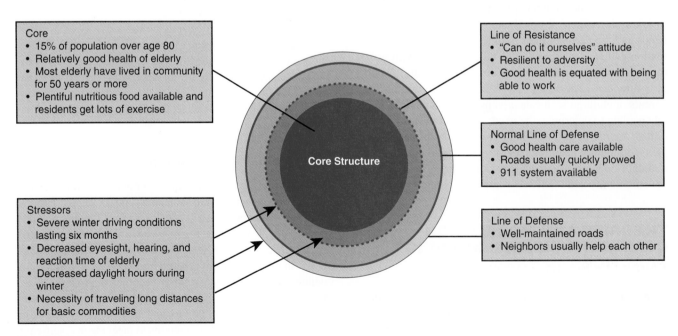

FIGURE 17–1.   Neuman's health care systems model applied to a rural county regarding traffic safety issues concerning the elderly. (Source: Derryl Block.)

Rogers' Model of the Science of Unitary Man

In 1970, Martha Rogers developed a nursing model based on systems theory. Her model emphasized that the whole is greater than the sum of its parts; that is, focusing on the parts of a community, such as its health care or housing, does not provide an adequate picture of its totality.

Rogers also incorporated developmental theory into her model by describing the development of "unitary" persons or systems according to three principles: (1) life proceeds in one direction along a rhythmic spiral, (2) energy fields follow a certain wave pattern and organization, and (3) human and environmental energy fields interact simultaneously and mutually, leading to completeness and unity (Rogers, 1990). Using this model, the community health nurse can focus on community–environment interaction; the community functions interdependently with others and with the environment. The goal of community health nursing is to promote holistic and healthful community–environment interaction.

Parse's Human Becoming Theory

Rosemarie Rizzo Parse developed her theory, initially called the "man-living-health" theory, in 1981. In 1992, she changed the name to "Human Becoming Theory" to better reflect all people. The theory posits quality of life from each person's own perspective as the goal of nursing practice. The theory is structured around three themes (Parse, 1981, 1998):

Meaning—people coparticipate in creating what is real for them through self-expression by living their values in their own chosen way.

Rhythmicity—the unity of life encompassess apparent opposites in rhythmic patterns of relating. While living moment-to-moment, one shows and does not show the self, creating both opportunities and limitations that emerge as moving with and moving apart from others.

Trancendence—moving beyond the moment and forging a unique personal path for oneself in the midst of ambiguity and continuous change.

These three themes apply effectively to the community. The nurse must know what the community means to its inhabitants, identify and be aware of the rhythmicity of the people as attempts are made to create positive health changes in the community, and realize the trancendence that occurs when people work in the presence of ambiguity and continuous change, characteristics inherent in a community. Use of this model as a guide enhances the ability of community members to work together to accomplish identified goals.

Pender's Health Promotion Model

As we have noted throughout this text, health promotion is a priority in community health nursing practice. Pender defined health promotion as actions that are directed toward increasing the level of well-being and self-actualization in individuals or groups (Pender, Murdaugh, & Parsons, 2002). It is a proactive set of behaviors in which people act on their environment rather than react to stressors arising from the environment.

Pender's *health promotion model* seeks to explain this proactive behavior. The model, based on social learning theory, stresses cognitive processes that help regulate behavior such as perceptions people have that directly influence their motivation to begin or continue health-promoting behaviors. These include, for example, perceptions of the following: control of health, health status, benefits of health-promoting behaviors, and barriers to engaging in health-promoting behaviors.

Five types of modifying factors influence people's perceptions about pursuing health-promoting behaviors:
- Demographic factors, such as age and race
- Biologic characteristics, such as height and weight
- Interpersonal influences, such as the expectations of others
- Situational factors, such as availability of healthful foods
- Behavioral factors, such as stress-coping patterns

Using Pender's model, a community health nurse might interview the residents of a low-income housing project to determine their perceptions about improving health and safety. Research of demographic, situational, and other factors that might influence the residents' motivation and ability to change their circumstances could then be conducted. Pender's model is further discussed in relation to client education in Chapter 12.

Roy's Adaptation Model

Sister Callista Roy's model describes people as open and adaptive systems that experience stimuli, develop coping mechanisms, and produce responses. These responses, which may be adaptive or maladaptive, provide feedback that influences the amount and type of stimuli that can be handled in the future (Andrews & Roy, 1991; Roy & Andrews, 1999).

Roy describes two response processes. In the *regulator* process, stimuli from the internal and external environments are received, and this combination of information is then processed to produce a response. In the *cognator* process, perceptions, learning, judgment, and emotion are considered in formulating a response to stimuli. For example, a regulator process might begin with a community's desire to keep adolescents from smoking (internal stimulus) and new state regulations prohibiting the sale of tobacco products to minors (external stimulus). These combined stimuli lead to a city ordinance that prevents the sale of cigarettes to minors (coping mechanism), resulting in reduced levels of smoking (response) among this population. A cognator process might begin with the stimulus of heavy rainfall in a riverside community. Residents' perceptions of the amount of rainfall, memories of past floods, insights about preventing or managing floods, and the level of anxiety all contribute to their plans for evacuation, sandbagging, and soliciting county or state assistance.

In applying Roy's model to community health nursing, it is important to remember that communities are made up of many parts and are influenced by many variables. The community's collective adaptation level is constantly changing. The community health nurse must assess a community's coping mechanisms and help its members use these collective abilities in adapting to challenges. For example, if a community is doing nothing to respond to the increased number of teen pregnancies, nursing actions can be designed to encourage more healthful coping patterns and adaptive responses.

Milio's Framework for Prevention

Nancy Milio, a nurse and leader in public health policy and public health education, developed a *Framework for Prevention* that includes concepts of community-oriented, population-focused care (Milio, 1981, 2001). Milio's basic treatise was that behavioral patterns of populations—and individuals who make up populations—are a result of habitual selection from limited choices. She challenged the common notion that a main determinant for unhealthful behavioral choice is lack of knowledge. Governmental and institutional policies, she said, set the range of options for personal choice. Milio's framework described a sometimes-neglected role of community health nursing—to examine the determinants of a community's health and attempt to influence those determinants through public policy.

Salmon White's Construct for Public Health Nursing

Marla Salmon White, a leader in public health nursing administration, nursing education, and public health policy in the United States, proposed a model to guide community health nursing practice. In "Construct for Public Health Nursing," Salmon White (1982) described public health as an organized societal effort to protect, promote, and restore the health of people, and public health nursing as focused on achieving and maintaining public health.

The model describes three practice priorities. Not surprisingly, these are prevention of disease and poor health, protection against disease and external agents, and promotion of health. There are three general categories of nursing intervention:

- Education directed toward voluntary change in the attitudes and behavior of the subjects
- Engineering directed at managing risk-related variables
- Enforcement directed at mandatory regulation to achieve better health

The scope of practice spans individual, family, community, and global care. Interventions target determinants in four categories: human/biologic, environmental, medical/technologic/organizational, and social. In Salmon White's view, a community health nurse attempting to reduce the transmission of tuberculosis should use education, engineering, and enforcement in working with the population of affected individuals and families. The nurse collaborates with the client community on a variety of interventions, from medications to teaching to social support, to prevent further disease in the community and to promote global health.

Minnesota Wheel—The Public Health Interventions Model

The Minnesota Department of Health, Division of Community Health Services, Public Health Nursing Section, has devised a model that depicts public health interventions and applications for public health practice. In the form of a wheel, the model shows 18 different interventions within three levels of public health practice: population-based community-focused practice, systems-focused practice, and individual-focused practice. The "Minnesota Wheel" (2001) is depicted in Figure 17–2. The wheel is a useful tool for community health nurses because it visually depicts the comprehensive list of interventions nurses must consider in the scope of practice. The model can assist the novice nurse as well as the expert practitioner.

TENETS OF PUBLIC HEALTH NURSING APPLIED TO COMMUNITY HEALTH NURSING

The word **tenet** stems from a Latin verb meaning "to hold," and can be defined as any principle or doctrine held as true. The goals of community health nursing to promote and protect the health of communities are facilitated by adhering to the eight tenets of public health nursing summarized in Display 17–1 (Quad Council, 1999).

Tenet 1: Use a Comprehensive and Systematic Process

The first tenet requires the use of a comprehensive and systematic process to assess population health, to plan or develop policies, and to ensure their implementation. A process is comprehensive when it considers all determinants of health. Additionally, when a sample of the population is being assessed or treated, a systematic process includes people who truly represent the entire population.

Tenet 2: Work in Partnership With the People

The second tenet requires the community health nurse to work in partnership with the community. The nurse and the community each bring their own values, beliefs, and expertise to the partnership. Policy development and assurance are more likely to be accepted and applied if there is mutual consideration of and respect for these elements. Developed policies need to be communicated in language that reflects an understanding of the community. For these reasons, an essential part of establishing a partnership with a community is getting to know the members and groups within that community.

Public Health Interventions
Applications for Public Health Nursing Practice

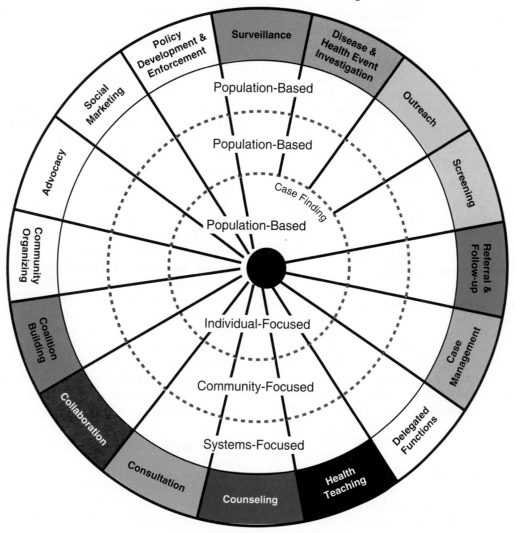

FIGURE 17–2.   The Minnesota Wheel. (Source: Minnesota Department of Health, Division of Community Health Services, Public Health Nursing Section.)

DISPLAY 17–1

Tenets of Public Health Applied to Community Health Nursing

1. The process of population-based assessment, policy development, and assurance is systematic and comprehensive.
2. In all processes, partnerships with representatives of the people are essential.
3. Primary prevention is given priority.
4. Creating healthful environmental, social, and economic conditions in which people can thrive guides selection of intervention strategies.
5. The practice incorporates an obligation to actively reach out to all who might benefit from an intervention or service.
6. The dominant concern and obligation are for the greater good of all of the people or the population as a whole.
7. The stewardship and allocation of available resources are supported to gain the maximum population health benefit from the use of those resources.
8. The health of the people is most effectively promoted and protected through collaboration with members of other professions and organizations.

(Quad Council of Public Health Nursing Organizations [1999]. *Scope and standards of public health nursing practice.* Washington, DC: American Nurses Publishing.)

Tenet 3: Focus on Primary Prevention

The third tenet of public health nursing underscores the importance of primary prevention in promoting the health of people. Most fields of medicine, including acute care nursing, are primarily concerned with illness, and with efforts to prevent complications from and reoccurrence of the illness. In contrast, community health nursing has an obligation to prevent health problems and to promote a higher level of wellness. Community health nurses take initiative to seek out high-risk groups, potential health problems, and situations that contribute to health problems. They then institute preventive programs. For example, if community assessment revealed a large number of new mothers with postpartum depression, community health nurses would address secondary prevention by establishing mental health programs. Equally as important, they would attend to primary prevention by working to change the conditions in the community that increase the risk for postpartum depression.

Tenet 4: Promote a Healthful Environment

The fourth tenet recognizes the importance of ensuring that people live in conditions conducive to health. Therefore, it is aligned with Nightingale's environmental theory of health. People are less likely to be healthy if they live in a community with high unemployment, crowded housing, and dirty air, or where it is difficult to obtain inexpensive, healthful food. They are also less likely to be healthy if the community's norms include acceptance or even encouragement of activities such as smoking, binge drinking, drug use, or unsafe sex. To change these conditions requires commitment, perseverance, patience, resourcefulness, and a long-range view (see Research: Bridge to Practice).

Tenet 5: Target All Who Might Benefit

The fifth tenet involves outreach strategies to meet the obligation to serve all people who might benefit from an intervention. This tenet requires that the nurse examine policies or programs to determine whether they are accessible and acceptable to the entire population in need and advocate for change if necessary.

In one community, families with young children had a high (80%) rate of compliance with regulations requiring the use of infant and toddler car seats, but assessment revealed that more than 90% of the seats were being used incorrectly. For example, the harness straps were too loose, the seats were not properly installed, or the model used had been recalled because of safety problems. A coalition of community health nurses and law enforcement officials implemented a summer-long, monthly car seat checkup service in the parking lot of a local mall and advertised the service in a media campaign. In evaluating the program, the coalition acknowledged that the campaign had not affected the transport of children born after the intervention period had expired, nor residents who were out of town for the summer, nor had it increased the knowledge of car seat safety among expectant parents or the community in general.

The questions in Display 17–2 can help the nurse evaluate a planned program's success in reaching people who might benefit. These questions should guide the design, implementation, and evaluation of outreach strategies.

Tenet 6: Give Priority to Community Needs

The sixth tenet deals with the ethical obligation of the community health nurse to give priority to the needs and preferences of the whole community over those of one individual.

RESEARCH: BRIDGE TO PRACTICE

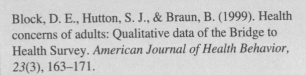

Block, D. E., Hutton, S. J., & Braun, B. (1999). Health concerns of adults: Qualitative data of the Bridge to Health Survey. *American Journal of Health Behavior, 23*(3), 163–171.

In a mostly rural upper Midwest region, community health nurses and other health care workers conducted a survey of more than 2000 randomly selected adult residents about their perceptions of the most important health concerns of their community and of the state and nation. The issue of insurance costs and access to insurance was most commonly mentioned, with 43% of the residents citing it as a most important state/national health concern and 21% of residents naming it as a most important local health concern. The high cost of health care was the next

most commonly mentioned issue. This included the high cost of medications and dental care and of caring for certain populations such as the elderly, poor, and single mothers. The high cost of care was mentioned by 30% of the residents as a most important state/national health concern and by 19% as a most important local concern.

These results were surprising because many community health nurses in the region expected more residents to mention issues of tobacco, cancer, heart disease, and protecting the environment.

- How do the Tenets of Public Health Nursing Applied to Community Health Nursing pertain to this survey?
- How might the community health nurses use the results of this survey to help plan population-focused care for this region?

D I S P L A Y   1 7 – 2

Determining Whether Programs Serve Intended Populations

- Is the service offered in a manner that encourages utilization?
    - Are the services located conveniently?
    - Do the hours of the service fit with the work or school life of the people?
    - Are the services offered in a manner that is respectful of the values, beliefs, mores, and traditions of the people?
    - What kind of marketing strategies have been used to inform the people of the service?
- What is the satisfaction level of users of the service?
- Why are some people not using services?

This means that the nurse must consider interventions that will lead to the greatest good for the most people. For example, programs that make mammograms for early detection of breast cancer available to all women regardless of income level are given priority over those that provide bone marrow transplantation for women with advanced metastatic breast cancer.

Tenet 7: Promote Optimum Allocation of Resources

The seventh tenet addresses resource-allocation decisions. In most communities, the available resources are not sufficient to meet all the needs of all the people. The nurse must ensure that the community is using limited resources in ways that lead to the greatest improvement in health. To promote optimum allocation of resources, the nurse must

- Know the latest research on the effectiveness of various programs in addressing needs
- Collect information about the short- and long-term costs of programs
- Evaluate existing programs and policies for ways to improve or discontinue them
- Communicate this information to community decision-makers so they can make resource-allocation decisions that are most likely to improve the community's health

Tenet 8: Collaborate with Others in the Community

The eighth tenet underlines the importance of collaboration with other nurses, health care providers, social workers, educators, spiritual leaders, business leaders, and government officials within the community. This interdisciplinary collaboration is essential to establish and maintain effective programs. Programs that are planned and implemented in isolation can lead to fragmentation, gaps, and overlaps in health services. For example, without collaboration, a well-child

clinic may be started in a community that already has a strong developmental screening program but does not have community prenatal services. Without collaboration, programs may also fail to be effective. For instance, a Saturday-morning cardiovascular fitness program designed without consultation with spiritual leaders may be totally ineffective in a devout Jewish community, where members devote Saturdays to religious observances.

SOCIETAL INFLUENCES ON COMMUNITY-ORIENTED, POPULATION-FOCUSED NURSING

Society is constantly changing. The community health nurse needs to stay abreast of these changes for several reasons.

Social changes influence a community's health. Community health nurses need to continually adapt their strategies to respond to changing conditions. For example, increased international air travel means increased levels of communicable disease in a small city with a new international airport. Community health nurses in this city must be proactive in developing strategies to control the spread of communicable disease.

Social changes affect the availability of resources necessary to ensure that effective intervention strategies are available. For example, a downturn in the stock market may prompt closure of a community business that once generously supported local community services.

Contemporary community health nurses must be especially aware of the mutual interaction between nursing and technology. The term **technology** refers to the application of science in order to change processes of production or industry. Ideally, technologic innovations lead to improvements in processes for creating products or services. The 20th century was filled with technologic innovations that simultaneously disrupted old patterns of production and created new opportunities to increase production. Two technologic changes that are highly relevant to contemporary community health nursing are communication technology and genetic engineering.

Communication Technology

Changes in communication technology present new opportunities and challenges for community-oriented, population-focused care. Because of advances in satellite and telecommunications chip technology, communication is possible anywhere in the world where resources are available to purchase equipment and services. This means that a community health nurse, whether working in the Australian outback or at a public health clinic in Anchorage, Alaska, can contact clients, consultants, and agencies worldwide, if resources are available to take advantage of the technologies.

In addition, Internet technology has made it possible to access local, state, national, and international data for community assessment, planning, and evaluation. Nurses who require data for a new intervention strategy, for example, can search the Internet for information from consumer groups, researchers, and other experts worldwide. To keep apprised of emerging issues and trends in public health, the nurse can join numerous Internet-based electronic discussion groups or listservs (electronic discussions distributed by way of e-mail). The challenge to the nurse is to manage the volume of information and to weigh its worth.

Health care consumers face similar opportunities and challenges. Most diseases and disabilities can be researched online; information is available on the Internet and consumers are increasingly searching the Net for health-related data. Certainly, the validity and reliability of information on the Internet vary widely. Research is needed to understand how people decide what information to use from the Internet, how they use it, and how its use affects their health. As health educators, community health nurses can provide guidelines to help people decide how to use health information found on the Internet (Display 17–3). Additionally, community health nurses need to participate in studies to determine whether regulation of health information on the Internet is feasible and desirable.

At the same time, community health nurses need to be actively involved in creating their own Internet sites to provide health information specific to their targeted communities. Such sites can include interactive chat sessions, listserv discussions, and asynchronous communications in which community health nurses interact with community members to improve their health (Goldsmith, 2001).

The Internet is a superb vehicle for rapidly tracing the international spread of infectious diseases. For example, the World Health Organization has developed an Internet site for countries to report epidemiologic and laboratory data on influenza. The Centers for Disease Control and Prevention (CDC) offers current data on communicable diseases through the online publication, *Morbidity and Mortality Weekly Report.*

Genetic Engineering

Genetic engineering can be defined as gene manipulation in a laboratory setting. The development of the field was made possible by the discovery of certain enzymes that can "cut" DNA from two or more different sources into pieces that can be recombined in a test tube. Gene manipulation also required the development of methods for inserting these recombinant DNA molecules into cells by the use of so-called *vectors* such as viruses.

Genetic engineering allows scientists to alter the herbicide-, pest-, and stress-resistance of crops and to increase the nutrition and attractiveness of the foods we eat. Genetic engineering also allows scientists to develop new kinds of medicines and to cure diseases by replacing absent or faulty genes. Mapping of the DNA sequence that makes up the "genetic blueprint" of human beings has provided new opportunities for protecting human health (Ellsworth & Manolio, 1999). In addition to increasing understanding of the contribution of genetic material to health and disease, it has created new opportunities for early identification, prevention, and treatment of people at risk for disease. For example, techniques for DNA screening of newborns allow early detection of risk for certain diseases and disabilities, thereby permitting early intervention.

Despite the enthusiasm of many groups, especially commercial concerns, genetic engineering has generated much controversy. The controversy emerges from a number of different concerns. One concern is the inability to know for certain the long-term consequences of genetic alteration of foods or organisms such as bacteria, insects, or human beings. For example, the release of a genetically altered weed or insect could be catastrophic if that weed or insect reproduces prolifically and damages the ecosystem. Fears of negative effects of engineered gene transfers between species in genetically engineered food include allergic reactions, spread of diseases across crop species, and emergence of new diseases because of unpredictable mutations in the genetic code.

The Human Genome Project, discussed in Chapter 1, has opened dramatic possibilites for health and well-being, as well as creating ethical challenges in the near future. The potential scientific capacity to alter methods of reproduction of humans raises concerns about creating unintended consequences for the human race. Another source of concern is that science is "playing God." For some people, the possibility of being able to select the gender, intelligence, or eye color of a child raises concerns about interfering with nature and creates conflict with religious or ethical views. In addition, genetic screening could be used to deny rights and opportunities to people. For example, someone who is found to carry a gene that increases the risk for heart disease might be denied health insurance coverage. Another source of concern

DISPLAY 17–3

Determining Worth of Health Information on the Internet

- What are the credentials and affiliation of the author?
- Is it easy to determine who is the publisher or sponsor of the web site? Evaluate how the publisher or sponsor might gain economically through your use of the information.
- Is the date of publication of the web site included? Is the information current?
- Are both sides of an issue described? Does the author discuss pros and cons of information presented?
- What references are included to substantiate the information in the article?

is the distrust many people have of government, large commercial enterprises, and the scientific community. Some people believe that they are not being told the truth about scientific or other issues. Because genetic alteration of food or humans can affect the survival of individuals, groups, or society as a whole, this distrust results in some strong opposition to any type of genetic engineering.

In dealing with these concerns, it is the community health nurse's responsibility to be aware of the latest scientific information when educating communities, so that the decisions made best fit the community's value system. Advocating for the highest scientific rigor in genetic engineering research is another important role of community health nurses. Community health nurses need to advocate for research that not only maps DNA but also identifies interventions that can change the outcome for people at risk for genetic disorders. Nurses need to balance what is good for the community as a whole against potential costs to people at risk, advocating for policies and regulations that ensure such a balance.

Global Economy

Hundreds of years ago, the economies of communities were largely local. If drought led to a reduction in crop yield in one region, only that region and perhaps its closest neighbors would be affected. Since World War II, however, there has been a consistent trend toward international trade, investment, travel, and ownership of information and ideas (Moller, 1999). This increasingly **global economy** is evidenced by the creation of the European Economic Community and passage of the North American Free Trade Agreement. It has contributed to a strong economy for many developed nations, including the United States, but has also led to increased instability of all economies as problems in markets in distant countries affect markets worldwide.

This interrelationship was made clear after the terrorist attacks in the United States on September 11, 2001. Key markets in the world experienced downturns, as did the economies of the United States and other nations. The United States and other countries are still experiencing the effects of that day, compounded by the effects of the "war on terrorism." The toll worldwide—a dramatic increase in refugees and poverty, and the long-term expense of infrastructure repair and redevelopment—is further evidence that national economies are interrelated. In addition, the international economy has been affected by the bankruptcy or closing of several major technology corporations in the United States. Corrupt management practices have forced companies across the country to close their doors, resulting in the loss of thousands of jobs and upheaval in the U.S. stock market, with subsequent effects on the entire international community.

A global economy also permits rich countries in need of skilled workers to recruit them from developing countries, causing a shortage of skilled labor in the countries that need it most. In countries able to recruit labor, the presence of new immigrant groups may be seen as a threat to the local culture or economy, causing an increase in ethnic, racial, and religious tensions (Moller, 1999). Even people with jobs that pay well may react negatively because they see their world changing and their own future as more uncertain. At the same time, when citizens in developing nations perceive their country or its citizens as suffering unjustly because of unfair economic changes, there may be an increase in nationalism and even international terrorism.

Finally, the economic trends of the late 20th century have contributed worldwide to greater disparities in wealth, health, and *relative poverty,* a measurement of an individual's income against the average for the society in which that individual lives (see What Do You Think?). In the United States, economic disparity has been fueled by increased demand for skilled workers and decreased demand for unskilled laborers. When the demand for skilled workers (eg, software engineers) exceeds the supply, these workers can demand increased wages, resulting ultimately in increased costs for housing, health care, products, and services, even for those unskilled laborers whose wages have decreased proportionately.

Another factor creating disparity in the United States has been the stock market. In the early 1990s, the "bull market" added tremendously to the wealth of those people already wealthy enough to invest, but left behind the people who were "just getting by." After the downslide of the stock market beginning in 2001, industries laid off skilled workers, and many people were out of work or underemployed for months or years. Older adults who thought their "nest egg" in the stock market would support them throughout retirement were forced to return to some form of work, because their investments were devalued by 50% or more. The entire economy became relatively stagnant, despite reductions of interest rates to historic lows. The low mortgage interest rates made new housing possible for many families, although the working poor still could not afford available homes. Wealthier families moved to more expensive homes, thereby maintaining or increasing the disparity between families in the United States.

Reducing income disparity and its numerous effects is a challenge for all people who work in service of humanity. Community health nurses have an obligation to read the latest research so that they can better understand the relationship of poverty to health. At the same time, they need to ad-

WHAT DO YOU THINK?

The world's 358 wealthiest people have a net worth equal to that of the world's 2.3 billion poorest people. How does this disparity in wealth affect the health of society?

(United Nations, 1996)

vocate for policies that will reduce adverse effects of poverty and income disparities. Chapter 32 addresses health issues related to poverty.

Migration

Migration is the act of moving from one region or country to another, either temporarily, seasonally, or permanently. Throughout history, people have migrated from place to place to seek improved opportunities or to escape intolerable conditions in their home countries. In the late 20th century and the early years of the 21st century, a dramatic increase occurred in the number of *refugees* who migrated from their homes to escape invasion, oppression, or persecution. We also saw an increased reliance on migrant farmworkers, people who move from one region to another seasonally, following the crops.

The health care needs of migrants and migrant refugees are enormous. Environmental factors are a primary reason for compromised health and include inadequate waste disposal, crowded and often unsanitary living conditions, lack of access to healthful foods, and air pollution from an increased concentration of vehicles used for moving refugees. The potential detriments to health associated with migration require that community health nurses ensure that surveillance systems able to detect emerging health problems are in place; programs to prevent health problems and treat existing conditions also need to be developed. The specific health care needs of migrant farmworkers are discussed in Chapter 33.

Terrorism and Bioterrorism

Terrorism is one way in which a small number of people who perceive that they have been unfairly treated can exert influence on a larger group or nation (Moller, 1999). Groups wishing to harm other countries need sophisticated skills and coordination for most conventional weapons. Terrorists may also use unconventional weapons when highly motivated such as flying planes into buildings, strapping bombs to their bodies, or hiding bombs in their shoes.

Some methods of bioterrorism may be even cheaper and easier to use. **Bioterrorism** is the use of living organisms, such as bacteria, viruses, or other organic materials, to harm or intimidate others, in order to achieve political ends. Some of the possible biologic agents used include *Bacillus anthracis*, smallpox virus, *Brucella,* and botulinum toxin (see Chapter 20).

Because of escalating concerns about bioterrorism, public health workers increasingly recognize the need for skills in dealing with a bioterrorist attack. They need to do the following (CDC, 2002):

- Ensure that adequate surveillance systems are in place for early detection
- Educate emergency and other health personnel about symptoms, treatment, and prevention of further spread
- Establish coordinated response plans with health and law-enforcement officials

Perhaps more importantly, community health nurses need to be involved in primary prevention of bioterrorism through advocating for the elimination of biologic weapons and addressing the root causes of terrorism, such as poverty, hunger, housing, clean water, and health care (Cohen, Gould, & Sidel, 1999).

Climate Changes

Climate changes can be considered societal changes because they may be influenced by economics. Since the Industrial Revolution, increased amounts of carbon dioxide, methane, and nitrous oxide created by manufacturing industries, automobile emissions, and consumer products have been introduced into the earth's atmosphere. These increases have contributed to climate changes that are expected to affect sea level; production of food, fiber, and medicines; and the spread of infectious diseases. Conversely, significant increases in fuel efficiency and efforts to reduce pollution could avoid millions of deaths around the world. Population-focused nurses need to educate the public about the potential dangers of continuing to contaminate the environment and to advocate for changes in public policy that reduce air and water contaminants. Chapter 10 explores health-related environmental issues in detail.

SUMMARY

Community health nursing is a community-oriented, population-focused nursing specialty that is based on interpersonal relationships. The unit of care is the community or population rather than the individual, and the goal is to promote healthy communities.

Theories and models of community health nursing aid the nurse in understanding the rationale behind community-oriented care. Florence Nightingale's environmental theory emphasizes the importance of improving environmental conditions to promote health. Orem's self-care model provides a framework, within which the community health nurse can promote a community's collective independence and self-care ability. Neuman's health care systems model describes the nurse's role as one of assisting clients to remain stable within their environment, whereas Rogers' model of the science of unitary man focuses on client–environment interaction and holistic health. Parse's Human Becoming Theory posits quality of life from each person's own perspective as the goal of nursing practice. Pender's model focuses on the promotion of health behaviors in people; the goal of nursing is to enhance the likelihood that people will engage in health-promoting behaviors by assessing and influencing perceptual and modifying factors. Roy's adaptation model describes the nurse's goal as one that promotes healthful coping mechanisms and adaptive responses to stressors. Milio's framework for prevention indicates that health-related behaviors are the result of habitual selection from limited choices. Salmon White's construct for public health nursing prescribes education, engineering, and enforcement with individuals, families, communities, and nations. Finally, the model used by the Minnesota Department of Health is presented in a "Wheel" that incorporates interventions and applications for public health nursing practice.

The eight tenets of public health nursing applied to community health nursing provide a framework within which the nurse works to promote and protect the health of populations. They emphasize the primacy of prevention, the need for outreach, and the importance of working in collaboration for the greatest good of the greatest number of people.

Nurses need to anticipate and adapt to societal changes in order to fulfill their mission of promoting the health of all people. Contemporary societal influences on community health nursing include communication technology, genetic engineering, the global economy, migration, terrorism, and climate changes.

ACTIVITIES TO PROMOTE CRITICAL THINKING

1. Interview a community health nursing director to determine what population-focused programs are offered in your locality. Explore nursing's role in the assessment, development, implementation, and evaluation of these programs. Discuss with the director how community health nurses might expand their population-focused interventions.

2. Describe a situation in community health nursing practice in which the use of an educational intervention would be most appropriate. Do the same with engineering and enforcement interventions. Discuss what made you match each situation with that intervention.

3. Assume you have been asked to make a home visit to a 75-year-old man, living alone, whose wife recently died. In addition to assessing his individual needs, what factors should you consider for assessment and intervention that would indicate an aggregate- or community-focused approach?

4. Select one of the societal influences on community or population. How would the theories or models for community health nursing practice that were discussed in this chapter guide your practice concerning that societal issue? Choose three models or theories to discuss.

5. Explore one of the societal influences on community or population using the Internet. Using the information in Display 17–3, try to determine the worth of the information available on several Internet sites.

REFERENCES

Andrews, H.A., & Roy, C. (1991). *The Roy adaptation model: The definitive statement*. Norwalk, CT: Appleton-Lange.

Block, D.E., Hutton, S.J., & Braun, B. (1999). Health concerns of adults: Qualitative data of the Bridge to Health Survey. *American Journal of Health Behavior, 23*(3), 163–171.

Centers for Disease Control and Prevention. (2002). *Overview: State and local preparedness—CDC's Bioterrorism Preparedness and Response Program*. Retrieved November 21, 2003, from *http://www.cdc.gov/od/oc/media/presskit/stateloc.htm*

Cohen, H.W., Gould, R.M., & Sidel, V.W. (1999). Bioterrorism initiatives: Public health in reverse? *American Journal of Public Health, 89*(11), 1629–1631.

Ellsworth, D.L., & Manolio, T.A. (1999). The emerging importance of genetics in epidemiologic research. I. Basic concepts in human genetics and laboratory technology. *Annals of Epidemiology, 9*(1), 1–16.

Goldsmith, J. (2001). How will the Internet change our health system? In E.C. Hein, *Nursing issues in the 21st century: Perspectives from the literature* (pp. 295–308). Philadelphia: Lippincott Williams & Wilkins.

Milio, N. (1981). *Promoting health through public policy*. Philadelphia: F.A. Davis.

Milio, N. (2001). *Public health in the market: Facing managed care, lean government, and health disparities*. Ann Arbor: University of Michigan Press.

Minnesota Wheel. (2001). *Public Health Interventions*. Minneapolis, MN: Minnesota Department of Health, Division of Commmunity Health Services, Public Health Nursing Section.

Moller, J.O. (1999). The growing challenge to internationalism. *The Futurist, 33*(3), 22–27.

Neuman, B. & Fawcett, J. (2002). *The Neuman systems model* (4th ed.). Upper Saddle River, NJ: Prentice Hall Health.

Neuman, B. (1982). *The Neuman systems model: Application to nursing education and practice*. Norwalk, CT: Appleton-Lange.

Nightingale, F. (1992). *Florence Nightingale's notes on nursing* [Edited with an introduction, notes, and guide to identification by V. Skretkowicz]. London: Scutari Press (Original work published in 1859).

Orem, D.E. (2001). *Nursing: Concepts of practice* (6th ed.). St Louis: Mosby.

Parse, R.R. (1981). *Man-living-health: A theory of nursing*. New York: Wiley & Sons.

Parse, R.R. (1998). *The human becoming school of thought: A perspective for nurses and other health professionals*. Thousand Oaks, CA: Sage.

Pender, N.J., Murdaugh, C.L., & Parsons, M.A. (2002). *Health promotion in nursing practice* (4th ed.). Norwalk, CT: Appleton-Lange.

Quad Council of Public Health Nursing Organization. (1999). *Scope and standards of public health nursing practice*. Washington, DC: American Nurses Publishing.

Rogers, M. (1990). Nursing: Science of unitary, irreducible human beings: Update 1990. In E.A.M. Barrett (Ed.). *Visions of Rogers' science-based nursing* (pp. 5–11). New York: National League for Nursing.

Roy, C., & Andrews, H.A. (1999). *The Roy adaptation model.* Stamford, CT: Appleton-Lange.

Salmon White, M.S. (1982). Construct for public health nursing. *Nursing Outlook, 30*(9), 527–530.

Shields, L.E., & Lindsey, A.E. (1998). Community health promotion nursing practice. *Advances in Nursing Science, 20*, 23–36.

SELECTED READINGS

American Nurses Association (2000). *Public health nursing: A partner for healthy populations.* Washington, D.C.: Author.

Boykin, A., & Schoenhover, S. (2001). *Nursing as caring: A model for transforming practice.* Sudbury, MA: Jones & Bartlett.

Clark, C.C. (2002). *Health promotion in communities: Holistic and wellness approaches.* New York: Springer Publishing Company.

Kenney, J.W. (2002). *Philosophical and theoretical perspectives for advanced nursing practice* (3rd ed.). Sudbury, MA: Jones & Bartlett.

Kim, H.S. (2000). *The nature of theoretical thinking in nursing* (2nd ed.). New York: Springer.

Kim, H.S., & Kollak, I. (2000). *Nursing theories: Conceptual and philosophical foundations.* New York: Springer.

Lee, P.R., & Estes, C.L. (2003). *The nation's health* (7th ed.). Sudbury, MA: Jones & Bartlett.

McCullough, C.S. (2001). *Creating responsive solutions to healthcare change.* New York: Springer.

Rappaport, J., & Seidman, E. (2000). *Handbook of community psychology.* Norwell, MA: Kluwer Plenum.

United Nations Development Programme. (1996). *Human development report.* New York: Oxford University Press.

United States Department of Health and Human Services (USDHHS). (2001). *Healthy people in healthy communities.* Washington, D.C.: U. S. Government Printing Office.

World Health Organization (WHO). (2002). *Healthy villages: A guide for communities and community health workers.* Geneva: Author.

Internet Resources

AACN's Institutional Data Systems and Research Center (IDS): *http://www.aacn.nche.edu/IDS/index.htm*

HealthWeb Nursing Page: *http://www.healthweb.org/ browse.cfm?subjectid=60*

Interagency Council on Information Resources for Nursing (ICIRN): *http://icirn.org*

National League for Nursing: *http://www.nln.org*

Nursing Theory and Theorists: *http://www.lib.flinders.edu.au/ resources/sub/healthsci/A-Zlist/nursingtheory.html*

18

The Community as Client: Assessment and Diagnosis

Key Terms

- Assets assessment
- Client myth
- Community as client
- Community collaboration
- Community diagnoses
- Community needs assessment
- Community subsystem assessment
- Comprehensive assessment
- Descriptive epidemiologic study
- Familiarization assessment
- Individualism
- Location myth
- Location variables
- Outcome criteria
- Population variables
- Problem-oriented assessment
- Skills myth
- Social class
- Social system variables
- Survey

Learning Objectives

Upon mastery of this chapter, you should be able to:

- Describe the meaning of community as client.
- Discuss how a key American value and three myths can undermine a nurses's intention to move beyond an individualistic focus to practice population-based community health nursing.
- Articulate specific considerations of each of the three dimensions of the community as client.
- Express the meaning and significance of community dynamics.
- Compare and contrast five types of community needs assessment.
- Discuss community needs assessment methods.
- Describe four sources of community data.
- Discuss the significance of formation of community diagnoses.
- Explain the characteristics of a healthy community.

C ommunity health nurses work with clients at several levels: as individuals, families, groups, subpopulations, populations, and communities. Table 18–1 presents the characteristics of these levels and describes typical nursing involvement at each.

Although community health nurses work at all six levels of practice, working with communities is a primary mission for two important reasons. First, the community directly influences the health of individuals, families, groups, subpopulations, and populations who are a part of it. For example, if a city fails to take aggressive action to stop air pollution, the health of all its citizens will be adversely affected. Second, provision of most health services occurs at the community level. Community agencies help develop specific health programs and disseminate health information to many types of groups and populations.

The community health nurse, then, must work with the community as the client (Clark, 2002). The **community as client** refers to the concept of a community-wide group of people as the focus of nursing service. Understanding the concept of the community as client is a prerequisite for effective service at every level of community nursing practice, as described in Chapter 17.

FACTORS OPPOSED TO THE CONCEPT OF COMMUNITY

A variety of factors can undermine a community health nurse's efforts to practice at the level of community. These include the American value of individualism and the myths that this value perpetuates about nursing practice.

The Value of Individualism

Every society has core values that give meaning to life and provide motivation for its people. The very existence of a society and its way of life depend on a deep commitment to these shared values. People learn them early in life and come to take for granted that these values determine the way things ought to be. Throughout the United States, individualism is one of these core values. **Individualism** refers to a belief that the interests of the individual are or ought to be paramount.

Almost every social observer who has written about American society has identified this value. "Protect the rights of the individual"; "Equal justice for all under the law"; "Life, liberty, and the pursuit of happiness for all individuals" are familiar cries. More than 65 years ago, the sociologist Robert Lynd described this value: "Individualism, 'the survival of the fittest,' is the law of nature and the secret of America's greatness; and restrictions on individual freedom are un-American and kill initiative" (Lynd, 1939, p. 60).

This basic premise underlies most American institutions. Individual effort and success are rewarded from kindergarten through graduate school by educational policies that evaluate and reward individual achievement. In the workplace, despite the recent focus on team building, individual awards, promotions, and bonuses are still the primary motivators. The criminal justice system punishes individual crimes far more harshly than corporate crimes: A woman who stole $5 in a Southern state was punished by several years in prison, whereas a large oil company that stole millions by overcharging customers paid a relatively small fine. Health care is also dominated by a commitment to the treatment of individuals. The vast majority of researchers, per-

T A B L E 18–1

Variations in Scope of Community Health Nursing Practice

	Client	Example	Health Characteristics	Nursing Assessment	Involvement
Individual	Individual	Kim Murphy	One person with various needs	Individual health assessment	A dyad; interaction with the individual
	Family	Murphy family (seven members)	A small group based on kin ties; specific roles	Family health assessment	Family visits; interaction with members as a group
	Group	Parenting group; Al-Anon club	Two or more people; face-to-face communication; inter-dependency	Assessment of group effectiveness in fulfilling its functions	Group participation; having a role in meetings
	Subpopulation	Unmarried pregnant adolescents in a school district	Large group sharing one or more characteristics (subset of a larger group)	Assessment of collective health problems and needs	Study of and planning for meeting specific health needs
	Population	Homeless people in Chicago	An aggregate of people who share one or more personal or environmental characteristics	Study of health needs and vital statistics	Membership in organizations such as a health planning council
Aggregate	Community	East Harlem, New York City; gay community in the United States	A large aggregate sharing geographic location or special interests	Study of community health characteristics and competence	Researching the community; planning and setting up services

sonnel, and health care institutions focus on the care of individual illness rather than promotion of community health.

This value profoundly influences the entire practice of nursing. All nurses are first educated to focus on the *individual* client in clinical nursing. In community health practice, the focus must shift to the community.

Myths Perpetuated by an Individualistic Focus

Three pervasive myths can hinder the nurse from focusing on aggregates or communities. They are the location myth, the skills myth, and the client myth.

Location Myth

The **location myth** defines community health nursing in terms of where it is practiced—in a specific setting or location such as outside the hospital. This myth silently influences nurses to define their practices based on the location of service rather than the nature of the service delivered. This myth supports the belief that community health nursing emphasizes care of individuals. Instead, community health nursing, past and present, focuses on assessing and treating the health needs of populations and aggregates wherever such groups are located—in the hospital, at home, in the workplace, or in the community (Clark, 2002; Williams, 1977).

Skills Myth

The **skills myth** states that community health nurses employ only the skills of basic clinical nursing when working with community clients. This myth leads many nurses to assume that their clinical skills are completely adequate for population-focused practice. Consequently, they may be unaware that sophisticated knowledge and competencies are required to define problems and develop solutions for populations (Williams, 1977). Community health nurses have always needed skills drawn from the public health sciences in measurement and analysis (epidemiology, environmental health, and biostatistics). Skills in social policy based on the history and philosophy of public health, and skills in management and organization for public health, are also necessary (Clark, 2002; Milbank Memorial Fund Commission, 1976). These skills have become more important as society and the environment have become more complex. At the baccalaureate level, nurses begin to build these skills; they strengthen and refine them at the masters and doctoral levels.

Client Myth

Community health nursing involves working with populations, but the **client myth** says that the primary clients are individuals and families. This myth can prevent the nurse from taking a broader focus on the health of aggregates and groups at risk, an approach that is central to community health nursing practice. It is population-focused practice that distinguishes community health nursing from other nursing specialties (American Public Health Association [APHA], 2003; Williams, 1977).

DIMENSIONS OF THE COMMUNITY AS CLIENT

Chapter 1 defined a *community* as having three features: (1) a location, (2) a population, and (3) a social system (Lynd, 1939). This three-dimensional view is especially appropriate for consideration of a local community, which can vary in location if the geographic boundaries are expanded or constricted (Fig. 18–1). For example, one might define the community of Seattle, Washington, as all the people living within the city limits, whereas the community of greater Seattle may include the city, its suburbs, and the other small towns located on its perimeter. To provide services or conduct a study, a community health nurse might want to restrict the size of the community to a specific district within Seattle. Although each of these three communities differs in size and geographic boundaries, they still share the three common denominators of an identified location, a population, and a social system. It is useful to think of these three dimensions of every community as providing a rough map that one can follow in assessing needs or planning for service provision. Further guidance in assessing the health of a community is provided in the Community Profile Inventory found in Tables 18–2, 18–3, and 18–4. In considering each dimension, one should pay particular attention to the questions that must be asked to assess the health of a community.

Location

Every physical community carries out its daily existence in a specific geographic location. The health of a community is affected by location, because placement of health services,

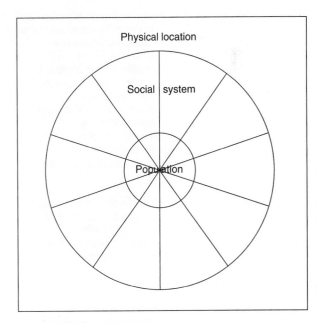

FIGURE 18–1. The community has (1) a physical location, represented here by the square boundary; (2) a population, shown here by the central circle; and (3) a social system, divided here into subsystems.

geographic features, climate, plants, animals, and the human-made environment are intrinsic to geographic location. The location of a community places it in an environment that offers resources and also poses threats (Skelly, et al., 2002; Neuman & Fawcett, 2001). The healthy community is one that makes wise use of its resources and is prepared to meet threats and dangers. In assessing the health of any community, it is necessary to collect information not only about variables specific to location but also about relationships between the community and its location. Do groups cooperate to identify threats? Do health agencies cooperate to prepare for an emergency such as a flood or earthquake? Does the community make certain that its members are given available information about resources and dangers? Table 18–2 describes the location perspective of the Community Profile Inventory, including the six **location variables**: community boundaries, location of health services, geographic features, climate, flora and fauna, and the human-made environment.

Community Boundaries

To talk about the community in any sense, one must first describe its boundaries (Shamansky & Pesznecker, 1981). Measurements of wellness and illness within a community depend on defining the outer geographic limits of the unit under con-

T A B L E 18–2

Community Profile Inventory: Location Perspective

Location Variables	Community Health Implications	Community Assessment Questions	Information Sources
			(For all—various Internet sites)
Boundary of community	Community boundaries serve as basis for measuring incidence of wellness and illness, and for determining spread of disease.	Where is the community located? What is its boundary? Is it a part of a larger community? What smaller communities does it include?	Atlas State maps County maps City maps Telephone book City directory Public library
Location of health services	Use of health services depends on availability and accessibility.	Where are the major health institutions located? What necessary health institutions are outside the community? Where are they?	Telephone book Chamber of commerce State health department County or local health departments Maps Public library
Geographic features	Injury, death, and destruction may be caused by floods, earthquakes, volcanoes, tornadoes, or hurricanes. Recreational opportunities at lakes, seashore, mountains promote health and fitness.	What major landforms are in or near the community? What geographic features pose possible threats? What geographic features offer opportunities for healthful activities?	Atlas Chamber of commerce Maps State health department Public library
Climate	Extremes of heat and cold affect health and illness. Extremes of temperature and precipitation may tax community's coping ability.	What are the average temperature and precipitation? What are the extremes? What climatic features affect health and fitness? Is the community prepared to cope with emergencies?	Weather atlas Chamber of commerce State health department Maps Local government Weather bureau Public library
Flora and fauna	Poisonous plants and disease-carrying animals can affect community health. Plants and animals offer resources as well as dangers.	What plants and animals pose possible threats to health?	State health department Poison control center Police department Emergency rooms Encyclopedia Public library
Human-made environment	All human influences on environment (housing, dams, farming, type of industry, chemical waste, air pollution, and so forth) can influence levels of community wellness.	What are the major industries? How have air, land, and water been affected by humans? What is the quality of housing? Do highways allow access to health institutions?	Chamber of commerce Local government City directory State health department University research reports Public library

sideration. Nurses need to be clear, for example, that a target community of the elderly includes a description of age and location (eg, all persons 65 years of age and older in a given city or county). Some communities are distinctly separate, such as an isolated rural town, whereas others are closely situated to one another, such as the suburbs of a large metropolis. Therefore, it is important for the nurse to know the nature of each location and explicitly define its boundary.

Location of Health Services

If the members of a town must travel 200 miles to the nearest clinic or dental office, the health of the community will be affected. When assessing a community, the community health nurse needs to identify the major health centers and know where they are located. For example, an alcoholism treatment center for indigent alcoholics was located 30 miles outside one city. This location presented transportation problems and profoundly affected the willingness of clients to voluntarily seek treatment and the length of time they remained at the center. If a well-baby clinic is located on the edge of a high-crime district, parents may be deterred from using it. It is often enlightening to plot the major health institutions, both inside and outside the community, on a map that shows their proximity and relation to the community as a whole.

Geographic Features

Communities have been constructed in every conceivable physical environment, and environment certainly can affect the health of a community (see Chapter 10). A healthy community is one that takes into consideration the geography of its location, identifies possible problems and likely resources, and responds in an adaptive fashion (Neuman & Fawcett, 2001). For example, both Anchorage, Alaska, and San Francisco, California, are located on a geologic fault line and subject to major earthquakes. In such places, the health of the community is determined, in part, by its preparedness for an earthquake and its ability to cope when such a crisis occurs. In Ontario, Canada, a series of lakes called the Lac la Croix is a valuable food resource for Ojibway Indian communities because they depend on fish from the lakes for their livelihood. Over the years, acid rain generated from coal-burning power plants in the United States and Canada has begun to affect the lakes and the fish, thus contaminating a major food supply of the Ojibway communities.

Climate

The climate also has a direct influence on the health of a community (Dixon, 2002; Kilbourne, 1998). When Buffalo, New York, is blanketed with deep winter snows, members of the community sometimes are immobilized for days. Deaths from coronary occlusion increase as people attempt to shovel their walks and uncover their cars. The intense summer heat of a location such as Phoenix, Arizona, can create other health problems. Asthma and other lung diseases are exacerbated in the Central Valley of California because the area is surrounded by mountains that create an air inversion, trap-

ping vehicle and agricultural byproducts and causing smog during many months of the year. Skin cancer is highest among people who spend much time outdoors in the Sun Belt states. A healthy community encourages physical activity among its members, but the climate affects this activity. Although long, cold winters can restrict activity, one community, St. Paul, Minnesota, holds an annual Winter Carnival. Sporting events, parades, ice sailing, dogsledding, a treasure hunt, and hot air balloon races bring thousands of Minnesotans outdoors at a time when they might otherwise be confined by the weather.

Flora and Fauna

Plant and animal populations in a community are often determined by location. The way a community responds to these populations, whether wild or domesticated, can affect the health of the community. In the Sierra foothill communities of central California, black widow and tarantula spiders, scorpions, and rattlesnakes are resident populations that pose potential health threats. The poison from a single bite may cause injury or death. In western Washington state, a bushy, attractive plant known as deadly nightshade thrives in backyards and vacant lots, but its appealing black berries are extremely poisonous. The community health nurse needs to know about the major sources of danger from plants and animals affecting the community under study. Are there community agencies that provide educational information about these dangers? Does the populace understand their significance? Are emergency services, such as a poison control center, available to community members?

Human-Made Environment

Every community is located in the midst of an environment created and transformed by human ingenuity. People build houses and factories, dump wastes into streams or vacant lots, fill the air with gases, and build dams to control streams. All of these human alterations of the environment have important implications for community health (Sattler & Lipscomb, 2003). A community health nurse might improve the health of a community by working for legislation to prevent disposal of waste chemicals into water or landfills. Such legislation might have prevented the disaster at Love Canal in New York state, where ground water contaminated with toxic wastes continued to seep into residential areas for many years, severely affecting the community's health.

Agricultural activity can alter the environment through chemical fertilizers and pesticide applications. The use of these chemicals can create potential health hazards to the community. Many farm communities attract migrant workers whose economic and health needs often pose a challenge to community resources (see Chapter 33). These are some of the many health implications of a community's physical location.

Population

When one considers the community as the client, the second dimension to examine is the total population of the community. Population consists not of a specialized aggregate but of all the diverse people who live within the boundaries of the community.

The health of any community is greatly influenced by the attributes of its population. Various features of the population suggest health needs and provide a basis for health planning (Oleske, 2001). A healthy community has leaders who are aware of the population's characteristics, know its various needs, and respond to those needs. Community health nurses can better understand any community by knowing about its **population variables**: size, density, composition, rate of growth or decline, cultural characteristics, social class structure, and mobility. Table 18–3 presents the population perspective section of the Community Profile Inventory.

T A B L E   18–3

Community Profile Inventory: Population Perspective

Population Variables	Community Health Implications	Community Assessment Questions	Information Sources
			(For all—various Internet sites)
Size	The number of people influences number and size of health care institutions. Size affects homogeneity of the population and its needs.	What is the population of the community? Is it an urban, suburban, or rural community?	State health department Census data Maps City or town officials Chamber of commerce
Density	Increased density may increase stress. High and low density often affect the availability of health services.	What is the density of the population per square mile?	Census data State health department
Composition	Composition of the population often determines types of health needs.	What is the age composition of the community? What is the sex composition of the community? What is the marital status of community members? What occupations are represented and in what percentages?	Census data State health department Chamber of Commerce U.S. Department of Labor Statistics
Rate of growth or decline	Rapidly growing communities may place excessive demands on health services. Marked decline in population may signal a poorly functioning community.	How has population size changed over the past two decades? What are the health implications of this change?	Census data State health department
Cultural differences	Health needs vary among sub-cultural and ethnic populations. Utilization of health services varies with culture. Health practices and extent of knowledge are affected by culture.	What is the ethnic breakdown of population? What racial groups are represented? What subcultural populations exist in the community? Do any of the subcultural groups have unique health needs and practices? Are different ethnic and cultural groups included in health planning?	Census data State health department Social and cultural research reports Human rights commission City government Health planning boards
Social class	Class differences influence the utilization of health services. Class composition influences cost of public health services.	What percentage of the population falls into each social class? What do class differences suggest for health needs and services?	State health department Census data Sociological reports
Mobility	Mobility of the population affects continuity of care. Mobility affects availability of service to highly mobile populations.	How frequently do members move into and out of the community? How frequently do members move within the community? Are there any specific populations, such as migrant workers, that are highly mobile? How does the pattern of mobility affect the health of the community? Is the community organized to meet the health needs of mobile groups?	State health department Census data Health agencies serving migrant workers Farm labor offices Program serving transients and the homeless

Size

The town of Dover, Delaware, with approximately 10,000 people, and the city of Los Angeles, California, with more than 4 million people, have radically different health problems. If a single case of *Salmonella* poisoning occurred in Dover, health officials would probably learn of it. It would be relatively easy to trace the course, check the few restaurants in town, and interview people about sanitation practices. However, many cases might occur in Los Angeles without the health department's knowledge. Moreover, once the cases were discovered, tracing the source of contamination might involve a long and complicated search. This is only one small way in which population size can affect the health of a community. The size of a community also influences the presence of inadequate housing, the heterogeneity of the population, and almost every conceivable aspect of health needs and services. Knowing a community's size provides community health nurses with important information for planning.

Density

In some communities, thousands of people are crowded into high-rise apartments. In others, such as farm communities, people live at great distances from one another. We do not yet know the full impact of living in high-density communities, but some research has already shown that crowding affects individual and community health. A classic study of Ohio farmers suggested that the absence of stress from crowding may have contributed to their reduced rate of coronary artery disease (Nagi, 1959).

A low-density community, however, may have problems. When people are spread out, health care provision can become difficult. There may not be enough resources in the form of taxes to support public health services. Rural communities often suffer from inadequate distribution of health care personnel, including private physicians and community health nurses (see Chapter 31). A healthy community takes into consideration the density of its population. It organizes to meet the differing needs created by its density levels (eg, it recognizes differences in density between the inner city and the suburbs and allocates services accordingly).

Composition

Communities differ in the types of people who live within their boundaries. A retirement community in Florida whose members are mostly older than 65 years of age has one set of interests and concerns. A city with a large number of women in their childbearing years will have another set of concerns. A healthy community is one that takes full account of its constituents and provides for their differences. Age, sex, educational level, occupation, and many other demographic variables affect health concerns. For example, in a town where 75% of the workers are employed in a textile mill, the community lives under the threat of brown lung disease, which is caused by cotton dust. Understanding a community's composition is an important early step in determining its level of health.

Rate of Growth or Decline

Community populations change over time. Some grow rapidly. The unparalleled recent growth of Las Vegas, Nevada, as a popular place to live has placed extreme demands on the provision of health care and other services. Others populations may experience a decline because of economic change. Any significant fluctuation in population size can affect the health of the community. As people leave to find new employment or better living conditions, consumption of goods and services drops. Community morale may suffer, and community leadership may decline. Even a stable community can have problems (eg, members may resist needed change because they see little fluctuation in their population).

Cultural Characteristics

A community may be composed of a single cultural group, such as Ojibway Indians on their reservation in Wisconsin, or it may be made up of many cultures or subcultures. If a city has a large population of Hispanics, a group of Native Americans living in the inner city, and a cluster of Vietnamese refugees, the cultural differences among these members will influence the health of the community. These differences can create conflicting or competing demands for resources and services or create intergroup hostility. A healthy community is aware of such cultural differences and acts to promote understanding among cultural subgroups.

Social Class and Educational Level

Social class refers to the ranking of groups within society by income, education, occupation, prestige, or a combination of these factors. There is no absolute agreement on income levels or other criteria to designate social class categories (upper, middle, lower), other than the government formula used to compute poverty level. Although class distinctions are not clearly defined, class rankings based on occupation, education, and wealth (income plus assets) seem to correlate with many different social patterns and are used frequently in research. Occupational level, in particular, has proved to be a reliable measure, with extraordinarily similar rankings among all societies for which there are data. It appears that people with higher occupational levels experience higher incomes, have more education, exert more political influence, and are more highly esteemed by others.

Educational level, which is closely associated with social class, is a powerful determinant of health-related behavior. Years of formal education are strongly related to age-adjusted mortality in countries as disparate as Hungary, Norway, and England (Institute of Medicine, 1997). In the United States, "adults with less than a high school education can be at increased risk for health problems because of illiteracy, low-paying jobs that do not provide health insurance, lack of health information, and poor living conditions" (Institute of Medicine, 1997, p. 157). People with higher educational attainment tend to be healthier, respond more readily to health professionals' interventions, and are more likely to modify their behavior in positive, health-enhancing ways. These modifications may include smoking cessation, weight control, exercise, dental care, and use of immunizations. People in the lower economic strata of society frequently have the worst health and are more difficult to reach with health information; they also tend to have a higher incidence of communicable diseases. Typically, health promotion and preventive health services are most needed by low-income groups and people with fewer years of education, although most members of a community will benefit from community health efforts.

It is generally known that different social classes have different health problems, different resources for coping with illness, and different ways of using health services. A healthy community recognizes these differences and creates health care services to meet these varied needs.

Mobility

Americans are a mobile population. People move to go to college, take a new job, or seek a new climate after retirement. This mobility has a direct effect on the health of communities. If the population turnover is extensive, continuity of services may suffer. Leadership for improving the health of the community may change so frequently that concerted action becomes difficult. High turnover may necessitate special attention to health education about local conditions.

Population groups may arrive and depart in seasonal swings; fluctuations in the number of migrant farm workers, tourists, or college students can affect a community. The community health nurse needs to identify those populations that are seasonally mobile. These subgroups present special health needs but also place an added burden on a community.

If a town of 3,000 people has an annual influx of 10,000 students who disappear in the summer, residents must prepare to meet this population instability. The small towns of the San Juan Islands in Puget Sound, Washington, can command such high prices for accommodations in the summer that some low-income, year-round residents camp in tents during those months because they are unable to pay the high rents. Thus, the lives of many families are disrupted each year. A healthy community neither ignores nor overreacts to this kind of mobility; rather, it identifies the nature of the population change, determines the needs created by such change, and organizes to meet those needs.

Social System

In addition to location and population, every community has a third dimension—a social system. The various parts of a community's social system that interact and influence the system are called **social system variables**. These variables include the following systems: health, family, economic, educational, religious, welfare, political, recreational, legal, and communication. Whether assessing a community's health, developing new services for the mentally ill within the community, or promoting the health of the elderly, the community health nurse needs to understand the community as a social system. A community health nurse working in a tiny village in Alaska needs to grasp the social system of that village no less than a nurse working in New York City. Table 18–4 guides the nurse in assessing a community's social system variables.

T A B L E   1 8 – 4

Community Profile Inventory: Social System Perspective

Social System Variables	Community Health Implications	Community Assessment Questions	Information Sources
Health system Family system Economic system Educational system Religious system Welfare system Political system Recreational system Legal system Communication system	Each system must fulfill its functions for a healthy community. Collaboration among the systems to identify goals and problems affects health of community. Undue influence of one system on another may lower the health of the community. Agreement on the means to achieve community goals affects community health. Communication among organizations in each system affects community health.	What are the functions of each major system? What are the major subsystems of each system? What are the major organizations in each subsystem? How well do the various organizations function? Are the subsystems in each major system in conflict? Is there adequate communication among the major systems? Is there agreement on community goals? Are there mechanisms for resolving conflict? Do any parts of the total system dominate the others? What community needs are not being met?	(For all—various Internet sites) Chamber of Commerce Telephone book City directory Organizational literature Officials in organizations Community self-study Community survey Local library Key informants

The Concept of a Social System

A social system is an abstract concept and can be more readily understood by first considering the people who make up the community's population. Each person enacts multiple roles, such as parent, spouse, employee, citizen, church member, and political volunteer. People in certain roles tend to interact more closely with others in related roles, such as a supervisor with a staff nurse or a customer with a sales clerk. The patterns and interactions that emerge from these interactions among roles form the basis of organizations. Some organizations are informal (eg, an extended family group). Other organizations, such as a city police department or a software business, are more formal. However, all organizations are constructed from roles that are enacted by individual citizens. Organizations, in turn, interact with one another, forming linkages. For example, a medical equipment company and a laboratory establish contracts (linkages) with a home care agency. When a group of organizations are linked and have similar functions, such as all those providing social services, they form a community system or subsystem (Fig. 18–2). The various community systems have a profound influence on one another. Because this interaction among parts determines the health of the whole, it is the total social system that concerns community health nurses.

The Health Care Delivery System as Part of the Social System

Although community health nurses must examine all the systems in a community and must understand how they interact, the health system is of particular importance. Studying the health system in a community can be compared with assessing an individual client. The latter involves a head-to-toe examination looking for indications of wellness and illness in the respiratory, musculoskeletal, glandular, skin, and circulatory systems, among others. Initial assessment of a community also begins with a survey of its ten major social systems. Before asking how well the specific parts are functioning, such as whether the police are doing their job or whether the mayor is an effective leader, the nurse inquires first about the political system as a whole: What are its constituent parts? Are there gross signs of health or illness? To answer questions about a system's level of functioning, one must first know its function (ie, the job it has to do as part of the larger system). The nurse might ask, for example, "How well does the communication system keep citizens informed about important matters?" This question implies that the communication system has a basic function: information dissemination. The nurse might also ask, "Does the educational system offer equal education to all children of the community?" This question implies that this system's function is to offer learning opportunities to everyone in a particular age group (see Clinical Corner I).

The major function of the health system is to promote the health of the community. Community assessment asks not merely whether, but also how well, the system is functioning. What is the level of health promotion carried out by the health system of a community? To answer this question, which can be applied to any system, one needs a clear notion about the subsystems, organizations, and roles that make up the system. Any evidence of inadequate functioning becomes a warning signal for more careful assessment. For example, a high rate of teenage pregnancies in a city may signal inadequate functioning of several systems (eg, family, educational, religious, health), so a closer look is in order. What community values influence sexual behavior among adolescents? What sex education programs are available to this population? Does the health system provide information and counseling?

The components of the health system, described in Figure 18–3, include eight major subsystems, each with one or more organizations. Although the community health nurse must be aware of all the systems in a community, the health system is of central importance.

COMMUNITY DYNAMICS

The discussion to this point may have suggested that the community is a rigid structure composed of a geographic location, a population, and a social system. Yet every community has a dynamic or changing quality. Think of the diagram in Figure 18–2 as a wheel that turns as the community changes. Three factors in particular affect community dynamics: (1) citizen participation in community health programs, (2) the power and decision-making structure, and (3) collaborative efforts of the community (Lynd, 1939).

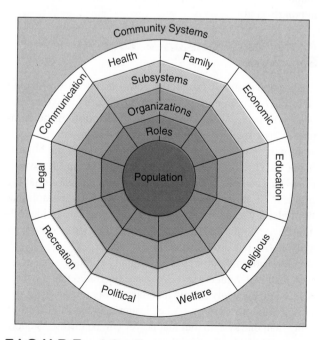

FIGURE 18–2. The community as a social system. Each of the ten major systems of a community includes a number of subsystems that are made up of organizations. Members of the community occupy roles in these organizations.

CLINICAL CORNER I

CENTERVILLE: INTERACTION OF SOCIAL SYSTEM VARIABLES

The health department of the city of Centerville reported more than 75 pregnancies in 1 year among teenage girls, a large number for the size of this community. The situation placed a marked strain on the families of the girls and caused increased demands for services from the health system. Because the vast majority of these pregnancies were unplanned, they presented a problem for the unmarried teenage parents, their families, and, eventually, the community. What would happen to the babies of these girls? Evidence from research suggested that, in the future, the girls were likely to have larger families, depend more frequently on the welfare system, and have a higher number of health problems than women who were not teenage mothers (Nakamura, 1999).

How should the community respond to this situation? The way it did respond gave clues to the overall health of the community. For one thing, the problem had been ignored, a sign of defense rather than adaptation. When it came to public attention, it divided various groups. Families blamed the schools; school officials, in turn, blamed the changing sexual mores represented in motion pictures and television shows. Some members of the health system asked Planned Parenthood to set up a clinic in the town to provide family planning education and services as a preventive measure. Almost immediately, however, the religious system entered the picture with groups forming to picket Planned Parenthood facilities because of the association's stand on abortion.

Planned Parenthood set up its clinic in an old restaurant on the edge of the business district. Individuals from the religious and economic system (local business-people) joined to file suit to prevent Planned Parenthood from occupying the old building. Within months, every major system of this community was involved in the problem, yet it was as far from solution as ever. Indeed, the original problem had almost fallen by the wayside as community members fought over the issues of abortion and the Planned Parenthood headquarters. Vandals set several fires that destroyed part of the building. Pickets daily called attention to what they considered to be an unwanted health agency. Moreover, in the midst of the trouble, more teenagers, some with parents who were deeply involved in the conflict, became pregnant.

What were the signs that this was an unhealthy community? How should the situation be handled? What role could community health nursing play in helping to resolve the problem of teen pregnancies?

Citizen Participation

In some communities, citizens show little concern about public health issues and rely on health officials to take the entire responsibility. When such apathy abounds, community health nurses need to promote community education and awareness. In other communities, participation may be widespread but is uninformed or obstructive; citizens may hamper or even try to block the development of some programs. It is much more difficult to work in a community where groups have become polarized by issues such as abortion or fluoridation. Assessing the type and extent of citizen participation is a necessary first step in community work.

The goal of encouraging responsible participation touches on the concept of self-care (discussed in earlier chapters). One goal of a community nurse when working with families or groups is to encourage people to participate and take responsibility for their own health care. They have the right to make decisions, to have adequate information, and to consult widely about their own health. The nurse's role is to encourage the full development of a self-care attitude. At the community level, self-care occurs when citizens become committed to the goal of a healthy community. Such a commitment includes responsible involvement in assessing, planning, conducting, and evaluating programs to meet community needs. Community self-care is community health nursing's goal.

Power and Decision-Making Structure

The second dynamic factor, the power and decision-making structure of a community, is a central concern to anyone who wishes to bring about change. The description of the community as a social system may suggest that power and decision-making reside primarily in the political system, but this is not the case. In their classic work, Sanders and Brownlee (1979) argued against oversimplifying the decision-making process: "In its naivest, simplest terms this [oversimplification] blandly states that (1) every community has an identifiable power clique and (2) that if you get the members on your side, all of your problems will be solved" (p. 421).

Decision-making in any community is much more complex than that. Sanders and Brownlee suggested that power is distributed unevenly among members of organizations in various community systems. A key leader may have influence in more than one system, but that power will be diffuse. Seldom does a public health official have power in the religious system or a member of the clergy in the legal system. A dominant leader is one who has specific power, but only within a single

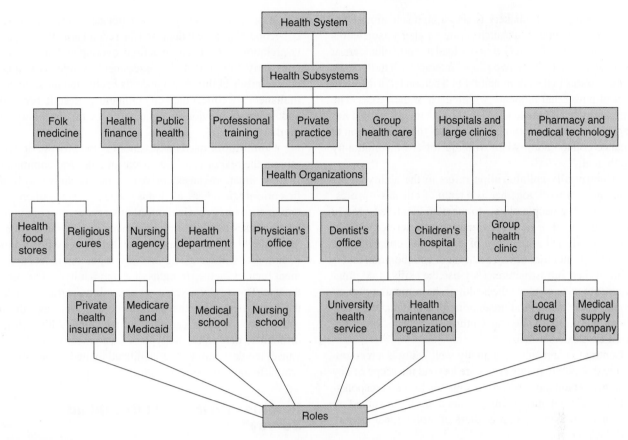

FIGURE 18-3.   Components of the health system. This figure shows some representative types of organizations for each of the major subsystems. In turn, each of these organizations also has members with many different roles, and the health of the entire system depends, in part, on how well these roles are carried out.

community system. An organizational leader has power, but usually within a single organization, not in the entire system. Sanders and Brownlee also stated that key and dominant leaders often work through other, less powerful leaders, called functionaries, issue leaders, or spokespersons. (The topic of leadership and types of leaders is explored in Chapter 13.)

Although power and decision-making in any community are complex, Sanders and Brownlee (1979) did suggest several general guidelines for understanding this aspect of a community's dynamics:

1. Because communities differ widely in their power structures, do not assume that what is known about one community will be true of another.
2. The leaders within the health system have different degrees of power and varying spheres of influence; knowledge of these differences is a prerequisite to effective community work.
3. Those leaders whose power is limited to the health system or to a health organization often have a network of contacts with similar leaders in other systems. Many of the decisions are made informally through this network.
4. Power does not automatically flow through established bureaucratic channels. Locate the informal patterns of power and decision-making.

5. Beware of leaders who speak authoritatively on issues outside their sphere of power. Their power may be more apparent than real.
6. Leaders from the health system may become key leaders with power that extends far beyond the health system.
7. Learn to distinguish between political, economic, and social power; then use the appropriate combination needed to promote community health issues.
8. Do not overestimate the support of key leaders or power cliques; their support may be helpful but still may leave much organizational work to be done.
9. Try to encourage participation in the decision-making process at every level, from average citizen to key leader.
10. One can assume that leaders in one part of a community are ignorant of needs and problems in other parts of the system. When one contacts such leaders, recognize that they will have to be educated in community health issues.

Community Collaboration Efforts

The third component of a functioning community social system is the degree to which the community collaborates. As mentioned earlier, people in a community have different roles. The owner of a bakery is also a high school baseball coach and a member of a church choir. Another person works as a legal secretary, is a Girl Scout leader, and volunteers at the local hospital. These two people interact with most of the major systems in the community. Each person has a different level of power and influence within each of their roles. The community health nurse keeps in mind that each person has many roles within a community and uses this information to enhance collaboration when working toward a community health goal.

Community collaboration refers to the ability of the community to work together as a team of citizens—professionals and lay people alike—to meet an identified need in the community. For example, Centerville, described in Clinical Corner I, had a low level of community collaboration. Healthy communities have a tradition of collaboration that is a part of their infrastructure. They use the skills of community members to enhance the health of the community for all people. There are several broad principles that underpin collaboration efforts (Anderson, Guthrie, & Schirle, 2002; Petersen & Alexander, 2001):

1. Central to client and community well-being is a recognition that public policy issues are beyond the scope of any single person's or profession's jurisdiction and responsibility. Community members need to be involved to change the status quo, regardless of professional identity or lack thereof.
2. The community needs results-based accountability that emphasizes programs' or projects' effectiveness as the goal.
3. Cultural competence is the norm. All programs (design, delivery, and evaluation) require respect for ethnic and linguistic identity and the reduction of marginalization, invisibility, and devaluation of people.
4. Ethical behavior is fundamental to collaborative relationships.
5. People work in teams that cross traditional lines of programs, agencies, disciplines, and professions.
6. Funding strategies need to be decategorized to give more flexibility at the community level, thereby providing a better way of allocating resources where they are needed.

Collaboration, a skill that community health nurses must have when working with communities, is discussed in detail in Chapter 11.

TYPES OF COMMUNITY NEEDS ASSESSMENT

After considering the importance of community dynamics, the community health nurse is ready to determine the community's needs. Assessment is the first step of the nursing process. Assessment for nurses means collecting and evaluating information about a community's health status to discover existing or potential needs as a basis for planning future action (Heinemann & Zeiss, 2002).

Assessment involves two major activities. The first is collection of pertinent data, and the second is analysis and interpretation of data. These actions overlap and are repeated constantly throughout the assessment. While assessing a community's ability to enhance its health, the nurse may simultaneously collect data on community lifestyle behaviors and interpret previously collected data on morbidity and mortality.

Community needs assessment is the process of determining the real or perceived needs of a defined community. In some situations, an extensive community study may be the first priority; in others, all that is needed is a study of one system or even one organization. At other times, the community health nurses may need to perform a cursory examination or "windshield survey" to familiarize themselves with an entire community without going into any depth. An assets assessment focuses on the strengths of a community and not on its deficits. The type of assessment depends on variables such as the needs that exist, the goals to be achieved, and the resources available for carrying out the study. Although it is difficult to determine the type of assessment needed in advance, the decision will be facilitated by understanding several different types of community assessment.

Familiarization or "Windshield Survey"

A familiarization assessment is the most necessary evaluation of a community. **Familiarization assessment** involves studying data already available on a community, and gathering a certain amount of firsthand data, to gain a working knowledge of the community. Such an approach, sometimes called a "windshield survey," is used by nursing students in community assessment courses and by new staff members in community health agencies. Nurses drive (or walk) around the community; find health, social, and governmental services; obtain literature; introduce themselves and explain that they are working in the area; and generally become familiar with the community. This type of assessment is needed whenever the community health nurse works with families, groups, organizations, or populations. Familiarization provides a knowledge of the context in which these aggregates exist and may enable the nurse to connect clients with community resources (see Clinical Corner II).

Problem-Oriented Assessment

A second type of community assessment, **problem-oriented assessment**, begins with a single problem and assesses the community in terms of that problem. Suppose that Jean, the nurse who explored services available for the Angelo family's deaf child in Clinical Corner II, had discovered that there were none. Confronted with this problem—one family with one deaf child—she could make a problem-oriented community assessment. Her first step would be to discover the incidence of childhood deafness, both in the community

CLINICAL CORNER II

THE ANGELO FAMILY AND A FAMILIARIZATION ASSESSMENT

A community health nurse named Jean visited the Angelo family on the outskirts of Philadelphia. During the initial visit, she gathered information, learning that the family was Italian American and that there were four children, ranging in age from 13 to 3. The father had been out of work for 6 months; the mother worked on weekends as a maid in a motel; the oldest boy had been in trouble with the juvenile authorities; a younger child was deaf; and their house appeared rundown. Jean assessed this family, trying to determine its coping ability and its level of health. Furthermore, because community health nursing is population focused, her concern was not only for the Angelo family but also for the population of families with similar problems that this family represented.

However, the nurse's assessment was almost impossible without further knowledge of the community. Was theirs an Italian-American neighborhood with specific cultural influences? What was the extent of unemployment in this city? What were the services for the deaf? Were all the houses in this part of town old and in need of repair? Once the nurse began working with the family, familiarity with the community became even more imperative. She discovered that, as a result of the Ange-

los' low income, family conflicts were intense. The family members seldom got out; they made almost no use of the community's recreational system. Before she could help them make use of it, however, the nurse had to find out what resources were available. As she familiarized herself with the community, she discovered Friends of the Deaf, which sponsored a group for parents of deaf children. The nurse could now help Mr. and Mrs. Angelo become part of that group. A quick survey of the religious system in the community revealed two job-transition support groups, one of which would welcome Mr. Angelo. In the meantime, the nurse chose to find out about the welfare system and how this family and other similar families could benefit from its services. Even her own attitude changed as she studied the community. For instance, she discovered that a strike had closed down the plant where Mr. Angelo worked for 20 years, and so could view his and others' unemployment from a broader perspective. Using a familiarization assessment helped this nurse to enhance her practice.

Whatever role nurses play in community health promotion, they will want to be making a continuous study, an ongoing assessment. Whether nurses become client advocates, work with the local government, or operate from a nursing agency serving the elderly, a familiarization assessment is prerequisite for their work.

and in the state. Second, she might begin interviewing officials in the schools and health institutions to find out what had been done in the past to assist deaf children. She could check the local library to locate available resources on the subject of deafness, such as the journal, *The Deaf American*. Are there interpreters available for adults who use sign language? How do hospitals and courts approach deafness? Are there any clubs or other organizations for deaf adults? Are there school programs for the deaf, and, if so, where are they located?

The problem-oriented assessment is commonly used when familiarization is not sufficient and a comprehensive assessment is too expensive. This type of assessment is responsive to a particular need. The data collected will be useful in any kind of planning for a community response to the problem.

Community Subsystem Assessment

In **community subsystem assessment**, the community health nurse focuses on a single dimension of community life. For example, the nurse might decide to survey churches and religious organizations to discover their roles in the community. What kinds of needs do the leaders in these or-

ganizations believe exist? What services do these organizations offer? To what extent are services coordinated within the religious system and between it and other systems in the community?

Community subsystem assessment can be a useful way for a team to conduct a more thorough community assessment. If five members of a nursing agency divide up the ten systems in the community and each person does an assessment of two systems, they could then share their findings to create a more comprehensive picture of the community and its needs.

Comprehensive Assessment

Comprehensive assessment seeks to discover all relevant community health information. It begins with a review of existing studies and all the data presently available on the community. A survey compiles all the demographic information on the population, such as its size, density, and composition. Key informants are interviewed in every major system—education, health, religious, economic, and others. Then, more detailed surveys and intensive interviews are performed to yield information on organizations and the various roles in each organization. A comprehensive assessment describes not only the systems of a community but also how power is distributed throughout the system, how decisions are made, and how change occurs (Plescia, Koontx, & Laurent, 2001; Williams & Yanoshik, 2001).

Because comprehensive assessment is an expensive, time-consuming process, it is seldom performed. Indeed, in many cases, such a thorough research plan might be a waste of resources and might repeat, in part, other studies. Performing a more focused study based on prior knowledge of needs is often a better strategy. Nevertheless, knowing how to conduct a comprehensive assessment is an important influence in the proper design of a more focused study.

Community Assets Assessment

The final form of assessment presented here is **assets assessment**, which focuses on the strengths and capacities of a community rather than its problems. Based on a model developed by McKnight and Kretzmann in the 1980s (McKnight, 1987), it provides tools with which to conduct a complete functional community assessment and serves as a guide to the community for the nurse. The previously mentioned methods are needs oriented and deficit based—in other words, they are "pathology" models, in which the assessment is performed in response to needs, barriers, weaknesses, problems, or scarcity in the community. This may result in a fragmented approach to solutions for the community's problems rather than an approach focused on the community's possibilities, strengths, and assets.

Assets assessment begins with what is present in the community. The capacities and skills of community members are identified, with a focus on creating or rebuilding relationships among local residents, associations, and institutions to multiply power and effectiveness. This approach requires that the assessor look for the positive, or see the glass as "half full." The nurse can then become a partner in community intervention efforts, rather than merely a provider of services.

Assets assessment has three levels: (1) specific skills, talents, interests, and experiences of individual community members; (2) local citizen associations and organizations; and (3) local institutions. The key, however, is linking these assets together to enhance the community from within.

COMMUNITY ASSESSMENT METHODS

Community health needs may be assessed by a variety of methods. Regardless of the assessment method used, data must be collected. Data collection in community health requires the exercise of sound professional judgment, effective communication techniques, and special investigative skills. Four important methods are discussed here: surveys, descriptive epidemiologic studies, community forums or town meetings, and focus groups.

Surveys

A **survey** is an assessment method in which a series of questions is used to collect data for analysis of a specific group or area. Surveys are commonly used to provide a broad range of data that will be helpful when used in conjunction with other sources or if other sources are not available. To plan and conduct community health surveys, the goal should be to determine the variables (selected environmental, socioeconomic, and behavioral conditions or needs) that affect a community's ability to control disease and promote wellness. The nurse may choose to conduct a survey to determine such things as health care use patterns and needs, immunization levels, demographic characteristics, or health beliefs and practices. The survey method involves three phases that are needed to ensure an adequate design and appropriate collection of data (Polit & Hungler, 2003):

1. Planning Phase
   a. Determine what information is needed and why.
   b. Determine precise data to be collected.
   c. Select population to be surveyed (eg, individuals, a household, a city block).
   d. Select survey method or instrument to be used (eg, interviews, telephone calls, questionnaires).
   e. Determine sampling size (eg, a percentage of the total population in question).
2. Data Collection Phase
   a. Identify and train data collectors (eg, interviewers).
   b. Pretest and adjust instrument.
   c. Supervise actual collection, including plans for nonresponses or refusals.
3. Data Analysis and Presentation Phase
   a. Organize data for tabulation and analysis.
   b. Apply appropriate statistical methods.
   c. Determine relationships and significance of analysis.
   d. Report results, including implications, recommendations, and next steps needed; provide feedback to the population surveyed through a community forum (discussed later).

Descriptive Epidemiologic Studies

A second assessment method is a **descriptive epidemiologic study**, which examines the amount and distribution of a disease or health condition in a population by person (Who is affected?), by place (Where does the condition occur?), and by time (When do the cases occur?). In addition to their value in assessing the health status of a population, descriptive epidemiologic studies are useful for suggesting which individuals are at greatest risk and where and when the condition might occur. They are also useful for health planning purposes and for suggesting hypotheses concerning disease etiology. Their design and use are detailed in Chapter 8.

The choice of assessment method varies depending on the reasons for data collection, the goals and objectives of the study, and the available resources. It also varies according to the theoretical framework or philosophical approach through which the nurse views the community. In other words, the community health nurse's theoretical basis for approaching community assessment influences the purposes for conducting the assessment and the selection of methodology. For example, Neuman's health care systems model forms the basis for the "community-as-partner" assessment model developed by Anderson and McFarlane (2004). Additional resources on methodologies for assessing community health are available in the list of References and Selected Readings at the end of this chapter.

Community Forums or Town Hall Meetings

The community forum or town hall meeting is a qualitative assessment method designed to obtain community opinions. It takes place in the neighborhood of the people involved, perhaps in a school gymnasium or an auditorium. The participants are selected to participate by invitation from the group organizing the forum. Members come from within the community and represent all segments of the community that are involved with the issue. For instance, if a community is contemplating building a swimming pool, the people invited to the community forum might include potential users of the pool (residents of the community without pools and special groups such as Scouts, elders, and disabled citizens), community planners, health and safety personnel, and other key people with vested interests. They are asked to give their views on the pool: Where should it be located? Who will use it? How will the cost of building it be assumed? What are the drawbacks to having the pool? Any other pertinent issues the participants may raise are included. This method is relatively inexpensive, and results are quickly obtained. A drawback of this method is that only the most vocal community members or those with the greatest vested interests in the issue may be heard. This format does not provide a representative voice to others in the community who also may be affected by the proposed decision.

This method is used to elicit public opinion on a variety of issues, including health care concerns, political views, and feelings about issues in the public eye, such as the verdict in a high-profile murder case. Frequently, local cable television channels air important city commissioner or school board meetings. Local news programs may hold town meetings, soliciting public opinion on regional issues. Other methods of opinion gathering include e-mailing (eg, to a television news program) to support a particular view and using a toll-free number set up especially for a "Yes" or "No" vote on an issue. Such electronic methods of data gathering are becoming more common and will continue to be so as technology advances. For instance, people can enter chat rooms from home on their personal computers. These "electronic town meetings" are designed to elicit grassroots opinions from local community members.

Focus Groups

This fourth assessment method, focus groups, is similar to the community forum or town hall meeting in that it is designed to obtain grassroots opinion. However, it has some differences. First, there is only a small group of participants, usually 5 to 15 people (Polit & Hungler, 2003). The members chosen for the group are homogeneous with respect to specific demographic variables. For example, a focus group may consist of female community health nurses, young women in their first pregnancy, or retired businessmen. Leadership skills are used in conjunction with the small group process to promote a supportive atmosphere and to accomplish set goals. The interviewer guides the discussion according to a predetermined set of questions or topics (see Voices from the Community).

Usually the group meets for 1 to 3 hours, and there may be a series of meetings. For example, community health nurses from each of six different agencies in a three-county area may meet with the same interviewer over the course of a month, or groups of pregnant women being served by three different agencies may meet over a period of weeks. In these examples, each group meets only once, but assessment data can be collected from several groups over a period of time. Major advantages of focus groups are their efficiency and low cost, similar to the community forum or town hall meeting format. A focus group can be organized "to represent a microcosm of an aggregate, to capture contingents or interest groups within a community, or to sample for diversity in the population by organizing several groups" (Stevens, 1996, p. 175). In each method, however, there may be some people who are uncomfortable expressing their views in a group situation (Polit & Hungler, 2003).

SOURCES OF COMMUNITY DATA

There are many places the community health nurse can look for data to enhance and complete a community assessment. Data sources can be primary or secondary, and they can be from international, national, state, or local sources. Web sites for many primary and secondary data sources are included at the end of this chapter.

Primary and Secondary Sources

Community health nurses make use of many sources in data collection. Community members, including formal leaders, informal leaders, and community inhabitants, can frequently offer the most accurate insights and comprehensive information. Information gathered by talking to people provides primary data, because the data are obtained directly from the community. Secondary sources of data include people who know the community well and the records such people create in the performance of their jobs. Specific examples are health team members, client records, community health sta-

VOICES FROM THE COMMUNITY

In this study, the researchers felt they needed participants to be able to define community with a level of consensus that would enhance community collaboration in planned human immunodeficiency virus (HIV) vaccine trials. Four groups of interviewees—25 African-Americans from Durham, NC; 25 gay men from San Francisco, CA; 25 injection drug users in Philadelphia, PA; and 42 HIV researchers across the US—were asked, "What does the word *community* mean to you?"

A Durham, NC, African-American: "I think community can be defined in two different ways. There's a community that you define as such because you are forced by where you live, by your upbringing, to be around those people. This isn't a voluntary type of thing. This is your community because you live there. And so you were molded and informed by that surrounding, by that society. . . . that's how I would describe my work community. It is my community because I have to work there and it is my workplace. But certainly, the people I choose to be sociable with most aren't people I share the same job with."

San Francisco gay man: "I lived alone for a while after [my partner] died and I really hated it. I really felt very lonely, and now I live in a situation with a good friend. . . . There's a sense of comfort in that. Because, you know, he's single and I'm single and we have a group of friends and there's a lot of connection, that we kind of create community. I think we as gay and lesbian people create family too, in a lot of ways that are not biological, and I think [in] some ways that sense of creat-

ing family is creating community; that's what we support ourselves and surround ourselves with."

Philadelphia injection drug user: "Well, in the drug culture, I wouldn't call that a community, you know. I would just call that a part of the community that's just tryin' to survive, but [what] community means to me is a way people look out for one another and they do things together, insofar as socializing together, praying together. You know, they have a mutual bond but see, you know, and some of that goes on in the community, you know, and that drug culture can be right here but you still have a group of people that tries to keep the neighborhood together and try to set the right values for the children."

A scientist: "A community is a fairly broad term in my mind that encompasses groups of people working together toward the same goal. . . . I would say I identify with the HIV research community, the HIV care community, my own personal community with my family, certainly my regional community. . . . I think that our communities are less dependent these days on actual physical adjacency, if you will, that the Internet has brought many people together, and when I say I'm part of the AIDS research community, I think of that as a worldwide community."

MacQueen, K.M., McLellan, E., Metzger, D.S., Jegeles, S., Strauss, R.P., Scotti, R., et al. (2001). What is community? An evidence-based definition for participatory public health. *American Journal of Public Health, 91*(12), 1929–1938.

tistics, Census Bureau data, reference books, research reports, and community health nurses. Because secondary data may not totally describe the community and do not necessarily reflect community self-perceptions, they may need augmentation or further validation (see Research: Bridge to Practice).

International Sources

International data are collected by several agencies, including the World Health Organization (WHO) and its six regional offices and health organizations, such as the Pan-American Health Organization. In addition, the United Nations and global specialty organizations that focus on certain populations or health problems, such as the United Nations Children's Fund, are major sources of international health-related data. WHO publishes an annual report of their activity (World Health Organization, 2003), and international statistics for diseases and illness trends can be found on the Internet. Information from these official sources can

give the nurse in the local community information about immigrant and refugee populations she or he serves.

National Sources

There are official and nonofficial sources of national data that community health nurses can access if needed. Official sources develop documents based on data compiled by the government. The following are the major agencies:

U. S. Public Health Service (USPHS).
This is the main agency from which data can be retrieved, and its agency, the National Center for Health Statistics, was specifically established for the collection and dissemination of health-related data. USPHS also published *Healthy People 2000* and the newer document *Healthy People 2010* (U.S. Department of Health and Human Services, 1991, 2000). These two comprehensive documents were designed to focus America's attention on the major health-related markers in the country, and they include realistic goals for national,

RESEARCH: BRIDGE TO PRACTICE

Muhib, F.B., Lin, L.S., Stueve, A., Miller, R.L., Ford, W.L., Johnson, W.D., et al. (2001). A venue-based method for sampling hard-to-reach populations. *Public Health Reports, 2001 supplement, 116,* 216–222.

A VENUE-BASED METHOD FOR SAMPLING HARD-TO-REACH POPULATIONS

The authors, in an attempt to sample hard-to-reach populations, describe a venue-based application of time-space sampling (TSS) that addresses the challenges of reaching these populations. Most communities are easy to access if we use a location approach, such as a city or town. Some population-based communities, however, can best be accessed at traditional non-home venues, such as senior citizens at a community center, student nurses in a university lounge area, or children at a specialty clinic.

These researchers wanted to sample young men (15 to 25 years old) who have sex with men. The TSS method identifies days and times when the hard-to-reach or "hidden" population gathers at specific venues. These researchers identify the steps of constructing a sampling frame of venue, day-time units (VDTs), randomly selecting and visiting VDTs; and systematically intercepting and collecting information from consenting members of the target population. Hidden populations can be located using the TSS method in many situations, environments,

and cultures. The value to these researchers came as they were attempting to generate a systematic sample of young men who have sex with men. Venues used to gather information in the Community Intervention Trial for Youth (CITY) project, funded by the Division of HIV/AIDS Prevention, of the Centers for Disease Control and Prevention and included 13 sites (communities or venues). Standardized time segments of 4-hour intervals were used by the researchers to sample the target population at clubs that frequented by young men who have sex with men. The clubs were open on Friday and Saturday evenings, and timeframes from 10 PM until 2 AM were selected, with subjects randomly selected from a sampling frame. The venue-based application of TSS allows researchers to use screener information to target specific populations and can generate a large and diverse sample. At such venues, a higher proportion of the people screened are members of the target population, so that the drawbacks of respondent-driven sampling are avoided.

This method of data gathering among hard-to-reach communities of people can be applied by many researchers when the research focus involves hidden population—the aged male alcoholic—the newly widowed woman—the preschooler with a speech defect. Beginning with a community such as a city, a neighborhood, or a school will take time, the sample will be small, and many of the target population will be missed. A venue-based approach reaches the targeted population.

---

state, and local agencies to work toward over the next decade.

U. S. Bureau of the Census. This agency undertakes a major survey of American families every 10 years, gathering data on health, socioeconomic, and environmental conditions. Since 1990, this information has been available on CD-ROM, allowing numerous variables to be viewed in combination and easier development of a community profile.

National Institutes of Health (NIH). This system of 17 biomedical research agencies focuses on improving the health of the nation. Employees of these agencies prevent, diagnose, and treat diseases and conduct and disseminate research findings.

Nonofficial agencies have data sources generated from research they conduct that focuses on the population, disease, or condition they were developed to serve. Each agency collects data at the national level; however, the more accessible arm for services functions at state and local levels. Examples of these agencies are the American Cancer Society

(ACS), the American Association of Retired Persons (AARP), and Mothers and Students Against Drunk Drivers (MADD and SADD). Information from such national sources allows community health assessment teams to compare local data with national and state statistics and trends.

State Sources

The most significant state source of assessment data comes from the state health department. This official agency is responsible for collecting state vital statistics and morbidity data. As a resource to local health departments, its support services are invaluable, and it is the main source of health-related data on the state level. Nonofficial agencies have state chapters or headquarters and compile their information at the state level. Local nonofficial agency chapters have documents of compiled state and national data on the population, disease, or condition they address. Individual states can be contacted on the World Wide Web in the ".gov" domain using the two-letter postal abbreviation for the state; for example, information from California can be found at http://www.ca.gov.

Local Sources

There are many sources of information at the local level. Some key sources are the local visitor's bureau, city Chamber of Commerce, city planner's office, health department, hospitals, social service agencies, county extension office, school districts, universities or colleges, libraries, clergy, business and service organizations, and community leaders and key informants. Some of these sources compile their own statistics, but all have views of the community particular to their discipline, interest, or knowledge base.

Some agencies at the local level develop city or county resource directories. These are updated periodically and are valuable resources for community health assessment teams and community health nurses.

Not to be overlooked is the usefulness of area maps. These are valuable tools for the community health nurse. Maps can be small and modest (eg, a free fold-up map from the Chamber of Commerce) or large and detailed (eg, one purchased from a discount or stationery store). Also available are the mapping services found on the Internet, such as MapQuest. At this site, the user identifies a beginning location and a destination; the site then produces specific directions and a map to the address. Many community health agencies have a large local on one of their walls. This might be used only to obtain directions to clients' and points of service, or it might be a "working" map. On working maps, such things as the numbers and types of diseases known to be in the community can be plotted, the location of clients presently being visited and the nurses serving them can be visualized with the use of different-colored pins, or places in the community that provide services especially needed by clients can be located. The most useful working map for community assessment data is one that is used to plot where people with known diseases or conditions live. For instance, red pins may be placed in the map at every location where a person with tuberculosis lives, yellow pins to locate clients with hepatitis, and so on. The result is a picture of the health of the community. The map can help monitor trends in illnesses that might be associated with population mobility patterns (Fig. 18–4).

DATA ANALYSIS AND DIAGNOSIS

This stage of assessment requires analysis of the information gathered, so that inferences or conclusions may be made about its meaning. Such inferences must be validated to determine their accuracy, after which a nursing diagnosis can be formed.

The Process of Analysis

First, the data must be validated: Are they accurate? Several validation procedures may be used: (1) data can be rechecked by the community assessment team, (2) data can be rechecked by others, (3) subjective and objective data can be compared,

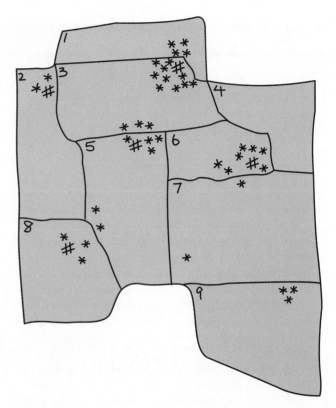

FIGURE 18–4.   A sample working map. Reported cases of tuberculosis in Harvard County, June through December 2000. * = cases of tuberculosis; # = cities over 5000 population; 1–9 = census tracts.

or (4) community members can consider the findings and verify them.

Validated data are then separated into categories such as physical, social, and environmental data. In many instances, data spreadsheets are used to provide a structure for data organization. Next, each category is examined to determine its significance. At this point, there may be a need to search for additional information to clarify the meaning of the data. Only then can inferences be made and a tentative conclusion about the meaning of the data be reached.

There are computer programs designed to analyze community assessment data. For large, complex, or ongoing community assessment plans, this may be the best method. For smaller, one-time assessments, the paper-and-pencil method may be sufficient and less unwieldy. Some communities may hire an outside professional assessment service. These teams often use the latest technology when analyzing data. Not all communities can afford such a service, and if key leaders become familiar with assessment, analysis, and diagnostic processes, an investment in a computer program may be worthwhile. Regardless of the analysis method used, data interpretation remains a critical phase of the process.

In data interpretation, there is an ever-present danger of making inaccurate assumptions and diagnoses. The importance of validation cannot be overemphasized. Before making a diagnosis, all assumptions must be validated: Are they sound? Community members should participate actively in validation efforts by clarifying perceptions, explaining the circumstances surrounding the situation, and acting as sounding boards for testing assumptions. Other resources, such as the health team members and community leaders, are used to explore and confirm inferences. Data collection, data interpretation, and nursing diagnosis are sequential activities, with validation serving as the bridges between them (Table 18–5). When performed thoroughly, these steps lead to accurate diagnoses.

Community Diagnosis Formation

The next step in the nursing process is a nursing diagnosis. Neufeld & Harrison (1994), based on the classic work of Mundinger and Jauron (1975) on developing nursing diagnoses, proposed the use of nursing diagnoses in the community by substituting the term *client, family, group,* or *aggregate* for the word *patient.* Their definition of a nursing diagnosis is the following (Neufeld & Harrison, 1996, p. 221):

> *The statement of a [client's] response which is actually or potentially unhealthful and which nursing intervention can help to change in the direction of health. It should also identify essential factors related to the unhealthful response.*

Neufeld and Harrison built on this work to form a wellness diagnosis by using the phrase *healthful response* instead of *unhealthful response.* Their definition of a wellness diagnosis is the following (p. 221):

> *The statement of a client's [community's] healthful response which nursing intervention can support or strengthen. It should also identify the essential factors related to the healthful response.*

By substituting the term *community* for client, family, group, or aggregate, the nursing or wellness diagnosis can be applied to the community as a whole. These diagnoses identify the conclusion the nurse draws from interpretation of collected data and describes a community's healthy or unhealthy responses that can be influenced or changed by nursing interventions. Change comes about through collaboration with other community and health team members.

In community health, nurses do not limit their focus to problems; they consider the community as a total system and look for evidence of all kinds of responses that may influence the community's level of wellness. Responses encompass the whole health–illness continuum, from specific deficits, such as a lack of senior centers or day care programs, to opportunities for maximizing a community's health, such as promoting improvement of police protection or the safety of the roadways. The statement of community response, the diagnosis, can focus on a wide range of topics.

Community Diagnoses

Data have been gathered from a variety of sources and have been validated by several means. The data have been recorded, tabulated, analyzed, and synthesized so that patterns and trends can be seen. The use of charts, graphs, and tables assists in visualizing the synthesized data. The community assessment team present the findings to peers and use their expertise to assist in the formulation of the community diagnoses.

Continuing with the nursing process format, nursing diagnoses for the community are developed. **Community diagnoses** refer to nursing diagnoses about a community's

T A B L E   1 8 – 5

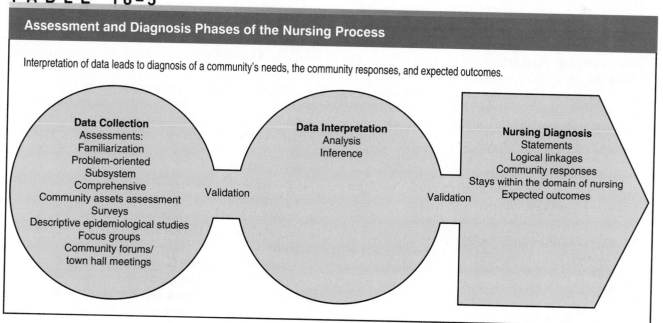

Assessment and Diagnosis Phases of the Nursing Process

Interpretation of data leads to diagnosis of a community's needs, the community responses, and expected outcomes.

Data Collection
Assessments:
Familiarization
Problem-oriented
Subsystem
Comprehensive
Community assets assessment
Surveys
Descriptive epidemiological studies
Focus groups
Community forums/
town hall meetings

Validation

Data Interpretation
Analysis
Inference

Validation

Nursing Diagnosis
Statements
Logical linkages
Community responses
Stays within the domain of nursing
Expected outcomes

ineffective coping ability and potential for enhanced coping. The statements about the community should include the strengths of the community and possible sources for community solutions, as well as the community's weaknesses or problem areas. Using the standard nursing diagnosis format, community-level diagnoses can be developed (Carpenito, 2002). These diagnoses are used as tools as the community begins to plan, intervene, and evaluate outcomes. Diagnostic categories for individuals (eg, knowledge deficit of senior services, high risk for injury or falls) can often be applied at the community level. Acceptable community level nursing diagnoses, adapted from Neufeld and Harrison (1996), do the following:

1. Portray a community focus
2. Include the community response (clause 1) and the related factors (clause 2) that have potential for change through community health nursing
3. Include response and related factors that are logically consistent

A wellness diagnosis may:

4. Include maintenance or potential change responses (due to growth and development) when no deficit is present

Community nursing diagnoses must also:

5. Include statements that are narrow enough to guide interventions
6. Have logical linkages between community responses (clause 1) and related factors (clause 2)
7. Use a community response instead of a risk, goal, or need statement
8. Include factors within the domain of community health nursing intervention

Two examples of wellness and deficit community nursing diagnoses and several diagnoses for a specific community follow.

1. *Wellness nursing diagnosis for an assisted living community of elders.* The senior residents of an assisted living center have the potential for achieving optimal functioning related to (host factors) their expressed interest in exercise, diet, and meaningful activities and to (environment factors) their access to exercise opportunities, nutritional information, and social outlets.
2. *Deficit community nursing diagnosis for a rural farmworker community.* The inhabitants of (name of the town) in (name of the state) are at risk for illness and injury related to (host factors) exposure to pesticides, a lack of motivation to add or use safety devices on farm machinery, lack of safety knowledge, and choice to take unnecessary risks and to (environment factors) lack of family income to purchase newer equipment and long hours of work that lead to stress and exhaustion.
3. *Community diagnoses for Anytown, Kansas.* Anytown, Kansas, is experiencing an increase in crime, a problem compounded by the small size of the police force and an influx of many new community members. The community has worked together constructively in the past, communicates well, and has strong recreational outlets for community members. The community

- Has expressed vulnerability and feels overwhelmed related to threats to community safety
- Has failed to meet its own expectations related to inadequate law enforcement services
- Has expressed difficulty in meeting the demands of change related to an influx of new community members
- Has a successful history in coping with a previous crisis of teenage pregnancy
- Has positive communication among community members
- Has a well-developed program for recreation and relaxation

Such diagnoses can guide communities toward maximizing or improving their health as they plan, implement, and evaluate changes to be measured by outcome criteria they have established for themselves. **Outcome criteria** are measurable standards that community members use to measure success as they work toward improving the health of their community. Outcome-based or evidence-based nursing practice applies to aggregates in the community as well as to patients in acute-care settings.

The nursing diagnosis changes over time because it reflects changes in the health status of the community; therefore, diagnoses need to be periodically reevaluated and redefined. The changing diagnosis can be a useful means of encouraging a community toward improved health because it gives community members a clear standard against which to measure progress.

WHAT IS A HEALTHY COMMUNITY?

What is a healthy community? To assess a community, develop nursing diagnoses, set goals based on outcome criteria for community health, plan health improvements, and work toward goals, health practitioners require some criteria that define a healthy community. Just as health for an individual is relative and will change, all aggregates exist in a relative state of health. New needs emerge every day; the system is threatened or weakened and must respond to maintain equilibrium.

Because of their complexity, criteria for healthy communities must be discussed cautiously. At present, there is not wide agreement on such criteria, but four important characteristics of a competent or healthy community were outlined by Cottrell (1976) and are still relevant today. A competent community can

1. Collaborate effectively in identifying community needs and problems
2. Achieve a working consensus on goals and priorities
3. Agree on ways and means to implement the agreed-upon goals
4. Collaborate effectively to take the required actions

These general requirements point to some of the characteristics of a healthy community. However, the factors that foster effective interaction among the community's systems must still be determined. Cottrell (1976) suggested several essential conditions for community competence:

1. Commitment of members
2. Self-awareness and awareness of others among groups
3. Clarity of situational (positional) definitions
4. Articulateness of various subgroups
5. Effective communication
6. Conflict containment and accommodation
7. Participation (community involvement)
8. Management of relations with the larger society
9. Machinery for effective decision-making.

The following descriptors can serve as a guide for assessing a healthy community. The healthy community

1. Is one in which members have a high degree of awareness that "we are a community."
2. Uses natural resources wisely while taking steps to conserve them for future generations.
3. Openly recognizes the existence of subgroups and welcomes their participation in community affairs.
4. Is prepared to meet crises.
5. Is a problem-solving community; it identifies, analyzes, and organizes to meet its own needs.
6. Has open channels of communication that allow information to flow among all subgroups of citizens in all directions.
7. Seeks to make each of its systems' resources available to all members of the community.
8. Has legitimate and effective ways to settle disputes that arise within the community.
9. Encourages maximum citizen participation in decision-making.
10. Promotes a high level of wellness among all its members.

SUMMARY

A major mission of community health nursing practice is to promote the health of aggregates of people. This focus conflicts with the strong value of individualism in the United States, which often distracts nurses from a broad focus. This emphasis on the individual has led to three pervading myths: (1) that community health nursing involves only clinical nursing in the community setting, (2) that community health nursing employs only the skills of basic nursing, and (3) that the primary client in community health nursing is the individual. In reality, community health nursing is practiced in many settings, employs not only basic nursing expertise but many important concepts and skills from the arena of public health, and focuses primarily on promoting the health of populations and aggregates, not only individuals.

In assessing the health needs of any geographic community, there are three important dimensions to consider: location, population, and social system. Location may be further analyzed by considering such variables as the community's boundaries, location of health services, geo-

graphic features, climate, flora and fauna, and human-made environment. Population, the second dimension, should be analyzed by determining population size, density, composition, rate of growth or decline, cultural differences, social class, and mobility. The social system includes ten major systems—health, family, economic, education, religious, welfare, political, recreation, legal, and communication—as well as many subsystems. Each subsystem is composed of organizations whose members assume various roles. A Community Profile Inventory guides the community health nurse in making thorough assessments of all of these important facets of a community.

The initial assessment of a community begins with a survey of the major systems to determine how well they are functioning. Evidence of malfunctioning in any part becomes a stimulus for further and more detailed analysis.

Community dynamics, the driving forces that govern a community's functioning, also must be considered when assessing community health. Three factors, in particular, affect community dynamics: citizen participation in community health programs, community collaboration efforts, and the power and decision-making structure. Community health nurses need to encourage community self-care by promoting the community's involvement in, commitment to, and responsibility for, its own health. Nurses also need to recognize the sources of community influence, so that they can use the system effectively to promote community health.

There are five primary types of community assessment: (1) familiarization assessment, in which available data are studied, and some firsthand data may be added, to gain a general understanding of the community; (2) problem-oriented assessment, in which the researcher focuses on a single problem and studies the community in terms of that problem; (3) community subsystem assessment, in which a single facet of community life is examined; (4) comprehensive assessment, in which the entire community is surveyed in depth; and (5) community assets assessment, in which a focus on the positive aspects of a community is used.

There are many methods for assessing a community's health. Four important ones are surveys, descriptive epidemiologic studies, community forum or town hall meetings, and focus groups. Once data have been collected from all available sources, they must be analyzed. This process can be done by hand or through the use of computer programs. After data analysis, the community health nurse can begin to form community-level nursing diagnoses. They need to be based on accurately analyzed data and can be deficit focused or wellness focused, either maximizing or improving the health of the community.

A healthy community has a number of characteristics that community health nurses look for when assessing its overall wellness. Among them are a sense of unity, the ability to collaborate and communicate effectively, a problem-solving orientation, the ability to judiciously use yet conserve resources, and the ability to handle crises and conflict.

ACTIVITIES TO PROMOTE CRITICAL THINKING

1. Explain to a colleague why it is important to understand and work with the community as a total entity.

2. How does defining the community as the client change the community health nurse's practice? List some specific examples of how this concept can be applied.

3. If you were part of a health planning team concerned about the health needs of the elderly in your community, what are some location, population, and social system variables you would want to assess? Name some of the sources from which you might collect the data.

4. Discuss under what circumstances you might choose to conduct a problem-oriented community health assessment. What method would you consider using to conduct this assessment, and how would you carry it out?

5. Interview someone from your state or local health department who has recently conducted a community needs assessment survey. Analyze the process used, and compare it with the steps for conducting a survey described in this chapter.

6. Use the Internet to contribute your ideas in response to a health-related survey taken by a television show, newspaper, or magazine, or share your opinions in a health-related chat room.

REFERENCES

American Public Health Association. (2003). *The definition of public health nursing: A statement of APHA Public Health Nursing Section.* Retrieved on 3/20/04 from *http://www.csuchico.edu/~horst/about/*

Anderson, D., Guthrie, T., & Schirle, R. (2002). A nursing model of community organization for change. *Public Health Nursing, 19*(1), 40–46.

Anderson, E.T., & McFarlane, J. (2004). *Community as partner: Theory and practice* (4th ed.). Philadelphia: Lippincott Williams & Wilkins.

Carpenito, L.J. (2002). *Handbook of nursing diagnosis* (9th ed.). Philadelphia: Lippincott Williams & Wilkins.

Clark, C.C. (Ed.). (2002). *Health promotion in communities: Holistic and wellness approaches.* New York: Springer.

Cottrell, L.S., Jr. (1976). *The competent community.* In B.H. Kaplan, R.N. Wilson, & A.H. Leighton (Eds.), *Further explorations in social psychiatry* (pp. 195–209). New York: Basic Books.

Dixon, J.K. (2002). Kids need clean air: Air pollution and children's health. *Family and Community Health, 24*(4), 9–26.

Heinemann, G.D., & Zeiss, A.M. (2002). *Team performance in health care assessment and development.* Norwell, MA: Kluwer Plenum.

Institute of Medicine. (1997). *Improving health in the community: A role for performance monitoring.* Washington, DC: National Academy Press.

Kilbourne, E.M. (1998). Illness due to thermal extremes. In R.B. Wallace (Ed.), *Maxcy-Rosenau-Last public health and preventive medicine* (14th ed.). Stamford, CT: Appleton & Lange.

Lynd, R. (1939). *Knowledge for what? The place of social science in American culture.* Princeton, NJ: Princeton University Press.

MacQueen, K.M., McLellan, E., Metzger, D.S., Jegeles, S., Strauss, R.P., Scotti, R., et al. (2001). What is community? An evidence-based definition for participatory public health. *American Journal of Public Health, 91*(12), 1929–1938.

McKnight, J. (1987). *The future of low-income neighborhoods and the people who reside there: A capacity-oriented strategy for neighborhood development.* Chicago: Center of Urban Affairs and Policy Research, Northwestern University.

Milbank Memorial Fund Commission. (1976). *Higher education for public health: A report.* New York: Prodist.

Muhib, F.B., Lin, L.S., Stueve, A., Miller, R.L., Ford, W.L., Johnson, W.D., et al. (2001). A venue-based method for sampling hard-to-reach populations. *Public Health Reports, 116*(Suppl. 1), 216–222.

Mundinger, M.O., & Jauron, G.D. (1975). Developing a nursing diagnosis. *Nursing Outlook, 23*(2), 94–98.

Nagi, S.Z. (1959, October). Factors related to heart disease among Ohio farmers. *Ohio Agricultural Experiment Station Research Bulletin,* 842.

Nakamura, R.M. (1999). *Health in America: A multicultural perspective.* Boston: Allyn & Bacon.

Neufeld, A., & Harrison, M.J. (1996). Educational issues in preparing community health nurses to use nursing diagnosis with population groups. *Nurse Education Today, 16,* 221–226.

Neuman, B., & Fawcett, J. (2001). *The Neuman systems model* (4th ed.). Stamford, CT: Appleton & Lange.

Oleske, D.M. (2001). *Epidemiology and the delivery of health care services: Methods and applications.* Norwell, MA: Kluwer Plenum.

Petersen, D.J., & Alexander, G.R. (2001). *Needs assessment in public health: A practical guide for students and professionals.* New York: Kluwer Plenum.

Plescia, M., Koontz, S., & Laurnet, S. (2001). Community assessment in a vertically integrated health care system. *American Journal of Public Health, 91*(5), 811–814.

Polit, D.F., & Hungler, B.P. (2003). *Nursing research: Principles and methods* (6th ed.). Philadelphia: Lippincott Williams & Wilkins.

Sanders, I.T., & Brownlee, A. (1979). Health in the community. In H.E. Freeman, S. Levine, & L.G. Reeder (Eds.), *Handbook of medical sociology* (3rd ed., pp. 412–433). Englewood Cliffs, NJ: Prentice-Hall.

Shamansky, S., & Pesznecker, B. (1981). A community is.... *Nursing Outlook, 29,* 182–185.

Skelly, A.H., Arcury, T.A., Gesler, W.M., Cravey, A.J., Dougherty, M.C., Washburn, S.A., et al. (2002). Sociospatial knowledge networks: Appraising community as place. *Research in Nursing and Health, 25,* 159–170.

Sattler, B., & Lipscomb, J. (Eds.). (2003). *Environmental health and nursing practice.* New York: Springer.

Stevens, P.E. (1996). Focus groups: Collecting aggregate-level data to understand community health phenomena. *Public Health Nursing, 13*(3), 170–176.

United States Department of Health and Human Services. (1991). *Healthy people 2000: National health promotion and disease prevention objectives* (S/N 017–001–00474–0). Washington, DC: U.S. Government Printing Office.

United States Department of Health and Human Services. (2000). *Healthy people 2010* (Conference ed., Vols. 1 & 2). Washington, DC: U.S. Government Printing Office.

Williams, C.A. (1977). Community health nursing: What is it? *Nursing Outlook, 25*(4), 250–254.

Williams, R.L., & Yanoshik, K. (2001). Can you do a community assessment without talking to the community? *Journal of Community Health, 26*(4), 233–247.

World Health Organization. (2003). *The world health report.* Geneva: Author.

SELECTED READINGS

Adams, C.F. (2000). Healthy communities and public policy: Four success stories. *Public Health Reports, 115,* 212–215.

Braveman, P., Cubbin, C., Marchi, K., Egerter, S., & Chavez, G. (2001). Measuring socioeconomic status/position in studies of racial/ethnic disparities: Maternal and infant health. *Public Health Reports, 116,* 449–463.

Clark, L., Barton, J.A., & Brown, N.J. (2002). Assessment of community contamination: A critical approach. *Public Health Nursing, 19*(5), 354–365.

Friedman, D.J., Anderka, M., Krieger, J.W., Land, G., & Solet, D. (2001). Accessing population health information through interactive systems: Lessons learned and future directions. *Public Health Reports, 116,* 132–141.

Krieger, N., Waterman, P., Chen, J.T., Soobader, M., Subramanian, S.V., & Carson, R. (2002). Zip code caveat: Bias due to spatiotemporal mismatches between zip codes and U. S. census-defined geographic areas—the Public Health Disparities Geocoding Project. *American Journal of Public Health, 92*(7), 1100–1102.

Mays, G.P., Miller, C.A., & Halverson, P.K. (2000). *Local public health practice: Trends and models.* Washington, DC: American Public Health Association.

Price, J.H., Dake, J.A., & Kucharewski, R. (2002). Assessing assets in racially diverse, inner-city youths: Psychometric properties of the search institute asset questionnaire. *Family Community Health, 25*(3), 1–9.

Rappaport, J., & Seidman, E. (2000). *Handbook of community psychology.* Norwell, MA: Kluwer Plenum.

Rosenblat, R.A., Casey, S., & Richardson, M. (2002). Rural-urban differences in the public health workforce: Local health departments in three rural western states. *American Journal of Public Health, 92*(7), 1102–1105.

Sharp, P.A., Greaney, M.L., Lee, P.R., & Royce, S.W. (2000). Assets-oriented community assessment. *Public Health Reports, 115,* 205–211.

Smith, S.K., & Swanson, D.A. (2001). *State and local population projections: Methodology and analysis.* Norwell, MA: Kluwer Plenum.

Strauss, R.P., Sengupta, S., Quinn, C., Goeppinger, J., Spaulding, C., Kegeles, S.M., et al. (2001). The role of community advisory boards: Involving communities in the informed consent process. *American Journal of Public Health, 91*(12), 1938–1943.

World Health Organization. (2002). *Healthy villages: A guide for communities and community health workers.* Geneva: Author.

Zust, B.L., & Moline, K. (2003). Identifying underserved ethnic populations within a community: The first step in eliminating health care disparities among racial and ethnic minorities. *Journal of Transcultural Nursing, 14*(1), 66–74.

Internet Resources

Agency for Toxic Substances and Disease Registry: *http://www.atsdr.cdc.gov*

The California Endowment—CommunitiesFirst-Grants: *http://www.calendow.org*

Centers for Disease Control and Prevention, National Center for Health Statistics: *http://www.cdc.gov/nchswww/*

Health Finder: *http://www.healthfinder.gov*

Hispanic Health Link: *http://www.cossmho.org*

National Health Information Center: *http://health.gov/nhic*

National Institute of Environmental Health Sciences: *http://www.niehs.nih.gov*

National Institutes of Health: *http://search.info.nih.gov*

National Library of Medicine: *http://www.nlm.nih.gov*

National Safety Council: *http://www.nsc.org*

Office of Disease Prevention: *http://www.odphp.osophs.dhhs.gov*

19

Planning, Intervention, and Evaluation of Health Care in Communities

| Key Terms | Learning Objectives |

Key Terms

- Coalition
- Community development
- Evaluation
- Goals
- Implementation
- Interaction
- Objectives
- Partnerships
- Planning
- Setting priorities

Learning Objectives

Upon mastery of this chapter, you should be able to:

- Describe the nursing process components of planning, implementation, and evaluation as they apply to community health nursing.
- Discuss methods the community health nurse uses to interact with the community.
- Identify the four phases of plan development for meeting health needs in a community.
- Identify actions required to implement health promotion activities with aggregates.
- Describe the process of evaluating aggregate health interventions.
- Discuss characteristics of the nursing process that affect nursing practice with the community as client.
- Describe the role of the community health nurse as a catalyst for community development.

Since starting in the nursing program, students have become familiar with one of the classic organizing systems underlying nursing practice—the nursing process. Does it continue to provide the community health nurse with the structure needed to work effectively with families and aggregates that have complex health care needs? Are there additional models and tools that can be used as guidelines when working in the community? These are some of the questions addressed in this chapter as the usefulness of the nursing process in the community is explored further.

Consisting of a systematic, purposeful set of interpersonal actions, the nursing process provides a structure for change that remains a viable tool employed by the community health nurse. In Chapter 18, the first two steps of this process, assessment and nursing diagnosis, were examined. This chapter examines the last three steps of the nursing process: planning, implementation, and evaluation as applied to the aggregate level. These five components give direction to the dynamics for solving problems, managing nursing actions, and improving the health of communities and community health nursing practice.

Three characteristics support the use of the nursing process in community health nursing. First, the nursing process is a problem-solving process that addresses community health problems at every aggregate level with the goals of preventing illness and promoting public health. Second, it is a management process that requires situational analysis, decision-making, planning, organization, direction and control of services, and outcome evaluation. As a management tool, the nursing process addresses all aggregate levels. Third, it is a process for implementing changes that improve the function of various health-related systems and the ways that people behave within those systems.

In this chapter, two other models for planning, intervention, and evaluation of health care delivered to aggregates are investigated. The models highlighted are the Health Planning Process and the Omaha Classification System, which was developed specifically for use in community health settings. In addition, the usefulness of the North American Nursing Diagnosis Association (NANDA) nursing diagnoses with families and aggregates is briefly explored in the context of planning, implementation, and evaluation of services.

NURSING PROCESS COMPONENTS APPLIED TO COMMUNITY AS CLIENT

In community health, the nursing process involves a series of components, or steps, that enable the nurse to work with aggregates in achieving optimal health. Process, the moving element of this tool, means forward progression in an orderly fashion toward some desired result. Nursing theorists attach different labels to the components, but all agree on the basic sequence of actions: assessment, diagnosis, planning, implementation, and evaluation.

Interacting With the Community

All steps of the nursing process depend on **interaction**, reciprocal exchange and influence among people. Although nurse—client interaction is often an implied or assumed element in the process, it is an essential first consideration for community health nursing. Listening to a group of elderly people, teaching a class of expectant mothers, lobbying in the legislature for the poor, working with parents to set up a dental screening program for children—all involve relationships, and relationships require interaction. Mutual give and take between nurse and clients—whether a family, a group of mothers on a Native American reservation, or a population of school children—is an expected and much needed skill that should be integrated throughout the nursing process (Fig. 19–1).

Need for Communication

Interaction Requires Communication. When a community health nurse initially contacts a group of community leaders, for example, any information the nurse may have in advance can give only partial clues to that group's needs and wants. Unless everyone involved talks and listens, the steps of the nursing process will go awry. By open, honest sharing, the nurse (and possibly others on the health team) will begin to develop trust and establish lines of effective communication. For instance, the nurse explains who he or she is and why he or she is there. The nurse encourages the group members to talk about themselves. Nurse and group members together discuss their relationship and clarify the desired na-

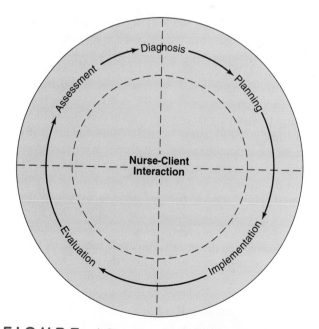

FIGURE 19–1. Nursing process components. Nurse–client interaction, a preamble structure, forms the core of the process. As a nurse and client maintain a reciprocal exchange of information and trust through interaction, they can effectively assess client needs; diagnose needs; and plan, implement, and evaluate care.

ture of that alliance. Does the group want help to identify and work on its health needs? Would its members like this nurse to continue regular contacts? What will their respective roles be? Effective communication, as a part of interaction, is essential to develop understanding and facilitate a free exchange of information between nurse and client.

Interaction Is Reciprocal. Sharing of information, ideas, feelings, concerns, and self goes both ways. Nurses must avoid the temptation either to do all the talking or merely to listen while group members monopolize the conversation. There is a dynamic exchange between two systems. The community health nurse (and other collaborating health professionals) represents one system and the client group represents the other. Whether the client is a parent group, a homeless population, or an entire community, this exchange involves a two-way sharing between the nurse and client group. The key elements of interaction are mutuality and cooperation.

Consider the following example: A dozen junior high school boys, most of whom were on the football team, met for several weeks with the school nurse to discuss physical fitness, nutrition, and other health topics. After their agreed-upon goals had been accomplished, the nurse wondered whether further meetings were needed. The nurse raised the question and offered several topics such as taking drugs and preventing injuries for possible future sessions. The boys were not interested in these suggestions but after more discussion, they decided that they did want help with talking to girls. Renewed interaction was a necessary first step in reapplying the nursing process and redefining the goals for the group.

Interaction Paves the Way for a Helping Relationship. As nurse and client interact, each is learning about the other. There is a period of testing before trust can be fully established. For the school nurse, establishing interaction was more difficult at the time of the initial contact with the boys. They had been reluctant to talk and had felt embarrassed to discuss personal subjects with an adult they did not know. Nonetheless, their interests in bodybuilding and personal appearance were strong enough to attract them to these optional sessions. Interaction began with a friendly exchange on nonthreatening topics and gradually deepened as the boys seemed ready to discuss personal subjects. Eventually it was relatively simple to talk about a new "problem" (and start the nursing process over again), because a helping relationship had already been developed. The nurse had a track record. The boys trusted, respected, and liked the nurse, so they were happy to interact around a newly stated need.

Aggregate Application

In her classic writings on community health nursing, Williams (1977) pointed out that community health practice focuses largely on the health of population groups; therefore, interaction goes beyond the one-to-one approach of clinical nursing. The challenge that the community health nurse faces is a one-to-aggregate approach. A group of parents concerned about teenage alcoholism, disabled people needing access ramps, and a neighborhood's elderly population frightened by muggings and theft are all aggregates of people with different concerns and opinions. As defined in previous chapters, the word *aggregate* refers to a mass or group of distinct individuals who are considered as a whole. Each person in an aggregate is influenced by the thoughts and behavior of other group members. Nursing interaction with an aggregate as the client demands an understanding of group behavior and group-level decision-making, and it requires interpersonal communication at the group level. Interaction is more complex with an aggregate than with an individual, but it also can be challenging and rewarding. Once community health nurses acquire an understanding of aggregate behavior, they can capitalize on the potential of group influence to make a far-reaching impact on the health of the total community. Chapter 11 examines communication and interaction with groups more closely.

Forming Partnerships and Building Coalitions

Another health-planning consideration is that aggregate-level nursing practice requires teamwork. The job of planning for the health of an entire community or a community subsystem requires that the nurse collaborate with other professionals. Usually, the nurse is part of an organized team, separate from the agency that employs the nurse. The team is brought together with the goal of improving the health of the community. Each group member brings expertise and a particular view of the problem. These interprofessional work groups are formed as either partnerships or coalitions.

Partnerships are agreements between people (and agencies) that support a joint purpose. A partnership can be large (eg, a multinational corporation and several high schools, a city government and the county jail system), or it can be a more modest endeavor (eg, a group of senior citizens and a preschool program, a Girl Scout troop and a community recycling program). Community-wide partnerships require more planning and coordination than do small partnerships. For example, because of increased student enrollment, a college may need two additional temporary and part-time faculty members who can teach the community health nursing course. The county public health department is interested in more new graduate nurses coming to work in the agency. The nursing program and the health department form a partnership and design a plan to solve both problems. The health department selects two staff nurses who have master's degrees and are qualified to instruct undergraduate clinical laboratories in community health nursing one day a week for two semesters. The benefits for everyone are numerous. The nursing program solves a temporary staffing problem; the nurses from the health department share their expertise with students, enhancing their practice and the students' learning experience; and the health department successfully introduces a pool of students who may be potential staff members to the agency and the services that it provides for the community.

A **coalition** is an alliance of individuals or groups that work together to influence outcomes of a specific problem (Green, Daniel, & Novick, 2001). Coalitions are an effective means to achieve a collaborative and coordinated approach to solving community problems. Steps to coalition building include defining goals and objectives, conducting a community assessment, identifying key players or leaders, and identifying potential coalition members.

Once these steps have been accomplished, the leader needs to keep the coalition active. This is best done by knowing and staying in touch with the coalition members, running effective meetings, and keeping every participant involved.

Sound public health practice depends on pooling resources—including people—in ways that will best serve the public. Whether health service is aimed at families, groups, subpopulations, populations, or communities, the consumers of that service are equally important members of the team. In planning for a community's health, the community (represented by appropriate individuals and agencies) must be involved. Community health nurses cannot lose sight of the need for client involvement at all levels and in all stages of community health practice.

PLANNING TO MEET THE HEALTH NEEDS IN THE COMMUNITY

Planning is the logical decision-making process used to design an orderly, detailed series of actions for accomplishing specific goals and objectives. Planning for community health is based on assessment of the community and the nursing diagnoses formulated, but assessment and diagnosis alone do not prescribe the specific actions necessary to meet clients' needs. Knowing that the group of mothers at the well-child clinic need emotional support does not tell the nurse what further action is indicated. A diagnosis of culture shock (adjustment deficit to a contrasting culture) for a family newly arrived from Cuba does not reveal what action to take. The nurse must plan (see Levels of Prevention Matrix).

Tools to Assist With Planning

Planning for community health caregiving and programs can be enhanced by the use of a variety of tools, including operational definitions of objectives and activities, conceptual

---

LEVELS OF PREVENTION MATRIX

SITUATION: Desire to reduce the incidence of child abuse in a given community by 50% within 2 years

GOAL: Using the three levels of prevention, negative health conditions are avoided, or promptly diagnosed and treated, and the fullest possible potential is restored.

PRIMARY PREVENTION		SECONDARY PREVENTION		TERTIARY PREVENTION		
Health Promotion and Education	*Health Protection*	*Early Diagnosis*	*Prompt Treatment*	*Rehabilitation*	*Primary Prevention*	
					Health Promotion and Education	*Health Protection*
• Assess factors contributing to child abuse • Institute family life education programs through schools and community groups • Develop community resources to support health promotion programs	• Identify families in the community who are at greatest risk (eg, parents with history of child abuse, families under great stress) • Develop community resources to support health protection programs	• Develop early detection programs through schools, clinics, and physicians' offices • Promote enforcement of child protection laws	• Establish programs to provide prompt treatment for abused children and abusing parents	• Establish rehabilitation programs for abused children, including safe home placement, physical and emotional treatment, and self-esteem building • Rebuild the family unit if appropriate or possible	• Provide family life education programs for families • Develop resources to support health promotion programs	• If unable or inappropriate to rehabilitate the abuser or family, keep abuser away from victim through incarceration or court order

frameworks, and models (Epstein et al., 2002). Such tools help to identify target population characteristics, clarify program goals, specify nursing interventions, and anticipate client outcomes. Tools that assist with planning also enable the nurse to test ideas and adjust solutions before actual implementation. Finally, use of tools enhances the planning process and promotes effectiveness of services, as well as professional standards of practice.

In addition to using tools, a systematic approach to planning guides the community health nurse to (1) list needs in order of priority, (2) establish goals and objectives, and (3) record the plan. As they do in the rest of the nursing process, community health nurses collaborate with clients and other appropriate professionals in each of these planning activities.

The Health Planning Process

The health planning process is a four-stage system used to design new health-related programs or services in the community. It is used by health educators when designing educational programs, by administrators in community health agencies when initiating new services, and by other people who are not nurses when developing services. The nursing process is very similar to the health planning process (Table 19–1). Each model helps to promote service effectiveness in addition to maintaining standards of practice. Community health nurses familiar with both the health planning process and the nursing process should be able to work collaboratively with community health professionals using either model.

The Omaha System

The Omaha System was developed in the 1970s by the Visiting Nursing Service of Omaha as a framework for caregiving. The Omaha system includes three schemes: problem classification, intervention, and the problem rating scale for outcomes. The Omaha system involves more than 40 client problems grouped into four domains: environmental, psychosocial, physiologic, and behavioral, a domain that includes health modifiers and signs and symptoms (Martin, Leak, & Aden, 1997). This model is outlined in detail in Chapter 15, where the focus is on quality measurement and improvement in the community. The Omaha system, along with other tools, can help the nurse organize assessment data so that client plans can be individualized. This creates a sound foundation from which outcomes can be measured and evaluated. Although the Omaha system is a useful tool for assessment of individuals, families, and small groups, it is not adaptable to the care of populations (ie, the primary focus of community health nursing).

The Omaha system addresses situations encountered by clients in the community more accurately than does the present taxonomy of the NANDA nursing diagnoses (approved by the 14th Conference, 2000). NANDA focuses on diagnoses for ill individuals with limited opportunity to focus on wellness nursing diagnoses. Health-promotion and diagnoses of more complex situations that arise within aggregates are not incorporated in the NANDA framework. How-

TABLE 19–1

Comparison Between the Health Planning Process and the Nursing Process

Health Planning Process	Nursing Process
1. ASSESSMENT STAGE	**1. ASSESSMENT**
	Determine data needed and collect data.
	Interpret data and identify needs.
	Set goals based on needs.
2. ANALYSIS AND DESIGN	**2. DIAGNOSIS**
	Analyze findings and set specific objectives.
	Design alternative interventions.
	Analyze and compare pros and cons of various solutions.
	Formulate nursing diagnoses.
	3. PLANNING
Create a plan.	List needs in order of priority.
	Establish goals and objectives.
	Write an action plan.
3. IMPLEMENTATION STAGE	**4. IMPLEMENTATION**
	Describe how to operationalize the plan.
	Design a method for monitoring progress.
4. EVALUATION STAGE	**5. EVALUATION**
	Examine costs and benefits of proposed solution.
	Judge the potential outputs, outcomes, and impact of plan.
	Modify to achieve the best plan.
	Present plan to sponsoring group or agency.
	Obtain acceptance (and funding).

ever, NANDA family diagnosis categories, such as altered family processes, parental role conflict, and compromised family coping have recently been developed and are now included (NANDA, 2000). Additional systems include the Nursing Interventions Classification System (NIC) and Nursing Outcomes Classification System (NOC); these can be used in conjunction with, or instead of, NANDA's nursing diagnoses, and they are more compatible with community health nursing care (Display 19–1). As health care continues to move into the community in the 21st century, there may be further development of the Omaha system, NANDA nursing diagnoses, NIC, and NOC, which will assist community health nurses in assessing, planning, implementing, and evaluating care of aggregates.

Nursing Interventions (NIC) and Nursing Outcomes (NOC) Classification Systems: Samples of Labels and Definitions Useful in Community Health Nursing

Examples of NIC

Abuse Protection Support: Domestic Partner—Identification of high-risk, dependent domestic relationships and actions to prevent possible or further infliction of physical, sexual, or emotional harm; neglect of basic necessities of life; or exploitation.

Infant Care—Provision of developmentally appropriate family-centered care to children younger than 1 year of age.

Surveillance: Community—Purposeful and ongoing acquisition, interpretation, and synthesis of data for decision-making in the community.

Teaching: Group—Development, implementation, and evaluation of a patient-teaching program for a group of individuals experiencing the same health condition.

Examples of NOC

Community Risk Control: Lead Exposure—Community actions to reduce lead exposure and poisoning.

Family Functioning—Ability of the family to meet the needs of its members through developmental transitions.

Risk Control: Drug Use—Actions to eliminate or reduce drug use that poses a threat to health.

Social Involvement—Frequency of an individual's social interactions with persons, groups, or organizations.

(Venes, D., & Thomas, C.L. [2001]. *Taber's Cyclopedic Medical Dictionary*. Philadelphia: FA Davis.)

Setting Priorities

Setting priorities involves assigning rank or importance to clients' needs to determine the order in which goals should be addressed. One way to order needs is to group them into three categories—immediate, intermediate, and long-range—and then prioritize those in each group. Immediate needs are more urgent but not necessarily more important. For example, a community health nurse and a group of senior citizens wanted a class on exercise techniques but did not have a place to meet. The goal of learning appropriate exercises was more important than finding a place to meet; however, the group had to first find a place to meet (immediate need) in order to accomplish its long-range goal. Some needs are ranked as immediate because they are potentially hazardous (eg, lack of eye protection in a school welding class). Some needs may even be life-threatening. Other needs are ranked first because they are of the greatest concern to clients. For example, a group of elderly people who were fearful of crime selected neighbor-

hood safety as their highest priority, although they had also identified many other needs.

Establishing Goals and Objectives

Goals and objectives are crucial to planning and should be accomplishable and specific (Anderson, Guthrie, & Schirle, 2002). The diagnosis that identifies needs must be translated into goals to give focus and meaning to the nursing plan. **Goals** are broad statements of desired end results. **Objectives** are specific statements of desired outcomes, phrased in behavioral terms that can be measured; target dates for expected completion of each objective are also stated. Objectives are the stepping stones to help one reach the end results of the larger goal. For the elderly group concerned about crime in their neighborhood, the need, the goal, and the objectives were defined as follows:

Need: The group of elderly people has altered coping ability related to their fear of crime.

Goal: Within 6 months, this group of elderly people will be free to walk the streets of their neighborhood without experiencing any incidents of criminal assault.

Objectives:
1. By the end of the first month, a safety committee (composed of seniors, nurses, police, and other appropriate community members) will be established to study the crime patterns in the neighborhood.
2. The safety committee will develop strategies for crime reduction and elder protection, which will be presented to the city council for approval by the end of the third month.
3. Safety strategies such as increased police surveillance and escort services will be implemented by the end of the fifth month.
4. By the end of the sixth month, nursing assessment will determine that seniors feel free to walk the streets.
5. By the sixth month, there will be no reported incidents of criminal assault.

Development of objectives depends on a careful analysis of all the ways in which one could accomplish the larger goal. One should first select the course of action that is best suited to meet the goal and then build objectives. For the group of elderly people, other alternatives, such as staying indoors or always walking in pairs, were considered and rejected. The choice was to find a way to make their environment safe and enjoyable.

Some rules of thumb are helpful when writing objectives. First, each objective should state a single idea. When more than one idea is expressed, as in an objective to obtain equipment and learn procedures, completion of the objective is much more difficult to measure. Second, each objective should describe one specific behavior that can be measured. For instance, the fourth objective from the list states that the seniors will report feeling free to walk outdoors within 6 months. It describes a behavior that can be measured at some point in time. One can more readily evaluate objectives that include specifics such as what will be done, who will do it, and when it will be accomplished. Then everyone knows exactly what has to be done and within what time frame. Writing measurable objectives makes a tremendous difference in the success of planning (Mager, 1975). (See Chapter 12 for more information on writing behavioral objectives).

Planning means thinking ahead. The nurse looks ahead toward the desired end and then decides what intermediate actions are necessary to meet that goal. Sometimes, an objective itself describes the intermediate actions. At other times, an objective may be further broken down into several activities. For example, the second objective states that the safety committee will be charged with developing strategies, presenting them to the city council, and gaining their approval. Good planning requires this kind of detail.

Making decisions is an important part of planning. Decisions must be made during the process of establishing priorities. Decisions are necessary for selecting goals and for choosing the best course of action from many possible courses. Further decision-making is involved in selecting objectives and taking action to accomplish the objectives.

To facilitate planning and decision-making, the community health nurse involves other people. Clients must be included at every step because they are the ones for whom the planning is being done. Without their insights and cooperation, the plan may not succeed. Additionally, the involvement of other nurses may be important. Team meetings, nurse-supervisor conferences, and nurse-expert consultant sessions are all useful resources for planning. In addition, the community health nurse frequently wishes to confer with members of other health and professional disciplines. Interdisciplinary team conferences are valuable for gaining a broader perspective and enlisting wider support for the evolving plan.

Recording the Plan

Recording the plan is the next step. Up to this point, the planning phase has been a series of intellectual exercises done jointly with clients and perhaps with other health team members. The nurse has probably written notes on the decisions made about priorities, goals, objectives, and actions. Now the nurse must clearly record the plan. One way to record the plan is to list items in columns with space for the nurse to record specifics. It is also helpful to share copies of the plan with clients. In many instances, having copies of the plan promotes a client's sense of equal partnership in and responsibility for meeting goals. It may also encourage clients to contribute more ideas once they see the plan in writing.

Regardless of the type of plan format used, certain items must be included in the written plan:

1. A *database* comprises all the subjective and objective information collected about clients—physical, psychological, social, and environmental. It includes background health information (past and present), aggregate health assessment, and group history or group systems review. The database is best kept in a format that allows space for ongoing entries and analysis. Various computer programs and applications can assist this process.

2. *Aggregate needs* are the specific areas related to clients' health that have been identified for intervention. Preferably, they are areas that both clients and nurse agree require action. They are drawn from the nursing diagnosis. *Goals* are statements that describe the resolution of needs. For clarity in planning, both a written need statement and a written goal statement are helpful.

3. *Objectives* are the specific statements that describe in behavioral and measurable terms what the nurse and clients hope to accomplish. It is often necessary to construct several objectives, sometimes around different categories of needs, to achieve comprehensive results. These objectives provide the nurse planner with specific targets at which to aim and around which to design actions.

4. *Planned actions* are the specific activities or methods of accomplishing the objectives or expected outcomes. Plans should include appropriate actions by the nurse, clients, and others.

5. *Outcome measurement* is judgment of the effectiveness of goal attainment. How and when was each objective met; if an objective was not met, why not? It is essential to include this type of outcome evaluation in the written plan. Progress notes are not the same as outcome measurements. Progress notes are useful periodic summaries that give a running account of what is occurring. Outcome measurement requires that analysis of these occurrences be conducted and conclusions drawn. Progress notes and outcome measurements may be combined if space is allowed on the plan format. Usually, it is best to enter progress notes in a separate space.

IMPLEMENTING PLANS FOR PROMOTING THE HEALTH OF AGGREGATES IN THE COMMUNITY

Implementation is putting the plan into action. The activities delineated in the plan must be carried out by the nurse, other professionals, or clients. Implementation is often referred to as the action phase of the nursing process. In community health nursing, implementation includes not just nursing action or nursing intervention but collaboration with clients and perhaps other professionals. When bringing about change in a community organization, "implementation involves preparing a timeline for completion of each program objective, obtaining the necessary funding, collaborating with agencies outside the community as needed, recruiting additional community volunteers needed for program implementation, and actually putting into action the interventions designed during the planning phase" (Anderson, Guthrie, & Schirle, 2002, p. 44). Certainly, the nurse's professional expertise and judgment provide a necessary resource to the client group. The nurse is also a catalyst and facilitator in planning and activating the action plan. However, a primary goal in community health is to help people learn to help themselves in achieving their optimal level of health (see The Global Community). To realize this goal, the nurse must con-

THE GLOBAL COMMUNITY

THE COPC SYSTEM IN ISRAEL: USING THE NURSING PROCESS

The Community-Oriented Primary Care (COPC) system, initiated in Jerusalem more than 30 years ago, was modeled after a successful program in rural South Africa in the 1950s. The concepts is "a continuous process by which primary health care is provided to a defined population on the basis of its defined health needs by the planned integration of public health with primary care practice" (p. 1717). The following model depicts the COPC cycle:

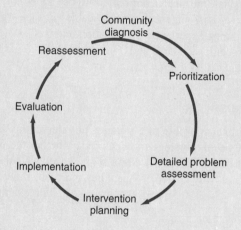

The cycle of care begins with a multistage community diagnosis (including the community's demographic characteristics, environment, health status, and available

health and social services). Problems are identified and then prioritized. A single health problem or set of problems with common risk factors is selected as the priority target for intervention. The targeted problem is then subjected to a detailed assessment to determine its precise nature. With this detailed information, an intervention program, which includes an evaluation component, can be developed and implemented. The stage is then set for later reassessment of the community's health status, with further prioritization, planning, implementation, and evaluation of intervention programs.

Through the use of graduate students in public health, medicine and nursing, they conducted health surveys, identified problems, and prioritized problem areas. From survey data, cardiovascular disease and child growth and development were identified and focused on in the medical clinics, in educational programs, and community outreach.

This Jerusalem experience has shown the feasibility and sustainability of primary care—public health integration in community health services and its positive impact on the health of a community. Since 1960, more than 1000 health professionals from Israel and 75 other countries have participated in field-based workshops to study the COPC approach and bring the techniques to the villages and towns in their countries.

Epstein, L., Gofin, J., Gofin, R., & Neumark, Y. (2002). The Jerusalem experience: Three decades of service, research, and training in community-oriented primary care. *American Journal of Public Health, 92*(11), 1717–1721.

---

stantly involve clients in the deliberative process and encourage their sense of responsibility and autonomy. Other health team members may also participate in carrying out the plan. All are partners in implementation.

Preparation

The actual course of implementation, outlined in the plan, should be fairly easy to follow if goals, expected outcomes, and planned actions have been designed carefully. Professionals and clients should have a clear idea of the "who, what, why, when, where, and how." Who will be involved in carrying out the plan? What are each person's responsibilities? Do all understand why and how to do their parts? Do they know when and where activities will occur? As implementation begins, nurses should review these questions for themselves as well as clients. This is the time to clarify any doubtful areas, thereby facilitating a smooth implementation phase.

Even the best planning may require adjustments. For example, some nurses who planned a health fair for seniors discovered that the target group would not have transportation to the site because the volunteering bus company had withdrawn its offer. Instead, the nurses arranged for volunteers from local churches to pick up the seniors, bring them to the health fair, and deliver them afterward to their homes. Implementation requires flexibility and adaptation to unanticipated events.

Activities or Actions

The process of implementation requires a series of nursing actions or activities:

1. The nurse applies appropriate theories, such as systems theory or change theory, to the actions being performed.
2. The nurse helps to facilitate an environment that is conducive to carrying out the plan (eg, a quiet room in which

to hold a group teaching session or solicitation of support from local officials for an environmental cleanup project).

3. The nurse and other health team members prepare clients to receive services by assessing their knowledge, understanding, and attitudes and by carefully interpreting the plan to clients. This interaction nurtures open communication and trust between nurse and clients. Professionals and clients (or representatives if the aggregate is large) form a contractual agreement about the content of the plan and how it is to be carried out.

4. The plan is carried out, or modified and then carried out, by professionals and clients. Modification requires constant observation and interchange during implementation, because these actions determine the success of the plan and the nature of needed changes.

5. The nurse and the team monitor and document the progress of the implementation phase by process evaluation, which measures the ongoing achievement of planned actions.

The Research: Bridge to Practice display describes a Healthy Communities (Health Communities Agenda campaign) success in California and the interventions undertaken from the ground up to promote health in one state.

EVALUATING IMPLEMENTED AGGREGATE HEALTH PLANS

Evaluation, the final component of the nursing process, is the last in a sequence of actions leading to the resolution of client health needs. As described before, **evaluation** refers to measuring and judging the effectiveness of goal attainment. The nursing process is not complete until evaluation takes place. Too often, emphasis is placed primarily on assessing client needs and on planning and implementing service (MacDonald, 2002). How effective was the service? Were client needs truly met? Professional practitioners owe it to their clients, themselves, and other health service providers to evaluate a program (see Clinical Corner).

Evaluation is an act of appraisal in which one judges value in relation to a standard and a set of criteria. For example, when eating dinner in a restaurant, diners evaluate the experience in terms of the standard of a satisfying meal. Their criteria for a "satisfying meal" may include qualities such as a wide variety of choices on the menu, reasonable price, tasty food, nice atmosphere, and good service. They also evaluate the meal in terms of a purpose: Does this restaurant serve satisfying meal at a reasonable price, desirable for future dining experiences? Evaluation requires a stated purpose, specific standards and criteria by which to judge, and judgment skills.

Purpose

The ultimate purpose of evaluating an intervention in community health nursing is to determine whether the planned actions met the client's needs. If so, how well were they met, and if not, why not? Were there any unexpected outcomes? Has the client's competence increased? For example, an

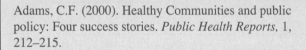

RESEARCH: BRIDGE TO PRACTICE

Adams, C.F. (2000). Healthy Communities and public policy: Four success stories. *Public Health Reports*, 1, 212–215.

FROM THE GROUND UP: CALIFORNIA SMOKE-FREE CITIES

The Healthy Communities initiatives are working to build community consensus for improving local health care and other quality-of-life issues. Many have had important effects on policy making at the county and state level in some cities and states.

California demonstrates a dramatic example of a Healthy Communities approach that is influencing policy, and improving health and quality of life. Beginning in 1990, funds generated by the tobacco tax were used to sponsor California Smoke-Free Cities (CSFC). This initiative used Healthy Communities tools to fight the health hazard of secondhand tobacco smoke.

The project relied on participation and education as tools to provide training and consultation with local offi-

cials and to pass smoke-free ordinances. This approach was unique, because most city officials do not usually deal directly with health issues, so education became crucial. The officials received information about the health threat of secondhand smoke, what other cities had done to fight it, availability of resources to begin a tobacco control campaign, and what could be expected from an organized opposition.

After some hard-won battles with the tobacco industry at the local level, officials emerged as leaders and educated others in municipal government. From 1990 to 1993, a wave of local ordinances led to passage in 1994 of a state law that banned smoking in all workplaces, including bars. This law continues today in California. A successful Healthy Communities approach capitalizes on the power of the local people taking control of their own health. CSFC coordinator Anne Klink stated, "One of the important side effects of this project was the creation of an opportunity for citizens to become involved in fighting for something important, something close to home, and winning" (p. 215).

CLINICAL CORNER

EVALUATING OUTCOMES OF A HOME CARE POSTPARTUM PROGRAM

Scenario

As a nurse working as the liaison between Capitol City Hospital and its home health agency, you are given the job of reviewing your early postpartum discharge program. Your program has been in effect for 18 months. Client satisfaction is high. The program has increased revenue for the hospital as many clients choose to deliver at Capitol City Hospital because of the early discharge program.

The protocol for your early discharge program includes a postpartum home visit by an RN from the home health agency. These visits are provided as a service to the client. In some cases, visits are billable to insurance companies. Medicaid authorizes payment for one postpartum visit.

You have gathered the following information about the early discharge program:

I. Protocol: Standard is one visit within 48 hours after discharge which includes:
   A. Education
      1. Newborn care
      2. Breastfeeding
      3. Warning signs warranting follow-up (mother and baby)
         —Infection
         —Hemorrhage
      4. Comfort
      5. Parenting
      6. Sexuality
         —Resumption of sexual activity
         —Contraception
      7. Community resources
      8. Nutrition
      9. Well and sick baby care
   B. Assessment
      1. Infant: Jaundice (heel stick performed if necessary)
         Mother: Hemorrhage, perineal lacerations, hematomas
         Both: Nutrition
         —Weight
         —Hydration
         —Breastfeeding
      2. Elimination
II. Cost:
   A. Fully reimbursed by some insurance companies

   B. All mother/baby dyads receive postpartum visits, regardless of insurance coverage
   C. Optional or additional methods of reimbursement have not been explored by the agency
   D. Agency makes money on reimbursed visits, loses money on non-reimbursed, but additional revenue generated by clients choosing the hospital because of the positive public perception. The program is thought to balance out cost of nonreimbursed visits.

Outcomes. Outcomes of postpartum early discharge with accompanying home visit (as compared to traditional length of postpartum stay)
I. Positive
   A. Higher percentage of successful (at least 2 months) breastfeeding
   B. Higher rate of immunization compliance
   C. Fewer inappropriate emergency room visits
   D. High client satisfaction
   E. Lower levels of maternal stress reported to pediatricians
II. Negative
   A. Higher incidence in jaundice in babies whose mothers participated in the early discharge program

Questions

1. What, if any, additional information do you need to make a recommendation regarding the program?
   • How will you obtain this information?
2. As the nurse making a recommendation for the continuation or termination of the postpartum early discharge program, what are your recommendations?
   • Should the program be abandoned?
   • Should the program be maintained?
3. What, if any, alterations would you make in the following areas:
   • Funding
   • Protocol
      —Client education
      —Assessment
      —Timing of visit
4. Outcome measurements are critical to demonstrate the efficacy of this program.
   • What will you evaluate?
   • How often?
   • Why?

evaluation is conducted to determine the effectiveness of a group health promotion program with community elders. Criteria for evaluation focus on health practices, psychological and spiritual well-being, and social integration. Outcomes are measured during weekly interventions with the group for a period of 3 months. What does the evaluation suggest? Do the participants continue with health promotion practices, or do the practices slowly erode away? What would an evaluation at 6 months or 1 year show?

Criteria

Sometimes, plans include individual goals and criteria as well as group goals and criteria. Goals are statements of desired outcomes, and criteria are the smaller increments or steps that must be taken to achieve the goals. For example, several diabetic women attending a clinic had a problem with obesity. A community health nurse working in the clinic helped them form a weight loss group. Each member developed individual weight loss goals to be accomplished within 6 months. The women planned to meet their individual goals by identifying specific criteria such as daily calorie limits (eg, 1500 calories per day) and regular exercise programs (eg, 20-minute exercise sessions performed three times a week). They evaluated their individual goals by determining whether they met these criteria.

To maximize group support and encourage healthy behavior patterns during weight loss, the nurse suggested having a group goal and objectives to measure group success.

Group Goal: The group will stay healthy while accomplishing 90% of member weight loss goals.

Group Objectives:

1. By the end of 6 months, the group will lose at least 90% of the sum of the expected individual weight losses.
2. The group will have no diabetes-related infections during the 6 months.
3. All of the group members will be exercising at least once a week by the end of 3 months.
4. No more than 10% of the group will have had an illness that keeps them in bed longer than 1 day during the 6 months.

The prepared set of criteria helped the group evaluate its success.

The previous examples emphasize the relationship of good planning to evaluation. When nurse and clients prepare clear, specific goals and objectives, there is no question about how or what to evaluate. It will be obvious whether the goal has been met.

Judgment Skills

Evaluation requires judgment skills that the nurse uses to compare real outcomes with expected outcomes so that discrepancies may be identified (Schalock, 2001). If actual client behavior matches the desired behavior, then the goal has been met. If goals are not met, the nurse needs to examine several possible explanations for the failure, which may include inadequate data collection, incorrect diagnosis, an unrealistic plan, ineffective implementation, or loss of enthusiasm. Circumstances or client motivation or both may have changed. There may not have been enough client participation in one or more parts of the process. After determining the cause of the failure, the nurse can reassess, plan, and initiate corrective action.

Types of Evaluations

To determine the success of their planning and intervention, community heath nurses use two main types of evaluation: structure-process evaluation and outcomes evaluation. Each type of evaluation has importance to the success of any plan.

Structure-Process Evaluation

Structure-process evaluation has as its emphasis the formation and operation of a plan or program. Established performance standards are used to determine what is working and what is not working throughout the process (Anderson, Guthrie, & Schirle, 2002). It is part of the structure-process-outcome model of quality improvement developed by Donabedian (1966), which is discussed in Chapter 15. In practice, agencies and professionals may develop two different evaluation systems, one for structure-process and the other for outcomes measurement.

Structure refers to the tools and resources in the health care environment that are beyond individual control. They include the physical and organizational structure of the agency, as well as community resources that provide a foundation for health care services. Such resources as staff qualifications, caseload, licensing, certification, compliance with state regulations, and available funding are part of the structural component. When conducting a structure-process evaluation, questions to be answered include the following: Are all professional staff members licensed? Do they hold the appropriate certifications? Does the facility meet state and local health department standards? Are there adequate and accessible resources in the community to meet client referral needs?

Process criteria refer to how caregiving is performed. These criteria focus on the delivery of services designed to achieve community health care outcomes. Process evaluation questions include the following: Are agency policies and procedures being followed? Are caregivers skilled in the latest technologies or caregiving practices required by the client mix? Do the staff nurses have adequate time for documentation? Is documentation done appropriately?

Outcomes Evaluation

The third part of the Donabedian model is outcomes evaluation (Donabedian, 1966). Although the term *outcomes evaluation* became recognized with Donabedian's conceptual framework in the 1960s, it has been used independently to measure the end results (quality) of service—the effect and the impact of services.

The *effect,* or degree to which an outcome objective has been met, informs the agency or program leader of the program's impact on clients' health. As an example, one manufacturing company had an 80% adherence rate for employees who were supposed to wear proper protective devices (goggles, safety shoes, and hard hats) in the plant. Noncompliance on the part of some workers was a concern to union representatives, the health and safety team, and the company management. They were concerned that 20% of their employees were at risk for injury that would cause pain, suffering, loss of work time, disruption to the manufacturing process, and reduced profitability. The occupational health nurse along with the safety officer began a month-long safety campaign that included safety miniclasses, posters, and incentives for departments with 100% safety equipment adherence. Three months after the program, 95% of the employees were adhering to the safety regulations. This 15% increase was attributed to the effect of the safety program.

The *impact* of a program determines how close it comes to attaining its goals. In the earlier example, the objective of the safety campaign was to increase safety equipment use, and use was significantly increased as a result of the program. However, if the goal of the program had been to decrease accidents and save the company money, the result could be determined only with additional information. Were there fewer injuries caused by accidents? Were there fewer days lost to injuries? Did the company save money as the direct result of employee safety adherence? Depending on the answers to these questions, the overall goal of the program may or may not have been met, even though the objective of the program was met. The full impact of the program cannot be determined without additional data.

Quality Measurement and Improvement

In community health nursing, evaluation is also performed to measure the quality of services, programs, and nurse performance. Programs that measure quality are known by several names—quality management programs (or systems), total quality management (TQM) programs, or quality assurance programs. Regardless of their names, they reflect nursing's increasing concern with measuring and improving quality. A sound quality management system includes the following:
1. An organizational entity created for assessing quality
2. Establishment of standards or criteria against which quality is assessed
3. A routine system of gathering information
4. Assurance that such information is based on the total population or a representative sample of clients or potential clients
5. A process that provides the results of review to clients, the public, providers, and sponsoring organizations and suggests methods to institute corrective actions

With the burgeoning emphasis on accountability in health services, community health nursing is being chal-

lenged to devise better ways of documenting service effectiveness and cost-efficiency. Methodologies and tools that provide guidelines are currently in use and are constantly expanded to facilitate these evaluative processes (Heinemann & Zeiss, 2002).

NURSING PROCESS CHARACTERISTICS APPLIED TO COMMUNITY AS CLIENT

The nursing process provides a framework or structure on which community health nursing actions are based. Application of the process varies with each situation, but the nature of the process remains the same. Certain characteristics of that process are important for community health nurses to emphasize in their practices (Fig. 19–2).

Deliberative

The nursing process is deliberative—purposefully, rationally, and carefully thought out. It requires the use of sound judgment that is based on adequate information. Community health nurses often practice in situations that demand the ability to think independently and make difficult decisions. Furthermore, thoughtful, deliberative problem-solving is a skill needed for working with the community health team to address the needs and problems of aggregates in the community. The nursing process is a decision-making tool to facilitate these determinations.

Adaptable

The nursing process is adaptable. Its dynamic nature enables the community health nurse to adjust appropriately to each situation and to be flexible in applying the process to aggregate health needs. Furthermore, its flexibility is a reminder to the nurse that each client group, each community situation is unique. The nursing process must be applied specifically to the individual situation and group of people. Based on assessment and sound planning, the nurse adapts and tailors services to meet the identified needs of each community client group.

Cyclic

The nursing process is cyclic and is in constant progression. Steps are repeated over and over in the nurse–aggregate client relationship. The nurse engages in continual interaction, data collection, analysis, intervention, and evaluation. As interactions between nurse and client group continue, various steps in the process overlap with one another and are used simultaneously. The cyclic nature of the nursing process enables the nurse to engage in a constant information feedback loop. That is, information gathered and lessons learned at each step of the process promote greater understanding of the group being served, the most effective way to

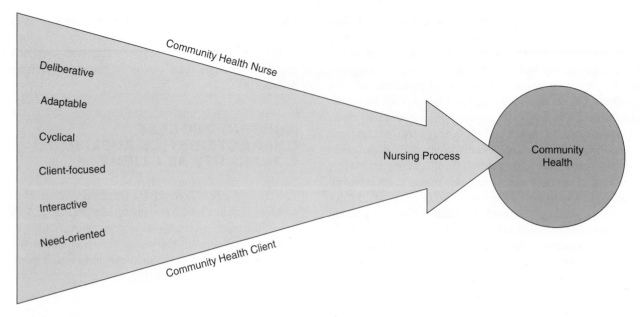

FIGURE 19-2.   Nursing process characteristics emphasized in community health nursing practice.

provide quality services, and the best methods of raising this group's level of health.

Client Focused

The nursing process is client focused; it is used for and with clients. Community health nurses use the nursing process for the express purpose of addressing the health of populations. They are helping aggregate clients, directly or indirectly, to achieve and maintain health. Clients as total systems—whether groups, populations, or communities—are the target of community health nursing's use of the nursing process.

Interactive

The nursing process is interactive in that nurse and clients are engaged in a process of ongoing interpersonal communication. Giving and receiving accurate information are necessary to promote understanding between nurse and clients and to foster effective use of the nursing process. Furthermore, because of the movement toward informed consumption of medical care, demands for clients' rights and the concept of self-care have gained emphasis. Client groups and community health nurses have increasingly joined forces to assume responsibility for promoting community health. The nurse–aggregate client relationship can and should be a partnership, a shared experience by professionals (nurses and others) and client groups.

Need Oriented

The nursing process is need oriented. Long association with problem-solving has tended to limit the focus of the nursing process to the correction of existing problems. Although problem-solving is certainly an appropriate use of the nurs-

ing process, the community health nurse can also use the nursing process to anticipate client needs and prevent problems. The nurse should think of nursing diagnoses as ranging from health problem identification to primary prevention and health promotion opportunities. This focus is needed if the goals of community health—to protect, promote, and restore the people's health—are to be realized.

THE COMMUNITY HEALTH NURSE AS CATALYST FOR COMMUNITY DEVELOPMENT

Regardless of the agency focus, inherent in the community health nurse role is improvement or development of the community. When individual clients become healthier, they bring their healthier state into the community. When a family's health is improved, their greater wellness improves the quality of their involvement in the community. When groups within the community improve their health (eg, pregnant teens follow up with prenatal care, third graders brush their teeth regularly), there is a positive effect on the community's health. Using community developmental theory, the community health nurse acts as a catalyst to promote safe and healthy communities.

Community Development Theory

Community development is the process of collaborating with community members to assess their collective needs and desires for positive change and to address these needs through problem-solving, the use of community experts, and resource development (Fawcett et al., 2000; Green, 2000; Green, Daniel, & Novick, 2001). A community development perspective assumes that community members participate in all aspects of change—assessment, planning, development, delivery of services, and evaluation. With this approach, the focus is on healthful community changes generated from within the community, as a partnership between health care providers and inhabitants, rather than a commodity dispensed by health care providers.

The outcomes are more positive when community members have a sense of "ownership" of health programs and services that address their needs. This enhances empowerment within the community and enables members to effectively control and participate in transforming their lives and environment (Bragg, 1997). This implies that health care agency infrastructures are appropriate additions to services that are planned and delivered in an acceptable manner to the community.

When applying community development theory, the agent of change (often the community health nurse) is considered a partner rather than an authority figure responsible for the community's health. To achieve acceptance as a partner, the nurse must listen and learn from the community members, because they are the "experts" with respect to their health care needs, culture, and values (Bragg, 1997; Kreuter, Lezin, & Young, 2000). They have mastered adaptation to the community, and they have firsthand knowledge of prevention methods and interventions that are appropriate to their lifestyles. For example, a study was conducted of 690 women from 18 impoverished inner-city neighborhoods in five cities. Women who were considered opinion leaders by their peers conducted human immunodeficiency virus (HIV) risk-reduction workshops and community HIV prevention events. There was evidence that significant changes in health behaviors to prevent HIV infection occurred among the women who attended these events. (Sikkema et al., 2000).

The outcomes of the services provided by any organization can be benchmarked against those of other groups. Benchmarking involves comparing an organization's outcomes against those of a similar organization or an organization that is known for its excellence in a particular area of client care (Nolan & Mock, 2000). The continuous comparison of outcomes involved in benchmarking is conducted by agency team members who have a vision of becoming the "best of the best" (Wojner, 2001). Information from this comparison can be used to identify an organization's areas of weakness and to focus attention on specific outcomes. The establishment of *best practice* activities entails "continuous, collaborative, and systematic processes for measuring and examining internal programs' strengths and weaknesses" (Lewis & Latney, 2002, p. 24).

From a global perspective, the Conference on Primary Health Care held at Alma-Ata in 1978 concluded that people have little control over their own health care services and that the emphasis should be on health problems identified by the members of the community in their attempts to attain a state of wellness (World Health Organization, 1998). Since that time, the World Health Organization has been providing leadership in the use of community development methods to improve global health.

Building Healthy and Safe Communities

What makes a community healthy? It is more than the health care services available in a community. It is the feeling of safety. It is being well informed, which gives the power to make choices. It is establishing lasting bonds with one another. It is having strong families. It is having a sense of meaning in one's life.

Community health nurses have a rich history in promoting health in communities. They are uniquely positioned to act as catalysts in the community. They are able to address major problems that affect the health of a given population and, as a result, the health of the community. Health problems such as infant mortality and acquired immunodeficiency syndrome (AIDS) are difficult to resolve at the individual level; they require community collaboration and action. Experts agree that the health of a community depends on its interconnectedness (see Voices from the Community).

The philosophical basis of community health nursing is grounded in the public health mission of promoting healthy communities. This requires collaboration with clients wherever they live, work, and go to school. The goal of community health nursing is to position the nurse as a central person in the community to improve accessibility of care for consumers.

A component of a healthy community is that the community is safe. Community member involvement is as essential to the success and stability of safety programs as it is to any community health program. For communities to be safe, there must

VOICES FROM THE COMMUNITY

Linda Bergthold (a principal in a human resource and benefits consulting firm)—"A healthy community would be dense with empowering organizations at the local level and is a community that has identified its own priorities and has set out to build them."

Hazel Henderson (anti-economist)—"A healthy community means shifting our value system away from compulsive individualism toward re-balancing the needs of communities."

Sean Sullivan (National Business Coalition)—"Housing, education, crime, or the community's vision of itself are not things that usually show up in conversations of healthcare reformers about ways of reducing healthcare costs . . . or that managed competition will have much impact on."

Drew Altman (Kaiser Family Foundation)—"A good job and a strong family is the best health and human services program."

be involvement by community participants, be they recent immigrants, ethnic minorities, parents of infants, elders, bicyclists, joggers, skaters, or schoolchildren. Different people perceive the world in different ways, and their observations can provide valuable insights for problem identification, program design, and solution development. These participants can act as "key informants" to provide qualitative data that can help prioritize the identified problems.

The community health nurse is in a position to initiate, promote, coordinate, and, at times, provide the beginning leadership as health and safety programs are developed in communities (El-Askari et al., 1998). Ideally, citizen participation will be developed and citizen control will emerge (Fig. 19–3).

SUMMARY

The effectiveness of community health nursing practice depends on how well the nursing process is used as a tool to enhance aggregate health. The nursing process involves appropriate application of a systematic series of actions with the goal of helping clients achieve their optimal level of health. The components of this process are assessment, diagnosis, planning, implementation, and evaluation.

Interaction is deeply integrated in the nursing process. Because nurse and clients must first establish a relationship of reciprocal influence and exchange before any change can take place, interaction could be considered the most essential step in the process. Effective communication is inherent in assessing needs and establishing trust between nurse and clients as partners in the nursing process.

The first two steps of the nursing process, assessment and formulation of nursing diagnoses, are covered in detail in Chapter 18. The third step, planning, includes designing a specific course of action to address the target group's diagnosis. It involves ranking a group's or aggregate's needs, establishing goals and measurable objectives, designing activities to meet the objectives, and developing a plan. The plan also includes a means to evaluate each objective.

Models are useful to community health nurses for organization of service delivery. Two models are mentioned, the health planning model and the Omaha system. They are discussed in light of the basic tools of the nursing process and with the help and limitations of the NANDA nursing diagnoses and the NIC and NOC systems. Community health nurses can judge the value of these models and tools when planning services with community members.

The fourth step, implementation, activates the plan and follows it through to completion. During implementation, the nurse applies appropriate theory, provides a facilitative environment, prepares clients for service, carries out or modifies and carries out a plan (with clients), and documents the implementation.

The last and very important step is evaluation, which measures and judges the effectiveness of the interventions. Well-prepared goals and objectives are essential for adequate evaluation. If goals are not met, the failure may have resulted from inadequate assessment or planning. Determining the cause of the failure can lead to corrective action. Evaluation does not end the nursing process; rather, it allows documentation of what has been accomplished and what needs to be done so that the process, a continuing cycle, can start again.

Certain characteristics are important to the nursing process and should be emphasized by community health nurses in their practices. The process is deliberative, requiring that judgment be exercised when making decisions. It is adaptable and encourages flexibility in practice. It is cyclic, fostering an ongoing use of the process. It is client focused and can help the nurse keep the proper client health target in view. It is interactive, promoting nurse–client communication and client participation. Finally, it is need oriented; it focuses on the client's current and future needs, including prevention and health promotion to help clients achieve optimal health.

Using the nursing process in the community would not be complete without looking at the role of the community health nurse as a catalyst for community development. Community development theory is the foundation that supports citizen empowerment and use of key players in the community to plan for the health and safety of the community.

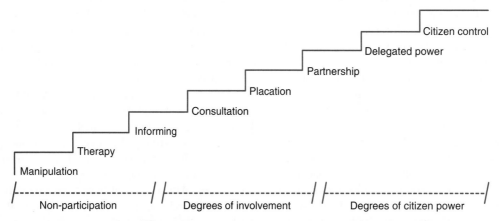

FIGURE 19–3. Eight steps of citizen participation. (Adapted from Arnstein, S.R. [1969]. A ladder of citizen participation. *Journal of the American Institute of Planners,* July, 217–224.)

ACTIVITIES TO PROMOTE CRITICAL THINKING

1. You have been using the nursing process with individuals to effect change in their health status. Now consider how you can expand that application to aggregates. Select a population group in your community, such as preschoolers, unwed mothers, a group of refugees, or homebound elderly people.
   a. How might you start the interaction phase with these potential clients?
   b. What specific areas would you want to assess? Make a list of hypothetical indicators that suggest a need.
   c. Invent a diagnosis for this group that would be supported by the data you collected in your assessment.
   d. What alternative courses of action should you consider for addressing this need? Select the most appropriate one.
   e. Start a plan for implementation, including an overall goal and at least one objective.
   f. List the activities needed to meet your objectives, and describe how you might carry them out.
   g. How would you evaluate your nursing interventions with this population group?
2. Search your own community for examples of healthy community practices in the form of programs, partnerships, coalitions, and so forth. Explore one such example and assess the degree of community involvement based on citizen leadership and control.
3. Use the Internet to locate community health nursing articles that highlight examples of community development in which the community health nurse assumes the role of catalyst.

REFERENCES

Adams, C.F. (2000). Healthy communities and public policy: Four success stories. *Public Health Reports, 115*(2–3), 212–215.

Anderson, D., Guthrie, T., & Schirle, R. (2002). A nursing model of community organization for change. *Public Health Nursing, 19*(1), 40–46.

Arnstein, S.R. (1969, July). A ladder of citizen participation. *Journal of the American Institute of Planners*, 217–224.

Bragg, M. (1997). An empowerment approach to community health education. In B.S. Spradley & J.A. Allender (Eds.), *Readings in community health nursing* (5th ed., pp. 504–510). Philadelphia: Lippincott-Raven.

Donabedian, A. (1966). Evaluating the quality of medical care. *Milbank Quarterly, 44,* 166–206.

El-Askari, G., Freestone, J., Irizarry, C., Kraut, K.L., Mashiyama, S.T., Morgan, M.A., et al. (1998). The healthy neighborhoods project: A local health department's role in catalyzing community development. *Health Education and Behavior, 25*(2), 146–159.

Epstein, L., Gofin, J., Gofin, R., & Neumark, Y. (2002). The Jerusalem experience: Three decades of service, research, and training in community-oriented primary care. *American Journal of Public Health, 92*(11), 1717–1721.

Fawcett, S.B., Francisco, V.T., Paine-Andrews, A., Schultz, J.A. (2000). A model memorandum of collaboration: A proposal. *Public Health Reports, 115,* 199–204.

Green, L.W. (2000). Caveats on coalitions: In praise of partnerships. *Health Promotion Practice, 1,* 191–197.

Green, L., Daniel, M., & Novick, L. (2001). Partnerships and coalitions for community-based research. *Public Health Reports, 116*(Suppl. 1), 20–31.

Heinemann, G.D., & Zeiss, A.M. (Eds.). (2002). *Team performance in health care assessment and development.* Norwell, MA: Kluwer Plenum.

Kreuter, M.W., Lezin, N.A., & Young, L.A. (2000). Evaluating community-based collaborative mechanisms: Implications for practitioners. *Health Promotion Practice, 1,* 49–63.

Lewis, P.S., & Latney, C. (2002). Achieve best practice with an evidence-based approach. *Nursing Management, 33*(12), 24–30.

MacDonald, S. (2002). Evaluating community health programs, In C.C. Clark, *Health promotion in communities: Holistic and wellness approaches.* New York: Springer.

Mager, R.F. (1975). *Preparing instructional objectives* (2nd ed.). Belmont, CA: Pitman Learning.

Martin, K., Leak, G., & Aden, C. (1997). The Omaha system: A research-based model for decision making. In B.W. Spradley & J.A. Allender (Eds.), *Readings in community health nursing* (5th ed., pp. 316–324). Philadelphia: Lippincott-Raven.

Nolan, M.T., & Mock, V. (2000). *Measuring patient outcomes.* Thousand Oaks, CA: Sage.

North American Nursing Diagnosis Association. (2000). *Nursing diagnoses: Definitions and classification.* 14th NANDA Conference. Philadelphia: NANDA.

Schalock, R.L. (2001). *Outcome-based evaluation* (2nd ed.). Norwell, MA: Kluwer Plenum.

Sikkema, K.J., Kelly, J.A., Winett, R.A., Solomon, L.J., Cargill, V.A., Roffman, R.A., et al. (2000). Outcomes of a randomized community-level HIV prevention intervention for women living in 18 low-income housing developments. *American Journal of Public Health, 90*(1), 57–63.

Venes, D., & Thomas, C.L. (2001). *Taber's Cyclopedic Medical Dictionary* (19th ed.). Philadelphia: F.A. Davis.

Williams, C.A. (1977). Community health nursing: What is it? *Nursing Outlook, 25,* 250–253.

Wojner, A.W. (2001). *Outcomes management: Applications to clinical practice.* St. Louis: Mosby.

World Health Organization. (1998). *Primary health care in the 21st century is everybody's business.* Geneva: Author.

SELECTED READINGS

Ahmed, S.M., & Maurana, C.A. (2000). Reaching out to the underserved: A successful volunteer program. *American Journal of Public Health, 90*(3), 439–440.

Altschuld, J.W., & Witkin, B.R. (1999). *From needs assessment to action: Transforming needs into solution strategies.* Thousand Oaks, CA: Sage.

Carter-Pokras, O. (2000). Toward a healthy Hispanic population: Healthy people 2010. In M. Bond, M. Jones, & J. Ashwill (Eds.), *Crossing borders in Hispanic health care: Implementing and evaluating cultural competence in the health workforce* (pp. 22–34). Arlington: University of Texas School of Nursing.

Clark, C.C. (Ed.). (2002). *Health promotion in communities: Holistic and wellness approaches.* New York: Springer.

Corrigan, D. (2000). The changing role of schools and higher education institutions with respect to community-based interagency collaboration and interprofessional partnerships. *Peabody Journal of Education, 75*(3), 176–195.

Hibbard, J.H. (2003). Engaging health care consumers to improve the quality of care, *Medical Care, 41*(Suppl. 1), I61–I70.

Hill, M. (1999). Outcomes measurement requires nursing to shift to outcome-based practice. *Nursing Administration Quarterly, 24*(1), 1–16.

MacQueen, K.M., McLellan, E., Metzger, D.S., Kegeles, S., Strauss, R.P., Scotti, R., et al. (2001).What is community? An evidence-based definition for participatory public health. *American Journal of Public Health, 91*(12), 1929–1938.

Mays, G.P., & Miller, C.A. (2000). *Local public health practice: Trends & models.* Washington, DC: American Public Health Association.

Minkler, M. (2000). Using participatory action research to build healthy communities. *Public Health Reports, 115,* 191–197.

Newman, B., & Fawcett, J. (2001). *The Neuman systems model* (4th ed.). Stamford, CT: Appleton & Lange.

Novick, L.F. (2000). A framework for public health administration and practice. In L.F. Novick & G.P. Mays (Eds.), *Public health administration: Principles for population-based management* (pp. 34–62). Gaithersburg, MD: Aspen.

Renders, C.M., Valk, G.D., Griffin, S.J., Wagner, E.H., van Eijk, J.T., & Assendelft, W.J.J. (2001). Interventions to improve the management of diabetes in primary care, outpatient, and community settings: A systematic review. *Diabetes Care, 24*(10), 1821–1833.

Wallerstein, N. (2000). A participatory evaluation model for healthier communities: Developing indicators for New Mexico. *Public Health Reports, 115,* 199–294.

20

Communities in Crisis: Disasters, Group Violence, and Terrorism

Key Terms

- Arson
- Assault and battery
- Biologic warfare
- Casualty
- Chemical warfare
- Critical incident stress debriefing (CISD)
- Direct victim
- Disaster
- Disaster planning
- Displaced person
- Gang
- Genocide
- Homicide
- Indirect victim
- Intensity
- Looting
- Lynching
- Manmade disaster
- Mass casualty
- Natural disaster
- Nuclear warfare
- Posttraumatic stress disorder (PTSD)
- Rape
- Refugee
- Riot
- Scope
- Terrorism
- Triage
- Violent crime

Learning Objectives

Upon mastery of this chapter, you should be able to:

- Describe a variety of characteristics of disasters, including causation, number of casualties, scope, and intensity.

- Discuss a variety of factors contributing to a community's potential for experiencing a disaster.

- Identify the four phases of disaster management.

- Describe factors involved in disaster planning.

- Describe the role of the community health nurse in preventing, preparing for, responding to, and supporting recovery from disasters.

- Compare and contrast the most common types of group violence.

- Discuss a variety of factors contributing to a community's potential for experiencing group violence.

- Describe the role of the community health nurse in preventing and responding to group violence.

- Distinguish terrorism from other types of group violence.

- Use the levels of prevention to describe the role of the community health nurse in relation to acts of chemical, biologic, or nuclear terrorism.

What would you do if your local news station broadcast an announcement that your community was directly in the path of a hurricane that earlier in the day had caused extensive damage and loss of life in a neighboring state? What would you do if you were shopping at a local mall, suddenly heard an explosive noise followed by shouts and cries for help, then noticed that a pungent odor was filling the air? What DID you do on the morning of September 11, 2001, when the world of each American, especially those in New York City, in Washington, D.C., and on a plane over rural Pennsylvania, changed forever? What did you do when you heard of multiple terrorist attacks on the United States? As distant as some of these scenarios might seem from your own life, disasters, group violence, and terrorism are ever-present possibilities, and nurses and other health care professionals have an obligation to respond appropriately. This chapter will increase your understanding of the community health nurse's role in preparing for, responding to, and recovering from disasters, group violence, and terrorism.

DISASTERS

A **disaster** is any natural or manmade event that causes a level of destruction or emotional trauma exceeding the abilities of those affected to respond without community assistance. The crash of a private plane over the Pacific Ocean in which no bodies are recovered and no environmental impact is felt is not a disaster by this definition, because no specific community-based response is required or even possible. Such a tragedy may, however, be felt for a lifetime by family members and friends, who need emotional support and possibly long-term financial assistance. If a plane with 150 passengers crashes over land, destroying several homes in its path, the community affected is unable to cope with the resulting injuries, deaths, and property destruction without assistance; by the definition used here, this constitutes a disaster.

The geographic distribution of disasters varies because certain types of disasters are more common in some parts of the world. For example, California is associated with earthquakes and Florida with hurricanes. Similarly, it is not surprising to hear of drought in Ethiopia or floods in India during the monsoon season. When certain types of disasters are anticipated, communities are usually better prepared for them. For instance, California has strict building codes to prevent destruction of structures in the event of earthquakes, but most California homes lack the basements and insulation that characterize homes in regions often visited by tornados or winter storms. Similarly, residents of Germany, Austria, and Russia are better prepared for blizzards than for heavy rain, which probably explains in part the devastation caused in some communities by floods there in 2002.

Because the local media in the United States do not typically report on disasters unless there are mass casualties, one may be unaware of the frequency and variety of both natural and technologic disasters worldwide. Here is a brief sampling of major disasters that occurred in 2002-2003:

- January 2002, Ipiales, Columbia—a Boeing 727 crashes into a mountain, resulting in 92 fatalities
- January 2002, Democratic Republic of Congo—a volcano engulfs the city of Goma; 300,000 to 500,000 people are displaced
- February 2002, Ayyat, Egypt—a fire engulfs a crowded passenger train and 361 people are killed
- March 2002, Afghanistan—a series of earthquakes leaves 1000 dead and 7000 homeless
- May 2002, Andhra Pradesh State, India—a brutal heat wave causes 600 deaths nationwide
- May 2002, Bangladesh—an overloaded ferry capsizes in a storm; 300 are drowned
- June 2002, Western United States—several major wildfires, including the worst fire in Colorado's history, with 137,760 acres and 600 structures consumed. In Arizona, another fire burns 468,638 acres and destroys 400 structures.
- June 2002, China—a coal mine gas explosion kills 111
- June 2002, Russia—the worst flooding in a decade leaves 93 dead and 87,000 homeless
- July 2002, Ukraine—a jet fighter crashes during an acrobatic maneuver at an air show, killing 83 people, including 23 children; it becomes the worst air show disaster in history
- September 2002, Dakar, Senegal—in one of Africa's deadliest ferry accidents, a vessel capsizes in heavy winds, resulting in the loss of almost 1000 lives
- October 2002, Moscow—gas kills 115 hostages in a raid on a theater
- December 2002, Mexico—New Year fireworks explosion kills 28
- February 2003, Daegu, South Korea—an arson attack on the subway system kills 182 people
- February 2003, Iran—a military plane crash kills 302
- May 2003, Algeria—a 6.7 earthquake kills more than 2000 people
- August 2003, France—a prolonged heat wave kills 10,000 people, mostly elderly
- September 2003, U.S.—Hurricane Isabel knocks out power to 2 million people
- December 2003, Bam, Iran—an earthquake kills 28,000 people and injures 30,000

Characteristics of Disasters

Disasters are often characterized by their cause. **Natural disasters** are caused by natural events, such as the floods in western Europe or the earthquakes in Afghanistan in 2002. **Manmade disasters** are caused by human activity, such as the bombing of the World Trade Center in New York City in 2001, the displacement of thousands of Kosovars during their war with Serbia in 1999, or the riots in Los Angeles in the early 1990s. Other manmade disasters include nuclear reactor meltdowns, industrial accidents, oil spills, construction accidents, and air, train, bus, and subway crashes.

A **casualty** is a human being who is injured or killed by or as a direct result of an incident. Although major disasters sometimes occur without any injury or loss of life, disasters are commonly characterized by the number of casualties involved. If casualties number more than 2 people but fewer than 100, the disaster is characterized as a *multiple-casualty incident*. Although multiple-casualty incidents may strain the health care systems of small or mid-sized communities, *mass-casualty incidents*—those involving 100 or more casualties—often completely overwhelm the resources of even large cities. Preparedness for mass-casualty incidents is essential for all communities.

The possibility of being prepared is another characteristic that varies with different types of disasters. For instance, the path and time of landfall of a hurricane can be tracked so that residents in the storm's path can be evacuated and families and businesses can be protected. Communities can also minimize devastation from flooding by building reservoirs or refusing to grant building permits in flood-prone areas, and sandbagging can be used during rainy weather. In fire-prone areas, communities can post notices to heighten awareness of fire danger and enforce regulations to cut back vegetation near structures in forested areas. On the other hand, some disasters strike without warning. For example, the terrorist attacks in New York City caught thousands of civilians unaware. They were trapped in buildings with limited escape routes and very little time to retreat to safety. For employees in the Pentagon on 9/11, survival depended on being in the right place at the right time. The number of fires in the western United States in 2002 was unanticipated and uncharacteristically large, and control was hindered by heat and high winds. Residents were stranded in rural areas or barred from re-entering their communities for weeks, without any knowledge of whether they would have homes when they were allowed to return.

The **scope** of a disaster is the range of its effect, either geographically or in terms of the number of victims. The collapse of a 500-unit high-rise apartment building has a greater scope than does the collapse of a bridge that occurs while only two cars are crossing.

The **intensity** of a disaster is the level of destruction and devastation it causes. For instance, an earthquake centered in a large metropolitan area and one centered in a desert may have the same numeric rating on the Richter scale, yet have very different intensities in terms of the destruction they cause.

Victims of Disasters

Because disasters are so variable, there is no typical victim in a disaster. Nor can anyone predict whether he or she will ever become a victim of a disaster. However, once disaster strikes, victims may be characterized by their level of involvement. **Direct victims** are the people who experience the event, whether fire, volcanic eruption, war, or bomb. They are the dead and the survivors, and even if they are without physical injuries, they are likely to have health effects from their experience. Some may be without shelter or food, and many experience serious psychological stress long after the event is over (Display 20-1).

Depending on the cause and characteristics of the disaster, some direct victims may become displaced persons or

DISPLAY 20-1

Direct and Indirect Victims of a Disaster

On September 11, 2001, almost 3000 people died in the terrorist attacks on the World Trade Center in New York City. All of the employees and visitors in the two buildings were direct victims of this disaster, and the entire population of Manhattan can be considered indirect victims.

Hotels, businesses, and apartments for blocks surrounding the Twin Towers suffered structural damage, blown-out windows, and interiors covered with inches of powdered cement and other debris. A year after this disaster, many residents in the surrounding areas still were unable to return home.

Many rescue workers who were survivors have lasting psychological effects from their own survival experiences and from losing close friends and colleagues. In addition, many rescuers breathed in the dust in the air for days and now have respiratory damage. As a result, their status changed from indirect victim to direct victim.

All people working or visiting Manhattan that day were affected by the closing of the bridges and tunnels and were stranded in New York City until transportation routes opened again, thus becoming indirect victims.

Other indirect victims included children attending school and living within sight of the Twin Towers. They received counseling in school for months, and in some cases years, after the disaster.

For 1 year after the attack, volunteer construction workers and rescue workers who lost fellow police officers, paramedics, or firefighters worked 24 hours a day. First, the efforts were geared to help look for survivors. Shortly after, workers knew that they were looking for the bodies or body parts of victims while removing thousands of tons of building pieces. Thousands of people who were involved in the recovery efforts can be considered indirect victims.

Family members of the 2833 deceased or missing victims, who have been affected for a lifetime, also are indirect victims. Thousands of children lost a parent, some parents lost multiple children, and, in some cases, both spouses were lost because husband and wife both worked in the World Trade Center. The ripples of tragedy extended beyond the borders of the United States, because there were hundreds of people working in the Twin Towers from many different countries whose family members are now indirect victims.

refugees. **Displaced persons** are forced to leave their homes to escape the effects of a disaster. Usually, displacement is a temporary condition and involves movement within the person's own country. A common example is relocation of residents of flooded areas to schools, churches, and other shelters on higher ground. Typically, the term **refugee** is reserved for people who are forced to leave their homeland because of war or persecution. For example, in early 2000, thousands of refugees fled Chechnya to escape advancing Russian troops opposed to the republic's separatist attempts. Often, the displacement of refugees is permanent. For example, many young people who fled Argentina during the "disappearances" between 1976 and 1982 did not return when a democratic government regained power in 1983. Thousands of young men and women who protested against the regime in power at the time simply disappeared.

    Indirect victims are the relatives and friends of direct victims. Although these people do not experience the stress of the event itself, they often undergo extreme anguish from trying to locate loved ones or accommodate their emergency needs. If bodies cannot be found or are unidentifiable, indirect victims experience even greater anguish and may not be able to accept that their loved one has died. For example, many of the mothers of young Argentineans who disappeared in the 1970s still march daily in downtown Buenos Aires, demanding public acknowledgment of the murders of their daughters and sons. Family members of victims from 9/11 in New York City have worked with architects to develop a complex of buildings and a memorial that meets the expectations of most of the indirect victims and honors their loved ones. This is a long and arduous task that, once completed, will help with the long healing process.

Factors Contributing to Disasters

It is useful to apply the host, agent, and environment model to understand the factors contributing to disasters, because manipulation of these factors can be instrumental in planning strategies to prevent or prepare for disasters.

Host Factors
The *host* is the human being who experiences the disaster. Host factors that contribute to the likelihood of experiencing a disaster include age, general health, mobility, psychological factors, and even socioeconomic factors. For instance, elderly residents of a mobile home community may be unable to evacuate independently in response to a tornado warning if they no longer can drive. Impoverished residents of a low-income apartment complex in a large city may notice that their building is not compliant with city fire codes but may avoid alerting authorities for fear of being forced to move to more expensive housing.

Agent Factors
The *agent* is the natural or technologic element that causes the disaster. For example, the high winds of a hurricane and the lava of an erupting volcano are agents, as are radiation, industrial chemicals, biologic agents, and bombs. The Station Nightclub fire and the apartment deck collapse in Chicago demonstrated that irresponsibility of contractors and inspectors and failure to adhere to safety policies can act as agents of disaster, resulting in death and destruction.

Environmental Factors
Environmental factors are those that could potentially contribute to or mitigate a disaster. Some of the most common environmental factors are a community's level of preparedness; the presence of industries that produce harmful chemicals or radiation; the presence of flood-prone rivers, lakes, or streams; average amount of rainfall or snowfall; average high and low temperatures; proximity to fault lines, coastal waters, or volcanoes; level of compliance with local building codes; and presence or absence of political unrest.

Agencies and Organizations for Disaster Management

Among disaster-relief organizations, perhaps none is as famous as the Red Cross, the name commonly used when referring to the American Red Cross, the Federation of Red Cross and Red Crescent Societies, and the International Committee of the Red Cross. The American Red Cross was founded in 1881 by Clara Barton and was chartered by the U. S. Congress in 1905. It is authorized to provide disaster assistance free of charge across the country through its more than 1 million volunteers.

    The Federal Emergency Management Agency (FEMA), established in 1979, is the federal agency responsible for assessment of and response to disaster events in the United States. It also provides training and guidance in all phases of disaster management.

    The World Health Organization's Emergency Relief Operations provide disaster assistance internationally, and the Pan American Health Organization works to coordinate relief efforts in Latin America and the Caribbean. In addition, various international nongovernmental organizations (such as Doctors Without Borders, the International Medical Corps, and Operation Blessing), religious groups, and other volunteer agencies provide needed emergency care.

    The newest safety-related agency in the United States is the Department of Homeland Security. Organized in 2002, it incorporates many of the nation's security, protection, and emergency response activities into a single federal department. As a relatively new department, it is undergoing many changes related to its scope of service. In June 2002, the American Public Health Association became concerned because some of the responsibilities of the Centers for Disease Control and Prevention and the Health Resources and Services Administration (such as the cache drugs, medical supplies, and equipment for emergencies through the National Pharmaceutical Stockpile) were being usurped by the Department of Homeland Security. Some experts see this department as fragmenting the nation's broad-based public health system, which may hinder overall responsiveness and compromise the public health system (Late, 2002). It is hoped that such serious concerns will be addressed as this department evolves.

Governments often send their military personnel and equipment in response to international disasters. For example, in March 2000, the governments of South Africa, England, Germany, France, and the United States, among other nations, responded to the floods in Mozambique with helicopters, planes, boats, and supplies.

When natural or manmade disasters within the United States are accompanied by civil disturbance, looting, or violent crime, the resources of local police departments may be overwhelmed. In such cases, the National Guard is often called in to restore order.

Phases of Disaster Management

In developing strategies to address the problem of disasters, it is helpful for the community health nurse to consider each of the four phases of disaster management: prevention, preparedness, response, and recovery.

Prevention Phase

During the *prevention phase,* no disaster is expected or anticipated. The task during this phase is to identify community risk factors and to develop and implement programs to prevent disasters from occurring. Task forces typically include representatives from the community's local government, health care providers, social services providers, police and fire departments, major industries, local media, and citizens' groups. Programs developed during the prevention phase may also focus on strategies to mitigate the effects of disasters that cannot be prevented, such as earthquakes, hurricanes, and tornadoes.

The United States has strengthened this phase of disaster management since September 2001. This can be seen especially at airports, where airline passengers must now go through a more rigorous security screening before boarding the plane. Nonpassengers cannot go beyond the security area. Photographic identification is required at two or more points before boarding. Random searches of hand-carried luggage occur, and passengers are screened with wands that detect metal. In some states, luggage is tested for radioactive material, police officials with trained dogs patrol the airport, or people are asked to take their shoes off for examination as part of the screening process. All of these measures have been initiated to prevent a disaster.

Preparedness Phase

Disaster *preparedness* involves improving community and individual reaction and responses so that the effects of a disaster are minimized. Disaster preparedness saves lives and minimizes injury and property damage. It includes plans for communication, evacuation, rescue, and victim care. Any plan must also address acquisition of equipment, supplies, medicine, and even food, clean water, blankets, and shelter.

Semiannual disaster drills and tests of the Emergency Broadcast System are examples of appropriate activities during the preparedness phase.

Disaster preparedness activities occur locally, regionally, and nationally. A town keeps its warning system working and tests it each month. Sections of the country coordinate larger warning systems to notify communities in the path of a tornado or hurricane, and the country has a plan to stockpile smallpox vaccine for mass immunization. The National Institute of Allergy and Infectious Diseases has tried diluting a few of the existing 86 million doses of vaccine and has tested the diluted dosage on 100 volunteers to see whether it still works. The results showed that this cache alone contained enough to vaccinate everyone in an emergency. Laboratories have been contracted to make more than 200 million doses in the event that biologic warfare becomes a threat. The last case of smallpox in the United States occurred in 1949, and routine immunization was halted in 1972, although many doctors refused to use the vaccine even before that date. With a largely unvaccinated population, most people in the nation would need the vaccine. Having the vaccine ready is a demonstration of disaster preparedness.

Response Phase

The *response phase* begins immediately after the onset of the disastrous event. Preparedness plans take effect immediately, with the goals of saving lives and preventing further injury or damage. Activities during the response phase include rescue, triage, on-site stabilization, transportation of victims, and treatment at local hospitals. Response also requires recovery, identification, and refrigeration of bodies so that notification of family members is possible and correct, even weeks after a disaster. This care of the dead is demanding and time-consuming work that is often overlooked by people unfamiliar with disaster response. Supportive care, including food, water, and shelter for victims and relief workers is also an essential element of the total disaster response.

Recovery Phase

During the *recovery phase,* the community takes actions to repair, rebuild, or relocate damaged homes and businesses and restore health and economic vitality to the community. Psychological recovery must also be addressed. The emotional scars from witnessing a traumatic event may last a lifetime. Both victims and relief workers should be offered mental health services to support their recovery (see Voices from the Community).

Role of the Community Health Nurse

The community health nurse has a pivotal role in preventing, preparing for, responding to, and supporting recovery from a disaster. After a thorough community assessment for risk factors, the community health nurse may initiate the formation of a multidisciplinary task force to address disaster prevention and preparedness in the community.

VOICES FROM THE COMMUNITY

"I saw the first plane hit the corner of the World Trade Center and explode from my kitchen window, which is 300 feet from the south tower. A blizzard of gray dust obliterated the bright blue of the sky. Paper floated through the dust, edges on fire and curling up. It was beautiful actually, and I couldn't take my eyes off of it.

In the aftermath, my life has been completely turned upside down. I lived in that apartment for 25 years. Until mid-May (2002), it was part of a police zone; I've been back only to clean up. I have thrown away all my possessions except for a few photographs and pieces of art. In effect, I'm starting over. I feel a kinship with the legions of displaced people in this world, made homeless by events beyond their control. They are incredibly strong and resilient. I hope that I will be too."

Kathleen, New York City resident (Cooper & Ianzito, 2002).

Preventing Disasters

Disaster prevention may be considered on three levels: primary, secondary, and tertiary. These are applied to a natural disaster in the Levels of Prevention Matrix.

Primary Prevention. Primary prevention of a disaster means keeping the disaster from ever happening by taking actions that completely eliminate its occurrence. This is the first aspect of primary disaster prevention. Although it is obviously the most effective level of intervention, both in terms of promoting clients' health and containing costs, it is not always possible. Tornadoes, earthquakes, and other disasters often strike without warning, despite the use of every available technologic device for prediction and tracking.

If possible, primary prevention of disasters can be practiced in all settings: in the workplace and home with programs to reduce safety hazards, and in the community with programs to monitor risk factors, reduce pollution, and encourage nonviolent conflict resolution. Primary disaster prevention efforts should take into account a community's physical, psychosocial, cultural, economic, and spiritual needs. The community health nurse has a role in each of these areas. As a teacher, the community health nurse educates people at home, at work, at school, or in a faith community about safety and security focused on preventing a disaster. The community health nurse can teach community members how to protect themselves from the effects of a natural disaster. The nurse can be a part of a safety team, if working as a school nurse or occupational health nurse. If working for a

health department, the nurse can determine during home visits whether a family has a personal disaster plan and help them develop one if none exists. There are many actions the nurse can initiate.

The second aspect of primary disaster prevention is anticipatory guidance. Disaster drills and other anticipatory exercises help relief workers experience some of the feelings of chaos and stress associated with a disaster before one occurs. It is much easier to do this when energy and intellectual processes are at a high level of functioning. Anticipatory work can dissipate the impact of a disastrous event. The community health nurse has a role in these disaster drills through committee membership, organization of drills at the place of employment, or activism at the grassroots level to assist in holding community-wide disaster drills on a regular basis.

Secondary Prevention. Secondary disaster prevention focuses on the earliest possible detection and treatment. For example, a mobile home community is devastated by a tornado, and the local health department's community health nurses work with the American Red Cross to provide emergency assistance. Secondary prevention corresponds to immediate and effective response.

Nurses at St. Vincent's Hospital, the closest Level I Trauma Center to the World Trade Center, prepared to respond to the victims of September 11, 2001, in New York City. They were expecting major trauma cases, but this area was quieter than usual. Triage was conducted both on the streets outside of the emergency department and inside, starting the process earlier and routing people for treatment more effectively. This system was developed after the 1993 terrorist attack on the World Trade Center. Because of the total devastation of the 2001 disaster, those who did survive emerged relatively uninjured and became rescuers of those they could free from the debris. Both rescuers and survivors suffered injuries from falling and flying debris outside of the buildings, but most of the survivors received less serious injuries than emergency personnel were expecting. There were many minor injuries, such as smoke inhalation, eye injuries, and fractures. In another area, heart attack, burn, and crushing injury victims were treated. With organization and preparedness, those needing hospitalization were admitted within 45 minutes after being triaged and stabilized. Most injuries occurred among rescuers, although a few civilians were also hurt. In the first 4 to 6 hours, 264 victims were seen. On a typical day, that number would have been 40 to 45 during the same time period. In the days after the disaster, some rescuers found body parts and had to transport them to the morgue. Rescuers came to the emergency department suffering from symptoms related to fatigue and emotional distress (Ostrowski, 2001).

Nurses from other hospitals offered to help, and volunteers brought food; the owners of a restaurant and coffee shop near the hospital closed their doors to the public and provided free food and beverages for hospital staff. Massage therapists came to the hospital and volunteered to give mas-

LEVELS OF PREVENTION MATRIX

SITUATION: A natural disaster—tornado.

GOAL: Using the three levels of prevention, negative health conditions are avoided, or promptly diagnosed and treated, and the fullest possible potential is restored.

PRIMARY PREVENTION		SECONDARY PREVENTION		TERTIARY PREVENTION		
Health Promotion and Education	*Health Protection*	*Early Diagnosis*	*Prompt Treatment*	*Rehabilitation*	*Primary Prevention*	
					Health Promotion and Education	*Health Protection*
• Increase community awareness • Increase community preparation through education • Each person is as prepared as possible both physically and emotionally	• Community members know what to do and where to go, whether at home, work, school, or elsewhere in the community • Get to safety before the impact—southwest corner of a home's basement or an interior room away from windows and under heavy furniture	• Remain in your position of safety until a community all-clear warning signal is sounded or until rescued • Leave a damaged building cautiously, if able and not seriously injured, and do not return until it is declared safe	• Rescue individuals promptly and get appropriate care for those injured as soon as possible • The infrastructure of the community becomes/remains intact, keeping community members safe from hazards such as live wires, broken gas lines, and fallen debris	• Remain safe during the immediate recovery period • Accept help from others—friends, family, and community services • Rebuild family lives through counseling and other services to restabilize life physically, emotionally, spiritually, and financially	• Educate community members about the need to enhance planning against damage from future natural disasters, based on experiences with the current disaster	• Keep recommended immunizations current • Community physical structures need rebuilding, with infrastructure planning and supports that improve ability to withstand natural disasters

sages. The nurses received tremendous support from strangers and peers across the country. This helped them keep up their spirits as they dealt with the direct victims, while being indirect victims themselves (Ostrowski, 2001).

Tertiary Prevention. Tertiary disaster prevention involves reducing the amount and degree of disability or damage resulting from the disaster. Although it involves rehabilitative work, it can help a community recover and reduce the risk of further disasters. In this sense, it becomes a preventive measure.

Another example from September 11, 2001, comes from a nurse living in the Boston area who, after that date, began to lose a sense of hope for her future. She often found it difficult to assist her patients with their needs because of her own insecurities and fears. She and a peer responded to a re-

quest from the Logan Airport Employee Assistance Program (EAP) asking for help with crisis counseling for United Airlines survivors of 9/11. The planes used in the attacks were from American and United Airlines, and the community of employees felt like survivors because they lived while fellow employees were lost in the disaster. Employees were in turmoil, and their ability to function was affected. "The terrorists had taken away their colleagues, friends and sense of security" (DiVitto, 2002, p. 21).

The most important interventions the nurses provided were a listening ear and validation that what the employees were feeling and experiencing was normal, and often essential, for healthy grieving. Some employees needed to talk about good times, others were quiet and sad, and others expressed a fear of flying again but did so with the support of family and friends. All demonstrated courage and an ability to continue their lives with a sense of strength and hope. Working with these employees enabled the nurse to recapture the essence and true meaning of her life (DiVitto, 2002).

Preparing for Disasters

Disaster planning is essential for a community, business, or hospital. It involves thinking about details of preparation and management by all involved, including community leaders, health and safety professionals, and lay people. A disaster plan need not be lengthy. Two weeks after the April 1995 Oklahoma City bombing of the Murrah Federal Building by two American citizens, one hospital distilled its 44-page manual into a 5-page disaster response guide. Such a concise plan should still contain information on the elements discussed in this and the following section. See Display 20–2 for a summary of these elements.

Personal Preparation. Before we discuss the preparation of a disaster plan for a community, we should consider the need for all nurses to address their own personal preparedness to respond in a disaster. Display 20–3 describes the tragic outcome of one nurse's lack of preparation when she attempted to provide nursing care at the scene of the Oklahoma City bombing. Personal preparedness means that the nurse has read and understood workplace and community disaster plans and has developed a disaster plan for her or his own family. The prepared nurse also has participated in disaster drills and knows cardiopulmonary resuscitation and first aid. Finally, nurses preparing to work in disaster areas should bring copies of their nursing license and driver's license, durable clothing, and basic equipment such as stethoscopes, flashlights, and cellular phones.

Assessment for Risk Factors and Disaster History. As noted earlier in the chapter, the community health nurse is uniquely qualified to perform a community assessment for risk factors that may contribute to disasters. In addition, the nurse should review the *disaster history* of the community.

DISPLAY 20-2

Elements of a Disaster Plan

A disaster plan should address all of the following:
Chain of authority
Lines of communication
Routes and modes of transport
Mobilization
Warning
Evacuation
Rescue and recovery
Triage
Treatment
Support of victims and families
Care of dead bodies
Disaster worker rehabilitation

DISPLAY 20-3

Nurses at Disaster Sites: Help or Hindrance?

On April 19, 1995, 37-year-old Rebecca Anderson, a registered nurse working in Oklahoma City, after hearing a televised report of the bombing of the Federal Building, went to the site wearing jeans and a sweatshirt. Along with firefighters and other rescue workers in hardhats and other protective gear, she was allowed to enter the scene. Within a short time, Rebecca was struck on the back of the head by a concrete slab that fell from the building's wreckage. She died 5 days later of massive cerebral edema. Nurses can learn the following lessons from this tragedy:

- Never enter a disaster scene unless you are directed to do so by an emergency medical technician, fire, or law enforcement official.
- Contact local hospitals and clinics to offer your help; your medical expertise is more useful in the clinical environment.
- Take courses in first aid and emergency care. Contact your local Red Cross for a list of courses.
- Contact your local health department to learn more about your community's disaster plan and how you can contribute in the event of a disaster in your area.

Have earthquakes, tornadoes, hurricanes, floods, blizzards, riots, or other disasters occurred in the past? If so, what (if any) were the warning signs? Were they heeded? Were people warned in time? Did evacuation efforts remove all people in danger? What were the community's on-site responses, and how effective were they? What programs were put in place to rehabilitate the community?

Establishing Authority, Communication, and Transportation. In addition to assessing for preparedness, the effective disaster plan establishes a clear chain of authority, develops lines of communication, and delineates routes of transport.

Establishing a clear and flexible chain of authority is critical for successful implementation of a disaster plan. Usually, the chain is hierarchical, with, for example, the community's governmental head (eg, mayor) initiating the plan, alerting the media to broadcast warnings, authorizing the police to begin evacuations, and so on. Within each level of the organization, the hierarchy continues. For example, at the local hospital, the hospital administrator may be responsible for alerting nurse managers to call in additional personnel. Flexibility is essential, because key authority figures may themselves be victims of the disaster. If the home of the chief of police is destroyed in an earthquake, his or her second-in-command must have equal knowledge of the community's disaster plan and be able to step in without delay.

Effective communication is often a point of breakdown for communities attempting to cope with major disasters. After the terrorist attacks in Oklahoma City and New York City, phone lines were damaged and cellular sites were overwhelmed, making communication difficult. Communication was possible only through handheld radios or by way of couriers on foot. At times of heightened chaos and stress, as well as after physical damage to communication facilities and equipment, misinformation and misinterpretation can flourish, leading to delayed treatment and increased loss of life.

Again, clarity and flexibility are the watchwords for establishing lines of communication. How will warnings be communicated? What backups are available if the normal communication systems are destroyed in the disaster? How will communication between relief workers at the disaster site, hospital personnel, police, and governmental authorities be maintained? What role will local media play, both in keeping information flowing to the outside world and in broadcasting needs for assistance and supplies? Finally, how will friends and family members of victims be informed of the whereabouts or health status of their loved ones? The characteristics of effective communication during disasters are summarized in Display 20–4.

Closed or inefficient routes of transportation can also increase injury and loss of life. For example, if a single, narrow mountainous road is the only means of transporting firefight-

DISPLAY 20–4

Effective Communication During Disasters

To be effective, communication during disasters must elicit action. Communication that elicits action provides information that is
- Believable
- Current
- Unambiguous
- Authoritative
- Predictive of the probability of future events (what is going to happen next?)

Effective communication is
- Interactive—it allows for and addresses questions
- Conclusive—it eliminates room for speculation and catastrophizing
- Urgent—conveys seriousness without resorting to fear tactics
- Clear, simple, and repetitive
- Characterized by solutions and suggestions for success
- Personal—it uses people's names if possible and addresses their real and perceived needs

Finally, because rumors can hinder effective action or provoke premature action, effective communication includes rumor control. It provides suggestions for constructive activity, reducing time and energy spent on rumor generation and perpetuation.

ers to or evacuating residents from the scene of a forest fire, then disaster planners should propose widening the road or clearing a second road. Disaster planners must also consider what routes emergency vehicles will take when transporting disaster victims to local and outlying hospitals or health care workers to the disaster site. What if the chosen routes are inaccessible because of floodwaters, advancing fires, mountain slides, or building rubble? Are alternative routes designated?

Mobilizing, Warning, and Evacuating. In many natural disasters, local weather service personnel, public works officials, police officers, or firefighters have the earliest information indicating an increasing potential for a disaster. These officials typically have a plan in place for providing community authorities with specific data indicating increased risk. They may also advise the mayor's office or other community leaders of their recommendations for warning or evacuating the public. Additionally, they may recommend actions the community can take to mitigate damage, such as spraying rooftops in the path of fires, sandbagging the banks of rising rivers, or imposing a curfew in times of civil unrest.

Disaster plans must specify the means of communicating warnings to the public, as well as the precise information that should be included in warnings. Planners should never assume that all citizens can be reached by radio or television or that broadcast systems will be unaffected by the disaster. Broadcast media may indeed be a primary means of communicating warnings, but alternative strategies, such as police or volunteers canvassing neighborhoods with loudspeakers, should also be in place. In multilingual communities, messages should be broadcast in multiple languages. Not only homes but also businesses must be informed. Information that should be communicated includes the nature of the disaster; the exact geographic region affected, including street names if appropriate, and the actions citizens should take to protect themselves and their property.

An evacuation plan is an essential component of the total disaster plan. The plan should cover notification of the police, local military personnel, or voluntary citizens' groups of the need to evacuate people, as well as methods of notifying and transporting the evacuees. A plan should also be made for responding to citizens who refuse to evacuate. For example, will police authorities forcibly remove an elderly citizen from his home to a shelter? Will evacuation plans include household pets? If farms or ranches are in the path of fires or floods, will animals be evacuated?

Responding to Disasters

At the disaster site, police, firefighters, nurses, and other relief workers develop a coordinated response to rescue, triage, and treat disaster victims.

Rescue. One of the first obligations of relief workers is to remove victims from danger. This job typically falls to firefighters and personnel with special training in search and rescue. Depending on the disaster agent, protective gear, heavy equipment, and special vehicles may be needed, and dogs trained to locate dead bodies may be brought in (Fig. 20-1). Usually, the immediate disaster site is not the best place for the disaster nurse, who can be far more effective in triage and treatment of victims. One of the lessons of the World Trade Center bombing was that the greatest need for medical professionals was at the local hospitals, not at the disaster site.

Rescue workers face the logistically and psychologically difficult task of determining when to cease rescue efforts. Some factors to consider include increasing danger to rescue workers, diminishing numbers of survivors, and diminishing possibilities for survival. For example, after a plane crash on a snowy mountain, rescue efforts may cease if it is deemed that anyone who might have survived the crash would subsequently have died from exposure.

Triage. Whereas emergency nurses daily determine which clients require priority care, the community health nurse may be at a loss as to where to start when faced with multiple victims of a disaster. Knowing the principles and practice of triage allows the nurse to offer her or his nursing skills most effectively.

Triage is the process of sorting multiple casualties in the event of a war or major disaster. It is required when the number of casualties exceeds immediate treatment resources. The goal of triage is to effect the greatest amount of good for the greatest number of people. Figure 20-2 shows the four basic categories of the international triage system, as well as a triage tag.

Prioritization of treatment may be very different in a mass-casualty event as opposed to an average day in a hospital emergency department. Under normal circumstances, a person presenting to a hospital emergency department with a myocardial infarction and showing no pulse or respirations would receive immediate treatment and have a chance of recovery. At a disaster site, a victim without a pulse or respi-

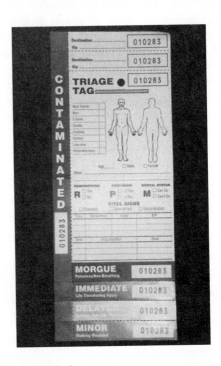

1. **Red:** Urgent/Critical
   Victims in this category have injuries or medical problems that will likely lead to death if not treated immediately (e.g., an unconscious victim with signs of internal bleeding).
2. **Yellow:** Delayed
   Victims in this category have injuries that will require medical attention; however, time to medical treatment is not yet critical (e.g., a conscious victim with a fractured femur).
3. **Green:** Minor/Walking Wounded
   Victims in this category have sustained minor injury or are presenting with minimal signs of illness. Prolonged delay in care most likely will not adversely effect their long-term outcome (e.g., a conscious victim with superficial cuts, scrapes, and bruises).
4. **Black:** Dead/Non-salvageable
   Victims in this category are obviously dead or have suffered mortal wounds because of which death is imminent (e.g., an unconscious victim with an open skull fracture with brain matter showing). Life-saving heroics on this group of victims will only delay medical care on more viable victims.

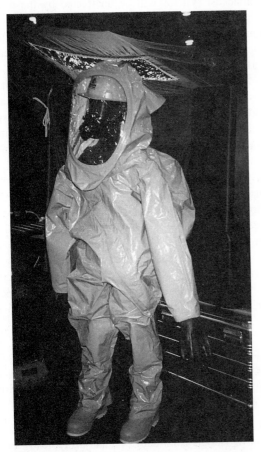

FIGURE 20-1.   Hazardous materials suit used by the military and most fire departments. (Photo by Cynthia Tait.)

FIGURE 20-2.   Victim triage tag recommended by the California Fire Chiefs Association. There are four basic categories that are all applied when a medical system is overwhelmed with victims. (Photo by Cynthia Tait.)

rations would most likely be placed in the nonsalvageable category.

Mass casualties refers to a number of victims that is greater than that which can be managed safely with the resources the community has to offer, such as rescue vehicles and emergency facilities available to serve disaster victims while also meeting the needs of the rest of the community. Frequently in mass casualty occurrences, the broader community needs to become involved, which necessitates calling in rescue vehicles, firefighters, and police officers from neighboring towns, or the use of neighboring hospitals. This adds another layer of disaster management coordination that must be considered.

Immediate Treatment and Support. Disaster nurses provide treatment on-site at emergency treatment stations, in shelters, or at local hospitals and clinics. In addition to direct nursing care, on-site interventions might include arranging for transport once victims are stabilized and managing the procurement, distribution, and replenishment of all supplies. Disposable items might be in short supply, requiring resterilization procedures that may be unfamiliar to a nurse not accustomed to field work. These procedures may pose a challenge even to an experienced nurse because of the field environment. The nurse may also manage provision or distribution of food and beverages, including infant formulas and rehydration fluids, and arrange for adequate, accessible, and safe sanitation facilities, either on-site or in a shelter. Finally, the nurse often must also arrange for psychological and spiritual care of victims of disasters.

Some victims who seem physically uninjured may, in fact, be suffering from major injuries but be unable to relate their symptoms to a relief worker because of shock or anxiety about injured, dead, or missing loved ones. For instance, a father pulling debris away from his collapsed house after a tornado may be so worried about a missing child that he does not realize that he has a broken arm.

Other victims may be so emotionally traumatized by a disaster that they act out, disrupting efforts to assist them and other victims and even engaging in dangerous activities. This may cause relief workers to focus on emotional care; however, such victims must be assessed for head trauma and internal injuries, because their behavior may have a physical cause. If they are physically able, such victims may be given a simple, repetitive task to perform, which serves as both a distraction and a means to restore, to a small extent, their sense of control over their environment.

Care of Bodies and Notification of Families. Identification and transport of the dead to a morgue or holding facility are crucial, especially if contagion is feared. Toe tags make documentation visible and accessible. Records of deaths must be made and maintained, and family members should be notified of their loved ones' deaths as quickly and compassionately as possible. If feasible, a representative from each of the area's faith communities should be available to assist families awaiting news of missing loved ones.

As stated earlier, a family's recovery from their loss is often delayed when notification of relatives (indirect victims) is not possible because the victims' bodies are badly damaged or not found. This was a major problem of the World Trade Center disaster, in which few of the victims were found. In some cases, only minute pieces of tissue were available for DNA processing. In other situations, just a piece of jewelry or clothing remained. And for some victims, no remains were found.

Supporting Recovery From Disasters

Disasters do not suddenly end when the rubble is cleared and the victims' wounds are healed. Rather, recovery is a long, complex process that often includes long-term medical treatment, physical rehabilitation, financial restitution, and psychological and spiritual support.

Long-Term Treatment. Long-term treatment may be required for many victims of disasters, straining the local rehabilitative-care facilities and resources. Children who were victims may have to deal with lifelong disabilities or scars from their ordeal, and families may be without adequate financial support for their child's medical care. Elderly citizens who may formerly have been in excellent health but who sustained serious injuries in the disaster might suddenly find that they can no longer live independently and must move to a long-term care facility. After floods, landslides, fires, or earthquakes, extensive property damage may cause some residents or businesses to relocate rather than rebuild on land they now deem to be disaster-prone. A disaster that creates numerous victims in a small community may alter the entire social fabric of that community permanently.

Long-Term Support. Victims of disasters may need funding to repair or rebuild their homes or to reopen businesses, such as stores, restaurants, and other services needed by the community. Insurance settlements, FEMA funding, and private donations may assist in financing community rehabilitation. Health care workers may be required to assist victims in filling out necessary paperwork. Immediately after a disaster, some victims may be unable to concentrate on anything beyond fulfilling their immediate needs and those of their family.

Psychological support is often required after a disaster, both for victims and for relief workers. Some individuals may experience **posttraumatic stress disorder (PTSD)**, a syndrome that may be marked by flashbacks, nightmares, disinterest in daily affairs, hypervigilance, survivor's guilt, or decreased concentration. The "traumatic event" criterion for PTSD, as set forth in the current edition of the *Diagnostic and Statistical Manual of Mental Disorders*, was undoubtedly met by the coordinated attacks on New York City, the Pentagon, and Flight 93 on September 11, 2001. Less dramatically, many victims, especially elderly persons displaced from their homes, may quietly lose their will to live and drift into apathy and malaise. Individuals whose belief in God was unshakable before the incident may now wonder how God could have let this happen, especially if they have lost a loved one. These victims often require not only empathic listening but also long-term skilled spiritual counseling before they can begin to regain their former faith. In assessing a community's citizens for counseling needs after a disaster, the nurse should not forget to include children. Often, children do not have words to express their feelings or fears and may act out in ways adults find difficult to understand, unless age-appropriate psychological intervention is provided.

Many studies were generated out of the unprecedented exposure to trauma in the United States on September 11, 2001. Some researchers examined mental health needs in New York State and the public costs of mental health response after the attacks (Jack & Glied, 2002; Herman, Felton, & Susser, 2002). Others studied immediate psychological reactions and reactions up to 6 months after the attacks. (Schlenger et al., 2002; Silver et al., 2002) (see Research: Bridge to Practice I).

Need for Self-Care. Self-care, including stress education for all relief workers after a disaster, helps to lower anxiety and put the situation into proper perspective. **Critical incident stress debriefing (CISD)** provides victims with professional debriefing in small groups or individually and becomes a mechanism for emotional reconciliation. The ideal time for CISD is between 24 and 72 hours after the disaster event. Positive effects of CISD include

- Accelerating the healing process
- Equipping participants with positive coping mechanisms
- Clearing up misconceptions and misunderstandings
- Restoring or reinforcing group cohesiveness
- Promoting a healthy, supportive work atmosphere
- Identifying individuals who require more extensive psychological assistance

CISD addresses all components of the human response to trauma, including physiologic effects, emotions, and cognition. Studies have shown that CISD allows individuals to regain a sense of normalcy much sooner than those not receiving CISD.

RESEARCH: BRIDGE TO PRACTICE I

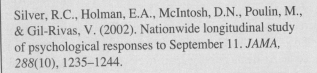

Silver, R.C., Holman, E.A., McIntosh, D.N., Poulin, M., & Gil-Rivas, V. (2002). Nationwide longitudinal study of psychological responses to September 11. *JAMA, 288*(10), 1235–1244.

On September 11, 2001 the United States experienced the most deadly terrorist attacks ever to occur on home soil. The traumatic events affected many people directly and the entire nation indirectly. Researchers found this to be a unique opportunity to examine longitudinally the process of adjustment.

A national probability sample of 3496 adults received a Web-based survey. The questionnaire focused on stress-related symptoms and behaviors that represent adjustment or maladjustment; respondents were polled initially and at 2 and 6 months after the event. Seventy-eight percent (2729 individuals) completed the survey within 23 days of the terrorist attacks; 1069 of the participants who resided outside New York City were selected from the first wave of respondents. The main outcome measures were September 11–related symptoms of acute stress, posttraumatic stress, and global distress. Seventeen percent of the U. S. population surveyed outside of New York City reported symptoms of September 11–related posttraumatic stress 2 months after the attacks, and 5.8% reported them at 6 months. High levels of posttraumatic stress symptoms were associated with

- Being female
- Marital separation
- Pre–September 11 physician-diagnosed depression or anxiety disorder or physical illness

- Severity of exposure to the attacks
- Early disengagement from coping efforts
- Denial

Global distress was associated with severity of loss due to the attacks, early coping strategies and giving up, which decreased with active coping.

Conclusions were that the psychological effects of a major national traumatic event are not limited to those who experience it directly. In addition, the degree of traumatic response is not predicted simply by exposure to or loss from the trauma. "Instead, use of specific coping strategies [seeking social support, active coping, denial, behavioral disengagement] shortly after an event is associated with symptoms over time. In particular, disengaging from coping efforts can signal the likelihood of psychological difficulties up to 6 months after a trauma" (p. 1235).

This study suggests that even individuals who are not directly exposed to a trauma may demonstrate potentially disturbing levels of trauma-related symptoms. Symptoms that appear in a large number of indirectly affected people may represent a normal response to an abnormal event. The study suggests that the use of coping strategies enhances recovery. A community health nurse needs to be cognizant of this relationship and prepared to enhance it in clients who experience a traumatic event. Rituals and activities that provide comfort—such as participation in faith community rituals, sharing fears and concerns with family and friends, and talking about feelings with others, lay and professional—are examples of healthy coping strategies.

Self-care comes in many forms and is part of a prescription for emotional healing after a traumatic event. Self-care is not just for rescue workers but for everyone touched by trauma. Keep in mind the following self-care points (Peeke, 2002):

- Give yourself time to heal. You need time to adjust. Even though you want the pain to be over immediately, it is healthier to realize that this is a long-term recovery process.
- Ask for emotional support. Talk with family and friends around the country. It feels good to be connected with others. You listen and support one another as you share your feelings.
- Take care of yourself; it will improve your ability to deal with stress. Eat regularly, avoid alcohol, maintain sleep patterns, follow your exercise routine, and embrace each day as a gift.
- Reestablish daily routines. Getting back to your regular routine is important and gives you a sense of security and normalcy.
- Use your time wisely. A significant traumatic event gives you an opportunity to reprioritize how you spend your time each day. Are you living your dreams and passions? Traumatic events remind us of our fragile nature and that each moment should be savored and enjoyed.
- Give something back. Your life goes on. Demonstrate your gratefulness by becoming part of a global healing process. Donate to charities and give time to causes you have ignored. Seek ways to reach out to those who are in need of help.

GROUP VIOLENCE

The rates of group violence and violent crime decreased in many U. S. cities at the end of the 1990s. The actual number of violent crimes peaked in 1993 at almost 4.2 million annually. By 1998, that number had dropped to less than 2.8 million (U. S. Department of Justice, 1999). The U. S. Department of Justice's National Crime Victimization Survey (NCVS) for 2000–2001 indicated that violent crime had decreased another 10%, making its incidence the lowest in NCVS history (since 1973) (U. S. Department of Justice, 2002). According to the Federal Bureau of Investigation's Uniform Crime Reports, the crime index rate fell for the 10th straight year in 2000, declining 3.3% from 1999, 18.8% from 1996, and 30.1% from 1991 (U. S. Department of Justice, 2002). However, violent crime is still an emotional and powerful public issue, often influencing our votes, our choices of where to live, work, shop, and vacation, and our decisions about where and how to educate our children. Indeed, the American Public Health Association (APHA) has worked for many years to turn the spotlight on violence as a public health issue. Gun violence in particular is both a public health emergency and a grave threat to an entire generation of young adults (USDHHS, 2000).

Types of Group Violence

The problem of family violence is discussed in more detail in Chapter 25, school and adolescent violence in Chapter 28, and workplace violence in Chapter 29. This chapter presents an overview of group violence and how it affects communities.

Gang Violence

The California Attorney General defines a **gang** as a loose-knit organization of individuals between the ages of 14 and 24 years that has a name, is usually territorial or claims a certain territory as being under its exclusive influence, and is involved in criminal acts. Its members associate together and commit crimes against other gangs or against the general population. Gangs are most commonly involved in drug distribution, aggravated assault, robbery, burglary, and motor vehicle theft (Huff, 2002). Some gangs focus on stealing, whereas others focus on fighting. Large cities are the most likely to have gang problems, and rural counties are the least likely.

There are theories on how gangs form. Hirschi's (2004) social bond theory proposed that criminal behavior results from the weakening (in youth) of the ties that bind the individual to society. He believed that the strong subcultural bonds insulate the individual from conventional behavior.

Gangs often require members to display symbols of their allegiance to one another. These symbols also serve to identify them to other gangs. They may include certain colors, special caps or coats, tattoos, handshakes or other signs, and terminology unique to the gang. Gangs may also require members to participate in rites of passage or "hazing" to test their loyalty, events that often involve committing a crime. Gang members usually share the same ethnicity or at least the same belief system. Many gangs today have sophisticated Web sites and are capable of equally sophisticated crimes (Huff, 2002; Miller, Maxson, & Klein, 2001).

Gang members consider themselves family and turn to each other for support. Often, members are searching for emotional intimacy in the gang as a substitute for a dysfunctional family that is unwilling or unable to provide that intimacy. Gangs also provide discipline and a structured environment to young people who, because of absent or unresponsive parents, may have a strong desire for an external locus of authority and a set of predictable rules and regulations.

Riots

A **riot** is a violent disturbance created by a large number of people assembled for a common purpose. It may or may not involve criminal activities, such as willful destruction of cars, stores, and other property; **looting** (stealing goods); **arson** (the deliberate burning of buildings); **lynching** (execution by hanging without due process of law); or physical attacks on a perceived enemy or on law enforcement officers.

Riots often erupt during times of war, political instability, racial inequity, and economic injustice. For example, in the United States, the decades of the 1960s and 1970s were marked by frequent demonstrations against the Vietnam

War, which occasionally escalated from peaceful marches and protests to full-scale riots. Riots have also been sparked during protests of racial inequities and are especially common after announcements of legal decisions that are perceived as racist. For example, when the officers accused of assaulting Rodney King in Los Angeles were acquitted in April 1992, violent riots caused 53 deaths, 2000 arrests, and more than 1 billion dollars in property damage. Internationally, riots often erupt over sporting events, especially if the fans are close to the action. Fans storm the field, assault officials, and attack the opposing team after a bad play or decision that negatively affects the outcome for their team. Such riots have caused multiple injuries and deaths. Inflated food prices or inequitable distribution of food or supplies can precipitate a riot. In 1999, for example, there were widespread riots in India in protest of the inflated price and limited availability of onions, a staple in the Indian diet.

Violent Crimes by Specific Groups of Perpetrators

Violent crimes are those involving physical or psychological injury or death, or the threat of injury or death. These crimes are often accompanied by destruction to or loss of property. For example, armed robbery is considered a violent crime, regardless of whether anyone is injured during the crime.

Assault and Battery. Legally, **assault and battery** refers to the threat to use force against another person, and the accomplishment of that threat. More loosely, *assault* can be used to refer to any violent attack such as assault with a deadly weapon or sexual assault. Domestic assault is discussed in Chapter 25.

One type of group assault that is becoming more prevalent is assault on the homeless. These assaults are usually perpetrated on individual homeless men, often by groups of three or more young men who beat the victim severely and sometimes fatally, sometimes for no other reason than that he asked them for money. Alcohol and drugs are often factors. In addition, abuse of the homeless is considered to be a new and underestimated hate crime (Bacque, 2000).

Rape. Legal definitions of **rape** vary, but the key elements include some form of sexual contact and a lack of consent. Consent is considered lacking under conditions of force, deception, or coercion, or when the victim is a minor or is drugged, unconscious, mentally retarded, or physically restrained.

Different categories of rape are commonly described. One of the most common is *date rape,* in which the assailant and victim meet by mutual consent but the assailant forces the victim to engage in a sexual act against the victim's will. *Stranger rape* is sudden and usually violent, involving the use of a knife, gun, or violent physical force. *Statutory rape* refers to sexual intercourse with a female who has not reached the statutory age of consent; in many states, this age is 14 years. Rape may also be perpetrated by a group, as when a group of college men drug and then rape a female student

or when a youth gang assaults and rapes a woman jogging on its "turf" after dark.

Both agent and environmental factors can contribute to rape. Some of the more common factors are an increased history of childhood sexual abuse among rapists, a patriarchal value system in which men are expected to prove their masculinity by dominating or "conquering" women, and an environment in which violence is explicitly or implicitly accepted or encouraged.

Homicide. Homicide is the killing of one person by another. Like the rates for group violence overall, the homicide rate is declining. In 1980, there were 10.2 homicides for every 100,000 people in the United States; by 1998, this rate had fallen to 6.2 per 100,000 (U.S. Department of Health and Human Services, 2000). However, homicide is still the leading cause of death for African-American youth aged 15 to 24 years. Their murder rate is an alarming 25.2 per 100,000 people (compared with 4.3 per 100,000 for white youths and 9.9 per 100,000 for Hispanic youths). Even though homicide rates in the United States have improved, the rate among males aged 15 to 24 years in the United States is 10 times higher than in Canada, 15 times higher than in Australia, and 28 times higher than in France or Germany (U.S. Department of Health and Human Services, 2000). Studies have shown that factors identified with violence include, but are not limited to "complex interactions between poverty, racism, excess consumption of alcohol, the plethora of illegal drugs, dysfunctional familial relations, abuse of children by adults, scarcity of viable employment and resources, lack of effective hand gun regulation, inadequate services from schools and other social agencies, stereotyping between peer groups and between adults and children, and a general erosion of respect for individual rights of freedom, security, and responsibility" (Benda & Turney, 2002, p. 7).

In addition, the 21st century has already been marred by numerous instances of multiple homicides in schools, universities, restaurants, and workplaces. For example, on March 1, 2000, a gunman in Pennsylvania went on a shooting spree at his apartment complex and at two fast-food restaurants, killing two people and critically wounding three. In the summer of 2002, a 10-year-old girl in the Bronx, New York, was fatally struck by a stray bullet after gang members looking for free food and beer crashed a baby's christening party at a church. In the fall of 2002, the areas around Silver Spring, Maryland; Washington, D.C.; and northern Virginia were terrorized by two snipers who randomly killed or injured 13 people engaged in everyday activities (see What Do You Think? I).

Genocide. The most notorious historical example of **genocide**, the killing of a group of people because of their racial, political, or cultural differences, was the murder of millions of Jews, Catholics, gypsies, homosexuals, intellectuals, and other "undesirables" by the Nazis before and during World War II. Tragically, genocide continues today. Recent

WHAT DO YOU THINK? I

One of the reasons our national homicide rates are going down may be the improvements in emergency care achieved over the past 30 years. Medical technology has helped to lower the death rate among assault victims by almost 70%, in the process decreasing the national murder rate. People who would have ended up in morgues 20 years ago are now simply treated and released by a hospital, often in a matter of a few days. As good as this news is, it artificially improves homicide statistics. Violence is still being committed, but the victims survive and do not become homicide statistics.

Associated Press. (2002, August 12). Medical advances, drop in death rate linked. *The Fresno Bee*, A5.

examples include the mass "ethnic cleansings" in Bosnia, Rwanda, and Kosovo in the last decade of the 20th century.

Factors Contributing to Group Violence

Violence among specific groups of perpetrators and violence directed toward selected groups of people often has its roots in the childhood or youth of the perpetrators. These forms of violence can be traced to many causes. The U. S. Department of Justice has identified a number of host causes or correlates of delinquency, including feelings of alienation or rebelliousness and lack of societal bonding (Wilson & Howell, 1993). Environmental factors include

- Parental conflict, lack of supervision, child abuse, or inconsistent parenting
- Negative school experiences, including early academic failure and lack of commitment to school
- Negative peer influence, including peers who engage in criminal activity
- Socioeconomic factors, such as high rates of substance abuse in the community, living in a high-crime neighborhood, and economic deprivation

The roots of youth gang problems are multifactorial. They may be related to lack of social opportunities, social disorganization, institutional racism, cultural maladaptation, deficiencies in social policy, and availability of criminal opportunities.

Additionally, frequent exposure to violence in the news, at sporting events, on television programs, in movies, on the Internet, in video games, and in violent pornography has been linked to an increase in aggression. Children seem to be especially vulnerable, and the link seems to be particularly strong if the subject matter glorifies violence as the ideal and appropriate solution to personal problems (Goode, 2000). For example,

Dr. James Garbarino, author of *Lost Boys: Why Our Sons Turn Violent and How We Can Save Them* (1999), observes that children "have ample opportunities to see on television and in the movies how you threaten people, what it means to shoot someone, and ample opportunities to learn about revenge and how desirable it is in this society. For the nation to be shocked and appalled . . . is either a kind of denial or hypocrisy."

Simple access to weapons cannot be discounted as a factor in criminal activity. The United States imposes fewer restrictions on the manufacture, sale, and licensure of guns than any other industrialized nation and, as a correlate, is faced with higher rates of gun-related injuries and murders. Many of the youths involved in school shootings in the United States in the 1990s had easy access to guns that belonged to parents, other relatives, or neighbors. Weapons such as simple bombs can be made from instructions found on the Internet. Increasingly, rifles and assault weapons, rather than handguns, are being used in acts of group violence. These weapons allow for more rapid firing of more bullets and tend to cause significantly higher numbers of casualties. The murders of 12 students and 1 teacher in the 1999 assault on Columbine High School in Colorado, for example, were made possible by the easy acquisition and use of these more sophisticated weapons (see Research: Bridge to Practice II).

Healthy People 2010 Goals for Reducing Group Violence

The *Healthy People 2010* document (U.S. Department of Health and Human Services, 2000) lists a number of goals for reducing youth violence, including the following:

- Reduce physical assaults among people aged 12 years and older to less than 25.5 per 1000 persons from a baseline in 1998 of 31.1 per 1000 persons.
- Reduce to 33.3% the prevalence of physical fighting among adolescents in grades 9 through 12, from a baseline in 1997 of 36.6%.
- Reduce to less than 6% the prevalence of weapon carrying by adolescents in grades 9 through 12, from a baseline in 1997 of 8.5%.

In addition, *Healthy People 2010* calls for a reduction in work-related homicides to no more than 0.4 per 100,000 workers, from a baseline in 1998 of 0.5 per 100,000. It also calls for a reduction in workplace assault to no more than 0.6 per 100 workers, from a baseline in 1987–1992 of 0.85 per 100.

Role of the Community Health Nurse

Community health nurses can play a key role in reducing group violence by interacting with students, parents, churches, law enforcement officials, local politicians, and community organizers.

Preventing Group Violence

The typical model for preventing or reducing group violence includes activities such as assessing the problem, developing

RESEARCH BRIDGE TO PRACTICE II

Schuster, M.A., Franke, T.M., Bastian, A.M., Sor, S., & Halfon, N. (2000). Firearm storage patterns in US homes with children. *American Journal of Public Health, 90*(4), 588–594.

SAFETY AND HOME FIREARM STORAGE PATTERNS

The researchers involved with this study used data from the 1994 National Health Interview Survey (NHIS) and the Year 2000 Objectives supplement to study the presence of firearms in the home and firearm storage patterns among families with children. The NHIS is an annual survey covering demographics, health, health care utilization, and insurance. One section of the Year 2000 supplement covers firearms.

Respondents from the 6990 sample homes with children younger than 18 years of age (representing more than 22 million children in more than 11 million homes) reported that they had at least one firearm (69% reported having more than one firearm), with 43% keeping at least one unlocked firearm. Overall, 4% kept

firearms unlocked, unloaded, and stored with ammunition, and 9% kept firearms unlocked and loaded. Therefore, a total of 13%—some 1.4 million homes with 2.6 million children—store firearms in a manner accessible to children.

The percentage of children living in homes with firearms increases with the child's age, from 28% for children younger than 1 year of age to 38% for children aged 13 to 17 years. The types of firearms included handguns (53%), shotguns (61%), rifles (65%), and other types (2%). With the accessibility of firearms increasing in households as children age, loading of firearms by older children is a possibility.

Community health nurses, of course, do not control what goes on in the homes of families with children. Ultimately, families decide what they believe is best. We can, however, make sure that when families make these decisions, they are informed about the risks associated with firearms and how to reduce those risks. Special efforts may be warranted to address firearm safety issues directly with adolescents.

---

policy based on established objectives, conducting research, procuring funding, and promoting offender accountability. For example, an increase in rapes on one university campus might prompt the nursing department to facilitate a university-wide open forum to discuss the issue, identify possible factors, initiate research, and develop solutions. Programs might include outreach to all students currently enrolled at the university through dormitory teaching sessions, church-group activities, involvement of team coaches for university sports, and even participation by teachers and student advisors.

Violence can be reduced in elementary and secondary schools by increasing supervision and surveillance. Examples of successful actions some schools have taken are listed in Display 20–5.

Community health nurses can influence the reduction of school violence by establishing strong cooperative relationships between adults and students, recognizing (and helping others, such as parents and teachers, to recognize) behaviors that could signal a problem, and identifying situations that may predispose teens to violence. The "Six Vs" can be used to help identify teens who may need evaluation, especially if the frequency or intensity of these behaviors increases (Steger, 2000):

- Venting—angry outbursts inappropriate for the child's age, frequent mood swings, and other behaviors indicating poor control of emotions

DISPLAY 20–5

Actions Schools Can Take to Reduce Violence

Schools can take the following actions to reduce their risk for violence:

- Improve environmental design
- Install surveillance cameras, metal detectors, and pay phones or dial-free access connections to emergency services
- Increase security personnel
- Decrease access by outsiders to campus
- Institute school-wide safety plans, drills, and codes
- Train administrators and teachers to identify potentially violent or psychologically impaired students
- Identify students who are associated with gangs
- Expel students who are caught with weapons on campus
- Suspend or expel students for threatened or real acts of violence
- Institute a policy that allows for searching students and lockers
- Hold parents accountable for students' actions and make them financially responsible for any damages incurred

- Vocalizing—threats by a teen to harm self or others, or use of inappropriate language or profanity
- Vandalizing—intentional damage of property or a history of vandalism, even targeting his or her own property
- Victimizing—teens who see themselves as victims, whether true or not, become just as prone to violence as those who have actually been abused; they blame others for their problems and do not take responsibility for their actions
- Vying (for attention)—being involved in gangs or fringe groups, acting out in class, bringing weapons or other contraband to school to show others, wearing outlandish or banned clothing, or purposefully getting suspended or expelled.
- Viewing—like actual victims of abuse, young people who witness the abuse of others are likely to display violent tendencies themselves.

Community health nurses can become involved through the following actions:

- Speaking about school violence at middle and high school assemblies, PTA meetings, parenting meetings, neighborhood watch meetings, and church meetings
- Encouraging parents to involve their children in youth group programs such as the Boy or Girl Scouts, Big Brothers/Big Sisters, faith community youth groups, and 4-H; donating time to these groups; or, if they do not exist in the community, working to establish them
- Participating in local and national crime-prevention councils
- Joining professional nursing organizations that engage in campaigns to reduce violence
- Writing, producing, or promoting public service announcements that aim to reduce violence
- Promoting the inclusion of articles about group violence in local newspapers, community newsletters, and faith-based community bulletins
- Offering ongoing anger management and conflict resolution courses

To reduce gang membership and associated violence, positive social development starting from infancy and an intensive focus on interactions within the school system are crucial. The school nurse or community health nurse working in education can sponsor programs to nurture social values and ethics and to help students dissociate from delinquent peers and role models. After-school programs in which youths have an opportunity to play sports; volunteer with the poor, the sick, or the elderly; or challenge their learning in math clubs and on debate teams can improve self-esteem and reduce the seduction of gang membership.

The community health nurse can also provide proactive leadership in preventing gang activity. Community mobilization and local organization are key components. Additionally, understanding of both the roots of specific gang issues and the community conditions that contribute to the problem is necessary for finding solutions and alternatives to youth gang involvement.

An effective school gang-suppression strategy should include the following:

- Development of guidelines for appropriate teacher and staff responses to a variety of gang behaviors and delinquency
- Application and enforcement of rules and regulations that support positive relationships and communication among school personnel, parents, students, and community agencies
- Development of parenting and gang-awareness classes
- Establishment of training programs for increasing knowledge about gangs and the community resources available for assistance

Finally, although community health nurses cannot prevent riots, they can be familiar persons in their neighborhoods, encouraging the sharing of feelings of anger or hostility or the exchange of information about criminal activities. Also, the nurse is usually familiar with the normal environment in the neighborhood—the flow of people, the degree of friendliness of neighbors and business owners, and the usual activities. The nurse can use this familiarity to detect when something feels "unusual." Part of continuous community assessment includes gathering such subconscious impressions or intuitions. If cues from the community indicate increased tensions or exaggerated negative feelings toward particular persons or groups, the nurse can share this information with the proper authorities. Many neighborhoods are served by community centers where there are social workers, educators, neighborhood-watch groups, probation officers, and other community service workers, all excellent resources with whom the nurse can share perceptions.

Assessing a Community's Level or Potential for Violence

School nurses are in an ideal position to identify behaviors that indicate an increased potential for youth violence and to initiate age-appropriate therapies. It is crucial to identify these behaviors early and to teach others to watch for them (National Crime Prevention Council, 2002). The following indicators can be used to identify potentially violent youths:

- Depression or mood swings
- Obsession with violent or pornographic games, Internet sites, television shows, or movies
- Absence of age-appropriate anger-management skills
- Artwork, writing, or language that displays violence, profanity, anger, association with gangs, or social isolation
- Evidence of cruelty to animals
- History of bullying or fighting
- Self-perception as a victim
- Obsession with violence or weapons

All riots begin with an altercation between two or more people that accelerates out of control. In assessing a community's potential for a riot, the nurse needs to be keenly and continually aware of interactions among individuals and small groups within the community. In some sharply divided communities, even disagreements at a school board or town council meeting can escalate into localized riots. In communities where drug dealing is common, riots between gangs can occur when drug deals "go bad" or police conduct large "sting" operations. Communities that are fraught with poverty, high levels of unemployment or ethnic or racial divisions also experience a high level of tension that can erupt into violence over seemingly minor events, such as a routine arrest of individuals in a barroom brawl. Even the number and quality of constructive after-school activities for older children and teens can be a predictor of group violence, because restless teens who roam neighborhood streets, drinking alcohol and "looking for fun," often end up engaged in violent fights and group crimes. The community health nurse has an obligation to assess the potential for group violence in all of these areas.

Responding to Group Violence

Community models for addressing the problem of group violence should involve as many community members as possible. Not only key legislators and law enforcement officials, but also former criminals, current gang members, and youth and adult offenders should be included. Community religious leaders, educators, members of social and cultural organizations, and criminologists can contribute significantly to the development of effective plans for action that the entire community can endorse. The community health nurse also should be integrally involved in these community actions to reduce group violence.

Supporting Recovery From Group Violence

Although the community health nurse should leave investigation and suppression of violent crime to law enforcement officials, an effective interface for community rehabilitation may involve education, community mobilization, and outreach. Comprehensive case management is paramount. Multiagency cooperation is required to provide needed services for mental health, drug treatment, family counseling, job training and placement, reentry to school or the workforce, formation of more positive social alliances, and expanded economic opportunities.

Counseling is the primary rehabilitative intervention for victims of rape. It may be necessary not only immediately after the attack but months or even years later, as new responses and reactions arise. In addition, options for pregnancy prevention and the prevention of sexually transmitted disease need to be discussed. Possible exposure to human immunodeficiency virus (HIV) is another harrowing aspect of rape with which women need medical and psychological support to cope.

TERRORISM

At the start of the 21st century, the world is a global community. This is particularly evident in the increased incidence and sophistication of terrorist threats and acts around the world. Incidents occurring on U.S. soil such as the bombing of the World Trade Center in 1993 and its destruction on September, 11, 2001, along with the other terrorist attacks that day, have alerted us to our vulnerability and dramatically emphasized the need for increased preparedness within our communities. The anthrax scares after September 11 confirmed that our vulnerability exists in many areas; biologic, chemical, and nuclear terrorist threats are possible.

The U. S. Federal Bureau of Investigation defines **terrorism** as "the unlawful use of force and violence against persons or property to intimidate or coerce a government, the civilian population, or any segment thereof, in furtherance of political or social objectives" (Evans et al, 2002). A terrorist is overzealous and obsessed with an idea. Terrorism and terrorist acts are not new; although the term *terrorism* can be traced back to 1798, the use of terrorist tactics precedes this date. A highly organized religious sect called the *sicarii* attacked crowds of people with knives during holiday celebrations in Palestine at about the time of Christ. During the French and Indian War of 1763, British forces gave smallpox-contaminated blankets to Native Americans. During World War I, the German bioweapons program developed anthrax, glanders, cholera, and wheat fungus as weapons targeting cavalry animals. In World War II, the Japanese tested biologic weapons on Chinese prisoners.

Three major countries operated offensive bioweapons programs in recent years: the United Kingdom until 1957, the United States until 1969, and the former Soviet Union until 1990. Iraq started its bioweapons program in 1985 and continued to develop weapons until 2003. At least 17 other nations are currently suspected of operating offensive bioweapons programs (Evans et al., 2002). Bioweapons include such things as mustard gas, materials to create sarin and VX gas, and anthrax.

Terrorists typically use nuclear, biologic, or chemical (NBC) agents and explosives or incendiary devices to deliver the agents to their targets.

Nuclear warfare involves the use of nuclear devices as weapons and can take several forms. Terrorists who gain access to nuclear power plants could cause a chain of events that lead to a meltdown of the nuclear core, thereby releasing radioactive particles for hundreds of miles around the site. Nuclear accidents have occurred, but no known terrorist attacks have yet involved the use of nuclear power plants as weapons. A terrorist attack using nuclear weapons or destruction of a nuclear plant would cause multiple and prolonged deaths with extensive damage and negative effects for decades.

Chemical warfare involves the use of chemicals such as explosives, nerve agents, blister agents, choking agents, and incapacitating or riot-control agents to cause confusion, debilitation, death, and destruction (Yergler, 2002). Terrorists in the Middle East, willing to sacrifice their own lives, strap bombs to themselves and detonate the explosives in or near targets. Others crash vehicles loaded with explosives into crowds of people or into a building. Many such incidents have occurred during the war in Iraq in 2003–2004.

The aircraft used on September 11, 2001, were huge chemical weapons because they were carrying thousands of tons of jet fuel. The success of the mission depended on the surprise of the attack, severe damage to recognizable buildings, and the deaths of many people. The collapse of the buildings was unplanned. If the planes had been low on fuel, the damage would not have been as severe. The liquid fuel burned at such a high temperature that the internal structure of the buildings was weakened.

Biologic warfare involves using biologic agents to cause multiple illnesses and deaths. Typical biologic agents are anthrax, botulinum, bubonic plague, Ebola, and smallpox. These agents could be used to contaminate food, water, or air. Deliberate food and water contamination remains the easiest way to distribute biologic agents for the purpose of terrorism (Khan, Swerdlow, & Juranek, 2001). In addition, the U. S. Office of Technology Assessment has speculated that the release of 220 pounds of anthrax spores from a crop-duster over the Washington, D.C., area on a calm, clear night could kill between 1 and 3 million people (U. S. Army Chemical and Biological Defense Command, 1998) (see Chapter 9).

The United States is very concerned about the possibility of biologic warfare or bioterrorism, as nations should be. The anthrax infections and deaths that occurred after September 11, 2001, have added to these concerns. However, it has not been confirmed that these incidents were committed by an organized foreign or domestic terrorist group. They could have been carried out by a single disturbed citizen, who would be a terrorist nevertheless, because the outcomes would be the same: fear, death, and destruction.

Factors Contributing to Terrorism

Political factors are the most common contributors to terrorism. Anti-American sentiment runs high in many foreign countries, especially those that perceive the United States as a threat to their military, economic, social, or religious self-determination. Terrorist acts against American military installations abroad, in airports, in airplanes, at American embassies, and even on American soil have occurred frequently in the last decade as an expression of political unrest. The war in Iraq in 2003–2004 was based on information about suspected bioterrorism weapons and reports that Iraq was harboring anti-Western terrorists; these two pieces of information resulted in the toppling of the Saddam Hussein political regime. However, hundreds of military lives were lost, and no weapons of mass destruction were found.

Within the United States, violence-prone members of militia movements, violent antiabortion activists, racial desegregation advocates, and other radical groups have performed terrorist acts, such as the bombing of health clinics offering abortions. In 1984, members of a religious cult, the Rajneeshees, lived in Wasco County, Oregon, and followed a self-proclaimed guru exiled from India. In an attempt to re-

duce voter turnout in an upcoming county election, they sprinkled *Salmonella* bacteria over items on salad bars in local restaurants and in the produce sections of grocery stores. They hoped that, with a reduced voter turnout, representatives friendlier to their group would win the election. Their attack failed to affect the election and killed no one; however, 751 people became sick. The media underreported this event because domestic terrorism was not a topic of concern at that time in U. S. history.

Role of the Community Health Nurse

Community health nurses need to be prepared for the possibility of terrorist activity. They have a role in primary, secondary, and tertiary prevention.

Primary Prevention

Community health nurses are in ideal situations within communities to participate in surveillance. They must look and listen within their communities for anti-group sentiments, which might reflect anti-religion, anti-gay, or anti-ethnic feelings. The nurse should report any untoward activities accordingly.

Nurses should be alert to signs of possible terrorist activity. Specific indicators of possible chemical or biologic terrorism include unusual numbers of dead or dying animals; unexplained serious illnesses or deaths; an unusual liquid, spray, vapor, or odor; and low-lying clouds or fog unrelated to weather. Unusual swarms of insects might also indicate the use of biologic agents for terrorism. "Many nurses currently employed have little knowledge regarding the potential pathogens that could be released, or how to respond to a chemical or biological attack" (Veenema, 2002, p. 63). Less subtle forms of terrorism include bombings, mass shootings, and hijackings, which are more difficult to uncover in time to prevent injury or death (see Clinical Corner).

Secondary and Tertiary Prevention

Although prevention of terrorist incidents is primarily the responsibility of the Department of Defense, the Department of Homeland Security, and public health and law enforcement agencies, community health nurses must be ready to handle the secondary and tertiary effects of such attacks. Knowing the lethal and incapacitating chemical weapons that may be used by terrorists is important. Many of the communicable disease organisms that could be used by terrorists are discussed in Chapter 9 (see What Do You Think? II).

Realizing that terrorist attacks may result in large numbers of casualties, the community health nurse must be prepared to act safely, access information rapidly, and use resources effectively. Specifically, the community health nurse may be called on to provide direct care to victims, to volunteer as a hospital-community liaison, to set up and administer mass immunizations, to make home visits to affected families, or to serve on committees responding to terrorist acts. Formu-

CLINICAL CORNER

A 1999 shooting at Columbine High School in Colorado left 15 people dead. National attention was focused on the issue of violence among teens. The public and the media looked to public health experts for answers to the problem of increasing violence in this population. Community health nurses are among those whose aim is to assess and address the problems surrounding individual and group violence in their communities.

Imagine that, as a community health nurse, you have just been named the head of a multidisciplinary task force whose objective is to prevent teen violence within your community. Your project has been funded for 3 years. Having worked in other nursing roles in your community over the past 10 years, you have developed excellent partnerships with resource persons within your community. After reading the information about your community, respond to the questions that follow.

COMMUNITY INFORMATION

You are in a desert suburban community of 40,000 individuals, who primarily commute to high-tech jobs in a nearby city. The average household income is $56,000 per year. The divorce rate in the community is 63%. The number of teens whose primary caregiver returns home after 5:30 PM is 78%. Ethnicity is as follows: 52% Anglo, 30% Asian, 12% Hispanic, 4% Black, and 2% other.

Identified problems among teens include racial division, gang violence, a high school dropout rate of 17%, and a high incidence of methamphetamine use. The incidence of violent crimes in this community is 28% higher than in neighboring communities. Besides organized sports, there are very few extracurricular activities available through the school or within the community.

QUESTIONS

1. Faced with this daunting task, where will you begin your efforts?
2. With what agencies and individuals will you need to develop partnerships to maximize the efficacy of the task force?
3. Brainstorm about possible ways to capitalize on the use of technology in your efforts to reduce the risk of violence in the community.
4. How will you disseminate the information you obtain to advance the cause of globalization of public health?
5. What ethical issues will you anticipate as you begin your efforts?

WHAT DO YOU THINK? II

THE AMERICAN RED CROSS—AMERICAN'S DISASTER RELIEF AGENCY

The American Red Cross (ARC) has responded to disasters of every shape and size for more than 100 years. In the 14 months after September 11, 2001, ARC chapters provided shelter or financial assistance for 67,000 separate disasters across the country. More than 2100 licensed mental health professionals are available for ARC assignments. In New York City, as a result of the September 11, 2001, terrorist attack, the ARC

- Opened 49,999 cases
- Served 13,171,855 meals/snacks
- Made 183,732 mental health contacts
- Opened 14 shelters
- Provided 41,898 relief workers for the disaster
- Opened 31 service delivery sites
- Received $933.2 million dollars in donations through June 2002.

The ARC has spent funds on a family gift program, aid for displaced workers or residents, immediate relief, and direct support, and for other purposes.

lating, updating, and following a disaster plan is one of the most effective community-based strategies to minimize injury and mortality from terrorism.

Most community health nurses will not be on the front line of uncovering or immediately responding to terrorist activities, but their skills will be needed with groups, families, or individuals who experience a terrorist-related event. Some of the activities listed earlier in this chapter to help people deal with the aftermath of a disaster would also be appropriate if terrorism is the cause of the disaster. In addition, community health nurses may work with people who need help coping or who want to do something to help.

After experiencing a traumatic event such as a terrorist attack, people do not know how to cope. We are warned to expect more attacks. We are told to be vigilant. The terror we are fighting is often our own. This is a new experience for most people, and assistance from the community health nurse can help them cope effectively. The following 10 tips were gathered from experts in many fields by Foley (2002) and are common-sense approaches to fight anxiety:

- Be a little afraid—a certain level of fear is healthy if you learn to use it as positive energy. Use your pinch of anxiety to be more vigilant about your safety and that of your family, especially when you travel, and in taking care of your health.
- Keep a courage journal—fear immobilizes, and courage

takes action. Every time you take action, you are getting past fear. Even small steps are an opportunity to build more courage. Every time you take a courageous step—getting on a plane, opening your mail—write it down.

- Reassure your children. In the act of reassuring your children, you will reassure yourself.
- Hang out with children. Do things with your children—most young people carry a charge of positive energy that is infectious. If you do not have young children, volunteer at a school or read to children at a nearby day care center.
- Cook something hearty, healthy, and large, and invite lots of people in to eat it. The process of cooking is good for the soul. The aromas are good for the soul. And the chopping and dicing make you feel that you are doing something useful and concrete.
- Give kindness to others. We all need each other now. Make a point of chatting with the woman at the checkout counter or letting a pedestrian cross the street when you are driving. Wave hello to strangers. You will be amazed how much it is true that in giving, we receive.
- Get spiritual. Reach out and participate in your faith community or get involved in one, if so inclined. Believing in a power greater than yourself can be comforting.
- Laugh. Laughter is the best medicine for fear. Spend evenings in good company—group laughter is better than laughing alone.
- Get back to nature. Spending interactive time with nature is a remedy for just about any soul sickness. Go to the park, take a walk, work in your garden.
- Find reasons to believe the sky is not falling. All the unpleasant facts and figures get our "anxiety juices" flowing. Seek out positive people, and read literature that encourages positive thinking. Do not feed the "dark side." Turn off the news and opt for a funny movie or an inspirational story.

Community health nurses can make major differences in grassroots efforts to bring about change, but on a day-to-day basis the little things they say and do with peers and clients can make just as big a difference.

SUMMARY

A disaster is any event that causes a level of destruction that exceeds the abilities of the affected community to respond without assistance. Disasters may be caused by natural or manmade/technologic events and may be classified as multiple-casualty incidents or mass-casualty incidents.

The scope of a disaster is its range of effect, and the intensity is the level of destruction it causes. Victims of disasters include direct victims, those injured or killed, and indirect victims, the loved ones of direct victims. Displaced persons are those who are forced to flee their homes because of the disaster, and refugees are those who are forced to leave their homelands, usually in response to war or political persecution.

Host factors that contribute to the likelihood of experiencing a disaster include age, general health, mobility, psychological factors, and socioeconomic factors. The disaster agent is the fire, flood, bomb, or other cause. Environmental factors are those that could potentially contribute to or mitigate a disaster.

In developing strategies to address the problem of disasters, it is helpful for the community health nurse to consider each of the four phases of disaster management: prevention, preparedness, response, and recovery.

Primary prevention of disasters means keeping the disaster from ever happening by taking actions to eliminate the possibility of its occurrence. Secondary prevention focuses on earliest possible detection and treatment. Tertiary prevention involves reducing the amount and degree of disability or damage resulting from the disaster.

In addition to assessing for preparedness, an effective disaster plan establishes a clear chain of authority, develops lines of communication, and delineates routes and modes of transport. Plans for mobilizing, warning, and evacuating people are also critical elements of the disaster plan. At the disaster site, police, firefighters, nurses, and other relief workers develop a coordinated response to rescue victims from further injury, triage victims by seriousness of injury, and treat victims on-site and in local hospitals. Care and transport of dead bodies must also be managed, as well as support for the loved ones of the injured, dead, or missing. Long-term support includes both financial assistance and physical and emotional rehabilitation.

Self-care, including stress education for all relief workers after a disaster, helps to lower anxiety and put the situation into proper perspective. CISD provides victims with a mechanism for emotional reconciliation and healing.

Problems of group violence include school violence, gangs, riots, and violent crimes. A gang is an organization of youths that has a name, is usually territorial or claims a certain territory as being under its exclusive influence, and is involved in criminal acts.

The roots of group violence are multifactorial and include inadequate parenting; socioeconomic and racial injustices; exposure to violence in media, cartoons, and pornography; and easy access to weapons.

The goals of *Healthy People 2010* for reducing violence include reductions in physical assaults and weapon carrying by schoolchildren and reduction of work-related assaults and homicides.

The role of the community health nurse in preventing and reducing group violence includes effective community organization and program development, as well as policy making to address the family and environmental factors that contribute to increased risk of group violence.

Terrorism is the unlawful use of force or violence against persons or property to intimidate or coerce a government or civilian population in the furtherance of political or social objectives. Terrorism may be nuclear, biologic, or chemical, including nerve agents and explosive devices. The community health nurse should be alert to signs of possible terrorist activity and prepared to address the secondary or tertiary effects of such attacks. Preparation includes knowledge of the effects of specific biologic or chemical agents and how to help people cope with the terror they personally feel.

ACTIVITIES TO PROMOTE CRITICAL THINKING

1. Think about your own community and its residents. What are some host factors that might increase its risk of experiencing a disaster? What environmental factors might be significant? In each case, identify the likely agent. What interventions could be included in a disaster plan to reduce these risk factors?

2. The nightly news shows that at least 200 people have been injured in an explosion in a neighboring community. At the disaster site, victims are still being recovered from the wreckage, and local hospitals are overwhelmed with patients who have fractures, lacerations, and burns. You want to offer your assistance as a registered nurse. How should you go about volunteering your services?

3. Your local high school is complaining of an increasing gang presence. Members have been recruiting and intimidating students, and fights with knives have broken out repeatedly in the past month. A random search of lockers revealed two guns and eight knives, and as many as 25% of students are staying out of school because of parents' fears of violence. Describe one possible response of a community health nurse to address the problem of gang violence in this situation.

4. Access one or more of the Internet sites listed in this chapter. Report on the change in statistics for disasters, group violence, or terrorism since the year 2003. Have rates increased or decreased? What factors might be involved in this change?

REFERENCES

Associated Press. (2002, August 12). Medical advances, drop in death rate linked. *The Fresno Bee*, p. 5.

Bacque, G. (2000). Advocates fear wave of homeless murders. *Toronto Star*. Retrieved December 15, 2003, from *http://projects.is.asu.edu/pipermail/hpn/2000-June/000849.html*

Benda, B.B., & Turney, H.M. (2002). Youthful violence: Problems and prospects. *Child and Adolescent Social Work Journal, 19*(1), 5–34.

Copper, M., & Ianzito, V. (2002). One year later.... *AARP: Modern Maturity, 45*(5), 88–93.

DeVitto, S. (2002). Giving hope, she found hope. *Reflections on Nursing Leadership, 28*(3), 21.

Evans, R.G., Crutcher, J.M., Shadel, B., Clements, B., & Bronze,

M.S. (2002). Terrorism from a public health perspective. *The American Journal of the Medical Sciences, 323*(6), 291–298.

Foley, D. (2002). Fight terror—your own. *Prevention, 54*(2), 126–133, 174–176.

Garbarino, J. (1999). *Lost boys: Why our sons turn violent and how we can save them.* New York: Free Press.

Goode, E. (2000, March 2). Struggling to make sense out of boy-turned-killer. *New York Times*. Available at: *http://www.nytimes.com/library/national/science/health/030200hth-behavior-children.html..* Accessed 3/24/04.

Herman, D., Felton, C., & Susser, E. (2002). Mental health needs in New York State following the September 11 attacks. *Journal of Urban Health: Bulletin of the New York Academy of Medicine, 79*(3), 322–331.

Hirschi, T. (2004). Travis Hirschi's social bond theory. Available at: *http://home.comcast.net/~ddemeio/crime/hirschi.html.*

Huff, R.C. (2002). *Gangs in America* (3rd ed.). Newbury Park, CA: Sage.

Jack, K., & Glied, S. (2002). The public costs of mental health response: Lessons from the New York City post-9/11 needs assessment. *Journal of Urban Health: Bulletin of the New York Academy of Medicine, 79*(3), 332–339.

Khan, A.S., Swerdlow, D.L., & Juranek, D.D. (2001). Precautions against biological and chemical terrorism directed at food and water supplies. *Public Health Reports, 116,* 3–14.

Late, M. (2002, August). Homeland department plan may undermine public health. *The Nation's Health,* pp. 1, 32.

Miller, J., Maxson, C.L., Klein, M.W. (Eds.). (2001). *The modern gang reader.* Los Angeles: Roxbury Press.

National Crime Prevention Council. (2002, October 8). Stopping school violence in its tracks. Watch for signs—Take action. Available at: *http://www.newsweek.com/ce/ce270a.htm.* Accessed on 3/26/04.

Ostrowski, M. (2001). A nurse's view from ground zero. *RN, 64*(11), 35–37.

Peeke, P.M. (2002). Reclaim your peace of mind. *Prevention, 54*(1), 92–97.

Schlenger, W.E., Caddell, J.M., Ebert, L., Jordan, B.K., Rourke, K.M., Wilson, D., et al. (2002). Psychological reactions to terrorist attacks: Findings from the national study of Americans' reactions to September 11. *JAMA: The Journal of the American Medical Association, 288*(5), 581–588.

Schuster, M.A., Franke, T.M., Bastian, A.M., Sor, S., & Halfron, N. (2000). Firearm storage patterns in U. S. homes with children. *American Journal of Public Health, 90*(4), 588–594.

Silver, R.C., Holman, E.A., McIntosh, D.N., Poulin, M., & Gil-Rivas, V. (2002). Nationwide longitudinal study of psychological responses to September 11. *JAMA: The Journal of the American Medical Association, 288*(10), 1235–1244.

Steger, S. (2000). Killed in school! *RN, 63*(4), 36–38.

U. S. Army Chemical and Biological Defense Command. (1998). *Domestic preparedness program: Hospital provider course.* McLean, VA: Booz-Allen & Hamilton, Inc. and SAIC, Inc.

U. S. Department of Health and Human Services. (2000). *Healthy people 2010* (Conference ed., Vols. 1 & 2). Washington, DC: U. S. Government Printing Office.

U. S. Department of Justice, Office of Juvenile Justice and Delinquency Prevention. (1999, March). *Highlights of the 1997 national youth gang survey.* Washington, DC: Author.

U. S. Department of Justice. (2002). National Crime Victimization

Survey (NCVS) for 2000–2001. Available at: *http://www.usdoj.gov/bjs/pub/pdf/cvol.pdf*

Veenema, T.G. (2002). Chemical and biological terrorism: Current updates for nurse educators. *Nursing Education Perspectives, 23*(2), 62–71.

Wilson, J. J., & Howell, J. C. (1993). *A comprehensive strategy for serious, violent, and chronic juvenile offenders.* Washington, DC: U. S. Department of Justice, Office of Juvenile Justice.

Yergler, M. (2002). Nerve gas attack. *The American Journal of Nursing, 102*(7), 57–60.

SELECTED READINGS

Chaffee, M., Conway-Welch, C., & Stephens, V. (2001). Bioterrorism in the United States: Take it seriously. *The American Journal of Nursing, 101*(11), 59, 61.

Charles, P. (2001). What I learned at ground zero. *RN, 64*(12), 42–44.

Cohen, H.W., Eolis, S.L., Gould, R.M., & Sidel, V.W. (2001). Hyping bioterrorism obscures real concerns. *The American Journal of Nursing, 101*(11), 58, 60.

Coleman, E.A., & Kearney, K. (2001). Anthrax: Know the guidelines for management. *The American Journal of Nursing, 101*(12), 48–52.

Ellickson, P.L., & McGuigan, K.A. (2000). Early predictors of adolescent violence. *American Journal of Public Health, 90*(4), 566–572.

Evison, D., Hinsley, D., & Rice, P. (2002). Regular review: Chemical weapons. *BMJ, 324,* 332–335.

Firshein, J. (2002). Public health preparedness for disaster: Perspective from Washington, DC. *Journal of Urban Health: Bulletin of the New York Academy of Medicine, 79*(1), 6–7.

Frattaroli, S., Webster, D.W., & Teret, S.P. (2002). Unintentional gun injuries, firearm design, and prevention: What we know, what we need to know, and what can be done. *Journal of Urban Health: Bulletin of the New York Academy of Medicine, 79*(1), 49–59.

Geiger, H.J. (2001). Terrorism, biological weapons, and bonanzas: Assessing the real threat to public health. *American Journal of Public Health, 91*(5), 708–709.

Glasser, J. (2002). Coming to grips with the pain. *U. S. News & World Report, 133*(10), 2730, 2732.

Keane, A., Houldin, A.D., Allison, P.D., Jepson, C., Shults, J., Nuamah, I.F., et al. (2002). Factors associated with distress in urban residential fire survivors. *Journal of Nursing Scholarship, 34*(1), 11–17.

Kennedy, M.S. (2002). Our worst disaster's first nurse. *The American Journal of Nursing, 102*(2), 102–103.

Landesman, L.Y. (2001). *Public health management of disasters: The practice guide.* Waldorf, MD: American Public Health Association.

Late, M. (2002, June/July). Partners improving community safety, emergency response. *The Nation's Health,* p. 4.

Levy, B.S., & Sidel, V.W. (2000). *War and public health.* Waldorf, MD: American Public Health Association.

Lutenbacher, M., Cooper, W.O., & Faccia, K. (2002). Planning youth violence prevention efforts: Decision-making across community sectors. *Journal of Adolescent Health, 30*(5), 346–354.

Miller, M., Azrael, D., & Hemenway, D. (2002). Firearm availability and suicide, homicide, and unintentional firearm deaths among women. *Journal of Urban Health: Bulletin of the New York Academy of Medicine, 79*(1), 26–38.

Murray, C.J.L., King, G., Lopez, A.D., Tomijima, N., & Krug, E.G. (2002). Armed conflict as a public health problem. *BMJ, 324,* 346–349.

Perez, M.A., Pinzon-Perez, H., & Sowby, S. (2002). The role of health educators in dealing with biological threats in the United States. *American Journal of Health Education, 33*(4), 216–224.

Slovak, K., & Singer, M.I. (2002). Children and violence: Findings and implications from a rural community. *Child and Adolescent Social Work Journal, 19*(1), 35–56.

St. John, R., & Giroux, C. (2002). Terrorism and public health: The little known equation. *Canadian Journal of Public Health, 93*(3), 165–166.

Internet Resources

Action Committee Against Violence: *http://www.acav.org*
Almanac of Disasters: *http://www.disasterium.com*
Bioterrorism: *http://bioterrorism.straws.com*
Bioterrorism Resources: *www.acponlone.org/bioterro/index.html*
Center for the Study and Prevention of Violence: *http://www.colorado.edu/cspv/*
Citizen Corps: *www.citizencorps.gov*
Men Against Domestic Violence (MADV)—Domestic Violence Resources: *http://www.silicom.com/~paladin/madv/*
National Coalition Against Domestic Violence (NCADVE): *http://www.healthtouch.com*
National Crime Prevention Council: *http://www.ncpc.org*
National School Board Association: *http://www.keepschoolssafe.org*
National School Safety Center: *http://www.nssc1.org*
National Youth Gang Center: *http://www.iir.com/nygc/*
Nursing World: Bioterrorism and Disaster Response: *www.NursingWorld.org/news/disaster*
Partnerships Against Violence Network (PAVNET): *http://www.pavnet.org*
Teens, Crime, and the Community: *http://www.nationaltcc.org*
United Nations Declaration of Human Rights—"A Life Free of Violence": *http://www.undp.org/rblac/gender/*
Youth Crime Watch of America: *http://www.ycwa.org*

21

The Global Community: International Health Concerns

Learning Objectives

Upon mastery of this chapter, you should be able to:

- Discuss the interrelationship of global health issues.
- Describe the pluralistic medical systems of the world.
- Differentiate between multilateral and bilateral agencies.
- Explain the role of nongovernmental agencies.
- Describe the purpose of the World Health Organization.
- Discuss the United States Agency for International Development (USAID).
- Analyze the implications of the Health for All movement.
- Be familiar with specific global health concerns.
- Describe what is meant by the global burden of disease and disability-adjusted life year.
- Differentiate between eradication, elimination, and control of communicable disease.
- Identify new and emerging diseases.
- Increase awareness of the role of the global nurse.
- Summarize global nursing opportunities.

he pictures taken of the earth from space a number of years ago were a graphic illustration that we belong to one small planet of interdependent nations. This interdependence relates to virtually all areas of life, including health. As systems theory suggests, what happens in one country affects many others in important ways. For example, air travel can transport health problems from a country halfway around the world to new communities in less than a day. Human immunodeficiency virus/acquired immunodeficiency disease (HIV/AIDS) began in Africa and is now pandemic because communicable diseases know no geographic boundaries. In New York in the fall of 1999, 61 severe cases and seven deaths were reported from a mysterious viral illness later identified as the West Nile virus, which had not previously been reported in the United States. Researchers now speculate that the virus may have traveled to the United States in smuggled exotic birds. The virus was closely related genetically to strains found in the Middle East (Centers for Disease Control and Prevention [CDC], 2000). Within 2 years, 3862 cases of West Nile Virus and 248 deaths had occurred in the U.S. Evidence of infections in birds, humans, mosquitoes and other animals has been documented in 43 states and the District of Columbia (CDC, 2002a). The globalization of food commodities and food safety also affects health. For example, there is strong evidence that a causal relationship exists between ongoing outbreaks in Europe of bovine spongiform encephalopathy ("mad cow disease") and the human disease called new variant Creutzfeldt-Jakob disease (vCJD). Between 1995 and 2002, 124 cases of vCJD were identified in the United Kingdom, 6 in France, and 1 case in Ireland, Italy, and the United States. The affected individuals from Ireland and the United States lived in the United Kingdom during the epidemic. Cattle are the only known food source of the disease (CDC, 2002b).

Global health issues become ours when they spread within our borders, when we commit resources to a country in need, when we make a personal commitment to improve the health of a population beyond our shores, and when we import or export food.

Much of this text focuses on community health nursing at the local, state, or national level. This chapter aims to help readers recognize the contributions of community health nurses internationally and perhaps investigate international nursing as a career option. Health care on a global level carries with it the allure of travel to foreign countries and offers the nurse exclusive views of the world and humanity. In addition, it provides unique opportunities to improve the health of the world that we inhabit and to help create a healthy global community. A sense of justice commonly compels nurses to enter the field of international health; many are concerned about the intolerable health conditions affecting one third of the world's population, especially when they realize that they are benefiting from the misfortunes of the poor (Lanza, 1996). Whatever their reasons for choosing global health as a focus, it is clear that nurses make a profound con-

tribution to the health of disenfranchised populations around the world.

This chapter describes how health issues are addressed throughout the world in terms of international responses, ideology, community development, and the establishment of health priorities. Some health care systems and agencies are described to illustrate both their differing goals and structures and their similar struggles and challenges. The main health concerns facing the world are then discussed. Lastly, career and service opportunities for nurses are suggested.

INTERNATIONAL HEALTH CARE SYSTEMS

Pluralistic medical systems are found in practically all developing countries. They often consist of traditional healing systems, lay practices, household remedies, transitional health workers, and Western medicine (Kloos, 1994). Traditional healing may be all that is available to populations in most rural areas and in some cities. Other than traditional birth attendants, it is not customary for national health systems to integrate traditional healing into the national health system, except in the United States, China, India, and some African countries. Western medicine was introduced to developing countries during colonial times, and systems were operated either by colonial administrations or by missions. After independence, health systems varied in their development. Some continued the colonial practices; others followed tax-financed government insurance or socialist health care systems. Curative health care expanded rapidly in urban areas, and the level of health care was raised in those locales. In the late 1970s, the Primary Health Care (PHC) approach was adopted in almost all of the developing countries as they sought to serve all populations, both urban and rural. It is common for such countries to expend a smaller percentage of their government budgets on health, compared with middle-income countries (Kloos, 1994). PHC helps provide affordable essential health services in developing countries.

Entrepreneurial, Welfare-Oriented, Comprehensive, and Socialist Systems

A country's health care system is based on its political economy. The worldwide economic recession in the 1980s was a barrier to the development of effective health services. Roemer (1993) developed the first typology of health systems based on political ideology. He categorized them as (1) entrepreneurial, (2) welfare-oriented, (3) comprehensive, or (4) socialist. He further described each category by the type of country in which it is found: industrialized, transitional, or very poor. Variations in these systems can be explained by differential growth in each country's economy and by differences in the redistribution of wealth and political will. It is commonly understood that economic growth is needed to increase the standard of living. Countries that also emphasize redistribution are characterized by better education, lower infant mortality, and higher life expectancy than countries focusing on growth alone. Therefore, the four types of health care systems have further variation depending on whether they are in industrialized, transitional, or very poor countries.

The entrepreneurial health system is typically found in industrialized countries. These countries have free-market economies, abundant resources, large amounts of money allocated to health care, and decentralized governments. Such countries have a highly individualistic perspective. The U.S. system of health care delivery is typical of the entrepreneurial system.

The welfare-oriented system is driven by statutory programs that support the cost of medical care for all, or almost all, of the population. Such programs are commonly referred to as "national health insurance." More than one half of the health-related expenditures are from government sources, but most physicians and dentists also remain in private practice. Western Europe, Japan, and Australia subscribe to the welfare-oriented health system.

A comprehensive system is a step further away from the welfare-oriented type. There are substantial modifications in delivery and financing that result in universal entitlements. This system abandons the separate and complex sources of financing found in the previous two systems. The Scandinavian countries, Great Britain, and New Zealand use a comprehensive health care delivery system.

The socialist system came about through social revolution that totally abolished free-market economies and replaced them with socialism. Under socialism, the health care system is also socialized. The first overthrow of capitalism was in Russia in 1917, followed by Eastern Europe, Albania, Bulgaria, Czechoslovakia, East Germany, Hungary, Poland, Romania, Yugoslavia, and later China. A socialist health care system views health services as a social entitlement and a government responsibility, emphasizes prevention, engages in central planning for health resources and services with one central health authority, gives priority to industrial workers and children, and bases health care work on scientific principles. Nonscientific and cultist practices are not permitted. Some of these countries are now in the process of democratization and are attempting to redesign their health care systems.

The four health systems that have been described apply to industrialized countries. Roemer applies the same typology to transitional and very poor countries. Countries that are in the process of development are referred to as transitional. Such countries and their health care systems are moving effectively toward economic and social development. The global median gross national product (GNP) of these countries is $1500 per capita.

Very poor countries are even less economically developed and have lower per-capita GNPs than do the industrialized or transitional countries. Examples of very poor countries are Ethiopia, Kenya, Ghana, Myanmar, Sri Lanka, Mozambique, and China.

Other countries that do not easily fit into the health care system matrix are the oil-rich developing countries. In just a few years, the wealth in such countries exploded upward, from low levels typical of Africa and some Asian countries to levels equal to or greater than those of highly industrialized countries. Examples are Gabon, Libya, Saudi Arabia, and Kuwait. The governments of these countries use their income to extend and improve health services for the general population. Entrepreneurial or socialist systems are not found in these countries. Gabon and Libya are classified as welfare-oriented because they have different schemes of social insurance for health services for a large percentage of the population. Saudi Arabia and Kuwait are universal and comprehensive systems that use government funding to provide complete health services to everyone.

Health systems are affected by broader social trends. The major social influences are urbanization, industrialization, education, government structure, international trade, and demographic changes. Since 1940, all national health systems have undergone significant changes resulting from increasing organization of health systems; expansion of resources (personnel, facilities, equipment); population demands for and increased use of health services; growth in health-related expenditures; collectivized financing; cost control; efficiency improvement; technology; preventive and primary health care; quality assurance; increased public responsibility; and community participation (Roemer, 1993).

GLOBAL HEALTH AGENCIES

Many different international agencies cooperate on world health matters. Historically, this cooperation has been erratic, although more recently it has improved greatly through the efforts of both intergovernmental and nongovernmental organizations.

Multilateral and **bilateral organizations** are mainly intergovernmental. The United Nations, the World Health Organization, and the World Bank are examples of **multilateral agencies**. These agencies are multinational organizations that support development efforts of governments and organizations in less-developed nations of the world. The U. S. Agency for International Development, the Peace Corps, and the CDC are examples of agencies that usually deal directly with other governments; therefore, they are called bilateral agencies.

In contrast, **nongovernmental organizations** (NGOs) are those not under government sponsorship or control. The U. S. government designates these as **private voluntary organizations** (PVOs). They include humanitarian and professional organizations concerned with global health. Examples of PVOs are the Global Health Council, the Center for International Health and Cooperation, CARE, the Carter Center, and the International Council of Nurses. NGOs are found in most countries.

The World Health Organization

The **World Health Organization** (WHO) promotes health on a global basis. Its mandate includes acting as the directing and coordinating authority for international health work and maintaining effective collaboration with United Nations specialized agencies and other national and international bodies responsible for health development (Grad, 2002; Wenzel, 1998). Fostering equitable human development, lifting populations out of poverty, and assisting men and women to realize their potential are all goals that the WHO shares with 192 member countries (Display 21–1).

The primary functions of WHO are to provide technical support for sustainable health care systems and to advise members on strategies to meet their health care needs. WHO serves as a catalyst to mobilize the resources of national governments, financial institutions and endowments, and bilateral partners for health development (WHO, 2002m). It is assisted in carrying out its mission by United Nations agencies, the private sector, NGOs, and leading service, training, and research centers worldwide.

In her address to the 1999 International Health Conference of the Global Health Council, Dr. Gro Harlem Brundtland, Director General of WHO, noted, "We are leaving a century of remarkable human progress. The health gains of the 20th century count as one of the biggest social transformations of our times. Living conditions have dramatically improved for the large majority of human beings. But the century also left a legacy. More than a billion fellow human beings have been left behind in the health revolution." She continued, "Health is key to reversing the downward spiral linking poverty, malnutrition and environmental degradation. Good health enhances the capabilities of the poor, builds social and human capabilities, which, in turn, advance the productivity of people, communities and societies. This is what development is all about" (Global Health Council, 1999a). Dr. Brundtland identified the burdens of excess mortality and morbidity that disproportionately affect poor people. Her organization primarily gives attention to known interventions that can achieve the greatest health gains possible with available resources.

History

WHO began in 1945 when three physicians serving as delegates from Brazil, China, and Norway to the founding General Assembly of the United Nations met at a San Francisco restaurant. Over lunch, they discussed the idea of global health as a peacekeeping strategy and envisioned a world body that would take the leading role in promoting global health. Just 1 year later, the WHO constitution was adopted in New York by the representatives of 61 countries (Grad, 2002; Wenzel, 1998). Although it has been closely associated with the United Nations since its inception, WHO has its own charter. It has taken the primary technical responsibility not only for its own programs, funded by regular and extrabudgetary funds, but also for health-related initiatives sponsored and funded by United Nations agencies and other international bodies.

Central and Regional Organization

The headquarters of WHO is in Geneva, Switzerland. It has a decentralized form of governance featuring six regional offices, each governed by a committee of delegates from that region's member countries. For example, the regional office in New Delhi, India, serves Southeast Asian members. Special offices have been established in Addis Ababa, Ethiopia, to work with the new African Union (formerly the Organization of African Unity) and in Moscow to work with Eastern European countries and the newly independent states of central Asia.

World Health Assembly

The World Health Assembly is the highest governing body within WHO. Made up of delegates from the 192 member countries, it meets annually to review the progress and performance of WHO and to give direction to its efforts. In 1999, the 52nd World Health Assembly resolved to promote equitable, accessible, and sustainable health care systems in developing countries based on PHC (see later discussion). The Assembly urged its members to take steps to meet the needs of the most vulnerable of their populations, including freeing the poor from the burden of infectious diseases and preventing noncommunicable diseases (WHO, 1999b, 1999c).

Major Programs

One of the greatest achievements of WHO has been the eradication of smallpox. In 1967, when smallpox was endemic in 31 countries, 13 million cases were estimated worldwide. It is projected that 20 million people would have died in the next two decades if smallpox had not been eradicated. Other important accomplishments include reduction of malaria, standardization of data-collection systems, adoption of international standards for the control and reporting of morbidity and mortality, and publication of classic works for the prevention and management of disease (Whaley & Hashim, 1995). In addition, the work of the WHO has been credited with preventing hundreds of millions of cases of tropical diseases.

As the 21st century begins, new eradication/elimination programs are under way for polio, leprosy, guinea worm, and measles. Other initiatives include

- Reducing transmission and incidence of HIV/AIDS
- Launching a "Roll Back Malaria" program
- Stopping the transmission of tuberculosis

D I S P L A Y   2 1 – 1

Definition of Health

Health is a state of complete physical, mental, and social well-being and not merely the absence of disease or infirmity.

Source: World Health Organization Constitution

- Increasing access to essential pharmaceuticals
- Reducing the poor quality of some pharmaceuticals
- Preventing and treating iron deficiency
- Reducing maternal morbidity and mortality
- Promoting healthful lifestyles for all age groups, including elders
- Establishing "Health Promoting Schools"

To achieve some of these initiatives, the WHO is involved in a number of significant partnerships. For example, the initiative for establishing Health Promoting Schools is a collaborative effort of WHO, the United Nations Educational, Scientific and Cultural Organization (UNESCO), and the United Nations Children's Fund (UNICEF). School Health Education is comprehensive when it does the following (WHO, 1997):

- Views health as more than the absence of disease
- Uses all available opportunities for health education (formal and informal, traditional and alternative, inside and outside school)
- Harmonizes the health messages that are delivered
- Enables students to promote conditions supportive of health services
- Encourages the development of a healthy environment

Another example of such partnerships is the Human Reproduction Program, a global research program on reproductive health. It collaborates with two programs of the United Nations as well as the World Bank. Similarly, the WHO has joined with several other organizations to fight hunger and improve food standards, and has collaborated in a "Solar Alert" campaign to alert people about the harmful effects of solar radiation (WHO, 1999d) (Display 21–2).

World Bank

The **World Bank (WB)** is a major health-related agency that collaborates with WHO and other global health organizations in health development. Founded in 1944, its goal is "a world free of poverty." Its threefold mission is

- To fight poverty with passion and professionalism for lasting results

DISPLAY 21–2

Health Promotion

Health is created and lived by people within the settings of their everyday life; where they learn, work, play and love. Health is created by caring for oneself and others, by being able to take decisions and have control over one's life circumstances; and by ensuring that the society one lives in creates conditions that allow the attainment of health by all its members.

(World Health Organization. [1997]. Promoting health through schools: Report of a WHO expert committee on comprehensive school health education and promotion. *WHO Technical Report Series, 180,* 5. Geneva: WHO.)

DISPLAY 21–3

World Bank

The fight against poverty is not a fight for glory. It is about equity and social justice, about the environment and resources we all share, and about peace and security. It is a fight for a better life for all of us and for our children who will live in this very interconnected world.

James D. Wolfensohn, 1999

- To help people help themselves and their environment by providing resources, sharing knowledge, building capacity, and forging partnerships in the public and private sectors
- To be an excellent institution that is able to attract, excite, and nurture committed staff with exceptional skills who know how to listen and learn.

The Bank's Population, Health, and Nutrition Department works to alleviate poverty and promote development through investments and partnerships with other organizations concerned with global health (World Bank, 2002) (Display 21–3).

The United States Agency for International Development

The **United States Agency for International Development (USAID)** is an independent, bilateral agency of the executive branch that, under the guidance of the Secretary of State, works to enhance long-term and equitable economic growth and to advance U. S. foreign policy by supporting countries in their efforts to recover from disaster, escape poverty, and engage in democratic reforms. The agency provides support to developing countries for economic development, agriculture and trade, global health, democracy, conflict prevention, and humanitarian assistance (Natsios, 2002). It collaborates with many governmental and private agencies to implement its programs.

American International Health Alliance

An example of USAID collaborating with other organizations to carry out its programs is the **American International Health Alliance (AIHA)**, which operates under a cooperative agreement with USAID. It establishes and manages hospital partnerships between health care institutions in the United States and their counterparts in central and eastern Europe and in the newly independent states of Central Asia. AIHA is reportedly the U. S. hospital sector's most coordinated response to health care issues in those areas. In 2002, AIHA managed more than 90 partnerships in 21 countries (American International Health Alliance, 2002).

Nongovernmental Organizations

NGOs operate in most countries of the world. Some of the organizations that are most significant to the work of community health nursing are discussed here.

Global Health Council

The Global Health Council (GHC), formerly known as the National Council for International Health, is the world's largest membership alliance dedicated to saving lives by improving health throughout the world. Its mission is to mobilize effective action by doing the following (Global Health Council, 1999b):

- Advocating for needed policies and resources
- Building networks and alliances among those working to improve health
- Communicating innovative ideas, knowledge and best practices in the health field

The membership of GHC includes hundreds of private and public organizations around the world as well as several thousand professionals involved in global health. It is staffed by a multidisciplinary, cross-cultural board of directors, health professionals, student interns, volunteers, and members (Global Health Council, 1999b).

Center for International Health and Cooperation

The Center for International Health and Cooperation (CIHC) was founded in 1992 to promote healing and peace in countries shattered by war, regional conflicts, and ethnic violence. Former U. S. Secretary of State Cyrus Vance, former U. N. Secretary General Boutros Boutros-Ghali, and many other distinguished men and women volunteer their services to the Center. They bring exceptional experience, knowledge, statesmanship, and insights to bear on the complex problems and opportunities associated with humanitarian efforts in international conflicts. The belief is that health and other basic humanitarian endeavors often provide the only common ground for initiating dialogue and cooperation among warring parties (Center for International Health and Cooperation, 2002).

CARE

The Cooperative for American Remittances to Europe (CARE) was founded in 1945 when 22 American organizations joined together to rush life-saving "care packages" from individual American citizens, churches, clubs, and businesses to survivors of World War II. Millions of CARE packages followed in the next two decades. In the 1950s, CARE expanded its program to developing nations, using surplus American food to feed the hungry. In the 1960s, it pioneered PHC. Now called the Cooperative for Assistance and Relief Everywhere, CARE is affiliated with an international confederation of 11 member organizations. It has responded to famines and disasters worldwide with emergency food, supplies, and rehabilitative efforts. In addition, it delivers programs in education, health, population, water and sanitation, agriculture,

---

DISPLAY 21–4

CARE

Every CARE package is a personal contribution to the world peace our nation seeks. It expresses America's concern and friendship in a language all peoples understand.

President John F. Kennedy, 1962

---

environmental preservation, economic development, and community building (CARE, 2002) (Display 21–4).

The Carter Center

Former President Jimmy Carter and his wife Roselyn founded the Carter Center in 1986 to help countries through a nongovernmental mechanism. The Center works in the fields of disease prevention and agriculture throughout the world. Two programs have succeeded in reaching their goals. Guinea worm disease has successfully been eradicated in Africa and parts of Asia in the areas served by the Carter Center, and river blindness has been eliminated in Africa and Latin America. The Trachoma Control Program continues to fight blindness in Africa and Yemen.

The Ethiopia Public Health Training Initiative strengthens teaching capacities of faculty members at five major universities of Ethiopia by collaborating with them to develop curriculum materials specifically created to meet the learning needs of rural and urban health center team personnel (Carter Center, 2002).

International Council of Nurses

The International Council of Nurses (ICN) represents the global interests and concerns of the nursing profession. Founded in 1899, its current membership includes nursing organizations from 120 countries and 1.5 million nurses. The mission of ICN is to maintain the role of nursing in health care through its global voice (Vance, 1999).

Because nurses and midwives constitute up to 80% of the qualified work force in most national health care systems, they represent a powerful force for bringing health care to all people. Nurses' contributions to health services cover the whole spectrum of primary care, promotion, and prevention, as well as health research, program planning, implementation, and innovation (International Council of Nurses, 1999).

HEALTH FOR ALL: A PRIMARY HEALTH CARE INITIATIVE

In 1977, the World Health Assembly determined that the major social goal of governments and WHO should be the attainment for all people by the year 2000 of a level of health that would allow them to lead socially and economically productive lives. This desire for **"Health for All"** was formally expressed in the *Declaration of Alma-Ata* in 1978. This document was produced by a WHO/UNICEF conference in Alma-Ata, Kazakhstan, in the former Soviet Union, and was attended by representatives of 134 nations. The *Declaration* promoted an ecologic/social concept of health and offered political and economic guidelines for achieving primary health care for all (Carlaw, 1988). In the United States, the *Healthy People 2010* initiative is based on the WHO Health for All model, as were the previous *Healthy People* agendas. (U.S. Department of Health and Human Services, 2000).

The Health for All initiative is a comprehensive approach to serving the most needy and remote populations through partnerships between national health services system and local communities. The communities take the leading responsibility for identifying their own priority health concerns and planning and implementing their own **primary health care (PHC)** service. They receive supportive guidance from their country's central health authority, generally the Ministry of Health (Carlaw, 1988). These PHC services include prevention, health promotion, and curative and rehabilitative care provided by the people themselves (WHO, 1998e) (Display 21–5).

Functions

Article VII, Section 3 of the *Declaration of Alma-Ata* lists the eight basic functions of PHC:
- Education concerning prevailing health problems and the methods of preventing and controlling them
- Promotion of food supply and proper nutrition
- An adequate supply of safe water and basic sanitation
- Maternal and child health, including family planning
- Immunization against major infectious diseases
- Prevention and control of locally endemic diseases
- Appropriate treatment of common diseases and injuries
- Provision of essential drugs

PHC goes beyond the health sector and, to be effective, must involve all related sectors concerned with national and community development, including agriculture, animal husbandry, food, industry, education, housing, public works, and communication (Article VII, sections 3–4; found in Carlaw, 1988, p. vii).

DISPLAY 21-5

Primary Health Care

Primary health care is not more medicine for the poor. Primary health care is essentially a call for a partnership in health, based on the concepts of equity and social justice, to enable communities, both rural and urban, to take intelligent responsibility for upgrading their health environment and health status.

Raymond W. Carlaw, 1988

Delivery Systems

Community-based PHC calls for a partnership between health professionals and communities and represents a striking change in responsibility and authority. The community becomes the initiator of action; the basic unit of PHC in most developing countries is a voluntary health service created at the village level. At least two components are commonly included: a local committee and a group of community health workers (CHWs). The committee accepts responsibility for health matters. The CHW is selected from the village and is approved by the committee to serve the village people in health matters. CHWs usually give 1 to 2 hours of health service per day, for which they may or may not be compensated by the community. Studies now have demonstrated that communities served by CHWs provide more effective service in controlling communicable diseases. This has been demonstrated particularly in malaria control programs in Ethiopia (Gebreyesus et al., 2000).

The CHW is trained in the fundamentals of promoting health and preventing and treating the most common diseases. This includes basic first aid, advice and assistance on simple treatments, and health teaching on personal hygiene, safe water supplies, safe disposal of human waste and refuse, and nutrition. The village midwife receives training in obstetrics and childcare. This person provides basic antenatal, intrapartum, and postnatal care and makes referrals as required. In some countries, traditional medical practitioners receive formal training and return to their villages to continue their services with new knowledge and skills to enhance their effectiveness. (See Figure 21–1 for an illustration of the organizational pattern of community-based PHC.)

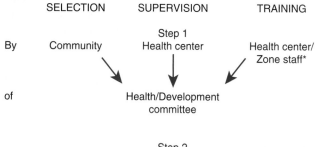

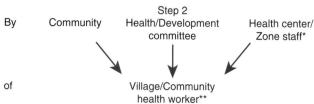

*Nurse, sanitarian, midwife, health education assistant
**Assistant midwife, traditional birth attendant, traditional practitioner

FIGURE 21-1. Community-based primary care. (Carlaw, R. [1988]. Community-based primary health care: Some factors in its development. In R.W. Carlaw & W.B. Ward [Eds.], *Primary health care: The African experience* [p. xx–xi]. Oakland, CA: Third Party Publishing Company.)

Achievements and Deterrents

PHC programs have resulted in the following significant and quantifiable improvements in the health status of people worldwide:

- The worldwide infant mortality rate decreased from 90 per 1000 live births in 1975 to 59 per 1000 in 1995—a 34% decrease.
- Immunization coverage for children younger than 1 year of age rose from 20% to 80% between 1980 and 1990.
- Access to safe drinking water in developing countries increased from 38% to 66%, and adequate sanitation from 32% to 38%, between the mid-1970s and 1990.

Some of the major deterrents to sustained effective PHC services include inadequate supervision and follow-up, failure to restock medical supplies on a regular basis, shortage of personnel, limited training, poor record keeping, and lack of cooperation on the part of health centers and nearby hospitals in receiving referrals from CHWs. Natural environmental phenomena such as rain, floods, and poor or absent communication facilities periodically isolate areas. Other problems arise when expensive drugs are dispensed in place of less expensive generic brands or are given first to family and friends of the health care workers in some cases, and when health centers fail to refer patients back to the referring CHW (see Research: Bridge to Practice).

Quality of service at the CHW level and its referral system and funding methods are critical determinants of effective PMC programs. The relation of these factors to demand for services and funding determined and provided by communities served by CHWs represents a powerful influence on productive PHC programs (Akin et al., 1985).

In acknowledgment of significant global accomplishments, there was a renewal of the strategy of Health for All by WHO members in 1994. Future action regarding PHC calls for strengthened collaboration across governmental agencies and NGOs in both the public and private sectors. Only then will the world have a realistic chance of achieving all the goals set out in the *Declaration of Alma-Ata* (Display 21–6).

GLOBAL HEALTH CONCERNS

Most of the agencies discussed in this chapter strive not only to fulfill a country's health-program priorities but also to protect the rest of the world from the spread of communicable diseases. To do so, reliable data on the global incidence and spread of communicable diseases are crucial. Such information is also critical for sound policy decisions related to the prevention of disease and injury. In any given year, only about 30% of deaths worldwide are medically certified, and until recently there were only limited standardized assessments of comparable information on morbidity, mortality, and disability in populations throughout the world. In 1992, at the request of the WB, WHO initiated a study on the global burden of disease (Murray & Lopez, 1996).

The Global Burden of Disease

The WHO's study of the **global burden of disease** (GBD) verified with quantifiable data numerous long-held assumptions about disparities in the burden of disease worldwide, especially in regard to children. Among other findings, it revealed the following (Murray & Lopez, 1997):

- Ninety-eight percent of all deaths in children younger than 15 years of age are in the developing world.
- Eighty-three percent of deaths of those aged 15 to 59 years are in the developing world.
- The probability of death before age 15 ranges from 22% in sub-Saharan Africa to only 1.1% in countries with established market economies.
- Five of the 10 leading causes of death are communicable, perinatal, and nutritional maladies that largely affect children.

Display 21–7 lists the top 10 causes of death worldwide and compares 1990 and 1998 data.

In addition to causes of mortality, the GBD study quantified the burden of disease with a measure that could be used for cost-effectiveness analysis. In order to compare across conditions and risk factors, a measure called the **disability-adjusted life year** (DALY) was developed. DALYs are the combination of years of life lost due to premature mortality and years of life lived with disability adjusted for the severity of disability. The GBD study ranked the leading causes of DALYs in 1990 and projected changes by the year 2020 (Table 21–1). Chronic disease, unipolar major depression, and accidents were expected to be the three top DALYs by that time, replacing respiratory infections, diarrheal diseases, and perinatal disorders.

Within the first 10 years of this period, changes in the rankings were evident. The three leading causes of DALYs in 2001 were acute respiratory infections, HIV/AIDS, and conditions related to the perinatal period (WHO, 2003d). The GBD study grouped diseases and injuries into three clusters: group 1 represents communicable diseases, maternal causes, conditions arising in the perinatal period, and nutritional conditions; group 2 consists of noncommunicable diseases; and group 3 lists all types of injuries (Table 21–2).

The information obtained from the GBD and its analysis guides current decisions related to investments in health, research, human resource development, and physical infrastructure. Reassessment of global and regional information on diseases and injuries is expected to occur every 3 to 5 years.

WHO researchers estimate that there will be dramatic changes in health-related needs within the next 20 years. There is evidence that noncommunicable diseases are rapidly replacing infectious diseases as the major causes of disability and premature death. Noncommunicable diseases are expected to account for 7 of every 10 deaths in developing countries, compared with fewer than 5 of every 10 today. The burden of mental illness was previously unseen. Now recognized, it accounts for almost 11% of disease burden worldwide. Unipolar major depression is expected to

RESEARCH: BRIDGE TO PRACTICE

Kirkpatrick, S.M. (2000). The Congo children's weeping sores. *Reflections on Nursing Leadership, 26*(2), 10–16, 45.

Despite an increasing number of high-technology assessments or interventions in developed countries, many villages throughout the world continue to rely on the creativity of nurses and the most basic of health care principles. This study of tropical leg ulcer treatment demonstrated one way in which village health workers can be taught by nurses to improve health in the community in an effective and economical manner.

Painful, debilitating leg ulcers are not uncommon for children in many developing countries. A group of five schoolchildren in the village of Chiba, in the Democratic Republic of Congo, requested treatment for such leg ulcers. Their request triggered a successful treatment project in 1996 that continues today.

Tropical leg ulcers primarily affect school age children and are painful and often debilitating. There is no causative organism for these ulcers; rather, they are caused by poor nutrition and lack of sanitation. Because they are more frequent in times of food scarcity, improved nutrition may not be available. Left untreated, tropical ulcers progress to open, weeping sores, 2 to 3 inches in diameter, that attract flies, eventually exposing tendons and bones. Such ulcers can remain for months or years. If healing occurs, it is often the site for future breakdown. These ulcers can lead to septicemia, osteomyelitis, or even death.

A house-to-house survey was conducted in the village to determine the underlying causes of the ulcers. Open-ended questions regarding overall health as well as the leg ulcers were included. The survey revealed an even higher incidence of ulcer than was initially projected.

Tissue biopsies were performed to diagnose the cases. If no causative organisms were found, the diagnosis of "tropical leg ulcers" was made. The design of the treatment plan included cost, availability of material, and sustainability for the project. The researcher served as a consultant to the village health workers who implemented the treatment. Pictures were designed for teaching children and mothers, and captions were translated into Swahili. Volunteers in the United States prepared bandages (made from sheets), washcloths, and bars of soap and raised money for antibiotic ointments that were subsequently sent to Africa.

Word of mouth alerted the villagers about the project. Parents and children were invited to a teaching session to learn about causes of the ulcers and intervention.

Each affected child was given supplies and an identification number. Once treatment began, a patient's response to treatment was tracked. The treatment consisted of cleaning the ulcers with a traditional tea made from guava leaves, applying antibiotic ointment to the most severe ulcers, and covering them with bandages. The traditional antiseptic solution made from guava tea has been reported to be effective in several nations, was readily available, and had no cost because villagers could make it themselves from local resources.

Mothers were taught to wash their hands and the wound with soap, apply the antiseptic solution, and cover each wound with a dressing and bandages. Each patient was given a replacement dressing for use while the other was washed and dried in the sun for "sterilization."

The sores responded rapidly to treatment. The ulcers were dubbed "uferi" after a local political party that had the same characteristics of "emerging and flourishing overnight." Many patients saw dramatic improvement in 1 week. A review of the records 6 months later revealed that volunteer health workers treated more than 600 uferi that had successfully healed. Eight failures were attributed to patients' lack of compliance.

News of the successful treatment traveled for several hundred miles and into the neighboring Zambia. Volunteer caregiver health care workers became consultants to neighboring communities. The development of self-esteem and leadership skills was a side benefit of the Uferi project. Both the treatment and the community leadership of health care workers continue today despite recent civil war and political difficulties. This is an excellent example of operationalization of the Primary Health Care model supported by the World Health Organization.

1. Do you think the results of the Uferi project would be the same if a nurse had conducted the intervention rather than the village health care worker? Why or why not?
2. How does the village health care worker fit into the Primary Health Care scheme? What were the advantages of the village health care workers in the Uferi project? Refer to Figure 21–1.
3. What factors do you think might affect a mother's compliance with the treatment of tropical leg ulcers?
4. If you were the nurse researcher, how would you go about determining indigenous, effective treatment interventions?
5. Could something like the Uferi project work in the United States?
6. Why do you think the health care workers developed increased self-esteem and leadership skills because of this project?

DISPLAY 21-6

WHO's Ten Goals Toward Health for All

- To increase the span of healthy life for all people in such a way that health disparities between social groups are reduced.
- To ensure universal access to an agreed upon set of essential health-care services of acceptable quality, comprising at least the eight essential elements of primary health care.
- To ensure survival and healthy development of children.
- To improve the health and well being of women.
- To ensure healthy population development.
- To eradicate, eliminate, or control major diseases constituting global health problems.
- To reduce avoidable disabilities through appropriate preventive and rehabilitative measures.
- To ensure continued improvements in nutritional status for all population groups.
- To enable universal access to safe and healthy environments and living conditions.
- To enable all people to adopt and maintain healthy lifestyles and health behavior.

(Lanza, R. [1996]. *One world: The health and survival of the human species in the 21st century.* Santa Fe, NM: Health Press.)

DISPLAY 21-7

Comparison of the Ten Leading Causes of Death Worldwide, 1990 and 1998

Rank/Cause of Death

1990 (Murray & Lopez, 1997)	1998 (Shannon, 2001)
Ischemic heart disease	Ischemic heart disease
Cerebrovascular disease	Cerebrovascular disease
Lower respiratory tract infection	Lower respiratory tract infection
Diarrheal diseases	HIV/AIDS
Perinatal disorders	Chronic obstructive pulmonary disease
Chronic obstructive pulmonary disease	Diarrheal disease
Tuberculosis (excluding HIV-seropositive individuals)	Perinatal conditions
	Tuberculosis
Measles	Cancer of the trachea, bronchus, and lung
Road traffic accidents	Road traffic accidents
Malaria	

TABLE 21-1

Seventeen Leading Causes of Disability-Adjusted Life Years (DALYs) in the World in 1990 and Projected to 2020

Disease or Injury	Rank: 1990	Rank: 2020
Lower respiratory tract infections	1	6
Diarrheal diseases	2	9
Conditions arising during the perinatal period	3	11
Unipolar major depression	4	2
Ischemic heart disease	5	1
Cerebrovascular disease	6	4
Tuberculosis	7	7
Measles	8	25
Road traffic accidents	9	3
Congenital anomalies	10	13
Malaria	11	24
Chronic obstructive pulmonary disease	12	5
Falls	13	19
Iron deficiency anemia	14	39
Protein-energy malnutrition	14	37
War	16	8
Self-inflicted injuries	17	14
Violence	19	12
Human immunodeficiency virus (HIV) infection	28	10
Trachea, bronchus, and lung cancers	33	15

(Murray, C.J. & Lopez, A.D. [1996]. Evidence-based health policy—Lessons from the Global Burden of Disease Study. *Science, 274,* 740–743.)

TABLE 21-2

Distribution of Death by Specific Causes in 1990

Group 1	Group 2	Group 3
Infectious and parasitic diseases	Malignant neoplasms	Unintentional injuries
Respiratory infections	Other neoplasms	Intentional injuries
Maternal disorders	Diabetes mellitus	
Perinatal disorders	Endocrine disorders	
Nutritional deficiencies	Neuropsychiatric disorders	
	Sense organ disorders	
	Cardiovascular disorders	
	Respiratory disorders	
	Digestive disorders	
	Genitourinary disorders	
	Skin disorders	
	Musculoskeletal disorders	
	Congenital anomalies	
	Oral disorders	

(Murray, C.J. & Lopez, A.D. [1996]. Evidence-based health policy—Lessons from the Global Burden of Disease Study. *Science, 274,* 740–743.)

D I S P L A Y 2 1 – 8

The Top Ten Preventable Health Risks Worldwide

Childhood and maternal underweight
Unsafe sex
High blood pressure
Tobacco
Alcohol
Unsafe water
Sanitation and hygiene
High cholesterol
Indoor smoke from solid fuels
Iron deficiency
Overweight/obesity

(World Health Organization. [2002h, October 28]. Years of life can be increased 5–10 years. *Press Release WHO/84.* Geneva. Author.)

be a leading cause of DALYS by 2020 (WHO, 2002h) (Display 21–8).

Eradication, Elimination, and Control of Communicable Diseases

A primary global health concern is communicable disease, and primary goals are **eradication, elimination, and control** of the leading communicable diseases worldwide. *Eradication* means interruption of person-to-person transmission and limitation of the reservoir of infection such that no further preventive efforts are required; it indicates a status whereby no further cases of a disease occur anywhere. At times, the term *elimination* is used when a disease has been interrupted in a defined geographic area. In 1991, WHO defined elimination as a reduction of prevalence to less than 1 case per 1 million population in a given area. In contrast, the term *control* indicates that a specific disease has ceased to be a public health threat. Control programs are aimed at reducing the incidence and prevalence of communicable and some noncommunicable conditions.

Although eradication is always the desired effect, extensive funding and much international cooperation are usually required to achieve such a goal (see What Do You Think?). The successful eradication of smallpox from the

world in 1977, as mentioned earlier, came about because of the leadership of WHO and was a tremendous accomplishment in public health. In 1967, smallpox was endemic in 31 countries, with 10 to 15 million individuals infected. Remarkably, within 10 years there were no cases in the world (Whaley & Hashim, 1995). A vital lesson of this multiregion effort was that, if global eradication programs are to be successful, interdependence is necessary (Foege, 1998). Certification of river blindness elimination has now joined the growing list of global public health accomplishments (WHO, 2002). These programs are dependent on commitment from involved governments, international bodies, NGOs, and the affected communities themselves.

Global eradication and elimination programs that are very close to being accomplished include poliomyelitis and guinea worm. Eradication programs for leprosy and measles are continuing. Additional major efforts have increased to reduce, control, and prevent malaria, tuberculosis, HIV/AIDS, diarrheal diseases, and respiratory infections.

International terrorism threatens to reintroduce smallpox through acts of bioterrorism. Smallpox vaccination is being re-established to protect health workers and the populations at risk as this edition goes to press (Connolly, 2003).

Poliomyelitis

In 1988, the World Health Assembly adopted the goal of global eradication of poliomyelitis by the end of the year 2000. At that time, there were an estimated 35,000 annual cases of polio in the world (WHO, 1999e). By 1991, the disease was eliminated from the Western hemisphere. Polio is now almost eliminated worldwide, even in densely populated and war-torn countries. This clearly illustrates the efficacy of eradication strategies. Since the inception of the Global Polio Eradication initiative, cases have fallen by 99.8% to only 483 (in 2001), and the number of polio-infected countries dropped from 125 to 10. These 10 polio-endemic countries are classified as areas of high-intensity or low-intensity transmission. India, Pakistan/Afghanistan, and Nigeria/Niger are the areas with high-intensity transmission, and together they accounted for 85% of new polio cases in 2001. All have large populations, low immunization rates, poor sanitation, and a wide distribution of the wild virus. Somalia, Sudan, Ethiopia, Angola, and Egypt are areas with low-intensity transmission; they have lower-density populations and focal areas of wild poliovirus. Global priorities for polio eradication include closing the funding gap, maintaining access and political commitment to the program, implementing the "polio endgame" strategies including laboratory containment, certificating polio eradication, and developing of a postcertification polio immunization policy. The estimated cost of eradication is $1 billion (WHO, 2002f).

Guinea Worm Disease (Dracunculiasis)

Guinea worm disease is the only additional parasitic disease that is expected to be completely eradicated soon. It is prevalent in 17 countries, 16 of which are in Africa. Cases de-

WHAT DO YOU THINK?

Imagine today's world without any international cooperation related to communicable disease knowledge or control. What would be some of the health, social, and economic consequences of such inaction?

creased from 1 million to 80,000 between 1989 and 1997, demonstrating that there is great promise for eradication.

Infection occurs when a person drinks water that contains the worm's intermediate host, a water flea that can ingest and harbor guinea worm larvae. Once in a human body, the larvae migrate through the tissue, and the mature adult worm attempts to emerge, usually from the lower leg. Farmers are the most commonly affected. Although there is no cure once the larvae are ingested, the eradication strategy includes interruption of transmission, surveillance, health education, and certification. Interruption of transmission includes measures such as protecting drinking water by keeping infected persons out of it, filtering drinking water, and chemically treating water to eliminate the intermediate host. The geographic information systems (GIS) monitor guinea worm cases. There is interagency collaboration for the Dracunculiasis Eradication Program; the estimated cost to reach the ultimate goal of eradication is $40 million (WHO, 1998a).

River Blindness (Onchocerciasis)

A landmark in public and private collaboration of thousands of people working together for the greater good was the official declaration of the elimination of river blindness at appropriate ceremonies in Ouagadougou, Burkina Faso, on December 6, 2002. The ceremony culminated a 30-year effort to eliminate this scourge as a public health threat in West Africa.

For centuries, this parasitic infection had been transmitted by the bites of black flies. Hundreds of thousands of people living near rivers had been infected, with resultant destruction of vision and significant damage to other tissues. When the program began, 10% of the infected population in high-impact areas were blind, and 30% had severe visual handicaps that caused loss of livelihood and autonomy (WHO, 2002k).

Massive aerial spraying of larvicide was undertaken to eliminate the vector, the black fly, in an area of 1.3 million square kilometers with a population of 30 million people. In 1991, the program set out to deliver ivermectin, the medication used to treat river blindness, to at least 80% of those living in endemic areas and to maintain coverage for 10 to 15 years (Miri, 1998).

With successful elimination of the disease, people began returning to fertile areas formerly left unoccupied because of the debilitating disease. The resulting economic benefits are now dramatically enhancing the well-being of the population.

Leprosy

Today, leprosy is a curable disease. In the last 2 decades of the 20th century, the prevalence rate of leprosy was reduced by 90%; today, it is found mainly in Africa, Asia, and Latin America, with 70% of the world's registered leprosy patients being in India (WHO, 2003a). All leprosy patients have had access to free effective drug treatment since 1995. The global health community has set a goal of leprosy elimination by 2005. Central to achievement of this goal is diagnosis and

treatment without stigma or isolation. Interventions require political commitment in affected countries, integration of treatment into the PHC systems, and a change in the image of leprosy so that patients will more readily present themselves for treatment (WHO, 2003b).

Measles

More than 30 million people contract measles every year, and about 1 million children subsequently die from the disease. Most of those deaths occur in sub-Saharan Africa and India (WHO, 1999g). Measles is a vaccine-preventable disease. **Integrated Management of Childhood Illness (IMCI)** is an intervention that is likely to have the greatest impact in reducing measles. This approach promotes wider immunization coverage; rapid referral of serious cases; prompt recognition of secondary conditions; improved nutrition, including breast feeding; and vitamin A supplementation (WHO, 1998c). A WHO/UNICEF Measles Mortality Reduction and Regional Elimination Strategic Plan is seeking a 50% reduction in measles mortality worldwide by 2005 and eventually hoping to eradicate the disease (WHO, 2002d).

Malaria

Fifty percent of the world's population live in malaria-endemic areas; 200 million new cases are diagnosed yearly, and 2 million deaths are reported (Kaneko, 1998). Malaria was originally targeted for eradication as far back as 1954. Although success was achieved in a certain places, malaria has not been eradicated in most of the developing world, and a number of areas have reverted to programs for control rather than eradication. High endemicity, dependence on pesticides such as DDT, resistance to multidrug therapy, lack of human and economic resources, and a tenacious vector have all contributed to this lack of worldwide success. Perhaps the major contributors to lack of success have been failure to integrate the malaria eradication effort into basic health services, inadequate efforts to exploit the effective involvement of communities, and an absence of necessary sustainable political commitment and funding.

These difficulties led the World Health Assembly to switch to a control strategy in 1993 (Trigg & Kondrachine, 1998). This strategy included the following elements (Jamison et al., 1993):

- Early case finding and treatment
- Reduction of contact with mosquitoes
- Destruction of adult mosquitoes and larvae
- Source detection
- Destruction of malaria parasites
- Community education programs

In May 1999, the World Health Assembly again launched a new initiative, the "Roll Back Malaria" (RBM) program, in partnership with the United Nations Development Program (UNDP), UNICEF, and the WB, with a goal of halving the incidence of malaria-related deaths throughout the world by 2010. The global disease burden from malaria is estimated to be greater than 300 million acute illnesses and 1 million deaths per year. Ninety percent of the world's malaria cases occur in Africa south of the Sahara. Malaria and the deaths it causes affect mainly two vulnerable groups: young children and pregnant women. The RBM initiative focuses on four major actions (WHO, 2002a):

* Prompt access to treatment
* Use of insecticide-treated bed nets
* Prevention and control of malaria in pregnant women
* Malaria epidemic and emergency response

The CDC, based in Atlanta, Georgia, continues work on developing an antimalaria vaccine with recombinant gene techniques. India and Kenya also have vaccine studies under way (WHO, 1999f).

Increased ineffectiveness of antimalaria drugs due to development of drug resistance, particularly for the parasite of the most deadly (*Plasmodium falciparum*) form of the disease, has brought attention to the need for new antimalaria medications. This problem is most acute on the Thai-Myanmar border in Southeast Asia, but it is also widespread in Africa.

The WHO Tropical Disease Research Program (TDR), the Swiss Medicines for Malaria Venture (MMV), and Shin Poong Pharmaceuticals, Co. Ltd. in Seoul, Korea, have collaborated in developing and producing a new combination antimalaria medicine, pyronaridine-artesunate, which is proving effective and affordable. One component of this medicine is a natural plant, *Artemesia annua,* whose antimalarial properties the Chinese first discovered centuries ago (WHO, 2002j).

Illustrating the spillover effect of disease from an endemic country to a nonendemic country are statistics on malaria in the United Kingdom. Of the estimated 2000 annual reported cases in a 10-year period, researchers found that 46% of the infected people had traveled to West or Central Africa on oil-related business (Nathwani & Spiteri, 1997).

Human Immunodeficiency Virus Infection and Acquired Immunodeficiency Syndrome

An estimated 42 million people worldwide are living with HIV/AIDS. Almost 95% of these people live in developing or transitional countries where health care, resources, and drugs are scarce (WHO/Food and Agriculture Organization, 2003). Asia and Eastern Europe are now poised for explosive increases in HIV/AIDS cases. Russia reported a 15-fold increase in just 3 years, and HIV is beginning to spread among high-risk populations in some Middle Eastern countries (WHO, 2001c). The pandemic could claim an additional 68 million lives by 2020, 55 million of them in Africa (Fleshman, 2002). It is predicted that life expectancy in those countries is likely to decline by as much as 27%. The disease attacks young adults in productive age groups, requiring older people to care for and support their terminally ill adult children and, later, the orphaned grandchildren. Often these elders are themselves impoverished and in poor health. Ultimately, the elders are left without caregivers when they

require assistance in their later years. The HIV/AIDS epidemic threatens to upset and destabilize entire societies in Africa. Reduced productivity of adult workers and early death are counterproductive to economic and social development (WHO, 2002l). However, there is some hope.

Recently, an expanded global response to the pandemic offered 12 essential interventions to reduce HIV transmission: mass media campaigns; public sector condom promotion and distribution; condom social marketing; voluntary counseling and testing programs; prevention of mother-to-child transmission; school-based programs; programs for out-of-school youth; workplace programs; treatment of sexually transmitted infections; peer counseling for sex workers; outreach to men who have sex with men; and harm reduction programs for injection drug users. It is estimated that if these interventions are enacted by 2005, 29 million new HIV infections among adults could be prevented by 2010. The estimated cost for the large-scale prevention program is $27 billion (WHO, 2002c).

There is also hope regarding treatment. In 2002, the International AIDS Society launched new international guidelines to treat AIDS in resource-poor areas. Simplified and now less expensive antiretroviral therapy has the potential to reach 3 million individuals by 2005. This breakthrough is expected to extend life expectancy and productivity of those persons living with AIDS (WHO, 2002b).

Tuberculosis

There is currently a worldwide tuberculosis (TB) epidemic:

* Someone in the world is newly infected with TB every second.
* More than 8 million people around the world become sick with TB each year.
* Almost 2 million TB cases per year occur in sub-Saharan Africa.
* Almost 3 million TB cases per year occur in Southeast Asia.
* More than a quarter-million TB cases per year occur in Eastern Europe.
* TB kills approximately 2 million people each year.
* TB accounts for more than one quarter of all preventable adult deaths in developing countries.
* Almost 1% of the world's population is infected with TB each year.
* Overall, one third of the world's population is infected with the TB bacillus.
* Between 5% and 10% of people who are infected with TB (but who are not infected with HIV) become sick or infectious at some time during life.

Each year the annual number of deaths from TB increases. HIV and TB form a lethal combination, each speeding the other's progress. TB is the leading cause of death among people who are HIV positive. Poorly managed TB programs are threatening to make TB incurable, and the movements of people through travel and relocation are helping spread the disease. In the United States, almost 40% of TB cases are among foreign-born people (WHO, 2002e). For a more detailed discussion of TB, see Chapter 9.

Diarrheal Diseases

The incidence of diarrheal diseases is somewhat elusive because it depends on the definition of diarrhea used, the frequency of surveillance, and the population. Recent studies have defined diarrhea as the passage of more than three stools during a 24-hour period for individuals older than 3 months of age. Sometimes public health professionals use the term *diarrhea* to mean dysentery, although the latter is usually characterized by the presence of blood in the stool with or without looseness or specified frequency. Among other causes, a host of enteric pathogens can result in diarrhea; these pathogens are most significant in developing countries. Poverty, poor personal and domestic hygiene, infected water, low maternal education, and lower occupational status have been associated with diarrheal morbidity and mortality (Martines et al., 1993). In the year 2000, an estimated 1.3 million children younger than 5 years of age in developing countries died from diarrheal diseases caused by unsafe water supply, lack of sanitation, and poor hygiene (WHO, 2002). The reduction of mortality was largely a result of the promotion of oral rehydration therapy, a simple treatment administered by mother to child that replaces fluid and electrolytes (Display 21–9). WHO recommendations for prevention of diarrheal disease include the promotion of personal and domestic hygiene, improvement of water supply and sanitation facilities, promotion of breast feeding, improvement in weaning practices, cholera immunization, and measles immunization (WHO, 2001a; 2002).

Acute Respiratory Tract Infections

The most common illness in the world, and a leading cause of mortality in the developing world, is acute respiratory tract infection (ARI). Three million deaths annually are attributed to ARI among children younger than 5 years of age, usually from pneumonia. Global commitment to reduction of ARI was realized by a resolution at the World Summit for Children in 1990 that called for a one-third reduction in deaths from ARI. This goal has been difficult to achieve because of the varying clinical symptoms and causative organisms of pneumonia. Risk factors include low birth weight, poverty, crowding, lower educational levels, poor nutrition, inadequate childcare practices, and a lack of health education about ARI. Additional risk factors include smoking and indoor and outdoor air pollution. Indoor air pollution is 20 times higher in villages in developing countries than in homes in the developed world where two packs of cigarettes are smoked per day (Stansfield & Shepard, 1993; WHO, 2002). The source is largely indoor cookstoves that use organic fuel. Immunizations, birth spacing, and improvement in nutrition and living conditions (including use of smokeless cooking stoves) will all assist in better control of ARI. A threat to the reduction of pneumonia, however, is the increase in drug-resistant organisms (see Levels of Prevention.)

Other Global Health Concerns

Immunization

Encouraged by the successful smallpox vaccination program and subsequent eradication of the disease, WHO and other partners launched the Expanded Program of Immunization in 1974 (Reingold & Phares, 2001). At that time, fewer than 5% of infants in the developing countries were fully immunized. Vaccines are one of the most cost-effective interventions found in public health. Today, almost three fourths of the children in the world are being reached with essential vaccines, but many barriers make it difficult to maintain high levels of immunization in low- and middle-income countries. In sub-Saharan Africa, for example, only one half of the children have access to basic immunization against common diseases (WHO, 2002i). WHO estimates that 3 million more lives could be saved with immunizations. Recognition of the barriers such as limited finances, lack of trained health care workers, physical obstacles to reaching remote areas, and civil wars, has prompted the development of an interagency vaccine initiative called the Global Alliance for Vaccine and Immunizations. This initiative seeks to protect every child against vaccine-preventable diseases (Reingold & Phares, 2001). Strategies include funding, research, development, distribution of vaccines, and program sustainability. It is anticipated that the use of such approaches will not only result in more immunized children but also move newer vaccines into developing countries more quickly.

Maternal and Perinatal Morbidity and Mortality

WHO estimates that 500,000 women die yearly from complications of pregnancy and childbirth. Ninety-nine percent of these deaths are in the developing world. Women living in parts of Africa face a 1-in-16 risk of death because they do not

---

DISPLAY 21–9

How to Prepare Homemade Oral Rehydration Solution (ORS)

If ORS sachets are available: dilute one sachet in 1 L of safe water.
Otherwise, use 1 L of safe water and add
  Salt—1/2 small teaspoon (3.5 g)
  Sugar—4 big spoons (40 g)
In addition, try to compensate for loss of potassium (eg, eat bananas or drink green coconut water).

(World Health Organization. [2003]. First steps for managing an outbreak of acute diarrhea. WHO Global Task Force on Cholera. Global health security: Epidemic alert and response, Box 2. Geneva: WHO.)

LEVELS OF PREVENTION MATRIX

SITUATION: Prevent acute respiratory tract infections (ARIs) in children in developing countries.

GOAL: Using the three levels of prevention negative health conditions are avoided, or promptly diagnosed and treated, and the fullest possible potential is restored.

PRIMARY PREVENTION		SECONDARY PREVENTION		TERTIARY PREVENTION		
Health Promotion and Education	*Health Protection*	*Early Diagnosis*	*Prompt Treatment*	*Rehabilitation*	*Primary Prevention*	
					Health Promotion and Education	*Health Protection*
• Promote general health education among community members • Good prenatal care • Advocacy of breast feeding, child spacing, and adequate nutrition • Teaching good hygiene and child care practices • Teach when to seek medical attention • Eliminate poverty and household crowding	• Administer appropriate immunizations • Eliminate indoor contaminants such as smoke from cookstoves without chimneys and cigarette, cigar, or pipe smoking • Ventilate rooms to eliminate indoor smoke and allow fresh air in	• Get a prompt diagnosis of an acute ARI	• Collaborate with families to combine the best of folk and home remedies with established Western medical practices • Treat early with antibiotics (if indicated and available) • Provide culturally appropriate symptomatic care • Teach caregiver signs and symptoms of complications	• Restore child to optimal level of functioning through the recovery period	• Continue to promote educational programs and individual teaching regarding practices that promote health and prevent diseases among family members	• Educate on the prevention of recurrence and spread of disease

receive needed prenatal care. In Europe and North America, the risk is 1 in 4000 (WHO, 1999g). The death of a mother profoundly affects the well-being of the entire family.

Early pregnancy, high fertility, and close child spacing are frequent in developing countries and are known to be major determinants of poor health for mothers and children. Poverty, illiteracy, poor nutrition, low weight gain, maternal age (younger than 20 or older than 34 years of age), infections, smoke in the home, smoking, and poor health care are some of the major determinants associated with high health risks to mothers and children in the poorest nations of the world.

Prevention strategies include better general health for women through poverty alleviation, education, guidance in family planning, prenatal care including food supplementation, immunization, local and regional care with referrals for complications, training of traditional birth attendants, and effective postpartum care (Walsh et al., 1993; WHO, 2001b).

Tobacco-Related Morbidity and Mortality

Tobacco is expected to develop into the single largest killer and to cause the greatest burden of disease in the 21st century, with deaths increasing from 4.9 million to 10 million per year by the late 2020s (WHO, 2002g). WHO has predicted that tobacco will be the leading cause of disease burden in the world by the year 2030, causing about one in eight deaths, with 70% of them in developing countries (WHO, 1999a). With a decline of tobacco use in Western countries, the tobacco industry has aggressively marketed in low- and middle-income countries (Kickbusch and Buse, 2001). As a result, the prevalence of smoking among adult men is high and troublesome. For example, more than 50% of men in Bangladesh, China, Japan, Korea, Russia, Indonesia, and Vietnam smoke tobacco (McQueen et al., 2001).

The Tobacco Free Initiative, launched by WHO in July 1998, began implementation of the WHO General Assembly's resolution to prevent and control the global spread of tobacco use in the 21st century. In early 2003, some 4 years later, 171 member states completed a groundbreaking public health treaty to control tobacco supply and consumption (WHO, 2003c). The treaty requires signatory parties to implement comprehensive tobacco control programs and strategies. Some of its central control components are tobacco taxation and pricing, health warning labels, restriction of advertising and promotion, holding the tobacco industry liable for tobacco-related costs, financial support for national tobacco control programs, and funding for treatment programs. This proposed legally binding treaty will be presented to the next World Health Assembly for adoption and can be put into effect after ratification. This international effort represents an important step in global public health and is expected to reduce the impact of tobacco use in the decades to come.

Chronic Disease

Despite the programs of control, many infectious diseases continue in the world. Compounding that challenge is the more recent emergence of chronic diseases in the developing world. For countries in development, an interesting transition occurs. As infectious diseases decrease, life expectancy lengthens and the population experiences the degenerative diseases that are seen in developed countries. The concept of epidemiologic transition explains the replacement of infectious disease morbidity and mortality with that of **chronic disease**. This phenomenon is occurring in many countries today. It requires a change in the response of the health care system in terms of provision of care, planning, and allocation of resources. Addressing these concerns is considered a cost-effective investment in a nation's human capital (McQueen et al., 2001).

Environmental Illness

In addition to disease and injury, the environment that people live in is also one of today's major health concerns. Air, climate, soil, and water all affect health, and environmental hazards are found throughout the world. There is a growing awareness of the effects of environmental pollution on human health. These factors include

- Environmental health risks from structural changes in developing country economics (shifts from rural to urban, mode of transportation, international trade)
- Role of socioeconomic status
- Impacts of major developments (dams, mines, waterways)
- Risks and benefits to producers and consumers from agricultural chemical use
- Impact of local climate changes on weather patterns and agriculture

The Blumenthal classification (Whaley & Hashim, 1995) lists classes of environmental hazards. They include

- Infectious agents (eg, bacteria and viruses)
- Respiratory fibrotic agents (eg, coal dust)
- Asphyxiates (eg, carbon monoxide)
- Poison (eg, pesticides)
- Physical agents (eg, noise)

- Psychological agents (stressful synergisms such as crowding combined with noise)
- Mutagens (eg, dioxin)
- Teratogens (eg, cadmium)
- Carcinogens (eg, cigarette smoke)

Humans are exposed to pollutants in two basic ways: by exposure to the source or by release of the pollutant into air or water. In places such as Peru, Egypt, and Thailand, raw sewage is directly released into rivers that are used for drinking and bathing. Such practices often result in diarrheal diseases, including cholera. In 1991 a cholera outbreak was identified at the port of Chancoy in Peru; it rapidly spread along the coast, over the Andes, and into the Amazon basin, resulting in 400,000 reported cases and 4000 reported deaths in 13 countries (Whaley & Hashim, 1995).

Annually, more than 5 million people die from illnesses linked to unsafe drinking water, poor household hygiene, and improper human and animal waste disposal. Every 8 seconds, a child dies of a water-related disease. One half of the population in the developing world suffers from one or more of the five main diseases associated with water and sanitation—diarrhea, ascariasis, hookworm, schistosomiasis, and trachoma—and one-fourth of the world's population is without proper access to water and sanitation (WHO, 1996).

Water-related diseases arise from the ingestion of pathogens in contaminated water or food and from insects or other water-associated vectors. Improvement of water and sanitation is estimated to reduce morbidity and mortality rates by 20% to 80% (WHO, 1996). No single type of intervention has greater overall impact on national development and public health than does the provision of safe drinking water and proper disposal of human excreta. However, overall progress in reaching people unserved by adequate water and sanitation services has been poor since 1990 (Display 21–10).

Another worldwide concern is the depletion of the ozone layer. Reduction of the ozone layer could result in increasing cataract and cancer rates (especially melanoma and basal cell

DISPLAY 21–10

Environmental Hazards that Kill Children

1. Inadequate drinking water and sanitation
2. Indoor air pollution and accidents
3. Injuries and poisonings

These are just three of the causes of the approximately 3 million deaths suffered annually by children younger than 5 years of age as a result of environmental hazards. Research suggests that more than 40% of the global burden of disease due to environmental risk factors may fall on such young children, who constitute only about 10% of the world's population.

(World Health Organization [2002, March 3]. Environmental hazards kill at least 3 million children aged under 5 every year. *Press Release WHO/12*. Geneva: WHO.)

carcinoma). It is believed that human activities are contributing to depletion of the ozone layer; these activities include the use of chlorofluorocarbons (CFCs; used in the manufacture of air conditioners, refrigerators, and aerosol propellants, and other products) and methyl bromides (found in pesticides and herbicides). Efforts are under way to phase out CFCs in 13 countries, including the United States.

New and Emerging Diseases

Most of the diseases discussed thus far have been present for many years, some for thousands of years. Twenty-five years ago, public health specialists believed that infectious diseases would soon play a minor role in health. However, they are still the world's leading cause of death, and some of the newly identified infectious agents have developed into public health problems on a local, regional, or global scale (WHO, 1998b).

Contributing factors in infectious disease mortality include a host of **new and emerging diseases** and resurgence of some that were previously thought to be under control. Since 1973, a number of previously unknown diseases have emerged, among them are HIV/AIDS, Ebola hemorrhagic fever, Lassa fever, Hantavirus, Lyme disease, Legionnaires'

disease, and toxic shock syndrome (Table 21–3). Most recently, severe acute respiratory syndrome (SARS), an atypical pneumonia thought to be caused by a coronavirus, has been recognized (WHO, 2003e). SARS has been reported to have a mortality rate of up to 15%, and up to 50% for seniors and infants.

The development of antimicrobial-resistant organisms, mainly as a result of the overuse and misuse of antibiotics, has fueled a resurgence of some diseases that were under control, such as TB. Anti-TB medications are no longer effective in up to 20% of patients in some parts of the world. Two leading antimalaria medicines have become ineffective in many Asian countries, and a third is effective in only half of the world. The easy availability of global air travel and subsequent rapid transmission of microbes poses real health threats.

Another cause of new and emerging diseases is urbanization, which serves to concentrate large numbers of people in small geographic areas. Deforestation may permit the movement of microbes into human populations, and humans who move into the cleared forests may encounter previously unknown pathogens. Changes in agricultural practices, such as new dams and irrigation schemes, also present potential trans-

T A B L E   21–3

Examples of Emerging Pathogens Identified Since 1973

Year	Microbe	Disease
1973	Rotavirus	Major cause of infantile diarrhea globally
1976	*Cryptosporidium parvum*	*Acute and chronic diarrhea*
1977	Ebola virus	Ebola hemorrhagic fever
1977	*Legionella pneumophilia*	*Legionnaires' disease*
1977	Hantaan virus	Hemorrhagic fever with renal syndrome
1977	*Campylobacter jejuni*	*Enteric diseases distributed globally*
1980	Human T-lymphotropic virus 1 (HTLV-1)	T-cell lymphoma-leukemia
1981	Toxin producing strains of *Staphylococcus aureus*	*Toxic shock syndrome*
1982	*Escherichia coli 0157:H7*	*Hemorrhagic colitis; hemolytic uremic syndrome*
1982	HTLV-II	Hairy cell leukemia
1982	*Borrelia burgdorfei*	*Lyme disease*
1983	HIV	AIDS
1983	*Helicobacter pylori*	*Peptic ulcer disease*
1988	Hepatitis E	Enterically transmitted non-A, non-B hepatitis
1990	Guanarito virus	Venezuelan hemorrhagic fever
1991	*Encephalitozzon hellem*	*Conjunctivitis, disseminated disease*
1992	*Vibrio cholerae 0139*	*New strain associated with epidemic cholera*
1992	*Bartonella henselae*	*Cat-scratch disease; bacillary angiomatosis*
1994	Sabia virus	Brazilian hemorrhagic fever
1995	Hepatitis G virus	Parenterally transmitted non-A, non-B hepatitis
1995	Human herpesvirus-8	Associated with Kaposi sarcoma in AIDS patients
1996	TSE-causing agent	New variant Creutzfeldt-Jakob disease
1997	Avian influenza (Type A [H5N1])	Influenza
1999	Nipah virus	Influenza-like symptoms, high fever, myalgia; may progress to encephalitis, convulsions, coma; 50% mortality rate
2002	SARS	Severe acute respiratory syndrome

(World Health Organization. [1998d]. Examples of pathogens recognized since 1973. *WHO Fact Sheet No. 97, 4.* Geneva: WHO; World Health Organization. [2001]. Nipah virus. WHO Fact Sheet, 262, 1–2. Geneva: WHO; World Health Organization [2003, 12 March]. WHO issues a global alert about cases of atypical pneumonia. *Press Release WHO/22.* Geneva: WHO.)

mission scenarios (Shannon, 2001). The ability of microbes to change and adapt rapidly is a persistent threat as well.

Armed Conflicts and Political Upheavals

Armed conflicts and political upheavals strongly influence both health status and health care needs of a country. They are extremely complex social phenomena, for which the most rooted causes are inequity, cultural and religious intolerance, and ethnic discrimination (Mulli, 1996). Between the end of World War II and the end of the Cold War, most conflicts occurred in developing countries in Africa, the Middle East, Asia, and Latin America. After the breakup of the Soviet Union, major conflicts occurred in the resulting countries and in Europe. Conflicts in other areas of the world also were reignited (eg, between Eritrea and Ethiopia), and Indonesia experienced unrest and violence after decades of relative stability. Most conflicts occur between states with the goal being economic and political power, but approximately 90% of those affected by such conflicts are civilians of all ages (Toole et al., 2001).

In 1999, the Carter Center reported 30 major armed conflicts in the world. (D. Congelio, personal communication, September 9, 1999). An armed conflict is defined as major if the number of deaths has reached 1000. Typically, armed conflicts and upheavals cause governments and agencies to place a high priority on health care initially, but their ability to sustain health care is reduced as time goes on. The health infrastructure becomes vulnerable because of the instability. Often, opposing factions raid hospitals and clinics. Health services become disorganized and experience decreased resources. Epidemics are almost inevitable. As conflict goes on, the medical needs of the combatants often take priority over those of civilians, which may leave thousands of children injured, orphaned, and at risk for disease. Additionally, conflict disrupts food cultivation, harvest, and distribution, leaving populations at risk for malnutrition and setting the stage for disease. Refugees from such events have special health and social needs. Often refugee camps are developed by international organizations on the fringe of such conflicts to temporarily assist refugees with shelter, food, and the rudiments of health care. Such camps place a strain on the resources of neighboring countries. All of these factors can lead to complex humanitarian emergencies. The CDC described complex humanitarian emergencies as "situations affecting large civilian populations which usually involve a combination of factors including war or civil strife, food shortages, and population displacement, resulting in significant excess mortality" (Burkholder & Toole, 1995).

Increasingly, conflicts are internal rather than between states. In their quest for economic and political power, the combatants target the lives and livelihoods of civilians associated with opposing factions. Recovery after conflict is a long-term project. Any postconflict recovery effort must deal with the disabled, the mentally ill, prisoners, widows, orphans, abandoned children, homeless and displaced persons, refugees, and the unemployed (Mulli, 1996). Additionally, land mines continue to injure or kill long after hostilities have ceased.

Human Development and Health

The relationship between development and health has been mentioned in previous sections. Development, in the broad sense, usually means investment by a country with the intent to improve its per capita income or gross national product. An improved economy is expected to result in better diets, better housing, social change, and a reduction in infectious diseases. Development can mean increased labor productivity, satisfaction of basic human needs, and modernization, including education and social and infrastructure changes. It can mean improving the status of women or other social groups. The United Nations Development Program (UNDP) is under the mandate of the United Nations Charter and is committed to the ideal that development is inseparable from the quest for peace and human security. The mission of UNDP is to assist countries in their own efforts to obtain sustainable human development by helping build their capacity to design and carry out development programs. It has long been thought that there is a reciprocal relationship between development and health. A healthy population is predisposed to economic development, whereas an unhealthy population is often characterized by poverty and underdevelopment (Phillips, 1990). This is the foundation on which the WB is based and is the principal reason that money is loaned to developing nations for development work. WHO also was founded on the concept that health was a necessary ingredient for socioeconomic development and peace.

THE ROLE OF NURSES IN GLOBAL HEALTH

The role of nurses in global health is multifaceted. Nurses can be involved in many of the organizations that have been mentioned in this chapter, through either volunteer or paid employment. **Global nursing** encompasses the full spectrum from nurse policy maker in an international organization to point-of-service delivery as an instructor of a village health worker or at one of the levels of PHC. To find out more about specific opportunities, the nurse should contact the organization of interest (see the listing of selected organizations at the end of the chapter). Some of the larger organizations, such as WHO, require graduate education and at least 5 years of experience, but many organizations do not. Nurses can participate in numerous smaller organizations that are involved in health programs. Among such groups seeking nurses are the U. S. Peace Corps, religious and lay organizations, private and governmental agencies, societies, and foundations. Health Volunteers Overseas (HVO) is an example of a private, nonprofit organization that seeks to improve health care quality and access in developing countries through education. Twelve professional organizations sponsor HVO, including the American Association of Colleges of Nursing (Health Volunteers Overseas, 2003). The GHC provides information on career opportunities in global health for community health nurses and others. It also offers career seminars and has noted some suggestions made by global health experts for nurses interested in entering the field (Global Health Council, 1999b):

- Be willing to accept unpaid work (internships/volunteer assignments) in return for valuable experience.
- Work on project administration/project management or participate in analytical work.
- Talk with others who have worked overseas.
- Volunteer at local nongovernmental offices or private organizations as a means of demonstrating your commitment to social action programs.
- Become involved with many cross-cultural opportunities in the United States.
- Get on mailing lists of projects and organizations that interest you.
- Organize informational interviews with people in your area of interest to establish a connection.
- Take a few risks.

University student nurses can also contact their campus Office of Global Affairs for opportunities available overseas (see Voices from the Community).

On a global basis, there are more community health nurses than any other professional group providing health services to people everywhere. They also are involved with and provide a wider range of services in multiple settings than any other health care professionals provide. They are responsible for health and medical services, teaching, and research in medical centers, health clinics, schools, workplaces, and other community settings ranging from the most remote areas of the least-developed countries to the most sophisticated of the world's renowned centers of excellence. In the most needy places in the world, nurses are the primary providers of preventive and curative services. This work includes providing training, guidance, and professional supervision to traditional midwives and practitioners. No other group is as involved in working with mothers, who are the most influential persons in all societies for development of health knowledge, beliefs, attitudes, and lifelong practices.

Former President Jimmy Carter and his wife, Roselyn, have been awarded the highest civilian honor in recognition of their worldwide work for peace and health through the Carter Center. Carter's comments encapsulate what global nursing is like when he describes such work as "satisfying, a joy, a pleasure, a challenge, and an adventure." Global nursing can be all of those things (see The Global Community).

VOICES FROM THE COMMUNITY

You cannot build a strong country on the backs of sick people.
> Dr. Mohammad Akhter, Executive Director, American Public Health Association

Nurses and midwives play a crucial and cost-effective role in reducing excess mortality, morbidity, and disability and in promotion of healthy lifestyles.
> Dr. Gro Harlem Brundtland, Director-General, World Health Organization

Global health nurses always receive far more than they give.
> Cydne, former Peace Corps nurse

The developing world may be poor materially, but it is rich in hope and spirit.
> Edith, missionary nurse

Nurses working in foreign lands make a big difference through their training and support of local nurses and others. Their professional dedication to quality health care and promotion of healthful living among their patients, families, and communities serves as an effective role model and has a profound impact on the well-being of the people they work with.
> Tom, physician

Living overseas for many years was a challenging and rewarding experience. Raising a family was not always easy, but our six children, now adults, value the exposure they had to other cultures and the many interesting friendships they made.
> Inez, spouse of a global health administrator

Nurses play an important role ministering to the health care needs of not only the indigenous population, but also the sometimes-sizable population of expatriates and their families.
> Jennifer, teacher

There is nothing so powerful as seeing a community that has changed through individuals taking responsibility for themselves and their own community.
> Lydia, volunteer PHN with Medical Ambassadors

SUMMARY

Our world is a complex one of interdependent nations. Health is an important part of that interdependency. What occurs in one country can have a profound health effect on other parts of the world, sometimes within less than 24 hours. Community health nurses often gravitate toward global practice because of their interest in the world as a larger community, the relationship of health in one part of the world to that in other parts, and a sense of justice for disenfranchised populations. Community health nurses make important contributions to international health.

THE GLOBAL COMMUNITY

Susan Purdin, RN, MPH, was the 1999 recipient of the Best Practices in Global Health Award from the Global Health Council. She has worked in the field of global health for 10 years and has worked in more than a dozen countries. Susan is currently with the Reproductive Health for Refugees Consortium as the global technical advisor and is based in Nigeria. Her insight in global health work is valuable for nurses who are interested in the field and is summarized below.

A lifelong interest in health led her to nursing and to study for an MPH degree. She found that a career in global health could combine her interests in nursing and travel. She finds wonder in the similarities and differences among people in the world and a great joy in learning from the accomplishments of health workers in each location as they tackle human problems with innovations born of good intentions coupled with hard work.

Susan finds that international health workers transfer effective measures to prevent and control illness from one location to another in a very practical way. They expose the local population to other caring people from other cultures, which brings insight to the universality of humanity in a world where often only differences are recognized. Any detrimental effects of international workers tend to be a matter of process more than content. Practices that disregard local cultural sensitivity in either professional or private arenas can cause new problems and rarely solve the ones they had targeted.

"International volunteering is great. There is plenty of work to be done, too little money, and a lot of learning available. The volunteer has to have a sensitive, almost self-effacing, approach. We always learn more than we teach."

Her advice to BSN graduates interested in the field:
- Learn a second language.
- Work with people from a culture other than your own, for example, in a local clinic serving an immigrant population.
- Work in a setting with low-income people.
- Live in an unfamiliar (foreign) situation for at least a year.
- Get overseas experience—Peace Corps or other.
- Be willing to work for low pay.
- Understand that the way something is done in the U.S. is not the only right way to do things.
- Be willing to volunteer for a few months to demonstrate your ability to be effective in the field—an "audition" before being hired.
- Clarify your expectations with the employer, and be sure you understand theirs.
- Consider an MPH with an international emphasis after a couple of years of work experience.

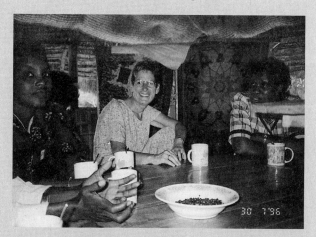

Susan Purdin in Nyagatare, Rwanda.

The world's communities deliver health care in different ways depending on their political economies. The entrepreneurial, welfare-oriented, comprehensive, and socialist systems provide for the health of their citizens in unique ways. Variations of these systems exist, depending on whether the country is considered industrialized, transitional, or very poor. Many global health agencies assist less-developed nations with areas of health. Some of these agencies are intergovernmental and multilateral, such as the United Nations and WHO; others are bilateral, such as the USAID and the Peace Corps. Many NGOs (or PVOs) also assist with global health. Each of these agencies plays a role in keeping the world healthy. WHO's "Health for All" movement, which utilizes PHC, has made a difference in many poor and remote populations.

The GBD study provided important quantifiable information about morbidity and mortality in the world, as well as disability measurements. Primary global health concerns include the eradication, elimination, or control of communicable disease, as well as immunization, maternal and perinatal morbidity and mortality, tobacco-related diseases, chronic disease, environmental illness, and malnutrition. In addition to these age-old health problems, there are new, emerging, and re-emerging diseases. Armed conflicts and political upheavals also adversely affect health; this is an important consideration because of the number of major armed conflicts occurring at any given time. There is important synergy between development and health: healthy populations promote economic development. Community health nurses are well represented in the global health arena. They provide important primary, secondary, and tertiary levels of care and prevention throughout the world. In the future, nurses will continue to be an important factor in the health of our interdependent nations.

ACTIVITIES TO PROMOTE CRITICAL THINKING

1. Go to the Internet and compare the three leading causes of mortality in the United States and several countries in sub-Saharan Africa, Asia, and the former Soviet Union. What do you think contributes to the differences?
2. Repeat the exercise, but examine the three leading causes of morbidity in each country. What do you think contributes to the differences?
3. Determine what kind of health care service each of these countries has. What relation do you think the health care system of each country has to its mortality and morbidity statistics?
4. Develop a plan to eradicate measles in the world.
5. What do you think the future holds for the "Health for All" movement?
6. Collect newspaper articles on issues of global health during the semester. What role does politics play in these health issues?

REFERENCES

Akin, J.S., Griffin, C.C., & Popkin, B.M. (1985). *The demand for primary health care services in the Third World* (pp. 165–177). Totowa, NJ: Rowan & Allanheld.

American International Health Alliance. (2002). About AIHA. Retrieved April 7, 2004, from *http://www.aiha.com/printversion.jsp?+=1081436351174*

Burkholder, H.H., & Toole, M.J. (1995). Evolution of complex disease. *Lancet, 346,* 1012–1015.

CARE. (2002). About CARE. Retrieved December 29, 2003, from *http://www.CARE.ORG/about/history.html*

Carlaw, R. (1988). Community-based primary health care: Some factors in its development. In R.W. Carlaw & W.B. Ward (Eds.), *Primary health care: The African experience* (p. iii). Oakland, CA: Third Party Publishing.

Carter Center. (2002). Health programs. Retrieved December 29, 2003, from *http://www.cartercenter.org/healthprograms/*

Center for International Health and Cooperation. (2002). About CIHC: The Center for International Health and Cooperation. New York: Author.

Centers for Disease Control and Prevention. (2000). Division of Vector-borne Infectious Diseases: West Nile virus. Retrieved February 24, 2000, from *http://www.cdc.gov/ncidod/dvbidarbpr/West_Nile_QA.htm*

Centers for Disease Control and Prevention. (2002a). Surveillance and control of the West Nile virus. Retrieved April 7, 2004, from *http//:www.CDC.gov/ncidoddvbid/westnile/conf/pdf/Campbell_surv_4th03.pdf*

Centers for Disease Control and Prevention. (2002b). Bovine spongiform encephalopathy and new variant Creutzfeld-Jakob disease. Retrieved December 29, 2003, from *http://www.cdc.gov/ncidod/diseases/cjd/bse_cjd.htm*

Connolly, C. (2003, March 16). Smallpox vaccine comes full circle: A trusty immunization is called out of retirement to face a new threat. *Washington Post*, p. A28.

Fleshman, M. (2002, September). A grim prognosis for AIDS in Africa. *Africa Recovery, 16*, 7–8.

Foege, W.H. (1998). Smallpox eradication in west and central Africa revisited. *Bulletin of the World Health Organization, 76*(3), 233–235.

Gebreyesus, A.M., Witten, K.H., Getachew, A., Yohannes, A.M., Tesfay, W., Minass, M., et al. (2000). The community-based malaria control programme in Tigray, Northern Ethiopia: A review of programme set-up, activities, outcomes, and impact. *Parassitologia, 42*(3–4), 255–290.

Global Health Council. (1999a). Speech delivered by Dr. Gro Harlem Brundtland, Director General, World Health Organization. Washington, DC: Global Health Council. Retrieved April 7, 2004, from *http://www.who.int/director-general/speechs/1999/english/19990621_arlington.html*

Global Health Council. (1999b). The Global Health Council, May 1, 1999. Retrieved April 7, 2004, from *http://www.globalhealth.org/view_top.php3?id+25*

Grad, F.P. (2002). Public health classics: The preamble of the constitution of the World Health Organization. *Bulletin of the World Health Organization, 80*(12), 981–984.

Health Volunteer Overseas. (2002). *Volunteering with HVO* [Brochure]. Washington, D.C.: Author.

International Council of Nurses. (1999). *Nursing N Line*. Retrieved December 29, 2003, from *http://www.icn.ch*

Jamison, D.T., Mosley, W.H., Measham, A.R., & Bobadilla, J.L. (Eds.). (1993). *Disease control priorities in developing countries*. New York: Oxford University Press.

Kaneko, A. (1998). Malaria on the global agenda: Control and chemotherapy of malaria in Vanuatu. *Rinsho Yori, 46*(7), 637–644.

Kickbusch, I., & Buse, K. (2001). Global influences and global responses: International health at the turn of the twenty-first century. In M.H. Merson, R.E. Black & A.J. Mills (Eds.), *International public health diseases, program, system, and policies* (pp. 710–711). Gaithersburg, MD: Aspen.

Kirkpatrick, S.M. (2000). The Congo children's weeping sores. *Reflections on Nursing Leadership, 26,* 10–16, 45.

Kloos, H. (1994). The poorer third world: Health and health care in areas that have yet to experience substantial development. In D.R. Phillips & Y. Verhasselt (Eds.), *Health and development* (pp. 199–215). New York: Routledge.

Lanza, R. (1996). *One world: The health and survival of the human species in the 21st century*. Santa Fe, NM: Health Press.

Martines, J., Phillips, M., & Feachem, R.G. (1993). Diarrheal diseases. In D.T. Jamison, W.H. Mosley, A.R. Measham & J.L. Bobdilla (Eds.), *Diseases control priorities in developing countries* (pp. 91–116). New York: Oxford University Press.

McQueen, D.V., McKenna, M.T., & Sleet, D.A. (2001). Chronic diseases and injury. In M.H. Merson, R.E. Black & A.J. Mills (Eds.), *International public health diseases, program, system, and policies* (p. 293). Gaithersburg, MD: Aspen.

Miri, E.S. (1998). Problems and perspectives of managing an onchocerciasis control programme: A case study from Plateau state, Nigeria. *Annals of Tropical Medicine and Parasitology, 68E*(92), 121–128.

Mulli, J.D. (1996). War and health. In R. Lanza (Ed.), *One world: The health and survival of the human species in the 21st century* (pp. 149–160). Santa Fe, NM: Health Press.

Murray, C.J., & Lopez, A.D. (1996). Evidence-based health policy: Lessons from the Global Burden of Disease Study. *Science, 274,* 740–743.

Murray, C.J., & Lopez, A.D. (1997). Mortality by cause for eight regions of the world: Global Burden of Disease Study. *Lancet, 349,* 1269–1347.

Nathwani, D., & Spiteri, J. (1997). Information about anti-malarial chemoprophylaxis in hospitalized patients: Is it adequate? *Scottish Medical Journal, 42*(1), 13–15.

Natsios, A.S. (2002). *This is USAID.* USAID, Washington, D. C. Retrieved December 29, 2002, from *http:/www./usaid.gov/about_usaid/*

Phillips, D.R. (1990). *Health and health care in the third world.* New York: Longman Scientific & Technical with Wiley and Sons.

Reingold, A.L. & Phares, C.R. (2001). Infectious diseases. In M.H. Merson, R.E. Black, & A.J. Mills (Eds.), *International public health diseases, program, system, and policies* (pp. 710–711). Gaithersburg, MD: Aspen.

Roemer, M.I. (1993). *National health systems of the world* (Vols. I & II). New York: Oxford University Press.

Shannon, J.B. (Ed.). (2001). *Worldwide health sourcebook* (pp. 104–113). Detroit, MI: Omnigraphics.

Stansfield, S.K. & Shepard, D.S. (1993). Acute respiratory infection. In D.T. Jamison, W.H. Mosley, A.R. Measham, & J.L. Bobadilla (Eds.), *Disease control priorities in developing countries* (pp. 67–90). Oxford: Oxford University Press.

Toole, M.J., Waldman, R.J., & Zwi, A. (2001). Complex humanitarian emergencies. In M.H. Merson, R.E. Black, & A.J. Mills (Eds.), *International public health: Diseases, programs, systems, policies* (pp. 439–513). Gaithersburg, MD: Aspen.

Trigg, P.I., & Kondrachine, A.V. (1998). Commentary: Malaria control in the 1990s. *Bulletin of the World Health Organization, 76*(1), 11–16.

United States Department of Health and Human Services. (2000). *Healthy people 2010: Understanding and improving health* (2nd ed.). Washington, D.C.: Author.

Vance, C. (1999). Nursing in the global arena. In E.J. Sullivan (Ed.), *Creating nursing's future* (p. 335). St. Louis: Mosby.

Walsh, J.A., Feifer, C.N., Measham, A.R., & Gertler, P.J. (1993). Maternal and perinatal health. In D.T. Jamison, W.H. Mosley, A.R. Measham, & J.L. Bobdilla (Eds.). *Disease control priorities in developing countries* (pp. 363–390). Oxford: Oxford University Press.

Wenzel, E. (1998, September 27). *WHO Constitution: Article 2.* Retrieved December 29, 2003, from *http://www.ldb.org/vl/top/whoconst.htm*

Whaley, R.F., & Hashim, T.J. (1995). *A textbook of world health: A practical guide to global health care.* New York: Parthenon.

World Bank. (2002, September). *What is the World Bank?* Retrieved December 29, 2003, from *http://www.worldbank.org*

World Health Organization. (1996, November). Water and sanitation. *WHO Fact Sheet, 112,* 2. Geneva: Author. Retrieved October 26, 1999, from *http://www.who.int/inf-fs/en/fact112.html*

World Health Organization. (1997). Promoting health through schools: Report of a WHO expert committee on comprehensive school health education and promotion. *WHO Technical Report Series, 180,* 5. Geneva: Author.

World Health Organization. (1998a, March). Dracunculiasis eradication. *WHO Fact Sheet, 98,* 1–2. Geneva: Author.

World Health Organization. (1998b, August Revised). Emerging and re-emerging infectious diseases. *WHO Fact Sheet, 97,* 1–7. Geneva: Author.

World Health Organization. (1998c, September). Reducing mortality from major killers of children. *WHO Fact Sheet, 178,* 3. Geneva: Author. Retrieved December 29, 2003, from *http://www.who.int/inf-fs/en/fact178.html*

World Health Organization. (1998d). Examples of pathogens recognized since 1973. *WHO Fact Sheet, 97,* 4. Geneva: Author.

World Health Organization. (1998e, November). Primary health care in the 21st century is everybody's business. *Press Release WHO/89,* 1–2. Geneva: Author.

World Health Organization. (1999a, February). WHO executive board gives green light to framework convention on tobacco control. *Press Release WHO/6.* Geneva: Author.

World Health Organization. (1999b). Highlights of the 52nd World Health Assembly. *Bulletin of the World Health Organization, 77*(7), 612–613. Geneva: WHO.

World Health Organization. (1999c, May 25). World Health Assembly gives resounding support to WHO technical programs. *Press Release WHA/18,* 1–3. Geneva: Author.

World Health Organization. (1999d, August 3). Solar alert '99. *Press Release WHO/40,* 1–2. Geneva: Author.

World Health Organization. (1999e, April 5). Polio outbreak in Central Africa. *Press Release WHO/21,* 102. Geneva: Author.

World Health Organization. (1999f). Malaria vaccine progress. *Bulletin of the World Health Organization, 77*(4), 361–362.

World Health Organization. (1999g, October 28). UN agencies issue joint statement for reducing maternal mortality. *WHO Press Release.* Geneva: Author.

World Health Organization. (2001). Nipah virus. *WHO Fact Sheet, 262,* 1–2. Geneva: Author.

World Health Organization. (2001a). Vaccines against diarrheal diseases. *WHO/GPV Strategic Plan 1998–2001.* Geneva: Author.

World Health Organization. (2001b). Surveillance for neonatal tetanus. *WHO/GPV Strategic Plan 1998–2001,* pp. 29, 46. Geneva: Author.

World Health Organization. (2001c, November). AIDS epidemic faster in eastern Europe than in rest of world: New figures. *Joint UNAIDS/WHO Press Release/53,* 1–2. Geneva: Author.

World Health Organization. (2002, March 3). Environmental hazards kill at least 3 million children aged under 5 every year. *WHO Press Release/12.* Geneva: Author.

World Health Organization. (2002a). Roll back malaria: 2001–2010 United Nations decade to roll back malaria. *RBM Infosheet 2 of 11, March 2002.* Geneva: Author. Retrieved December 29, 2003, from *http://www.rbm.who.int*

World Health Organization. (2002b, July 9). 3 million HIV/AIDS sufferers could receive antiretroviral therapy by 2005. *WHO Press Release/58,* 1–2. Geneva: Author.

World Health Organization. (2002c, July 4). Scaling up interventions could prevent 29 million new HIV infections among adults by 2010. *WHO Press Release/57,* 1–2. Geneva: Author.

World Health Organization. (2002d, July 12). WHO-UNICEF measles mortality reduction and regional elimination strategic plan 2001-2005. Geneva: Author. Retrieved March 20, 2003, from *http://www.who.int/mediacentre/releases/2003/pr76/en/*

World Health Organization. (2002e, August Revised). Tuberculosis. *WHO Fact Sheet, 104,* 1–3. Retrieved December 29, 2003, from *http://www.who.int/mediacentre/factsheets/who104/en/*

World Health Organization. (2002f, August). Poliomyelitis. *WHO Fact Sheet, 114,* 1–5. Retrieved December 29, 2003, from *http://www.who.int/mediacentre/factsheets/fs114/en/*

World Health Organization. (2002g, October). WHO atlas maps global tobacco epidemic. *Press Release WHO/82.* Geneva: Author.

World Health Organization. (2002h, October 28). Years of life can be increased 5–10 years. *Press Release WHO/84.* Geneva: Author.

World Health Organization. (2002i, November). Low investment in immunization and vaccines threatens global health. *Press Release WHO/87.* Geneva: Author.

World Health Organization. (2002j, November 25). TDR, Medicines for Malaria Venture and Shin Poong Pharmaceuticals sign agreement for development of pyronaridine-artesunate for treatment of malaria. *Notes for the Press WHO/8.* Geneva: Author.

World Health Organization. (2002k, December 6). River blindness campaign ends: West Africans return to fertile farmlands. *Press Release WHO/93.* Geneva: Author.

World Health Organization. (2002l, December 11). WHO study reveals harsh realities for older persons caring for orphans and people living with AIDS. *Press Release WHO/95,* 1–2. Geneva: Author.

World Health Organization. (2002m, December). About WHO. Retrieved December 29, 2003, from *http://www.who.int/about/en/*

World Health Organization. (2003a, January). Leprosy. *WHO Fact Sheet, 101,* 1–3. Retrieved December 29, 2003, from *http://www.who.int/mediacentre/factsheets/fs101/en/*

World Health Organization. (2003b, February). Leprosy: Urgent need to end stigma and isolation. *Press Release WHO/7,* 1–2. Geneva: Author.

World Health Organization. (2003c, March). Agreement reached on global framework convention on tobacco control. *Press Release WHO/21.* Geneva: Author.

World Health Organization (2003, 12 March). WHO issues a global alert about cases of atypical pneumonia. *Press Release WHO/22.* Geneva: W.H.O.

World Health Organization. (2003d, March). *Burden of disease project.* Geneva: Author. Retrieved March 21, 2003 from *http://www.who.int/whr/2003/en/Annex3-en.pdf*

World Health Organization. (2003e, May). Severe acute respiratory syndrome (SARS). Retrieved December 29, 2003, from *http://www.who.int/csr/sars/en/*

World Health Organization. (2003). First steps for managing an outbreak of acute diarrhea. WHO global task force on cholera. Global health security: Epidemic alert and response, Box 2. Geneva: WHO.

World Health Organization/Food and Agriculture Organization. (2003, February 25). Feeding hope: Nutrition plays key role in HIV/AIDS care. *Joint Press Release WHO/FAO/18.* Geneva: Author.

SELECTED READINGS

Abell, H. (1998, Summer). Globalization causes a world of health problems. *Hesperian Foundation News,* 1–3.

Berlinguer, G. (1999). Health and equity as a primary global goal. *Development, 42,* 17–21.

Berman, P. (1997). National health accounts in developing countries: Appropriate methods and recent applications. *Health Economics, 6,* 11–30.

Chin, J. (Ed.) (2000). *Control of communicable diseases manual.* Washington, DC: American Public Health Association.

Deen, J.L., Vos, T., Huttly, S.R., & Tulloch, J. (1999). Injuries and noncommunicable diseases: Emerging health problems of children in developing countries. *Bulletin of the World Health Organization, 77*(6), 518–523.

Garrett, L. (2000). *Betrayal of trust: The collapse of global public health.* New York: Hyperion.

Hammer, J.S., & Berman, P. (1995). Ends and means in public health policy in developing countries. *Health Policy, 32,* 29–45.

Hart, G. (1997). From "rotten wives" to "good mothers": Household models and the limits of economism. *IDS Bulletin, 28*(3), 14–25.

Hsiao, W.C. (1995). The Chinese health care system: Lessons for other nations. *Social Science and Medicine, 41*(2), 171–220.

Kalache, A., & Keller, I. (1999). The WHO perspective on active aging. *Promotion and Education Quarterly, VI* (4), 20–23.

Mayer, K.H., & Pizer, H.F. (Eds.). (2000). *The emergence of AIDS: The impact on immunology, microbiology and public health.* Washington DC: American Public Health Association.

Merson, M.H., Black, R.E. & Mills, A.J. (Eds.). (2001). *International public health: Diseases, programs, systems and policies.* Gaithersburg, MD: Aspen.

Ministry of Health. (1998). *AIDS in Ethiopia: Background, projections, impacts and interventions.* Addis Ababa, Ethiopia: Ministry of Health.

Murray, C., & Chen, L. (1993). In search of a contemporary theory for understanding mortality and change. *Social Science and Medicine, 36*(2), 143–155.

Nyamu, J. (1998). Target: A stronger health sector: Special initiative gives priority to preventive and primary care. *Africa Recovery, 11*(4), 18–20.

Salvatierra-Gonzalez, R., & Benguigui, Y. (Eds.). (2000). *Antimicrobial resistance in the Americas: Magnitude and containment of the problem.* Washington, DC: Pan American Health Organization.

Schuler, S.R., Hashemi, S.M., & Riley, A.P. (1997). The influence of women's changing roles and status in Bangladesh's fertility transition: Evidence from a study of credit programs and contraceptive use. *World Development, 25*(4), 563–575.

Schuermann, L. (1999, September). American Society for Microbiology supports PAHO efforts to strengthen region-wide network of public health laboratories. *PAHO Today,* 3.

Van Grinneken, J.K., Lob-Levyt, J., & Gove, S. (1996). Potential interventions for preventing pneumonia among children in development countries: Promoting maternal education. *Tropical Medicine and International Health, 1*(3), 283–294.

Varmus, H., & Satcher, D. (1997). Ethics are local: Engaging cross-cultural variation in the ethics for clinical research. *Social Science and Medicine, 35*(9), 1070–1091.

Walt, G. (1998). Globalization of international health. *Lancet*, 351, 434–437.

World Health Organization. (1978). *Alma-Ata 1978: Primary health care*. Geneva: Author.

World Health Organization. (1986). *The Ottawa charter for health promotion*. Geneva: Author.

World Health Organization. (1998). *Fifty facts from the World Health Report 1998: Global health situations and trends 1955 to 2025*. Geneva: Author.

World Health Organization. (2003, March). Severe acute respiratory syndrome (SARS): Multi-count outbreak update. Retrieved March 16, 2003, from *http://www.who.int/csr/don/ 2003_03_16/en/*

Related Resources

American Red Cross, and International Red Cross and Red Crescent Societies: *http://www.red-cross.org*

Career Network: Global Health Council (GHC), 1701 K St. NW, Suite 600, Washington, DC 20006; telephone 202-833-5900, fax 202-833-0075; *http://www.globalhealth.org*

Culture Grants: 333 S. 520 West, Suite 360, London, UT 84042; telephone: 1-800-528-6279.

Doctors of the World: 375 West Broadway, New York, NY 10012; telephone 212-226-9890 or toll-free 1-888-817-4357. Doctors of the World mobilizes the American health sector to promote and protect physical and mental health, the right to equality before the law, and the right to be free from torture in the United States and abroad.

Health Volunteers Overseas (HVO): P.O. Box 65157, Washington, DC 20035-5157; telephone 202-296-0928; *http://www.hvousa.org*. A private, nonprofit organization dedicated to improving the quality and availability of health care in developing countries through education. AACN is a sponsor of HVO.

International Career Opportunities: Rt. 2, Box 305, Standardsville, VA 22973; telephone: 804-985-6444. Bimonthly.

International Employment Hotline: Will Cantrell, (Ed.), PO Box 3030, Oakton, VA 22124; telephone 703-620-1972. Monthly.

International Jobs Bulletin: University Placement Center, Woody Hall B208, Southern Illinois University, Carbondale, IL 62901. Biweekly.

International Opportunities: A Career Guide for Students: published by the Kennedy Center for International Studies, Brigham Young University, 280 Herald, Clark Building, P.O. Box 24538, Provo, UT 84602-4538; telephone 1-800-528-6279. $10.95. Information on internships and employment opportunities with nonprofit and volunteer organizations, private agencies, the United Nations, the U. S. Government, and educational organizations.

Medical Ambassadors International: P.O. Box 576645, Modesto, CA 95357; telephone 209-524-0600. Nondenominational.

Monday Developments: Interaction, 1717 Massachusetts Ave., NW, 8th floor, Washington, DC 20006; telephone 202-667-8227. Employment opportunities listed; biweekly.

Options: Project Concern, 3550 Afton Road, San Diego, CA 92123; telephone 619-279-9690. Information on professional volunteer opportunities in programs, hospitals, and clinics worldwide.

PDRC Placement Hotline: School for International Training, 1 Kippling Rd., Brattleboro, VT 05302; telephone 802-257-7751.

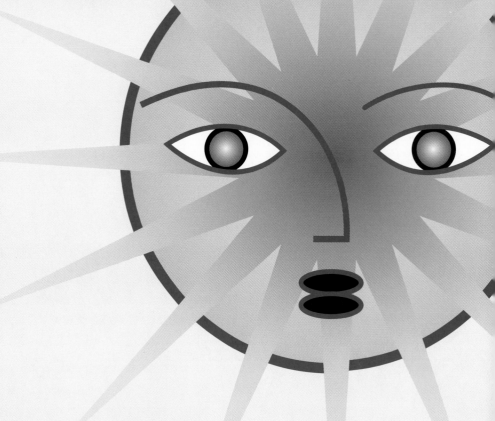

The Family as Client

22

Theoretical Bases for Promoting Family Health

Key Terms

- Adoptive family
- Augmented family
- Blended family
- Cohabitating couples
- Commune family
- Commuter family
- Contemporary family
- Energy exchange
- Family
- Family culture
- Family functioning
- Family map
- Family structure
- Family system boundary
- Foster families
- Gangs
- Group-marriage family
- Group-network family
- Homeless family
- Intrarole functioning
- Kin-network
- Multigenerational family
- Nontraditional family
- Nuclear-dyad family
- Nuclear family
- Primary relationship
- Roles
- Single-adult family
- Single-parent family
- Stepfamily
- Traditional family
- Wider family

Learning Objectives

Upon mastery of this chapter, you should be able to:

- Analyze changing definitions of family.

- Discuss characteristics all families have in common.

- Identify five attributes that help explain how families function as social systems.

- Discuss how a family's culture influences its values, behaviors, prescribed roles, and distribution of power.

- Compare and contrast the variety of structures that make up families.

- Describe the functions of a family.

- Identify the stages of the family life cycle and the developmental tasks of a family as it grows.

- Analyze the role of the community health nurse in promoting the health of the family unit.

When you hear the word *family,* what do you think of? How would you define you own family? Is your grandfather a member of your family? Your niece? Your neighbor? A friend? A family pet? Although many different definitions exist, most family theorists agree that a **family** consists of two or more individuals who share a residence or live near one another; possess some common emotional bond; engage in interrelated social positions, roles, and tasks; and share a sense of affection and belonging (Friedman, Bowden, & Jones 2003; Murray & Zentner, 2000).

The family is a separate entity with its own structure, functions, and needs. In every society throughout history, the family is the most basic unit; so, too, in community health. It is the family, more than any other societal institution, that nurtures and shapes a society's members.

Today's community health nurse needs to understand and work with many types of families, each of which has different health problems and needs. For example, a young single mother who is homeless seeks help in caring for her sick infant. A 55-year-old grandfather provides care for his elderly mother, who was recently discharged from the hospital after a stroke. A group of parents, siblings, cousins, and children, all refugees from Laos, need instruction on the purchase and preparation of food. Why is it important for the community health nurse to understand and respect the unique characteristics, cultures, structures, and functions of each of these families? Do families as basic units of a community have characteristics that affect community health nursing service? The answer is an unqualified yes. The effectiveness of the community health nurse depends on knowing how to work with a family as a unit of care. This chapter examines the nature of families, family functioning, and family health. It draws from various theories to strengthen the student's understanding and appreciation of families as clients. This information will increase the effectiveness of interventions with families at the primary, secondary, and tertiary levels of prevention (see Levels of Prevention Matrix). **Family functioning** is defined as those behaviors or activities by family members that maintain the family and meet family needs, individual member needs, and society's views of family. The interdependence of family members involves a set of internal relationships that influence the effectiveness of family

---

LEVELS OF PREVENTION MATRIX

SITUATION: The family will provide the emotional and material resources necessary for its members' growth and well-being.

GOAL: Using the three levels of prevention, negative health conditions are avoided, or promptly diagnosed and treated, and the fullest possible potential is restored.

PRIMARY PREVENTION		SECONDARY PREVENTION		TERTIARY PREVENTION		
Health Promotion and Education	*Health Protection*	*Early Diagnosis*	*Prompt Treatment*	*Rehabilitation*	*Primary Prevention*	
					Health Promotion and Education	*Health Protection*
• Adults are well prepared for the responsibilities of their union • Adults enter the relationship with the personal resources necessary to promote the growth and development of their family unit		• Identification of a family member's personal problems that affect the family as a whole • Early recognition that problems exist in the relationships among family members	• The family seeks out the appropriate resources that brings the family to the highest level of wellness possible	• After the family suffers a crisis, the members recognize the need for help and accept that help • Families draw on personal resources to rebuild relationships and heal the family unit	• The family continues using resources that enhance the growth and well-being of individuals and the family as a unit	• Engage in family strengthening practices to protect the family from possible inhibitors to growth and well-being

functioning (Friedman, Bowden, & Jones, 2003). There is a complex communication pattern of functioning among family members, and the quality of the pattern contributes to the health of the family.

Family health is concerned with how well the family functions together as a unit. It involves not only the health of the members and how they relate to other members, but also how well they relate to and cope with the community outside the family. In fact, family health, like individual health, ranges along a continuum from wellness to illness. A family may be at one point on that continuum now and at a much different point 6 months from now. Family health refers to the health status of a given family at a given point in time (Hanson, 2001).

UNIVERSAL CHARACTERISTICS OF FAMILIES

Several observations can be made about families in general. First, each family is unique. The families mentioned earlier each have their own distinct problems and strengths. When you approach the door of a house or push the buzzer of an apartment, you cannot assume what the family inside will be like. Consequently, you will have to gather information about each particular family in order to achieve nursing objectives.

Second, every family shares some universal characteristics with every other family. These universal characteristics provide an important key to understanding each family's uniqueness. Five of the most important family universals for community health nursing are

1. Every family is a small social system.
2. Every family has its own cultural values and rules.
3. Every family has structure.
4. Every family has certain basic functions.
5. Every family moves through stages in its life cycle.

No matter how many families a nurse might visit or serve in the course of a year, each one will have these universal features; it is important for community health nurses to know each family's unique manifestation of these features and their effects on family health. These five universals of family life, which provide the framework of this chapter, are based on systems theory, sociologic theories, and theories of family development. In addition to considering the universals of family life, this chapter covers the unique family features and structures that characterize our changing world (see The Global Community).

ATTRIBUTES OF FAMILIES AS SOCIAL SYSTEMS

Many Americans fall into the habit of viewing families merely as collections of individuals. Caused partly by the strong cultural emphasis on individualism, this error also occurs because families are often encountered through the individual members. When a community health nurse sits in a living room talking with a young mother about her new infant, it is difficult to keep in mind that all the other family members are present by way of their influence. Systems theory offers some insights about how families operate as social systems. Knowing the attributes of living systems or open systems can help strengthen understanding of family structure and function. There are five attributes of open systems that help explain how families function: (1) families are interdependent, (2) families maintain boundaries, (3) families exchange energy with their environments, (4) families are adaptive, and (5) families are goal-oriented.

Interdependence Among Members

All the members of a family are interdependent; each member's actions affect the other members. For example, consider the changes a father might make to reduce his risk of coronary heart disease. If he cuts back on working overtime, the family's income will be reduced. If he begins to eat different foods, food preparation and eating patterns in the family will be altered. If he starts a new exercise program three evenings a week, this may upset other family routines. Even his ability to carry out his usual roles as husband and father may be affected if, for instance, he has less time to help his children with their homework or share household chores with his wife.

It is possible to illustrate the pattern of interactions between members using a **family map** (Fig. 22–1). This tool can reveal a great deal about the interdependence of family members. The way parents relate to each other, for instance, influences the quality of their parenting. When the interactions between them are frequent, honest, and nurturing, they have more to offer their children. Marital, parent–child, and sibling relationships all significantly influence family functioning. They determine how well the family as a system handles conflict, provides a support system for its members, copes with crises, solves daily problems, and capitalizes on its own resources.

Family Boundaries

Families as systems set and maintain boundaries: ego-boundaries, generation boundaries, and family–community boundaries (Barker, 1998). These boundaries, which result from shared experiences and expectations, link family members together in a bond that excludes the rest of the world. Also, a greater concentration of energy exists within the family than between the family and its external environment, thereby creating a **family system boundary**.

For example, the Salazar extended family gathers for a Sunday afternoon backyard cookout. The distinctiveness of this family from all the others in the neighborhood is noticeable, as would be that of any other family. The elders in the family were born in Mexico, and they sit together reminiscing in Spanish. The food is traditional and plentiful. It is

THE GLOBAL COMMUNITY

Shyu, Y.L. (2002). A conceptual framework for understanding the process of family caregiving to frail elders in Taiwan. *Research in Nursing and Health, 25,* 111–121.

In this study of family caregiving to frail elders in Taiwan, the author tested a framework of "finding a balance point," which means a balance among care receiver characteristics, caregiver factors, and caregiver consequences. The percentage of elders in Taiwan has more than tripled in the past 50 years—from 2.5% of the population in 1951 to 8.6% in 2000. Because 90% of all caregiving is provided by family in Taiwan, it is an issue needing exploration.

A total of 125 families served by 11 home-nursing agencies in greater Taipei participated in this study. The median age of care receivers was 76.7 years; 54.4% of the participants were women, and 69.6% of them had severe to moderate cognitive impairment. All care receivers required assistance with at least three activities of daily living (ADLs). All families lived with the care receiver, and 74.4% of the caregivers were women, ranging in age from 18 to 76 years (37.6% were spouses, 20% were daughters-in-law, 19.2% were daughters, 14.4% were sons, and 8.8% were friends or other relatives). Most of the care receivers ($n=118$) were severely dependent; 76% of the caregivers admitted to having a very good or good relationship with the care receiver, and the other 24% had a neutral to poor relationship.

Several scales were used to measure qualitative data: the Family Caregiving Factors Inventory (FCFI) with four subscales, The Family Caregiving Process of Finding a Balance Point Scale, and the Family Caregiving Consequences Scales with three subscales. All scales had good to excellent content validity and significant test-retest reliability.

The following model depicts the conceptual framework for understanding the caregiving process in Taiwan:

The findings from this study included the following:
- Caregivers who were younger had a better relationship with the care receiver.
- Younger caregivers had more caregiving resources.
- Younger caregivers had more realistic self-expectations, more knowledge of the care receiver, and better overall caregiving consequences.
- Caregivers who tended to find a balance point among competing needs also appeared to have significantly better overall caregiving consequences.
- The quality of the relationship appeared to predict all caregiving factors but not the process of finding a balance point.
- Caregivers who scored higher in knowledge about the care receiver scored higher for degree of perceived balance among competing needs.
- Very little of the variance in finding a balance point was explained by caregiving characteristics and caregiving factors.

Implications from this study can assist with caregiving decisions among the Chinese in Taiwan and may be applicable to other countries with Chinese populations and to health care providers in the United States who are working with Chinese and Taiwanese immigrants.

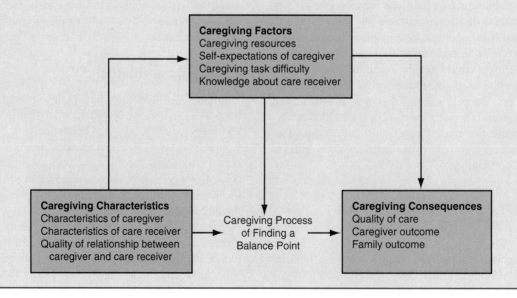

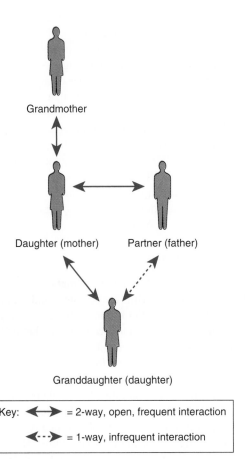

Grandmother

Daughter (mother)   Partner (father)

Granddaughter (daughter)

Key: ←→ = 2-way, open, frequent interaction

←- -→ = 1-way, infrequent interaction

FIGURE 22-1.
This map indicates that the mother is a key figure for family interaction. The maternal grandmother, father, and daughter communicate primarily to her rather than directly to one another.

prepared and served by the women: Aunt Rosa's tamales, Cousin Teresa's tortillas, and flan for dessert from Grandma Lupe's own recipe. While the women prepare the food, some of the men play ball and others listen to Uncle Gilberto play the guitar and discuss the future of the family grape-growing business. The children gather in small groups and play loudly. Several of them, prompted by their parents, display their musical talent later in the day by singing some old favorite songs and doing some traditional Mexican dances. Because of the things they have in common, the Salazars set and maintain boundaries that unite them and also differentiate them from others.

Energy Exchange

Family boundaries are semipermeable; although they provide protection and preservation of the family unit, they also allow selective linkage with the outside world. As open systems, in order to function adequately, families exchange materials or information with their environment (Friedman, Bowden, & Jones, 2003). This process is called **energy exchange**. All normally functioning living systems engage in such an input–output relationship. This energy exchange

serves to promote a healthy ecologic balance between the family system and the environment that is its immediate community.

A family's successful progress through its developmental stages depends on how well the family manages this energy exchange. For example, a child-bearing family needs adequate food, shelter, and emotional support, as well as information on how to accomplish its developmental tasks. The family also needs community resources such as health care, education, and employment, all of which are forms of environmental input. In return, the family contributes to the community by working and by consuming goods and services. If a family does not have adequate income or emotional support or does not use community resources, that family does not experience a proper energy exchange with its environment. An inadequate exchange can lead to dysfunction and poor health (Neuman, 2001).

Adaptive Behavior

Families are adaptive, equilibrium-seeking systems. In accordance with their nature, families never stay the same. They shift and change in response to internal and external forces. Internally, the family composition changes as new members are added or members leave through death or divorce. Roles and relationships change as members advance in age and experience; normative expectations change as members resolve their tensions and differing points of view. Externally, families are bombarded by influences from sources such as school, work, peers, neighbors, religion, and government; consequently, they are forced to accommodate to new demands. Adapting to these influences may require a family to change its behaviors, its goals, and even its values. Like any system, the family needs a state of quasi-equilibrium to function (Neuman, 2001). With each new set of pressures, the family shifts and accommodates to regain balance and maintain a normal lifestyle.

There are times when a family's capacity for adaptation is stressed beyond its limits. At this point, the system may be in danger of disintegrating; that is, family members may leave or become dysfunctional because of unresolved stress. This is an indication that some form of intervention may be needed to help restore family equilibrium. These interventions may take the form of extended family mediation or external professional help.

Community health nurses play an influential role in family equilibrium-seeking. Neuman described the major goal of nursing as keeping the individual and family client systems stabilized within their environments (Neuman, 2001). Chapter 24 explores the community health nurse's stabilizing interventions with families in detail.

Goal-Directed Behavior

Families as social systems are goal directed. Families exist for a purpose—to establish and maintain a milieu that promotes the development of their members. To fulfill this purpose, a family must perform basic functions such as providing love, security, identity, a sense of belonging; assisting with preparation for adult roles in society; and maintaining order and control. In addition to these functions, each family member engages in tasks to maintain the family as a viable unit. Duvall and Miller (1985) described specific functions and tasks for each stage of the family's development. These functions and tasks are examined in more detail later in this chapter.

FAMILY CULTURE

Families are social systems with cultural dimensions; families are also tied biologically through kinship and socially through choice. This structure exists for a purpose. Duvall's definition nicely summarizes these aspects of the family: "The family is a unity of interacting persons related by ties of marriage, birth, or adoption, whose central purpose is to create and maintain a common culture which promotes the physical, mental, emotional, and social development of each of its members" (Duvall & Miller, 1985, p. 6).

Family culture is the acquired knowledge that family members use to interpret their experiences and to generate behaviors that influence family structure and function. The concept of family culture arises from a significant body of literature in the social and behavioral sciences; cross-cultural comparisons and in-depth analyses demonstrate that each family has a "culture" that strongly influences its structure and function. Culture explains why families behave as they do (Leininger, 2001; Pender, 2001; Spector, 2000). Family culture also gives the community health nurse a basis for assessing family health and designing appropriate interventions.

Three aspects of family culture deserve special consideration: (1) family members share certain values that affect family behavior; (2) certain roles are prescribed and defined for family members; and (3) a family's culture determines its distribution and use of power.

Shared Values and Their Effect on Behavior

Although families share many broad cultural values drawn from the larger society in which they live, they also develop unique variants. Every family has its own set of values and rules for operation that can be considered as family culture (Barker, 1998). Some values are explicitly stated: "Family matters must always stay within the family." Such values may give rise to specific operating rules: "Don't tell anyone about our problems."

Like all cultural values, many family values remain outside the conscious awareness of family members. These values, often not verbalized, become powerful determinants of what the family believes, feels, thinks, and does. Family values include those beliefs transmitted by previous genera-

tions, religious influences, immediate social pressures, and the larger society. Values become an integral part of a family's life and are very difficult to change. A family that values free expression for every member engages comfortably in loud, noisy debates. Another family that values quietness, order, and control does not tolerate its members' raising their voices. One family uses birth control based on beliefs about human life and parental responsibility; another family chooses not to use birth control because the members hold a different set of values. How a family views education, health care, lifestyle, courtship, marriage, child-rearing, sex roles, or any of the myriad other issues requiring choices depends on the cultural values of that family.

Prescribed Roles

Roles, the assigned or assumed parts that members play during day-to-day family living, are bestowed and defined by the family (Hanson, 2001). For instance, in one family the father role may be defined as an authoritative one that includes establishing rules, judging behavior, and administering punishment for violation of rules. In another family, the father role may be defined primarily as that of a loving benefactor. If there is an absence of an immediate male parent, a grandfather, uncle, friend, or mother may take over the father role. Selection of specific roles to be played in any given family varies depending on the family's structure, needs, and patterns of functioning. In a single-parent family, the parent may need to assume the roles of mother, father, and breadwinner, as well as others.

Families distribute among their members all the responsibilities and tasks necessary to conduct family living. The responsibilities of breadwinner and homemaker, with their accompanying tasks, may belong to husband and wife, respectively, or may be shared if both husband and wife hold jobs outside the home. Older children may help younger ones with homework or entertain them. This releases parents for other tasks and increases the responsibility of older children.

Family members play several roles at the same time. This **intrarole functioning** can be exceptionally taxing. A woman, may play the role of wife to her husband, daughter to her mother who lives with her, and mother to each of her children. The mother role may involve taking on several additional roles and responsibilities and varies with each child's needs. In a family in which the mother is seriously ill, many of the roles she held must be assumed by others. This places new demands on other family members during the treatment and healing process or throughout a terminal illness (Fitch, Bunston, & Elliot, 1999). A single parent often takes on the roles of both father and mother but may distribute responsibilities and tasks more widely. A grandmother or a child may assume responsibility for some chores and thereby relieve the demands placed on the single parent. Among families, there is great variation in expectations for each role and in the degree of flexibility in role prescriptions. A family may place great demands on some members, but those same members may interpret the expectations placed on them and their roles differently. Confusion and conflict can develop unless roles are clarified.

Other roles of family members extend beyond the immediate family. There may be extended family members nearby who interact with the family on a regular basis or only on special occasions such as birthdays. If both parents are employed, they may have an expansive social network from work or from within the neighborhood. Friendships are often made with the parents of the childrens' friends, particularly if their children participate in the same extracurricular activities. Many families enjoy the fellowship of organized religious or cultural groups. This fellowship can be a source of support and comfort, as well as an additional role function for the family members. Another intrarole function is that of community participant in activities separate from the family. These roles may involve local or regional politics, community improvement, volunteerism for nonprofit agencies, or any other service outside the home that the community may offer. These diverse role relationships should enrich and energize the participants. However, many people become overcommitted, creating an imbalance of role responsibilities that is draining and causes friction and stress. The community health nurse must work with families to achieve a balance of activities and roles that promotes family health.

Power Distribution

Power–the possession of control, authority, or influence over others–assumes different patterns in each family. In some families, power is concentrated primarily in one member; in others, it is distributed on a more egalitarian basis. The traditional patriarchal family, in which the father holds absolute authority over the other members, is rare in American society. However, the pattern of husband as head of the household and dominant member of the family is still frequently seen. Whether male or female, the dominant partner holds the majority of the decision-making power, particularly over more important family matters such as employment and finances. Other areas of decision-making, including choices about vacations, housing, leisure activities, household purchases, and child rearing, may be shared or delegated. With changing societal influences, however, the present trend among American families is toward egalitarian power distribution.

Rudolf Dreikurs (1964) advocated that families form a "family council" for shared decision-making and distribution of tasks. Today, many families practice joint decision-making and equal participation by all members. However, the community health nurse can suggest this activity for families not using such a method. Role-playing this technique can be incorporated during a home visit or as a teaching technique with an aggregate group. Specific educational interventions are discussed in Chapter 12.

Roles often influence power distribution within the family. Along with the responsibilities attached to a role, a family may assign decision-making authority. The mother role frequently includes decision-making with respect to household management. Responsibility related to a son's role such as lawn-mowing may be enhanced as a learning activity, if he is allowed to decide when and how often he does the job.

Family power structure is also influenced by the amount of personal power residing in each member (Friedman, Bowden, & Jones, 2002). A mother or eldest son, for example, can exercise considerable influence over the family by virtue of personality and position, rather than by delegated authority. Even a child who throws temper tantrums can wield considerable power in a family.

FAMILY STRUCTURES

Globally, families—in all their varied forms—are the basic social unit. The meaning of family among the Hmong of northern Laos may include hundreds of people who make up a clan. In Mexico, families remain close, are large, and extend into multiple generations. In Germany and Japan, families are small and tend to the needs of their elders at home. In the United States, where families come from many cultural groups, many variations coexist within communities.

For many people in the United States, the term *family* evokes a picture of a husband, wife, and children living under one roof with the male as breadwinner and the female as homemaker. In the past, this nuclear family was often seen as the norm for everyone. Changes in social values and cultural lifestyles (eg, women working outside the home) combined with acceptance of alternative lifestyles has changed the definition of family. Today, definitions of family include unmarried adults living together with or without children, single-parent households, divorced couples who combine households with children from previous marriages (the blended family), and homosexual couples with or without children.

It must be considered a privilege to gain entrance into a family's home. This is a uniquely private space belonging to the family. The people who are members of this household interact, care for one another, and bond in ways that may never be fully understood by anyone outside the family. Therefore, being granted entrance into this system gives the community health nurse an opportunity to work with the family that few other professionals experience. Each type of household requires recognition and acceptance by community health nurses, who must help families achieve optimal health.

Families come in many shapes and sizes. The varying **family structures** or compositions comprise the collective characteristics of individuals who make up a family unit (age, gender, and number). A growing body of research on family structure and function shows that families have changed dramatically since the nuclear family was the dominant form. Family structures fall into two general categories: traditional and nontraditional (see What Do You Think?).

Traditional Families

Traditional family structures are those that are most familiar to us and that are most readily accepted by society. They include the **nuclear family**—husband, wife, and children living together in the same household. In nuclear families, the workload distribution between the two adults can vary. Both adults may work outside the home; one adult may work outside the home while the other stays at home and assumes primary responsibilities for the household; or partners may alternate, constantly renegotiating work and domestic responsibilities. A **nuclear-dyad family** consists of a husband and wife living together who have no children or who have grown children living outside the home. Traditional families also include **single-adult families** in which one adult is living alone by choice or because of separation from a spouse or children or both. Separation may be the result of divorce, death, or distance from children. Some 4% of U.S. households are **multigenerational families**, in which several generations or age-groups live together in the same household (Cohn, 2001). A household in which a widowed woman lives with her divorced daughter and two young grandchildren is an example of a multigenerational family, as is one in which adult children live with aging parents. Such arrangements are increasing in number, according to the 2000 U. S. census. Sometimes, particularly in close-knit ethnic communities, families form a **kin-network**, in which several nuclear families live in the same household or near one another and share goods and services. They may own and operate a family business, sharing work and child care responsibilities, income and expenses, and even meals. Variations of this trend are increasing among all groups as children postpone leaving home because of economic conditions or educational plans or an elderly parent moves into an adult child's home to recover from a recent illness. A variation of the kin-network is the **augmented family**. This is a family group in which extended family members or nonrelatives or both live with and provide significant care to the children (Barnes, 2001).

Another variation of the traditional nuclear family is the **blended family**. In this structure, single parents marry and raise the children from each of their previous relationships together. They may be custodial parents who have the children except during planned visits with the noncustodial parent, or they may share custody so that the children live in the blended arrangement only part-time. This family may include children from the couple's union, in addition to the children brought into this relationship.

Single-parent families include one adult (either father or mother) caring for a child or children as a result of a temporary relationship, a legal separation or divorce, or the death of a spouse. In single-parent families, the parent may or may not be employed. Other nontraditional single-parent family situations are described in the next section.

One contemporary variant of the traditional family is the **commuter family**. Both partners in this family work, but their jobs are in different cities. The pattern is usually for one partner to live, work, and perhaps raise children in the "home" city, while the second partner lives in the other city and commutes home. Sometimes this arrangement is short-term; for example, one partner may be transferred through work and the couple chooses not to move the rest of the family for one or several reasons (eg, waiting until the end of the school year, making sure the new job is secure, locating the right housing, or selling the old home). At other times, commuting may continue for years. For example, the family home may be in a town where the cost of living is reasonable, but one parent works in a financially and personally rewarding career several hundred miles away and commutes home on weekends. In other instances, one parent may be on military assignment in another country for 6 months or longer, leaving the other parent alone for months at a time. Clearly, these arrangements influence family roles and functions, challenging a family's ability to maintain healthy relationships. A traditional family in which one partner is required to travel often (eg, for business, to care for an ill family member at a distant location) may experience similar problems and stressors. Table 22–1 lists a number of traditional family structures.

Nontraditional or Contemporary Families

The traditional nuclear family has been a fundamental part of the European cultural heritage shared by many Americans, reinforced by religion, education, and other influential social institutions. Variations from this pattern often were treated as deviant and abnormal, even in relatively recent studies of the family (Olson et al., 1983). Nonetheless, infants born to unwed mothers made up 26.6% of the births in 1990 and 33% in 2000 (U. S. Statistical Abstract, 2001). The number of unmarried people living together continues to increase, as does the never-married population. In 1980, 20.3% of the population were never married, increasing to 22.2% in 1990 and

T A B L E 22–1

The Traditional and Nontraditional American Family

Structure	Participants	Living Arrangements
TRADITIONAL		
Nuclear dyad	Husband Wife	Common household
Nuclear family	Husband Wife Child(ren)	Common household
Commuter family	Husband Wife Children (sometimes)	Household divided between two cities
Single-parent family	One adult (separated, divorced, widowed) Children	Common household
Divorced family (shared custody of children)	One adult parent, children part-time	Two separate households
Blended family	Husband Wife (His and/or hers, and possibly their children)	Common household
Single adult	One adult (at times not considered a "Family")	Living alone
Multigenerational family	Any combination of the traditional family structures	Common household
Kin network	Two or more reciprocal households (related by birth or marriage)	Close geographic proximity
Augmented family	Extended family group or nonrelatives who provide significant child care	Common household or close geographic proximity
NONTRADITIONAL		
Unmarried single-parent family	One parent (never married) Children	Common household
Cohabiting partners	Two adults (heterosexual, homosexual, or "just friends") Children (possibly)	Common household
Commune family	Two or more monogamous couples Sharing children	Common household
Group marriage commune family	Several adults "married" to each other Sharing childrearing	Common household
Group network	Reciprocal nuclear households or single members	Close geographic proximity
Homeless families	Any combination of family members previously mentioned	The streets and shelters
Foster families	Husband and wife or single adult Natural children (possibly) Foster children	Common household
Gangs	Males and females usually of same cultural or ethnic background	Close geographic proximity (same neighborhood)
"Loose shirt" families	Parents work from home via the personal computer (word processing, e-mail, faxing, cellular telephone—"telecommuting")	Common household

23.9% in 2000 (U. S. Statistical Abstract, 2001). In addition, the proportion of single-parent families has continued steady over the past decade. In both 1990 and 2000, 12% of family households were headed by a single woman caring for 3.17 family members. During the same period, 3% of family households (with an average of 3.16 household members) in 1990 were headed by a single man; this increased to 4% in 2000. Furthermore, between 1980 and 2000, one-parent families with a female head of household were more frequently black than white, Hispanic, Asian, or any other identified race (U. S. Statistical Abstract, 2001). There is every indication that the upward trend for unmarried family units, single parent households, and female heads of households (especially among blacks) will continue in the 21st century and will represent important contemporary family units in American society.

Society has begun to accept nontraditional definitions of family. The concept of **wider family** was initially presented by Marciano (1991) and is defined as a family that "emerges from lifestyle, is voluntary, and independent of necessary biological or kin connections" (p. 160). "With today's wide variety of family types and structures, the most advanced definition of family may be 'the family is who the client says it is'" (Bell & Wright, 1993, p. 391).

Families that do not fit the traditional nuclear model make up an increasing proportion of the American population (U. S. Statistical Abstract, 2001). For instance:

- In 1960, legally married couples made up 75% of American households; in 2000, that number had dropped to 59.9% (which now includes blended, remarried families).
- In 1970, 12% of children younger than 18 years of age lived with one parent; in 1990, the percentage was 25%; 40% of all children will live part of their lives before adulthood with a single parent (Coleman et al., 1998).
- In 1980, 20.3% of all people in the United States were single and never married; in 2000, the percentage was 23.9%.
- In 1980, single-parent households headed by men represented 2.1% of all families; this figure rose to 3% in 1990 and 4% in 2000, almost doubling in 20 years.
- In 2000, American families composed of a husband, wife, and children made up 36.2% of the white population and 24.2% of the black population.
- In 2000, 8.1% of white families and 27.8% of black families were headed by a single woman; for black families, this was a greater percentage than that of married couples with children.

Divorce changes family structures. Half of all marriages now end in divorce (the rate is higher for teenage marriages), and the median duration of marriages is approximately 7 years. In the United States, 20 of every 1000 women divorce each year. This number has remained steady since 1990, but it is twice the rate of other industrialized nations (Germany, 9 per 1000; Canada, 11 per 1000; Japan, 10 per 1000) (U. S. Department of Commerce, 1998). Display 22–1 describes one nontraditional American family.

DISPLAY 22–1

A Look at One Nontraditional American Family

Baby boomer families experience divorce and other contemporary family phenomena in unique ways, as demonstrated in the following example:

Our granddaughter, Susan (a Harvard alumna), cohabits with Ted (an astrophysicist at Harvard). They are not married, but they have a baby (our first great-grandson). Ted has been twice divorced and has a daughter nearly as old as Susan. Susan has close bonds to this daughter and to both of Ted's ex-wives and often travels from Massachusetts to Texas to visit them. The question is: How is Susan related to all these "ex's"? Even more intriguing: Suppose one of us were suddenly stranded alone in Texas and needed a supportive relationship. It is not unimaginable that Susan's grandparent might seek out one of Ted's ex-wives for help—indeed, might eventually develop a close relationship with her. And what would that relationship be called?

(Riley, M.W., & Riley, L.W. [1996]. Generational relations: A future perspective. In T.K. Hareven [Ed.], *Aging and intergenerational relations: Life course and cross-cultural perspectives.* Hawthorne, NY: Aldine de Gruyter, pp. 288–289.)

Some **nontraditional** and **contemporary family** structures are becoming more common and are generally accepted by society. Other arrangements are still regarded as unacceptable or even dangerous to society. Table 22–1 lists some of the more common nontraditional and contemporary family structures.

The approach used by Scanzoni and colleagues (1989) is to consider the **primary relationship** of two or more persons interacting in a continuing manner within the greater environment. This primary relationship encompasses all the possible family structures. In 1981, Stein suggested the idea of a "life spiral," rather than a life cycle, to describe the fluctuations of contemporary nontraditional families. The spiral more realistically depicts the fluid movement within family structures than does a cycle, which suggests continuous linear movement along a path. Traditional functions and structures of the family continue to evolve as new combinations of people live together and consider themselves a "family."

One of the most common nontraditional family structures is the single-parent family headed by a woman. Sometimes, single women choose to adopt or have children without being married. More often, an unplanned pregnancy without marriage creates this family unit. Statistics indicate that single-parent families are being headed increasingly by teenagers, some of whom become pregnant while in junior high school. Among teens 15 to 19 years old, 1 in 10 becomes pregnant each year, resulting in 1,100,000 pregnancies annually (U. S. Statistical Abstract, 2001). The implications for the role of the community health nurse are greatest with this population. For example, nurses work with young teens through schools or clinics to ensure healthy pregnancies and to teach parenting skills to the youthful parents and grandparenting skills to the teen's parents. Nurses can also ensure that the infant receives immunizations and primary health care services as needed and can provide family planning information to the new parents. On a broader scale, community health nurses collaborate with other professionals to make sure that the community has resources for all levels of prevention, focusing on primary prevention.

Many adult couples form a family alliance outside of marriage or in a private ceremony not legally recognized as marriage. **Cohabitating couples** may range from young adults living together to an elderly couple sharing their lives outside of marriage to avoid tax penalties or inheritance issues. Cohabitating couples may be heterosexual or homosexual; they may or may not share a sexual relationship. In some instances, these couples have their own biologic or adopted children.

Another nontraditional family form is the **commune family**, a group of unrelated couples who are monogamous (married or committed to one person) but who live together and collectively rear their children. Perhaps more popular in the 1960s and 1970s, this type of family may presently exist among people with similar life-views or spiritual beliefs. A **group-marriage family** involves several adults who share a common household and consider that all are married to one another; they share everything, including sex and child rearing. Group-marriage families usually center on a patriarch who designates responsibilities and dictates to the other members some religious or social ideology. The Branch Davidians, who lived together outside of Waco, Texas, until their compound was destroyed by fire in 1993, were a tragic example of this family type.

A **group-network family** is made up of unrelated nuclear families that are bound by a common set of values such as a religious system. These families live close to one another and share goods, services, and child-rearing responsibilities. Some commune and group-network families select one of their members, usually a man, to be their leader or head.

Many children are removed from their homes of origin because of abuse, violence, or neglect. In most communities, these children are housed with families known as **foster families**. These families take a variety of forms, but all foster families have had formal training to accept unrelated children into their homes on a temporary basis, while the children's parents receive the help necessary to reunify the original family. Although this arrangement is not ideal, most foster families provide safe and loving homes for these children in transition. Often foster children have emotional and physical health problems, and they may never have experienced the positive structure that foster families provide. These problems, which can cause stress for everyone involved, are typically ones that the community health nurse can help to solve. In 1999, the state of California appropriated $2.48 million to provide pub-

lic health nursing expertise so that the health care needs of children in foster care could be effectively met. State funds were matched (25%/75%) with federal funds, making a total of $9.9 million available for health promotion of foster children. The nurses are located at county welfare offices but are hired, funded, and supervised by local health departments (Department of Social Services, 1999).

Some families, because of lack of marketable skills, negative economic changes, or chronic mental health problems including substance abuse, find themselves without permanent shelter. **Homeless families** are increasing in numbers, and their characteristics are changing. "Each year of this decade, homeless service providers have reported that single women with dependent children are the fastest growing segment of the homeless population, at approximately 20%" (Gillis & Singer, 1997, p. 30). The homeless population is also increasingly made up of nuclear families. The community health nurse may provide services to shelters or drop-in clinics frequented by the homeless. Because this population is increasing, it has many implications for the nurse.

A destructive form of "family" that occurs in many cities is gangs. **Gangs** are formed by young people who are searching for emotional ties and turn to one another as a substitute for an absent or dysfunctional family. Gang members consider themselves family; they rely on one another and the group for support that they do not receive from their families of origin. Obviously, gangs are a dysfunctional and destructive form of family. Typically, members are drawn into drugs and violence; frequent injury, abuse, and even death to gang members, their associates, and innocent bystanders may be the result. Gangs are discussed in more detail in Chapter 20. Nurses who serve urban areas may be working with families and groups who are involved with gangs, and they should be prepared to deal with the issues that gangs create.

Implications for the Community Health Nurse

The variety of family structures raises three important issues for consideration. First, community health nurses can no longer hold to a myth that idealizes the traditional nuclear family. They must be prepared to work with all types of families and accept them as valid. Unless the community health nurse is able to accept the full array of family lifestyles and address the special problems and needs of each, she or he may not be able to help the family and may even create additional problems.

Second, the structure of an individual's family may change several times over a lifetime. A girl may be born into a kin-network, shift to a nuclear family when her parents move, and become part of a single-parent family when her parents are divorced. As she matures, she may become a single adult living alone, then become a part of a cohabitating couple. Still later, she may marry and have children in a nuclear family. For the individual, each family form involves changes in roles, interaction patterns, socialization processes, and links with external resources. The community health nurse must learn to address clients' needs throughout these life changes, equipping people with the skills needed to deal with the inevitability of changing structures.

Finally, each type of family structure creates different issues and problems that, in turn, influence a family's ability to perform basic functions. Each particular structure determines the kind of support needed from nursing or other human service systems (Eliopoulos, 2001). A single adult living alone may lack companionship or a sense of being needed by other family members. A kin-network family provides extended family support and security but may have problems with power distribution and decision making. An unmarried couple raising a child may be parenting well but may feel isolated from married couples in the community; they may need more peer support and socialization. Variations in structure create variations in family strengths and needs, an important consideration for community health nurses. Display 22–2 lists additional facts about families in America.

FAMILY FUNCTIONS

Families in every culture throughout history have engaged in similar functions: families always have produced children,

DISPLAY 22–2

Facts About Families in America

- On any given night in the United States, there are 500,000 to 600,000 homeless men, women, and children (Gillis & Singer, 1997).
- Some 500,000 children go missing each year.
- More than 3 million children live with their grandparents as the primary care providers.
- Approximately 500,000 children are in foster homes.
- Ten percent of girls between 15 and 19 years of age get pregnant each year, producing 1,100,000 pregnancies annually (U. S. Statistical Abstract, 2001).
- There are 5 million migrant farmworkers in the United States, with an infant mortality rate 2.5 times higher than the national average; a life expectancy of 49 years, compared with the national average of 75 years; and a parasitic infection rate 11 to 59 times higher than in the general population (Sandhaus, 1998).
- Ten percent of the population has significant problems related to substance abuse (Reilly, 1998).
- At least 4% of U. S. households include three generations; approximately 78,000 homes include four generations (Cohn, 2001).
- In California, gay adoptions, or "second-parent" adoptions, number 10,000 (Kravets, 2003).

physically maintained their members, protected their health, encouraged their education or training, given emotional support and acceptance, and provided supportive and nurturing care during illness. Some societies have experimented with separation of these functions, allocating activities such as child care, socialization, or social control to a larger group. The Israeli kibbutz and Chinese commune are examples. In American society, certain social institutions help perform some aspects of traditional family functions. Schools, for example, help socialize children; professionals supervise health care; and religious organizations influence values.

Six functions are typical of American families today and are essential for maintenance and promotion of family health: (1) providing affection, (2) providing security, (3) instilling identity, (4) promoting affiliation, (5) providing socialization, and (6) establishing controls (Duvall & Miller, 1985). These tasks help promote the growth and development of family members. Understanding these functions and how well individual families provide them enables the community health nurse to work effectively with each family at its level of functioning.

Providing Affection

The family functions to give members affection and emotional support. In Western societies, love brings couples together. In some other cultures, affection comes after marriage. Continued affection creates an atmosphere of nurturance and care for all family members that is necessary for health, development, and survival. It is common knowledge that infants require love to thrive. Indeed, human beings of any age require love as sustenance for growth and find it most often in the family. Families, unlike many other social groups, are bound by affectionate ties, the strength of which determines family happiness and closeness. Consider how sharing of gifts on a holiday or loving concern for a sick member draws a family together.

Positive sexual identity and sexual fulfillment are also influenced by a loving atmosphere. Early students of the family emphasized sexual access and procreation as basic family functions. It is now recognized that families exist not only to regulate the sex drive and perpetuate the species, but also to sustain life and foster human potential through a strong affectional climate.

Providing Security and Acceptance

Families meet their members' physical needs by providing food, shelter, clothing, health care, and other necessities; in so doing, they create a secure environment. Members need to know that these basics will be available and that the family is committed to providing them.

The stability of the family unit also gives members a sense of security. The family offers a safe retreat from the competition of the outside world and provides a place where its members are accepted for themselves. They can learn, make mistakes, and grow in a secure environment. Where else does a toddler, after repeated falls, receive the encouragement to keep trying to walk; or a child, teased by a bully, regain his courage; or a parent, feeling burned out by a job, find comfort and renewal? The dependability of the family unit promotes confidence and self-assurance among its members. This contributes to their mental and emotional health and equips them with the skills necessary to cope with the outside world.

Instilling Identity and Satisfaction

The family functions to give members a sense of social and personal identity. Like a mirror, the family reflects back to its members a picture of who they are and how valuable they are to others. Positive reflections provide the individual with a sense of satisfaction and worth such as that experienced by a girl when her family applauds her efforts in a swim meet or by a boy whose family praises the bird house he builds in Cub Scouts. Needs fulfillment in the home determines satisfaction in the outside world; it particularly affects other interpersonal relationships and career choices. Roles learned within the family also give members a sense of identity. A boy growing up and learning his family's expectations for the male role quickly develops a sense of the kind of person he must strive to be; often, he is expected to be strong, competitive, successful, and unemotional. As a girl grows up, she often learns what is expected of her from her mother: to defer her needs to those of the family, be flexible and nurturing, and have homemaking skills. In other families, all children may have equal expectations of achievement and success. Families influence their members' positions in society by instilling values and goals. For some families, the emphasis may be on higher education; for others, it may be to work at a skill or trade. Still other families may be influenced by religious or political affiliations. Whatever the family influence, it is certain to shape each member's identity.

Promoting Affiliation and Companionship

The family functions to give members a sense of belonging throughout life. Because families provide associational bonds and group membership, they help satisfy their members' needs for belonging. Each person knows that he or she is integral—that he or she belongs—to the family. However, the quality of a family's communication influences its closeness. If communication patterns are effective, then affiliation ties are strong and needs for belonging are met. One family handles conflict over financial expenditures, for instance, by discussing differences and making compromises; this promotes affiliation. In another family, financial conflicts go unacknowledged; members keep spending selfishly and never discuss compromises.

The family, unlike other social institutions, involves permanent relationships. Long after friends from school, the old neighborhood, work, or the religious center have come and gone, there is still the family. The family provides its members with affiliation and fellowship that remain unbroken by distance or time. Even if scattered across the country, family members gather to support one another and to share a holiday, wedding, graduation, or funeral. It is to the family that its members turn in times of happiness, tragedy, or need. This family affiliation remains a resource for life.

Providing Socialization

The family functions to socialize the young. Families transmit their culture—their values, attitudes, goals, and behavior patterns—to their members. Members, socialized into a way of life that reflects and preserves the family's cultural heritage, pass that heritage on, in turn, to the next generation. From infancy on, children learn to control their bowels, eat with utensils, dress themselves, manage emotions, and behave according to sociocultural prescriptions for their age and sex. Through this process, members also learn their roles in the family. Lifestyle, food preferences, relationships with other people, ideas about child rearing, and attitudes about religion, abortion, equal rights, or euthanasia are all strongly influenced by the family. Although experiences outside the family also have a strong influence, they are filtered through the perceptions acquired during early socialization.

The socialization process also influences the degree of independence experienced by growing children. Some families release their maturing members by degrees, preparing them gradually but steadily for adult roles. Other families promote dependent roles and find release painful and difficult.

Establishing Controls

The family functions to maintain social control. Families maintain order through establishment of social controls both within the family and between family members and outsiders. Conduct of members is controlled by the family's definition of acceptable and unacceptable behaviors. From minor etiquette rules such as keeping elbows off the table to larger issues such as standards of home cleanliness, appropriate attire, children's behavior toward adults, or a teenager's curfew, the family imposes limits. It then maintains those limits by a system of rewards for conformity and punishments for violations. Children growing up in a family quickly learn what is "right" and what is "wrong" by family standards. Gradually, family control shifts to self-control as members learn to discipline their own behaviors; later on, they adopt or modify many of the same standards to use with their own children.

Division of labor is another aspect of the family's control function. Families allocate various roles, responsibilities, and tasks to their members in order to ensure the provision of income, household management, child care, and other essentials. Families also regulate the use of internal and external resources. The family identifies and directs the use of internal resources, such as member abilities, financial income, or material assets. For instance, if a man has artistic skills, he may be chosen to landscape the yard; if a woman has mechanical aptitude, she may be designated to repair appliances. One family may choose to drive an old car, rather than buy a new one, in order to spend more on entertainment.

Families also determine the external resources used by their members. Some families take advantage of the religious, health, and social services available to them in the community. They seek regular medical care, encourage their children to use the public library, become involved in religious activities, or join a bowling league. Other families, either because they do not know about potential external resources or because they do not recognize those resources as having any value, limit their members' use of them.

FAMILY LIFE CYCLE

Many of the characteristics and defined developmental stages of individual growth also apply to families. For example, it is known that families, while maintaining themselves as entities, change continuously. Families inevitably grow and develop as the individuals within them mature and adapt to the demands of successive life changes. A family's composition, set of roles, and network of interpersonal relationships change with the passage of time (Friedman, Bowden, & Jones, 2002). Family structures, too, vary with each stage of the family life cycle.

Consider the following example. The Jordans, a young married couple, concentrated on learning their respective roles of husband and wife and building a mutually satisfying marriage. With the birth of their first child, Scott, the family composition and relationships changed and role transitions occurred. The Jordans were not only husband and wife but also father, mother, and son; the family had added three new roles. Within the next 4 years, two daughters, Lisa and Tammy, were born. The introduction of each new member not only increased family size but also significantly reorganized family living. As Duvall and Miller (1985) pointed out, no two children are ever born into precisely the same family. The children entered school; Mrs. Jordan returned to work as a florist; and soon, Scott was leaving for college. The Jordans, like every family, were moving through a predictable and sequential pattern of stages known as the *family life cycle*. Community nurses who are knowledgeable about this cycle can provide anticipatory guidance to families. For instance, while teaching prenatal care to a pregnant teen, the nurse can help the soon-to-be mother anticipate the responsibility and costs of raising her child by helping her calculate child care needs that must be met while she finishes school. The nurse can suggest that she figure out the monthly costs of breast feeding versus buying formula; disposable diapers versus cloth or a diaper service; and the clothing, equipment, and medical costs of infant care. When working with the middle-aged parents of a brain-injured adult son living at home, the nurse can discuss what arrangements the parents have made for their son's care after they are older and unable to provide care themselves, or after one or both of them die.

Stages of the Family Life Cycle

There are two broad stages in the family life cycle: one of *expansion* as new members are added and roles and relationships are increased, and one of *contraction* as family members leave to start lives of their own or age and die. Within this framework of the expanding-contracting family are more specific phases, such as launching of children and retirement of parents. In some families, expansion and contraction are repeated as various members are added, return home with their children and perhaps a partner, or leave home permanently.

Family Developmental Tasks

To progress through the stages of the life cycle, a family must carry out its basic functions and the developmental tasks associated with those functions. Unlike individual developmental tasks, which are specific to each age level, family developmental tasks are ongoing throughout the life cycle. All families, for instance, must provide for the physical needs of their members at every stage. The manner and degree to which each function is carried out varies depending on how well members accomplish individual developmental tasks and meet the demands of each particular stage. Physical maintenance, for example, is affected by the parents' ability to accept responsibility and procure the necessary resources to provide food, clothing, and shelter for their children. At early stages, children are dependent on their parents for meeting these needs; at the school, teenage, and launching stages, children may increasingly contribute to home management and family income. The responsibility for these tasks shifts from just the parents to other family members as well.

Some functions require greater emphasis at certain stages. Socialization, for example, consumes much of a family's time during the early years of child development. These same functions and their associated developmental tasks can be further broken down into actions specific to certain stages. While carrying out its function of maintaining controls, a family sets clearly defined limits for children at the preschool stage: "Do not cross the street." "You may have dessert only after you finish your vegetables." "Bedtime is at 8 o'clock." During the school stage, control activities may center on allocating responsibilities and division of labor within the family: "Feed the dog." "Clean your room." "Take out the trash." When a family reaches the teenage stage, its control function increasingly focuses on the relationships between family members and outsiders. The family may regulate some activities by setting limits: "Be home by midnight." In areas such as moral conduct, controls may involve family values and therefore may be more subtle. A family at this stage must recognize the need for young people to assume increasing responsibility for their own behavior and acknowledge its own diminishing control over members who are exploring independence. Duvall and Miller (1985) described these activities as "stage-critical" family developmental tasks. Sample community health nursing actions with the family at different stages are presented in Table 22–2.

EMERGING FAMILY PATTERNS

Up to this point, the discussion of the family life cycle has focused primarily on the nuclear family. Because the nurse encounters many nuclear families in community health, the family life cycle provides a useful means of analyzing their growth and development.

Because of gradual changes in American society, community health nurses face increasing numbers of adolescent unmarried mothers, gay and lesbian families, blended families, elderly couples, and individuals living alone. They need to know the impact that emerging family patterns have on society and available resources. To be effective, nurses must equip themselves with an appropriate knowledge base to provide needed services.

Adolescent Unmarried Parents

Teen parenthood is an important social issue with distinct medical and nursing ramifications. Teens are still undergoing emotional development themselves. They have limited

TABLE 22–2

Selected Stage-Critical Family Developmental Tasks

Stage of Family Life Cycle	Family Position	Stage-Critical Family Developmental Tasks	Role of the Community Health Nurse
Forming a partnership	Female partner Male partner	Establishing a mutually satisfying relationship	Interact with family where they are at
Childbearing	Partner-mother Partner-father Infant child(ren)	Adjusting to pregnancy and the promise of parenthood Fitting into the kin network Having and adjusting to infants, and encouraging their development Establishing a satisfying home for both parents and infant(s)	Assist them in developing strong relationships
Preschool-age	Partner-mother Partner-father Child, siblings	Adapting to the critical needs and interests of preschool children in stimulating, growth-promoting ways Coping with energy depletion and lack of privacy as parents	Assist in preparing for family expansion through education and anticipatory guidance
School-age	Partner-mother Partner-father Child, siblings	Fitting into the community of school-age families in constructive ways Encouraging children's educational achievement	Encourage time for each other as adults in a relationship separate from parenting role
Teenage	Partner-mother Partner-father Child, siblings	Balancing freedom with responsibility as teenagers mature and emancipate themselves Establishing outside interests and careers as growing parents	Provide anticipatory guidance for the school-age children as they grow into adulthood
Launching center	Partner-mother-grandmother Partner-father-grandfather Child, sibling, aunt or uncle	Releasing young adults into work, military service, college, marriage, etc., with appropriate rituals and assistance Maintaining a supportive home base	Provide anticipatory guidance for the contracting family as children leave home
Middle-aged parents	Partner-mother-grandmother Partner-father-grandfather	Rebuilding the relationship Maintaining kin ties with older and younger generations	Prepare adults for grandparenting role
Aging family members	Widow or widower Partner-mother-grandmother Partner-father-grandfather	Adjusting to retirement Coping with bereavement and living alone Closing the family home or adapting it to aging	Assist aging adults with emotional and financial security as they approach retirement Prepare the aging adults with ways to cope with the losses of old age, including changes in space, work, health, status, and loss of friends and family members

parenting skills and need a tremendous amount of education and support. Even with much media attention, availability of family planning methods, and a social environment open to discussing sexuality and pregnancy, teen pregnancy rates have remained high, especially among teens of color and those in lower socioeconomic situations.

Infants born to teen mothers are at risk for low birth weight, developmental delay, and death before 1 year of age. The infant mortality rate among mothers younger than 15 years of age is twice as high as for women ages 20 to 24 years, and 20% higher among teens ages 15 to 19 years than for women in their 20s (U. S. Department of Health and Human Services, 2000). In addition, children born to teen mothers face high rates of poverty, educational underachievement, and inadequate health care.

Teen fathers are often left out of the bevy of services that communities provide for the teen mother and infant. However, paternal involvement contributes positively to the physical, social, and cognitive development of children. Children with absent fathers are at increased risk for behavioral difficulties and poor academic performance. A father who is emotionally supportive of the mother and provides child care and financial support directly and indirectly affects the well-being of his child.

With so many high-risk factors for pregnant teens and their children, it is imperative that community health nurses be knowledgeable about needed services, available resources, and the accessibility of each. In addition, because of the high-risk nature of teen pregnancy, prevention should be a priority. Nurses must collaborate in caregiving with other professionals and key players in teens' lives to provide the supportive services that young families need.

Gay and Lesbian Families

Another emerging family pattern is the gay or lesbian family. Whether the unions between two same-sex individuals are legitimate in the eyes of the law (such civil unions are legal in some states) or are based on strong emotional attachments without legal sanction, gay and lesbian families may include natural children from previous heterosexual relationships, artificial insemination, or adoption (Kravets, 2003).

This emerging family pattern is not as numerically significant as adolescent or blended families, but it is increasing. Community health nurses may provide services to these clients in many communities. It is important to recognize that much progress has been made in accepting people with values and beliefs different from those of the mainstream. However, pervasive homophobia and heterosexism continue to exist in our society (Kravets, 2003; Silvestre, 2001). Nurses must confront and set aside their own biases in order to provide nonjudgmental and comprehensive care to these emerging families.

Gay and lesbian families have all the fears and concerns regarding parenting that any family a community health nurse visits may have. In addition, they experience the stress that accompanies being stigmatized by much of society. The nurse can become a valued resource for the family. Through education and anticipatory guidance, the nurse can assist the parents to successfully navigate the growth and developmental stages of their children, as well as the varied issues faced by families.

Divorced and Blended Families

Divorce and remarriage are more frequent occurrences today than in previous generations. Divorces have gone from fewer than 20% of all marriages in the 1960s to almost 50% in 2000 (U. S. Statistical Abstract, 2001). It is estimated that 40% of all children will experience living with divorced or single parents before they reach adulthood (Coleman et al., 1998).

Adjusting to divorce involves a series of transitions and reorganizations for all family members. For children, it may require coping with a new geographic location and a new school, as well as adjusting to changes in mental and physical health of family members. Children must adjust to a single-parent household and, possibly, to remarriage and the addition of new family members (Thompson, 1998). In addition to the normal growth and developmental changes, children of divorce face (1) an absent father or mother, (2) interparental conflict, (3) economic distress, (4) parent adjustment, (5) multiple life stressors, and (6) short-term crisis.

Not all divorced adults stay single. Most remarry or cohabitate with another adult who may or may not have children. This new couple may have children from their union, creating an even more complex family. Merged or blended families require considerable adjustment and relearning of roles, tasks, communication patterns, and relationships (Friedman, Bowden, & Jones, 2002).

There are identifiable phases that occur in divorce, remarriage, and the blending of families; each phase has its own emotional transitions and developmental issues. Table 22–3 shows the phases of a divorce, and Table 22–4 shows the phases of remarriage and blending families.

Because this emerging family pattern has become so prominent in such a short period, it is very possible that the community health nurse is familiar with this pattern or lives in such a family. Nursing skills that are needed when working with divorced or blended families include the ability to listen and be empathic, as well as a nonjudgmental attitude. The nurse can be a rich resource for the family. Support groups for adults and children are excellent resources and provide invaluable services at a time of emotional instability in the family. Peer support groups for children and adolescents and support from within the schools should be used, if available, or started if they do not exist. The community health nurse can have a significant role in community-wide planning if there are services that are needed but unavailable.

Older Adults

Elderly individuals are the fastest growing segment of the population. It is estimated that this group will represent 20% of the population by 2030 (Miller, 1999). There are 76 mil-

T A B L E 22–3

When Families Divorce

Phase	Emotional Responses	Transitional Issues
1. Stressor leading to marital differences	Reveal the fact that the marriage has major problems	Accepting fact that marriage has major problems
2. Decision to divorce	Accepting the inability to resolve marital differences	Accepting one's own contribution to the failed marriage
3. Planning the dissolution of the family system	Negotiating viable arrangements for all members within the system	Cooperating on custody visitation, and financial issues Informing and dealing with extended family members and friends
4. Separation	Mourning loss of intact family Working on resolving attachment to spouse	Develop coparental arrangements/relationships Restructure living arrangements Adapt to living apart Realign relationship with extended family and friends Begin to rebuild own social network
5. Divorce	Continue working on emotional recovery by overcoming hurt, anger or guilt	Giving up fantasies of reunion Staying connected with extended families Rebuild and strengthen own social network
6. Post-divorce	Separate feeling about ex-spouse from parenting role Prepare self for possibility of changes in custody as child(ren) get older, be open to their needs Risk developing a new intimate relationship	Make flexible and generous visitation arrangements for child(ren) and non-custodial parent and extended family members Deal with possibilities of changing custody arrangements as child(ren) get older Deal with child(ren)s reaction to parents establishing relationships with new partners

T A B L E 22–4

Remarriage and Blending Families

Phases	Emotional Responses	Developmental Issues
1. Meeting new people	Allowing for the possibility of developing a new intimate relationship	Dealing with child(ren) and exfamily members reactions to a parent "dating"
2. Entering a new relationship	Completing an "emotional recovery" from past divorce Accepting one's fears about developing a new relationship Working on feeling good about what the future may bring	Recovery from loss of marriage is adequate Discovering what you want from a new relationship Working on openness in a new relationship
3. Planing a new marriage	Accepting one's fears about the ambiguity and complexity of entering a new relationship such as: New roles and responsibilities Boundaries; space, time, and authority Affective issues: guilt, loyalty, conflicts, unresolvable past hurts	Recommitment to marriage and forming a new family unit. Dealing with stepchild(ren) as custodial or non-custodial parent Planning for maintenance of coparental relationships with ex-spouses Planning to help child(ren) deal with fears, loyalty conflicts and memberships in two systems Realignment of relationships with ex-family to include new spouse and child(ren)
4. Remarriage and blending of families	Final resolution of attachment to previous spouse Acceptance of new family unit with different boundaries	Restructuring family boundaries to allow for new spouse or stepparent Realignment of relationships to allow inter-mingling of systems Expanding relationships to include all new family members Sharing family memories and histories to enrich members lives

lion baby boomers heading toward maturity, and our society is already experiencing the beginning of this "age wave" (Dychtwald, 1997).

Most elders live independently well into their 80s and maintain healthy contacts with family and friends. Others feel isolated because of chronic health problems that limit mobility, thereby reducing or eliminating the ability to interact or contribute meaningfully in society. Aging is a relatively new phenomenon, and many aging families do not understand or practice the appropriate stage-specific functions and developmental tasks that would help them adjust and experience positive aging (Miller, 1999).

The community health nurse needs to understand the complex dynamics of such situations and offer support and encouragement as family members work through these problems. Often, a nurse serves an entire community of elders, in a senior apartment complex, an assisted living center, or a mobile home community, for whom maintaining wellness is the focus. Keeping physically active, eating healthy meals regularly, receiving appropriate medical care and immunizations, and establishing and maintaining social contacts are some of the tasks elders should focus on to stay healthy well into old age. These are some of the areas in which the community health nurse can intervene as teacher, counselor, and clinician (Gavan, 2003). Reaching 100 years of age is not an unusual occurrence today, and more people will live to see advanced age in the 21st century.

SUMMARY

The family as the unit of service has received increasing emphasis in nursing over the years. Today, family nursing has an important place in nursing practice, particularly in community health nursing. Its significance results from recognition that the family itself must be a focus of service, that family health and individual health strongly influence each other, and that family health affects community health. A community health nurse's effectiveness in working with families depends on an understanding of family theory and characteristics, in addition to changing family structures.

Every family on the globe is unique; its needs and strengths are different from those of every other family. At the same time, each family is alike because of certain shared universal characteristics. Five of these universals have particular significance for community health nursing: every family is a small social system, has its own cultural values and rules, has structure, has certain basic functions, and moves through stages in its life cycle.

Every family is a small social system. The members within a family are interdependent; what one does affects the others and, ultimately, influences total family health. Families, as social systems, set and maintain boundaries that unite them and preserve their autonomy, while also differentiating them from others. Because these boundaries are semipermeable, families engage in an input–output energy exchange with external resources. Families are equilibrium-seeking, adaptive systems

that strive to adjust to internal and external life changes. Like other systems, families are goal directed. They exist for the purpose of promoting their members' development.

Every family has its own culture, its own set of values, and rules for operation. Family values influence member beliefs and behaviors. These same values prescribe the types of roles that each member assumes. A family's culture also determines its power distribution and decision-making patterns.

Every family has a structure that can be categorized as either traditional or nontraditional (contemporary). The most common traditional family structure is the nuclear family, consisting of husband, wife, and one or more children living together. Other traditional structures include husband and wife living as a couple alone, single-parent families, single-adult families, multigenerational families, kin-networks, and blended families. Nontraditional family structures incorporate many family forms, some not all of which are readily accepted by society. These variations include commune families, group marriages, and group networks. Unmarried single parent families, unmarried gay or straight couples living together with or without children, and umarried older adults living together are examples of emerging nontraditional family structures. As less typical families become more common, they receive more recognition and acceptance. These variant family structures remind us that the nuclear family is now in the minority, that people experience many family structures during their lifetimes, and that a family's ability to perform its basic functions is influenced by its structure.

Every family has certain basic functions: (1) to provide members with affection and emotional support; (2) to promote security by providing members with an accepting, stable environment in which physical needs are met; (3) to provide members with a sense of social and personal identity and influence their placement in the social order; (4) to provide members with affiliation, a sense of belonging; (5) to socialize members by teaching basic values and attitudes that determine behavior; and (6) to establish social controls to maintain order. Community health nurses use this information to assess a family's functioning. This information enables the nurse to work with the family and assist in improving the quality of its functioning.

Every family moves through stages in its life cycle. Families develop in two broad stages: a period of expansion when new members and roles are added, and a period of contraction when members leave. Some families demonstrate a spiraling pattern with repeated expansion and contraction.

There are emerging family patterns that influence the role of the community health nurse. The single adolescent parent in particular needs the community health nurse's knowledge of family developmental theory. Gay and lesbian families with children may also have special needs. More complex interaction patterns and living arrangements are created by divorce, remarriage, the blending of families, and the unique relationships these arrangements create. Older adults are living longer and will soon make up 20% of the population. The multiple needs of elders from age 65 to 100 years or older are more varied than those of any other population group. Community health nurses see many more families today in one of these four emerging family patterns. Understanding their different needs will help the nurse provide appropriate services.

ACTIVITIES TO PROMOTE CRITICAL THINKING

1. Within a small group of your peers, individually define *family* and then compare each of your definitions. How alike and how different is each definition? What in each person's background contributes to the differences in the definitions? Was each of the peers in nursing? If not, how did that contribute to any differences in the definitions?

2. Analyze two families (other than your own) that you know well, one traditional and the other nontraditional (contemporary), and answer the following questions:
   a. If the major breadwinner in this family became permanently disabled and unable to work or lost his or her income, how would the family most likely respond immediately and in the long term?
   b. What are some of this family's rules for operation and the values underlying the rules?
   c. Structurally, what kind of family is this?
   d. What are the strongest and weakest functions performed by this family, and why do you think this is so?
   e. In what developmental stage is this family, and how does it affect their functioning?

3. Talk with the members of a blended family and discuss with each member his or her relationships with stepchildren or siblings, half-siblings, and stepparents. What problems can they identify? What problems have they overcome? What do they see as the positive elements of the union?

4. Gay and lesbian couples often seek parenting opportunities. How do you feel about this? What makes you feel this way? What are the positive and negative aspects of a child's being raised by a homosexual couple?

5. Use the Internet and find information at various Web sites on family structural patterns in other countries. Many families in developing and some industrialized countries live in clans, tribes, groups, and kin-networks. In what countries do you find such family structures? What are the benefits and drawbacks of such systems?

REFERENCES

Barker, P. (1998). *Basic family therapy* (4th ed.). New York: Oxford University Press.

Bell, J.M., & Wright, L.M. (1993). Flaws in family nursing education. In G. Wegner & R. Alexander (Eds.), *Readings in family nursing* (pp. 390–394). Philadelphia: Lippincott.

Barnes, S.L. (2001). Stressors and strengths: A theoretical and practical examination of nuclear, single-parent, and augmented African American families. *Families in Society: The Journal of Contemporary Human Service, 82*(5), 449–460.

Cohn, D. (2001, September 7). 4% of U. S. homes are multigenerational: Culture, finances dictate lifestyles. *Washington Post,* p. A8.

Coleman, M., Ganong, L.H., Killian, T.S., & McDaniel, A.K. (1998). Mom's house? Dad's house? Attitudes toward physical custody changes. *Families in Society: The Journal of Contemporary Human Services, 79*(2), 112–122.

Department of Social Services. (1999). *New foster care public health nurse program in county welfare department.* Sacramento, CA: Health and Human Services Agency.

Dreikurs, R. (1964). *Children: The challenge.* New York: Meredith.

Duvall, E.M., & Miller, B. (1985). *Marriage and family development* (6th ed.). New York: Harper & Row.

Dychtwald, K. (1997). The 10 physical, social, spiritual, economic, and political crises the boomers will face as they age in the 21st century. *Critical Issues in Aging, 1,* 11–13.

Eliopoulos, C. (2001). *Gerontological nursing* (5th ed.). Philadelphia: Lippincott Williams & Wilkins.

Fitch, M.I., Bunston, T., & Elliot, T. (1999). When mom's sick: Changes in a mother's role and in the family after her diagnosis of cancer. *Cancer Nursing, 22*(1), 58–63.

Friedman, M.M., Bowden, V.R., & Jones, E. (2003). *Family nursing: Research, theory, and practice* (5th ed.). Upper Saddle River, NJ: Prentice-Hall.

Gavan, C.S. (2003). Successful aging families: A challenge for nurses. *Holistic Nursing Practice, 17*(1), 1–18.

Gillis, L.M. & Singer, J. (1997). Breaking through the barriers: Healthcare for the homeless. *Journal of Nursing Administration, 27*(6), 30–34.

Hanson, S.M.H. (Ed.). (2001). *Family health care nursing: Theory, practice, and research* (2nd ed). Philadelphia: F.A. Davis.

Kravets, D. (2003, May 8). High court weighs gay adoptions. *The Fresno Bee,* p. B3.

Leininger, M.M. (2001). *Culture, care, diversity, and universality: A theory of nursing.* New York: NLN Press.

Marciano, T. (1991). A postscript on wider families: Traditional family assumptions and cautionary notes. *Marriage and Family Review, 17,* 159–163.

Miller, C.A. (1999). *Nursing care of older adults: Theory and practice* (3rd ed.). Philadelphia: Lippincott Williams & Wilkins.

Murray, R.B., & Zentner, J.P. (2000). *Health promotion strategies through the life span* (7th ed.). Upper Saddle River, NJ: Prentice-Hall.

Neuman, B. (2001). *The Neuman systems model* (4th ed.). Upper Saddle River, NJ: Prentice-Hall.

Olson, D., McCubbin, H.I., et al. (1983). *Families: What makes them work.* Beverly Hills, CA: Sage.

Pender, N.J. (2001). *Health promotion in nursing practice* (3rd ed.) Upper Saddle River, NJ: Prentice-Hall.

Reilly, C.E. (1998). A satisfaction survey on distance education: A model for educating nurses in the cognitive treatment of patients with addictive disorders. *Journal of Psychosocial Nursing, 36*(7), 38–41.

Riley, M.W., & Riley, J.W. (1996). Generational relations: A future perspective. In T.K. Hareven (Ed.), *Aging and intergenerational relations: Life course and cross-cultural perspectives*. Hawthorne, NY: Aldine de Gruyter.

Sandhaus, S. (1998). Migrant health: A harvest of poverty. *American Journal of Nursing, 98*(9), 52, 54.

Scanzoni, J., Polonko, K., Teachman, J., & Thompson, L. (1989). *The sexual bond: Rethinking family and close relationships*. Newbury Park, CA: Sage.

Silvestre, A.J. (Ed.). (2001). *Lesbian, gay, bisexual, and transgender health issues*. Washington, DC: American Public Health Association.

Spector, R.W. (2000). *Cultural diversity in health and illness* (5th ed.). Upper Saddle River, NJ: Prentice-Hall.

Stein, P.J. (Ed.). (1981). *Single life: Unmarried adults in social context*. New York: St. Martin's.

Thompson, P. (1998). Adolescents from families of divorce: Vulnerability to physiological and psychological disturbances. *Journal of Psychosocial Nursing, 36*(3), 34–39.

United States Department of Commerce. (1998). *Statistical abstract of the United States* (118th ed.). Washington, DC: U. S. Government Printing Office.

United States Department of Health and Human Services. (2000). *Healthy people 2010* (Conference ed., Vols. 1 & 2). Washington, DC: U. S. Government Printing Office.

United States Statistical Abstract. (2001). Retrieved May 5, 2003, from *http://www.census.gov/prod/statistical-abstract-us.html*

SELECTED READINGS

Baris, M.A., Coates, C.A., Duvall, B.B., Garrity, C.B., Johnson, E.T., Lacrosse, E.R. (2001). *Working with high-conflict families of divorce: A guide for professionals*. Northvale, NJ: Jason Aronson.

Denham, S.A. (2002). *Family health: A framework for nursing*. Philadelphia: F.A. Davis.

Erikson, E. (1963). *Childhood and society* (2nd ed.). New York: Norton.

Gottman, J.M., & Notarius, C.I. (2002). Marital research in the 20th century and a research agenda for the 21st century. *Family Process, 41*(2), 159–197.

Havighurst, R.J. (1972). *Developmental tasks and education* (3rd ed.). New York: McKay.

Higgins, P.A., & Moore, S.M. (2000). Levels of theoretical thinking in nursing. *Nursing Outlook, 48*, 179–183.

Im, E., & Meleis, A.I. (2001). An international imperative for gender-sensitive theories in women's health. *Journal of Nursing Scholarship, 33*(4), 309–314.

Linn, R. (2001). *Mature unwed mothers: Narratives of moral resistance*. Norwell, MA: Kluwer Plenum.

Long, M.V., & Martin, P. (2000). Personality, relationship closeness, and loneliness of oldest old adults and their children. *Journal of Gerontological Social Science, 55B*(5), P311–P319.

Lynch, M., & Cicchetti, D. (2002). Links between community violence and the family system: Evidence from children's feelings of relatedness and perceptions of parent behavior. *Family Process, 41*(3), 519–532.

Pan American Health Organization. (2000). *Why should we invest in adolescents?* Washington, DC: Author.

Phipps, M.G., & Sowers, M. (2002). Defining early adolescent childbearing. *American Journal of Public Health, 92*(1), 125–128.

Piaget, J. (1973). *The psychology of intelligence*. Totowa, NJ: Littlefield Adams.

Renpenning, K.M., Taylor, S.G., & Eisenhandler, S.A. (2003). Self-care theory in nursing: Selected papers of Dorothea Orem. New York: Springer.

Scanzoni, J. (1999). *Designing families: The search for self and community in the information age*. Thousand Oaks, CA: Pine Forge.

Spradley, J.P., & McCurdy, D.W. (1989). *Anthropology: The cultural perspective* (2nd ed.). Chicago: Waveland Press.

United States Department of Health and Human Services, Administration on Aging. (2001). *A profile of older Americans: 2001*. Washington, DC: Author.

Wegner, G.D., & Alexander, R.J. (1999). *Readings in family nursing* (2nd ed). Philadelphia: Lippincott Williams & Wilkins.

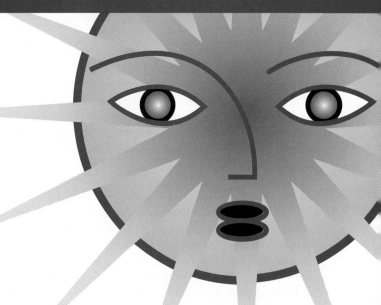

23

Assessment of Families

Learning Objectives

Upon mastery of this chapter, you should be able to:

- Describe the effect of family health on individual health and community health.

- Describe individual and group characteristics of a healthy family.

- Identify five family health practice guidelines.

- Describe three conceptual frameworks that can be used to assess a family.

- Describe the 12 major assessment categories for families.

- List the five basic principles the community health nurse should follow when assessing family health.

Chapter 22 explored the theoretical basis of family formation and the variety of family structures. The next important step in the process of working with families as a unit of service is to develop family assessment skills. This is foundational to the development of a database on which to formulate nursing diagnoses, an essential step before planning, implementation, and evaluation of services can occur.

Assessment is a challenging experience because families are complex and because assessment takes place in the family's environment, where members feel "at home" and the nurse may feel like a stranger. The reverse of this situation is the acute-care setting, in which the nurse may feel at home and the family feels out of place.

Although community health nursing emphasizes the family as a unit of service, a gap exists between family nursing theory, development, and practice (Friedman, Bowden, & Jones, 2003). The problem derives in part from a health care system that fosters individualistic orientation, often to the exclusion of the family. Programs geared to individuals in specific age groups or with specific health problems are numerous. Many third-party payers and reimbursement policies impose limits on the kinds of services funded, most of which are for individuals. Even public health agencies tend to organize services around individuals. In keeping with governmental requirements, agencies keep statistics for specific disease or service categories, a practice that reflects individual rather than family or aggregate orientation. Family-level problem-solving techniques are needed to deal with many important health issues, including health promotion, pregnancy and childbirth, acute life-threatening illness, chronic illness, substance abuse, and terminal illness (Gavan, 2003; Kitzman et al., 2000; Pinelli, 2000; Saunders, 2003). Community health nurses need to focus their practices on families and aggregates, an approach that benefits both individual clients and the community at large.

EFFECTS OF FAMILY HEALTH ON INDIVIDUALS AND COMMUNITIES

The health of each family member affects the other members and contributes to the level of **family health**. For example, a woman whose husband has had a stroke may cope successfully with the resulting physical and emotional demands of his care but may have inadequate reserves for effectively meeting the needs of her children. The level at which a family functions—how well it is able to solve problems and help its members reach their potential—significantly affects the individual's level of health (Early, 2001). A healthy family fosters individual growth and resistance to ill health and sustains members during times of crisis such as serious illness, emotional dilemmas, divorce, or death of a family member. On the other hand, a family with limited coping skills or an underdeveloped capacity for problem solving, self-manage-

ment, or self-care is often unable to promote the potential of its members or assist them in times of need (Barnes, 2001; Donnelly, 2002; Reutter, 1997).

Family health standards and practices also influence each member's health. For instance, many individuals, even as adults, adhere to cultural and family patterns of eating, exercise, and communication. Cultural and family values influence decisions about health services, such as whether a child receives immunizations or has access to preventive measures such as regular visits to the doctor or birth control. Family health patterns also dictate whether members participate in their own health care, follow through, and comply with professional advice. Individuals influence family health, and the family can either obstruct or facilitate individual health. The family, then, becomes an important focus for community health nursing assessment and intervention.

Just as families influence individual health, they also influence the health of communities. Rarely do families live in isolation from one another. Even in the most uncommunicative of neighborhoods, one family's noisy children, another family's trash-littered yard, and another's barking dog all affect the surrounding families. The level at which each family functions determines whether it can participate in the promotion of a healthy community and support other families and groups or whether it will be a liability (Tapia, 1997).

Healthy families influence community health positively. Some families, for example, have become foster parents. Some have temporarily housed Southeast Asian or Cuban refugees and assisted them in finding employment. Others have formed community groups to encourage neighborhood safety and beautification. Many families are regularly involved in church, scouting programs, or various civic activities, such as parent-teacher-student associations, all of which work toward the common good.

Conversely, families with a low level of health have a negative influence on community health. Because they lack the resources to manage their own affairs, they may create problems and even health hazards for others. Garbage left to accumulate in a backyard attracts rats; loaded guns left unsecured may find their way into playmates' hands; abandoned appliances may become death traps for playing children; and children subjected to physical or emotional abuse may lash out at others. Regardless of socioeconomic level, a poorly functioning family may become a drain on community resources and a threat to community health. Consider the large proportion of tax dollars and private funds that go into remedial programs for children with learning and behavioral difficulties caused by problems at home, for adults with mental health problems, for the chemically dependent, and for victims of family violence. Because family health affects the health of other families, groups, and communities, nurses who help families develop and maintain positive health patterns and practices are also promoting community health (Lia-Hoaberg et al., 2001).

CHARACTERISTICS OF HEALTHY FAMILIES

How does the community health nurse determine family health status? Analysis of how basic functions are met does not give a satisfactory picture of a family's health status. More definitive criteria are needed. Although it is difficult to define a "normal" family, studies have provided some standards that characterize a healthy family (Barker, 1998; Thompson, 1998). Over the years, research on families and on family health behavior has produced a growing body of data with which to assess family health.

In looking at families over the years, researchers have found many similar characteristics. Otto (1973) identified characteristics of family unity, loyalty and interfamily cooperation, support and security, role flexibility, and constructive relationships with community. Olson, McCubbin, Barnes, et al. (1983) identified seven major family strengths that are important for family functioning and coping with crises: family pride, family support, cohesion, adaptability, communication, religious orientation, and social support. Becvar and Becvar (1996) listed the following characteristics: (1) a legitimate source of authority that is supported and consistent over time, (2) a stable and consistent system of rules, (3) consistent and regular nurturing behaviors, (4) effective child-rearing practices, (5) stable and well-maintained marriages, (6) a set of agreed-upon goals toward which the family and individuals work, and (7) sufficient flexibility to change in the face of both expected and unexpected stressors. More recently, Parachin (1997) identified six signs of a healthy family: maintaining a spiritual foundation, making the family a top priority, asking for and giving respect, communicating and listening, valuing service to others, and expecting and offering acceptance. Rucibwa, Modeste, & Montgomery (2003) found significant relationships between family characteristics and sexual attitudes and behaviors among Black and Hispanic adolescent males.

This chapter explores six important characteristics of healthy families that consistently emerge in the literature (Becvar & Becvar, 2003; Friedman, Bowden, & Jones 2003; Parachin, 1997):

1. A facilitative process of interaction exists among family members.
2. Individual member development is enhanced.
3. Role relationships are structured effectively.
4. Active attempts are made to cope with problems.
5. There is a healthy home environment and lifestyle.
6. Regular links with the broader community are established.

Healthy Interaction Among Members

Healthy families communicate. Their patterns of interaction are regular, varied, and supportive. Adults communicate with adults, children with children, and adults with children (Anderson & Sabatelli, 2003). These interactions are frequent and assume many forms. Healthy families use frequent verbal communication. They discuss problems, confront each other when angry, share ideas and concerns, and write or call each other when separated. They also communicate frequently through nonverbal means, particularly those families from cultural or subcultural groups that are less verbal. There are innumerable ways to convey feelings and thoughts without words, including smiling encouragingly, embracing warmly, frowning disapprovingly, being available, withdrawing for privacy, doing an unsolicited favor, serving refreshments, and giving a gift. The family that has learned to communicate effectively has members who are sensitive to one another. They watch for cues and verify messages to ensure understanding. This kind of family recognizes and deals with conflicts as they arise. Its members have learned to share and to work collaboratively with each other.

Effective communication is necessary for a family to carry out basic functions. Family members must communicate to demonstrate affection and acceptance, to promote identity and affiliation, and to guide behavior through socialization and social controls. Just as there is a correlation between a high degree of communication and a high degree of effectiveness in organizational functioning, facilitative communication patterns within a family promote the health and development of its members. Healthy families are more likely than unhealthy families to negotiate topics for discussion, use humor, show respect for differences of opinion, and clarify the meaning of one another's communications.

Enhancement of Individual Development

Healthy families are responsive to the needs of individual members and provide the freedom and support necessary to promote each member's growth. If a father in a healthy family loses his job, the family will work to support his ego and help him use his energy constructively to adjust and find new work. The healthy family recognizes and fosters the growing child's need for independence by increasing opportunities for the child to try new things alone. This kind of family can tolerate differences of opinion or lifestyle. Each member is accepted unconditionally, and the right to be an individual is respected. Within an appropriate framework of stability and structure, the healthy family encourages freedom and autonomy for its members (Friedman, Bowden, & Jones, 2003).

Patterns for promoting individual member development vary from one family to another, depending on cultural orientation. The way in which autonomy is expressed in an Italian-American family differs from its expression in a Native American family, yet each family can promote freedom and autonomy. The result is an increase in competence, self-reliance, social skills, intellectual growth, and overall capacity for self-management among family members (Wright & Leahey, 2000) (see Clinical Corner).

CLINICAL CORNER

A FAMILY ASSESSMENT: MEETING HECTOR'S NEEDS

You are a home health nurse working in Smithville. You have been given a referral for a new client, Hector. Hector is being released from the rehabilitation unit of Metropolis Hospital. Although he lives in Smithville, Metropolis Hospital was the only facility willing to accept a Medicaid client with a severe spinal cord injury.

Hector is a 19-year-old Hispanic man who sustained major injury to his spinal cord (T-4 injury) in a motorcycle accident. The injury occurred approximately 6 weeks ago. Hector has been diagnosed as paraplegic with some residual limitation of upper body strength and mobility.

Your job is to facilitate Hector's transition from the hospital to the home environment. You will be teaching Hector and his caregivers about the following:
1. Nutrition and fluid intake
2. Signs and symptoms warranting follow-up
3. Medication administration
4. Bowel and bladder care
5. Skin care
6. Activities of daily living (ADLs), self-care with sensory-motor deficits
7. Safety/injury prevention
8. Community resources
9. Rehabilitative services
10. Anticipatory guidance about grief, anger, and suicidal ideations; sexual function; fear of abandonment, role change, and social isolation; and altered family processes.

Following is a synopsis of information obtained during your initial visit with Hector and his family in their home.

Visit One. Hector lives in a migrant labor camp located on the outskirts of Smithville. His family has resided in the camp for 18 years. Living in the two-bedroom cabin-like home are:
- Hector
- Hector's uncle Manuel (32 years old). Manuel's job is seasonal; he has been offered a temporary job for a much higher salary, working out of state.
- Hector's brother Efran (16 years old). Efran is considering dropping out of high school in order to assist with the care of his family. His goal is to become an auto mechanic. He is fluent in both Spanish and English.
- Manuel's wife Micaela (29 years old). Micaela was a teacher in Mexico. She is extremely supportive of her family. She is concerned about the possibility of another pregnancy but does not believe in the use of birth control.

- Manuel and Micaela's children, Arturo (5 years old) and Jasmin (6 months old). Arturo begins a Head Start Program soon and will be gone for 5 hours each day. Jasmin is a healthy baby; she continues to be breast fed and is thriving at home.
- Hector's 74-year-old paternal grandmother (Abuela), who has recently arrived from Mexico and plans on assisting in Hector's care. Abuela has congestive heart failure and arthritis. She is not a legal resident of the U.S. and is not eligible for medical assistance.

The whereabouts of Hector's mother are unknown; she moved from their village in Mexico shortly after Efran was born. She has remarried and started another family. She has had no contact with Hector or Efran. Hector's father lives in their home village in Mexico. Although he lived in the migrant camp in Smithville for many years, he recently remarried and has two young daughters in Mexico. Hector's father is aware of Hector's injury and has no plans to return to the U.S.

Your ability to speak fluent Spanish has enabled you to solicit the above information. Manuel has provided you with most of the information. He has been very involved in Hector's recovery through daily visits to the rehabilitation unit and frequent discussions with Hector's health care providers. Manuel tells you that "Hector is like a son to me...I have a responsibility to my older brother to watch over his son. My brother watched out for me when I was young...he even left school to work to help support our family." Manuel adds, "We don't have much but we will take care of Hector...we'll all work together."

You begin your discussion by explaining your role as home health nurse. You inform the family about the type of education and interventions you are able to provide. You ask Hector and the family to tell you what they have learned from the health care team at the rehabilitation unit and what plans have been developed by the family to address Hector's medical and psychosocial needs. As you begin the visit you notice that Hector's grandmother is sitting quietly in the corner of the room rocking Jasmin. You learn that Efran is working in the fields. Arturo is in school. Manuel, Micaela, and Abuela are participating in the home visit this morning.

The conversation is as follows.

Nurse: Hector, can you tell me how you feel about being home?

Hector (looks at Micaela): Okay, I guess.

Micaela: He's a little scared, I think. He feels like it's going to be too much for us to deal with.

Nurse (looking at Hector): There's so much happening right now, so much to think about...

Hector: Uh-huh.

CLINICAL CORNER (Continued)

(Hector is maintaining eye contact with Manuel and Micaela only; since this is your initial visit to the home you feel that Hector may be more comfortable in the role of observer.)

Nurse (looking at Manuel and Micaela): Do you have any questions before we begin?

Micaela: They gave us a lot of information at the hospital... I'm most afraid about if the phone doesn't work and Hector needs help. What if something happens to Hector and I can't call anyone? That's the only thing I worry about.

Abuela: If anything happens to him I'll be right here with you, "mija." We can do this, we can take care of Hector if we work together.

Manuel: There is a store with a phone only two blocks away, if you needed to you could call from there. What I want to know is how we can get Hector into school or something that will help him to be around kids his own age. His English is good enough, he even finished high school. He needs to be ready to make a future for himself.

Hector (grins and looks at Manuel): Right, uncle, that is what I want, too.

You continue the conversation by revisiting Micaela's concerns about access to a telephone in case of an emergency. You ask specific questions about her concerns and use this as an opportunity to educate the family about circumstances warranting immediate follow-up. Together you decide that Micaela will develop a list of specific concerns that you will review together at a subsequent visit planned for 2 days from today.

Today's visit consists of:

I. Assessment
  A. Home environment
    1. Safety
    2. ADLs
  B. Knowledge of disease processes
  C. Fluid volume balance
  D. Nutritional resources of family
    1. Food availability
    2. Food preparation
  E. Insurance and financial status
II. Education
  A. Medications
  B. Warning signs and symptoms and appropriate follow-up procedures
  C. Bowel and bladder care
  D. Hygiene prior to and following patient care

The plan for your visit in 2 days includes:

I. Referrals
  A. Community resources
  B. Educational opportunities
  C. Support groups (Spanish speaking)
  D. Peer group opportunities for Hector
II. Assessment
  A. Continuation of above
III. Education
  A. Continuation of above

Questions

1. What is the social structure of this family (traditional versus nontraditional)? Be specific about the type of traditional or nontraditional family system that exists in this scenario.
2. Discuss an example of triangulation in this scenario.
3. What essential functions are present within this family system?
4. What developmental stages appear to have been achieved?
5. What steps will you take in order to empower the family to make their own decisions?
6. List the strengths of the family.
7. Prioritize Hector's issues—medical and psychosocial.
8. Prioritize issues facing the other family members.
9. Identify mutual goals for this family:
   Immediate
   Mid-range
   Long-term
10. What community health nursing interventions will you utilize to achieve these mutual goals?

Effective Structuring of Relationships

Healthy families structure role relationships to meet changing family needs over time (Hanson, 2001). In a stable social context, some families establish member roles and tasks (eg, breadwinner, primary decision-maker, homemaker) that are maintained as workable patterns throughout the life of the family. Families in rural areas, isolated communities, or religious and subcultural groups are more likely than others to retain role consistency, because they face little or no external pressure or need to change. The Amish communities in Pennsylvania and other midwestern states have maintained marked differentiation in family roles for more than 100 years.

In a technologically advanced society such as the United States, most families must adapt their roles to changing family needs created by external forces. As women enter the work force, family roles, relationships, and tasks must change to meet the demands of the new situation. Many husbands assume more homemaking responsibilities; fathers engage in child rearing; children, along with the adults in their families, share decision-making and a more equal distribution of power. The latter may be essential for the survival of a single-parent family in which the children must assume adult responsibilities while the parent works to support the family (Baris et al., 2001).

Changing life cycle stages require alterations in the structure of relationships. The healthy family recognizes members' changing developmental needs and adapts parenting roles, family tasks, and controls to fit each stage (Anderson & Sabatelli, 2003). For example, household chores of increasing complexity and responsibility are assigned as children become capable of handling them. Rules of conduct relax as members learn to govern their own behavior.

Active Coping Effort

Healthy families actively attempt to overcome life's problems and issues. When faced with change, they assume responsibility for coping and seek energetically and creatively to meet the demands of the situation (Becvar & Becvar, 2003; Olson et al., 1983). Coping skills are needed to deal with emotional tragedies such as substance abuse problems, serious illness, or death. If a family member has a substance abuse problem, the family may seek counseling and treatment opportunities involving all family members. If a family member is seriously ill, the family may ask for and accept assistance from extended family members or community health care workers. In the event of a death in the family, receiving consolation and support from one another and from relatives and friends is an important step in the healing process. The healthy family recognizes the need for assistance, accepts help, and pursues opportunities to eliminate or decrease the stressors that affect it.

More frequently, healthy families cope with less dramatic, day-to-day changes. For instance, one family may cope with the increased cost of food by cutting down on meat consumption, substituting other protein foods, and eating less frequently at restaurants. Healthy families are open to innovation, support new ideas, and find ways to solve problems. One family may try to solve the problem of spending too much on transportation by cutting down on daily travel; this may cause additional problems if three members have jobs in different areas of town or need to go to school functions and meetings. Another family, responding to environmental concerns and a personal need for a healthier lifestyle, may explore and arrive at new ways to reach destinations by walking, bicycling, skating, or car-pooling to school or work. Healthy coping may go beyond finding a simple, obvious solution. Members may try to rearrange schedules to avoid frequent trips to regular destinations and plan ahead to avoid last-minute trips to stores. Healthy families actively seek and use a variety of resources to solve problems. They may discover these resources within the family or externally; they engage in self-care. For example, a professional couple, faced with the unaffordable expense of daytime baby-sitting, arranged their work schedules

so that they could share child care during the first 2 years. Later, they joined a cooperative preschool that allowed their child to attend daily but required parental participation only 1 day a week. In another example, a single parent of five children, who was also a full-time nursing student, was able to finance two or three family outings each year by recycling aluminum cans that everyone in the family collected.

Healthy Environment and Lifestyle

Another sign of a healthy family is a healthy home environment and lifestyle. Healthy families create safe and hygienic living conditions for their members. For instance, a healthy family with young children childproofs the home by removing such potential hazards as exposed electric outlets and cleaning solvents from a child's reach. A healthy family with an older adult who is prone to falls installs good lighting and sturdy handrails (Farren, 1999). A healthy home environment is one that is clean and reduces the spread of disease-causing organisms.

A healthy family lifestyle encourages appropriate balance in the lives of its members. In an ideal family, there is activity and rest sufficient for the energy needs of daily living; the diet offered is varied and nutritionally sound; physical activity maintains ideal weight while promoting cardiac health; preventive hygiene habits are taught and followed by family members; emotional and mental health are encouraged through a supportive network of caring others; and family members seek out and use health care services and demonstrate adherence to recommended regimens.

The emotional climate of a healthy family is positive and supportive of growth. Contributing to this healthful emotional climate is a strong sense of shared values, often combined with a strong religious orientation (Olson et al., 1983; Parachin, 1997). A healthy family demonstrates caring, encourages and accepts expression of feelings, and respects divergent ideas. Members can express their individuality in the way they dress or decorate their rooms. The home environment makes family members feel welcome and accepted.

Regular Links With the Broader Community

Healthy families maintain dynamic ties with the broader community. They participate regularly in external groups and activities, often in a leadership capacity. They may join in local politics, participate in a church bazaar, or promote the school's paper drive to raise money for science equipment. They use external resources suited to family needs. For example, a farm family with teenagers, recognizing the importance of peer group influence on adolescents, becomes very active in the local 4-H Club. Another family, in which the father is out of work, joins a job transition support group. Healthy families also know what is going on in the world around them. They show an interest in current events and attempt to understand significant social, economic, and political issues. This ever-broadening outreach gives families knowledge of external forces that might influence their lives. It exposes them to a wide range of alternatives and a variety of contacts, which can increase options for finding resources and strengthen coping skills.

An unhealthy family has not recognized the value of establishing links with the broader community. This may be because of (1) a knowledge deficit regarding community resources, (2) previous negative experiences with community services, or (3) a lack of connection with the community because of family expectations or cultural practices.

It is important for the community health nurse to assess the family's relationship with the broader community, in addition to structural and developmental variations, interaction, coping strategies, and lifestyle. With a comprehensive family assessment, the nurse has a base from which to begin a plan of care.

FAMILY HEALTH PRACTICE GUIDELINES

Family nursing is a kind of nursing practice in which the family is the unit of service (Friedman, Bowden, & Jones, 2003). It is not merely a family-oriented approach in which family concerns that affect the health of an individual are taken into account. Family nursing asks how one provides health care to a collection of people. It does not mean that nursing must relinquish service to individuals. On the contrary, one of the distinctive contributions of nursing as a profession is its holistic approach to individual needs. Community health nurses rise to the challenge of adding a service to populations that include families.

Five principles guide and enhance family nursing practice: (1) work with the family collectively, (2) start where the family is, (3) adapt nursing intervention to the family's stage of development, (4) recognize the validity of family structural variations, and (5) emphasize family strengths.

Work With the Family Collectively

To practice family nursing, nurses must set aside their usual focus on individuals and remind themselves that several people together have a collective personality, collective interests, and a collective set of needs. Viewing a group of people as one unit may seem less strange if one considers the way in which business organizations are perceived. For example, you may think of a particular corporation as conservative or liberal. You may hear that a women's group has taken a stand on abortion or that a government agency needs to become better organized. In each case, the group is viewed collectively as a single entity with attributes and activities in common. So it is with families. A family has its own personality, interests, and needs.

As much as possible, community health nurses want to involve all of the family's members during nurse–client in-

teraction (Wright & Leahey, 2000; Wallace et al., 1999). This approach reinforces the importance of each individual member's contribution to total family functioning. Nurses want to encourage everyone's participation in the work that the nurse and the family jointly agree to do. Like a coach, the nurse wants to help family members work together as a team for their collective benefit.

Consider how a nurse might work collectively with the Beck family (Display 23–1).

Start Where the Family Is

When working with families, community health nurses begin at the present, not the ideal, level of functioning. To discover where a family is, the community health nurse first conducts a family assessment to ascertain the members' needs and level of health and then determines collective interests, concerns, and priorities. The accompanying description of the Kovac family illustrates this principle (Display 23–2).

Adapt Nursing Intervention to the Family's Stage of Development

Although every family engages in the same basic functions, the tasks necessary to accomplish these functions vary with

DISPLAY 23–1

The Beck Family

A community health nurse had an initial contact with Mr. and Mrs. Beck and their youngest child at the well-baby clinic. The 9-month-old child was over the 95th percentile for weight and at the 40th percentile for height. The nurse also noted that both parents were obese. The nurse asked about the eating patterns in the family and of the baby in particular and suggested a home visit to determine whether the Becks were interested in family nursing. The nurse explained the purpose of home visits (to assess all family members, coping patterns, eating patterns, and food purchasing choices) and the importance of including all family members and asked for a time that would be good for the family as a whole. The nurse explained that each person should be involved and committed to the agreed-upon goals; that, like a team of oarsmen, the family would have to pull together to accomplish the purpose of the visits. To help the Beck family improve its nutritional status, the nurse might suggest a session of brainstorming to uncover many causes of poor nutrition. More brainstorming might result in solutions and plans for action. On each visit the nurse would view the Becks as a group. Group responses and actions would be expected. Evaluation of outcomes would be based on what the family did collectively. The Becks were interested and a home visit date was made.

DISPLAY 23-2

The Kovac Family

Marcia Kovac brought her baby, Tiffany, to the well-child clinic once but failed to keep further appointments. Concerned that the family might be having other difficulties, Sara Villa, a community health nurse, made a home visit. The mobile home was cluttered and dirty; the baby was crying in her playpen. Marcia seemed uninterested in the nurse's visit. She listened politely but had little to say. She repeated that everything was okay and that the baby was doing fine, explaining that she was just fussy because she was teething. As they talked, Marcia's husband Henry, a delivery van driver, stopped by to pick up a sports magazine to read on his lunch hour. The three of them discussed the problems of inflation and how expensive it was to raise a child. Sara reminded them that the clinic was free and that they could at least get good health care without extra cost. They agreed without enthusiasm. After Henry left, the nurse spent the remainder of the visit discussing infant care with Marcia, particularly emphasizing regular checkups and immunizations.

The next visit also focused on the baby, but Sara had an uncomfortable feeling that this family was not really interested in her help. After consulting her supervisor, the nurse did what she wished she had done in the first place. She asked to talk with Marcia and Henry together and explained frankly why she had come to their home and what she could offer in the way of counseling, teaching, support, and referral to other community resources. She then asked them what problems or concerns they had. The Kovacs were more than responsive and described their financial difficulties and feelings of isolation from family and friends. They were new in the city, and both their families lived some distance away on farms. The neighbors were friendly but not close enough to confide in. They believed they would eventually overcome their problems if they just had "someone to lean on," as they put it.

Now Sara could address the Kovacs' primary needs and concerns for friends and emotional support. The nurse began to address the Kovacs' social needs first and introduced them to a young couples' group that met at the community center. Sara continued to make periodic home visits and shared additional information about community services that the Kovacs might find helpful. She praised Marcia and Henry for following up on immunizations for Tiffany. Over time, Sara saw differences in the family's interest in their relationship with the community and their connection to its services. Sara realized that before she could address the issue of Tiffany's health, she needed to address the emotional health of the parents.

---

each stage of the family's development. A young family, for instance, can appropriately meet its members' affiliation needs by establishing mutually satisfying relationships and meaningful communication patterns. As the family enters later stages, bonds change with the release of some members into new families and the loss of others through death. Awareness of the family's developmental stage enables the nurse to assess the appropriateness of the family's level of functioning and to tailor intervention accordingly. Nurses are becoming adept at family assessment, but intervention needs to be the focus (Wright & Leahy, 2000; Hanson, 2001). A nurse's work with the Ravina family illustrates this need (Display 23-3).

Recognize the Validity of Family Structural Variations

Many families seen by community health nurses are nontraditional, such as single-parent families and unmarried couples (Baris et al., 2001; Scanzoni, 1999). Other families are organized around nontraditional patterns; for example, both parents may have careers, a husband may care for children at home while his wife financially supports the family, or both parents may telecommute and work at home. Such variations in structure and organizational patterns have resulted from social and technologic changes in employment practices, welfare programs, economic conditions, sex roles, status of women and minorities, birth control, incidence of divorce, even war. Such variations in family structure and organization lead to revised patterns of family functioning. Member roles and tasks often differ dramatically from our expectations. Examples are a family with a single parent who works full-time while raising children or a dual-career marriage in which both partners have undifferentiated roles. Community health nurses, many of whom are accustomed to traditional family patterns, must learn to understand and accept these variations in family structure and organization in order to address the needs of the families. (See Chapter 22 for more information on changing family structure.)

There are two important principles to remember. First, what is normal for one family is not necessarily normal for another. Each family is unique in its combination of structure, composition, roles, and behaviors. As long as a family carries out its functions effectively and demonstrates the characteristics of a healthy family, one must agree that its form, no matter how variant, is valid.

Second, families are constantly changing. Marriage transforms two people into a married couple without children. Adding children changes the family structure. Divorce alters structure and roles. Remarriage with the addition of children from another family changes the family again. Chil-

DISPLAY 23-3

The Ravina Family

The Ravinas, a couple in their early 70s, recently moved to a retirement complex. They received nursing visits after Mrs. Ravina's stroke 3 years earlier but requested service now because Mr. Ravina was feeling "poorly" all the time. He thought that perhaps his diet and lack of activity might be the cause and hoped the nurse would have some helpful suggestions. The couple had eagerly awaited Mr. Ravina's retirement from teaching, planning to be lazy, travel, visit all their children, and do all those things they never had time to do when they were young. Now neither of them seemed to have enough energy or the capacity to enjoy their new life. The move from their home of 28 years had been difficult; they were still trying to find space in the tiny apartment for their cherished books and mementos, although they had given many of them away.

Ronald Bell, a community health nurse, recognized that the Ravinas were experiencing a situational crisis (leaving their home of 28 years), a developmental crisis (aging and entering retirement), and perhaps some underlying health problems. Many of the Ravinas' expectations for this new life stage were unrealistic; they had not adequately prepared themselves for the adjustments that the loss of their home and retirement would demand. Through discussion, Ronald was able to help the Ravinas understand their situation and express their feelings. He completed physical assessments on the Ravinas and encouraged regular follow-up with their health care provider. He also helped them join a support group of retired persons who were experiencing some of the same difficulties. Because this nurse was able to help the Ravinas through their crisis in a supportive and nonjudgmental manner, he found them receptive later to discussing preparation for the inevitable loss and bereavement that would occur when one of them died. He was adapting his nursing intervention to this family's stage of development.

dren grow up and leave the home while the parents, together or singly, are left to adjust to yet another family structure. Throughout the life cycle, a family seldom stays the same for very long. Each of these changes forces a family to adapt to its circumstances. Consider the young woman with a baby whose husband deserts her. She has no choice but to assume a single-parent role. Each change also creates varying degrees of stress and demands considerable adaptive energy on the family's part. Many family changes are predictable; they are part of normal life-cycle growth. Some are not. The nurse's responsibility is to help families cope with the changes while remaining nonjudgmental and accepting of the various forms encountered.

Homosexual unions may be difficult for some nurses to deal with, particularly if they conflict with the nurse's own set of religious or cultural ideas. Yet the nurse's responsibility remains the same—to help promote the collective health. Consider the nurse's work with James Cutler and Brian Hoag (Display 23–4).

Nurses should view all families as unique groups, each with its own set of needs, whose interests can best be served through unbiased care. The Global Community display discusses the efforts to engage Romanian families and children in an aggressive immunization campaign to eliminate measles by 2007.

Emphasize Family Strengths

Too often, community health nurses tend to focus their attention on family weaknesses, looking for and referring to them as needs or problems. This negative emphasis can be devastating to a family and can undermine any hope of a truly therapeutic relationship between nurse and client. Instead, families need their strengths reinforced. Emphasizing a family's strengths makes people feel better about themselves. It

DISPLAY 23-4

James Cutler and Brian Hoag

James Cutler and Brian Hoag have a 6-year monogamous relationship. A homosexual couple, they worked with an attorney to privately adopt a child. The arrangements were completed and their 2-week-old son, Adrian, arrived in their home last week. Helen Jeffers, a community health nurse, receives a referral from the county hospital where Adrian was born. The request is for an assessment of the home situation and parenting skills. The baby tested positive for cocaine with Apgar scores of 6 and 8 and had some initial difficulty sucking. Birth weight was 2900 g. Discharge weight, at 3 days, was 2850 g. At her first home visit, Helen finds a neat and orderly two-bedroom condominium, well-equipped with baby supplies. The infant has gained 200 g and is being well cared for by two fatigued parents who had had limited contact with infants previously. James and Brian have many questions and are anxious learners. Helen plans with the couple to make weekly home visits to assess infant growth and development, provide support, and answer questions. She also suggests a neighborhood parenting class and finding a reliable babysitter, and she helps James and Brian develop an infant care work schedule. After 6 weeks of intervention, Adrian is thriving; Helen closes the case to home visits, feeling confident that the parents' goal of becoming knowledgeable and confident has been achieved.

THE GLOBAL COMMUNITY

Keeping Families Healthy

Romania suffered a large measles outbreak in the 1990s and consequently initiated a country-wide immunization campaign to eliminate the disease. The goal of the World Health Organization's European region is to eliminate measles by 2007, and organizations are closely watching Romania's experience.

The Romanian Ministry of Health initiated a national immunization program in 1998–1999 affecting all families with children in the country. The mass immunization campaign was to include all school-aged children (7 to 18 years old); girls aged 15 to 18 years were to receive a combined measles-rubella vaccine as the first step in a rubella vaccination program designed to prevent congenital rubella syndrome in future cohorts. It is estimated that 2.1 million children, or 76% to 93% of the children in the target age group, were reached.

For such an ambitious campaign to be successful, collaboration among several agencies and all families was necessary. Intensive efforts were made to locate all children. Many families lived in inaccessible communities or had moved out of the district or the country (itinerant families seeking work), so many agencies became involved in the effort to reach all families with children, including the Romanian Red Cross, the World Health Organization, Centers for Disease Control and Prevention, Red Crescent Society, and UNICEF.

Romania is being observed as a possible model for other eastern European countries as they plan similar campaigns. Romania's government, national and international agencies, and the families are to be commended for their efforts to create a successful campaign to eliminate measles.

Ion-Nedulcu, N., Cracium, D., Pitigoi, D., et al. (2001). Measles elimination: A mass immunization campaign in Romania. *American Journal of Public Health, 91*(7), 1042–1045.

---

erage of two times a week in the previous month); or the mother is awake with a robe on at 1 PM (not asleep as on other home visits made in the early afternoon). Each represents a positive change. If there is nothing positive the nurse can honestly say, he or she may be able to say that the family seems to be managing as best it can. This strengthening technique helps the nurse approach clients positively rather than with a condescending or punitive approach. This is not to say that nurses should ignore problems. On the contrary, assessment should explore all aspects of family functioning to determine both strengths and weaknesses. The nurse needs a total picture to achieve an adequate perspective in nursing care planning and to know when the family is ready to begin work on problems. Even as the nurse becomes more aware of a family's unhealthy behaviors, the emphasis should remain on the positive ones. Emphasizing strengths proves to the clients, in effect, that they are important to the nurse.

Family strengths are traits that facilitate the ability of the family to meet the members' needs and the demands made by systems outside the family unit. Not all traits that appear positive are necessarily strengths. Before the nurse selects a trait to emphasize, the behavior should be examined closely to determine whether it is actually facilitating family functioning. A strong work orientation may be a strength when balanced with play and relaxation, but a family obsessed by work experiences this trait as a weakness. Whether a trait is a strength or a weakness is determined by the amount of free choice, as opposed to compulsive drive, being exercised.

Some traits a nurse may consider as possible strengths are basic family functions, family developmental tasks, and characteristics of family health. For instance, a nurse might wish to commend a family that meets its members' physical, emotional, and spiritual needs; shows respect for members' various points of view; or fosters self-discipline in its children. A vivid illustration of this principle is found in the family nursing care of the Stevensons (Display 23–5).

FAMILY HEALTH ASSESSMENT

To assess a family's level of health in a systematic fashion, three tools are needed: (1) a conceptual framework on which to base the assessment, (2) a clearly defined set of assessment categories for data collection, and (3) a method for measuring a family's level of functioning.

Conceptual Frameworks

A **conceptual framework** is a set of concepts integrated into a meaningful explanation that helps one interpret human behavior or situations. Several conceptual frameworks have been used historically to study families (Hill & Hansen, 1960; Kantor & Lehr, 1975; Reiss, 1981). More recently, Beavers and Hampton (1990) and Anderson & Sabatelli (2003) published models describing family functioning.

---

fosters a positive self-image, promotes self-confidence, and often helps the family address other problems.

One helpful communication technique is **strengthening**. Verbally or in writing, the nurse lists positive points about an otherwise negative situation. For example, these points might include the fact that the baby is kept warmly dressed (the clothing might be filthy, but the baby is warm); the 2-year-old is taking a nap (albeit on the dirty floor); the 5-year-old got to school three times last week (up from an av-

DISPLAY 23-5

The Stevenson Family

The community health nurse, Keith Dow, made an initial home visit after referral by an outpatient physician who was concerned about possible child abuse. Alice Stevenson had brought her baby to the emergency room for treatment of a laceration on the baby's forehead. He had fallen off the table while she was changing him, she claimed. A bruise on his arm made the physician suspicious, but Alice explained it was caused by his older brother's rough play. The nurse opened the visit by stating that he was simply following up on the emergency room treatment and wanted to see how the baby was progressing. Keith made no mention of child abuse. He observed the mother and children closely, looking for small things to compliment Alice on (strengthening) while learning all he could about the family's background. Because the nurse appeared approving rather than suspicious or judgmental, Alice agreed to further visits. During a later visit, Alice admitted to the nurse that she had slapped the baby and her ring cut his forehead. She could not get him to stop crying, no matter what she did; she just could not endure it any longer, she said. There had been other times when she grabbed him roughly to pull him away from things he wasn't allowed to touch, causing bruises on his arms. Alice told the nurse that she had not planned this baby; when her husband found out she was pregnant, he had left her shortly before the baby was born. Like many abusive parents, Alice had unrealistic expectations of her children's behavior as well as very inadequate self-esteem (Ryan, 1997; Taylor & Kemper, 1998). Realizing that Alice would be particularly vulnerable to any criticism, the nurse concentrated on her strengths. Keith complimented her on how well she managed her home and dressed the children, on maintaining her job, and on reading to her 3-year-old son. It took many visits before Alice trusted the nurse, but in time they were able to discuss her feelings frankly and work toward improving this family's health. Keith got her to attend a support group for single parents and she began counseling. Emphasizing strengths had provided a bridge for Alice and assisted in bringing her into a helping relationship.

Three frameworks that are particularly useful in community health nursing are presented here: the interactional, structural-functional, and developmental frameworks.

The **interactional framework** describes the family as a unit of interacting personalities and emphasizes communication, roles, conflict, coping patterns, and decision-making processes. This framework focuses on internal relationships but neglects the family's interactions with the external environment.

The **structural-functional framework** describes the family as a social system relating to other social systems in the external environment, such as church, school, work, and the health care system. This framework examines the interacting functions of society and the family, considers family structure, and analyzes how a family's structure affects its function.

The **developmental framework** studies families from a life-cycle perspective by examining members' changing roles and tasks in each progressive life-cycle stage. This framework incorporates elements from interactional and structural-functional approaches so that family structure, function, and interaction are viewed in the context of the environment at each stage of family development.

Others have combined these concepts in various ways to design family assessment and intervention models that focus on human-environmental interactions, interactional and structural-functional frameworks, self-care, responses to stressors, and a developmental framework.

The six characteristics of healthy families already discussed serve as an initial framework for assessing family health by a combination of interactional, structural-functional, and developmental concepts.

Data Collection Categories

When using a conceptual framework for family health assessment, the community health nurse selects specific categories for data collection. The amount of data that one can collect about any given family may be voluminous, perhaps more than necessary for the purposes of the assessment. Certain basic information is needed, however, to determine a family's health status and to design appropriate nursing interventions. From many sources in the family health literature, particularly Turk and Kerns (1985), Edelman and Mandle (2002), and Friedman, Bowden, & Jones (2003), a list of 12 data collection categories has been generated. Table 23-1 lists the 12 categories, each grouped into one of three data sets: (1) family strengths and self-care capabilities, (2) family stresses and problems, and (3) family resources.

1. *Family demographics* refers to such descriptive variables as a family's composition, its socioeconomic status, and the ages, education, occupation, ethnicity, and religious affiliations of members.
2. *Physical environment* data describe the geography, climate, housing, space, social and political structures, food availability and dietary patterns, and any other elements in the internal or external physical environment that influence a family's health status.
3. *Psychological and spiritual environment* refers to affectional relationships, mutual respect, support, promotion of members' self-esteem and spiritual development, and life satisfaction and goals.
4. *Family structure and roles* include family organization, socialization processes, division of labor, and allocation and use of authority and power.

T A B L E   23–1

Categories of Data Collection for Family Health Assessment

Assessment Categories	Family Strengths and Self-Care Abilities	Family Stresses and Problems	Family Resources
1. Family demographics			
2. Physical environment			
3. Psychological and spiritual environment			
4. Family structure/roles			
5. Family functions			
6. Family values and beliefs			
7. Family communication patterns			
8. Family decision-making patterns			
9. Family problem-solving patterns			
10. Family coping patterns			
11. Family health behavior			
12. Family social and cultural patterns			

5. *Family functions* refer to a family's ability to carry out appropriate developmental tasks and provide for members' needs.

6. *Family values and beliefs* influence all aspects of family life. Values and beliefs might deal with raising children, making and spending money, education, religion, work, health, and community involvement.

7. *Family communication patterns* include the frequency and quality of communication within a family and between the family and its environment.

8. *Family decision-making patterns* refer to how decisions are made in a family, by whom they are made, and how they are implemented.

9. *Family problem-solving patterns* describe how a family handles problems, who deals with them, the flexibility of a family's approach to problem-solving, and the nature of solutions.

10. *Family coping patterns* encompass how a family handles conflict and life changes, the nature and quality of family support systems, and family perceptions and responses to stressors.

11. *Family health behavior* refers to familial health history, current physical health status of family members, family use of health resources, and family health beliefs.

12. *Family social and cultural patterns* comprise family discipline and limit-setting practices; promotion of initiative, creativity, and leadership; family goal setting; family culture; cultural adaptations to present circumstances; and development of meaningful relationships within and outside the family.

Assessment Methods

Many different methods are used to assess families. These methods serve to generate information about selected aspects of family structure and function; the methods must match the purpose for assessment.

Three well-known graphic assessment tools are the eco-map, the genogram, and the social network support map or grid (Meyer, 1993; Tracy & Whittaker, 1990). The **eco-map** is a diagram of the connections between a family and the other systems in its ecologic environment. It was originally devised to depict the complexity of the client's story. Developed by Ann Hartman in 1975 to help child welfare workers study family needs, the tool visually depicts dynamic family–environment interactions. The nurse involves family members in the map's development. A central circle is drawn to represent the family, and smaller circles on the periphery represent people and systems, such as school or work, whose relationships with the family are significant (Fig. 23–1). The map is used to discuss and analyze these relationships (Hartman, 1978; Meyer, 1993).

The **genogram** displays family information graphically in a way that provides a quick view of complex family patterns. It is a rich source of hypotheses about a family over a significant period of time, usually three or more generations (McGoldrick & Gerson, 1985). Family relationships are delineated by genealogic methods, and significant life events are included (eg, birth, death, marriage, divorce, illness). Identifying characteristics (eg, race, religion, social class), occupations, and places of family residence are also noted (Meyer, 1993). Again, this tool is used jointly with the family. It encourages family expression and sheds light on family behavior and problems (Fig. 23–2).

A **social network support map** or grid gives details about the quality and quantity of social connections. Strengths within the system can be elaborated with words, checks, or numbers, or a combination of these (Tracy & Whittaker, 1990). The nurse uses this tool to help the family understand its sources of support and relationships and to form a basis for nursing care planning and intervention. Figures 23–3 and 23–4 show samples of a social network support map and grid.

Tapia (1997) depicted her concept of levels of family functioning through her classic model for family nursing.

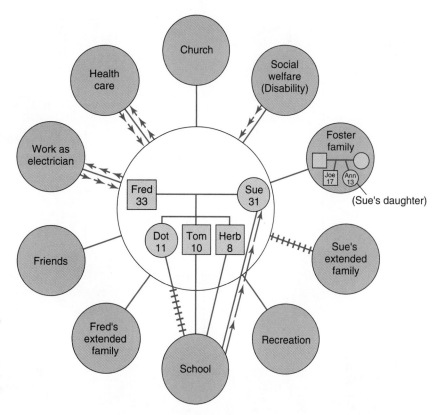

FIGURE 23–1. Eco-map of a family's relationship to its environment. Lines indicate types of connections: *solid lines,* strong; *dotted line,* tenuous; *lines with cross-bars,* stressful. *Arrows* signify energy or resource flow, and absence of lines indicates no connection.

This model, which has been in use for more than 30 years, is based on a continuum of five levels of family functioning:

- Infancy (level I—a very chaotic family)
- Childhood (level II—an intermediate family)
- Adolescence (level III—the normal family with many conflicts and problems)
- Adult (level IV—the family with solutions to its problems)
- Maturity (level V—the ideal independent family)

Tapia provided specific behaviors of families at each level, the family's expectations of the nurse, and, most importantly, the nurse's specific skill needed at each level to best meet the family needs and help them reach a higher level of function. This visualization of family strengths, weaknesses, expectations of the nurse, and needed nursing skills (Fig. 23–5) is a helpful assessment tool for the novice nurse when working with families in the community.

Community health nurses use several different family assessment instruments to gather data on family structure, function, and development. Public health nursing agencies usually develop their own tools, often in the form of questionnaires, checklists, flow sheets, or interview guides. The format varies to fit organizational needs. For example, most agencies have changed to computerized information management systems and have adjusted data collection to be technologically compatible. Two sample assessment tools are shown in Figures 23–6 and 23–7. Figure 23–6 shows a checklist format with scores and dates of assessment gathering. It is useful over a span of time for observing family growth or decline, especially for the novice community health nurse, who can document assessment data as rapport

with the family is established or as the comfort level with home visits increases.

Figure 23–7 offers an open-ended assessment tool. Such a tool may be useful in a teen perinatal program or a senior support program where a primary nurse makes the home visits and an additional nurse visits occasionally. The open-ended format is brief and lends itself to subjectivity. The goal is to create a document that is informative for all who use it while limiting subjective observations—a difficult task with open-ended tools. However, there may be an agency or program for which this tool fits best.

Other methods may use assessment tools or technology (eg, videotaping family interactions, structured observation, analysis of life-changing events). Examples include the Holmes-Rahe scale (Holmes & Rahe, 1967), a classic tool to measure a person's degree of stress, and the Self-Care Assessment Guide (Cleveland & Allender, 1999), which measures a family member's ability to provide self-care (Fig. 23–8). In a public health nursing agency or other community-based agency, documentation is completed for individuals after family assessment information data are gathered. Useful information can be gathered about stressors and self-care practices, including prescription medicines, over-the-counter (OTC) medicines, herbal remedies, nutritional supplements, and other complementary therapies. Such tools are useful adjuncts, especially for families coming from cultural groups different from that of the health care provider. They are often used in combination with other tools to enhance breadth of data collection and understanding of the family.

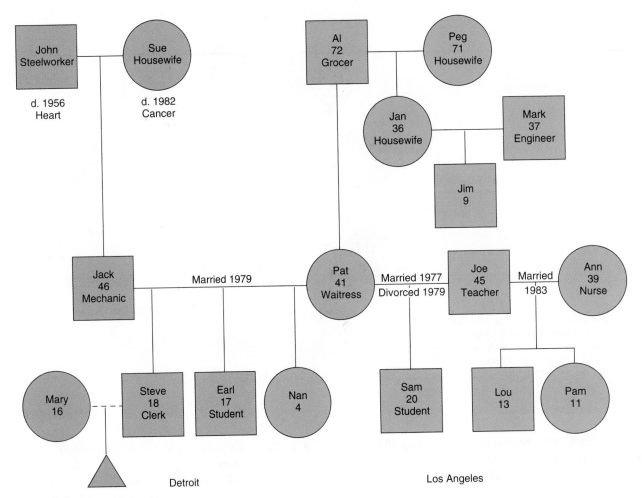

FIGURE 23-2. A genogram depicting three generations of family history. *Square*, male; *circle*, female; *triangle*, infant; *solid line*, married; *broken line*, not married.

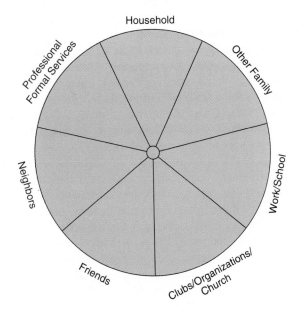

FIGURE 23-3. Social network support map.

	Area of Life	Concrete support	Emotional support	Information/ advice	Critical	Direction of help	Closeness	How often seen	How long known
ID _____ Respondent _____	1. Household 2. Other family 3. Work/school 4. Organizations 5. Friends 6. Neighbors 7. Professionals 8. Other	1. Hardly ever 2. Sometimes 3. Almost always	1. Hardly ever 2. Sometimes 3. Almost always	1. Hardly ever 2. Sometimes 3. Almost always	1. Hardly ever 2. Sometimes 3. Almost always	1. Goes both ways 2. You to them 3. They to you	1. Not very close 2. Sort of close 3. Very close	0. Does not see 1. Few times/yr. 2. Monthly 3. Weekly 4. Daily	1. Less than 1yr. 2. 1–5 yrs. 3. More than 5 yrs.
Name #									
01									
02									
03									
04									
05									
06									
07									
08									
09									
10									
11									
12									
13									
14									
15									
1–6	7	8	9	10	11	12	13	14	15

Social Support Network Grid. SOURCE: Tracy and Whittaker 1990.

FIGURE 23–4.   Social network support grid.

Nursing activities	Trust	Counseling	Complex of skills	Prevention	None
Continuum of Nursing Skills	Nurse and Family Partners	Partnership	Partnership Stressing Family's Ability		Family Independent Nurse not Needed
	Acceptance and trust, maturity and patience, clarification of role, limit setting, constant evaluation of relationship and progress.	Based on trust relationship, uses counseling and interpersonal skills to help family begin to understand itself and define its problems. Nurse uses honesty and genuineness, and self-evaluation.	Information, coordination, teamwork, teaching; uses special skills, helps family in making decisions and finding solutions.	Nurse—Expert and Partner Nurse—Expert and Partner with Family Anticipated problem areas studied, teaching of available resources, assistance in family-group understanding, maturity and foresight.	Ideal family, homeostatic, balance between individual and group goals and activities. Family meets its tasks and roles well, and are able to seek appropriate help when needed.
	Nurse—"Good Mother" to Family	Nurse and Family–Siblings	Nurse—Adult Helper to Family		
Continuum of Family Functioning	Chaotic family, barely surviving, inadequate provision of physical and emotional supports. Alienation from community, deviant behavior, distortion and confusion of roles, immaturity, child neglect, depression-failure.	Intermediate family, slightly above survival level, variation in economic provisions, alienation but with more ability to trust. Child neglect not as great, defensive but slightly more willingness to accept help.	Normal family but with many conflicts and problems, variation in economic levels, greater trust and ability to seek and use help. Parents more mature, but still have emotional conflicts. Do have successes and achievements, and are more willing to seek solutions to problems, future oriented.	Family has solutions, are stable, healthy with fewer conflicts or problems, very capable providers of physical and emotional supports. Parents mature and confident, fewer difficulties in training of children, able to seek help, future oriented, enjoy present.	
Family Levels	**I. Infancy**	**II. Childhood**	**III. Adolescence**	**IV. Adulthood**	**V. Maturity**

FIGURE 23–5. Tapia's model of family nursing.

Family Assessment

Family Name _____

Family Constellation

Member	Birth Date	Sex	Marital Status	Education	Occupation	Community Involvement

Financial Status _____

Using the following scale, score the family based on your professional observations and judgement:

0 = Never   3 = Frequently
1 = Seldom   4 = Most of the time
2 = Occasionally   N = Not observed

	score	date	score	date	score	date	score	date
Facilitative Interaction among Members								
a. Is there frequent communication among all members?								
b. Do conflicts get resolved?								
c. Are relationships supportive?								
d. Are love and caring shown among members?								
e. Do members work collaboratively?								

Comments _____

_____

Totals

	score	date	score	date	score	date	score	date
Enhancement of Individual Development								
a. Does family respond appropriately to members' developmental needs?								
b. Does it tolerate disagreement?								
c. Does it accept members as they are?								
d. Does it promote member autonomy?								

Comments _____

_____

Totals

F I G U R E   2 3 – 6 .   Family assessment using questions based on characteristics of healthy families.

	score	date	score	date	score	date	score	date

Effective Structuring of Relationships
  a. Is decision making allocated to appropriate members?
  b. Do member roles meet family needs?
  c. Is there flexible distribution of tasks?
  d. Are controls appropriate for family stage of development?

Comments _____

_____   Totals

Active Coping Effort
  a. Is family aware when there is a need for change?
  b. Is it receptive to new ideas?
  c. Does it actively seek resources?
  d. Does it make good use of resources?
  e. Does it creatively solve problems?

Comments _____

_____   Totals

Healthy Environment and Life-style
  a. Is family life-style health promoting?
  b. Are living conditions safe and hygienic?
  c. Is emotional climate conductive to good health?
  d. Do members practice good health measures?

Comments _____

_____   Totals

Regular Links with Broader Community
  a. Is family involved regularly in the community?
  b. Does it select and use external resources?
  c. Is it aware of external affairs?
  d. Does it attempt to understand external issues?

Comments _____

_____   Totals

FIGURE 23–6.   (*continued*)

GUIDELINES FOR FAMILY HEALTH ASSESSMENT

An assessment of family health will be most accurate if it incorporates the following five guidelines:
1. Focus on the family as a total unit.
2. Ask goal-directed questions.
3. Collect data over time.
4. Combine quantitative and qualitative data.
5. Exercise professional judgment.

Focus on the Family, Not the Member

Family health is more than the sum of its individual members' health. If the health of each person in a family were rated and the scores combined, the total would not show how healthy that family is. To assess a family's health, the nurse must consider the family as a single entity and appraise its aggregate behavior (Centers for Disease Control and Prevention, 1998; Wright & Leahey, 2000). As each criterion in the assessment process is considered, the community health nurse asks, "Is this typical of the family as a whole?" Assume that the nurse is assessing the communication patterns of a family. The nurse observes supportive interaction between two members in the family. What about the others? Further observation shows good communication among all but one member. It may be decided that, despite that one person, the family as a whole has good communication. If individual behavior deviates from that of the aggregate, the nurse notes the differences. They can influence

```
┌─────────────────────────────────────────────────────────────────────────────┐
│                          FAMILY ASSESSMENT                                    │
│   Family Name _____                                   │
│                                                                               │
│   Family Constellation                                                        │
│                                                                               │
│   Member names                Occupation              Educational background  │
│   _____ │
│   _____ │
│   _____ │
│   _____ │
│   _____ │
│                                                                               │
│   Significant change in family life —                                         │
│                                                                               │
│   Coping ability of family —                                                  │
│                                                                               │
│   Energy level —                                                              │
│                                                                               │
│   Decision-making process within the family —                                 │
│                                                                               │
│   Parenting skills —                                                          │
│                                                                               │
│   Support systems of the family —                                             │
│                                                                               │
│   Use of health care (include plans for emergencies) —                        │
│                                                                               │
│   Financial status —                                                          │
│                                                                               │
│   Other impressions —                                                         │
│                                                                               │
│   Signature of Nurse _____      Date _____        │
└─────────────────────────────────────────────────────────────────────────────┘
```

FIGURE 23–7.   Open-ended family assessment.

total family functioning and need to be considered in nursing care planning.

Ask Goal-Directed Questions

The activities of any investigator, if fruitful, are guided by goal-directed questions. When solving a crime, a detective has many specific questions in mind. So, too, does the physician attempting a diagnosis, the teacher trying to discern a student's knowledge level, or the mechanic repairing a car. Similarly, the nurse determining a family's level of health has specific questions in mind. It is not enough to make family visits and merely ask members how they are. If relevant data are to be gathered, relevant questions must be asked. The family assessment tool shown in Figure 23–6 provides a sample set of questions that community health nurses may use to assess a family's health. Built on the framework of the characteristics of a healthy family, these questions guide thinking and observations. They direct attention to specific aspects of family behavior to facilitate the goal of discovering a family's level of health.

Consider the characteristic, "Active Coping Effort" (Fig. 23–6). When visiting a family, the community health nurse watches for signs of its response to change and its problem-solving ability. The nurse asks, "Does this family rec-

ognize when it needs to make a change?" or "How does it respond when a change is imposed?" Perhaps a health problem has arisen; for instance, the baby has diarrhea. Does the family assume responsibility for dealing with the problem? Do family members consider a variety of ways to solve it? How do they respond to the nurse's suggestions? Do they seek out resources on their own, such as reading about causes of infant diarrhea, using home remedies, or consulting with the community health nurse, the doctor, or a nurse practitioner? How well do they use resources, once identified? Do they try creative methods for solving the problem and see it through to resolution? As the nurse focuses on these behaviors, he or she is asking goal-directed questions aimed at finding out the family's coping skills. This investigation is one part of the nurse's assessment of the family's total health picture.

The set of questions presented in Figure 23–6 is one useful way to appraise family health. Another, more open-ended format is used by some community health nursing agencies. This approach, displayed in Figure 23–7, proposes assessment categories as stimuli for nursing questions. When exploring family support systems, for example, the nurse asks, "What internal resources or strengths does this family have?" "Who outside the family can they and do they turn to for help?" "What agencies such as churches, clubs, or community services do they use?" The open-ended style of this

SELF-CARE ASSESSMENT GUIDE

Name _____ Birth date _____

Address _____ Phone number _____

Names of health care providers visited in past year:

Name	Discipline	Address	Phone number	Times visited past year
1.				
2.				

Surgeries (Include date)

1. _____

2. _____

Major acute illnesses (Include date; indicate whether hospitalization was necessary)

1. _____

2. _____

Chronic illnesses (Include date)

1. _____

2. _____

Age of parents (If deceased, indicate date of death, age at death, and cause of death)

Mother _____ Father _____

Age of grandparents (If deceased, indicate age at death and cause of death)

MGM _____ MGF _____ PGM _____ PGF _____

Natural teeth Y N

Dentures or partials Y N

Dental care: ___ Brush teeth/Frequency _____
                 ___ Floss teeth/Frequency _____

Women/men over 50 Sigmoidoscopy/colonoscopy Date _____

Women

Breast self-exam Y N Frequency _____
Mammograms   Y N Frequency _____
Pap smears   Y N Frequency _____

Men

Testicular self-exam Y N Frequency _____

PSA   Y N Date _____ Results _____

TB skin test (Date) _____ Results _____

Immunizations

Adult DT (or tetanus) _____
Flu vaccine _____
Hepatitis vaccine _____
Other _____

Weight (At age 25) ____Current weight ____Normal weight ____

Height (At age 25) ____Current height ____

Dietary practices (24-hour dietary recall)

First meal (Time) _____ Contents (Include amount) _____

_____

Second meal (Time) _____ Contents (Include amount) _____

_____

Third meal (Time) _____ Contents (Include amount) _____

_____

Snacks (Include time, contents, and amount) _____

_____

Usual food eaten (not mentioned above) _____

Foods not eaten at all (by preference) _____

Food allergies _____

Medicine allergies _____

Food taboos _____

Religious practices that affect health (prayer, special practices or services) _____

_____

Exercise patterns (Include sample activities, duration, frequency, problems or side effects):

1. _____

2. _____

Medications and therapies

OTC drugs (Include name, length of treatment, frequency of use, side effects):

1. _____
2. _____
3. _____
4. _____

Prescription drugs (Include name, length of treatment, frequency of use, side effects):

1. _____
2. _____
3. _____
4. _____

Folk medicine/home remedies (eg, postpartum isolation, mustard poultice for chest congestion):

1. _____
2. _____
3. _____
4. _____

Complementary therapies (eg, biofeedback, imagery, herbalism)

1. _____
2. _____
3. _____
4. _____

Plan for self-care improvement

Overall goal _____

_____

Areas needing modification (e.g., enhancement, moderation, deletion; include short- and long-term goal for each area):

1. _____
STG: _____
LTG: _____
2. _____
STG: _____
LTG: _____

Client role to reach long-term goals

_____

Nurse's role(s) to reach long-term goals (eg, collaboration, teaching, evaluation)

_____

_____

Others' roles in reaching goals (Include discipline, name, address and phone number)

1. _____
2. _____

Comments

_____

_____

_____

F I G U R E 2 3 – 8 .   Self-care assessment guide. (Adapted from Cleveland, L., & Allender, J. A. [1999]. Environment: Self-care issues. In L. Cleveland, D. S. Aschenbrenner, S. J. Veneable, & J. A. P. Yensen, *Nursing management in drug therapy*. Philadelphia: Lippincott Williams & Wilkins. Used with permission.)

assessment tool allows questions aimed at determining family health to be raised.

Allow Adequate Time for Data Collection

Accurate family assessment takes time. An appraisal done on the first or second visit will most likely give only a partial picture of how a family is functioning. Time is needed to accumulate observations, make notes, and see all the family members interacting together in order to make a thorough assessment. To appraise family communication patterns, for instance, the nurse needs to observe the family as a group, perhaps at mealtime or during some family activity. The family needs to feel comfortable in the nurse's presence, so that they will respond freely; time and patience are needed for such rapport to develop.

Consider one nurse's experience. Jolene Burns had talked with the Olson family twice, first in the clinic, and then at home. Because Mr. Olson had not been present either time, Jolene asked to see the family together and arranged an early evening visit. The Olsons were receiving nursing service for health promotion. They were particularly interested in discussing discipline of their young children. They contracted with Jolene for six weekly visits to be held in the late afternoon, when Mr. Olson was home from work. Jolene's assessment began with her first contact with the Olsons. She made notes on their chart and, guided by questions similar to those in Figure 23–6, kept a brief log. After the fourth visit, she filled out an assessment form to keep as a part of the family record. It was not until then that Jolene felt she had collected enough data to make valid judgments about this family's level of health.

Combine Quantitative With Qualitative Data

Any appraisal of family health must be qualitative. That is, the nurse must determine the presence or absence of essential characteristics in order to have a database for planning nursing action. To guide planning more specifically, the nurse can also determine the degree to which various signs of health are present. This is a quantitative measure. The nurse asks whether a family does or does not engage in some behaviors and how often. Is this behavior fairly typical of the family, or does it occur infrequently? Figures 23–6 and 23–8 demonstrate ways to measure family health quantitatively.

For example, if the nurse were to use the tool in Figure 23–6 to assess the Beck family's ability to enhance individuality, he or she could score behavior on a scale from 0 (never) to 4 (most of the time). After several observations, the nurse would probably conclude that responses to the members' developmental needs were appropriate most of the time (*a* under "Enhancement of Individual Development"). Opposite *a* on the assessment form, the nurse would write the numeral 4 and the date of assessment.

The value of developing a quantitative measure is to have some basis for comparison. The nurse can assess a family's progression or regression by comparing its present score with its previous scores. For instance, had the nurse conducted a family health assessment of the Kovacs 6 months ago and compared it with their present level of health, he or she would probably have discovered a drop in their scores in several areas. Many of their communication patterns, role relationships, and coping skills, in particular, would show signs of deterioration. A scored assessment gives a vivid picture of exactly which areas need intervention. For this reason, it is useful to conduct periodic assessments when a case is reopened, or every 3 to 6 months if it is kept open for an extended period. The nurse can monitor the progress of high-risk families through early introduction of preventive measures when a trend or regressive behavior is observed. Periodic quantitative assessments also provide a means of evaluating the effectiveness of nursing action and can point to documented signs of growth.

Quantitative data serve another useful purpose. The nurse can compare one family's health status with that of another family as a basis for priority setting and nursing care planning. The difference in the level of health between the Becks and the Kovacs, for example, shows that the Kovacs need considerably more attention right now. (See Research: Bridge to Practice.)

Exercise Professional Judgment

Although nurses seek to validate data, their assessment of families is still based primarily on their own professional judgment. Assessment tools can guide observations and even quantify those judgments, but, ultimately, any assessment is subjective. Even though it may be observed that a family makes good use of a community agency, the decision that use of this external resource contributes to the health of the family is a subjective one. This determination is not bad. Indeed, effective health care practice depends on sound professional judgment. However, nurses must be cautious about overemphasizing the value or infallibility of an assessment tool. It is only a tool and should be used as a guide for planning, not as an absolute and irrevocable statement about a family's health status. Caution is particularly important when dealing with quantitative scores, which may seem to be objective.

Ordinarily, assessment of a family is best conducted unobtrusively. An assessment tool used by the nurse is not a questionnaire to be filled out in the family's presence but rather a way to guide the nurse's observations and judgments. Before going into a family's home, the community health nurse may wish to review the questions. He or she may find it helpful to keep the assessment tool in a folder for easy reference during the visit. Depending on the nurse's relationship with the family, notes may be made during or immediately after the encounter. Like Jolene, the nurse may choose to keep a short log—an accumulation of notes—until

RESEARCH: BRIDGE TO PRACTICE

Gottman, J.M., & Notarius, C.I. (2003). Marital research in the 20th century and a research agenda for the 21st century. *Family Process, 41*(2), 159–197.

MARITAL RESEARCH—THEN AND NOW

The progress in marital research over the last half-century is documented in this study. Research in this area has included the following developments:

1940s–1950s—A focus on personality traits that promote a successful marriage

1950s–1970s—Studying partner interactions and the influence of the general systems theory (first recognized in these decades)

1970s–1980s—Development of more sophisticated observational measures, particularly the study of affect and self-report perceptual data

1980s–1990s—Research focus on secular changes occurring in America, such as the changing role of women, violence and incest in the family, cultural variation in marriages, longevity, health, and physiology.

The future agenda in the 21st century will include:
   More observation in naturalistic settings
   Continued focus on sequences or patterns of interaction
   Recognition of the importance of positive affect
   Need to revisit personality and effects on marriages
   Study of the management of stress spillover into the marriage

Over the decades, marital research has been dominated by social scientists. There is a need for community health nurses to be more present in this research area. They have a vested interest in successful marriages and families and have access to them. All of the focus areas for the future fit with community health nursing practice.

---

enough data have been collected to complete the assessment form.

Occasionally, a family with high self-care capability may be involved in the assessment. The nurse should introduce the idea carefully and use professional judgment to determine when the family is ready to engage in this kind of self-examination.

SUMMARY

The family unit remains the focus of service in community health nursing. Family health and individual health strongly influence each other, and family health also affects community health. It is important for the nurse to understand healthy family characteristics and to use a variety of tools so that family assessments are thorough.

Healthy families demonstrate six important characteristics:

1. A facilitative process of interaction exists among family members.
2. Individual member development is enhanced.
3. Role relationships are structured effectively.
4. Active attempts are made to cope with problems.
5. There is a healthy home environment and lifestyle.
6. Regular links with the broader community are established.

To assess a family's health systematically, the nurse needs a conceptual framework on which to base the assessment, a clearly defined set of categories for data collection, and a method for measuring the family's level of functioning. The six characteristics of a healthy family provide one assessment framework that community health nurses can use. Assessment tools to aid the nurse in appraising the health of families include the eco-map, the genogram, and the social network support map or grid. There are 12 main categories of family dynamics for which the nurse must collect data: family demographics, physical environment, psychological/spiritual environment, family structure and roles, family functions, family values and beliefs, family communication patterns, family decision-making patterns, family problem-solving patterns, family coping patterns, family health behaviors, and family social and cultural patterns.

Community health nurses enhance their practices with families by observing five principles: (1) work with the family collectively, (2) start where the family is now, (3) fit nursing intervention to the family's stage of development, (4) recognize the validity of family structural variation, and (5) emphasize family strengths.

During assessment, the nurse should focus on the family as a total unit, use goal-directed assessment questions, allow adequate time for data collection, combine quantitative with qualitative data, and exercise professional judgment.

ACTIVITIES TO PROMOTE CRITICAL THINKING

1. Construct an eco-map of your family. Ask a peer to do the same thing. Assess the balance between your family and the resources in its environment. How does your eco-map compare with that of your peer? What changes are needed in each family system? Are you able to influence the changes that are needed?

2. Draw a genogram of your family and ask a peer to discuss it with you. Make your drawing of the genogram as complete as possible. Then analyze your thoughts and feelings. How did you feel while tracing your family history? Did you learn anything new about your family? Did any family trends or traits appear? Did any uncomfortable or suppressed information come to the surface? Do you have any new insights about your family?

3. Complete a social network support map or grid on yourself. Discuss it with a peer. Did any of the data surprise you? What areas need to be worked on?

4. Assess a family (other than your own) that you know well by completing a family assessment guide. You may use one of the forms in this chapter or an available form from another source. Based on your assessment, determine as many nursing interventions as you can think of that could be used to promote this family's health as practically as possible.

REFERENCES

Anderson, S.A., & Sabatelli, R.M. (2003). *Family interaction: A multigenerational developmental perspective* (3rd ed.). Boston: Allyn & Bacon.

Baris, M.A., Coates, C.A., Duvall, B.B., Garrity, C.B., Johnson, E.T., & Lacrosse, E.R. (2001). *Working with high-conflict families of divorce: A guide for professionals*. Northvale, NJ: Jason Aronson.

Barker, P. (1998). *Basic family therapy* (4th ed.). New York: Oxford University Press.

Barnes, S.L. (2001). Stressors and strengths: A theoretical and practical examination of nuclear, single-parent, and augmented African American families. *Families in Society: The Journal of Contemporary Human Services, 82*(5), 449–460.

Beavers, W.R., & Hampton, R.B. (1990). *Successful families: Assessment and intervention*. New York: Basic Books.

Becvar, D.S., & Becvar, R.J. (2003). *Family therapy: A systematic integration* (5th ed.). Boston, MA: Allyn & Bacon.

Cleveland, L., & Allender, J.A. (1999). Environment: Self-care issues. In L. Cleveland, D.S. Aschenbrenner, S.J. Veneable, & J.A.P. Yensen (Eds.), *Nursing management in drug therapy*. Philadelphia: Lippincott Williams & Wilkins.

Centers for Disease Control and Prevention. (1998). *Assessing health risks in America: The behavioral risk factor surveillance system (BRFSS)*. Washington, DC: U. S. Department of Health and Human Services.

Donnelly, T.T. (2002). Contextual analysis of coping: Implications for immigrants' mental health care. *Mental Health Nursing, 23*, 715–732.

Early, T.J. (2001). Measures for practice with families from a strengths perspective. *Families in Society: The Journal of Contemporary Human Services, 82*(3), 225–232.

Edelman, C., & Mandle, C.L. (Eds.). (2002). *Health promotion throughout the life span* (5th ed.). St. Louis: Mosby.

Farren, M. (1999). Ensuring safety for the elderly client at home. In S. Zang & J.A. Allender (Eds.), *Home care of the elderly* (pp. 59–77). Philadelphia: Lippincott Williams & Wilkins.

Friedman, M.M., Bowden, V.R., & Jones, W. (2003). *Family nursing: Research, theory and practice* (5th ed.). Upper Saddle River, NJ: Prentice-Hall.

Gavan, C.S. (2003). Successful aging families: A challenge for nurses. *Holistic Nursing Practice, 17*(1), 11–18.

Gottman, J.M., & Notarius, C.I. (2003). Marital research in the 20th century and a research agenda for the 21st century. *Family Process, 41*(2), 159–197.

Hanson, S.M.H. (Ed.). (2001). *Family health care nursing: Theory, practice, and research* (2nd ed.). Philadelphia: F.A. Davis.

Hartman, A. (1978). Diagrammatic assessment of family relationships. *Social Casework, 59*(10), 59–64.

Hill, R., & Hansen, D. (1960). The identification of conceptual frameworks utilized in family study. *Marriage and Family Living, 22*, 299–311.

Holmes, T., & Rahe, R. (1967). The social readjustment rating scale. *Journal of Psychosomatic Research, 11*, 213–217.

Ion-Nedulcu, N., Cracium, D., Pitigoi, D., Popa, M., Hennessey, K., Roure, C., et al. (2001). Measles elimination: A mass immunization campaign in Romania. *American Journal of Public Health, 91*(7), 1042–1045.

Kantor, D., & Lehr, W. (1975). *Inside the family: Toward a theory of family process*. San Francisco: Jossey-Bass.

Kitzman, H., Olds, D.L., Sidora, K., Henderson, C.R., Hanks, C., Cole, R., et al. (2000). Enduring effects of nurse home visitation on maternal life course: A 3-year follow-up of a randomized trial. *Journal of the American Medical Association, 283*(15), 1983–1989.

Lia-Hoagberg, B., Kragthorpe, C., Schaffer, M., & Hill, D.L. (2001). Community interdisciplinary education to promote partnerships in family violence prevention. *Family and Community Health, 24*(1), 15–27.

McGoldrick, M., & Gersen, R. (1985). *Genograms in family assessment*. New York: Norton.

Meyer, C.H. (1993). *Assessment in social work practice*. New York: Columbia.

Olson, D., McCubbin, H.I., Barnes, H., et al. (1983). *Families: What makes them work?* Beverly Hills, CA: Sage.

Otto, H.A. (1973). A framework for assessing family strengths. In A. Reinhardt & M. Quinn (Eds.), *Family-centered community nursing: A socio-cultural framework*. St. Louis: Mosby.

Parachin, V.M. (1997, March/April). Six signs of a healthy family. *Vibrant Life*, 5–6.

Pinelli, J. (2000). Effects of family coping and resources on family adjustment and parental stress in the acute phase of the NICU experience. *Neonatal Network, 19*(6), 27–37.

Reiss, D. (1981). *The family's construction of reality.* Cambridge, MA: Harvard University Press.

Reutter, L. (1997). Family health assessment: An integrated approach. In B.W. Spradley & J.A. Allender (Eds.), *Readings in community health nursing* (5th ed., pp. 329–342). Philadelphia: Lippincott Raven.

Rucibwa, N.K., Modeste, N., & Montgomery, S. (2003). Exploring family factors and sexual behaviors in a group of Black and Hispanic adolescent males. *American Journal of Health Behavior, 27*(1), 63–74.

Ryan, J.M. (1997). Child abuse and the community health nurse. In B.W. Spradley & J.A. Allender (Eds.), *Readings in community health nursing* (5th ed., pp. 371–376). Philadelphia: Lippincott-Raven.

Saunders, J.C. (2003). Families living with severe mental illness: A literature review. *Mental Health Nursing, 24,* 175–198.

Scanzoni, J. (1999). *Designing families: The search for self and community in the information age.* Thousand Oaks, CA: Pine Forge.

Tapia, J.A. (1997). The nursing process in family health. In B.W. Spradley & J.A. Allender (Eds.), *Readings in community health nursing* (5th ed., pp. 343–350). Philadelphia: Lippincott Raven.

Taylor, J.A., & Kemper, K.J. (1998). Group well-child care for high-risk families. *Archives of Pediatric and Adolescent Medicine, 152,* 579–584.

Thompson, P. (1998). Adolescents from families of divorce: Vulnerability to physiological and psychological disturbances. *Journal of Psychosocial Nursing and Mental Health Services, 36*(3), 34–39.

Tracy, E.M., & Whittaker, J.J. (1990). The social network map: Assessing social support in clinical practice. *Families in Society, 71,* 461–470.

Turk, D.C., & Kerns, R.D. (Eds.). (1985). *Health, illness and families: A life span perspective.* New York: John Wiley.

Wallace, H.M., Green, G., Jaros, K., Paine, L., & Story, M. (1999). *Health and welfare for families in the 21st century.* Boston: Jones & Bartlett.

Wright, L.M., & Leahey, M. (2000). *Nurses and families: A guide to family assessment and intervention* (3rd ed.). Philadelphia: F.A. Davis.

SELECTED READINGS

Broome, M.E., Knafl, K., Pridham, K., & Feetham, S. (Eds.). (1998). *Children and families in health and illness.* Thousand Oaks, CA: Sage.

Bulechek, G.M., & McCloskey, J.C. (Eds.). (1999). *Nursing interventions: Essential nursing treatments* (3rd ed.). Philadelphia: W.B. Saunders.

Chatterjee, P., & D'Aprix, A. (2002). Two tails of justice. *Families in Society: The Journal of Contemporary Human Service, 83*(4), 374–386.

Denham, S.A. (2002). *Family health: A framework for nursing.* Philadelphia: F.A. Davis.

Glasser, P.H., & Glasser, L.N. (1970). *Families in crisis.* New York: Harper & Row.

Lotas, M., Penticuff, J., Medoff-Cooper, B., Brooten, D., & Brown, L. (1992). The HOME SCALE: The influence of socioeconomic status on the evaluation of the home environment. *Nursing Research, 41,* 338–341.

Lynch, M., & Cicchetti, D. (2002). Links between community violence and the family system: Evidence from children's feelings of relatedness and perceptions of parent behavior. *Family Process, 41*(3), 519–532.

McCroskey, J., Sladen, A., & Meezan, W. (1997). *The family assessment form: A practice-based approach to assessing family functioning developed by the Children's Bureau of Southern California.* Washington, DC: Child Welfare League of America.

Meyer, I.H. (2001). Why lesbian, gay, bisexual, and transgender public health? *American Journal of Public Health, 91*(6), 856–859.

Minuchin, S. (1974). *Families and family therapy.* Cambridge: Harvard University Press.

Moules, N.J., & Tapp, D.M. (2003). Family nursing labs: Shifts, changes, and innovations. *Journal of Family Nursing, 9*(1), 101–117.

Murray, R.B., & Zentner, J.P. (2000). *Health assessment and promotion strategies through the life span* (7th ed.). Upper Saddle River, NJ: Prentice-Hall.

Neuman, B. (2001). *The Neuman systems model* (4th ed.). Upper Saddle River, NJ: Prentice-Hall.

Pender, N.J. (2001). *Health promotion in nursing practice* (4th ed.). Upper Saddle River, NJ: Prentice-Hall.

Phipps, M.G., & Sowers, M. (2002). Defining early adolescent childbearing. *American Journal of Public Health, 92*(1), 125–128.

Renpenning, K.M., Taylor, S.G., & Eisenhandler, S.A. (2003). *Self-care theory in nursing: Selected papers of Dorothea Orem.* New York: Springer.

Sanfilippo, J.G., & Forker, J.E. (2003). Creating family: A holistic milieu at a geriatric adult day center. *Holistic Nursing Practice, 17*(1), 19–21.

Simonsen, S.M. (2001). *Telephone health assessment: Guidelines for practice.* Upper Saddle River, NJ: Prentice-Hall.

Spector, R.E. (2000). *Cultural diversity in health and illness* (5th ed.). Upper Saddle River, NJ: Prentice-Hall.

Wegner, G.D., & Alexander, R.J. (1999). *Readings in family nursing* (2nd ed.). Philadelphia: Lippincott-Raven.

24

Planning, Intervening, and Evaluating Health Care for Families

Key Terms

- Home visit
- Mutual goals
- Nursing bag
- Outcome evaluation
- Referral
- Resource directory

Learning Objectives

Upon mastery of this chapter, you should be able to:

- Describe the components of the nursing process as they apply to enhancing family health.
- Identify the steps in a successful family health intervention.
- Discuss the two foci of family health visits: education and health promotion.
- List at least six specific safety measures the community health nurse should take when traveling to a home or making a home visit.
- Describe useful activities and actions when intervening on family health visits.
- Describe three types of evaluations that are necessary after family health intervention.

Have you ever thought about how your family has influenced you? Did family members influence you in your career choice, where you are attending school, your value system, your level of health, or the friends you have? How different do you think your life would be if you had grown up with vegetarian parents, or with a parent who took you out every fall to hunt deer? No two families are alike. Community health nurses primarily work with families—in their own homes, classrooms, support groups, clinics, outpatient departments, neighborhood centers, homeless shelters, or relatives' homes.

Families are the main unit of service in the community and have been for more than a century (Schoor & Kennedy, 1999). It is with the family in mind that the bulk of health care and related services are provided in the community. Immunization programs exist for infants and children; parks, recreation services, organized team sports, and social centers are there for the physical and emotional well-being of families. Pregnant women can attend childbirth education classes and receive medical care from their health care providers. Growing families can access parenting classes and support groups for developmental crises and management of chronic illness. For the older adults in the family, there are senior centers and a myriad of social and recreational activities that offer senior discounts. What all of these clients have in common is the fact that they are members of families.

Other chapters have stressed that families come in all sizes; they consist of members of many ages and biologic relationships, and they experience life filtered through unique cultures (see Chapter 23). There are many theoretical approaches and roles to consider when caring for families (see Chapter 22). This chapter explores how community health nursing services are planned for and delivered to families in clinics, homes, work settings, and schools.

Just as each family is unique, so is each family's home and neighborhood. Some families live in homes that look very much like yours, and you will feel comfortable there almost immediately. Others live in places that do not feel so comfortable, including small, cluttered apartments; farm labor camps; sparsely furnished single rooms; houses in disrepair; mobile homes; high-rise inner-city apartments; rural cabins; and inner-city neighborhoods. Each setting brings a different challenge. Assessing, planning, implementing, and evaluating care for families in their own environments can be a daunting task to the novice community health nurse. This chapter focuses on the planning, implementing, and evaluating phases of the nursing process that are used to enhance family health.

NURSING PROCESS COMPONENTS APPLIED TO FAMILIES AS CLIENTS

Assessing, planning, implementing, and evaluating nursing care are steps used to deliver care to clients in acute care settings and in the extensive clinic system. These same steps are used with families and aggregates in community health nursing. The steps do not change, but because the context and client focus are different, external variables that have not been encountered in other contexts must now be considered.

Working With Families in Community Health Settings

Family visits need not be limited to homes. Family members may be visited in school or at work during a lunch break, in a day care or senior center, in a group home, or in a myriad of after-work or after-school and recreational settings. The nurse must be creative to accommodate various family schedules and routines. In general, if a visit is all right with the family, school, or employer, it should be all right with the nurse (see Voices From the Community). Families appreciate the individualized effort and respond more positively when nurses are willing to work with family member schedules.

When making visits in public places such as worksites or schools, be mindful of confidentiality and respect the family's wishes. A client may agree to your visit during lunch break in the department store on a Tuesday, which is the boss's day off, or after the lunch crowd in a fast-food restaurant disperses and the client can take a break. Seek out a place for the visit where other employees or customers cannot overhear your conversation with the client.

Sometimes, visiting clients during the day helps to enhance family assessment. In families with a child in day care or an older adult in an adult day care program, your assessment of the individual's ability to manage, participate, and interact can give insight into problems the family is referring to when you make a home visit.

Visiting children during the school day often gives insight into health problems the parents may be concerned about. Such a visit offers the community health nurse an excellent opportunity to consult with the principal, teachers, school nurse (see Chapter 28), counselor, and school psychologist. The community health nurse may suggest a team

VOICES FROM THE COMMUNITY

"I couldn't believe it when she [the community health nurse] said she could visit me during my lunch break. I have been so worried about Ben's hearing and with my new work hours I kept missing her—I got her notes she left in the screen door. She actually drove all the way out to my work to tell me about his hearing test at school and the teacher's classroom changes. I can't afford to lose this job—and she came here!"

Beth, 34, Ben's mother

meeting of school professionals and the parents, coordinate the meeting, and act as liaison and client advocate during the meeting.

Working With Families Where They Live

Depending on the setting for community health nursing practice, the nurse encounters most clients in their homes and in their neighborhoods. Some see families in transition, who are living on the street, in a homeless shelter, or with other relatives. Regardless of the family's location, the client is the family; the family is the unit of service in family nursing (Friedman, Bowden, & Jones, 2003).

The Home Visit

Working in the community and being able to visit families in their homes is a privilege. In this unique setting you are permitted into the most intimate of spaces we, as human beings, have. Our homes are our creations, our private spaces; they hold our personal treasures, our memories. To let a stranger into our home takes a certain amount of trust. To enter a client family's home also takes trust on the part of the nurse. Once the door is shut behind you, you are in the client's world. The rules have changed; they are the experts, you are the guest. You must respond to the family with this "switch" in mind. A **home visit** is conducted to visit clients where they live in order to assist them in their efforts to achieve as high a level of wellness as possible. Later sections in this chapter discuss the components of a family health intervention that are included in a home visit and how the community health nurse can best use the phases of the nursing process to enhance family health.

Nursing Skills Used During Home Visits

There are many skills, in addition to expert nursing skills, that are needed when assessing, planning, implementing, and evaluating service in the home to families at a variety of levels of functioning (Tapia, 1997). Expert interviewing skills and effective communication techniques are essential for effective family intervention (see Chapter 11). Special skills required when making home visits are described in the following paragraphs.

Acute Observation Skills

The environment is new to you, and observation of environment and client are equally important. In addition to focusing on the family members' concerns and the purpose of the visit, you need to be observant about neighborhood, travel safety, home environmental conditions, number of household members, client demeanor and body language, and other nonverbal cues.

Travel in new neighborhoods and attempts to locate a family can cause distress to even the most experienced nurse. Often clients are difficult to locate because the house or apartment number is missing. The residence may be situated behind another house or it may be a basement apartment without a number. Many anomalies in the layout of a building or a neighborhood may make it difficult for the nurse to locate a client. Addresses on referrals may have numbers transposed such as 123 Hickory instead of 132 Hickory. Perhaps there is a North Hickory–miles away from South Hickory—or there are different streets called Hickory, such as Boulevard, Drive, Street, Road, Court, Lane, and Way. In some communities, house numbers such as $132\frac{1}{2}$ or street numbers such as $13\frac{1}{2}$ Avenue or $12\frac{1}{4}$ Street may be used. There is always the chance that the address is fictitious–given by clients who, for whatever reason, prefer to remain as anonymous as possible.

Assessment of Home Environmental Conditions

Conditions in the neighborhood and home environments reveal important assessment information that can guide planning and intervention with families. While traveling to and arriving at the family home, you have been gathering information about resources and barriers encountered by the family. This information is used during planning with the family. It is important to remember that neighborhood conditions and even the physical appearance of the apartment or house may belie the family's values, resources, and goals. They have little control over the neighborhood or, frequently, the building they live in, especially if they are renting. For instance, the family may be a young couple with a baby who can afford $475 in rent; the only apartment available to them for that amount is in a deteriorating low-income neighborhood with dilapidated buildings occupied by renters and owned by absentee landlords. These landlords do not live in the neighborhood and may own several buildings, mainly for profit. Properties are handled by managers who may not know the landlord and are employed through the owner's management company. Yet when you enter the apartment, you may see a well-furnished, neat, clean home that is opened to you, with pride by the family.

In another situation, you may plan to visit an older couple who live in their own home in an upscale suburban neighborhood. On approaching the house, however, you may see an overgrown yard and a house in need of painting and repairs. Inside the home, you barely manage to squeeze through a pathway made in the living room, which is piled ceiling-high with boxes, newspapers, and furniture. This continues throughout the house and even into a back bedroom, where half the bed is covered with papers, books, and a few cats. An older woman is in the bed. The husband moves very slowly, and after showing you in, he leaves the bedroom and heads toward the back yard.

There are many environmental clues in each of these situations that help the nurse begin an assessment that will lead to a plan to assist each family. Most neighborhoods and homes do not present such extremes. However, if you are unprepared for the extremes, they may overwhelm you, and you may become so distracted that you cannot focus wholly on the family and incorporate these important observations into the plans.

Assessment of Household Members' Demeanor, Body Language, and Other Nonverbal Cues

After you have knocked on the door or rung the doorbell and are in the home (see What Do You Think?), or even while greeting the people in the doorway, you are gathering data. Being human, you may form opinions or make judgments about the family from the initial meeting. Know that they are doing the same thing. Be aware of all household members; acknowledge and greet them. If some are absent, inquire about them. Make this a habit on all visits. Each member of the family is important and has opinions and health care needs, even if you only see parts of the family on each visit.

Be observant of family body language and demeanor. These nonverbal cues provide information that must not be overlooked. Observations such as, "You seem anxious today," or "Did I come at a bad time? You seem distracted" are openings that allow family members to express what is on their minds. If you are not open to body language while making a visit, you may overlook important cues and continue with your agenda, without realizing that the family is distracted by another, more pressing issue.

On a related note, it is important for the nurse to be aware of her or his own body language or demeanor. If you fidget with your car keys during the entire visit, noisily chew gum, give minimal eye contact while continuously looking at your paperwork, appear rushed, or refuse to sit on any of the family's furniture, your behavior will tell the family a great deal about you, including how you feel about being in their home.

PLANNING TO MEET THE HEALTH NEEDS OF FAMILIES DURING HOME VISITS

The greatest barrier to a successful family health visit is a lack of planning and preparation. A visit is not successful just because the nurse enters a home or other setting where clients are present. A successful family health visit takes much planning and preparation and requires accurate documentation and follow-up. In addition, safety measures must be followed, not only while traveling in the neighborhood, but also in the home.

Components of the Family Health Visit

The structure of family health visits can be divided into four components that follow the nursing process (Display 24–1). Previsit preparation steps (assessment and planning) are necessary to ensure that the actual family health visit (implementation) is complete. The documentation and planning for the next visit (evaluation) concludes the responsibilities for one visit and prepares the nurse for the next action needed.

Previsit Preparation

Community health nurses design a plan for the initial family health visit based on a referral coming into the agency. A **referral** is a request for service from another agency or person. This request is formalized by the use of a form or information that the originating agency has transferred to the receiving agency. Referrals may be formal coming from complementary agencies, or they may be informal, resulting from verbal or telephone referrals from friends or relatives who believe that someone is in need. Referrals are the source of new cases for agencies, and they need timely responses. Referrals could be from labor and delivery units, requesting service for low-birth-weight babies and teen mothers, aged 17 years and younger. They could be from social service agencies requesting a home assessment for a child being returned to parents after previous removal from the home. A referral could come via a telephone call from a woman in a city 500 miles away, requesting that a nurse check on an elderly relative who lives alone in the community and has recently exhibited slurred speech. Follow-up visits are made to these families based on need and agency protocol.

Nurses must have a physical place to work, with access to a telephone and any other supportive resources deemed necessary such as educational materials (pamphlets, brochures, computer and related Web site addresses to access educational

WHAT DO YOU THINK?

HOW YOU KNOCK HELPS FAMILIES OPEN THE DOOR

At first this may seem trite, but how do you knock on the door when you visit a family? Do you use the "I don't want to be here and if they don't hear the knock I can quietly leave" type of knock that even Superman can't hear? Or do you knock like, "I'm a bill collector and YOU BETTER open this door!" During this knock the entire family is leaving through the back door! We suggest a knock that is loud enough to be heard, yet friendly and nonthreatening. If necessary, practice "your knock" until you can create this beneficial combination.

With some families, it is helpful to call toward the door as you knock or ring the bell with, "Mrs. Smith, this is Jenny from the Health Department—remember I was coming by today" or, "Ms. Jiminez, it's the student community health nurse, Terry Guara, and I brought those pamphlets for you" or, "Hello, it's James from the neighborhood clinic, we planned to meet today." Using such a greeting allows the family to know who is at the door and choose to open the door if they want. It will get you into more homes than the "quiet-as-a-mouse" or "bill-collector" knocks.

DISPLAY 24-1

Guidelines for Making Home Visits: 30 Steps to Success

The following guidelines can be followed to evaluate yourself after making a home visit; or it can be a tool used when you are evaluated by another nurse (peer or instructor). Rate yourself using the following scale: 0 = does not apply, 1 = unsatisfactory, 2 = satisfactory.

Rating Assessment
_____ 1. Studies referral, record, or other available data about the family.
_____ 2. Gathers community resource information potentially appropriate to the family.
_____ 3. Obtains appropriate supplies or educational material in anticipation of family needs.

Planning
_____ 4. Contacts family to set up an appropriate time for the home visit.
_____ 5. Ascertains correct address and directions to the family for the home visit.
_____ 6. Formulates a written plan for nursing intervention with each family member.
_____ 7. Organizes a chart with forms and charting tools based on the focus of the visit.
_____ 8. Plans a route to the family's home that is the most direct, being resource efficient.

Implementation
_____ 9. Travels the community with safety, locating the family home with ease.
_____ 10. Knock on the door loudly enough to be heard and in a friendly manner.
_____ 11. Introduces self to family members in an appropriate manner.
_____ 12. Clearly states the reason for the visit.
_____ 13. Allows a few moments of socialization before beginning the visit.

_____ 14. Smiles, speaks in a pleasant, friendly tone of voice, and maintains eye contact.
_____ 15. Uses aseptic technique when providing nursing care.
_____ 16. Respects the dignity, privacy, safety, and comfort of family members.
_____ 17. Listens attentively to ascertain what family members are saying or implying.
_____ 18. Converses with family members during the home visit.
_____ 19. Communicates accurate and meaningful information to family members.
_____ 20. Responds to family members in a way that encourages them to continue talking.
_____ 21. Uses appropriate words of explanation for family member understanding.
_____ 22. Utilizes opportunities for incidental teaching.
_____ 23. Commends progress made by individual family members.
_____ 24. Explains nursing measures before, during, and after each procedure.
_____ 25. Shares the results of nursing measures with family members when indicated.
_____ 26. Closes the home visit by summarizing the main points of the visit.
_____ 27. Makes plans for the next visit, considering family member wishes.

Evaluation
_____ 28. Utilizes information gathered on the home visit to plan care for next visit.
_____ 29. Documents home visit in an appropriate and timely manner.
_____ 30. Completes a self-evaluation of the home visit.

information), charting tools, and other supplies required for home visits. Nurses also need a **resource directory**, which is a published list of resources for the broader community, or a nurse-made directory of resources created over years of working with people in the community.

Some agencies issue a **nursing bag** to their nurses. This bag, traditionally black leather with two handles, now may be made of canvas with an agency or program logo on it. Such a bag serves to carry the materials a nurse may need on a home visit and can identify where the person carrying it comes from. Not all agencies provide a nursing bag, so many nurses become creative and devise their own carry-all for supplies. Canvas "conference" totes, briefcases, or small molded plastic carriers may be used. The supplies community health nurses need are minimal and depend on the type of visit; some nurses have several totes for different kinds of

visits. If the focus is educational, such as a Denver Developmental Screening Test (DDST) or a newborn assessment, each tote should have the appropriate materials in it. Basic supplies for any visit include disposable gloves, paper towels, and soap packets or a waterless hand cleanser. Nurses engaged in home health nursing are prepared with more supplies for each visit, because the focus is on treatment in most of the visits (see Chapter 37).

Once the nurse is prepared, contact with the family is needed. For a home visit, ideally the referral contains a correct telephone number for the family, a relative, or a neighbor. If the referral or chart does not contain this information, the nurse makes an unannounced visit. During this visit, it is important to get a telephone number of the client family, or of a relative or neighbor if there is currently no telephone in the residence. When calling for the first time, the nurse must introduce herself or himself, explain the reason for the call and why this family was selected for a visit, tell what the visit consists of, and determine a time when a visit would be convenient for the family and the nurse. Some people become defensive or suspicious of the nurse's intentions. For example, a new young mother may think, "What did they see me doing wrong with my baby in the hospital?" In this kind of situation, it is very important that the nurse explain that

- The visit is a service provided by the agency to all young mothers.
- The visit is paid for by taxes (or donations) or by the client's health maintenance organization (if applicable), so there is no direct charge to the family.
- Young mothers often have lots of questions about their new babies. Having a nurse come to the home provides an opportunity for the mother to ask questions. It is an opportunity for the nurse to show the mother things about her baby that she may not know.

The nurse needs to ask explicit directions to where the family is staying. The referral may have a different address, and the family may forget to mention that they are staying with an aunt until the nurse requests the directions.

Making the Visit

On locating and meeting the family, the following guidelines for initial contact should be used (Allender, 1998):

- Introduce yourself and explain the value to the family of the nursing services provided by the agency.
- Spend the first few minutes of the visit establishing cordiality and getting acquainted (a mutual discovery or "feeling out" time).
- Use acute observational skills.
- Be sensitive to verbal and nonverbal cues.
- Be adaptable and flexible (you may be planning a prenatal visit, but the woman delivered her baby the day after you made the appointment and there is a newborn now).
- Use your "sixth sense" as a guide regarding family responses, questions they ask, and your personal safety (trust your feelings).
- Be aware of your own personality; balance talking and listening, and be aware of your nonverbal behaviors.
- Be aware that most clients are not acutely ill and have higher levels of wellness than are usually seen in acute care settings.
- Become acquainted with all family members and household members if you are making a home visit.
- Encourage each person to speak for himself or herself.
- Be accepting and listen carefully.
- Help the family focus on issues and move toward desired goals.
- After the body of the visit is over, review the important points, emphasizing family strengths.
- Plan with the family for the next visit.

The length and primary focus of the visit vary depending on its purpose. As a general guide, if the visit is shorter than 20 minutes, it probably should be folded into another visit (unless you are offering a piece of very important information, providing supplies, or have come by family request). On the other hand, if the visit exceeds 1 hour, it should be conducted over two visits. Families have routines that are important to them, and taking a large portion of time out of their day may lead to resentment, putting future visits in jeopardy. Similarly, if nothing of value (according to the family) occurs on a visit, family members may not continue to make themselves available for future visits. This becomes a balancing act for the family and the nurse, and it is an area in which using your sixth sense and picking up on nonverbal cues is helpful (Zerwekh, 1997). In addition, home visits are an expensive way to provide community health nursing services, which are population based. The outcome of better health for family members must be demonstrated in order to support the value of such costly services (see Bridging Financial Gaps).

Concluding and Documenting the Visit

After planning for the next visit, saying goodbye to the family members terminates the home visit. This is a good time to put away the paperwork, materials, and supplies from this visit and retrieve items needed for the next visit on your schedule. It is always safer to open your car trunk in front of this home and get out what is needed for the next family's visit than to open your trunk in front of the next family's home. You do not want to give community members information about what is stored in your car's trunk while it is unattended and you are in the family's home.

Most typically, the documentation of each home visit is completed as soon as the nurse returns to the agency. Some agencies provide their nurses with laptop computers with electronic charting forms, and charting is encouraged at the end of the visit before leaving for the next one. Sometimes, time is allowed for the nurse to chart at home after the last visit of the day. For the most part, you will be expected to complete the charting by hand, using agency forms, as soon as is practically possible. Most agencies expect all charting to be completed by the end of each work day or no later than the end of the work week.

Agencies use a variety of forms that assist the nurse to document fully and succinctly. On some forms, the nurse uses code numbers, letters, or checkmarks on developmental or disease-specific care plans that are devised in a checklist format. For example, a packet of four pages may be used to document a postpartum visit and newborn assessment—two narrative forms to chart the exceptions for mother and baby, and postpartum and newborn assessment forms on which head-to-toe assessment information is documented. These forms have a place to document parent or client teaching according to expected parameters and a place for listing other professionals involved with the family. Similar developmentally focused forms may be used in the agency for high-risk infants, high-risk children, adolescents, and older adults. Other packets of forms may focus

BRIDGING FINANCIAL GAPS

Karoly, L.A., Everingham, S.S., Hoube, J., et al. (1998). *Investing in our children: What we know and don't know about the costs and benefits of early childhood interventions.* MR—898. Santa Monica, CA: RAND.

A 1998 RAND study of nine early intervention models found that the Prenatal and Early Childhood Nurse Home Visitation model (the Olds model) yielded cost savings much greater than program costs; documented the program's high success rate in meeting its goals; and demonstrated significant benefits compared with other models. Benefits achieved are based on 15 years of research and evaluation of families served in Elmira, NY.

In the years since this study, many health departments across the country have adopted the Olds model and find that they are reaching the high-risk families and keeping parents and children healthier. Research data on these replication programs are anxiously awaited. The following benefits to families were found in the RAND study:

30 fewer months' use of welfare after the birth of the first child

2 years' interval or greater between the birth of the first and second child

69% fewer arrests among the mothers

44% fewer behavioral problems among the mothers due to substance abuse

79% fewer verified reports of child abuse and neglect through the first child's 15th birthday

56% fewer arrests among the 15-year-old children

69% fewer convictions and probation violations among the 15-year-old children

58% fewer sexual partners among these 15-year-old children

56% fewer days of consuming alcohol by the 15-year-old children

28% fewer cigarettes smoked by the 15-year-old children

The following benefits to the community were found:

Cumulative costs (per child) of the program by age 15 = $5,000

Cumulative savings (per child) of the program by age 15 = $15,000*

Sources of the $10,000 net savings:

Welfare	= $5,600
Taxes	= $2,300
Criminal justice	= $2,000
Emergency room visits	= $100

*As these savings are projected over the child's life, the savings are much greater.

---

on chronic illnesses, such as chronic obstructive pulmonary disease, hypertension, diabetes, alcoholism, acquired immunodeficiency syndrome (AIDS), or cancer, that are common in the agency client base.

Focus of Family Health Visits

The focus of family health visits depends on the mission and resources of the agency providing the service and the needs of the families being served. Some agencies provide education, recreational activities such as summer camps, and support groups for families of people with specific health problems such as Alzheimer's disease, asthma, diabetes, or neurologic disorders. Other agencies provide services directed toward those with special social or economic needs, such as immigrant families, people living in poverty, or the homeless. Home visits may be a part of the services when family members are unable to come to an agency or the service being provided is best conducted and received in the comfort and privacy of a family's home. In general, family health visits are designed to be educational, to provide anticipatory guidance, and to focus on health promotion or prevention.

Family Education and Anticipatory Guidance

Official agencies, such as county or city health departments, distribute their services based on the broader community's needs. For example, if there is a large population of teen pregnancies and high-risk infants, the health department may contract with hospitals and private doctors' offices to provide home or clinic visits to all teens or women with high-risk pregnancies and their newborns after delivery. On these visits, the community health nurse teaches prenatal, postpartum, and newborn care and provides anticipatory guidance (information needed in the future regarding the child and the need for regular infant health care provider visits, immunizations, and safety awareness). Another community may have a significant number of older adults who need to learn how to manage a chronic illness, enhance their nutrition, and practice safety measures to prevent injuries and falls.

Family Health Promotion and Illness Prevention

All populations, regardless of age, income, culture, or nation of origin, need the fundamental protection immunization gives to protect themselves and the health of the larger community. In addition, providing the means for families to receive required immunizations is a responsibility of health departments. Usually, immunization services are not brought into the home, but the nurse can provide information about immunizations, teach the importance of following an immunization schedule, and follow up with the client during home visits.

Teaching people how to prevent illness and how to remain healthy is basic to community health nursing (see Chapter 12). Even within the limitations of chronic illnesses, family members can be taught health promotion activities to live as healthfully as possible (Denham, 2002; Pender, 2001). Health promotion activities may include screening for hypertension and elevated cholesterol, performing a physical assessment, and teaching about nutrition and safety.

Such activities can occur during a family health visit; while family members are at their places of work, school, or recreation; or at self-help group meetings. Community health nurses often provide health promotion services to couples during prenatal classes by teaching about the expected changes during pregnancy and providing anticipatory guidance for safe infant care. They may also screen older adults at senior centers for hypertension or elevated cholesterol or teach family members who attend support groups, such as Alcoholics Anonymous or Gamblers Anonymous (see Chapter 35).

Personal Safety on the Home Visit

As mentioned earlier in this chapter, personal safety while traveling throughout the community is essential. In addition, continuation of personal safety while on the home visit must be considered.

Neighborhood, Travel, and Personal Safety.
On leaving your "base of operation," such as the health department office, neighborhood clinic, homeless shelter, or campus classroom, have with you all the necessary tools to travel in the community with safety. Most importantly, leave an itinerary of your planned travels, the telephone numbers of the families you will attempt to visit, and your cellular phone number. Traveling in the community takes a variety of forms and means different things to different people.

If you are traveling in an agency or private car, you need
- A full gas tank
- A city/county map
- A cellular phone
- The family addresses
- Money for lunch or telephone calls (in case you are in an area where your cellular phone does not work)
  If you are using public transportation, plan to
- Have exact change for each bus trip
- Carry a bus schedule
- Exit the bus as near as possible to your client's home
- Know where to get the bus for the return trip or to the next home visit
- Carry a cellular phone

If you are walking or riding a bicycle to a home visit, you still need to travel safely. All the rules of the road pertain to you as a pedestrian and when on a bicycle. Do not jaywalk or ride the bicycle on the sidewalk; cross streets at crosswalks and at traffic lights. In some neighborhoods, it is best to call ahead to the family you plan to visit, give them an approximate time of your arrival, and, if necessary, have them look out a window or door for your arrival. When walking in neighborhoods, walk with direction and purpose; do not look lost even if you are. Use neighborhood shopkeepers as resources for direction and information and as havens of refuge if you feel uncomfortable or threatened. If you need to ask for directions and you are not near any stores, look for another professional, such as a social worker, a public service employee (a postal worker or utility worker), or an apartment manager. If you need to approach a stranger for information, select a woman. If you see a group of teenagers or adults that makes you feel uncomfortable, cross the street, limit eye contact, and continue to the home you are intending to visit. Always avoid walking through alleys or along buildings that open onto alleys, and stay in the middle of the sidewalk or closer to the street. It might be useful to carry a whistle on your key ring.

It is always safest to avoid compromising situations by staying alert and using safe traveling methods whenever you are in public, no matter how "safe" an area appears. However, if you are ever accosted by an individual or a group, immediately try to break free and run to a public place while making loud noises. Yell "Fire!" This response gets more attention than "Help!" If a criminal wants your nursing bag, purse, or wallet, freely give it up—the contents are not worth your safety. Some nurses feel safer after they have attended self-defense classes, which are offered by police departments, as employee in-service programs in some agencies, and on some university campuses.

In some rough inner-city neighborhoods, professionals visiting families travel only in pairs (usually with at least one man in the pair) or with a security guard or police escort. Know whether these resources are necessary or available to you before venturing into a crime-ridden community. In some inner-city neighborhoods, community health nurses refuse to visit people living on one block or in one apartment building. Know and do not challenge important safety measures that are used by expert nurses and are followed for personal safety. They are unique to each community.

Another focus of concern is the perceived risk to self when making a home visit. An individual's cognition and perception of a situation, his or her views on risks and risk taking, and the time, setting, and coping process all factor into feelings of safety when traveling in a community, entering a family's home, or conducting a home visit (Kendra & George, 2001). What one person sees as a risk, another sees as a challenge or an opportunity. Yet another may see nothing. We each perceive risks differently based on knowledge, experience, and personality.

Arriving at the Home. Make sure you are at the right house, and do not go into the home until you are assured that the family you are intending to visit does live there and is home. For example, you may be planning to visit 16-year-old Jennifer and her 5-day-old infant, Marcus. However, when you knock on the door, it is answered by a 50-year-old man. Do not enter the home without asking whether Jennifer can come to the door, or unless you see her in the house through the door, even if the man answering the door invites you in. Remain outside the home and go inside only after you talk to Jennifer at the door. This precaution ensures that the family members you want to visit are really home and that this is the right address.

Friction Between Family Members. During a home visit, two or more family members may begin to argue or physically fight with one another. Immediately remove yourself from the home visit and tell the family members that you will visit at another time when the family differences are resolved. You must let the family know that it is not a good time to visit when there are such distractions and you must leave. Depending on the type of altercation, it may be appropriate to discuss the friction in the family on a later visit or to call 911 from your cellular phone when you are out of the house. Never step in and offer to assist an adult family member when two people are physically fighting; you may be the next victim.

Family Members Under the Influence. If the focus of the visit is on two family members and a third member is demonstrating behaviors that indicate drug or alcohol use, you must use your judgment as to your best action. The agency you work for or the school you attend has guidelines you should follow. If the intoxicated person goes to another room and falls asleep, it might be appropriate to continue the visit and perhaps discuss your observations with the remaining family members. On the other hand, if the person becomes abusive, remains in the room, or interrupts the home visit, it is best to terminate the visit and reschedule when this member is not under the influence or is not present. Again, you do not want to put yourself in the middle of a situation that could deteriorate rapidly and could compromise your safety.

The Presence of Strangers. In some families, the coming and going of many extended family members, neighbors, and friends is commonplace; it is the norm and is not distracting to them. However, a busy environment or the presence of too many people can create an uncomfortable environment for the nurse. For example, what would you do if you arrived at a home and five teenage boys were sitting on the front porch steps, so that you had to sidle your way through to knock on the door? What if you found three men sleeping on the living room floor in the small apartment of a teenage mother and her infant, or four neighbor children riding tricycles inside the house during a teaching visit to two young parents who do not seem fazed by the commotion?

Such situations may not be indicative of danger, but they can make you feel vulnerable, uncomfortable, or distracted. It is best to ask the family when would be a better time to visit, move the visit to another room, or go for a walk with the clients, continuing the visit while outside. In some way, take control of the environment so that you feel safe and comfortable and your attention can focus on the family members who are a part of the visit. Certainly, inquire about the other people you see on the periphery of the home visit. Ask about their relationships to the family, their general health, and whether they should be included in the visit. Be prepared for the family to suggest that you ignore the other people or to say that they are transient family members whom you may never see again. On the other hand, it may be important to learn who they are, because they may have unmet health care needs.

IMPLEMENTING PLANS FOR PROMOTING THE HEALTH OF FAMILIES

Once you have received a referral, contacted the family for a visit appointment, prepared for the visit, and met the family, you are ready to implement the plan. As the visit progresses, there are specific activities and actions that you can take to enhance the effectiveness of the visit and improve family health outcomes. These include contracting with the family and promoting the strengths of the family.

Assessing, Teaching, and Referring

The focus of each family visit is different. On a first visit, initial assessment data must be obtained in addition to helping the family set goals that they want to accomplish. On subsequent visits, actions and activities are taken to reach the goals. Specific actions fall mainly in the categories of assessing, teaching, and referring.

Assessing family health may be done informally through observation and occasional questioning, or it can take a more formal approach. Specific questions may be asked of each family member, and such information as health data and family history may be included. Physical data such as height, weight, pulses, temperature, and blood pressure are recorded on an assessment tool. (Chapter 23 describes family assessment in greater detail.)

With young children, specific assessment questionnaires or tests may be conducted to measure how well they are meeting growth and developmental tasks. One familiar test that has been used for decades is the Denver Developmental Screening Test (DDST). The results of this gross assessment screening test provide the nurse with information about the child's growth and developmental progress and can be used to teach families anticipatory guidance, as well as how to provide growth-enhancing experiences. This easily administered test can be purchased and comes with a training manual, test kit, and score sheets. There are also videos demonstrating the correct way to administer the DDST to children of different ages. The DDST items can be ordered from DDM, Inc., P. O. Box 6919, Denver, CO 80203.

If an adult family member has an identified disease (eg, diabetes, congestive heart failure, substance abuse, hypertension, chronic obstructive pulmonary disease) or a child has the potential for or has an identified health problem (eg, a high-risk newborn, a drug-exposed infant, failure to thrive, a birth defect), a flow sheet developed by the agency can be used to guide the nurse in obtaining standard assessment information during the home visit (Fig. 24–1). From this, an individualized approach to gathering additional information can be developed. In addition, older adults may be assessed through observation of activities of daily living (ADL) and instrumental activities of daily living (IADL) (Farren, 1999) (see Chapter 30).

While on a home visit, the community health nurse should also conduct a home and family assessment that includes all aspects of the home environment, such as adequacy and permanency. Education, employment, income, furnishings, support systems, and other agencies involved in family care are some of the family resources that should be assessed (Murry & Zentner, 2000).

The assessment process is lengthy, time-consuming, and ongoing. The nurse must gather the most essential assessment information on the first visit. By selecting one or two concerns of priority to the family and nurse, it is possible to focus assessment on these areas. The nurse then uses this information as a guide to additional assessments needed on subsequent visits. The selected assessment tools, when complete, provide family information; these data can be used to assist the family during future visits by offering instruction or referral to appropriate services available in the community.

Teaching health promotion activities to the family should begin only after members express an interest and recognize a need. If the family is not at a level of functioning that enables members to use anticipatory guidance and teaching, the nurse can provide more basic services, such as gathering resources and acting as a counselor (Tapia, 1997). If family members are ready to learn ways to improve their health status, the nurse needs to assess the best teaching approach to use (see Chapter 12). Consideration of language barriers, previous knowledge and experience, family and community resources, and time available influence the choice of approach.

Often, the community health nurse discovers that the family has needs beyond those met by teaching and that there are others in the community with the skills and services to meet those needs. In such cases, the nurse can initiate the referral process. Referring families to appropriate resources is discussed in detail later in this chapter.

Contracting

Contracting is a method of formalizing the relationship between the family and the community health nurse and in-

cludes a verbal or written commitment on the part of the family and the nurse for the development and accomplishment of goals (see Chapter 11). Such a contract contains **mutual goals**—goals that the family and the nurse plan and take action on together. It is easy to go into a family's home, see exactly what is wrong, and set about "making it right" according to your values. You might think, "If only the family would wash their dishes each evening, keep the floors uncluttered, put sheets on the bed, set an alarm and get up in the morning to get the children off to school, and spend their money on milk and orange juice instead of beer and cigarettes, most of their problems would be solved." It is easy to criticize from the outside and make blanket judgments and decisions about what others should do. As an observer, you may value clean dishes, swept floors, sleeping on sheets, getting children to school, and drinking milk and orange juice. However, not all of these values are essential to the family's functioning. Instead, your role as a nurse is to influence the choices a family makes that affect health, safety, and comfort. If the cluttered floors cause falls or the dirty dishes attract roaches and rats, you might find that intervening by teaching the family about the connection between these factors is important. If the family decides that a change in behavior is one of its goals and you agree to assist with the change, this mutual goal could be formalized through a contract (Display 24–2).

Empowering Families

Throughout the family visit, you must remember that the ultimate goal is to assist the family in becoming independent of your services. This is accomplished by the approach used in conducting the visit. How you structure the nurse–client relationship also influences the outcomes. Four thoughts will help to clarify your working relationship with families:

- The family functioned in a manner that worked for them before you ever met them.
- If you ever feel obliged to do something for a family, consider who did this before you were available.
- Find family strengths even in the most deprived family situation.
- If you were in a similar situation, would you manage, cope, or function as well as the members of this family?

Families have strengths that some middle-class nurses may overlook or interpret as weaknesses. It is the nurse's job to recognize the strengths in families and to help families recognize them as well. For example, some families borrow needed items (diapers, food, clothes) from each other, whereas others do not even recognize their next-door neighbors by sight. Children from large families often learn to physically care for one another and entertain themselves, whereas in some families with only one or two children, the youngsters must constantly be entertained. The members of one family may take public transportation or walk to accomplish errands, whereas members of a family with a reliable car may use it for the closest of errands and may never

FLOW SHEET
HIGH RISK INFANT

Pt's Name _____ Address _____ Phone _____

At Birth: Weight _____   Length _____   Head Circ. _____   APGARS _____

	Date										
Irritability											
Lethargic											
Vomiting											
Diarrhea											
Feedings											
• Amount											
• Frequency											
• Suck											
Seizures/Convulsions											
Stools											
• Color											
• Consistency											
• Frequency											
Urine Output											
Edema											
Eyes Roll											
Temperature											
Pulse											
Respiration											
Weight											
Length											
Femoral Pulses											
Reflexes											
Muscle Tone											
Skin											
• Color											
• Condition											
Auscultate Chest											
Edema											
Output-Concentration											
Respiratory Function											
• Nasal Flaring											
• Grunting											
• Sternal Retracting											
• Tachycardia											
Head Circumference											
Chest Circumference											
Initials											

O - Normal   X - Problem (See Narrative)   C - Counseled for prevention

FIGURE 24-1.   High-risk infant flow sheet.

Immunization (Circle & Date)

DPT 1 2 3 4 5 _____ PPD _____ MMR _____ Hib _____

Polio 1 2 3 4 5 _____ Hep B _____ Varicella _____

Instruction	Instruction Date	Pt. Understanding Date	Pamphlets Given Date	Comments	Initials
Review Disease Process					
Temperature Technique					
Feeding & Technique					
Bonding					
General Care					
• Bath					
• Hygiene					
• Formula Preparation					
• Cord Care					
Prevention of Infection					
Environment - Temperature Control					
Position					
Growth & Development					
Safety					
Stimulation					
Immunizations					
Referred to:					
Medical App./Date/M.D.					
S/S of Sick Child					

Initials	Signature

FIGURE 24-1.   *(continued)*

have been on a bus or subway. These are examples of strengths that some middle-class families have forgotten or never developed.

At times, community health nurses want to help families by taking one of the members to a doctor or to the store or by bringing a supply of formula or diapers. It might be a simple task, because you will be driving by the clinic anyway or because there are extra cans of formula in the agency office, but will it promote the family's independence and self-sufficiency? It is a much better gift to promote the skill of planning ahead so that the family may meet its own transportation needs (neighbors, family members, loose change saved for the bus, or even walking) or find ways to use formula supplies wisely. For example, bottles can be filled with only the amount the baby consumes, so that ounces are not wasted at each feeding. Unused formula should be kept refrigerated so

that it does not spoil, and care should be taken to make sure that infants are not overfed. The amount of formula consumed in 24 hours by the baby can be determined to ensure that the correct quantity is being provided. After a child reaches the appropriate age, foods and fluids other than formula may be provided. A can of powdered formula may be kept on hand for emergencies, and families may wish to switch to powdered formula if they are using the more expensive premixed or concentrated formulas. Once families learn these skills, crises will occur less frequently or will be managed more effectively.

Finally, you should always look for ways to genuinely praise families for managing in difficult situations. On a home visit, you can empower families by pointing out the positive aspects of their self-care and caregiving, rather than pointing out what they do not do or have (Renpenning, Tay-

DISPLAY 24-2

Sample Family Contract

Ramona Davenport, community health nurse, is agreeing to visit Sonia Jeffers two times a month between 1/2/05 and 4/4/05 to work together toward helping Brian, aged 3, become toilet trained by April, 2005. Ramona Davenport will

1. Make seven home visits during the next 3 months, focusing on toilet training.
2. Bring Sonia a pamphlet about successful toilet training and use it as a teaching guide.
3. Reinforce progress on each visit and make suggestions for improvement.
4. Praise the successful accomplishment of toilet training or renegotiate the contract if needed.

Sonia Jeffers will

1. Purchase a potty-seat and underpants for Brian during the first 2 weeks of working together.
2. Read a story to Brian about toilet training and a little boy his age.
3. Be consistent in following the successful toilet-training steps.
4. Discuss her feelings about progress and setbacks with Ramona Davenport on each visit.
5. Celebrate toilet training success with Brian (a toy or underwear with super heros on them) or work with Ramona to renegotiate the contract.

Ramona Davenport, signature _____
Sonia Jeffers, signature _____
Date _____

lor, & Eisenhandler, 2003). Verbally list the positive aspects in a natural and conversational manner. For example, a young woman, who is holding her baby, greets you at the door. You note that she has a dresser drawer on the floor next to her mattress for the baby to sleep in. They live in a sparsely furnished one-room apartment. She has two baby bottles and a limited assortment of baby clothes. Later during the first visit, you say, "Carlo looks so happy when you cuddle him in your arms, and you are considering his safety by letting him sleep in the dresser drawer next to your mattress. I notice you wash each bottle before making the formula, and you keep him warm in the sleeper and blanket. I think you are managing Carlo very well." In this brief scenario, you have mentioned, in a positive way, bonding, infant health and safety, and proper infant clothing. You have not mentioned the absence of furniture, a full set of bottles, or a layette of clothing. During the remainder of the visit, you discuss the services your agency can provide and assess whether any of them would be of interest to the young mother. You allow her to make decisions for her family and to use you as a resource and guide (Wright & Leahey, 2000). This encourages empowerment.

EVALUATING IMPLEMENTED FAMILY HEALTH PLANS

The final step in the nursing process is evaluation. The evaluation process leads to a reassessment of your work with the family and a determination of what is needed in preparation for the next visit. This reassessment helps you in further individualizing services to the family. Evaluation of the structure-process of the visit and your self-evaluation can be done informally in a reflective manner. Outcomes are documented in the client record, and the evaluation becomes formalized. A thorough evaluation also assists you in making the most appropriate referrals and contacting key resources to meet family needs.

Types of Evaluations

Each family visit should be evaluated in three ways: structure-process, outcome, and self-evaluation. Each provides a different piece of information about the success of the visit. If the visit was not successful, what part made it less than successful? Most importantly, were the outcomes achieved? If not, is there something about the structure-process or your own preparedness or behavior that needs to be changed? When conducting an evaluation of the home visit, you are looking for answers to these questions.

Structure-Process

The structure-process of a visit should be analyzed first. Were there aspects of the organization, timing, environment, or sequencing of the components that needed to be changed or modified to make it a more effective visit? What could you have done about these factors? Were you organized? Would better preparation help with your organization? Were there distractions in the home that influenced organization? Ask yourself questions such as these, and then make plans to avoid or reduce disorganizing distractions. For example, if you made the visit based on limited information from a referral, you now have additional family data and can be better prepared for the next visit. If transportation schedules made the family late to the clinic, perhaps other transportation could be arranged. If the distraction on a home visit occurred because children were arriving home from school, visits could be made earlier in the day. If the television was playing loudly, you could make it a point to ask the family whether they would mind turning down the volume, or visit at a time when they do not watch television. Make the modifications that you can to assist with the visit process.

Outcome Evaluation

Second and most important is evaluation of the outcomes of the visit. Were the anticipated outcomes achieved? If not, why not? If so, what made it possible? The **outcome evaluation**, or the assessment of change in the family's (client's) health status based on mutually agreed activities, is a formal process demonstrated in the documentation of the home visit.

The agency may use the Nursing Outcomes Classification (NOC) System along with the Nursing Intervention Classification (NIC) System. Alternatively, there may be agency-driven criteria for success and expectations for each client category or visit type. On a visit-by-visit basis, the changes observed in the family may be small; progress toward an expected outcome is noted. At the conclusion of agency services to the family, the cumulative changes in the client's health and the success or failure to achieve various outcomes are evaluated. Depending on the conclusions that can be drawn, the decision to terminate services may need to be reevaluated. It is possible that continuance of service is required and the terms must be renegotiated. Whatever the decision, the family must be included in the decision-making process.

Self-Evaluation

The third component of evaluation is self-evaluation. What aspect of your performance as a community health nurse during the home visit facilitated the achievement of a desired outcome? Were you prepared? Did you gather all the data needed to assist the family on the next visit? What would you do differently if you could do the visit over? What went right? What went wrong? What are you going to do on the next visit to make it better? This close look at yourself is important for your own growth and effectiveness as a community health nurse.

Sometimes we cannot see our own strengths or flaws, and evaluations by others are helpful. In some agencies, regular peer evaluations are conducted. An agency staff nurse makes a family visit with the community health nurse and provides feedback based on her or his observations. This is a useful technique to use even at times other than planned evaluations of all staff members in the agency. You might ask a colleague to accompany you on a home visit to a family that has not made progress toward outcome achievement or to a family you have not been able to "reach" or find difficult to work with (Drummond, Weir, & Kysela, 2002). For a variety of reasons, consultation with peers regarding certain visits and how best to conduct them can assist you in being better prepared or more focused. It can improve your interaction with families from different cultures or in difficult situations (Spector, 2000; Walsh, 1999).

Planning for the Next Visit

Part of the evaluation of one family visit is planning for the next. Use what occurred on the previous visit to guide you toward activities on subsequent visits. Goals may need to be modified, or family situations may change and specific outcomes become irrelevant. For example, you may plan to visit a prenatal family one last time before the baby is born to reinforce prior teaching about when to leave for the hospital with a second pregnancy. You intend to remind the parents to arrange babysitting for the older child and to assess the pregnant woman's rising blood pressure and complaints of backache. When you arrive for the visit, the husband is home alone with the younger child and is about to leave to bring his wife and new baby home from the hospital. He asks you about the diaper rash that just appeared on the 2-year-old. He also asks how to secure the new car seat into the car, because the instructions do not seem to make sense for his make of car. Outcomes for a problem-free pregnancy and healthy birth are not relevant; there are new outcomes to be formulated and worked on with this young family.

More frequently, planning for subsequent visits is relatively predictable and is done to ensure that steps toward outcome accomplishment are achieved on the visit. Being totally prepared each time is the best predictor of a successful family visit. Once you have met and gotten to know a family during a visit, the planning can be individualized and tailored to meet the family's unique needs. This information is not available from a paper referral, which makes planning for a first home visit important. The tone set during the first visit can affect your continued success with the family.

Referrals

A referral in written or verbal form (by agency-created form, telephone, fax, or e-mail) initiates contact with a family. In addition to responding to a referral, which begins the relationship with a family, the nurse makes referrals on behalf of the family. Families often need access to services beyond the agency's scope, and the nurse's knowledge of other resources can mean the difference between their having and not having access to additional services. Therefore, nurses must have information available to them about the eligibility requirements and availability of services provided by a bevy of official, voluntary, religious, and neighborhood organizations. If this information is not readily at hand, community health nurses need to know how to locate needed services. This is a daunting challenge, because the services are many, and organizations frequently change telephone numbers, services, and the populations they serve. Networking with colleagues on a regular basis helps keep nurses up to date with community services from which they can generate referrals for clients.

Contacting Resources

At times, community health nurses implement their roles as client advocates by helping families gain services in a more timely manner than they could by themselves. Community health nurses know how to access key personnel in agencies and can eliminate some of the red tape involved in obtaining services. Nurses can provide pointers that may help families procure needed services; for example, clients may have an advantage if they go to an agency early in the morning in the middle of the week. The fact that they should have all forms completely filled out and should bring their last 3 months' rent and utility receipts, or that they should ask to speak with a certain worker, may also be helpful information.

When nurses seek informal services for families, a relationship with the director of the agency can help them gain

Two Community Programs for Pregnant Teens

In two programs, pregnant teens are the target population for community health nursing intervention.

1. In Madera County Health Department in Madera, California, pregnant teens are followed throughout their pregnancy and the first year of the infant's life with home visits and educational programs and materials. They are provided with an extensive referral network and incentives for participation in the program in the form of infant toys and a car seat.

2. A series of prenatal classes at Kaiser Permanente Northern California managed care organization is open to the public for "women who are pregnant and will deliver before their 20th birthday." Family members and significant others are invited to attend along with the teen. The eight classes are offered weekly in the afternoon for 90 minutes, and each class stands alone in that a teen can begin at any time. After all eight separate classes have been attended, the teen mother receives an infant car seat.

services for the clients. For example, a client family has a personal crisis and needs a donation of food and a volunteer to stay with a handicapped child for 3 days while a spouse undergoes surgery. The nurse telephones the religious leader of a neighborhood church and shares the family's requests, clarifies the situation, and gets a donation of food from the church's food pantry. The name of a member of the church who can stay with the child is also provided. The family may not have been aware that such services were available to them, and the links provided by the nurse are as important as other community health nursing functions (Display 24–3).

SUMMARY

Making family health visits is a unique role for nurses and is one of the activities common to most community health nurses. In some agencies, family health visits are conducted for only the most high-risk families. In other agencies, a visit is the method of choice for most care.

When nurses visit families, they must use acute observation skills, good verbal and nonverbal communication, assessment skills, and a "sixth sense" to guide them safely in the community and with the families. Some visits are conducted with families in settings other than their homes. Neighborhood clinics, schools, work places, or recreational settings may be the preferred or the only locations in which you can gather most of the family members for the visit. Other families may be in transition and living in homeless shelters or with relatives or neighbors. These settings are familiar to the family and provide a unique environment for the nurse in which to visit the family.

Previsit preparation, conducting the visit, and postvisit documentation are the main components of a family health visit. Each step is important and has value for the success of the next step. Being well prepared for a visit is the first concern (eg, know the location, have family health status information and needed materials). The visit should be conducted in an orderly and organized fashion. Time should be allowed for getting acquainted, for the body of the visit, including teaching and anticipatory guidance, and for any other nursing care that may be a part of the visit. Concluding with a summary of the important parts of the visit and planning for the next visit ensures an appropriate ending.

Being safe in a neighborhood is important for all people. Community health nurses spend a great part of the day in the community, and safe travel is of constant importance. Use of a personal or agency car, public transportation, or walking to visit families each has its own set of precautions for personal safety. Even in a family's home, personal safety must be a consideration. If family members are arguing or under the influence of drugs or alcohol, the situation may deteriorate rapidly and become unsafe; at this point, it is best to terminate the visit.

During the implementation phase of the family health visit, the nurse establishes a verbal or written contract with the family. This permits understanding by both the family and the nurse of the personal roles and responsibilities in the relationship. Empowerment of family members is significant for clients. People who are empowered can help themselves for a lifetime and can make independent decisions about their own health.

Evaluation and preparation for the next visit completes the family health visit cycle. Three types of evaluation can be conducted at the end of a visit. Recall of the structure-process assists the nurse in reflecting on the physical aspects of the visit that were positive or negative. Discovering these factors can help enhance the positive and eliminate the negative. Evaluating whether the outcomes of the visit were achieved is done in a more formal way with agency documentation. Because the purpose of conducting family health visits is to bring about positive changes in family behaviors, it is necessary to evaluate the achievement of mutual goals made by the nurse and the family. The hardest part of evaluation is looking at yourself and how you conduct home visits. Often, peer evaluation is a helpful way to obtain feedback, because people tend to minimize their own strengths and overlook their weaknesses.

Conducting family health visits involves making referrals to other agencies and services on behalf of the family. One agency cannot provide all the services that a family needs. Written or verbal forms of communicating a need involve contacting resources available in the community. Community health nurses have unique skills in knowing and locating both official and voluntary services within their community. Such skills come with experience.

ACTIVITIES TO PROMOTE CRITICAL THINKING

1. Invite a peer to go on a family health visit with you, and be open to feedback regarding your strengths and weaknesses. How does it make you feel to have someone else on a family health visit with you, knowing that they are observing your skills? Offer to do the same for a peer and provide him or her with feedback. Discuss your experiences.

2. Go on several family health visits with an experienced community health nurse and observe the nurse's visiting techniques. Observe how he or she contacts the family, knocks on the door, greets the family, conducts, summarizes, and concludes the visit, and makes plans for the next visit. Discuss the various techniques used, and ask questions about your observations to get a better idea of why things are done as they are. Use some of this information on your next home visit.

3. Initiate a small group discussion among your peers about safety on your school campus and in your community. Encourage each person to share the safety habits used. How are these techniques different from safety techniques used when making family visits in the community? If they are different, why are they? Should they be different?

4. Locate nursing Web sites on the Internet and look for the following studies on family health: Olds et al., 1999; Eckenrode et al., 2000; Kitzman et al., 2000; and Kearney, York, & Deatrick, 2000. All four studies included intensive home visits to high-risk families. How did intensive family health visiting make a difference in the lives of the participants in these studies? Do you know any communities where the Olds model of home visiting to families or other models are being replicated? If so, how do the results of visiting these families compare with the results found in these studies?

REFERENCES

Allender, J.A. (1998). *Community and home health nursing.* Philadelphia: Lippincott-Raven.

Denham, S.A. (2002). *Family health: A framework for nursing.* Philadelphia: F.A. Davis.

Drummond, J.E., Weir, A.E., & Kysela, G.M. (2002). Home visitation practice: Models, documentation, and evaluation. *Public Health Nursing, 19*(1), 24–29.

Eckenrode, J., Ganzel, B., Henderson, C.R., Smith, E., Olds, D.L., Powers, J., et al. (2000). Preventing child abuse and neglect with a program of nurse home visitation: The limiting effects of domestic violence. *Journal of the American Medical Association, 284*(11), 1385–1391.

Farren, M. (1999). Ensuring safety for the elderly client at home. In S. Zang & J.A. Allender, *Home care of the elderly* (pp. 59–77). Philadelphia: Lippincott Williams & Wilkins.

Friedman, M.M., Bowden, V.R., & Jones, E. (2003). *Family nursing: Research, theory, and practice* (5th ed.). Upper Saddle River, NJ: Prentice-Hall.

Karoly, L.A., Everingham, S.S., Hoube, J., et al. (1998). *Investing in our children: What we know and don't know about the costs and benefits of early childhood interventions.* MR—898, Santa Monica, CA: RAND.

Kearney, M.H., York, R., & Deatrick, J.A. (2000). Effects of home visits to vulnerable young families. *Journal of Nursing Scholarship, 32*(4), 369–376.

Kendra, M.A., & George, V.D. (2001). Defining risk in home visiting. *Public Health Nursing, 18*(2), 128–137.

Kitzman, H., Olds, D.L., Sidora, K., Henderson, C.R., Hanks, C., Cole, R., et al. (2000). Enduring effects of nurse home visitation on maternal life course: A 3-year follow-up of a randomized trial. *Journal of the American Medical Association, 283*(15), 1983–1989.

Murray, R.B., & Zentner, J.P. (2000). *Health assessment and promotion strategies through the life span* (7th ed.). Upper Saddle River, NJ: Prentice-Hall.

Olds, D.L., Henderson, C.R., Kitzman, H.J., Eckenrode, J.J., Cole, R.E., & Tatelbaum, R.C. (1999). Prenatal and infancy home visitation by nurses: Recent findings. *The future of children, 9*(1), 44–65.

Pender, N.J. (2001). *Health promotion in nursing practice* (4th ed.). Upper Saddle River, NJ: Prentice-Hall.

Renpenning, K.M., Taylor, S.G., & Eisenhandler, S.A. (2003). *Self-care theory in nursing: Selected papers of Dorothea Orem.* New York: Springer.

Schorr, T.M., & Kennedy, M.S. (1999). *100 years of American nursing.* Philadelphia: Lippincott Williams & Wilkins.

Spector, R.E. (2000). *Cultural diversity in health and illness* (5th ed.). Upper Saddle River, NJ: Prentice-Hall.

Tapia, J.A. (1997). The nursing process in family health. In B.W. Spradley & J.A. Allender, *Readings in community health nursing* (5th ed., pp. 343–350). Philadelphia: Lippincott-Raven.

Walsh, M. (1999). Dealing effectively with physically and verbally abusive elderly clients and families. In S. Zang & J.A. Allender (Eds.), *Home care of the elderly* (pp. 190–206). Philadelphia: Lippincott Williams & Wilkins.

Wright, L.M., & Leahey, M. (2000). *Nurses and families: A guide to family assessment and intervention* (3rd ed.). Philadelphia: F.A. Davis.

Zerwekh, J.V. (1997). Making the connection during home visits: Narratives of expert nurses. *International Journal for Human Caring, 1*(1), 25–29.

SELECTED READINGS

Baltazar, V., Ibe, O.B., & Allender, J.A. (1999). Maintaining optimum nutrition among elderly clients at home. In S. Zang &

J.A. Allender (Eds.), *Home care of the elderly* (pp. 98–121). Philadelphia: Lippincott Williams & Wilkins.

Barnes, S.L. (2001). Stressors and strengths: A theoretical and practical examination of nuclear, single-parent, and augmented African American families. *Families in Society: The Journal of Contemporary Human Services, 82*(5), 449–460.

Becvar, D.S., & Becvar, R. (2003). *Family therapy: A systematic integration* (5th ed.). Boston: Allyn & Bacon.

Bulechek, G.M., & McCloskey, J.C. (Eds.). (1999). *Nursing interventions: Essential nursing treatments* (3rd ed.). Philadelphia: W.B. Saunders.

Early, T.J. (2001). Measures for practice with families from a strengths perspective. *Families in Society: The Journal of Contemporary Human Services. 82*(3), 225–232.

Gottman, J.M., & Notarius, C.I. (2002). Marital research in the 20th century and a research agenda for the 21st century. *Family Process, 41*(2), 159–197.

Koniak-Griffin, D., Anderson, N.L.R., Verzemnieks, I., & Brecht, M. (2000). A public health nursing early intervention program for adolescent mothers: Outcomes from pregnancy through 6 weeks postpartum. *Nursing Research, 49*(3), 130–138.

Linn, R. (2001). *Mature unwed mothers: Narratives of moral resistance.* Norwell, MA: Kluwer Plenum.

Lynch, M., & Cicchetti, D. (2002). Links between community violence and the family system: Evidence from children's feelings of relatedness and perceptions of parent behavior. *Family Process, 41*(3), 519–532.

McNaughton, D.B. (2000). A synthesis of qualitative home visiting research. *Public Health Nursing, 17*(6), 405–414.

Navaie-Waliser, M., Martin, S.L., Campbell, M.K., Tessaro, I., Kotelchuck, M., & Cross, A.W. (2000). Factors predicting completion of a home visitation program by high-risk pregnant women: The North Carolina maternal outreach worker program. *American Journal of Public Health, 90*(1), 121–124.

Phipps, M.G., & Sowers, M. (2002). Defining early adolescent childbearing. *American Journal of Public Health, 92*(1), 125–128.

Rucibwa, N.J., Modeste, N., Montgomery, S., & Fox, C.A. (2003). Exploring family factors and sexual behaviors in a group of Black and Hispanic adolescent males. *American Journal of Health Behavior, 27*(1), 63–74.

Wagner, M.M., & Clayton, S.L. (1999). The parents as teachers program: Results from two demonstrations. *The Future of Children, 9*(19), 91–115.

Wallace, H.M., Green, G., Jaros, K., Paine, L., & Story, M. (1999). *Health and welfare for families in the 21st century.* Boston: Jones & Bartlett.

Wegner, G.D., & Alexander, R.J. (1999). *Readings in family nursing* (2nd ed.). Philadelphia: Lippincott Williams & Wilkins.

25

Families in Crisis: Facing Violence from Within and Outside the Family

Learning Objectives

Upon mastery of this chapter, you should be able to:

- Explain the difference between developmental crises and situational crises and give several examples of each within families.

- Discuss strategies to prevent the impact of a situational crisis and a developmental crisis at each level of prevention.

- Discuss the global incidence and prevalence of family violence.

- Describe how the United States has historically responded to family violence.

- Describe three main categories of family violence.

- Identify characteristics of five forms of abuse against infants, children, and adolescents.

- Describe the "cycle of violence" seen in partner/spousal abuse.

- Explain the types of mistreatment common to the elderly.

- Discuss the preparation a family can make for a community-wide situational crisis such as a natural disaster or an act of terrorism.

- Describe the role of a community health nurse with families in crisis at each level of prevention.

- Use the steps of the nursing process to outline nursing actions in developmental and situational crises.

A **family crisis** is a stressful and disruptive event (or series of events) that comes with or without warning and disturbs the equilibrium of the family. A family crisis can also result when usual problem-solving methods fail. All families experience periods of crisis: a toddler is diagnosed with a serious illness; a teenager discovers she is pregnant; a father and sole breadwinner in a family loses his job; a mother's social drinking becomes habitual after her children go off to college; a family's home is destroyed in a hurricane, earthquake, flood, or fire; a family prepares for a potential terrorist attack. If you think back on your own family's history, you probably can identify one or more periods of crisis that you and your family members have experienced. If so, how directly were you affected? How did the crisis resolve? As a result of the crisis, were there any permanent changes in your family's dynamics or individual behaviors?

People respond to crises differently. Some approach them as a challenge, an event to be reckoned with; others are overwhelmed and feel defeated or give up. Some seek help if needed and come through the experience unscathed or as survivors, perhaps even stronger than before. Others who are unable to cope with the crisis, or do not cope well, may suffer severe psychological damage or may inflict their feelings of rage, frustration, or powerlessness on their children, partners, or elders. This chapter focuses on families that have responded to stressors with violence, neglect, or abuse and those that have experienced stress and losses during a national disaster or war or the threat of violence through terrorism.

Regardless of their responses, families in crisis need help, and community health nurses have a unique opportunity and responsibility to provide that help in a broad variety of situations. For example, in one family, an 8-year-old boy begins doing poorly in school; he wets his pants during class twice in 1 week and starts a small fire in the schoolyard. The school nurse is astute enough to begin an investigation into the family dynamics that may be contributing to these symptoms. In another family, a pregnant woman reschedules her appointment at a community clinic twice, then arrives with multiple faded bruises on her face and arms. The clinic nurse uses sensitivity and caring to screen her for domestic violence. In addition to assessment, community health nurses provide direct assistance during times of crisis, and they help prevent crises by teaching families parenting skills, coping strategies, and primary/secondary preparation and tertiary responses in times of national crises. This chapter examines how nurses can sharpen their knowledge and skills in the practice of crisis prevention and intervention in order to promote the health of families in the community.

DYNAMICS AND CHARACTERISTICS OF A CRISIS

Researchers have studied the nature of crises and have developed a body of knowledge called **crisis theory**. Initially limited to the field of mental health, crisis theory now influences every field of health care, helping to explain why people respond in certain ways and to predict the phases that people go through in a crisis of any kind. These are important ideas for the community health nurse to understand before crises can be prevented or managed.

How does a crisis occur? Each of us is a dynamic system living within a given environment under circumstances unique to us alone. Our behavior—both consciously and subconsciously—is gauged to maintain a balance within ourselves and in our relations with others. When some internal or external force disrupts our system's balance and alters its functioning, loss of equilibrium occurs. We then attempt to restore equilibrium by using whatever resources are available to us, in an effort to cope with the situation. **Coping** refers to those actions and ways of thinking that assist people in dealing with and surviving difficult situations. If we cannot readily cope with a stressful event—for example, if our home is destroyed by fire, or we fail a final examination—we experience crisis.

Crises are precipitated by specific identifiable events that become too much for the usual problem-solving skills of those involved. Often, a single distressing event follows a host of previous difficulties and becomes the "straw that breaks the camel's back." For example, a wife who suffers years of spousal abuse finally becomes unable to cope and shoots her husband during a violent attack. Occasionally, tragic events occur suddenly without previous stressors, as when a father is killed in a plane crash or a child drowns in the family swimming pool.

Crises are normal in that all people feel overwhelmed occasionally. A person who intervenes in today's crisis may very well be tomorrow's crisis victim. No individual is immune from sudden overwhelming difficulties. For example, a hospice nurse assists families through crises as part of her job. Suddenly the nurse learns that her own spouse is diagnosed with cancer.

Often a crisis is not an event per se, but rather a person's perception of the event. Each person reacts in his or her own individual way. A situation that throws one person off course may merely create an interesting detour for another (Display 25–1). It is usually the individual's interpretation of the event, rather than the event itself, that is crucial. At other times, a community crisis occurs on a large scale or is so unexpected that it directly involves people who are known by others hundreds of miles away, causing distant friends and relatives personal shock and sorrow. Examples are a nightclub fire that kills dozens of people and the terrorist attacks on September 11, 2001. Even strangers, knowing no one involved directly, are affected and experience signs and symptoms of stress (Levy & Sidel, 2002).

Crises are resolved, either positively or negatively, within a brief period, usually 4 to 8 weeks (Aguilera, 1998; Hoff, 2001). People's strong need to regain homeostasis and the intense nature of crises both work to make them temporary conditions that cannot continue indefinitely. In the fam-

D I S P L A Y   2 5 – 1

Two Families' Response to Crisis

The Redondos and the Fosters will be moving to a town in another state, 900 miles away, because of a job change. The Redondos are in crisis over the move. They have never lived in any other town. They will have to leave relatives and lifelong friends who live nearby and a community in which they have been very involved. Mrs. Redondo is the secretary at her family's house of worship. Their teenage daughter, a cheerleader, just started high school. Their son is in kindergarten; Grandma happily watches him in the mornings before school. Everyone is upset because of how the move will affect them. The family is stressed and argues each evening. They don't want to put their house up for sale or even to visit the new community to which they will be moving. Mr. Redondo is second guessing his decision to move, but his choices were limited as his company is relocating. The Redondos, in crisis, are not exploring alternatives that may allow them to stay in their present community. One possible alternative might be for Mrs. Redondo to work while Mr. Redondo looks for another job. When people perceive that they are in crisis, decision making and problem solving become more difficult.

The Fosters, however, are excitedly looking forward to their move. They have two young children who are not yet in school. The move will bring them only 50 miles from old college friends. They hope to realize a significant profit on their house, which they recently remodeled. They can't wait to go "house hunting" in the new town. Everyone is enjoying planning the anticipated move; their two children, aged 3 and 4, have been playing "moving day" with their favorite toys.

Both families are experiencing the same event. The difference is each person's situation and perception of the event. The Redondos' equilibrium is being disrupted. They have not developed previous coping skills and do not see the move as a positive experience. They are at a different time in their family life cycle than are the Fosters. Although the move upsets their equilibrium, too, the Fosters experience it as an exciting event that conjures positive feelings; they are passing these feelings on to their children. They see this move as an opportunity.

resulting in illness or even death. The battered wife reevaluates her life, gets divorced, learns employment skills in jail, becomes more assertive with stronger self-esteem, and returns to her children able to support them financially and emotionally after she is paroled. She finds growth and health while successfully resolving the crisis. The children settle into their aunt's home with minimal difficulty, start a new school, and visit their mother and father regularly. After their mother is released, she finds an apartment near her sister's home so that the children can continue in the same school district. The husband recovers from his wounds, gets counseling, relocates to another town, and sees his children frequently. The crisis situation is resolved at a higher level of wellness for all members than existed before the crisis. In this example, the members are determined to improve their situation by working with skilled health care professionals. By using the resources within the community, this family is healthier after their crisis.

Developmental Crises

Developmental crises are periods of disruption that occur at transition points during normal growth and development (Display 25–2). When developmental crises occur, people feel threatened by the demands placed on them and have difficulty making the changes necessary to fit the new stage of development.

During the process of normal biopsychosocial growth, people go through a succession of life cycle stages, from birth through old age. Each stage is quite different from the previous one, and transitions from one stage to the next require changes in roles and behavior. There are periods of upset and disequilibrium. Popular and classic authors such as Levinson (1978), Bridges (1980, 2001), Sheehy (1976, 1992, 1999), and Sheehy and Delbourgo (1996) have called these periods "passages" and "transitions." They are the times when developmental or maturational crises occur.

D I S P L A Y   2 5 – 2

Major Differences Between Types of Crises

Developmental Crisis
Part of normal growth and development that can upset normalcy
Precipitated by a life transition point
Gradual onset
Response to developmental demands and society's expectations

Situational Crisis
Unexpected period of upset in normalcy
Precipitated by a hazardous event
Sudden onset
Externally imposed "accident"

ily of the wife who shot her abusive husband, as shocking as the event might seem, life returns to a recognizable pattern within a few weeks. Although the members will feel the change for years, the crisis soon disappears. The husband is hospitalized and recovers from his wound; the wife's case goes to trial, and she is sentenced to 2 years in prison; the children stay with relatives and attend school.

Crisis resolution can be an adaptive process in which growth and improved health occur, or it can be maladaptive,

Most family developmental crises have a gradual onset. The change is evolutionary rather than revolutionary. People usually anticipate and even prepare to start school, enter adolescence, leave home, marry, have a baby, retire, or die. They move into and through each transitional period knowing in advance that some kind of change will be required. In many instances, people have already seen others experience these transitions. As a result, developmental crises have a degree of predictability. They offer the possibility of a period of time for anticipation and adjustment.

Developmental crises arise from both physical and social changes. Each new life stage confronts people with changed relationships, responsibilities, and roles. The transition to parenthood, for example, demands a change in role from caring for oneself and one's mate to include nurturing, caring for, and protecting a completely helpless infant. Relationships with adults, children, and even one's own parents also change. Parenthood is an entrance into a previously unexperienced part of the adult world. New parents may fear the unknown. Will this infant develop normally? Can I give adequate care? Parents often feel anxiety about the responsibility of shaping this new person's life, satisfying society's expectations for their child's proper education and training, or bringing children into a world that is in crisis and already overpopulated. They may worry about the increased financial burden and struggle with mixed feelings about giving up a large measure of freedom. These transitions put people under considerable stress, which contributes to tension, feelings of helplessness, and resultant crisis. Some people adapt quickly; others cannot cope, probably because earlier developmental crises went unresolved. If people lack a repertoire of adaptive skills, even positive and planned changes can develop into crises (Display 25–3).

Situational Crises

A **situational crisis** is a stressful, disruptive, event arising from external circumstances that occurs suddenly, often without warning, to a person, group, aggregate, or community. Typically, the external event requires behavioral changes and coping mechanisms beyond the abilities of the people involved.

Such events are not predicted, expected, or planned. They occur to people because of where they are in time and space. For instance, a baby grabs her mother's hot cup of tea and burns her chest; a college student is raped in the library parking lot; an older adult falls and fractures a hip; a mother with a van full of Little League baseball players has a crash at a busy intersection; a couple, after 25 years of marriage, gets divorced; a hurricane devastates a town; or a terrorist sends anthrax spores through the mail. These kinds of events, which involve loss or the threat of loss, represent life hazards to those affected. Some crisis-precipitating events can be positive, such as a significant job promotion or sudden acquisition of great wealth; however, they still make increased

DISPLAY 25–3

A Developmental Crisis

Marcia Sand is 39 years old. Married for 22 years, she has been a capable homemaker and mother of four children. Her husband, Lou, a construction worker for the past 20 years, thinks Marcia does a "super job at home." In the past, Marcia's time was filled with cooking, laundry, cleaning, shopping, and meeting the endless demands of the family. Their limited income prompted her to adopt many money-saving strategies. She made most of her own and the children's clothes, did all her own baking, and raised vegetables in her backyard garden. Now the youngest of the children, Tommy, has just left home to join the Navy. Her husband spends much of his spare time at the local bar with his friends, leaving Marcia alone. With a nearly empty house and little need for cooking, baking, and sewing, Marcia has lost her sense of usefulness. She thinks of taking a job, but knows her choices are limited because she has only a high school education. Marcia has not slept well in weeks; she wakes up tired and drags through the day barely able to manage the simplest task. She cries frequently but does not know why. Her hair, always neat and attractive in the past, looks bedraggled, and her shoulders slump. "I just can't seem to get on top of things any more," she complains.

Marcia has entered a developmental crisis that is sometimes called the "empty nest syndrome." She faces a turning point in her life, a time when parenting has seemingly ended. Leaving her satisfying homemaker role, she faces a new life stage filled with unknowns, changes, and a seeming lack of purpose. The transition came about gradually, almost imperceptibly, but now she must deal with it. Yet she feels unable to cope and wishes to turn to someone who would understand and lend her strength. She can be helped, but her crisis could also have been prevented at the pre-crisis phase. Anticipatory planning could have prevented the dilemma Marcia finds herself in now.

demands on individuals who must make major life adjustments. Even positive events involve a modified grieving process, because the individuals involved may be losing or giving up old, familiar, and comfortable situations and facing stressful changes.

Community health nurses see an almost infinite variety of situational crises, including debilitating disease, economic misfortune, unemployment, physical abuse, divorce, unwanted pregnancy, chemical abuse, sudden death of a loved one, tragic accidents such as drownings or plane crashes, and many others. In each situation, people feel overwhelmed and need help to cope. Skilled intervention can make the difference between a healthy and an unhealthy outcome.

Multiple Crises

Different kinds of crises can overlap in actual experience, compounding the stress felt by the persons involved. For example, a couple could experience a developmental crisis (birth) and a situational crisis (birth defect) simultaneously, with the resulting stress being compounded. The developmental crisis of midlife may be complicated by situational crises such as divorce or job change. With older adults, the developmental crisis of retirement may be compounded by the situational crisis of a fire that destroys the family home. The transition a child faces entering school may occur at the same time the family moves to a new neighborhood and a new infant joins the family. The child must share the parents' attention and affection with a new sibling at a time when all the child's resources are needed to cope with starting school and adjusting to the new neighborhood. Classic research has shown that these accumulated stresses can lead to ill health (Holmes & Rahe, 1967). Those who might normally work through one crisis in a healthy way may find that compound events overwhelm them and cause more stress than they can handle.

HISTORY OF FAMILY VIOLENCE

Family crisis is not limited to the developmental crises that we all experience or the situational crises that come upon us suddenly, usually from forces—such as nature—that are external to the family. Many women and children in the world also experience the crisis of domestic violence. The terms **domestic violence, family violence**, and **interpersonal violence** refer to morbidity and mortality attributable to violence within the home setting, involving action by a family member or intimate partner. They involve "a systematic pattern of assaultive and coercive behaviors, including physical, sexual, and psychologic attacks and economic coercion, that adults or adolescents use against their intimate partners" (Kramer, 2002, p. 190). This type of violence is becoming more of a global burden.

Global History

Family violence is not new. For centuries, children were thought of as the property of their parents, and any treatment doled out by the parents was their prerogative. In fact, most countries had animal welfare laws long before child welfare laws were adopted. In addition, the ideology of childhood that emerged in the Western world in the late 1800s assumed that only "abnormal" children needed protection. These children were casualties of urban industrial society who were abandoned, dependent, and delinquent or products of social dislocation, such as orphaned or refugee children.

In the early 1900s, sensitive leaders concerned with child welfare issues emerged. Several international agencies were created that were designed to positively affect the health of children. The British Children's Act was passed in

1908, and the first White House Conference was held in 1909. These were early attempts to define a role for the state. The U. S. conference was the forerunner of the United States Children's Bureau (USCB) and a national voluntary organization, later known as the Child Welfare League of America, that would complement any federal agency (Bolen, 2001). The USCB became a model for other countries, with well-developed programs targeting infant mortality. In one innovative program of the early 1900s, a heated mobile child welfare center was used in rural communities and was staffed by a female physician and a public health nurse.

Other international organizations that emerged in the early 1900s were the International Association for the Promotion of Child Welfare (IAPCW), League of Red Cross Societies (LRCS), Save the Children Fund (SCF), and Save the Children International Union (SCIU). The latter two were immensely successful in raising funds for children in Germany, Austria, France, Hungary, and Serbia. As these organizations began serving the needs of children internationally, they moved from a sentimental depiction of victims to a medicosocial scientific view of children at risk that expanded the concepts of victimization, exploitation, and abuse (Bolen, 2001).

By the mid-1920s, the work of these agencies began to focus on children from non-European countries. The first conference on children from non-European countries focused on African children in 1931 and included such issues as infant mortality, child labor, education, and child slavery. In 1924, the League of Nations adopted the Declaration of the Rights of the Child, which would influence the League of Nation's successor, the United Nations, in years to come in the form of the Declaration of the Rights of the Child in 1959 and the Convention on the Rights of the Child in 1989.

Children are not the only victims of family morbidity and mortality from violence. Historically, women too were treated as property and often suffered physical and psychological damage. Huge numbers of women (between 16% and 52% of women in some parts of the world) experience domestic violence and other forms of violence ranging from emotional abuse to rape and genital mutilation. One in five women worldwide experience rape or attempted rape in their lifetimes, and an estimated 130 million girls and women alive today have undergone genital mutiliation (World Health Organization [WHO], 1998). As with children, the rights of women are socially, culturally, and religiously motivated, with change coming slowly.

United States History

The history of treatment of children, women, and elders in the United States began with emigration in the 1500s and has been influenced by the cultural and religious practices of the early settlers. In addition, necessity, attitudes of the time, and the stress and hardship of life in the colonies and on the frontier influenced how people were treated.

Children were born into families to help with the chores of an agricultural society. Families had many children, again out of necessity: infant mortality rates were high, and it was not uncommon for half of the children in a family to die before their second birthday. Older people did not retire; they contributed to family survival until they died. There were no special considerations for children, women, or elders. The best a woman could hope for was that the man she married would not abuse her emotionally, physically, sexually, or fiducially (taking advantage of a person's financial resources). Women had limited or no education, resources, or rights, and children had none. If a woman married "poorly," she would have to live with the consequences. Separation and divorce were either unheard of or were a "death sentence" for the woman and her children, because there was nowhere she could go and no way for her to support her family.

It took many years for the United States to establish laws that benefited women and children. Nonetheless, we did so earlier than many other countries. The Childrens's Bureau began to focus on child abuse in the 1960s, and in 1962 a child abuse mandatory reporting law was developed to be used by the states as a model. The law required health professionals and child care workers to report suspected child abuse to appropriate officials.

In 1974, the Child Abuse Prevention and Treatment Act was passed, becoming Public Law 93-247. It served to reinforce the earlier mandatory reporting law model and was aimed at solving the growing problem of child abuse in the country. Public Law 93-247 has been amended several times since 1974. The Child Abuse Prevention and Treatment and Adoption Reform Act of 1978 was followed by the Family Violence Prevention and Services Act of 1984. Later, all three acts were consolidated into The Child Abuse Prevention, Adoption, and Family Services Act of 1988 (Public Law 100-294).

Public Law 100-294 mandates funding designed to support states in their efforts to prevent violence in families and to identify and treat the victims. Funding from this act supports the work of the National Center on Child Abuse and Neglect, a national commission on childhood deaths. This center studies the national incidence of family violence. It focuses on eliminating barriers to the adoption of older children, minority children, and children with physical and mental disabilities, in addition to supporting professional training and research. Each state acts on Public Law 100-294 in ways that best meet its needs. The newer elder abuse laws are modeled after the Family Services Act of 1988.

In 1997, the Child Maltreatment Report from the States to the National Child Abuse and Neglect Data System found that there were approximately 948,000 child victims of maltreatment. This was a decrease from the more than 1 million victims in 1996 in the 50 states, the District of Columbia, Puerto Rico, the Virgin Islands, and Guam. However, the rate of 13.9 per 1000 children in the general population in 1997 was slightly higher than the rate of 13.4 victims per 1000 children in 1990 (U. S. Department of Health and Human Services [USDHHS], 2000).

Healthy People 2000 Goals

Of the more than 300 national objectives of *Healthy People 2000,* 19 were directed toward violent and abusive behavior. As of 1998, the year 2000 targets had been surpassed for three of the objectives: reduction of weapon carrying, implementation of child death review systems, and an increase in nonviolent conflict resolution programs in schools. Six objectives had progressed toward their year 2000 targets: reducing suicides; reducing firearm-related deaths; reducing physical fighting and weapon-carrying among adolescents aged 14 to 17 years; increasing the proportion of elementary and secondary schools that teach nonviolent conflict resolution skills, preferably as part of comprehensive school health education; and enacting laws requiring that firearms be properly stored to minimize access and the likelihood of discharge by minors (USDHHS, 1998).

Disappointingly, there was movement away from the year 2000 targets for eight objectives: homicide; maltreatment of children younger than 18 years of age; physical abuse directed at women by male partners; assault injuries among people aged 12 years and older; rape and attempted rape of women aged 12 years and older; suicide attempts among adolescents aged 14 to 17 years; battered women and their children turned away from emergency housing due to lack of space; and the number of states with protocols to facilitate identification and appropriate intervention for the prevention of suicides in jails (USDHHS, 1998). Six of these eight objectives are related to violence against women and children. Many reasons account for these disturbing results. Youth continue to be involved as both *perpetrators,* those people committing the violence, and victims of violence. Women, including their children, continue to be the targets of both physical and sexual assault perpetrated by individuals known to them, specifically the women's current and former intimate partners. Other issues, including the lack of comparable data sources, definitional issues, and the lack of resources to adequately establish consistent tracking systems, contribute to the negative data trends (USDHHS, 2000).

Healthy People 2010 Goals

The goal for *Healthy People 2010* regarding violence and abuse is to reduce injuries, disabilities, and death due to violence among all people of the United States. On an average day in America, 70 people die from homicide, 87 people commit suicide, as many as 3000 people attempt suicide, and a minimum of 18,000 people survive interpersonal assaults. The problem is pervasive, affecting the victim directly and all the family members indirectly. Selected violence and abuse objectives for 2010 include the following (USDHHS, 2000):

- Reduce maltreatment and maltreatment fatalities of children from 13.9 victims per 1000 to 1.1 per 1000 by 2010.
- Reduce physical assault by current or former intimate partners from 4.5 per 1000 people to 3.6 per 1000 by 2010.
- Reduce the annual rate of rape or attempted rape of persons aged 12 years and older to less than 0.7 per 1000 persons in 2010, from 0.9 per 1000 in 1998.

- Reduce sexual assault other than rape to less than 0.2 per 1000 people in 2010, from 0.6 in 1998.
- Reduce weapon carrying by adolescents on school property (grades 9 through 12) from 8.5% in 1997 to 6% by 2010.

Myths and Truths About Family Violence

There are many beliefs or myths about family violence that need to be dispelled because they may influence violent behavior in families. Strongly held myths by members of society, including community health nurses and other health care providers, may interfere with getting families in crisis the help they need. Table 25–1 displays some common myths and truths about family violence.

FAMILY VIOLENCE AGAINST CHILDREN

As a cause of morbidity among children, communicable diseases "are coming under control through a combination of health promotion, prevention and simplified standard treatment regimens. But at the same time, the healthy growth and development of many children is threatened by very rapid, often disruptive social, cultural and economic changes" (WHO, 1998, p. 71). This emerging new morbidity is of a psychosocial nature, is associated with behavioral problems, and is much more difficult to prevent than diseases known for centuries.

Child abuse is the maltreatment of children. It may include any of the following: physical, emotional, medical, or educational neglect; physical punishment or battering; and emotional or sexual maltreatment and exploitation. Types can occur alone or in combination.

Child abuse and psychosocial developmental problems are taking a toll globally. It is estimated that the child abuse mortality rates for infants in most countries is 7 per 100,000 live births (WHO, 1998). This provides a rough global estimate and indicates only the "tip of the iceberg." There are abuses against children in many countries where accurate data are hard to uncover. Very young children are expected to aid the family financially. Their "chores" may include spending the whole day scrounging around city dumps for bits of food, clothing, or other useful or saleable items. Some children are sold for sexual favors to whoever asks. Still others spend all day working in fields, home businesses, or "sweat shops" for the equivalent of pennies a day. In some societies, female children are not valued and are killed at birth, given away, or sold into slavery for a pittance.

More than 3 million cases of suspected child abuse are reported in the United States each year. This is a 20-fold increase since the 150,000 suspected cases reported in 1963 (Besharov, 1998). In 1999, 826,000 suspected cases were substantiated. "While there were 10.6 cases of substantiated maltreatment for every 1000 white children, the rates for black, Hispanic, and Indian/Alaskan Native children were 25.2, 12.6, and 20.1 cases/1000 children, respectively" (Lane, et al., 2002, p. 1603). These rates may be giving a false picture of the actual rates among racial groups. It may

T A B L E 25–1

Common Myths and Truths About Abuse in Families

Myth	Truth
Violence in families is rare	Family violence is common and increasing
Violence occurs most frequently among low-income families	Family violence occurs across all incomes
Violence occurs more frequently in some racial and cultural groups	Family violence occurs across all racial and cultural groups
Violence in families does not coexist with love	Love may exist but is unable to be displayed appropriately due to conflicting emotions
Men who batter women are mentally ill	The percentage of batterers who are mentally ill is the same as in the general population
Women who accept battering are mentally ill	The percentage of battered women who are mentally ill is the same as in the general population; however, they have low-esteem and a damaged spirit
Violence occurs only in heterosexual relationships	Domestic violence has no gender or sexual boundaries; it can occur among all people
Abused women instigate the battering	Quite the contrary, they go out of their way not to agitate or confront the abuser
Abuse occurs when the abuser is under the influence of drugs or alcohol	It can, but many abusers do not drink or use drugs
Children should not be taken from their parents	In some violent families, the safest place for the child is with another family member or a foster home (temporarily or permanently)
Even abusive parents are better for a child than a child living elsewhere	Children must be protected, and living away from abusive parents may save their lives
Abused children become abusive adults	Some may, but most can learn how to channel their emotions positively if the cycle of violence is broken

be that minority children are abused more frequently, or that minority children are more likely to be reported for abuse, or that reports among minority groups are more likely to be substantiated. Mandated reporters may have biases that contribute to the differences.

With the release of *Healthy People 2010* goals in 2000, the nation remained without a clear baseline for child abuse cases, mainly because of evaluation and follow-up documentation issues among the states (USDHHS, 2000). However, in 1997 there were 13.9 child victims per 1000 children in the general population. The types of maltreatment were general neglect (55.9%), physical abuse (24.6%), sexual abuse (12.5%), and emotional abuse (6.1%) (USDHHS, 2000).

Child Neglect

Neglect occurs when the physical, emotional, or educational resources necessary for healthy growth and development are withheld or unavailable. Neglect is obvious to an observer if a very young child is playing unattended outside, is not dressed appropriately for the weather, or has an unkempt appearance. However, neglect is not always so obvious. Parents may refuse to buy eyeglasses for a child who needs them (medical neglect). An 8-year-old may get to school only 3 days a week, usually without breakfast and with no lunch money or packed lunch (educational neglect). A family with three children may live in a sparsely furnished apartment, with very little food available and only intermittent heat, and the children may appear at school unwashed and without coats in winter weather (general neglect).

Thousands of children in the United States experience neglect each day. They are frequently "invisible" victims. At times, stories of severe child neglect are reported in the media and cause a sensation. Examples include 12 children found among piles of garbage in an abandoned apartment building during a drug raid; parents vacationing in Florida while their two daughters, aged 6 and 4, are left unattended at home; and three young children found barely alive, kept in a basement closet. However, most children suffering from neglect do not make newspaper headlines or television reports. They go to school like others. If they are fortunate, their plight is uncovered by a community health nurse, teacher, or counselor. Because of the invisibility of neglect, its prevalence is hard to estimate. Often cases of neglect are brought to the attention of the proper authority only during the exploration of another form of abuse (Display 25–4).

Physical Abuse

Physical abuse is intentional harm to a child by another person that results in pain, physical injury, or death. The abuse may include striking, biting, poking, burning, shaking, or throwing the child. **Corporal punishment**, which involves violence against a child as a form of discipline, was an acceptable form of discipline earlier in our country's history

DISPLAY 25-4

Signs and Symptoms of Neglect

Neglect may be suspected if one or more of the following conditions exist:

- The child lacks adequate medical or dental care.
- The child is often sleepy or hungry.
- The child is often dirty, demonstrates poor personal hygiene, or is inadequately dressed for weather conditions.
- There is evidence of poor or inadequate supervision for the child's age.
- The conditions in the home are unsafe or unsanitary.
- The child appears to be malnourished.
- The child is depressed, withdrawn, or apathetic; exhibits antisocial or destructive behavior; shows fearfulness; or suffers from substance abuse or speech, eating, or habit disorders (eg, biting, rocking, whining).

and is still condoned in some subgroups. Many parents today were raised in families in which physical punishment was used as a form of discipline. Even today it is not unusual to see a parent slap the hand of a toddler to get his attention after he has been told not to do something several times or to prevent him from touching something that would hurt him more than the slap on the hand. Some families know where to draw the line. Others—especially if they were raised with "the belt" or "the switch"—see no harm in using the same disciplinary practices with their children.

Some parents cannot control the degree of physical punishment they give their child. In one case in 2002, a mother repeatedly physically assaulted her young daughter while getting her into the car. This behavior was caught by the store's parking lot surveillance camera, and intervention and follow-up occurred, including incarceration and counseling for the mother and foster home placement for the child. If physical punishment is administered in anger, while the parent is under the influence of mind-altering substances, or out of a sense of frustration, the punishment may cross over to battering. **Battered child syndrome** refers to the collection of injuries that are sustained by a child as a result of repeated mistreatment or beatings. Display 25–5 lists physical and behavioral indicators of physical abuse (U. S. Department of Justice [USDOJ], 2003a).

Sexual Abuse

Sexual abuse of children includes acts of sexual assault or sexual exploitation of a minor and may consist of a single incident or many acts over a long period. Sexual assault includes rape, gang rape, incest, sodomy, lewd or lascivious acts with a child younger than 14 years of age (in most states), oral copulation, penetration of the genital or anal

DISPLAY 25-5

Signs and Symptoms of Physical Abuse

Types of Injuries

Types of physical abuse injuries include bruises, burns, bite marks, abrasions, lacerations, head injuries, internal injuries, and fractures.

Behavioral Indicators of Physical Abuse

The following behaviors are often exhibited by physically abused children:

- The child is frightened of parents/caretakers or, at the other extreme, is overprotective of parent or caretakers.
- The child is excessively passive, overly compliant, apathetic, withdrawn or fearful or, at the other extreme, excessively aggressive, destructive, or physically violent.
- The child and/or parent or caretaker attempts to hide injuries; child wears excessive layers of clothing, especially in hot weather; child is frequently absent from school or misses physical education classes if changing into gym clothes is required; child has difficulty sitting or walking.
- The child is frightened of going home.
- The child is clingy and forms indiscriminate attachments.
- The child is apprehensive when other children cry.

- The child is wary of physical contact with adults.
- The child exhibits drastic behavioral changes in and out of parental/caretaker presence.
- The child is hypervigilant.
- The child suffers from seizures or vomiting.
- The adolescent exhibits depression, self-mutilation, suicide attempts, substance abuse, or sleeping and eating disorders.

Other indicators of physical abuse may include the following:

- A statement by the child that the injury was caused by abuse. (Chronically abused children may deny abuse.)
- Knowledge that the child's injury is unusual for the child's specific age group (eg, any fracture in an infant).
- Knowledge of the child's history of previous or recurrent injuries.
- Unexplained injuries (eg, parent is unable to explain reason for injury; there are discrepancies in explanations; blame is placed on a third party; explanations are inconsistent with medical diagnosis).
- A parent or caretaker who delays seeking or fails to seek medical care for the child's injury.

---

opening by a foreign object, and child molestation. **Sexual exploitation** of children includes conduct or activities related to pornography that depict minors in sexually explicit situations and promotion of prostitution by minors (USDOJ, 2003b). **Incest** is sexual abuse among family members who are related by blood (eg, parents, grandparents, older siblings, aunts and uncles); it constitutes the most hidden form of child abuse. **Intrafamilial sexual abuse** refers to sexual activity involving family members who are not related by blood (eg, step-parents, boyfriends).

In most reported cases, the father or male caretaker is the initiator and the victim is a female child; however, boys are victims more often than previously believed. It is estimated that one in every four girls is sexually abused, as are one in every seven boys, a much higher percentage for boys than reported numbers indicate. The initial sexual abuse may occur at any age, from infancy through adolescence. However, the largest number of cases involves girls younger than 11 years of age. Regardless of how gentle, trivial, or coincidental the first approach may have seemed, sexual coercion tends to be repeated and to escalate over a period of years. The child may eventually accept blame for tempting or provoking the abuser.

The mother in the family, who would usually be expected to protect the child, may purposely try to stay isolated from a problem of sexual abuse. Sometimes the mother is distant, uncommunicative, or so disapproving of sexual matters that the child is afraid to speak up. Sometimes she is extremely insecure, and the potential loss of her husband or boyfriend, together with the economic security he provides, is so threatening that she cannot allow herself to believe or even to suspect that her child is at risk. She may have been a victim herself of child abuse and may not trust her judgment or her right to challenge the man in authority in the home. Some mothers consciously acknowledge that their children are being sexually abused but, for whatever reason, "look the other way."

Until the victim is old enough to realize that incest or intrafamilial sexual abuse is not a common occurrence or is strong enough to obtain help outside the family, there is no escape unless the abuse is reported (Crime and Violence Prevention Center, 2003b).

Indicators of sexual abuse, including the history, sexual behavioral indicators of children, behavioral indicators of sexual abuse in younger children, behavioral indicators of sexual abuse in older children and adolescents, and physical symptoms, provide information to assist community health nurses in their mandated reporter role (Display 25–6). It should be noted that sexual abuse of a child may surface through a broad range of physical, behavioral, and social symptoms. Some of these indicators, taken separately, may not be symptomatic of sexual abuse. They are presented here as a guide and should be examined in the context of other behaviors or situational factors.

Community health nurses can be part of the sexual abuse response team (SART). This group's responsibilities include obtaining the evidence and supplying the support for the

DISPLAY 25-6

Indicators of Sexual Abuse

I. History of Sexual Abuse

- A child confides to a friend, classmate, teacher, a friend's mother, or other trusted adult that she/he has experienced sexual abuse.
- A child may disclose information indirectly by such statements as:
  "I know someone . . ."
  "What would you do if . . . ?"
  "I heard something about somebody . . ."
- The child has torn, stained, or bloody underclothing (among her/his clothing or is wearing it).
- Knowledge that a child's injury/disease (vaginal trauma, sexually transmitted disease) is unusual for the specific age group.
- Unexplained injuries/diseases (parent/caretaker unable to explain reason for injury/disease); there are discrepancies in explanation; blame is placed on a third party; explanations are inconsistent with medical diagnosis.
- A very young girl is pregnant or has a sexually transmitted disease. Pregnancy alone does not constitute sexual abuse, but if there are indications of coercion or significant age disparity between the minor and her partner, this may lead to reasonable suspicion of sexual abuse that must be reported.

II. Sexual Behavioral Indicators of Sexually Abused Children

- Detailed and age-inappropriate understanding of sexual behavior (especially among very young children).
- Sexually explicit language.
- Inappropriate, unusual, or aggressive sexual behavior with peers or toys.
- Compulsive indiscreet masturbation.
- Excessive curiosity about sexual matters or genitalia (self or others).
- Unusually seductive or flirtatious behavior with classmates, teachers, and other adults.
- Excessive concern about homosexuality, especially by boys.

III. Behavioral Indicators of Sexual Abuse in Younger Children

- Enuresis (wetting pants or bedwetting).
- Fecal soiling.
- Eating disturbances such as overeating or undereating.
- Fears or phobias.
- Overly compulsive behavior.
- School problems or significant change in school performance (attitude and grades).
- Age-inappropriate behavior that includes pseudomaturity or regressive behavior such as bedwetting or thumb sucking.
- Inability to concentrate.

- Sleeping disturbances (nightmares, fear of falling asleep, fretful sleep pattern, sleeping long hours).
- Drastic behavior changes.
- Speech disorders.
- Frightened of parents/caretaker or of going home or being at home.

IV. Behavioral Indicators of Sexual Abuse in Older Children and Adolescents

- Withdrawal.
- Chronic fatigue.
- Clinical depression, apathy.
- Overly compliant behavior.
- Over or under reaction (hysteria or cavalier attitude) to a genital exam.
- Poor hygiene or excessive bathing.
- Poor peer relations and social skills; inability to make friends.
- Acting out, running away, aggressive, antisocial or delinquent behavior.
- Alcohol or drug abuse.
- Prostitution or excessive promiscuity.
- School problems, frequent absences, sudden drop in school performance.
- Refusal to change clothes for physical education class.
- Non-participation in sports and social activities.
- Fearful of showers or restrooms.
- Fearful of home life as demonstrated by arriving at school early and leaving late.
- Suddenly fearful of other things (going outside or participating in familiar activities).
- Extraordinary fear of males (in cases of male perpetrator and female victim).
- Self-consciousness of body beyond that expected for age.
- Sudden acquisition of money, new clothes, or gifts with no reasonable explanation.
- Suicide attempt or other self-destructive behavior.
- Crying without provocation.
- Setting fires.

V. Physical Symptoms of Sexual Abuse

- Sexually transmitted diseases, especially in pre-pubescent girls.
- Genital discharge or infection.
- Physical trauma or irritation to the anal/genital area (pain, itching, swelling, bruising, bleeding, lacerations, abrasions), especially if injuries are unexplained or there is an inconsistent explanation.
- Pain during urination or defecation.
- Difficulty in walking or sitting due to genital or anal pain.
- Psychosomatic symptoms (stomach aches, headaches, chronic pain).

(Adapted from the Crime and Violence Prevention Center. [1996]. *Child abuse: Educator's responsibilities.* Sacramento, CA: California Attorney General's Office.)

victim and family after an episode of sexual abuse has been reported. Team members include nurses, physicians, social workers, police, laboratory personnel, and lawyers and district attorney staff. They work to provide care, discover and protect evidence, investigate the incident, and act as liaisons between the victim and media. Their continuation in the situation goes beyond the home or emergency room and continues into the courts.

The sexual assault nurse examiner (SANE) role is more specific to the victim and appropriate family members immediately after the victim presents to the police or to an emergency department setting. The nurse has very specific actions to take to promote trust, obtain needed specimen evidence, and treat the sexual abuse victim. The victim has already been significantly traumatized, and the nurse can be effective in this role only if trust can be established during this critical time after the sexual assault. The nurse works with victims of all ages and both genders and under all sexual abuse situations.

Although there are several classifications of child molesters, pedophiles present the greatest danger. A **pedophile** is an adult whose main sexual interest is a child. A pedophile tends to be well-liked by children. Pedophiles, who most often are men, frequently choose to work in professions or volunteer organizations that allow them easy access to children, where they can develop the trust and respect of children and their parents. The pedophile believes that sex with children is appropriate and often lures children into sexual relationships with love, rewards, promises, and gifts. He may be among a child's family members (eg, grandfather, father, uncle, cousin) or a trusted community leader the child knows (eg, next-door neighbor, teacher, scout or religious leader). Recently, reports of pedophiles among clergy in the Catholic Church have clearly rocked the church's status and stability.

Emotional Abuse

Emotional abuse of children involves psychological mistreatment or neglect, such as when parents do not provide the normal experiences that produce feelings of being loved, wanted, secure, and worthy (Crime and Violence Prevention Center, 2003c). This too can take several different forms. It may involve verbal abuse, such as calling the child names, belittling, or threatening. A mother may shout at the child, "You're just like your father, a real good-for-nothing lazy bum." A father may say, "You're ugly. You look just like your mother." If the child spills some juice, a parent may scream, "Everything you do you do wrong. Can't you do anything right?"

Emotional abuse may also take the form of emotional abandonment. Some parents "shun" their children as a form of punishment. They will not speak to them and do not look at them; they behave as if their children do not exist. This may continue for a day or longer, whenever a child displeases the parent. In some cases, the shunning lasts for days.

Verbal threats, although a common discipline practice among many parents, are a form of emotional abuse. Exam-

ples of verbal threats include, "Take your feet off the furniture or I'll chop your feet off" and "Do that again and you'll really know what my belt feels like." In the first instance, the child might realize that the parent wouldn't really chop her feet off, but hearing the parent say such a violent thing can be emotionally scarring. In the second instance, the parent may have beaten the child with a belt in the past, so that merely threatening to use it again causes emotional trauma. Emotional abuse often accompanies other forms of abuse. Emotional abuse alone is rarely reported, because it is another "hidden" form of abuse. However, **mandated reporters**, people who have responsibility for the welfare of children, including nurses, doctors, teachers, counselors, and certain other professionals, such as animal protection workers and those who develop photographs, are required by law to report *suspected* cases of severe emotional neglect, abuse, or deprivation in addition to *suspected* neglect and physical or sexual abuse (Crime and Violence Prevention Center, 2003a, 2003c) (Display 25–7).

DISPLAY 25–7

Signs and Symptoms of Emotional Abuse or Deprivation

Emotional abuse should be suspected if the child displays the following behavioral indicators:
- Is withdrawn, depressed or apathetic.
- Is clingy and forms indiscriminate attachments.
- "Acts out" and is considered a behavior problem.
- Exhibits exaggerated fearfulness.
- Is overly rigid in conforming to instructions of teachers, doctors, and other adults.
- Suffers from sleep, speech, or eating disorders.
- Displays signs of emotional turmoil that include repetitive, rhythmic movements (rocking, whining, picking at scabs).
- Pays inordinate attention to details or exhibits little or no verbal or physical communication with others.
- Suffers from enuresis and fecal soiling.
- Unwittingly makes comments such as "Mommy always tells me I'm bad."
- Experiences substance abuse problems.

Emotional deprivation should be suspected if the child
- Refuses to eat adequate amounts of food and therefore is very frail.
- Is unable to perform normal learned functions for a given age (eg, walking, talking).
- Displays antisocial behavior (aggression, disruption) or obvious delinquent behavior (drug abuse, vandalism); conversely, the child may be abnormally unresponsive, sad, or withdrawn.
- Constantly "seeks out" and "pesters" other adults such as teachers or neighbors for attention and affection.
- Displays exaggerated fears.

Specific Abusive Situations

Although the previous information has presented the major types of violence occurring in families, two specific patterns of abuse against children should be discussed here. Shaken baby syndrome and Munchausen syndrome by proxy are fairly rare, but by the time they are discovered it is often too late, with the diagnosis being made during a visit to the emergency department or at autopsy.

In addition, Internet crimes against children, child abduction, and crimes against children by babysitters are increasingly common issues feared by parents. They are occurring more often as computers are becoming common household appliances, millions of children go missing, and both parents (or a single parent) are working, causing children to spend more time alone or with babysitters.

Shaken Baby Syndrome

Shaken baby syndrome is the intentional abusive action of violently shaking an infant or toddler, usually one younger than 18 months of age. The type of damage that occurs to these infants very seldom occurs through play, as in the minor falls a baby at play may experience, or as a result of parents' tossing a baby in the air. The classic medical symptoms associated with infant shaking are bilateral retinal hemorrhage, subdural or subarachnoid hematomas, absence of other external signs of abuse, and symptoms including breathing difficulties, seizures, dilated pupils, lethargy, and unconsciousness (USDOJ, 2003a). These injuries are caused by a violent, sustained action in which the infant's head, which lacks muscular control, is violently whipped forward and backward, hitting the chest and shoulders. According to experts, it is shaking that an observer would describe as being "as hard as the shaker was humanly capable of shaking the baby" or "hard enough that it appeared the baby's head would come off." (USDOJ, 2003a). Within minutes to hours after the injury, the baby begins to show symptoms, such as seizures or unconsciousness. A typical explanation given by the parents or caretakers is that the baby was "fine" and then suddenly went into respiratory arrest or began having seizures—both common symptoms of shaken baby syndrome.

Munchausen Syndrome by Proxy

Munchausen syndrome is a psychological disorder in which a client fabricates the symptoms of a disease in order to undergo medical tests, hospitalization, or even medical or surgical treatment. Clients with this disorder may intentionally injure themselves or induce illness in themselves. In cases of **Munchausen syndrome by proxy**, a parent or caretaker suffering from Munchausen syndrome attempts to bring medical attention to himself or herself by injuring or inducing illness in his or her children. The following scenarios are typical of these cases:

- The child's parent or caretaker brings the child to the emergency department or calls paramedics repeatedly for alleged problems that have no medical basis.

- The child experiences "seizures" or "respiratory arrest" only when the parent or caretaker is present—never in the presence of a neutral third party or when hospitalized, unless the parent or caretaker reports that the incident occurred in his or her presence.

- While the child is hospitalized, the parent or caretaker shuts off intravenous tubes or life-support equipment, causing the child distress, and then turns everything back on and summons help.

- The parent or caretaker induces illness by introducing a mild irritant or poison into the child's body; chronic ingestion of such substances may cause the child's death.

Internet Crimes Against Children

Internet crimes are insidious because they come right into the home. Either unintentionally or intentionally, a minor accesses an Internet chat room or Web site developed or used by pedophiles. The perpetrator establishes contact, usually passing himself off as a teen or young man who has similar interests, and states affection for and understanding of the youth's "problems." Eventually the pedophile either sets up a meeting time and place or engages in sexually explicit dialogue with the minor (USDOJ, 2001c). Many minors find the attention from this stranger inviting or exciting and plan to meet the person. When this happens, the minor falls victim to this individual who preys on children, and most often the outcomes are not good.

Community health nurses can assist families to prevent such crimes by placing "blocks" on computers in the home through their Internet server, keeping the family computer in a high-traffic area in the home so that the parents can always be aware of the sites accessed by their children, and limiting access to the computer to specific sites or times of day when the parents are home. Certainly, talking with their children about the risks of chat rooms or specific Internet sites and developing strong and open channels of communication are important and will help the children and parents to bond more strongly, much needed for successful child rearing.

Child Abduction

Child abduction is a crime that every parent fears. Although stranger abduction happens infrequently, it remains an uppermost fear. Massive and immediate media coverage through systems such as the Amber Alert program, adopted in 2003 by about half the states in the country, has been very successful in locating recently abducted children (USDOJ, 2002). However, this intense media coverage gives the impression that such crimes occur frequently and causes stress among parents.

Child abduction by family members or intimate partners, such as a divorced mother, father, step-parent, boyfriend, or grandparents, is much more common. Nonetheless, the parent from whom the child was taken may be unaware that the abduction was by a relative or known person and may experience the same type of stress and loss as parents who lose a child by stranger abduction. In some cases, knowing the relative or person who abducted the child causes just as much fear, because the abductor may have a history of violence or sexual abuse crimes.

Prevention of child abduction is difficult, and at times parents who think they have taught their children well may have only a false sense of security. In some studies, children have been observed taking a "stranger awareness" class that included lessons on avoiding strangers, not talking to strangers, what is a stranger, saying "no" to strangers, running away and screaming, and so forth, and then going out the classroom door with an unknown person (a stranger sent in by the researcher) who asked them to help them find a lost puppy or go with them to get candy. Parents who watched their own children on tapes of these studies could not believe what they saw. Children are trusting and curious, and they may not consider people who look like their parents as *strangers*.

Community health nurses can help parents by promoting close supervision of young children and practice of behaviors that promote anonimity. Ideas include holding the child's hand while in malls or stores or keeping the child in the seat of a shopping cart, keeping a young child in sight at all times when playing outside, sharing parental supervision with another mother when children play so that an adult is always supervising the children, not putting the child's name or initials on clothing or backpack, and teaching the child a "password" that only the parents and child know to use when a different person is picking them up from a neighborhood activity.

With older children and teens who go outside the home unattended by parents, the following behaviors help promote safety: staying with groups of other children or teens, having a cell phone, leaving an itinerary with parents and not changing it without the parents' knowledge, attending a self-defense class, and carrying a whistle and pepper spray.

Crimes Against Children by Babysitters

Crimes against infants and young children by babysitters have been given attention by the media in recent years (USDOJ, 2001b). Some parents who have suspected mistreatment of their children by caretakers have used hidden cameras and revealed the problem. Abuse by caretakers is a fear of parents who must work and leave children with others.

The community health nurse can help parents assess day care settings by providing them with a list of descriptors of good programs. Parents who use neighbors as babysitters should get references and should drop by the home or day care setting at various times during the day. They should assess their infants and follow-up on bruises, rashes, burns, or any conditions or behaviors they observe that are not normal for their child. With older children, the parents need to listen to them and ask about their day and activities. They must not ignore signs such as a child's fear of going to the babysitter or reports of spankings, being shouted at, or other inappropriate treatment. Day care centers and many home day care programs are licensed by the state. Programs for which parental complaints have been filed with licensing agencies

are monitored more closely, and the state is mandated to make changes or to close the facility if necessary. Parents need to feel empowered in such situations as they leave their children while they pursue their employment or educational activities.

PARTNER/SPOUSAL VIOLENCE

Adult violence is rooted in childhood violence. A father hits a mother. The mother hits her son. The son hits his sister. The sister hits her little brother. The little brother sets fire to the cat, pulls wings off butterflies, and grows up to be a spouse batterer. Although abused girls may grow up to be abusing mothers, more often they grow up to be abused wives. Researchers operationalize domestic violence as pushing, grabbing, shoving, slapping, choking, kicking, biting, hitting with a fist or some other object, being beaten, or being threatened with a knife or gun by a spouse or cohabiting partner.

Partner violence often begins during adolescent dating, or dating at any age, with a push or shove that at first is overlooked by the girlfriend (Hanson, 2002). As these "minor" episodes of violence continue, the victim typically feels that she is doing something wrong and attempts to modify her behavior. She also assumes wrongly that once she and her boyfriend are married, these physical assaults will stop automatically or that in time she will be able to "change" him. The cycle of violence has begun.

Cycle of Violence

The **cycle of violence** is the repetitive, cyclic pattern of abuse seen in domestic violence situations. This theory of family violence was first described as a three-phase cycle by Walker in 1979, after she studied more than 1000 battered women and a smaller group of battering men. The cycle includes the tension-building phase, the acute battering incident, and the loving reconciliation (Jenkins & Davidson, 2001). The psychological dynamics of these three phases help explain why women feel so guilty and ashamed of their partner's violence toward them and why they find it so difficult to leave, even when their lives are in danger (Display 25–8).

The Domestic Abuse Intervention Project in Duluth, Minnesota, has developed a wheel of violence, identifying power and control at the center, with eight categories of perpetrator behaviors. This model is a useful tool for visualizing the dimensions of abuse (Fig. 25–1).

Dating Violence

Dating violence in adolescent relationships is a serious and prevalent problem. Because of its prevalence, community health nurses should include screening for dating violence in all encounters with teens. **Adolescent dating violence (ADV)** includes physical, sexual, emotional, and verbal abuse between teenaged persons who are or have been in a

DISPLAY 25-8

The Cycle of Violence

Acute battering
incident phase

Tension-building
phase

Loving reconciliation
phase

Tension-Building Phase

The woman senses her partner's increasing tension. She may or may not know what is wrong. The partner is "edgy" and lashes out in anger. He challenges her, calls her names, and tells her she is stupid, incompetent, and unconcerned about him. She "tries hard" not to make any "mistakes" that may upset him. She takes the responsibility for making him feel better, and begins to set herself up to feel guilt when he eventually explodes in spite of her best efforts to calm and please him. During the increasing tension, the woman is rarely angry even at the most outrageous demands or blame. Rather, she internalizes her appropriate anger at the partner's unfairness and, instead, experiences depression, anxiety, and a sense of helplessness. As the tension in the relationship increases, minor episodes of violence increase, such as pinching, tripping, or slapping. The batterer knows his behavior is inappropriate, and he fears the woman will leave him. This fear of rejection and loss increases his rage at the woman and his need to control her.

Acute Battering Incident

The tension-building phase ends in an explosion of violence. The incident that sets off the man's violence is often trivial or unknown, leaving the woman confused and feeling helpless. The woman may or may not fight back. She may try to escape the violence or call for help. If she cannot escape the beating, she may have a sense of unreality—as if it is a dream. Following the battering, the woman is in a state of physical and psychological shock. She may be passive and withdrawn or hysterical and incoherent. She may not be aware of the seriousness of her injuries and may resist help. The man discounts the episode and also underestimates the woman's injuries.

He may not summon medical help even when her injuries are life-threatening.

Loving Reconciliation

The loving reconciliation phase may begin a few hours to several days following the acute battering incident. Both partners have a profound sense of relief that "it's over." Although the woman is initially angry at the man, he begins an intense campaign to "win her back." Just as his tension and violence were overdone, his apologies, gifts, and gestures of love may also be excessive. Showering her with love and praise helps her repair her shattered self-esteem. It is nearly impossible for her to leave him during this phase as he is meeting her desperate need to see herself as a competent and lovable woman. The woman's feelings of power and romantic ideals are nurtured. She believes this gentle, loving person is her "real" lover. She believes that if only she can find the key, she can stop him from further violent episodes. She believes that, no matter how often it has happened before, somehow this episode seems different this time and it will never happen again.

The Increasing Spiral of Violence

One aspect of the cycle of violence of particular concern is its progressive and spiraling nature. Once violence has begun, every study indicates that it not only continues but over time increases in both frequency and severity. As the violence continues, the three-phase cycle begins to change. The tension-building phase becomes shorter and more intense, the acute battering incidents become more frequent and severe, and the loving reconciliation phase becomes shorter and less intense. After many years of battering, the man may not apologize at all.

---

casual or serious dating relationship (Hanson, 2002). ADV begins on average at age 15 years. About 50% of rape victims are between 10 and 19 years old, which indicates that teenage girls are vulnerable to the violence of sexual abuse (Jackson, Cram, & Seymour, 2000).

Partner/Spousal Abuse

Spousal abuse is violence against an intimate partner. Because of the nature of intimate partner violence, the problems

are difficult to study. Much remains unknown about the factors that increase or decrease the likelihood that men will behave violently toward women, the factors that endanger or protect women from violence, and the physical and emotional consequences of such violence for women and their children.

Domestic violence is a leading cause of morbidity and mortality in women. Nationwide, battering exceeds rapes, muggings, and motor vehicle crashes combined as the leading cause of injury to women age 15 to 44 years (Sheehy,

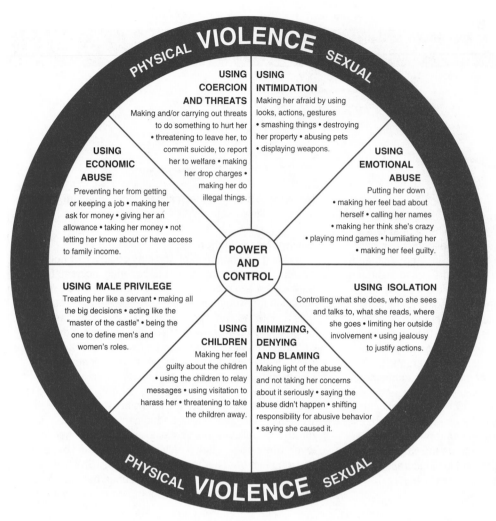

FIGURE 25-1. Wheel of violence. (Adapted from the Domestic Abuse Intervention Project, Duluth, MN.)

2000a). *Healthy People 2010* identified the reduction of physical assault by current or former intimate partners as one of our nation's health objectives (USDHHS, 2000). In a 1998 survey by The Commonwealth Fund, almost one third of American women (31%) reported having been physically or sexually abused by a husband or male partner at some point in their lives (Kramer, 2002). Each year, 6% of all pregnant women in the United States are battered by the men in their lives. For women with disabilities, the abuse ranges from 33% to 83%. Two thirds of elder domestic abuse victims are women, and more than half of elder abuse is perpetrated by family members (Kramer, 2002). Additionally, more than 25% of female homicide victims in the general population are killed by a husband, ex-husband, boyfriend, or ex-boyfriend.

In Oklahoma, the number of domestic violence reports rose 42% between 1989 and 1998. Almost 88,000 women and children sought shelter or crisis intervention between 1993 and 1997. Because of these alarming trends, through a grant from the Centers for Disease Control and Prevention, the state is conducting intimate partner violence injury surveillance in an attempt to determine the prevalence of intimate partner violence and the extent of injuries resulting in hospital treatment (Sheehy, 2000a).

Physical or sexual violence, or both, are used as a tactic to maintain power and control over another. Behaviors often include the following:

- Physical violence
- Sexual violence or intimidation
- Coercion and threats
- Emotional abuse
- Isolating the victim
- Using issues around children to harass or threaten
- Rigid imposition of beliefs in male superiority and privilege
- Economic abuse

Although victims may be of either sex and any sexual orientation, 95% of victims are women (see Voices from the Community).

Effects of Violence on Children

If children live in a home where a parent (usually the mother) is being emotionally, physically, or sexually abused, whether the children are being assaulted or not, they are still suffering from the tension they feel and the trauma they witness. Most often, wife abuse and child abuse occur together. Literature reviews consistently suggest that there is a positive

VOICES FROM THE COMMUNITY

"It would erupt, as it always did, over nothing. Some little trigger would start an outburst, and the outburst would turn into taunting, and the taunting into a spiral of viciousness. I remember thinking, in one of those moments of clarity when the world stands still, and your heart seems to stop, and you look at yourself from afar, that it was like a bullfight, and that I was cornered like an animal for the slaughter, with nowhere to hide, It was either him or me. . . . I was one of the lucky ones. I got out. After all these years, I finally managed to get out."

Jane

(Adapted from Locsin, R.C., & Purnell, M.J. [2002]. Intimate partner violence, culture-centrism, and nursing. *Holistic Nursing Practice, 16*(3), 1–4.)

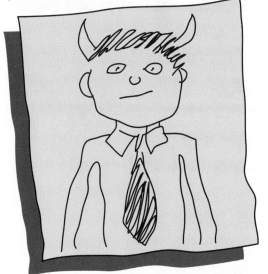

National Coalition Against Domestic Violence • P.O. Box 34103 • Washington, DC 20043-4103 • 1-800-799-SAFE

FIGURE 25–2. Poster of "My Daddy is a Monster." (National Coalition Against Domestic Violence.)

correlation between children's witnessing intimate partner violence and some aspects of impaired child development (Lemmey et al., 2001), in addition to the additional risk to their lives. These children are at risk for depression, negative mental health effects, and long-term consequences that last far into adulthood. Maladjustments may be behavioral (aggression and conduct problems), emotional (withdrawal, anxiousness, fearfulness), social, cognitive (learning disabilities), and physical (Fig. 25–2).

Violence During Pregnancy

Domestic violence continues through childhood and adolescence and follows a woman into long-term relationships and into pregnancy. Studies show that between 4% and 14% of adult pregnant women experience physical violence from an intimate partner (Campbell, 1999). Abuse is more likely to be reported by pregnant adolescents than pregnant adults, and by women with unplanned pregnancies compared with other pregnant women.

Abuse during pregnancy has been linked with maternal health problems such as smoking, decreased weight gain, and substance use (Cokkinides & Coker, 1998). The fetus is also endangered, with spontaneous abortion, preterm delivery, fetal distress, and lower birth weight often seen. Curry, Doyle, & Gilhooley (1998) found that pregnant teens who were abused were more likely to be high school dropouts, smoked more, and experienced more second-trimester bleeding. Once born, the infant of an abused teen or adult is at risk for child abuse.

The most serious aspect of domestic violence as a threat to a woman's safety is the link between abuse during pregnancy and homicide, called femicide. Femicide is now the leading cause of maternal mortality (rather than medical complications of pregnancy) in several cities in the United States. Men who abuse their partners during pregnancy are more likely to own guns or knives or both, which puts the women at greater risk, and the batterings that occur during pregnancy tend to have increased severity (Campbell, 1998, 1999).

Studies have found that the prenatal care visit is one of the few times when women are seen by the helping professions. This visit is an important opportunity to identify women who are abused and therefore at risk for homicide. It is imperative that nurses conduct an assessment for danger and lethality so that the women can be aware of their own level of risk and take safety precautions as needed. A series of questions requiring a "Yes" or "No" response and inquiries about occurrences of abuse, escalation of abuse, frequency, severity, weapons, drugs or alcohol use by the perpetrator, and safety of other children should be incorporated into prenatal home visit assessments. This is especially important with women who have not followed through with

DISPLAY 25-9

Domestic Violence Risk Assessment Tool

Frame the Questions

"Because abuse and violence are common in the lives of women, I have begun to ask about it with all women (or all pregnant women). I don't know if this is a problem for you, but I would like to ask you some questions, talk about ways to reduce your risk of being hurt, and give you some information and phone numbers that might be helpful to you."

Universal Questions

	Yes	No
1. Do you feel safe in your current relationships? Comments: _____	_____	_____
2. Have you ever been physically abused (pushed, shoved, hit, punched, bitten, burned, etc.)? Comments: _____	_____	_____
3. Have you ever been emotionally abused (neglected, called names, controlled, threatened, had your activities or decisions hindered, been denied	_____	_____

resources to meet your physical or financial needs)?
Comments: _____

4. Have you ever been sexually abused (forced to have an unwanted sexual act)? Comments: _____	_____	_____
5. Do you want to talk to someone about receiving help? Comments: _____	_____	_____

Resources

National Domestic Violence Hotline: 1-800-799-SAFE (7233)
Local Battered Women's Shelter _____
Local Department of Women's Health Services _____
Other resources _____
_____

(Adapted from Sheehy, G. [2000b]. *Violence against women.* Fairfax, VA; The National Women's Health Information Center; Kramer, A. [2001]. Domestic violence: How to ask and how to listen. *Nursing Clinics of North America, 37*(1), 189–210; and Davis, R.E., & Harsh, K.E. [2001]. Confronting barriers to universal screening for domestic violence. *Journal of Professional Nursing, 17*(6), 313–320.)

prenatal care during which health care professionals can monitor the progress of their pregnancies (Display 25–9).

Batterer Characteristics

Although men who batter come from all walks of life educationally, culturally, and socioeconomically, they have certain characteristics in common. The following list represents some characteristics of batterers:

1. They have low self-esteem.
2. They believe all myths regarding battering relationships, such as the myth that the woman "asks for it" or that "if she would do what the man says it wouldn't happen" or that "abuse doesn't happen in the suburbs but only among low-income people in the inner city."
3. They are traditionalists who believe in male supremacy and stereotyped male sex roles in the family.
4. They blame others for their actions.
5. They are pathologically jealous.
6. They have severe stress reactions.
7. They use sex as an act of aggression to enhance self-esteem.
8. They do not believe their violent behavior should have negative consequences.
9. They have a low frustration threshold; poor impulse control; a violent, explosive temper; and an external locus of control.
10. They present a dual personality.

11. They are emotionally dependent on their partner/spouse and children.
12. They have a family history of domestic violence.
13. They see violence as a viable method of problem-solving.
14. They use threats of violence as a control mechanism.
15. They were physically and/or sexually abused as a child or saw their mothers abused.
16. They have a high level of job dissatisfaction, underemployment, or unemployment.
17. They have unrealistic expectations of the relationship.
18. They are preoccupied with weapons.

MISTREATMENT OF ELDERS

It is estimated that as many as 10% of older adults are victims of abuse (Gray-Vickrey, 2001). **Elder abuse**, the mistreatment or exploitation of older adults, may involve neglect; physical, sexual, emotional, or fiduciary abuse; or any combination of these. Among substantiated cases, 25% involve physical abuse, 49% intentional or unintentional neglect, 35% emotional abuse, and 30% financial or material exploitation. Elders are abused by family members in similar ways that younger family members are abused: by abandon or neglect (physical or emotional); by physical, sexual, or emotional abuse; or by exploitation. Adult children, divided between males and females equally, are the most frequent abusers of the elderly. However, spouses who were batterers do not stop at age 65; they commit about 14% of the reported cases of elder abuse in the United States. The victims of elder abuse have a median age of 76.5 years, and 65% of them are white.

Abuse against elders is not new, but research on elder abuse is new. Until recently, the reasons for elder abuse were extrapolated from the literature on abuse in younger populations. By the mid-1980s, more research was being conducted, and the findings indicated that elder abuse results from multiple, interrelated variables associated with the perpetrator or the victim (Menzey, 2001).

Forms of physical abuse include rough handling during caregiving, pinching, hitting, and slapping. Emotional abuse can take many forms, including being shouted at or threatened and having needed care withheld. More rarely, elders are sexually abused, which may include rape. Some elders are neglected by those they depend on to meet their caregiving needs. In this form of abuse, the elder may appear unwashed and unkempt and may be suffering from malnutrition, dehydration, and ultimately pressure sores. Elders who are dependent on the care of others often do not report such abuses for fear of being abandoned. They feel powerless and at a loss about how to change a bad situation, and they fear reprisal from the perpetrators if they tell others about the abuse.

Older adults are frequently exploited in a variety of ways. Family members may take their Social Security retirement money, savings, or investments and use it on themselves. Criminals who approach elders with get-rich-quick schemes, sham investment opportunities, or illegitimate charities often prey on the trusting nature of older adults.

Perpetrator and Victim Characteristics

The dominant underlying factors that contribute to abuse of an elder by a family member are social isolation and pathology on the part of the perpetrator. Research has identified emotional or financial dependence on the victim, alcohol use, and isolation or few external contacts as major contributing factors. Men are more likely to exploit or physically abuse elders, whereas women are more likely to neglect elders physically or abuse them psychologically. Because women are more frequently the caretakers of elders, they are in a position to provide either appropriate or neglectful care to frail older adults (Menzey, 2001). Frequently caregiver "burnout" contributes to the too-casual, neglectful, or obvious hurtful practices some family member or employed caregivers may impose on the elder.

Some characteristics of older people appear to increase their risk of abuse. They include dementia and poor health (Menzey, 2001). Newly diagnosed cognitive impairment correlates with occurrences of abuse. If violence or threats of violence by the elder toward the caregiver accompany dementia, this contributes to elder abuse. The failing health of an elder may contribute to self-neglect or diminished ability for self-defense or escape from maltreatment. Finally, if the abuser and victim live together, the close proximity can bring up unresolved family conflicts or create new conflicts when the expectations of cohabitating are not met (Menzey, 2001).

Risk Factors

Regardless of the type of abuse an elder suffers or the motivation of the abuser in the family, two factors are common to all elder abuse situations. The first is the *invisibility* of elders in general and of the abused elder specifically. It is estimated that fewer than 10% of elder abuse cases are reported. In 1988, Pillemer and Finkelhor found that only 1 of every 14 cases of elder abuse came to public attention in Massachusetts, a state with model reporting laws. Reasons for invisibility among the elderly are multifaceted. Older people usually have less contact with the community. They are no longer in the workforce or in public on a regular basis, which keeps their problems hidden longer. In addition, older adults are reticent to admit to being abused or neglected. Because the abuser is most often a family member, the elder desires to protect the abuser; without this abusing family member, the elder would be entirely alone. On the other hand, the elder may fear reprisal from the abuser for coming forward with a self-report of abuse or telling another about the home situation.

The second risk factor is the *vulnerability* of older adults. Many elders who are becoming frail are dependent on others for some aspect of their day-to-day survival. At first they may need to rely on others for transportation, shopping, and housekeeping. Later they may need help with financial affairs, cooking, and laundry. In time, they may need help managing their medications, bathing, and eating. The degree to which an elder needs assistance is often kept hidden from others because they fear being removed from their present living situation and placed in a more restrictive environment. This contributes to vulnerability, and they can become easy victims for abusive family members. In addition, vulnerability in elders is increased when the following four sets of characteristics are present: (1) impairment and isolation; (2) poverty and pathologic caregivers; (3) learned helplessness and living in a violent subculture; and (4) deteriorating housing and crime-ridden neighborhoods.

OTHER FORMS OF FAMILY VIOLENCE

There are three forms of family violence not previously discussed in detail: suicide, homicide, and rape. These three forms of violence demonstrate the ultimate extreme of violence to the victim and are the most traumatic to the surviving family members.

Suicide

Suicide is taking action that causes one's own death. Globally, 820,000 people commit suicide each year (WHO,

1998). In the United States, on an average day 87 people successfully commit suicide and more than 3000 attempt suicide (USDHHS, 2000). The *Healthy People 2010* goal is to reduce sucides to no more than 6.0 per 100,000 people. White men older than 65 years of age are at highest risk, with 35.5 deaths per 100,000 in 1997. In 1996, suicide was the third leading killer of those between the ages of 15 and 24 years in the United States (USDHHS, 2000).

Parasuicidal acts are deliberate acts with nonfatal outcomes that attempt to cause or actually cause self-harm. The yearly prevalence of parasuicidal acts varies between 2% and 20%. The prevalence of parasuicide is estimated to be 10 to 20 times higher than that of completed suicides. Three times more women than men attempt suicide, whereas three times more men than women succeed. Cutting one's wrists is often dramatized on television, but it is not an effective way to die. People who attempt suicide, or commit a parasuicidal act, may use this method.

Completed suicides are carried out in a variety of ways, some more violent than others. Women usually choose less violent methods, such as overdosing on medications. Men choose more violent forms of suicide, such as hanging, use of firearms, or vehicle crashes. Deaths from suicide are underreported because of a tendency to group them as accidental deaths or deaths from undetermined causes.

Any verbalization of suicide ideation from clients (or others) should be taken seriously, with appropriate intervention steps taken immediately. Intervention strategies, including early recognition of depression, elimination or treatment of drug or alcohol abuse, and violence prevention programs, are available. Many more are being developed, implemented, and evaluated for effectiveness.

Homicide

Homicide is any non–war-related action taken to cause the death of another person. Globally, some 560,000 homicides occur each year. In many developed and developing countries, 20% to 40% of deaths among men aged 15 to 34 years are the result of homicide or suicide (WHO, 1998). In the United States in 1997, 53 people died each day from homicide. A goal for *Healthy People 2010* is to reduce homicides to less than 3.2 per 100,000 people; the baseline was 16.2 in 1998 (USDHHS, 2000).

Many homicide casualties are victims of domestic abuse. The cycle of violence escalates and the partner is killed, most often in a violent episode, or by arrangement with the homicide committed by a third party. Of all women seen in hospital emergency departments, 20% to 50% are victims of partner violence (Davis & Harsh, 2001), and 25% of female homicides result from injuries inflicted by spouses, ex-spouses, or nonmarital partners, not strangers (USDOJ, 2001a).

Rape

Rape is an act of aggression in which the perpetrator is motivated by a desire to dominate, control, and degrade the victim. It was once considered an act of sexuality. It is now believed that it is a combination of the two, with rape defined as the "sexual expression of aggression."

The USDOJ reported that more than 407,000 females aged 12 years and older were victims of rape, attempted rape, or sexual assault in 1994. These are conservative figures, with other studies reporting that more than 683,000 women experience forcible rape in a year and that 12.1 million American women have been the victim of forcible rape at some time in their lives (USDHHS, 2000).

LEVELS OF PREVENTION: CRISIS INTERVENTION AND FAMILY VIOLENCE

Family violence is a family crisis and needs interruption. Community health nurses are in a unique position to prevent, detect, and intervene during crisis situations. They encounter people in their own settings, where direct observation, discussion, and intervention can occur. Because of their assessment skills, familiarity with the community, access to resources, and opportunity to go into the homes of families, community health nurses are ideally situated to help families in crisis. By implementing the three levels of prevention, the nurse can begin to put back together the lives of family members encountering domestic violence (see Levels of Prevention Matrix).

Primary Prevention

The cycle of violence within the family can be interrupted. Even when partners, spouses, or parents have been brought up in violent homes by abusive parents, they can learn to rechannel and control their emotions and behaviors to be appropriate. Primary prevention is obviously the most effective level of intervention, in terms of both promoting clients' health and containing costs. Primary prevention reflects a fundamental human concern for well-being and includes planned activities, undertaken by the nurse, to prevent an unwanted event from occurring, to protect current states of health and healthy functioning, and to promote desired states of health for the members of a particular community. For the community health nurse, any activity that fosters healthful practices, counteracts unhealthful influences, and increases empowerment can help prevent a crisis. Health promotion should take into account physical, psychological, sociocultural, and spiritual needs.

Several opportunities exist for families who want to improve relationships with their partner or spouse and children. First, social problem-solving skills for both partners and assertiveness skills for women provide a foundation on which additional programs can build. Many people have not learned positive problem-solving skills that are socially acceptable. Women have learned passivity and submissiveness, perhaps in response to their own inadequate parenting or abusive upbringing. Men and women can benefit from these two types of skill development.

LEVELS OF PREVENTION MATRIX

SITUATION: Promotion of crisis resolution.

GOAL: Using the three levels of prevention negative health conditions are avoided, or promptly diagnosed and treated, and the fullest possible potential is restored.

PRIMARY PREVENTION		SECONDARY PREVENTION		TERTIARY PREVENTION		
Health Promotion and Education	*Health Protection*	*Early Diagnosis*	*Prompt Treatment*	*Rehabilitation*	*Primary Prevention*	
					Health Promotion and Education	*Health Protection*
• Anticipatory guidance • Reinforce positive coping strategies • Mobilize social support and other resources	• Reduce factors that increase vulnerability • Reduce hazards in some events (safety and multiplicity of stressors)	• Recognize signs and symptoms of the crisis	• Provide necessary assistance including emergency medical and emotional support, and assist with reaction to the event and functioning • Allow behavior (eg, dependence, grief) • Refer to resources • Set goals with client	• Promote adaptation to a changed level of wellness • Promote interdependence • Reinforce newly learned behaviors, lifestyle changes, coping strategies • Explore application of learned behaviors to new situations • Identify and use of additional resources	• Continue with primary health promotion activities to enhance healthy response to future crises	• Continue with primary health protection activities to enhance healthy response to future crises

Second, people need to have the self-esteem that improved education and occupational success can bring. If poverty is a related factor to the violence, educational preparation and a successful employee role may eliminate this stressor. As stated earlier, violence occurs across all socioeconomic levels of society; however, if a family is so impoverished that their basic needs cannot be met, stress can lead the more vulnerable family members to seek out illegal ways to solve their financial problems. This happens especially in neighborhoods in which criminal activity is easily accessed.

People must take lessons or pass tests in order to drive; to get into college; to become nurses, attorneys, teachers, and other licensed professionals; and to join the military. The most important job an adult will ever have is that of parent, yet no lessons are required and there are no tests to pass. Parenting training is something all parents would benefit from, but especially those potential parents who are at high risk: teens, people with no exposure to children in their upbringing, and people raised in violent and abusive families.

Community health nurses often make home visits to

families based on referrals from hospital perinatal departments. During the mother's postpartum stay, a nurse may have noted some inappropriate parenting behaviors or the parents may meet high-risk parameters set by the hospital, such as being 17 years old or younger, being single, or having a history of substance abuse. On the first few visits to the family, the nurse can assess parenting skills and any need for training. If a parenting class is recommended, it should cover age-appropriate content, such as safety, breast-feeding, formula preparation, food progression, anticipatory guidance for growth and development, discipline techniques including behavior modification and time-out, well-baby care and immunizations, and so on. An additional benefit for the parents is the social support they get from other attending parents.

The opportunity for home visiting has been formalized into model programs around the country, based on 2 decades of work by David Old and others, that have been shown to effectively prevent abuse (Olds et al., 1997, 1999). In such programs, the nurse visits on a regular basis over several years, teaching and role-modeling many parenting techniques, providing needed support, and initiating necessary referrals.

The interrelatedness between families and communities cannot be overlooked or underestimated. Neighborhoods need to be enfranchised; they need to be developed; they need to be safe for all members; they need to be healthy. Empowered families can take back their neighborhoods from criminals, and they can be sources of growth for families.

Secondary Prevention

Early diagnosis and prompt treatment of the effects of family crisis or violence is the focus of the secondary level of prevention. It seeks to reduce the intensity and duration of a crisis and to promote adaptive behavior. By creating a positive relationship with family members and seeing them in their homes, the community health nurse can often uncover and intervene in a crisis or stop abusive situations.

People in crisis need help. They often desperately want help. The crisis or violence and its associated disequilibrium has a twofold effect on the individuals involved: (1) it renders them temporarily helpless and unable to cope on their own, and (2) it makes them especially receptive to outside influence. There are crisis resolution models that community health nurses can use to help clients at the secondary level. The following steps have been used successfully by people in the mental health field working on crisis hot lines, in mental health centers, and in emergency departments (Aguilera, 1998):

1. Establish rapport
2. Assess the individual and the problem for lethality
3. Identify major problems and intervene
4. Deal with feelings
5. Explore alternatives and coping mechanisms
6. Develop action plan
7. Follow up, including anticipatory planning for coping with future crises

People in crisis will seek and generally receive some kind of help, but the nature of that help can rule in favor of or against a healthy outcome in which the participants can grow and evolve. Clients' desires for assistance give the helping professional a prime opportunity to intervene; this opportunity also presents a challenge to make the intervention as effective as possible. Some behaviors found to be helpful include the following (Davis & Harsh, 2001; Kramer, 2002):

1. Respect confidentiality—Discussions must occur in private, without other family members present or in hearing distance. This is essential to build trust and ensure the woman's safety.
2. Believe and validate her experiences—Listen to her and believe her. Acknowledge her feelings and let her know that she is not alone that many women have similar experiences.
3. Acknowledge the injustice—The violence perpetrated against her is not her fault. No one deserves to be abused.
4. Respect her autonomy—Respect her right to make decisions in her life. She must decide whether to involve the police. Validate and respect her choice. She is the expert in her life.
5. Help her plan for her future safety—What has she tried in the past to protect herself? Does she have a safe place to go if she needs to escape? What plans does she have to protect her children? Help her recognize the danger in her life.
6. Promote access to community services—Know the resources in your community. Is there a battered women's shelter, a domestic violence hotline, or a rape crisis center? Give her the phone numbers.

One goal of crisis intervention should be to help clients reestablish a sense of safety and security while allowing them to ventilate their feelings and be validated. This helps to reestablish equilibrium at as healthy a level as possible and can result in client change and growth. Minimally, that goal involves resolving the immediate crisis and restoring clients to their precrisis levels of functioning. Ultimately, however, intervention seeks to raise that functioning to a healthier, more mature level that will enable clients to cope with and prevent future crises. As discussed earlier, crises tend to be self-limited; intervention time lasts from 4 to 8 weeks, with resolution, one way or another, within 2 to 3 months (Aguilera, 1998). The urgency of the situation represents a window of opportunity that invites the prompt, focused attention of clients and nurse working together to achieve intervention goals.

Special programs for children living in homes where crises and violence are chronic include Head Start programs for prekindergarten children meeting certain socioeconomic characteristics. These programs give children the social and academic stimulation to be on a par with peers when they enter kindergarten. Other programs include those for social skills development and Special Friends Programs explicitly for children who have survived abusive situations. Survivors experience multiple developmental and psychological problems. Assessment of children who are experiencing learning and social failure should be an ongoing service in both elementary and high schools. Just as important is the early identification of and intervention with conduct-disordered youth. School nurses can be important interprofessional team members in such programs.

Intervention at the secondary level for adults who experience abuse focuses on women and their children. Shelters for women and children are available in most communities and offer a bevy of services, including counseling for the woman, classes in self-esteem building and assertiveness training, referrals to or programs for job acquisition training, even money and time management classes. Some shelters offer programs that last for up to 2 years of progressive independence and employment skill development while the women and their children live in protective home environments with addresses being kept confidential from abusers.

Depending on the situation that brings the woman to a

shelter, the perpetrator may or may not be incarcerated or on probation. If the abuser was arrested during the most recent violent episode, he may be released, on parole, or incarcerated. Even while incarcerated, the abuser may be able to take part in an anger-management class, psychological counseling, substance abuse treatment, Alcohol Anonymous (AA) meetings, or Narcotics Anonymous (NA) meetings. Visits between the abuser and his children are supervised if they are part of a court order.

At times, the nurse may be responding to a referral regarding suspected abuse; at other times, an abusive or neglectful situation is uncovered on a home visit that is made for another reason. In any case, the community health nurse has an important role in reporting the suspected abuse and encouraging the child, partner/spouse, or elder to go to the appropriate facility for care and documentation of the abuse.

Reporting Abuse

All states have reporting laws for suspected abuse. The particulars regarding timing, who is notified, and the sequence of events may differ from state to state. The following steps represent one state's guidelines for reporting suspected child abuse (Crime and Violence Prevention Center, 2003b):

1. All mandated reporters must report known or suspected abuse. (Mandated reporters include public and private school employees; administrators and employees of youth centers and recreation programs; child welfare employees; foster parents; group home and residential facility personnel; social workers; probation workers; health care workers including nurses, doctors, and chiropractics; animal control workers; and personnel working in film development laboratories.)
2. Immediately, or as soon as reasonably possible, a local child protective agency (police department after normal working hours) must be contacted and given a verbal report. During this verbal report, mandated reporters must give their name, which is kept confidential and may be revealed only in court or if the reporter waives confidentiality (others can give information anonymously), the name and age of the child, the present location of the child, the nature and characteristics of the injury, and any other facts that led the reporter to suspect abuse or would be helpful to the investigator.
3. Within 2 working days, a written report must be completed by the mandated reporter and filed. If a mandated reporter fails to report known or suspected instances of child abuse, she or he may be subject to criminal liability, punishable by up to 6 months in jail or a fine of $1000.

Similar steps are required for nurses to report elder abuse. Cases of maltreatment and neglect among elders are reported to a local office of the Area Agency on Aging (or to the police), and a screening/documentation form is used to gather and record the pertinent information.

In cases of partner/spousal abuse, adults who are mentally competent cannot be removed involuntarily from the abusive situation. The community health nurse can encourage the victim to leave the perpetrator for her safety until he gets professional help and can give information regarding community resources, such as a shelter for women and children. If the adult has a life-threatening injury or illness, medical follow-up must be encouraged; however, the victim may still be reluctant to seek help. At times, another family member or neighbor who witnesses the abusive event calls 911; when the police and paramedics arrive, the victim may have support to seek the care and protection needed. A domestic violence screening/documentation form is completed and filed by the nurse as a part of the official health records for the client.

Tools

Assessment of suspected abuse cannot be overemphasized. The community health nurse may be the only person entering the home of a family in crisis where abuse is occurring. Asking the right questions, being a careful observer, and following the right reporting and recording procedures may mean the difference between life and death for the victims of the cycle of violence.

Displays 25–10, 25–11, and 25–12 at the end of this chapter consist of three sample tools that the community health nurse and other advocates use in their role of mandated reporter. They include a Suspected Child Abuse Report, a two-page medical report of suspected child abuse, and a Domestic Violence Screening/Documentation Form.

Tertiary Prevention

Tertiary prevention of family violence focuses on the rehabilitation of the family. The family may never again be the same unit of service, because the partners may separate—by choice, motivated by fear or hate; by court order, if the perpetrator is incarcerated; or by death. If the family chooses to stay together, long-term intervention for all family members is needed to establish a climate conducive to family normalcy. Many of the services discussed as part of the secondary level of prevention are continued into tertiary prevention to heal, restore, and promote the growth of the family.

If incarceration is a part of tertiary prevention, the effects of having one family member living in this environment must be factored into the services and support provided by the community health nurse to the family as a whole (see Chapter 36). Even if the partner/spouse has separated from the perpetrator emotionally or legally, or both, the perpetrator usually has legal rights to see his children. This means that other family members, usually from the abuser's side of the family, may bring the children to the prison to visit their father. Just making these arrangements can cause stress for the mother and the children. The community health nurse needs to be aware of the complicated dynamics and emotional stress such difficult situations can produce for all family members. The victim–perpetrator relationship is as complex as the forces that created the violence and abuse.

FAMILIES FACING VIOLENCE FROM OUTSIDE THE FAMILY

The concern of violence coming into the family from outside the home, often beyond the family's control, is a relatively new phenomonon in the United States. There has always been some degree of violence that makes its way into the home in the form of burglaries and, at times, murder or abduction. Increasingly, however, home invasion as a form of forced entry has been a violent crime perpetrated most frequently by strangers. Other forms of violence of which families are newly aware include the potential for biologic, chemical and radioactive homeland terrorist activities.

Home Invasion

This form of violence is a new form of terror and is increasing. Home invasion occurs mainly in large cities, although rural areas are not immune. **Home invasion** is the purposeful and sudden entry into a home by force while the family is home and awake. The effectiveness of this form of terror relies on surprise. Motivation may be material or thrill; household belongings are frequently stolen while family members are incapacitated by being bound, blindfolded, and/or gagged. In other cases, family members are killed. Often the perpetrators are under the influence of drugs or alcohol, and at times the violence may be gang related.

The community health nurse most likely will not encounter families who have experienced such violence. However, nurses may work with extended family members of the victims or families who have reported such a happening in their neighborhood and are now fearful. Fear of violence can create psychological and physiologic stress reactions similar to those that occur when one actually experiences the violence. These fears should not be ignored. The role of the nurse includes the four steps suggested in the generic approach to crisis intervention (see later discussion).

Homeland Terrorist Activities

In 2002 and 2003, fear of and preparation against homeland terrorist activities from outside the country became a reality in the United States. **Homeland terrorist activities** include the use of biologic, chemical, or radioactive agents against civilians during peace or war designed to create fear, terror, and death. In 2002, a new department was established at the federal level, the Department of Homeland Security. In addition, the government established a terrorism alert rating scale to warn the population through a color code about the present risk of terrorist activity (low to extremely high). States, regions, and local authorities put into place plans to thwart bioterrorist activities. Security was increased at water purification plants and water sources. A program of administration of smallpox immunizations to "first responders" also began, because smallpox, anthrax and tularemia are possible biologic terrorist weapons (Spake, 2003). The potential

WHAT DO YOU THINK?

"Israeli parents, when they take their newborns home from the maternity ward, are given a special gift for the little one: a blue plastic case that looks as if it might hold a violin. It's courtesy not of the Israel Philharmonic but of the Israel Defense Forces; inside is a gas mask kit made especially for babies. Duct tape and other such gear may be a novelty for Americans, but Israeli hospitals have been handing out these gifts since the 1991 Gulf War, when Israelis donned gas masks and huddled inside 'sealed rooms' in their homes. Indeed, since the war, all new homes and buildings must have 'security rooms' that seal shut with rubber."

L. Derfner

(From Spake, A. [2003]. Are you ready? *U. S. News & World Report, 134*[6], 24, 26, 27.)

use of radioactive agents in the form of "dirty bombs," which throw off radiation by an explosive device and cannot be seen or smelled, left families feeling very vulnerable. Families were encouraged to obtain a supply of potassium iodine pills to counteract the effects of the radioactive material. As protection against chemical agents, such as the gases sarin and VX or the poison ricin, that may be introduced into the air, families were encouraged to buy plastic sheeting and duct tape to seal themselves into their homes. Some stores sold out of plastic, tape, packaged foods and bottled water within hours after this advice was given (see What Do You Think?)

Making preparations for acts of terrorism and planning ways to prevent or survive the effects of agents used as terrorism weapons can themselves create fears and can become all-encompassing. Unanswered questions remain: Should I get my family vaccinated against smallpox? Should we stock up on potassium iodine? How effective will it be and when should we take it? How useful are the government's new guidelines to help families prepare for a possible attack? It is likely that our children will be in schools when an attack occurs—Are the schools prepared? Have hospitals made improvements since the anthrax scare of 2001–2002? Perhaps these questions will be asked of the community health nurse. What responses are appropriate? How can the nurse provide support, education, and counseling for families struggling with the potential of violence coming into their homes?

METHODS OF INTERVENTION

Crisis intervention in community health nursing uses either or both of two approaches: generic and individual. For the

CLINICAL CORNER

COMMUNITY HEALTH NURSING AND A POTENTIAL FAMILY IN CRISIS

You are a community health nurse working for Smithville Health Department. You are following up on a referral from a community clinic's family planning clinic. The referral was made for a 19-year-old woman, Sandy, who presented in clinic and exhibited inappropriate behaviors with her 6-month-old daughter. In their referral, staff stated that they observed the mother shouting at the child, accusing her of "being spoiled rotten." They added that the mother appeared quite anxious and seemed to have difficulty waiting the 15 minutes for her examination. Although the behaviors described in this referral were insufficient to warrant a report to social services, the staff felt that this young mother would benefit from intervention on the part of the nurse.

You prepare for this home visit by reviewing the medical records of both Sandy and her child to determine whether the family has had previous involvement with social service agencies such as child protective services. You find that the maternal grandparents made a referral to Child Welfare on behalf of Sandy when she was 15. They were concerned about the relationship between Sandy and her step-father. The report cited suspected sexual involvement between the two. An investigation occurred but was inconclusive, and the charges were never pursued.

You also discuss the case with family planning and immunization clinic staff, since the family receives services at both clinics. The staff advise you that they are familiar with Sandy and her husband Nick. They state that their only interaction with Nick was during a family planning clinic 2 months ago. They report that Sandy appeared anxious and in a hurry on that day, stating, "I really need to hurry, Nick is waiting in the car and he gets impatient." Shortly after that, the staff tells you, Nick came running into the clinic shouting, "What the hell is taking you people so long?" He reportedly glared at Sandy, and the two quickly exited the clinic.

You phone the client and advise her that you are a nurse with the local health department. You inform her that nurses often visit new mothers to assist them in finding resources. You add that as a community health nurse, you will be available to talk with her about her child's growth and development.

The client expresses interest in the visit and states, "I want you to show me some things about feeding her and stuff. I need help figuring out what to do at night, she still isn't sleeping much and it's driving me crazy." You advise the client that you will be happy to discuss those issues with her, that you will bring information which you will review with her. You add that you noted in her medical record that the father of the baby is living in the home and assure her that she may involve other family members, including the father of the baby, in the home visit. You jointly decide that the visit will occur the following day at 10:30 AM and that the father of the baby will be present if his work schedule allows.

On the day of the visit, as you walk up the stairs toward the apartment, you notice someone looking at you through the curtains. As you near the apartment door the curtains close. Your repeated knocking on the door is met with no response. You call the client's name but there is no answer.

QUESTIONS

1. Would this scenario provoke anxiety for you? How would you deal with your reaction?
2. How is this different from a scenario in the acute care setting in which a supervisor would be readily available?
3. Given this scenario, what actions will you take?
4. If you had been working in the family planning clinic on the day that Nick came in, what, if anything, would you have done differently?
5. As young parents, Nick and Sandy are part of an aggregate that has unique risk factors for parenting. List as many of these risk factors as you can think of and brainstorm about possible community health nursing interventions for each.
6. What methods would you suggest the clinic staff utilize to detect signs and symptoms of physical, sexual, or emotional abuse among this aggregate?

---

majority of crisis encounters, the generic approach is more appropriate. Family violence is a major situational crisis in which community health nurses intervene. However, many other situational and developmental crises affect families, who are benefited by the skills of the community health nurse. Newly recognized crises include community violence coming into the home and the potential of terrorism at home.

Generic Approach

The generic approach designs interventions to fit a particular type of crisis, focusing on the nature and course of the crisis rather than on the psychodynamics of each client (Aguilera, 1998). Crisis intervention using the generic approach is tailored to a specific kind of crisis, situational or developmental, and comprises four important elements: (1) encouraging use of adaptive behavior and coping strategies, (2) support, (3) preparation for the practical and emotional future, and (4) anticipatory guidance.

As an example, the generic approach is used with families experiencing child abuse. The child may be in foster care while the family receives needed services and rebuilds itself. The nurse encourages the parents to discuss and analyze their feelings, teaches stress-reduction techniques and positive coping skills, and creates a supportive, caring atmosphere, especially through self-help groups such as Parents Anonymous. The nurse can help individual family members strengthen self-esteem by encouraging positive interpersonal relationships. The community health nurse also teaches the parents needed parenting skills and provides anticipatory guidance so that they are prepared to raise their children with the use of consistent and appropriate discipline techniques that are age appropriate.

The generic approach does not require advanced professional psychotherapy skills. More important for community health practice, it works well with families, groups, and even communities in crisis. The community health nurse may work with a group of cancer clients, abused elders, adolescents struggling with developmental crisis, or an entire community recovering from some natural or manmade disaster. The generic approach allows the nurse to intervene with any group of people who have a crisis in common. It offers a broad base of support, because such a group can provide resources for its members beyond those brought by the nurse (see Clinical Corner).

Individual Approach

The individual approach is used for clients who do not respond to the generic approach or who need special therapy. Individual crisis intervention should not be confused with individual psychotherapy, which tends to focus on a client's developmental past. In contrast, crisis intervention directs treatment toward the immediate state of disequilibrium, identifying its causes and developing coping mechanisms. Family members or significant others are included during the process of crisis resolution. An entire group may need this type of intervention. If this approach is needed, clients are usually referred to a professional with specialized training.

ROLE OF THE COMMUNITY HEALTH NURSE IN CARING FOR FAMILIES IN CRISIS

Crisis intervention in community health assumes that clients have resources. If their potential for managing stressful events can be tapped, people in crisis will need minimal direct assistance. In accordance with the self-care concept, crisis intervention seeks to identify and build on client strengths. Aguilera (1998) outlined a series of four steps for intervention during crisis: assessment, planning, intervention, and resolution. Interventions to promote crisis resolution are presented using the three levels of prevention in Table 25–2 (see also Levels of Prevention Matrix).

T A B L E   2 5 – 2

Levels of Prevention to Promote Crisis Resolution

Phase	Goals	Interventions
		PRIMARY PREVENTION
Precrisis	Health promotion Disease prevention Education	Anticipatory guidance Reduce factors that increase vunerability Reduce hazards in some events (safety and multiplicity of stressors) Reinforce positive coping strategies Mobilize social support and other resources
		SECONDARY PREVENTION
Crisis	Reduction of stress load Cure or restoration of function	Assist with reaction to the event and functioning Allow behavior: dependence, grief Set goals with client Refer to resources
		TERTIARY PREVENTION
Postcrisis	Rehabilitation and maintenance	Promote adaptation to a changed level of wellness Promote interdependence Reinforce newly learned behaviors, lifestyle changes, coping strategies Explore application of learned behaviors to new situations Identification and use of additional resources

Assessment and Nursing Diagnosis

Initially, the nurse must assess the nature of the crisis and the clients' response to it. How severe is the problem, and what risks do the clients face? Are other people also at risk? Assessment must be rapid but thorough, focusing on certain specific areas.

First, the nurse concentrates on the immediate problem during the assessment. Why have clients asked for help right now? How do they define the problem? What precipitated the crisis? When did it occur? Was it a sudden accidental or situational event, or a slower developmental one?

Next, the nurse focuses on the clients' perceptions of the event. What does the crisis mean to them, and how do they think it will affect their future? Are they viewing the situation realistically? When a crisis occurs to a family or group, some members see the situation differently from others. During intervention, all should be encouraged to express themselves, to talk about the crisis, and to share their feelings about its meaning. Acceptance of the range of feelings is important.

Determine what persons are available for support. Consider family, friends, clergy, other professionals, community members, and agencies. With whom are the clients close, and whom do they trust? One advantage of group intervention is that the members provide some of this support for one another. In subsequent sessions, the quality of support should be evaluated. Sometimes a well-meaning individual can worsen the situation or deter clients from facing and coping with reality.

Finally, the nurse assesses the clients' coping abilities. Have they had similar kinds of experiences in the past? What techniques have they previously used to relieve tension and anxiety? Which techniques have they tried in this situation, and if they did not work, why not? Clients should be encouraged to think of other stress-relieving techniques, perhaps ones they have used in the past, and to try them.

The nurse gathers all of these data and mentally begins to form nursing diagnoses. As a plan of care is developed for the client, these nursing diagnoses are formalized in writing. Standardized nursing diagnoses are available for reference, or the agency for whom the nurse works may have a format of nursing diagnoses that it prefers. These nursing diagnoses are effective tools as the nurse begins planning intervention (see Using the Nursing Process).

Planning Therapeutic Intervention

Several factors influence clients' reaction to crises. Nurses should try to determine what factors are affecting clients before making intervention plans. The major balancing factors—clients' perceptions of the event, situational supports, human resources, and clients' coping skills—have been assessed in the first step (Aguilera, 1998). While continuing to explore these, the nurse now also considers the clients' general health status, age, past experiences with similar types of situations, sociocultural and religious influences, and the actual assets and liabilities of the situation. This helps to clarify the situation and gives the nurse the opportunity to further encourage clients' participation in the resolution process. If clients are defensive, resistant, and rigid, they are not processing clearly and can complete only simple tasks. It will take time before clients can begin to problem-solve the effects of the crisis on themselves and the loss they are experiencing, but they need to be encouraged by the nurse to reach this level.

The plan is based on the kind of crisis (situational or developmental, acute or chronically recurring), the effect the crisis is having on clients' lives (can they still work, go to school, and keep house, or are they secured within their home for an indefinite period, not knowing whether other family members have survived a major natural or manmade crisis?), where they are in coming to resolution of the crisis, the ways in which significant others are affected and respond, their level of preparation for such a crisis, and the clients' strengths and available resources.

Using the problem-solving process, nurse and clients develop a plan. They review the event that precipitated the crisis, obvious symptoms, and the disruption in the clients' lives. The plan may focus on one or several areas. For instance, clients may need to grasp intellectually the meaning of the crisis, to engage in greater expression of feelings, or both. Part of the plan may be directed toward finding appropriate and safe shelter, counseling, or physical care. Another part may focus on helping clients identify and use more effective coping techniques or locate supportive agencies and resource people. The plan also includes the development of realistic goals for the future. Planning to protect the family in the event of a terrorist attack may be the family's first attempt at preparing for such an unknown occurrence, and the community health nurse may be the first and only resource the family is relying on for information.

Implementation

During implementation, it is important for nurse and clients to continue to communicate. They should discuss what is happening, review the plan and the rationale behind its elements, and make appropriate changes when indicated. It is helpful to assign definite activities at the end of each session so that clients can try out different solutions and evaluate various coping behaviors. The implementation step is enhanced by use of the following guidelines (Levy & Sidel, 2002; Vastag, 2001):

1. Demonstrate acceptance of clients. A crisis often shatters the ego. Clients need to feel the support of a positive, caring person who does not judge their feelings or behavior. Some negative expressions, such as anger, withdrawal, and denial, are normal aspects of the crisis phase. Accept them as normal.
2. Help clients confront crisis. Clients need to face and discuss the situation. Expressing their feelings reduces tension and improves reality perception. Recounting what has actually occurred may be painful, but it helps clients confront the crisis. Do not assume that once clients have told about the event, no further recounting is necessary. Each time the story is told, they come closer to dealing realistically with the crisis.

USING THE NURSING PROCESS

Preparing for a Terrorist Attack

The Reyes family live in a large urban community on the east coast of the United States. The country has been at odds with nations supporting terrorism and is at code red, the highest terrorist alert level. Families are to prepare for possible terrorist attacks by remaining alert, having needed supplies for being homebound if necessary, and preparing a "safe room" in their homes. The Reyes family have been visited regularly by a community health nurse since the 8-week-premature birth of their youngest child. They have asked the nurse about the preparations needed and specifically how should they prepare their three children, aged 8 years, 6 years, and 6 months.

NURSING DIAGNOSIS

1. Lack of sufficient knowledge related to family protection in the event of a terrorist attack.
2. At risk for potential altered parenting related to the unnatural conditions of securing the family in a "safe room" for an undetermined period with unpredictable outcomes, while maintaining a safe, secure, and comforting nature with children.

ASSESSMENT

The family is preparing physically and emotionally for the possibility of a terrorist event. They have the financial means to purchase needed supplies and have the physical space in the basement of their home to secure the family as suggested. The parents are concerned about informing the children without unnecessarily alarming them. The nurse assesses that the family is calm and in control while preparing to face the possibility of a terrorist attack.

IMPLEMENTATION

1. The nurse provides the family with informational brochures prepared by the terrorism preparedness program of the health department, which outline how to prepare the home and family for a terrorist act. The brochures highlight the facts that the "safe room" must be sealed, that no water source coming into the home may be used, and that the family needs to prepare for a 1-month stay. Because the family's basement has no windows, they need only seal the doorway leading to the kitchen.
2. The nurse tours the basement with the parents and helps them determine additional preparations needed to promote security and livability, including bedding with extra blankets for warmth, adequate seating for comfort and eating, and a disposable toilet system (the type used for camping).

3. Supplies needed for 1 month include canned and packaged food items, many bottles of water (for drinking, bathing, and food preparation), powdered/canned milk, flashlights, cell phone, candles, batteries, portable radio, first-aid kit, medicines that family members take (including children's vitamins), bedding, changes of clothing, waterless soap products, dental hygiene products and toilet articles, disposable diapers for the infant, and several sealed containers in which to place the soiled diapers, and diversional activities for all family members that do not rely on a light source or electricity (eg, battery-operated CD player, Game Boy–like hand held games that are battery operated and light up, favorite soft toys, "old-fashioned" forms of entertainment such as singing, hand games, and storytelling). Important or useful items that can be used if there is electricity are also included (eg, books, board games, coloring books, cards). The family may be comforted by some religious items or books such as prayer beads, a prayer book, the Bible, or Koran.
4. The nurse suggests that the parents share limited information with the children. The older, school-aged children should be informed that the family needs to prepare for any emergency that may happen to the community and affect them (eg, hurricane, tornado) and that being prepared is the best way to feel safe. The children's help may be enlisted by asking them to choose favorite items they want to have in the basement. Television viewing or radio listening of news broadcasts that provide detailed descriptions of the ongoing conflict and may be disturbing to the children should be limited. The nurse also reminds the parents of the importance of their attitude and how it will affect the children. They should try to keep up-beat, stick with usual routines as much as possible, and stay calm. Children pick up on the parent's fears, and this compounds their fears.

EVALUATION

1. The parents are informed and are making the necessary preparations.
2. The children have helped to make some decisions about favorite food items and toys they want to keep in the basement.
3. The family states they are keeping more viligent and feel calmer now that they are more infomed and getting prepared.
4. The children are going about their usual routine while the parents keep alert and protective of the older children, who come and go from the home for school and other activities.

3. Help clients find facts. Distorted ideas and unknown factors of the situation create additional tension and may lead to maladaptive responses. For instance, it would help inexperienced parents to know that children younger than 2 years of age cannot deliberately misbehave. Facts about childhood development and parenting training may be important for preventing crisis. Likewise, sharing the facts about smallpox disease versus vaccination, or the value of having a secure place in their home for the family to survive an earthquake or tornado, is part of the community health nurse's role depending on the region or state of civilian preparedness recommended.

4. Help clients express feelings openly. Suppressed feelings can be harmful. For instance, a widow may feel guilty that she is glad her husband is gone. Expression of such feelings helps reduce tension and gives clients an opportunity to deal with them.

5. Do not offer false reassurance. Clients need to face reality, not avoid it. A statement such as "Don't worry, it will all work out" is demeaning and meaningless. Instead, make positive statements about faith in the clients' ability to cope: "It is a very difficult situation, but I believe you will be able to deal with it."

6. Discourage clients from blaming others. Clients often blame others as a way to avoid reality and the responsibility for problem solving. Withhold judgment when they blame others, but point out other causal factors and avenues for dealing with the situation.

7. Help clients seek out coping mechanisms. Explore and test old and new techniques to reduce stress and anxiety. Ask questions. What are all the things the client and nurse might do together to resolve the problem? What are the things that need to be done? What do clients think they can do? This assistance gives clients more adaptive energy to work toward resolution.

8. Encourage clients to accept help. Denial in the early phases of crisis cuts off help. Encouraging clients to acknowledge the problem, which is a first step toward acceptance of help. Often, clients fear the loss of their independence and the invasion of their privacy. They may say, "We ought to be able to handle this problem." At this point, the community health nurse can reassure clients that people in a crisis of this sort almost always need help. Preparing people to accept help enables them to make the best use of what others have to offer.

9. Promote development of new positive relationships. Clients who have lost significant persons through unintentional or intentional death, divorce, incarceration, or an act of terrorism, war, or perpetrated violence should be encouraged to find new connections, purpose, and people to fill the void and provide needed supports and satisfactions.

Evaluation of Crisis Resolution and Anticipatory Planning

In the final step, clients and nurse evaluate, stabilize, and plan for the future. First, evaluate the outcome of the intervention.

Are the clients using effective coping skills and exhibiting appropriate behavior? Are adequate resources and support persons available? Is the diagnosed problem solved, and have the desired results been accomplished? Analysis of these outcomes provides a greater understanding for coping with future crises.

To stabilize the change, identify and reinforce all the positive coping mechanisms and behaviors. Discuss why they are effective, and explore ways to use them in future stressful situations. Summarize the crisis experience, emphasizing the clients' successes with coping, to reconfirm progress and reinforce self-confidence. Point to evidence that they have reached their pre-crisis level, or an even higher level of functioning.

Clients' plans for the future should include setting realistic goals and means to implement them. Review with clients how their handling of the present crisis can help them cope with, minimize, or preferably prevent future crises.

SUMMARY

Crisis is a temporary state of severe disequilibrium for persons who face a threatening situation. It is a state that they can neither avoid nor solve with their usual coping abilities. A crisis occurs when some force disrupts normal functioning and thereby causes a loss of balance or normalcy in life. A crisis creates tension; subsequently, efforts are made to solve the problem and reduce the tension. If such efforts meet with failure, people feel upset, redefine the situation, try other solutions, and, if failure continues, eventually reach the breaking point.

There are two main types of crisis: developmental and situational. Developmental crises are disruptions that occur during transitional periods in normal growth and development. They usually have a gradual onset and are often predictable. Situational crises are precipitated by an unexpected external event and occur suddenly, sometimes without warning.

Family violence constitutes a unique crisis for the victim and the entire family and is becoming disturbingly prevalent in the United States. Historically, family violence is not new. Until recently in our nation's history, there were no laws or societal concerns about the treatment of spouses/partners or children. Although advances in human rights have been made, abuses against women and children remain socially and culturally accepted in some countries in the world.

Abuse can be physical, emotional, and/or sexual. Neglect and sexual exploitation are additional forms of abuse. Neglect can be general or specific, such as medical or educational neglect. Child abuse occurs among children of all ages, from infancy through the teen years. Some specific forms of abuse sometimes are identified only on autopsy: shaken baby syndrome and Munchausen syndrome by proxy. Teen dating violence, violence during pregnancy, and violence against women in general constitute partner/spousal abuse. Finally, a most unsettling form of violence—elder abuse, neglect, and exploitation—occurs more frequently than previously suspected.

New and unexpected forms of violence are becoming a reality in our unsettled world. Within communities, violence comes into the home in the form of Internet crimes against children, child abductions, and home invasions. Globally, there are terrorist groups threatening biologic, chemical, and nuclear attacks on civilians in the United States and abroad. For people in the United States this is a new reality since September 11, 2001, and the anthrax scares later that same year. Preparation against and survival of such attacks is a new concern for most Americans, and the community health nurse can play an important role.

Community health nurses use three levels of prevention when working with families. Primary prevention focuses on providing people with the skills and resources to prevent violent situations. Secondary prevention involves immediate intervention at the time of the violent episode. This includes providing different services for each family member, such as medical attention, emotional support, and police involvement. Tertiary prevention offers family rebuilding services and helps the family establish equilibrium with a structure that may be different, but healthier.

People in crisis need and often seek help. Crisis intervention builds on these two phenomena to achieve its primary goal—reestablishment of equilibrium. The two major methods of crisis intervention are the generic and the individual approaches. The generic approach is used with groups of people involved in the same type of crisis, such as rape victims, mothers who have lost children because of drunken driving, or a family experiencing child abuse. The individual approach is used if clients do not respond to the generic approach or need additional therapy. Crisis intervention begins with assessment of the situation. Then a therapeutic intervention is planned. Next, the nurse carries out the intervention, building on the strengths and self-care ability of clients. Crisis intervention concludes with resolution and anticipatory planning to avert possible future crises.

Regardless of the method of intervention the community health nurse uses, the steps of the nursing process provide a framework within which to intervene. Assessing the family's assets and liabilities, their willingness to change, and the nature of the violence helps the nurse form a nursing diagnosis. With this diagnosis, the nurse can begin to plan appropriate interventions and implement plans in concert with the family. Evaluation of the intervention techniques provides the nurse with new data to assist with ongoing assessment of the family's progress and additional anticipatory guidance needs.

ACTIVITIES TO PROMOTE CRITICAL THINKING

1. What are the major differences between a developmental and a situational crisis? Give examples of each from personal experiences.
2. Describe a developmental crisis experienced by a family. What was this family's response? Describe some actions a community health nurse might have taken (alone or within an interdisciplinary team) to help the family cope with the crisis.
3. Children, even the very young, are becoming more violent. What preventive actions can the community health nurse take? Design actions at each level of prevention.
4. Watch a news station on television. Listen for examples of developmental or situational crises occurring to families in the world. Analyze the situations and anticipate what the role of a community health nurse would be during the crises selected.
5. Family violence is a significant public health problem. Assume that a battered wife becomes a community health nurse's client, and the nurse suspects there may be more women with this problem in the community. Describe how the nurse might provide assistance using the crisis intervention steps. Then discuss how a three-level preventive program might be instituted in the community.
6. Using the Internet, select a situational crisis, such as spousal abuse, adolescent sexual exploitation, neglect of the elderly, or terrorist weapons used against civilians and read the most current information on this topic. Depending on your personal interests or current community health nursing experiences, develop a file of articles you have uncovered using the Internet. This file can be useful to you, to agency staff in your clinical setting, and to families you visit.
7. The Using the Nursing Process display focused on preparing the home for a chemical terrorist attack. Develop a nursing care plan using the nursing process for families in other crisis situations (nuclear or biologic) that involve terrorism. How do you and your family feel about such preparations? Are they necessary or helpful, or do they provide a sense of false security? Read more on these issues using current literature or the Internet.

DISPLAY 25–10

Suspected Child Abuse Report

SUSPECTED CHILD ABUSE REPORT
To Be Completed by Reporting Party
Pursuant to Penal Code Section 11166

A. CASE IDENTIFICATION

TO BE COMPLETED BY INVESTIGATING CPA

VICTIM NAME: _____

REPORT NO./CASE NAME: _____

DATE OF REPORT: _____

B. REPORTING PARTY

NAME/TITLE

ADDRESS

PHONE ( )   DATE OF REPORT   SIGNATURE

C. REPORT SENT TO

☐ POLICE DEPARTMENT   ☐ SHERIFF'S OFFICE   ☐ COUNTY WELFARE   ☐ COUNTY PROBATION

AGENCY   ADDRESS

OFFICIAL CONTACTED   PHONE ( )   DATE/TIME

D. INVOLVED PARTIES

VICTIM

NAME (LAST, FIRST, MIDDLE)   ADDRESS   BIRTHDATE   SEX   RACE

PRESENT LOCATION OF CHILD   PHONE ( )

SIBLINGS

NAME	BIRTHDATE	SEX	RACE	NAME	BIRTHDATE	SEX	RACE
1.				4.			
2.				5.			
3.				6.			

PARENTS

NAME (LAST, FIRST, MIDDLE)   BIRTHDATE   SEX   RACE   NAME (LAST, FIRST, MIDDLE)   BIRTHDATE   SEX   RACE

ADDRESS   ADDRESS

HOME PHONE ( )   BUSINESS PHONE ( )   HOME PHONE ( )   BUSINESS PHONE ( )

E. INCIDENT INFORMATION

IF NECESSARY, ATTACH EXTRA SHEET OR OTHER FORM AND CHECK THIS BOX. ☐

1. DATE/TIME OF INCIDENT   PLACE OF INCIDENT   *(CHECK ONE)*   ☐ OCCURRED   ☐ OBSERVED

IF CHILD WAS IN OUT-OF-HOME CARE AT TIME OF INCIDENT, CHECK TYPE OF CARE:

☐ FAMILY DAY CARE   ☐ CHILD CARE CENTER   ☐ FOSTER FAMILY HOME   ☐ SMALL FAMILY HOME   ☐ GROUP HOME OR INSTITUTION

2. TYPE OF ABUSE: *(CHECK ONE OR MORE)*   ☐ PHYSICAL   ☐ MENTAL   ☐ SEXUAL ASSAULT   ☐ NEGLECT   ☐ OTHER

3. NARRATIVE DESCRIPTION:

4. SUMMARIZE WHAT THE ABUSED CHILD OR PERSON ACCOMPANYING THE CHILD SAID HAPPENED:

5. EXPLAIN KNOWN HISTORY OF SIMILAR INCIDENT(S) FOR THIS CHILD:

SS 8572 (Rev. 1/93)

INSTRUCTIONS AND DISTRIBUTION ON REVERSE

DO NOT submit a copy of this form to the Department of Justice (DOJ). A CPA is required under Penal Code Section 11169 to submit to DOJ a Child Abuse Investigation Report Form SS-8583 if (1) an active investigation has been conducted and (2) the incident is **not** unfounded.

Police or Sheriff-WHITE Copy;   County Welfare or Probation-BLUE Copy;   District Attorney-GREEN Copy;   Reporting Party-YELLOW Copy

D I S P L A Y 25–11

Medical Report—Suspected Child Abuse

DOJ 900   84 89220

HOSPITAL

MEDICAL REPORT—SUSPECTED CHILD ABUSE

INSTRUCTIONS: ALL PROFESSIONAL MEDICAL PERSONNEL ARE REQUIRED BY SECTION 11166 OF THE PENAL CODE TO COMPLETE THIS FORM IN CONJUNCTION WITH THE SS 8572 SUSPECTED CHILD ABUSE REPORT WHERE CHILD ABUSE, AS DEFINED BY SECTION 11165 OF THE PENAL CODE, IS SUSPECTED. THE REPORTS, DOJ 900 AND SS 8572, MUST BE SUBMITTED TO A POLICE OR SHERIFF'S DEPARTMENT, OR A COUNTY PROBATION OR WELFARE DEPARTMENT WITHIN 36 HOURS. PROFESSIONAL MEDICAL PERSONNEL MEANS ANY PHYSICIAN AND SURGEON, PSYCHIATRIST, PSYCHOLOGIST, DENTIST, RESIDENT, INTERN, PODIATRIST, CHIROPRACTOR, LICENSED NURSE, DENTAL HYGIENIST OR ANY OTHER PERSON WHO IS CURRENTLY LICENSED UNDER DIVISION 2 (COMMENCING WITH SECTION 500) OF THE BUSINESS AND PROFESSIONS CODE. EACH PART OF THE FORM MUST BE COMPLETED UNLESS INAPPLICABLE. IN FILLING OUT THIS FORM, NO CIVIL LIABILITY ATTACHES AND NO CONFIDENTIALITY IS BREACHED.

I. GENERAL INFORMATION   Print or type

PATIENT'S NAME   HOSPITAL ID NO.

ADDRESS   CITY   COUNTY   STATE   PHONE

AGE | BIRTHDATE | RACE | SEX | DATE AND TIME OF ARRIVAL | MODE OF TRANSPORTATION | DATE AND TIME OF DISCHARGE

ACCOMPANIED TO HOSPITAL BY: NAME   ADDRESS   CITY   STATE   RELATIONSHIP

PHONE REPORT MADE TO   ID NO.   DEPARTMENT   PHONE   RESPONDING OFFICER/AGENCY

NAME OF: ☐ FATHER ☐ STEPFATHER   ADDRESS   CITY   COUNTY   HOME PHONE   BUS. PHONE   AGE/DOB

NAME OF: ☐ MOTHER ☐ STEPMOTHER   ADDRESS   CITY   COUNTY   HOME PHONE   BUS. PHONE   AGE/DOB

SIBLINGS: LAST NAME, FIRST   DOB   LAST NAME, FIRST   DOB   LAST NAME, FIRST   DOB

II. MEDICAL EXAMINATION

A. History   1. EXPLANATION OF INJURIES BY PARENT OR PERSON ACCOMPANYING CHILD (LOCATION; DATE, TIME AND CIRCUMSTANCES)

2. PATIENT'S STATEMENT EXPLAINING INJURY (PARAPHRASE)

3. PATIENT'S EMOTIONAL REACTION TO EXAMINATION (SUBMISSIVE, COMPLIANT, ETC.)

4. PREVIOUS HISTORY OF CHILD ABUSE (IF KNOWN)

B. Sexual Assault   Perform exam only if necessary.

1. ACTS COMMITTED: NOTE—COITUS, FELLATIO, CUNNILINGUS, SODOMY

2. DURING ASSAULT
☐ VAGINAL PENETRATION (HOW)   EJACULATION: ☐ VAGINAL ☐ ORAL ☐ ANAL ☐ OTHER:

☐ ANAL PENETRATION (HOW)   ☐ CONDOM USED ☐ VOMITED ☐ LOSS OF CONSCIOUSNESS ☐ OTHER:

3. AFTER ASSAULT: ☐ WIPED/WASHED ☐ BATHED ☐ DOUCHED ☐ VOMITED ☐ CHANGED CLOTHES ☐ BRUSHED TEETH ☐ DEFECATED ☐ OTHER:

C. Physical Examination   DATE AND TIME OF EXAM   DATE AND TIME OF ASSAULT   BP | PULSE | RESP. | TEMP

HEIGHT | WEIGHT | HEAD CIRCUM | LAST TETANUS | KNOWN ALLERGIES   CURRENT MEDICATION

DIAGNOSTIC DATA

Check if indicated and incorporate results in written examination at left

☐ X-rays (skull, chest, longbone, full skeletal)

☐ Bleeding, coagulation, tourniquet, tests

☐ Funduscopic

☐ Other

DISPLAY 25-11

Medical Report—Suspected Child Abuse (continued)

DATE	HOSPITAL ID NO.	HOSPITAL	DOJ 900

PHYSICAL EXAMINATION (CONTINUED) LOCATE AND DESCRIBE IN DETAIL ANY INJURIES OR FINDINGS: TRAUMA, BRUISES, ERYTHEMA, EXCORIATIONS, LACERATIONS, WOUNDS. TRACE OUTLINE USED AND INDICATE LOCATION OF WOUNDS/LACERATIONS USING 'X' FOR SUPERFICIAL, 'O' FOR DEEP; SHADE FOR BRUISES OR BURNS. BESIDE EACH INJURY INDICATED NOTE COLOR, SIZE, PATTERN, TEXTURE, AND SENSATION. WRITE OVER UNUSED OUTLINES. DESCRIBE IN DETAIL SHAPE OF ARM OR OTHER BRUISES WHICH MAY INDICATE FORCE.

D. PELVIC A PELVIC EXAMINATION SHOULD NOT BE PERFORMED UNLESS THE PARENT, GUARDIAN OR MINOR CONSENT OR UNLESS NECESSARY AS PART OF TREATMENT. SEE DEPARTMENT OF HEALTH REGULATIONS TITLE 22, DIVISION 2, VICTIMS OF SEXUAL ASSAULT. SAME INSTRUCTIONS AS GENERAL PHYSICAL; IN ADDITION, NOTE PUBIC HAIR COMBINGS WHERE INDICATED, DRIED SECRETIONS AND RECENT INJURIES TO HYMEN, TRACE AND OUTLINE AS ABOVE.

V. SPECIMENS

STAINS/FOREIGN MATERIALS
(WHEN INDICATED)

LOOSE HAIR	___	FINGERNAIL SCRAPINGS	___
BLOOD	___	DIRT OR GRAVEL	___
THREADS	___	VEGETATION	___
GRASS	___	CLOTHING	___
DRIED SECRETIONS	___		

	SLIDES	SWABS
VAGINAL	___	___
RECTAL	___	___
ORAL	___	
ASPIRATES/ WASHINGS	___	___
BITE MARKS	___	___
OTHER:	___	___

III. DIAGNOSTIC IMPRESSION OF TRAUMA AND INJURIES

IV. TREATMENT/DISPOSITION OF PATIENT

A. ☐ GC CULTURE   ☐ VDRL   ☐ PREGNANCY TEST   ☐ POST COITAL ESTROGEN   ☐ VD PRO-PHYLAXIS   ☐ OTHER:

☐ MOTILE SPERM: ☐ PRESENCE   ☐ ABSENCE   ☐ NOT TAKEN   ☐ FAMILY ASSESSMENT BY: ☐ NOT ORDERED

B. ORDERS:

PATIENT'S SAMPLES. TIME OF COLLECTION AT MD DISCRETION

BLOOD	___
HAIR FROM HEAD	___
SALIVA	___
HAIR FROM PUBIC AREA	___

C. DISPOSITION: ☐ ADMIT   TRANSFERRED TO:

☐ RELEASED   ACCOMPANIED BY: NAME   ADDRESS   RELATIONSHIP

D. FOLLOW-UP WITHIN:

☐ MEDICAL

☐ SOCIAL SERVICES   ___ HRS   ___ DAYS

☐ PRIVATE MD   ___ HRS   ___ DAYS

☐ OTHER   ___ HRS   ___ DAYS

___ HRS   ___ DAYS

I HAVE RECEIVED THE INDICATED ITEMS AS EVIDENCE AND A COPY OF THIS REPORT.

OFFICER: ID NO.:   DATE:

NURSE   SIGNATURE OF EXAMINATION PHYSICIAN

D I S P L A Y   2 5 – 1 2

Domestic Violence Screening/Documentation Form

DV SCREEN
- ☐ Screened
  - ☐ Yes
  - ☐ No
  - ☐ Probable/Suspected DV
- ☐ Not Screened

Date _____   Patient ID# _____
Patient Name _____
Provider Name _____
Patient Pregnant? Yes _____ No _____

Describe frequency and severity of present and past abuse (use direct quotes as much as possible)

_____
_____
_____
_____
_____
_____

Underline Routinely Screen at Each Visit
"Because violence is so common in women's lives, I've begun to ask about it routinely."

Ask Direct Questions
"I'm concerned that your injuries/symptoms may have been caused by someone hurting you. Is this what happened to you?"
            -OR-
"Has your intimate partner or ex-partner ever physically hurt you? Have they ever *threatened* to hurt you or someone close to you?"

Describe location and extent of injury

_____
_____
_____
_____
_____
_____

Assess Patient Safety

- ☐ Yes ☐ No Is patient afraid to go home?
- ☐ Yes ☐ No Has physical violence increased in severity over past years?
- ☐ Yes ☐ No Have threats of homicide been made?
- ☐ Yes ☐ No Have threats of suicide been made?
- ☐ Yes ☐ No Is alcohol or substance abuse also a problem?
- ☐ Yes ☐ No Is there a gun in the house?
- ☐ Yes ☐ No Is patient afraid of their partner?
- ☐ Yes ☐ No Was safety plan discussed?

Indicate where injury was observed

Referrals
- ☐ hotline number given
- ☐ legal referral made
- ☐ shelter number given
- ☐ in-house referral made
- ☐ discharge instructions given

☐ Yes ☐ No Photographs taken?
☐ Yes ☐ No Consent to be photographed?
(Attach Photographs) + Appropriate Form

REFERENCES

Aguilera, D.C. (1998). *Crisis intervention: Theory and methodology* (8th ed.). St. Louis: Mosby.

Besharov, D.J. (1998). Four commentaries: How we can better protect children from abuse and neglect. *The Future of Children: Protecting Children from Abuse and Neglect, 8*(1), 120–123.

Bolen, R.M. (2001). *Child sexual abuse: Its scope and our failure.* Norwell, MA: Kluwer Plenum.

Bridges, W. (1980). *Transitions: Making sense of life's changes* (2nd ed.). Cambridge, MA: Perseus Publishing.

Bridges, W. (2001). *The way of transition: Embracing life's most difficult moments.* Cambridge, MA: Perseus Publishing.

Campbell, J. (1998). *Empowering survivors of abuse: Health care, battered women and their children.* Thousand Oaks, CA: Sage.

Campbell, J.C. (1999). If I can't have you no one can: Murder linked to battery during pregnancy. *Reflections, 25*(3), 8–12.

Cokkinides, V.E., & Coker, A.L. (1998). Experiencing physical violence during pregnancy: Prevalence and correlates. *Family Community Health, 20*(4), 19–37.

Crime and Violence Prevention Center. (2003a). *Child abuse: Educator's responsibilities.* Sacramento, CA: California Attorney General's Office. Publication accessed online and available for downloading from *http://www.safestate.org/shop/files/CAEd.Resp.pdf*

Crime and Violence Prevention Center. (2003b). *Child abuse and neglect reporting law, condensed version.* Sacramento, CA: California Attorney General's Office. Publication accessed online January 16, 2004, and available for downloading from *http://www.safestate.org/shop/files/CA_Child_Abuse_Rep.pdf*

Crime and Violence Prevention Center. (2003c). *Child abuse prevention handbook.* Sacramento, CA: California Attorney General's Office. Publication accessed online January 16, 2004, and available for downloading from *http://www.safestate.org/shop/files/child abuse handbook chap_1-3.pdf, .../child abuse handbook chap_4-6.pdf, and .../child abuse handbook appen3-7.pdf*

Curry, M.A., Doyle, B.A., & Gilhooley, J. (1998). Abuse among pregnant adolescents: Differences by developmental age. *Maternal and Child Nursing, 23*(3), 144–150.

Davis, R.E., & Harsh, K.E. (2001). Confronting barriers to universal screening for domestic violence. *Journal of Professional Nursing, 17*(6), 313–320.

Gray-Vickrey, P. (2001). Protecting the older adult. *Nursing Management, 32*(10), 36–40.

Hanson, R.F. (2002). Adolescent dating violence: Prevalence and psycholological outcomes. *Child Abuse and Neglect, 26,* 449–453.

Hoff, L.A. (2001). *People in crisis: Clinical and public health perspectives* (5th ed.). Indianapolis, IN: Jossey-Bass.

Holmes, T., & Rahe, R. (1967). The social readjustment rating scale. *Journal of Psychosomatic Research, 11,* 213–217.

Jackson, S.M., Cram, F., & Seymour, F.W. (2000). Violence and sexual coercion in high school students' dating relationships. *Journal of Family Violence, 15,* 23–36.

Jenkins, P.J., & Davidson, B.P. (2001). *Stopping domestic violence: How a community can prevent spousal abuse.* Norwell, MA: Kluwer Academic/Plenum.

Kramer, A. (2002). Domestic violence: How to ask and how to listen. *Nursing Clinics of North America, 37*(1), 189–210.

Lane, W.G., Rubin, D.M., Monteith, R., & Christian, C.W. (2002). Racial differences in the evaluation of pediatric fractures for physical abuse. *JAMA, 288*(13), 1603–1609.

Lemmey, D., Malecha, A., McFarlane, J., et al. (2001). Severity of violence against women correlates with behavioral problems in their children. *Pediatric Nursing, 27*(3), 265–270.

Levinson, D.J. (1978). *The seasons of a man's life.* New York: Knopf.

Levy, B.S., & Sidel, V.W. (2002). *Terrorism and public health: A balanced approach to strengthening systems and protecting people.* New York: Oxford University Press.

Locsin, R.C., & Purnell, M.J. (2002). Intimate partner violence, culture-centrism, and nursing. *Holistic Nursing Practice, 16*(3), 1–4.

Menzey, M.D. (Ed.). (2001). *The encyclopedia of elder care: The comprehensive resource on geriatric and social care.* New York: Springer Publishing.

Olds, D.L., Eckenrode, J., Henderson, C.R., et al. (1997). Long-term effects of home visitation on maternal life course and child abuse and neglect: Fifteen-year follow-up of a randomized trial. *Journal of the American Medical Association, 276*(8), 637–643.

Olds, D.L., et al. (1999). Prenatal and infancy home visitation by nurses: Recent findings. *The Future of Children, Home Visiting: Recent Program Evaluations, 9*(1), 44–65.

Pillemer, K., & Finkelhor, A. (1988). The prevalence of elder abuse: A random sample survey. *The Gerontologist, 28,* 51–57.

Sheehy, G. (1976). *Passages: Predictable crises of adult life.* New York: Dutton.

Sheehy, G. (1992). *The silent passage.* New York: Ballantine Books.

Sheehy, G. (1999). *Understanding men's passages: Discovering the new map of men's lives.* New York: Ballantine Books.

Sheehy, G. (March, 2000a). Oklahoma monitors intimate partner violence. *The Nation's Health, 30*(2), 1, 7.

Sheehy, G. (2000b). *Violence against women.* Fairfax, VA: U. S. Department of Health and Human Services, National Women's Health Information Center.

Sheehy, G., & Delbourgo, J. (1996). *New passages: Mapping your life across time.* New York: Ballantine Books.

Spake, A. (2003). Are you ready? *U. S. News & World Report, 134*(6), 24, 26, 27.

United States Department of Health and Human Services. (1998). *Healthy people 2010 objectives: Draft for public comment.* Washington, DC: Author.

United States Department of Health and Human Services. (2000). *Healthy people 2010* (Conference ed., Vols. 1 & 2). Washington, DC: Author.

U. S. Department of Justice. (2001a). *An update on the cycle of violence* (NCJ 184894). Washington, DC: U. S. Department of Justice, Office of Justice Programs.

U. S. Department of Justice. (2001b). *Crimes against children by babysitters* (NCJ 189102). Washington, DC: U. S. Department of Justice, Office of Justice Programs.

U. S. Department of Justice. (2001c). *Internet crimes against children* (NCJ 184931). Washington, DC: U. S. Department of Justice, Office of Justice Programs.

U. S. Department of Justice. (2002). *When your child is missing* (NCJ 170022). Washington, DC: U. S. Department of Justice, Office of Justice Programs.

U. S. Department of Justice. (2003a). *Battered child syndrome: Investigating physical abuse and homicide.* Washington, DC: Office of Justice Programs.

U. S. Department of Justice. (2003b). *Understanding and investigating child sexual exploitation.* Washington, DC: Office of Justice Programs.

Vastag, B. (2001). Experts urge bioterrorism readiness. *JAMA, 285,* 30–31.

Walker, L.E. (1979). *The battered woman.* New York: Harper & Row.

World Health Organization. (1998). *Report of the Director-General: The world health report 1998. Life in the 21st century: A vision for all.* Geneva: World Health Organization.

SELECTED READINGS

Cohen, M., Deamant, C., Barkan, S., et al. (2000). Domestic violence and childhood sexual abuse in HIV-infected women and women at risk for HIV. *American Journal of Public Health, 90(4),* 560–565.

Davis, K.E., Frieze, I.H., & Maiuro, R.D. (2002). *Stalking: Perspectives on victims and perpetrators.* New York: Springer.

Geiger, H.J. (2001). Terrorism, biological weapon, and bonanzas: Assessing the real threat to public health. *American Journal of Public Health, 91(5),* 708–709.

Glasser, J. (2002). Coming to grips with the pain. *U. S. News & World Report, 133(10),* 27–30, 32.

Humphreys, J. (2000). Spirituality and distress in sheltered battered women. *Journal of Nursing Scholarship, 32(3),* 273–278.

Landesman, L.Y. (2001). *Public health management of disasters: The practice guide.* Washington, DC: American Public Health Association.

Lemmey, D., McFarlane, J., Willson, P., & Malecha, A. (2001). Intimate partner violence: Mothers' perspectives of effects on their children. *MCN, 26(2),* 98–103.

Lewis, F., & Fremouw, W. (2001). Dating violence: A critical review of the literature. *Clinical Psychology Review, 21,* 105–127.

Loue, S. (2000). *Intimate partner violence: Societal, medical, legal and individual responses.* Norwell, MA: Kluwer Plenum.

Martinez, M. (2001). *Prevention and control of aggression and the impact on its victims.* Norwell, MA: Kluwer Academic/Plenum.

Miller, M., Azrael, D., & Hemenway, D. (2002). Firearm availability and suicide, homicide, and unintentional firearm deaths among women. *Journal of Urban Health, 79(1),* 26–38.

Ottens, A.J., & Hotelling, K. (2001). *Sexual violence on campus: Policies, programs and perspectives.* New York: Springer.

Rice, V.H. (2000). *Handbook of stress, coping, and health: Implications for nursing research, theory, and practice.* Thousand Oaks, CA: Sage.

Scott, S. (2001). *The politics and experience of ritual abuse: Beyond disbelief.* Philadelphia, PA: Open University Press.

Sidel, V.W., Cohen, H.W., & Gould, R.M. (2001). Good intentions and the road to bioterrorism preparedness. *American Journal of Public Health, 91(5),* 716–718.

Underwood, T.L., & Edmunds, C., (2003). *Victim assistance: Exploring individual practice, organizational policy, and societal responses.* New York: Springer.

Community Resources

Child Abuse Councils. Provide information and referral; educational services including book and film library. Usually are multidisciplinary in nature, and help coordinate service delivery. Provide visibility to the problem of child abuse.

Child Care Resource Centers. Provide valuable child care information to parents who may be overwhelmed by the demands of parenting. Information and referral.

Community Mental Health Departments. Provide low-fee therapeutic services to families and children. Available in every community. Frequently serve a broad range of abusive families.

Emergency Family Care. In-home based services. Workers literally "move in" with the family to provide concrete services. Frequently work with neglectful parents whose children might be removed without this service.

Family Service Agencies. Many of these agencies have taken a leadership role in child abuse prevention/treatment services. Therapeutic services are available on a sliding-fee scale.

Parent Discussion Groups. Provide a forum in which parents may discuss childrearing problems, gain peer support, and minimize their isolation.

Parent Education Classes. Designed to help parents gain better understanding of child development and learn skills for disciplining their children in a safe way.

Parent-Infant Bonding (Perinatal Programs). Designed to help new parents with bonding skills; provide parent education regarding the child's needs. Provide early intervention services.

Parental Stress Hotlines. 24-hour crisis telephone assistance for persons under stress. Telephone counseling primarily, but can also provide home visiting program and respite care. Usually offer parent rap groups and other services.

Parents Anonymous. Self-help groups for potentially abusive or abusive parents. Facilitators consist of a professional and a formerly abusive parent. Usually no fee/low fee; child care and transportation provided.

Parents United. Self-help groups for sexually abusive families. Consists of groups for offenders, children, and mothers. Also have groups for Adults Molested as Children (MAC). Comprehensive child sexual abuse program.

Private Mental Health Clinics/Therapist Groups. There are many private therapists who specialize in working with child abuse. Child Abuse Councils or Child Protective Agencies are usually familiar with good referral possibilities.

Respite Care Programs. Licensed homes that provide care for children when their parents "need a break." Not a baby-sitting service. Designed for high-risk parents. Voluntary.

National Resources

National Center on Child Abuse and Neglect (NCCAN), National Center on Family Violence Clearinghouse, P.O. Box 1182, Washington, D.C. 20013; 1-800-FYI-3366.

National Committee for the Prevention of Child Abuse (NCPCA), 332 S. Michigan Avenue, Suite 1600, Chicago, IL 60604; 312-663-3520.

American Professional Society on the Abuse of Children (APSAC), 332 S. Michigan Avenue, Suite 1600, Chicago, IL 60604; 312-554-0166; accessed January 16, 2004, at *http://www.apsac.org*

National Center for the Prosecution of Child Abuse, American Prosecutors Research Institute, 1033 North Fairfax Street, Suite 200, Alexandria, VA 22314; 703-739-0321.

Regional Poison Control Center: 1-800-222-1222.

Internet Resources

Centers for Disease Control and Prevention, Division of Violence Prevention: *http://www.cdc.gov/ncipc/dvp/dvp.htm*

Child Abuse Prevention Network: *http://www.child.cornell.edu*

Domestic Violence Resources:
   http://www.growing.com/nonviolent/

Mothers Against Guns: *http://mothersagainstguns.org/*

National Criminal Justice Reference Service:
   http://www.ncjrs.org/

The Convention on the Rights of the Child:
   http://www.unicef.org/crc/

National Latino Alliance for the Elimination of Domestic Violence: *http://www.dvalianza.org*

United Nations Background Note on Children's Rights:
   http://www.un.org/rights/dpi1765e.htm

Violence Research Resources on the Web:
   http://www1.umn.edu/cvpc/linksviolence.html

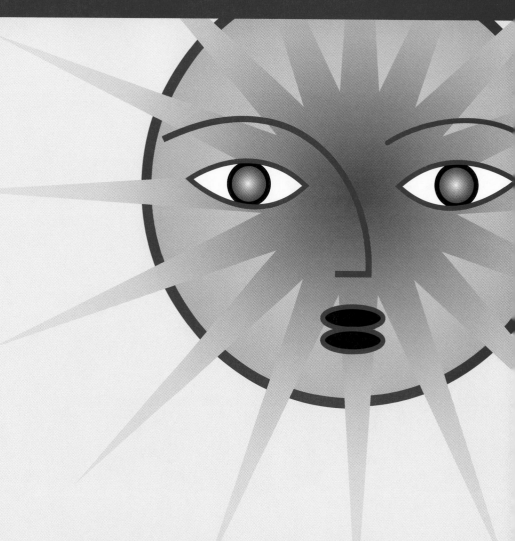

Promoting and Protecting the Health of Aggregates With Developmental Needs

26

Maternal, Prenatal, and Newborn Populations

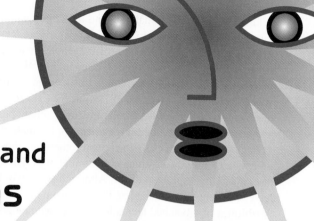

Key Terms

- Developmental disability
- Drug dependent
- Drug exposed
- Fetal alcohol effects
- Fetal alcohol syndrome
- Gestational diabetes mellitus
- Low birth weight
- Passive smoking
- Self-help groups
- Smokeless tobacco products
- Sudden infant death syndrome (SIDS)
- Very low birth weight

Learning Objectives

Upon mastery of this chapter, you should be able to:

- Discuss the global view of maternal and infant health.
- Identify the *Healthy People 2010* goals established for the maternal–infant population.
- Discuss major risk factors and special complications for child-bearing families.
- Describe the important considerations in designing effective health promotion programs to fit the needs of diverse maternal–infant populations.
- List several features of a typical health promotion program for maternal–infant populations.
- Identify six methods of delivering services to maternal–infant populations.
- Describe various roles of a community health nurse in serving the maternal–infant population.

The majority of the community health nurse's clients are pregnant teens; women who are pregnant with a third, fourth, or fifth child; and infants and young children. Working with maternal and infant populations is a primary facet of community health nursing. More than 70% of nursing practice in official health agencies involves primary preventive work with mothers and infants. Why should maternal–infant populations require this amount of attention from community health nursing? Despite the existence of advanced technology and the availability of excellent perinatal services in our society, certain segments of the maternal and infant populations such as adolescent mothers and those who are economically disadvantaged remain at high risk for disease, disability, and even death. Although some women receive excellent prenatal care and benefit from the diagnostic capabilities of advanced technology, other women go without prenatal care and even without proper nutrition.

Historically, the health needs of pregnant women and their newborns began to receive priority status in the public health arena after some degree of control over communicable diseases was achieved. By the mid-20th century, many health programs had been established at the local level. In the 1970s, funding from state and federal revenues enhanced existing prenatal and newborn services. The community health nurse has always had a prominent role in planning, implementation, and evaluation of these programs.

This chapter addresses three major areas in the health of maternal–infant populations: (1) health status and needs; (2) design, implementation, and evaluation of maternal–infant health programs; and (3) availability of community resources.

HEALTH STATUS AND NEEDS OF PREGNANT WOMEN AND INFANTS

Community health nurses constitute a key group of health care workers involved in both the planning of programs and the actual delivery of services to mothers and babies. A solid understanding of vital statistics and other data regarding maternal–infant populations serves nurses as they determine both the appropriateness and the effectiveness of programs and services. A review of some of the global and national vital statistics of the past decade provides insight into the problem areas in maternal–infant health and gives direction for the future.

Global Overview

It is estimated that 515,000 women die each year of pregnancy-related causes (World Health Organization [WHO], 2001). More than half of the deaths (273,000) occur in Africa, where the rate is 1 death for every 16 pregnancies; 42% (217,000) occur in Asia, about 4% in Latin American and the Caribbean, and less than 1% (2800) in the more developed regions of the world including Europe and North

America. The maternal mortality rate (MMR) is highest in Africa with 1000 per 100,000 live births, followed by Asia (280), Oceania (260), Latin American and the Caribbean (190), Europe (28), and North America (11) (WHO, 2001). On a risk per birth basis, the countries with the highest MMRs are all in Africa; the top 11 countries, with MMRs of 1000 or greater, are Rwanda, Sierra Leone, Burundi, Ethiopia, Somalia, Chad, Sudan, Burkina Faso, Equatorial Guinea, Angola, and Kenya. About 80% of maternal deaths are the result of direct causes (complications of pregnancy, labor, and delivery), interventions, omissions, or incorrect treatment; or the chain of events resulting from any one of these. Postpartum hemorrhage accounts for 25% of the maternal deaths.

Globally, 7.1 million neonatal deaths and stillbirths occur each year; they are largely caused by the same factors that result in death and disability of the mothers, including poor maternal health, inadequate care, poor hygiene, and inefficient management of delivery, as well as lack of essential newborn care (WHO, 2000). Worldwide infant mortality rate (IMR) has decreased over the past decades, from 148 per 1000 live births in 1955 to 90 per 1000 in 1980 and 59 per 1000 in 1995. Overall, the number of countries with an IMR lower than 50 per 1000 live births increased to 102 in 1995, compared with only 23 in 1955; these countries accounted for 34% of global live births in 1995. It is expected that the global IMR will continue to decline, to 32 per 1000 live births by the year 2025. However, in 1995 there were 24 countries, 20 of them in Africa, in which 1 of every 10 children died before the first birthday. On the other end of the spectrum, among those countries with greater than 250,000 inhabitants in 1999, 23 had lower IMRs than the United States (MacDorman et al., 2002). In the U. S. IMR was 7.1 per 1000 live births in 1999, compared with 3.1 in Hong Kong, 3.2 in Japan, 3.4 in Sweden, 5.5 in Greece, and even 6.4 in Cuba.

Adolescent mothers have increased maternal–infant mortality risk. In 1997, adolescents aged 15 to 19 years gave birth to 17 million infants. Sixteen million of these births occurred in developing areas: Asia, Africa, Latin America, and the Caribbean (WHO, 2001). With the exception of Asia, in which every country has reported a decline, other regions report only modest decreases in the number of women experiencing pregnancy at an early age. Both the teenage mother and the infant are at risk. Teenage mothers have a higher rate of pregnancy-related complications, and their infants are more likely to have low birth weight or to be premature, injured at birth, or stillborn. Mortality rates for infants born to adolescent mothers are higher than for those born to older women. It is expected that the global rate of childbirth among adolescents will decrease to 16 million infants annually by 2025 (WHO, 2001).

Perinatal transmission of human immunodeficiency virus (HIV) is an emerging global health crisis. The majority of children with acquired immunodeficiency syndrome (AIDS) are children of HIV-positive mothers. Mother-to-child transmission (MTCT) of HIV can be reduced by a stunning 67% with a single antiretroviral drug taken for a short time (Bassett, 2001). However, the drug is unavailable in many countries. In addition, women must seek out prenatal care early enough in their pregnancies for the antiretroviral drug to be effective. These limiting factors are especially important in developing countries, in underserved areas, and among certain groups (eg, those involved in the drug culture). The result is that AIDS is seen in 15% to 35% of the children of HIV-positive mothers. Virtually all of the HIV-infected children younger than 10 years of age live in developing countries and acquired HIV from their mothers (Bassett, 2001). A significant number of these children are born to HIV-infected adolescent mothers, especially in sub-Saharan Africa, where the rates of both adolescent pregnancy and HIV are the highest in the world. Pediatric AIDS will increase accordingly in the future.

National Overview

More than 4 million women in the United States gave birth in 2001, down about 1% from 2000. In 2001, 21% of all births were to Hispanic women, with Mexican-American women having the highest fertility rate and the highest age-specific birth rate among women younger than 30 years of age. In contrast, Asian and Pacific Islander women had the highest birth and fertility rates among women age 30 and older. Overall, rates in 2001 were considerably lower for black, Native American, and non-Hispanic white women (MacDorman et al., 2002). In 2001, 33% of all births were to unmarried women, similar to the 33.2% in 2000. Many of these women do not have the financial or social resources to sustain minimal health levels for themselves and their infants.

In 1991, the United States reached a 20-year high in the number of children born to teen mothers (aged 15 to 19 years), with a rate of 62.1 per 1000 teen girls. Data for 2000 indicated a 10-year low of 48.5 births per 1000 adolescents, and preliminary data for 2001 pointed to a further reduction to 45.9 per 1000 (MacDorman et al., 2002). Although the majority of pregnant adolescents are of European-American descent, the proportion of pregnant adolescents is higher in the African-American and especially in the Hispanic-American populations, and pregnant adolescents in both groups are more likely to be teens 18 and older. The pregnancy rate for younger teens, those 17 and younger, has declined much more than for those 18 and older. Additionally, there is an increasing trend in recent decades for unwed teenage mothers to keep their babies. These "children having children" with limited educational and economic advantages will affect the health of society well into the future.

Another area of concern is substance use and abuse among the child-bearing population. The range of adverse consequences associated with the use of tobacco, alcohol, and illicit drugs during pregnancy is wide and includes preterm birth, low birth weight, and fetal alcohol syndrome, described later in this chapter. Two studies have shown that many women who abuse drugs while pregnant do not receive prenatal care (Armstrong et al., 2003; Chasnoff et al., 2001). This puts these women and their unborn children in "double jeopardy." Not only are they at risk from the consequences of alcohol or drug use, but they also do not receive the preventive prenatal care that can eliminate or reduce other obstetric complications.

Healthy People 2000 included specific goals for the maternal–infant population along with significant vital statistics and baseline information. The *Healthy People 2010* objectives for this population are based on the previous achievements in the same or similar areas (U. S. Department of Health and Human Services [USDHHS], 2000) (Table 26–1).

After years of working toward improving maternal–infant health, the United States has made very limited progress. Although the U. S. IMR (deaths for all babies up to 1 year of age) has dropped substantially, from 20.0 per 1000 live births in 1970 to 7.1 per 1000 in 1999, it remains higher than in many other industrialized nations. In addition, the rate for African-American infants remains more than twice that of white infants (USDHHS, 2000).

Low-birth-weight (LBW) babies are those weighing less than 2500 g at birth; **very-low-birth-weight** (VLBW) babies weigh less than 1500 g at birth. Maternal mortality, LBW, and VLBW births are three areas in which work is needed. Birth weight is one of the most important predictors of infant mortality. Infants weighing 3500 to 4499 g have the lowest IMR. In 2000, LBW infants accounted for 7.6% of all births but 66% of all infant deaths; VLBW infants were 1.4% of all births but accounted for 52% of all infant deaths. These statistics worsened between 1994 and 1998 but since then have leveled off. The number of LBW babies for the total U. S. population increased from a low of 6.8% in 1985 to 7.6% in 2000 (MacDorman et al., 2001; USDHHS, 2000). The rate of VLBW births was 1.4% in 2000 and has remained fairly stable since 1990; however, within this framework, the VLBW rate has risen among African-Americans while falling slightly among whites. Table 26–2 lists the percentages of LBW and VLBW babies for selected populations in 2000 and states the goals for 2010.

In addition to infant deaths and low birth weights, the effects of pregnancy and childbirth on women are other important indicators of health and access to reproductive health care. The reported number of maternal deaths in the United States in 1999 was 525. In 1986, the number of infant deaths was 6.6 per 100,000 live births; a disparity existed between African-American and white women. In the years from 1991 to 1998, the pregnancy-related mortality rate was 11.8 deaths per 100,000 live births. During this period, the ratio for black women was 30.0 deaths per 100,000 live births, compared with 8.1 per 100,000 for white women (Centers for Disease Control and Prevention, 2003). The maternal mortality ratio among African-American women has consistently been three to four times that of white women, and the gap has continued to widen (USDHHS, 2000). Ectopic pregnancy is the leading cause of maternal mortality in the first trimester. Pregnancy-related death risk increases with age and with

T A B L E 26-1

Selected Maternal and Infant *Healthy People 2010* Target Objectives

Objective	Baseline
Reduce infant mortality rate from all birth defects to 1.1 per 1,000 live births.	1.6 (1998)
Reduce the sudden infant death syndrome (SIDS) mortality rate to 0.3 per 1,000 live births.	0.77 (1997)
Reduce the rate of child mortality to 25 per 100,000 children aged 1 to 4.	34.2 (1998)
Reduce the rate of child mortality to 14.3 per 100,000 children aged 5 to 9.	17.6 (1998)
Reduce the perinatal mortality rate per 1,000 live births plus fetal deaths as follows:	
Deaths of infants from 28 weeks' gestation to 7 days after birth to 4.5	7.5 (1997)
Deaths of infants from 20 weeks' gestation to 7 days after birth to 4.1	6.8 (1997)
Reduce to less than 20% the proportion of pregnant women who experience maternal complications during labor and delivery.	32.1% (1997)
Increase to at least 90% the proportion of all pregnant women who begin prenatal care in the first trimester of pregnancy.	83% (1998)
Reduce the prevalance of serious developmental disabilities arising from events in the prenatal and infant periods for:	
Mental retardation to 124 per 10,000	131 (1991–1994)
Cerebral palsy to 31.5 per 10,000	32.2 (1991–1994)
Reduce cesarean deliveries:	
Primary (first time) cesarean delivery to 12.5%	17.8 (1997)
Repeat cesarean deliveries to 63%	71% (1997)
Increase to 70% the percentage of infants who are put to sleep on their backs.	35% (1996)
Increase abstinence from alcohol use by pregnant women as follows:	
No use in the past month—increase to 94%	86% (1996–1997)
No binge drinking in the past month—increase to 100%	99% (1996–1997)
Increase abstinence from tobacco use by pregnant women to 98%.	87% (1996–1997)
Eliminate use of illicit drugs by pregnant women to 100%.	98% (1996–1997)
Reduce the incidence of spina bifida and other neural tube defects to 3 per 10,000 live births.	6 (1996)
Increase to at least 80% the proportion of women of childbearing age who take a vitamin with the recommended 0.4 mg of folic acid daily.	21 (1991–1994)
Increase breastfeeding among mothers as follows:	
To at least 75% in the early postpartum period	64% (1998)
To at least 50% until babies are 6 months old	29% (1998)
To at least 25% until babies are 1 year old	16% (1998)
(Retain *Healthy People 2000* target)	

(Adapted from U.S. Department of Health and Human Services [2000]. *Healthy people 2010* [Conference ed., Vols. 1 & 2]. Washington, DC: Author.)

lack of prenatal care for women of every race. Other major causes of maternal morbidity are hemorrhage, pregnancy-induced hypertension, embolism, and infection (USDHHS, 2000).

There are several areas in which great progress has been made toward the year 2010 goals. The neonatal mortality rate (deaths for all infants up to 28 days old) decreased from 15.1 per 1000 live births in 1970, to 5.8 per 1000 in 1990 and 4.6 per 1000 in 2000—a considerable reduction.

Progress in other areas has been mixed. The percentage of cesarean section deliveries has increased from 22.7% in 1990, to 22.9% in 2000, and to 24.4% in 2001. The goal set by *Healthy People 2010* is 17.8% of all deliveries (USDHHS, 2000). The increase rather than decrease in the last decade is attributed to an increase in the primary cesarean rate and to a sharp decline in the rate of vaginal births after previous cesarean (VBAC) delivery (MacDorman et al., 2001).

Breast feeding during the early postpartum period has increased. There has been progress in this area among racial and ethnic minorities, with gains of 48% and 20% among African-Americans and Hispanics, respectively. However, little progress has been shown among all women in breast feeding at 5 and 6 months after delivery.

Progress is also being made in early prenatal care, with 83.4% of women entering care during the first trimester in 2001, up from 75.8% in 1990. Disparity still exists between races, but prenatal care increased 6% for non-Hispanic white women, 23% for black women, and 26% for Hispanic women during the same period.

The success in reaching the year 2010 objectives for abstinence from alcohol, tobacco, and drug use during pregnancy has been mixed. The rate of abstinence from tobacco has declined steadily since 1989. In 2000, 12.2% of women reported smoking during pregnancy. The percentage was highest for non-Hispanic white women (15.6%), moderate for black women (9.1%), and lowest for Hispanic women (3.5%). The rates of abstinence from alcohol (from a baseline of 86% for use and 99% for binge drinking in 1996–1997) and illicit drug use (from a baseline of 98% in

T A B L E   2 6 – 2

LBW and VLBW Statistics in Selected Populations for 2000 and *Healthy People 2010* Goals

Healthy People 2010 target goal is to reduce the incidence of LBW babies to no more than 5% of live births and VLBW babies to no more than 0.9% of live births.

Selected Population	2000 Statistics (%)	
	LBW	VLBW
All races	7.6	1.4
African American	13.0	3.0
American Indian/Alaska Native	6.8	1.2
Asian/Pacific Islander	7.2	1.1
Hispanic	6.4	1.1
White	6.5	1.1
Mothers <15 yr	13.6	3.1
Mothers 15–19 yr	9.5	1.8
Mothers ≥35 yr	8.6	1.7

LBW, low-birth-weight; VLBW, very-low-birth-weight.

(Adapted from U.S. Department of Health and Human Services [2000]. *Healthy people 2010* [Conference ed., Vols. 1 & 2]. Washington, DC: Author; MacDorman, et al., 2001.)

1996–1997) have remained almost unchanged, despite efforts to achieve 100% abstinence in 2010 for drugs and alcohol and 98% abstinence for tobacco.

Risk Factors for Pregnant Women and Infants

Most pregnant women in the United States are healthy; they have normal pregnancies and produce healthy babies. Many factors contribute to the health problems of those mothers and babies who figure in the statistics on infant mortality and low birth weight. The factors associated with low birth weight and infant mortality can be grouped into three categories (MacDorman et al., 2001; USDHHS, 2000):

1. Lifestyle—smoking, inadequate nutrition, low prepregnancy weight, high alcohol consumption, narcotic addiction, environmental toxins, prolonged standing, strenuous work, stress, and lack of social support
2. Sociodemographic—low maternal age, low educational level, poverty, and unmarried status
3. Medical and gestational history—primiparity, multiple gestation, short interpregnancy intervals, premature rupture of the membranes, uterine abnormality, febrile illness during pregnancy, abortion, genetic factors, gestation-induced hypertension, and diabetes

It is in the realm of lifestyle choices that the work of community health nurses can have the most significant impact.

Drug Use

Cities, suburbs, and rural areas are being overwhelmed with drug-related problems. Substance abuse during pregnancy is a problem of enormous scope and staggering social and medical implications, because the VLBW infant is primarily associated with preterm birth, which may itself be associated with the use of illicit drugs during pregnancy (USDHHS, 2000). According to *Healthy People 2010,* two thirds of LBW and 98% of VLBW births are attributable to preterm delivery. Preterm birth is associated with a number of modifiable risk factors, including the use of illicit drugs during pregnancy (Armstrong et al., 2003; Chasnoff et al., 2001) (see Clinical Corner).

In the last 3 decades, when the IMR should have been decreasing, an increasing number of women were using illicit drugs during pregnancy. This increased the proportion of women entering pregnancy at a greater risk for poor outcomes. Many of these women had unintended pregnancies attributable to prostitution to support a drug habit or to inconsistent contraceptive protection while under the influence of drugs. Their focus on drug acquisition and use superseded everything and everyone else in their lives.

Associated with drug use are limited prenatal care, inadequate nutrition, low prepregnancy weight, alcohol consumption, and smoking (Alexander & Kotelchuck, 2001). In addition, cocaine use during pregnancy is associated with impaired fetal growth, neonatal seizures, and congenital anomalies. Neonatal withdrawal is characterized by abnormal functions of the gastrointestinal tract, the central nervous system, and the respiratory system. Poor feeding, abnormal sleep patterns, long-term learning disabilities, and delayed language development in the infant are observable results of maternal drug use. In addition, the child faces a high risk of infectious diseases, including hepatitis B and HIV (March of Dimes, 2003; Singer et al., 2001). Infants exposed to heroin or cocaine prenatally are also more likely to succumb to **sudden infant death syndrome (SIDS)** (USDHHS, 2000).

It is difficult to determine precisely the rates of substance abuse among pregnant women. Nevertheless, current estimates of the number of women who are **drug exposed** (use drugs intermittently) and give birth to crack- or cocaine-exposed newborns range from 30,000 to 100,000 or greater annually. Other illicit substances may be abused in combination, contributing to higher numbers of exposed women and infants. Another 5000 to 10,000 infants each year are born to women who are **drug dependent** (physically and psychologically require use of drugs to function). Many pregnant addicts do not receive prenatal care, and it is not until their newborns exhibit signs of withdrawal after birth that many of these women are identified (USDHHS, 2000).

All these factors contribute to the birth of LBW infants at a time when technologic advancement is approaching its maximum capabilities to provide neonatal intensive care. There is only so much care that can be given extra utero for the VLBW infant. The decrease in IMR has slowed, leveling off in 2000 at 6.9 deaths per 1000 live births. The year 2010

CLINICAL CORNER

MATERNAL, PERINATAL AND NEWBORN CLIENTS

You are a public health nurse working in the high-risk infant follow-up program in Capitol City. You are responsible for home visits to families whose infants have been exposed, in utero, to illicit drugs. The determination of perinatal substance abuse may be made prenatally but is primarily identified in routine postpartum toxicology screening. Both of your clients today tested positive for methamphetamines while in the immediate postpartum period.

Mrs. Boyle is your first client of the day. She is a 35-year-old Anglo woman. She lives in an exclusive gated community north of Capitol City. She has private insurance and is employed by a local software company. Her husband is an architect. This is the couple's first child. Prenatal records indicate that this child was the result of artificial insemination. The pregnancy was without complications. There was no toxicology screen performed prenatally. When you phoned Mrs. Boyle to arrange for the visit, she seemed surprised and initially reluctant to agree to the visit. She stated, "I know they said there was something wrong with my tests, but I don't do drugs and I'm very upset about their accusations." She agreed to the visit after your assurances that you had information for her about infant development and parenting classes in her community.

Next, you will visit *Ms. Craig*. She is a 21-year-old Anglo woman who lives in a low-income housing complex downtown. Ms. Craig is single, and prenatal records indicate involvement by the father of the baby. Ms. Craig's medical costs were covered by Medicaid for this pregnancy. Ms. Craig is gravida three, para one. She has had two therapeutic abortions. Prenatal records document a toxicology screen performed at 7 months' gestation, which was also positive for methamphetamines. At that time, Ms. Craig stated that her boyfriend was a "dealer" and that she was cutting down and would eventually attempt to discontinue drug usage. When you telephoned to schedule an appointment for the visit, she stated, "I know why you're coming . . . it's okay with me but we have to do it when my boyfriend is at work or he'll get mad."

Questions

1. What considerations must be made for safety in preparation for these visits?

- Mrs. Boyle
- Ms. Craig

Discuss the following issues as they relate to the initial visit with each client:

2. "Getting in the door"
   - Mrs. Boyle
   - Ms. Craig
3. Establishing a trusting relationship, empathy, and rapport
   - Mrs. Boyle
   - Ms. Craig
4. Assessing for drug usage
   - Mrs. Boyle
   - Ms. Craig
5. Involving significant family members
   - Mrs. Boyle
   - Ms. Craig
6. Making appropriate referrals
   - Mrs. Boyle
   - Ms. Craig

After you complete your visits with Mrs. Boyle and Ms. Craig, your supervisor asks you to develop a postpartum visitation protocol for women who have tested "toxicology positive" and their children. You will be allowed four to six visits postpartum. Your aggregate will consist of all women testing positive who deliver at any of the three Capitol City hospitals. An average of eight to twelve women each month fit this category. Your aggregate's average age is 23. Most are single women with limited involvement by the father of the baby or the woman's extended family. The ethnicity breakdown for this aggregate is 12% African-American, 38% Anglo, 18% Asian, 30% Hispanic, and 2% other. Most of your aggregate falls at or below poverty level for income, and most have completed high school.

Questions

1. What additional information do you need to plan an effective program? How will you go about obtaining this information?
2. Identify the components of a program that will lead to effective home visits with this aggregate.
3. How will you accommodate for individual variances within your aggregate?

---

goal of 4.2 deaths per 1000 live births is ambitious and will require transcending the limitations of present-day neonatal intensive care (MacDorman et al., 2002).

A lifestyle choice that includes the use of drugs during pregnancy has placed millions of children at risk. These chil-

dren are seen in neonatal intensive care units, foster care, special-education programs in the public schools, and later in the juvenile court system. Family structure patterns are altered because grandparents find themselves primary caregivers for their grandchildren. A woman who is an intravenous drug user introduces another public health problem, that of acquisition of HIV infection and possible spread of the virus to the fetus or others (Minkoff, 2003; USDHHS, 2000). The primary, secondary, and tertiary prevention roles of the community health nurse cannot be underestimated when drug use takes such a high toll on every aspect of society (see Voices in the Community I).

Alcohol Use

Use and especially addiction to alcohol as the substance of choice is another problem in society. Because alcohol is a legal and socially acceptable substance, it is the drug most commonly abused by pregnant women (Weber et al., 2002). It is difficult to establish accurate statistics on the number of women who drink during pregnancy, because inquiries about drinking habits trigger denial or minimization of intake, especially in heavy drinkers (Barr & Streissguth, 2001).

Alcohol use can cause devastating effects in the fetus, even when limited to early pregnancy and in the absence of addiction. For example, regular intake of alcohol during pregnancy, especially in the first trimester can cause **fetal alcohol syndrome** (FAS), which is characterized by structural abnormalities of the head and face (microcephaly and flattening of the maxillary area), intrauterine growth retardation,

decreased birth weight and length, developmental delays, intellectual impairment, hyperactivity, altered sleep patterns, feeding problems, perceptual difficulties, impaired concentration, mood problems, and language dysfunction. It is a national health problem that was first identified in 1968 by Lemoine and colleagues (Hankin, McCaul, & Heussner, 2000). FAS is the primary cause of mental retardation in the Western world, with an estimated incidence of 0.2 to 1.5 per 1000 live births, yet it is 100% preventable (USDHHS, 2000; Weber et al., 2002). Among the Native American population, the incidence of FAS is four times higher than in the general U. S. public; among African-Americans, the incidence of FAS has risen steeply to 5.4 cases per 1000. Common in alcohol consumption research is the underreporting of consumption by subjects (Hankin, McCaul, & Heussner, 2000; Kaskutas, 2000). For example, participants may report one or two drinks a day, but when asked to show the vessel used, it is frequently a beverage container of large capacity. (Standard measurements of alcohol are 1 beer = 12 oz, 1 glass of wine = 4 oz, 1 drink of liquor = 1 oz.) The containers they drink from may hold 16 to 24 oz per "drink." Worldwide, the estimated rate of FAS among pregnant women who are heavy drinkers is greater than 40 cases per 1000 live births. Kaskutas (2000) conducted a study in California among 321 pregnant women (185 African-Americans, 102 Native Americans, and 34 whites). She found that 83% of the subjects reported seeing an advertisement about drinking during pregnancy, yet the risk drinkers (those consuming one or more standard-sized drinks per day while pregnant) saw the federally mandated warning label on alcoholic beverage containers less frequently (77%) than did the nondrinkers (97%). Those who saw alcohol and pregnancy messages but continued to drink during pregnancy stated that the messages did not change their behavior but made them feel bad about themselves. This information reinforces the importance of primary prevention before pregnancy and the necessity of efforts to reach women before a lifestyle of drinking becomes such a strong part of their lives that they are unable or unwilling to abstain during pregnancy.

Fetal alcohol effects (FAE) syndrome causes some but not all of the symptoms of FAS. It occurs in children whose mothers have used varying amounts of alcohol while pregnant, including those who have engaged only in occasional binge drinking. FAE is seen three times more often than FAS. "There seems to be no safe threshold below which pregnant women can safely drink" (Kaskutas, 2000, p. 1241).

Alcohol use during pregnancy also increases the risks for abruptio placentae, stillbirth, spontaneous abortion, congenital anomalies, prematurity, postmaturity, and infections (Kaskutas, 2000). Mothers who drank heavily and also smoked during pregnancy delivered babies that weighed 500 g less than babies of mothers who abstained from both. The combined effects of drinking and smoking are important factors in infant mortality and impaired mental and physical development. Research studies indicate demographic markers

VOICES FROM THE COMMUNITY I

Voices of pregnant women in a focus group in a drug rehabilitation program:

"I started drinking to escape my parents. They were so abusive. The school knew it, but they didn't do anything about it."

"I remember being 9 years old and thinking everything that was going on in my house was my fault and that the drugs, pimps, and lifestyle in my house was OK because that's what my mother did. For so long I thought that lifestyle was OK."

"My baby's father is an addict. He's been in and out of detox seven times since I've been here, and I've been here 2 months. And my mom drinks, but not when I'm around. I say she's an addict, but she doesn't agree. My father, he's in jail in New York. He's an addict."

"After I was sober for a year, I went to a bar. My boyfriend's friend kept saying, 'Oh, it's so good, just taste it. Taste it.' And I was drinking again from that day on. You need new friends, a new environment."

(Howell, E.M., & Chasnoff, I.J. [1999]. Perinatal substance abuse treatment: Findings from focus groups with clients and providers. *Journal of Substance Abuse Treatment, 17*[1–2], 139–148.)

strongly linking use of alcohol and tobacco, thus placing the woman and fetus at twice the risk (Britton, 1998).

Tobacco Use

Tobacco use increased dramatically among women in the last third of the 20th century, inevitably affecting maternal and newborn health. The nicotine in tobacco is a major addictive substance, and smoking is an addiction that many people find difficult to stop. Although the risk factors of smoking are well documented, many pregnant women continue to smoke. Smoking during pregnancy is one of the most studied risk factors in obstetric history. It has been associated with ectopic pregnancy, spontaneous abortions, intrauterine growth retardation, preterm birth, stillbirths, higher perinatal mortality, small-for-gestational-age (SGA) birth, LBW birth, neonatal anomalies, and lower Apgar scores (Duncan, 2002). Health problems do not end once the infant is born. Infants of women who smoked during pregnancy continue to be at higher risk for SIDS, respiratory infections, asthma, ear infections, and decreased lung function (Britton, 1998; Duncan, 2002). As the children get older, they are at higher risk for learning disabilities and behavioral problems as preteens.

Passive smoking, which is exposure to tobacco smoke from other people smoking in one's environment, also puts a person at risk for smoking-related disease. The smoke from a burning cigarette sitting on an ashtray, inhaled passively by the nonsmoker, contains a higher concentration of toxins and carcinogens than the smoke inhaled directly by the smoker; physical distance between infant and smoker correlates with the amount of cotinine in the baby's urine (Blizzard et al., 2003). If a pregnant woman lives with a smoker, she and her fetus can be negatively affected by the other person's addiction. Blizzard and associates (2003) found in a study of 4486 infants in Tasmania, Australia, that the number of infant hospitalizations with respiratory infection during the first year of life was 56% higher if the mother smoked in the same room with the infant, 73% higher if she smoked while holding the infant, and 95% higher if she smoked while feeding the infant.

The use of **smokeless tobacco products**, such as snuff and chewing tobacco, has led to an increase in oral cancers related to tobacco exposure. Any form of tobacco is extremely hazardous to health. At this time, it is not known whether the use of smokeless tobacco has any direct adverse effects on the fetus.

Community health nurses and other health care professionals must be involved in the control of tobacco products on many levels, especially in health policy development; client assessment, planning, and intervention; as positive role models; and in research implementation. Health policy development has made important strides at the grassroots level. Seventeen states have received funding since 1992 through the American Stop Smoking Intervention Study Program, which is supported by the Centers for Disease Control and Prevention, the National Cancer Institute, and the American Cancer Society. A top priority of health care policy development is to reduce access of youth to tobacco products by re-stricting tobacco product advertising and promotion. Imposing dramatic cigarette excise taxes, requiring that public places such as malls and restaurants be smoke free, monitoring tobacco retailers for illegal sales to minors, and keeping cigarettes in locked cases are some of the significant steps that have been taken to discourage young people from smoking. Most smokers begin their addiction in their early teens. If fewer adolescents begin smoking, there will be fewer women of child-bearing age who smoke in the future.

An initial health history of a pregnant woman should always include the assessment of tobacco use, smoking status, and smoke in the personal environment. The nurse must not only advise clients to quit smoking but also offer supportive and empathetic approaches to smoking cessation, including methods or interventions that can help. For example, the nurse may counsel clients individually, suggest behavioral therapy, provide self-help manuals, or recommend nicotine replacement therapy. Studies of nicotine patches have indicated varying levels of success, similar to unsolicited advice without other supportive measures from a physician or nurse. Other approaches such as support groups or even controlled use of tobacco can be helpful. Any permanent reduction in the number of cigarettes smoked, amount of secondhand smoke inhaled, or amount of smokeless tobacco used can only improve the health of the mother and her fetus.

Nurses can be positive role models for health and demonstrate health-promotion strategies to clients by their own behavior. In addition, if you have struggled with smoking cessation, your admission of failures or explanation of successful strategies offers an opportunity to enhance your believability with clients. They recognize that you struggle with some of the same health issues that they deal with.

Finally, there is a need for more research on the reasons why women smoke. Specific attention is needed to address the effects of depression and social isolation on the initiation and continuation of smoking by women. Studies are also needed on the effectiveness of various nursing interventions on a woman's smoking behaviors.

Sexually Transmitted Diseases

The public has been lulled into a false sense of security with respect to the risk of contracting sexually transmitted diseases (STDs) other than AIDS. Because the major media sources have focused on HIV and AIDS for the last 2 decades, information about the effects of other STDs has been essentially ignored. However, Wingood and DiClemente (2002) indicated that STDs represent a growing threat to women's health and that national action is urgently needed.

Globally, the prevalence of syphilis in developing countries is up to 100 times that in developed countries; rates are 10 to 15 times higher for gonorrhea, and 3 times higher for chlamydial infection (WHO, 1998). The age at initiation of sexual activity is between 16 and 20 years for a majority of men and women in most parts of the world. Although contraceptive use has increased in most countries in the last 25 years, many sexually active people do not protect themselves against STDs. WHO estimates that 1 in 20 teenagers contracts an STD each year. Teens are less likely to seek care for STDs, and this delay can contribute to permanent health effects, including sterility and death. If the teen becomes pregnant, there may be negative health effects for the fetus or infant.

In the United States, herpes affects 20 million people every year, and almost 2 million cases of gonorrhea are reported annually. Other common STDs include syphilis, chancroid, lymphogranuloma venereum, granuloma inguinale, and human papillomavirus (HPV), the infectious agent that causes venereal warts and is associated with cervical cancer. In a study by Southwick and colleagues (1999), researchers investigated an epidemic of congenital syphilis in Texas between 1994 and 1995 to determine the cause of the outbreak. They found that inadequate prenatal testing for syphilis after an outbreak in adults contributed to the epidemic. In other studies, bacterial vaginosis has been associated with spontaneous preterm birth in the United States, especially among African-American women, and it may account for as many as 40% of early preterm births (Goldenberg et al., 1998). Two thirds of all STDs occur in persons 15 to 24 years old—the same age group in which more than one third of all births occur (U. S. Census Bureau, 1999).

Women who discover that they have an STD often feel ashamed, betrayed, embarrassed, and angry. Those who are asymptomatic may deny the existence of the disease and not carry out the treatment plan. Although educating the pregnant client about the effects of STDs is critical, providing information alone is not enough. The community health nurse has a pivotal role in enhancing the empowerment of women so they can act on the information they receive. The nurse talks with the women and helps them understand that they have control over their bodies. Usually, STDs are first discovered in pregnancy during routine prenatal screening, which places the clinic nurse and the nurse who may make home visits in the position to take an affirmative approach to treatment and follow-up.

HIV and AIDS

The HIV epidemic is the great tragedy of the last 2 decades of the 20th century. An HIV-positive woman who is pregnant or has delivered a baby requires special nursing management of the pregnancy and of the family after the birth of the newborn. There are many teaching opportunities for the community health nurse during a high-risk pregnancy such as helping the client identify, change, or curtail high-risk behaviors. Success in changing behaviors often requires an interdisciplinary approach of health care, social, emotional, and financial resources. What follows is a discussion of some of the pregnancy-management issues (see The Global Community).

Antepartum Management. Evidence suggests that there is a higher rate of genitourinary tract infections and an increased incidence of STDs in HIV-positive women during pregnancy. The nurse should advise clients to see their health providers for immediate evaluation if they develop fever,

THE GLOBAL COMMUNITY

DETERMINANTS OF LBW AMONG HIV-INFECTED PREGNANT WOMEN IN TANZANIA

Low birth weight (LBW) increases the risk of infant death, but little is known about its cause among women infected with the human immunodeficiency virus (HIV) in sub-Saharan Africa, where 90% of the world's cases of HIV exist.

Sociodemographic, nutritional, immunologic, parasitic, and infant risk factors for birth weight, LBW, and small-for-gestational-age (SGA) status were assessed in 822 HIV-positive women enrolled in a clinical trial of vitamin supplementation and pregnancy outcomes in Dar es Salaam, Tanzania. Blood, stool, urine, genital specimens collected, and anthropometric measurements and sociodemographic data were recorded at a prenatal care clinic during their second trimester of pregnancy. At hospital delivery, birth weight was measured.

Among this cohort of 822 women, the mean birth weight was 3015 g, 11.1% of newborns weighed less than 2500 g (LBW), and 11.5% were SGA. Maternal weight at enrollment and low CD8 cell count were inversely associated with LBW. Advanced-stage HIV disease, previous history of preterm birth, *Plasmodium falciparum* malaria, and any helmintic infection were factors associated with higher risk of LBW.

The conclusion of the study indicates that prevention of HIV disease progression and vertical transmission, improved nutrional status, and better management of malaria are likely to reduce the incidence of LBW infants in Tanzania.

These results support the value of early prenatal care and use of antiretroviral drugs to reduce HIV transmission to the fetus. In addition, the availability of nutritious foods and elimination of infectious diseases, both primary prevention methods, can significantly decrease the number of LBW infants. Such information is useful for other countries in sub-Saharan Africa, where HIV is at epidemic proportions and a generation of children are at risk.

(Dreyfuss, M.L., Msamanga, G.I., Spiegelman, D., Hunter, D.J., Urassa, E.J.N., Hertzmark, E., et al. [2001]. Determinants of low birth weight among HIV-infected pregnant women in Tanzania. *American Journal of Clinical Nutrition, 74,* 814–826.)

sweats, cough, or diarrhea. HIV-positive clients should also receive nutritional counseling and should be encouraged to gain weight appropriately. It should not be overlooked that a woman who is HIV negative at the beginning of a pregnancy can seroconvert, especially if she continues high-risk behaviors. HIV can be acquired at any time during pregnancy.

The first effective intervention to reduce the perinatal transmission of HIV was developed in the United States in AIDS Clinical Trials Group (ACTG) Study 076 in 1994. In that study, zidovudine was administered orally to HIV-positive pregnant women beginning in the second trimester of pregnancy. During labor, the drug was administered intravenously to the mother, and newborns received oral medication for 6 weeks. This regimen reduced the incidence of HIV infection among newborns by two thirds, from about 25% to 8%. Within 6 months after the study was completed, the U. S. Public Health Service recommended the ACTG 076 regimen as the standard of care in the United States (Annas & Grodin, 1998). In 1996, it became the standard (Minkoff, 2003).

Postpartum Management. There is no clear evidence that an HIV-positive woman experiences increased rates of postpartum or postoperative morbidity. Some studies show that other STDs coexist in HIV-positive women more frequently than in non–HIV-positive women. Therefore, HIV-positive women should be monitored for the development of any signs and symptoms of infection. If a community health nurse is doing a newborn assessment, performing a lochia check, or coming into contact with maternal or infant blood, he or she should use universal precautions. The use of universal precautions is no longer the "ideal to be achieved" but the standard under which all nurses must practice.

Breast-Feeding. HIV-infected women are advised not to breast feed their infants, because approximately 20% of the infants will become infected with HIV from breast milk (Venes & Thomas, 2001). The community health nurse focuses teaching on providing a safe, available form of infant formula. In developing countries, the lack of clean water still makes formula feeding dangerous, and breast feeding is overwhelmingly recommended. The infection rate for HIV from breast feeding and the mortality rate from formula made with impure water are about the same, resulting in a dilemma for women and health care providers in developing countries. The best immediate intervention would be to put increased effort into providing clean water and sanitation (Annas & Grodin, 1998). In the long term, the nurse must focus on preventing and eliminating HIV infection. Additional information on the role of the community health nurse who works with HIV-positive clients is found in Chapter 9.

Poor Nutrition and Weight Gain

Research has demonstrated a positive correlation between weight gain during pregnancy and normal birth weight in the babies. Weight gain of 25 to 35 lb during pregnancy is recommended for women of normal body weight; the recommendation is 28 to 40 lb for underweight women and 15 to 25 lb for obese women (USDHHS, 2000). Obese women have a higher incidence of gestational diabetes, urinary tract infections, wound infection, thromboembolism, pregnancy-induced hypertension, fetal monitoring difficulties, prolonged labor, and birth trauma (Sherwen, Scoloveno, & Weingarten, 2001). Brown and colleagues (2002) found that maternal weight change in the first trimester of pregnancy more strongly influenced newborn size than did weight change in the second or third trimester. These findings were very different from those of other studies and should be considered when community health nurses teach clients about nutrition early in a pregnancy. Recent studies have found that, compared with women of normal weight, women who were obese or overweight before pregnancy faced double the risk of having babies with heart defects and double the risk of multiple birth defects (Watkins et al., 2003). Community health nurses who work with morbidly obese pregnant women can help them most by emphasizing good nutrition and by encouraging them to maintain their prepregnant weight without reducing caloric intake. This can be accomplished primarily by a marked decrease in consumption of "empty calories" from junk food. Pregnancy is never a time for dieting, and eating foods from the Food Guide Pyramid (U. S. Department of Agriculture, 1992) or the Vegetarian Food Pyramid (Health Connection, 1994; see Chapter 1) ensures the proper number of servings and portion sizes. Nutritional counseling can have an additional benefit in that it may ultimately decrease the risk of obesity or eating disorders in the client's children.

Underweight women have twice as many LBW babies as women whose weight is within normal range. There is a correlation between weight gain (excessive or low) in pregnancy and poor obstetric outcomes (Sherwen, Scoloveno, & Weingarten, 2001). Low maternal weight gain is associated with LBW infants who have higher incidences of growth problems, developmental delays, central nervous system disorders, and mental retardation (USDHHS, 2000).

Nutritional teaching is part of the community health nurse's role when working with a pregnant woman who has difficulty gaining the recommended 25 to 35 lb during pregnancy. Finding ways to add calories to foods and increasing the woman's desire to eat are effective methods to improve maternal weight gain. Insufficient caloric intake in pregnant adolescents (who themselves are still growing) is an additional concern. For women who are prone to gaining too much weight, nutrition-rich, low-calorie foods are recommended. After assessment, the community health nurse determines whether the unwanted weight gain is related to the consumption of additional calories with limited activity or to fluid retention. Each cause must be managed differently.

Teenage Pregnancy

Each year, more than 1 million American teenagers become pregnant. There is a strong association between young maternal age and high IMR, and infants born to teenagers are at increased risk for preterm delivery, neonatal, and postneonatal mortality (Jolly et al., 2000). Infants born to African-American adolescents are more likely to be LBW babies than are infants of white teens. Infants born to very young adolescents (aged 10 to 14 years) are at very high risk for neonatal mortality. Teen mothers have increased psychological risks, such as isolation, powerlessness, depressive disorders, lowered self-concept, and increased somatic complaints. Developmental and maturational processes are disrupted or compromised; and young mothers face diminished prospects for completing their education.

The markers for successful pregnancy outcomes and future life events are more complex. The mother's educational attainment, marital experiences, subsequent fertility behavior, labor force experience, occupational attainment, and experiences with poverty and public assistance are all directly related to the adolescent pregnancy.

The issues of adolescent parenting are complex. They encompass many areas, including emotional, physical, and social issues. The community health nurse has a unique challenge when teaching teens about pregnancy-related changes, accompanying needs, and preparation for the important role of parent to the infant.

Emotional Needs. Teenagers who become pregnant deal with this change in their life in a variety of ways. Some have such a strong denial system that they deny the pregnancy, even to themselves. It may take 3 or 4 months into the pregnancy before they can admit it and seek out a physician's diagnosis. Often, their parents are the last to know.

What is difficult about this scenario is that prenatal care is delayed into the second trimester of pregnancy. If the teen chooses to continue with the pregnancy, the delayed prenatal care could compromise the well-being of both the young mother and the fetus.

What the teen needs at this time is supportive caring parents and professionals. Teen parents have difficult choices to make; most continue with the pregnancy, although some may later choose to give the baby up for adoption. Others choose abortion. These choices are difficult and are fraught with emotion. Supportive parents along with their teens, in consultation with professionals, can explore all options. This may be the time that the community health nurse first begins to work with the teen, perhaps at school in a school-based clinic. First contact may also occur in a clinic or physician's office, or on a home visit resulting from a referral from a health care provider. The nurse can offer educational services, emotional support, and referrals for services as needed. Adolescent parenting programs set up in some communities have positive effects. In one program, paraprofessionals indigenous to the community made intensive home visits to pregnant teens. This program, implemented by a visiting nursing service, demonstrated that mentorship and social support improved pregnancy outcomes by reducing the percentage of LBW babies born to participating teens to 4.6%, compared with the national average of 13.5% (Flynn, 1999).

The goal of any pregnancy is positive maternal–infant outcomes, including a positive relationship. For some teen mothers, positive relationships are more difficult to achieve than for older mothers. The importance of positive relationships and self-esteem has an impact on the quality of mothering and positive responses to infant distress. Typically, older adolescents have higher self-esteem than younger mothers do; this was observed in classic studies by Olds and colleagues (1999; 2000) and by Koniack-Griffin and colleagues (2000; 2002; 2003). These significant studies demonstrated the benefits of intensive intervention programs. Community health nurses who have special training are able to provide each participant with services that promote overall health of the mother and maternal-infant bonding. Results of these studies can guide nurses in their work with pregnant adolescents.

Physical Needs. Pregnant teens have a gamut of physical needs that can be addressed by routine prenatal care and education, but there is need for continuity if such endeavors are to be successful. Routine prenatal care is one of the most important needs, and teens may require assistance in recognizing the value of monitoring the pregnancy. Some may feel embarrassed and uncomfortable with male health care providers and refuse to keep appointments. If she is able to make her discomfort known, adjustments can be made so that the teen is seen by female professionals or is allowed to bring the baby's father or a girlfriend. Whatever it takes to get the teen to prenatal appointments should be encouraged, including making arrangements for transportation—procuring bus tokens, calling a taxi, or arranging for a friend or social worker to drive the teen to her appointments.

The pregnant teen needs education regarding changes in her emotional state and her body, the growth and development of the fetus, dietary requirements, rest and relaxation needs, and anticipatory guidance for infant caregiving and parenting. Teaching can take place as part of each prenatal appointment, in specific classes at school for pregnant teens, in the health department clinic, or during home visits. In each setting, the community health nurse can modify the teaching methods to the setting and the individual needs of the teen. Changing teen behavior during pregnancy can be challenging. The community health nurse may focus on one important and seemingly less complex issue of nutrition during pregnancy. However, it is a more difficult task to change the eating habits of teens than it is with adults. In their stage of development, they usually are more concerned with body image than with fetal growth and development. Fad diets, peer pressure, and personal control are all issues with which the pregnant teen is struggling. If a teen has been raised in poverty, a multiplicity of other issues can affect her motivation to make dietary changes during pregnancy.

Social Needs. Pregnant teens are dealing with two stages of their own growth and development at the same time, which makes their social needs complex. They are struggling with the normal adolescent challenges along with the responsibilities of pregnancy and parenting (young adulthood stage of development).

There may be changes in acceptance by social groups or in types of activities (eg, surfboarding, mountain climbing).

The group may participate in activities that the pregnant teen should not participate in, such as smoking, drinking, or taking illicit drugs. This causes conflict for a pregnant teen who has a strong need to be accepted by her peer group and also knows that she has a responsibility to her unborn child. The community health nurse can help the teen solve her dilemma by providing a social support system among the attendees at prenatal classes. The nurse can also convince the teen's parents or other adults in her life to offer her more support. Often, a developmental crisis such as a teen pregnancy can help cement the mother–daughter relationship. It takes time and work on the part of the parents and the teen. The teen will need the support of her parents after the baby is born, and strengthening the relationship during pregnancy is an important start.

Another social outlet and an important resource is school. The teen should be encouraged to continue her studies, with the goal of graduation. The health and welfare of children are related to the educational levels of their parents. Higher educational levels increase the likelihood that children will receive adequate medical care and live in a safe and supportive environment with adults who are responsive to their needs (Koniack-Griffin et al., 2000). Teen pregnancy and education are discussed more thoroughly in Chapter 28 (see Using the Nursing Process).

Maternal Developmental Disability

The maternal–infant relationship is of utmost importance, regardless of whether this relationship exists between adolescent mothers and their babies, mothers and babies in ideal circumstances, or developmentally disabled mothers and their infants. **Developmental disability** is the preferred term for a broad scope of limitations that includes intellectual limitations identified before 22 years of age and limitations in the ability to perform certain activities of daily living. The disability may be mild, moderate, or severe (see Chapter 34). For couples who are developmentally disabled, having a child puts increased stress on a system that is already burdened. Studies have shown that child abuse, neglect, and developmental delays; intergenerational disability; and inadequate home environments accompany the parenting style of developmentally disabled parents.

Much of the pediatric literature discusses the needs of developmentally disabled infants and children and the roles of nurses and other health care professionals in assisting families of these children. Developmentally disabled adults, however, are rarely represented in studies of disability, so there is limited information about their success as parents. Over the past 20 years, studies identified that a primary problem affecting the children of developmentally disabled mothers is the poor quality of maternal–infant or maternal–child interaction. The parenting style of mothers with developmental disabilities is often nonstimulating, punitive, and restrictive. In addition, unusual and sometimes bizarre behaviors such as locking a toddler out of the house or hitting a child for asking a question have been documented.

How does the community health nurse work with developmentally disabled parents effectively? Most importantly, nursing support must enhance the natural resilience of the family. The success of family support depends on immediate and continuing health promotion visits. The goal is to establish safe parenting routines that will serve as a foundation for parenting skills needed when the infant begins to walk and explore—a time when the infant's safety is in jeopardy.

The establishment of a trusting relationship between the nurse and the family is of foremost importance. Teaching by using demonstration, many visual aids, and prompts can challenge the nurse's creativity. Modeling of appropriate parenting behavior needs to occur on each visit. Supervision and monitoring of family functioning must continue until the child reaches adulthood. Many agencies for which community health nurses work cannot provide the intensive follow-up that such a family requires. It is then necessary to make referrals to organizations that can provide the support such as the American Association of Retarded Citizens (AARC) or Exceptional Parents. The nurse may stay involved as a consultant to the paraprofessionals or make periodic home visits at times of developmental or situational crises.

Complications of Child Bearing

Although some major risk factors among pregnant women and infants have been covered, several common complications of child bearing need to be mentioned. The effects of hypertensive disease in pregnancy, gestational diabetes, postpartum depression, and grief in families who have lost a child are important areas in which the community health nurse can intervene successfully.

Hypertensive Disease in Pregnancy

Blood pressure measurements in all people shows daily variation, regardless of physical and mental activities. At times, people demonstrate elevated blood pressure during clinic visits, a phenomenon known as "white coat syndrome"; excessive blood pressure readings might not be observed at other times. However, 10% of pregnant women are diagnosed with hypertension, and if this condition is left untreated, there can be negative effects on the health and safety of the fetus and the outcome of the pregnancy (Garovic, 2000).

Preterm birth is a frequent and negative occurrence in a pregnancy that is associated with maternal infection, smoking, drinking, or hypertension. Additional maternal risk factors associated with hypertensive disease in pregnancy include lung disease, age older than 30 years, and proteinuria.

A variety of methods are employed to prevent and control hypertension during pregnancy, namely, a diet high in fresh fruits and vegetables, weight gain limitations, sodium restriction, rest, and regular exercise. These remain the most

USING THE NURSING PROCESS

Working with Pregnant Teenagers

BETH MAKES A LIFELONG DECISION

BACKGROUND DATA AND ASSESSMENT

Beth is 15 years old. She lives with her divorced mother and is dating 17-year-old Kevin, a best friend of Beth's older brother. Her mother asked if "sex was an issue" between them, and when Beth adamantly said "no" her mother did not pursue the subject any more. Within a few months, Beth was pregnant. She will deliver 1 month after her 16th birthday. This is devastating to the family structure. Beth's mother takes her to a woman's health clinic for counseling (and possible abortion). Corrina Adams, a community health nurse, who works with women contemplating abortion or adoption, meets with Beth, Kevin, and Beth's mother; alone with Beth; and with Beth and Kevin alone. She finds out that Beth strongly wants to keep her baby, that she's "wanted a baby since she was 9 years old." Kevin pretty much will go along with whatever Beth says, but he has a job opportunity 200 miles away, and the mother sobs as she realizes she will need to support her young daughter and boyfriend in this lifelong decision Beth is making. Corrina assesses the disruption to family functioning, recognizable family strengths, areas of growth needed, and a strong desire for a healthy pregnancy outcome, because abortion and adoption are not options Beth is willing to consider.

NURSING DIAGNOSES

1. Altered family functioning related to an unplanned young adolescent's pregnancy and intention to raise her infant.
2. Family coping: Potential for growth related to situational/maturational crisis with anticipated changes in family structure/roles/needs.
3. At risk for altered role performance due to maturational level of pregnant teen.

PLAN/INTERVENTION

Corrina and the family work on plans for each person involved, make the following suggestions, and will meet again in 2 weeks:

1. The teens are to go to stores and keep a record that includes all the costs of having a baby and raising a baby: formula/food, age-appropriate clothing, diapers, furniture, bedding, medical bills, educational costs, and so on. (The teens complete the task and are amazed at the cost over 18 years of raising a child.)
2. Beth wants to continue with school, and will check on doubling up on gym classes this semester so she won't have gym in her last trimester. (She has doubled up her gym classes and is staying in school.)
3. Beth's mother will check with her health insurance plan at work to see if it covers the pregnancy of a single dependent and will make an appointment for Beth with her gynecologist. (Mother checked on her policy and Beth's entire pregnancy costs are covered if she delivers in the hospital where mother works. She attended the first prenatal visit with her MD, and when he said, "Beth is quite a grown-up young lady," the mother sobbed again.)
4. Kevin will talk with his parents about the pregnancy and explore job opportunities. (He talked with his parents and they did not want to participate in "Beth's problems." They encouraged their son to take the out-of-town job since he has graduated from high school.)

EVALUATION

Kevin will not be as involved and supportive as Beth and her mother would like. He plans to keep in touch with Beth and "come home" when Beth delivers. Beth and her mother are strengthening their bonds, talking positively about the pregnancy, planning for Beth's staying in school, and exploring prenatal classes and babysitting arrangements in the future. They are trying to make the best of a situation that is not desirable but can be resolved positively.

common preventive suggestions that community health nurses, in collaboration with the clients' primary health care providers, can give to their pregnant clients. Additional assessment data may guide the nurse to focus teaching on stress reduction techniques and modification or elimination of smoking. These modifications have a very limited effect for some clients in reducing blood pressure during pregnancy, and medication or even hospitalization may be necessary. The nurse can offer support and understanding while contin-

uing to be a resource for the client as the pregnancy progresses and the infant is born.

Gestational Diabetes

Gestational diabetes mellitus (GDM) is defined as glucose intolerance of variable degree with onset or first recognition during pregnancy. For the mother with GDM, there is a higher risk of hypertension, preeclampsia, urinary tract infections, cesarean section, and future diabetes (Venes &

Thomas, 2001). The infant is at increased risk for fetal death because GDM has been associated with large-for-gestational-age (LGA) babies, which puts them at risk especially during delivery (Mondestin et al., 2002). The prevalence of GDM varies worldwide partly because different criteria and screening regimens exist. In the United States, the prevalence rate is usually between 1% and 4% of pregnancies. Pathophysiologically, GDM is similar to type 2 diabetes, and more than one third of women with GDM eventually develop type 2 diabetes during their lifetimes (Venes & Thomas, 2001).

Because growth and maturation of the fetus are closely associated with the delivery of maternal nutrients, particularly glucose, maintenance of appropriate glucose levels is essential to the health of the fetus. This is most crucial in the third trimester and is directly related to the duration and degree of maternal glucose elevation. The negative impact is as diverse as the degree of carbohydrate intolerance that women bring to pregnancy.

The community health nurse can help in the control of GDM by encouraging early prenatal care, adequate nutrition, rest and exercise, and adherence to the particular regimen suggested by the woman's health care provider. The infants of GDM women often weigh significantly more than other full-term infants. Some infants have weighed 12 lb or more. Some women who have such large babies may expect more of the infant because at birth the baby weighs the same as a 2- to 3-month-old child. Teaching and provision of anticipatory guidance become particularly important for these women.

Postpartum Depression

Depression during a woman's lifetime is a fairly common phenomenon; 17.3% of women experience depression in their lifetimes, and a 12-month prevalence of 10.3% has been reported (Barrio & Burt, 2000). In the postpartum period, 10% of the population suffers from major or minor depression. It occurs in primiparas as well as in women with several children, and in some cases, depression can last for 1 year or longer. Depressive symptoms may not indicate major clinical depression; nevertheless, symptoms may cause considerable psychological distress (see Voices From the Community II).

Through numerous studies over the years, researchers have identified specific risk factors associated with postpartum depression and have developed a profile of women with postpartum depression (Barrio & Burt, 2000; Beck, 1996; 2002). Risk factors include a personal or family history of depression, young age at the time of pregnancy, marital discord, lack of social support, first pregnancy, unwanted pregnancy, and recent adverse life events such as the death of a parent. Most depressed postpartum women have low self-esteem, which can be reinforced by the infant's temperament; the demands of an irritable infant on a new mother who is fatigued and has limited support from a spouse or significant other can increase the depressive symptoms. Other mothers, who have a "good" baby feel guilty for the apathy they feel toward their infants. This affects maternal–infant

VOICES FROM THE COMMUNITY II

Voices of three women experiencing postpartum depression:

"I had no control of my own self-being, nothing, mind, soul, nothing. It basically controlled me. I wanted to reach out to my baby, yet I couldn't."

"Every time my baby cried when she woke up, I'd feel a chill go up my body, and I wanted her to stay asleep because I knew it was so hard when she woke up. The fear of the baby needing you or crying for your help. . . ."

"After 4 months of suffering from postpartum depression, I do remember my very first moment of clarity and total joy in the whole depression. I was sitting with my daughter and rocking in a chair, giving her a bottle. I realized that I was feeling incredibly close to her. I remember this totally piercing sense of okay. We will be okay."

(Beck, C.T. [1996]. Postpartum depressed mothers' experiences interacting with their children. *Nursing Research, 45*[2], 98–104.)

bonding. In addition, stressful life events combined with a lack of social support and everyday stressors, the greatest of which is interpersonal conflict, are etiologic factors in postpartum depressive symptoms. The value of confidants to new mothers is evident, because studies show that depressed new mothers do not perceive their spouses or others as confidants.

There are several nonpharmacologic interventions the community health nurse can initiate in addition to helping the woman identify someone she can rely on as a confidant. First, caffeine can lead to sleep disturbance, and alcohol is a depressant that has been implicated in depression. The elimination of both is a simple yet helpful suggestion. Getting adequate sleep is important—sleep deprivation exacerbates psychiatric symptoms. Napping when baby naps, resting when possible throughout the day, and going to bed early (albeit with the knowledge that sleep may be interrupted two or more times to feed the infant) will provide more hours of rest and sleep in 24 hours for the new mother. Anxiety symptoms often coexist with depression. Relaxation techniques that reduce anxiety can be helpful, including listening to relaxing music, doing yoga, or performing a simple exercise routine. Participation in a support group allows women to identify with others who may be experiencing similar difficulties. Through discussion, women provide each other with both emotional and practical support. A final area of assistance is client education. A woman with postpartum depression is more likely to manage her depression successfully if she is aware of the symptoms of depression; the need for a support system; the importance of adequate rest, sleep, and nutrition; and the possibility of supportive psychological or pharmacologic therapy. The critical nature of postpartum depressive symptoms and the potential negative ramifications for mothers and their children are evident. Community health nurses can intervene by initiating primary preventive measures that promote health throughout pregnancy and the postpartum period. Assessment of the pregnant woman for factors that contribute to depression with standardized questionnaires or one developed by the nursing agency is a beginning (Beck & Gable, 2001). If women with compromised mental health resources can be identified, positive mental health outcomes may be fostered by supporting their self-esteem, optimizing the quality of their primary intimate relationships, and reducing day-to-day stressors. At times, the nurse's efforts alone are not sufficient and a referral to community mental health services is essential for the women and their children.

Fetal or Infant Death

An infrequent role for community health nurses in maternal–infant care is that of grief counselor. A couple may experience a miscarriage, stillbirth, or the death of an infant. In each situation, the nurse has an important and supportive role.

People respond to grief in a variety of ways. Some express deep sadness, shock, or disbelief. Some weep and are unable to talk; others talk incessantly about regrets or guilt. Even if a miscarriage occurs early in a pregnancy, the bonding between the mother and fetus has begun and expressions of grief may be as intense as with the loss of an infant or child. The nurse should encourage the parents to express their feelings by using supportive statements and open-ended questions. The parents may have doubts about actions or behaviors that they believe may have caused the miscarriage. Reassurance and rectification of any misconceptions may alleviate the parents' feelings of guilt and help them cope with their grief in a healthy manner.

For couples who have delivered a stillborn baby, the shock is compounded by the experience of the entire length of the pregnancy, the anticipation of an imminent delivery, and the expectation of an addition to the family, especially if all signs before the birthing event itself were positive. They may say such things as, "We felt him move just yesterday and now he's dead—what did I do wrong?" or "I did everything right during this pregnancy. Why did this happen?" These are questions for which there may be no answers, even from the family's health care provider. Frequently, a stillbirth is related to fetal entanglement in the umbilical cord or to an infection. Mostly, the family needs reassurance that they did nothing wrong or that there is nothing they could have done differently to prevent the stillbirth. Tenderly encouraging the family to talk about the baby and the sadness they feel is important. Therapeutic touch; the offer of food, a beverage, tissues, or a blanket; and simply being there for the family and listening well are invaluable nursing interventions. Not allowing the parents to accept blame will help them through the grieving process.

When a family experiences the loss of an infant after the baby has been brought home from the hospital, grief and guilt are compounded by the loss of an anticipated future and the continuity in the lives of family members. An infant may die from SIDS, a congenital anomaly, an infection, or an accident. There are constant reminders of the infant's presence in the home from memories, photos, videos, and accumulated possessions. This death disrupts family homeostasis and the psychological and physiologic equilibrium of the family. In many cases, the police are involved and an autopsy is required, contributing to the anguish of the grieving family. This promotes both guilt and loss of self-esteem and can even threaten the marriage. The nurse's presence at this time is important. Often, families are inundated with visits from supporters immediately after a death and during the burial ceremony. Thereafter, the parents are visited less frequently or not at all, although this is usually a very lonely and critical time for them. Providing continuity and support to the family for months after the death of an infant gives the nurse an opportunity to assess the family for signs of healthy or unhealthy grief resolution. In addition, grieving families may find comfort, support, and helpful information from support groups such as The Compassionate Friends or the SIDS Alliance. If the grief is protracted with no degree of resolution, referral to the appropriate support group is more than important—it is crucial (see What Do You Think?).

WHAT DO YOU THINK?

"Since the recommendation of an American Academy of Pediatrics task force in 1992 that infants not be placed in the prone position to sleep and the implementation of the national public education campaign, 'Back to Sleep,' in 1994, the incidence of sudden infant death syndrome (SIDS) in the United States has declined by 44%, from 1.2 per 1000 live births in 1992 to 0.67 per 1000 in 1999 (De-Kun, et al., [2003], p. 446).

Note: There are times when a baby can be placed on his or her stomach for "tummy time," when he or she is awake and someone is watching. When the baby is awake, tummy time is good because it helps develop the baby's neck and shoulder muscles.

The "Back to Sleep" campaign sponsors include
The National Institute of Child Health and Human
 Development
Maternal and Child Health Bureau
American Academy of Pediatrics
SIDS Alliance
Association of SIDS and Infant Mortality Programs

For more information about the "Back to Sleep" campaign, call 1-800-505-CRIB or write Back to Sleep/NICHD, 31 Center Drive, Room 2A32, Bethesda, MD, 20892-2425.

PLANNING FOR THE HEALTH OF MATERNAL–INFANT POPULATIONS

To design programs and services for maternal–infant populations, planners need to have a sound understanding of the population they wish to serve. Specific aggregates of pregnant women have needs that the community health nurse should assess and incorporate into a prenatal program. Two important considerations are the specific needs identified through data collection and client input and the developmental stage of the population being served.

Vital statistics assist planners in identifying problems and pinpointing segments of the population in which problems are more likely to occur, yet statistics alone cannot fully characterize the populations they represent. Society has witnessed numerous ineffective community, health care, and public works projects. Programs often have failed because the targeted populations were assessed incompletely or were not involved in the planning process (see Chapter 19).

Most nurses realize that a predetermined, generalized plan may not meet the needs of any one specific client. To increase effectiveness, the nurse involves the client in designing a plan that meets individual needs. Such a plan must consider the client's level of education, previous life experiences, level of motivation, culture, and developmental stage. A prenatal program planned for a group of college-educated career women would be very different from one planned for pregnant adolescents, or women in rural Appalachia, or Hispanic migrant farm workers. The needs of the women in each of these subpopulations are very different, and programs should be adjusted accordingly. The career women may want information on nurse-midwives, alternative birthing methods, and sources of literature on pregnancy, birthing, and newborn care. Pregnant teens may benefit from special teen pregnancy clinics, group classes on parenting, and assistance with selecting supplies needed for the baby. Women living in rural Appalachia may respond best to a mobile health clinic staffed by a female nurse practitioner, a social worker to assist with completing the application process for social services, and someone to watch their other children during the appointments. The migrant workers may best be served by bilingual health care workers who offer a clinic in the evenings at a migrant camp or one that is mobile and can come to the workers in the fields. Women from each of these groups can provide valuable information to planners regarding their specific needs. As with programs for individual clients, input from the target population increases the program's chances for success.

As people grow and mature, they continually experience physiologic changes, personality changes as new psychosocial issues are met (Erikson, 1968), and increasingly sophisticated thought processes (Piaget, 1950). Consequently, a person's most pressing concerns at one stage in life may seem insignificant at the next stage of development. When planning maternal–infant health programs, the community health nurse must consider the developmental stages of the women being served. For example, adolescents are in a stage of intellectual development in which they are beginning to move from concrete to abstract thinking patterns (Piaget, 1950). Concrete thinking is based on what the person has actually experienced or is experiencing. Abstract thinking involves the ability to hear or read something and apply it to a future problem or dilemma. Some adolescents have difficulty comprehending the complex psychosocial issues and problems with which they are faced when caring for an infant and young child. Nurses must use innovative and creative approaches when helping adolescents to understand the complex and demanding nature of child care. Some maternal–infant health programs and high schools involve pregnant adolescents (and those judged to be at risk of becoming pregnant) in child day care programs in which the adolescents participate in the day-to-day care of infants and toddlers. In some health education classes, young teens are given a life-like doll to parent for 24 to 48 hours (Baby Think-It-Over). It comes with a computer inside, which causes the doll to cry intermittently and if it is not handled properly. One minute of crying with no attention is recorded as a neglectful event. Students experience firsthand the intense demands and heavy responsibility of being a parent.

The needs of pregnant women in the developmental stages of young and middle adulthood differ substantially from those of adolescents; variation also exists among individuals (Erikson, 1968). Women in young and middle adulthood more frequently have planned their pregnancies, and they more often make realistic decisions regarding their expanding responsibilities. The community health nurse's most valuable skills are as teacher, coordinator, resource manager, counselor, and collaborator. The nurse uses these skills to design programs that meet the needs of the more mature prenatal client. Thorough understanding of the developmental tasks and psychosocial issues confronting each population should be the cornerstone of solid, well-developed programs. Such programs can be adapted to the developmental needs of clients in adolescence, young adulthood, or middle adulthood (see Levels of Prevention Matrix).

HEALTH PROGRAMS FOR MATERNAL–INFANT POPULATIONS

For more than a half century, the federal government has granted money to states for the promotion of maternal and child health. Through the Maternal and Child Health Block Grant Program, millions of dollars come to individual states each year. This money supplements state funds to meet maternal and child health care needs for people at the local level. With this money, each state provides basic services to its maternal–child population. An additional companion program provides services to special needs children. Community health nurses need to become familiar with the Maternal and

LEVELS OF PREVENTION MATRIX

SITUATION: DESIRE FOR A HEALTHY FULL-TERM INFANT.

GOAL: Using the three levels of prevention, negative health conditions are avoided, or promptly diagnosed and treated, and the fullest possible potential is restored.

PRIMARY PREVENTION		SECONDARY PREVENTION		TERTIARY PREVENTION		
Health Promotion and Education	*Health Protection*	*Early Diagnosis*	*Prompt Treatment*	*Rehabilitation*	*Primary Prevention*	
					Health Promotion and Education	*Health Protection*
• The pregnancy is planned • Pregnancies are spaced 2 years (or more) apart • Mother has a positive attitude going into the pregnancy • A health care provider is chosen • There are financial resources to meet the expanding family's needs • Family and significant others are supportive • Mother's weight is as close to ideal as possible before conception	• Parents do not use alcohol, tobacco, or other mood-altering substances when planning to conceive • The mother begins a vitamin regimen containing folic acid before the pregnancy	• The mother starts prenatal care early in the first trimester, and it is continuous	• The mother does not use alcohol, tobacco, or other mood-altering substances during the pregnancy • The mother takes a daily prenatal vitamin with folic acid • Parents avoid exposure to people with infectious disease • The mother has adequate nutrition, rest, sleep, and exercise • The mother begins supportive services if eligible (AFDC, WIC) • Family and significant others continue to be supportive • The parents attend labor preparation, infant care, and parenting classes • Names are selected for the infant • Delivery method and location are selected • The home is prepared for the infant—adequate infant furnishings and supplies are acquired within the parents' budget • Preparations and plans are made regarding breast or bottle feeding • A pediatrician or pediatric nurse practitioner is selected • An infant car seat is acquired • Plans are made to get to the chosen health care facility when in labor	• The parents and significant others begin to bond with the newborn • Parents get to know the newborn and establish a successful breast- or bottle-feeding routine • The infant returns home in an age-appropriate infant car seat, which is used properly whenever traveling • The infant's birth is celebrated according to cultural and religious preferences • Parents resume sexual intercourse using a family planning method of their choice • The parents enjoy the new life they have created	• Appointments are made and kept for postpartum and newborn visits to health care provider	• Exposure to people with infectious diseases is avoided • Infant immunization schedule begins on time and continues through childhood

Child Health Programs in their states and the services provided by the programs.

Program plans for maternal–infant populations across the country include many typical features. For example, there are concerted efforts to educate clients during the antepartum and postpartum periods and to assess their specific needs. A major focus of community health nurses is teaching. Nurses introduce new information or reinforce existing knowledge of pregnancy, delivery, and postpartum health considerations (Display 26–1). Through teaching, nurses help mothers to adapt to the physiologic and emotional changes they experience with pregnancy and to anticipate and plan for the impact their infants will have on their daily lives.

During the comprehensive, ongoing client assessments, in addition to considering their clients' physiologic and emotional status, nurses must assess the clients' social support systems, access to medical care, financial status, housing needs, and ability to provide for their babies. If clients need assistance in any or all of these areas, nurses must intervene and refer them to other appropriate community resources. Nurses often must serve as advocates for their clients in the referral process and should continue to work collaboratively with other professionals during follow-up services to meet clients' needs.

Types of Health Programs

Methods of delivering services vary based on the population and its specific needs. The geographic distribution of clients and the size of the nursing staff available to deliver the services also play significant roles. For example, in rural areas where clients are scattered over a large area, it may be appropriate to deliver services to the population on a one-to-one basis through nurse-run clinics (stationary or mobile) or home visits.

Clinic Programs

In the clinic setting, each client receives an individualized examination, immunizations, and health teaching. Because of time constraints placed on the nurse, the actual time spent in teaching clients is relatively short. Clinics may be effective on Native American reservations, where the population is centrally located, and on sites where migrant farm workers and their families are temporarily located.

A motor home, bus, or van converted to serve as a mobile clinic may be the resource needed in some rural or isolated areas that are populated by groups who experience physical barriers to health care services. Often, the community health nurse in a mobile health clinic provides routine prenatal, postpartum, and newborn care, including teaching

D I S P L A Y 2 6 – 1

Typical Features of Maternal–Infant Health Programs

I. Antepartum teaching
   A. Significance of prenatal care
   B. Self-responsibility
   C. Physiologic/emotional changes during pregnancy
   D. Fetal growth and development
   E. Nutrition
   F. Proper exercise
   G. Hazards of substance use: Drugs/alcohol/tobacco
   H. Breastfeeding techniques and problem solving
   I. Stages of labor
   J. Delivery—Process and options available
   K. Future birth control
II. Introduction to community resources for prenatal care
   A. Childbirth classes
   B. Self-help groups (pregnant teens, parents of twins, and so forth)
   C. WIC
   D. Department of Social Services
   E. Family planning services
   F. School-based clinics
   G. High-risk clinics
III. Postpartum teaching
   A. Newborn assessments
   B. Care of the newborn
   C. Growth and development of the infant

   D. Infant immunization schedule/health care follow-up
   E. Mother–infant bonding
   F. Postpartum physiologic changes in the mother
   G. Breast/bottle feeding techniques
   H. Postpartum health care follow-up
   I. Exercise to regain muscle tone
   J. Family planning
   K. Returning to work (balancing home, family, and work)
   L. Child care
IV. Delivery of services for prenatal/postnatal care
   A. Clinic/private health care provider visits
   B. Home visits
   C. Formal classes
   D. Emotional support
   E. Self-help groups
   F. Community education
V. Client advocacy and coordination with other community resources
   A. Physicians/nurse practitioners/nurse midwives
   B. Clinics
   C. Hospitals
   D. High schools
   E. Industries
   F. WIC
   G. Department of Social Services

and administering scheduled immunizations. These are much-needed services in some areas, and ones that cannot be provided as cost-effectively by other methods. The recommended immunization schedule for children, which starts in infancy, is discussed in detail in Chapter 27.

Home Visits

Home visits provide a one-to-one opportunity for the community health nurse to provide client teaching. There are two major benefits to home visits. First, the client is in the comfortable, familiar surroundings of her own home. Second, the nurse's assessment is enhanced by observations in the home setting of such things as family interactions, values, and priorities. Chapter 24 provides detailed information about how to make home visits.

Home visits to clients are costly for an agency. One-to-one delivery of service is becoming a luxury for some agencies with limited finances. In such agencies, the nurses provide most of the routine care in clinic or group settings. Home visits are made in the most serious of cases only. If clients are not at home at scheduled visit times and a visit must be rescheduled, this increases an already strained agency budget.

In metropolitan areas where community health nurses and clients are located near one another, nurse-run clinics and home visits may still be appropriate mechanisms for the delivery of services. In these cases, clients can visit the clinic frequently, and nurses can make more home visits with less distance to travel between clients. In addition, metropolitan areas afford community health nurses an opportunity to use a group approach with clients. This may include small, informal group discussions or larger, more formal classes. Whether small or large, groups can provide a vehicle for teaching by the nurse as well as a means for clients to teach and learn from one another. Group discussions can complement clinic and home visits and can be ongoing at both neighborhood clinics and Special Supplemental Food Program for Women, Infants, and Children (WIC) clinics.

Self-Help Groups

Self-help groups are usually formed by peers who have come together for mutual assistance to satisfy a common need, such as overcoming a handicap or life-disrupting problem. The group goal is to bring about specific desired behavior changes. Although many groups are formed by peers, the community health nurse can often facilitate the formation, function, and direction of the group. The nurse's role is that of facilitator.

Community health nurses should be familiar with the concept of self-help groups, because it is a concept that needs to be integrated consistently into community health nursing practice. The role of the nurse varies depending on the size, interests, and level of sophistication of the group. For example, with a group of well-educated women who are effective problem solvers, the nurse may initiate formation of the group and then serve primarily as a resource person. In contrast, if the group consists of adolescents, the nurse may need to be present at each meeting to facilitate group process and to clarify information shared within the group. In Chapter 11, group work is described in greater detail.

Self-help groups provide many benefits to participants. Within the present health care system, clients often express feelings of insignificance and loss of control. However, in a self-help group environment, individuals regain their sense of identity and control. Acceptance of responsibility for health-promoting behaviors is a key concept supported by the majority of self-help groups. Members who lose sight of their responsibility are readily confronted by the group. Individuals reach out to help other members and, in the process, help themselves to become better informed and stronger in their own beliefs.

Self-help groups have been successfully developed for the prenatal population to address common concerns such as prenatal changes, adapting to pregnancy, fetal growth and development, and labor and delivery. For postpartum women, groups have been established for breast-feeding mothers, mothers of infants, mothers of toddlers, and mothers of twins. In each instance, members of healthy populations help one another to remain healthy and prevent potential problems.

The term *peer counseling* is used in some settings for the self-help group process. For instance, in a high school, an informed and respected group of peers is identified and trained. These students then work with their classmates in small groups to discuss safe sex, saying no to drugs, self-esteem, conflict resolution, or teen parenting. The topics vary to meet the needs of the peers. The concept of peer counselor and self-help groups can be initiated by the innovative and creative community health nurse.

School-Based Programs

Delivery of maternal and child health care programs in the school setting has become more common over the last 2 decades. Many high schools offer special courses for pregnant teens, as well as at-home study programs after delivery, followed by on-site day care for the infants and toddlers. All of these services may be part of school-based programs. Some schools have initiated innovative programs that include additional health care services for their pregnant teens. This type of care may include family planning services, immunizations, and primary health care for illness and injury. Each community and school district needs to decide, in consultation with community health nurses, school nurses, community leaders, parents, teens, and the board of education, what services the community desires and needs.

High-Risk Clinics

High-risk clinics are established especially to meet the needs of women whose pregnancy is considered to be high risk. The risk may be related to a multiple pregnancy, a primipara client younger than 15 years or older than 40 years of age, a grand multipara client, hypertension, or GDM. The high-risk clinic is staffed by health care providers with special maternal–child health skills and advanced diagnostic equipment.

They see clients with a variety of conditions that might lead to fetal distress and therefore require special monitoring. In some communities, health care facilities have several types of high-risk clinics. Some see only teens or substance abusers. In smaller communities, there may be one high-risk clinic that meets the needs of all those experiencing a special pregnancy. A community health nurse often becomes involved in the referral to such clinics or may work in one as part of the job description in a small health department. The nurse needs to be knowledgeable about clinic services so potential clients can be referred if necessary.

Information Services

Providing safe and cost-effective prenatal and postpartum care is an increasing focus of the health care delivery system. Shortened hospital stays for childbirth and limited community health agency budgets affect the services available for new mothers and their families. Routine home visits are becoming rare and are reserved for high-risk families. Such conditions make a telephone service or health education center viable options.

A telephone line that is staffed by community health nurses can assess client concerns and link parents and professionals with information and community resources (Simonsen, 2001). Staffers of an information line can help parents adjust to the postpartum period, address concerns regarding infant care and nutrition, make referrals for home visits, provide information regarding services available within the larger system, and refer to other community agencies. Telephone lines can be specialized by using a bank of numbers on a touch-tone phone, and parents can get recorded information on such topics as breast feeding or other postpartum concerns. Other telephone lines can be answered by specialists in contact through a paging system (eg, lactation specialist) or by an on-call community health nurse who could make a home visit if needed. Parents often find these types of services reassuring, and health care practitioners find that they reduce the number of office visits for minor problems and thereby help to keep costs down.

The Kaiser Permanente Health Maintenance Organization system, the largest HMO in the country, uses such a method to assist clients in solving their health concerns. In addition to this service, they provide their members with a comprehensive *Healthwise Handbook,* and in each region they have a health education center where members can obtain written materials, videos, and information about classes and other programs (Kaiser Permanente, 2000).

Both types of services, telephone lines and handbooks, rely on clients' self-care capacity. Clients take the initiative to seek the information they need to optimize their health. Community health nurses can link clients to such services if they are available in the community. If they are not available, the community health nurse can help to establish such services in collaboration with public or private health care agencies. Such services can prove to be beneficial for all involved—client as well as health care provider.

Another form of information services was part of a 4-year project in Detroit. The program, called INREACH, was designed to meet the needs of maternal walk-ins (women who did not receive prenatal care from the hospital systems in which they delivered their infants or who received five or fewer prenatal visits) and their newborns, to provide them with a comprehensive needs assessment, and to link them with community-based agencies, such as substance abuse treatment or mental health treatment programs. INREACH nurses remained in contact with both the mother and the agency to which they were referred for 12 weeks to monitor effectiveness. More than 80% of the women were linked to an agency, and one third of this group remained with the agency for 12 weeks. Benefits of the program were many. It was influential in the development of health and social service policies at the local and state levels; agencies demonstrated more willingness to coordinate services and became open to adopting new approaches to client care; and participants, who had previously had negative experiences with the health care system, appreciated the caring interventions (McComish, Lawlor, & Laken, 1996).

The Community Health Nurse and Maternal–Infant Health

The maternal–child population makes up a major portion of a community health nurse's caseload. There is a need for commitment to excellence in service to this special aggregate within the community. The reality is that the future health of the nation lies within each woman who is pregnant. The challenges are great for the nurses who work with this vulnerable group. Three roles of the community health nurse are particularly important when working with the maternal–child population: (1) special professional qualities, (2) the role of educator, and (3) the role of client advocate and liaison with community resources. In addition, the community health nurse has an important role in the evaluation of maternal–infant health programs and as a facilitator to influence government policies for the maternal–infant population (see Voices From the Community III).

Special Professional Qualities

Nurses working with maternal–infant health populations require special qualities and education. It is recommended that nurses have the following qualifications:

1. A sound educational background with the minimum of a baccalaureate degree in nursing
2. A solid understanding of the nursing process and the ability to use it in working with individuals, families, and groups
3. Knowledge of and willingness to work with other community resources
4. Effective communication skills
5. Effective organizational and leadership skills
6. A sincere, nonjudgmental approach to clients

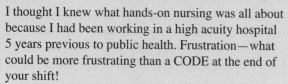

I thought I knew what hands-on nursing was all about because I had been working in a high acuity hospital 5 years previous to public health. Frustration—what could be more frustrating than a CODE at the end of your shift!

Upon entering my young pregnant client's home, armed with my college degree and prepared to teach her everything she needed to know in a very short time, I soon became frustrated and angry when not only were her blood sugars not coming down but she was not following my perfect 2400 calorie diabetic diet plan. She was frustrated too, thinking she was doing the right things for her baby. I conferred with her MD, and, after much deliberation, we came up with a diet plan to 'squeeze' out the fat in her current diet.

My next visit was to behold. I drove up to her home, left my starched, bleached nurse's jacket, stethoscope, charts, etc. in the car, rolled up my sleeves, sat my client on a stool in her kitchen, and began cooking class 101. I showed her how to cook her favorite foods in as healthy a manner as possible, including removing fat by washing the Mexican sausage under warm water after thoroughly cooking it and using a spray oil instead of lard when she made tortillas. I also kept my fingers crossed when I lifted the lid to a pot of steamed rice that I would not encounter any steamed bugs! Environmental health and safety principles were included in the cooking classes as well.

After several visits of cooking instruction, reinforcement of positive health changes, and encouragement, we noticed, together, a decrease in her blood sugars to the 150s from 200+. Needless to say, we were both highly pleased. The visits continued and focused on her gestational diabetes along with preparation for delivery and infant care. Her pregnancy proceeded without complications, and she delivered a healthy 8-lb baby at 38 weeks' gestation. She is early in a second pregnancy and maintaining good blood sugar levels using the techniques taught the year before. The foci of the visits with this pregnancy are broader because we have developed rapport, and because she had a healthy outcome with her first pregnancy, she is very interested in making changes to ensure success again.

Until I was a public health nurse, I had no clue what hands-on nursing and frustration were all about.

Barbara, RN, BSN, PHN
Public Health Nurse

Role of Educator

Because teaching is such an integral part of any maternal–infant program, nurses working in this area must possess good communication and teaching skills. For teaching to be effective, however, the content and methods must reflect the needs, characteristics, and developmental stage of each population. For example, when teaching nutrition to pregnant women, the nurse must alter the recommended calorie intake according to the woman's height and weight, age group, culture, and lifestyle. Nutrition information would be presented in one way to a group of college graduates who are already familiar with the basics of the Food Guide Pyramid and in another way to pregnant teens who need basic nutritional information.

In addition to tailoring subject matter to fit the client population, community health nurses should select teaching methodologies that are appropriate to the client group. Some groups such as couples attending childbirth education classes may respond positively to structured classes; others, such as teens, may prefer a less formal discussion format. Peer counseling and self-help support groups may be appropriate formats for clients who respond to the structure and support this format provides.

Teaching aids should be appropriate for each audience. It is important to remember that many of the available teaching aids are in English and depict white, middle-class women and infants. Although these are appropriate for some populations, not all people are able to identify with the mothers and babies portrayed. If possible, teaching aids should be congruent with the language, race, and culture of the population being served so that clients can understand and identify with them. For example, pamphlets on infant care need to be available in appropriate languages, with pictures portraying people from that cultural group who are using supplies and equipment available in all homes. Pamphlets that show infant room monitors, expensive educational toys, or fancy cribs with canopies may not depict the environment of the audience the nurse is trying to reach.

Teaching and motivating women to promote their own health and the health of their babies are major challenges, and there is no single correct way to approach the task. Community health nurses need to be innovative and creative in their approaches to teaching and to be aware that not all women are interested in their pregnancies. In Chapter 12, further information and resources, including appropriate teaching methods and materials for community health settings, are presented in more detail. In Chapter 11, the client with whom it is difficult to communicate is discussed.

Role of Client Advocate and Liaison With Community Resources

The maternal–infant population has complex needs. It is not unusual for community health nurses to see multiple personal and family problems in this group. Because community health nurses clearly cannot meet all needs of these clients, they must act as advocates in referring clients to other community resources. The nurse must have a working knowledge of available community resources for maternal–infant health, including family planning services, community childbirth education classes, resources available through the state Department of Social Services, and WIC, a federal program administered by the states. A clear understanding of the services available and a positive working relationship with agency personnel facilitate effective provision of services to this population.

Department of Social Services. The Department of Social Services assigns each family a trained social worker. After interviewing the family, the social worker determines whether the family or individual members of the family meet eligibility criteria for programs administered by the Department of Social Services, such as Medicaid (health insurance for low-income families), food stamps (a program to increase low-income families' buying power of most foods), and Aid to Families with Dependent Children (financial grants to low-income and unemployed families with dependent children for a combined lifetime limit of 5 years). If family or individual eligibility can be established, the social worker starts the process of applying for benefits. These benefits are essential for the basic survival of many families, and it may be the community health nurse who first identifies a family in need and makes the initial referral (see Bridging Financial Gaps).

Special Supplemental Food Program for Women, Infants, and Children. WIC is a federal program that provides nutrition education for low-income women and children and vouchers for the purchase of specific supplemental foods and infant formula. Pregnant, breast-feeding, and postpartum women, infants, and children up to 5 years of age who are at medical or nutritional risk are eligible. The food provided by the program helps pregnant women produce healthy, normal-birth-weight babies. WIC also refers participants to prenatal care, well-child care, and other services. Established in 1972 as a pilot program, WIC receives its funding from the Food and Nutrition Service of the U. S. Department of Agriculture.

Eligibility for WIC is based on income level, geographic area, and nutritional risk. Determining income eligibility is relatively uncomplicated, because guidelines are clearly defined by each state. Geographic eligibility varies because many states offer services in all areas whereas others do not. Clients must live in an area that has been designated to receive funding. Nutritional risk is determined by the nurse or nutritionist through interviews with individual clients and reviews of their previous medical and nutritional histories. Eligibility factors for pregnant or postpartum women include age (ie, adolescents or older than 40 years), poor obstetric history (eg, previous LBW infants, miscarriages, short periods between pregnancies, GDM), anemia, inappropriate weight gain (low or high), and inadequate consumption of food. Risk factors for infants and children include poor growth, anemia, obesity, chronic illness, and nutrition-related disease.

BRIDGING FINANCIAL GAPS

Today, when more than half the mothers in the country work, it is an important find to discover companies that are family-friendly. Such companies provide unique components that demonstrate their recognition of the financial and professional need for both parents to work. Below are samples of creative services some companies offer parents with infants and children. These companies are some of the 2002 awardees of the National Healthy Mothers, Healthy Babies Coalition's (HMHB) Workplace Models of Excellence.

COMPANY	FAMILY/FINANCIALLY FRIENDLY SERVICES
Wendy's International, Inc.	Full-time employees with 1 year of service are eligible for financial assistance and paid leave of absence for the adoption of a child.
Sigma-Tau Pharmaceuticals, Inc.	This pharmaceutical company pays for information and testing kits for screening for metabolic disorders in employees' newborns.
Highmark, Inc.	This health insurance products and services company has created a center for grieving children, adolescents, and their families. Children come to The Caring Place and benefit from age-specific groups.
Fannie Mae	This nationwide mortgage lender has a corporate culture that supports breast-feeding among its female employees or partners of employees. It includes equipped lactation rooms, and personal breast-feeding consultations with weekly on-site office hours. Their committment to family also includes 10 weeks of paid maternity leave.
Sears, Roebuck and Co.	Pays for up to 50% of neighborhood child care costs for employees who want culturally appropriate caregiving in their neighborhood as Sears attempts to find workable child care solutions.

Based on these risk factors, the health professional identifies areas of strength and areas for change. The program then offers supplemental food to clients. The food offered contains high-quality protein, iron, calcium, and vitamins A and C. The specific foods offered tend to be combinations of fruit juice fortified with vitamin C, eggs, milk (low-fat or whole), cheese, beans, fortified cereals, and fortified infant formula. Distribution of food varies. In some states, local dairies deliver the food to the home; in other states, clients receive vouchers and exchange them for food at local grocery stores. The WIC program reevaluates clients at predetermined intervals. It reassesses needs, continues nutrition education, and recertifies food distribution if appropriate.

Family Planning Services. Family planning may be an integral part of the comprehensive services of a local health department or community clinic, or specialized services may be provided by separate organizations such as Planned Parenthood. Depending on the prevailing attitudes and needs in the community, family planning services may include teen counseling, abortions, and long-term family planning methods (eg, Depo-Provera injections, Norplant inserts). Family planning service agencies provide counseling, gynecologic examinations that include Pap smears, breast examinations, and mammograms. Some agencies provide a broader range of services for which there is a need, such as genetic counseling, infertility counseling, or diagnosis and treatment of problems related to male and female sexual dysfunction.

Childbirth Education Classes. Most community clinics or health departments that provide maternal–child health care services also hold childbirth education classes. However, many community groups, such as religious centers, YWCAs, and hospitals, develop and provide their own classes. If the agency for which the nurse is working does not provide such a service, it is the nurse's responsibility to be aware of community resources and refer interested women and their significant others to childbirth education classes. Women find these classes very helpful in preparing for the birthing experience and the demands of parenthood. Group support from other pregnant women in the class is also rewarding. For childbirth education classes to be useful, they must be accessible; this means they must be held at convenient times and locations. For some clients, the availability of public transportation is a factor in accessing classes.

Evaluation of Maternal–Infant Health Programs

Evaluation is a critical aspect of maternal–infant health program planning, as it is with any health planning. Four questions in particular should be addressed: (1) Did the program meet the identified needs of this particular population? (2) Did the program meet its goals and objectives? (3) Was the program cost-effective, or did the outcomes justify the resources used? and (4) What was the program's long-term impact on the health of this population?

Community health nurses find the answers to these questions through a carefully designed, systematic evaluation plan. Program evaluation is discussed in detail in Chapter 19. For the purposes of this chapter, three useful methods for obtaining evaluation data are examined.

Vital statistics provide an important database for evaluating maternal–infant programs. Local, state, or national figures can help agency personnel determine whether their own statistics are improving, remaining constant, or worsening. Using vital statistics, nurses can make comparisons between or within population groups. For instance, they might compare the incidence of LBW babies born to their clients with rates reported by similar agencies in other urban areas or the rates for their own agencies in previous years. One disadvantage of using vital statistics is that the time required to compile these data can make it difficult to have the most current figures.

A second mechanism for evaluation within individual maternal–infant programs is measuring quality through performance improvement programs. Such programs are used by health care agencies to monitor and maintain or improve delivery of service and care to clients. The quality management and improvement process looks at maternal–infant program goals and raises questions such as the following:

How soon after receiving the referral were clients seen?
Was the database complete?
Was the plan of care appropriate?
Were the established outcomes reasonable and achievable?
Were clients involved in the planning process?
Were appropriate referrals made?
Was there follow-up on the referrals?
Was discharge of the client appropriate?

Quality management systems use various methods to gather this type of information, such as feedback from clients through periodic questionnaires and personal interviews or telephone surveys. Disadvantages of these methods include the time consumed, the expense for the agency, and the questionable reliability of self-reported feedback rather than more objective data obtained from client records and health outcomes. Chapter 15 discusses quality management and improvement and the role of the nurse in more detail.

Finally, a cost-effective mechanism for assessing a program and the client care delivered is auditing of client records. It is not feasible for an agency to review every client record, but random sampling can be done at predetermined times each year. If clearly defined criteria are established, those conducting the audit can easily review a record and determine, in their professional judgment, whether the criteria have been met. Auditing client records can be a positive learning experience, and agency staff should be encouraged to participate in the process. Reading through another nurse's documentation can be a positive reminder of the impact that the community health nurse has on the effectiveness of services delivered.

Role as Facilitator to Influence Government Policies

Another responsibility of the nurse in maternal–infant health programs is the role of client advocate. This is done for clients at the local level on a daily basis; however, changes are often needed at the state or federal level. The community health nurse can influence legislation and policies that affect the services provided at the local level. Funding of maternal–child programs occurs through actions of the state legislature. By giving testimony on behalf of the maternal–infant population, the community health nurse can attest to the needs of this population and promote the funding of additional programs at the local level. However, this takes time; meanwhile, funding may dwindle and other sources must be found.

The role of facilitator may include writing grants to obtain funding for new projects or to maintain existing programs. Writing grants and getting them funded is becoming an important skill of nurses in agencies that are experiencing fiscal constraints. Public and private grants, both large and small, can supplement shrinking state support. Limited funding and increasing client needs will continue into the 21st century, and the programs provided through local agencies may depend on grant monies generated by proposals written by community health nurses.

SUMMARY

Global and national vital statistics indicate that the status of maternal–infant health in the world has improved but is still of major concern. Significant numbers of pregnancies are unplanned, and unwanted children are born to families already burdened by multiple socioeconomic stressors. The vital statistics for the maternal–infant population in the United States leave room for improvement in comparison with those of other industrialized nations. Both the knowledge and the resources to improve the quality of life for mothers and babies are available in this country. However, the issues and importance of maternal–infant well-being extend beyond the borders of any single country.

Factors influencing the health of pregnant women and infants may be related to their obstetric history, genetics, socioeconomic status, or lifestyle choices. The latter category is a prime target for community health nursing intervention. Lifestyle-related factors that influence the health status of

pregnant women and infants include use of illicit drugs, alcohol, or tobacco; presence of STDs, HIV/AIDS, or other infectious diseases during pregnancy; and weight gain during pregnancy. Pregnancy during adolescence, especially early adolescence, adds additional risk. Emotional, physical, and social needs of pregnant teens require special consideration. In addition, the special circumstances caused by hypertensive disease in pregnancy, GDM, developmental disability, postpartum depression, and fetal or infant death can be addressed through community health nursing intervention.

In planning effective maternal–infant programs, community health nurses must consider needs identified by the populations themselves as well as vital statistics. Maternal–infant programs across the country have certain features in common, including perinatal follow-up and teaching, client assessment, service delivery, coordination with other community resources, and client advocacy. These common features assist community health nurses in designing maternal–infant programs. Two other planning considerations include specific needs identified through data and client input and the developmental stage of the population being served.

Creative and innovative methods of implementation, such as discussion and self-help groups, should be used more widely for teaching and working with maternal–infant populations. Effective implementation of health programs also depends on having appropriately qualified staff members. The nature of the maternal–infant population is complex and diverse; the community health nurse must be appropriately prepared with highly developed professional skills and knowledge and use of community resources.

To evaluate the effectiveness of maternal–infant health programs, the community health nurse needs to ask the following questions: (1) Was the program relevant? (2) Did it meet identified goals and objectives? (3) Was it cost-effective? and (4) What was its long-term impact on the health of the population of mothers and infants? Three methods for obtaining evaluation data are collection of vital statistics, use of quality management processes, and use of the auditing process.

There is an increased need for the community health nurse to influence government policies and funding at the local level. More often, the nurse is called on to acquire grant funding to maintain or promote needed programs that were once automatically funded. The development of programs to serve complex client needs may also fall to the community health nurse.

ACTIVITIES TO PROMOTE CRITICAL THINKING

1. What specific objectives has your local health department developed for mothers and infants to help achieve the goals listed in the U.S. *Healthy People 2010* document? How do your county's statistics compare with those of others in your state on (1) infant death rates (collectively and by specific ethnic groups [eg, Asian, African-American, white, Hispanic]), (2) incidence of LBW and VLBW infants, and (3) incidence of birth defects?

2. Describe three different maternal–infant populations in your county. What are their most pressing health needs? Do any existing services target these populations? How well, in your judgment, are clients' needs being met? Interview a city or county community health nurse and other public health professionals to help you find answers.

3. Select one lifestyle-related factor that affects pregnant women and infants (eg, use of drugs, alcohol, or tobacco; nutritional status) and design a health program to deal with it. Be sure to include the main factors discussed in this chapter for planning and evaluating a maternal–infant program.

4. Sonia, an 18-year-old woman, is single and 14 weeks pregnant. Her first prenatal visit was made at the urging of her aunt, who uses the clinic. Sonia reluctantly admitted to the clinic nurse that the pregnancy was unplanned. She consumes alcohol two to three times a week, frequently as much as six 12-oz cans of beer and 16 oz of wine, and she smokes one pack of cigarettes a day. She has tried a variety of street drugs in the last 3 months but does not use any regularly. The clinic nurse believed that Sonia might not return for regular prenatal care and made a referral to the community health nurse for follow-up home visits to assess Sonia's home environment and teach prenatal care and preparation for the infant. You have been given the case. Design a plan of care to address Sonia's needs. What specific services and programs might you recommend? What barriers might exist? How would the prenatal and postpartum teaching delivered to Sonia differ from care needed by other single teens?

5. Use the Internet to locate international maternal–infant vital statistics. In which countries are the statistics the worst? In which countries are the statistics the best? What do you think accounts for these dramatic differences? What do you know about each group of countries that may account for the differences (eg, economic level, type of government, overall physical environment)? What activities could a community health nurse become involved in within the countries with the worst statistics to help to improve them?

REFERENCES

Alexander, G.R., & Kotelchuck, M. (2001). Assessing the role and effectiveness of prenatal care: History, challenges, and directions for future research. *Public Health Reports, 116,* 306–316.

Annas, G.J., & Grodin, M.A. (1998). Human rights and maternal–fetal HIV transmission prevention trials in Africa. *American Journal of Public Health, 88*(4), 560–563.

Armstrong, M.A., Osejo, V.G., Lieberman, L., Carpenter, D.M., Pantoja, P.M., & Escobar, G.J. (2003). Perinatal substance abuse intervention in obstetric clinics decreases adverse neonatal outcomes. *Journal of Perinatology, 23,* 3–9.

Barr, H.M., & Streissguth, A.P. (2001). Identifying maternal self-reported alcohol use associated with fetal alcohol spectrum disorders. *Alcoholism: Clinical and Experimental Research, 25*(2), 283–287.

Barrio, L.M., & Burt, V.K. (2000). Depression in pregnancy: Strategies for primary care management. *Women's Health in Primary Care, 3*(7), 490–498.

Bassett, M.T. (2001). Keeping the M in MTCT: Women, mothers, and HIV prevention. *American Journal of Public Health, 91*(5), 701–703.

Beck, C.T. (1996). Postpartum depressed mothers' experiences interacting with their children. *Nursing Research, 45*(2), 98–104.

Beck, C.T. (2002). Predictors of postpartum depression: An update. *Nursing Research 59*(5), 275–285.

Beck, C.T., & Gable, R.K. (2001). Further validation of the postpartum depression screening scale. *Nursing Research 50*(3), 155–164.

Blizzard, L., Ponsonby, A., Dwyer, T., Venn, A., & Cochrane, J.A. (2003). Parental smoking and infant respiratory infection: How important is not smoking in the same room with the baby? *American Journal of Public Health, 93*(3), 482–488.

Britton, G.A. (1998). A review of women and tobacco: Have we come such a long way? *Journal of Obstetric, Gynecologic, and Neonatal Nursing, 27,* 241–249.

Brown, J. E., Murtaugh, M. A., Jacobs, D. R. Jr., & Margellos, H. C. (2002). Variation in newborn size according to pregnancy weight change by trimester. *American Journal of Clinical Nutrition, 76*(1), 205–209.

Centers for Disease Control and Prevention. (2003, February 20). *CDC reports pregnancy-related deaths still higher in black women than white women* [Press release]. Atlanta, GA: Author.

Chasnoff, I.J., Neuman, K., Thornton, C., & Callaghan, M.A. (2001). Screening for substance use in pregnancy: A practical approach for the primary care physician. *American Journal of Obstetrics and Gynecology, 184,* 752–758.

De-Kun, L., Petitti, D.B., Willinger, M., McMahon, R., Odouli, R., Vu, H., et al. (2003). Infant sleeping position and the risk of sudden infant death syndrome in California, 1997–2000. *American Journal of Epidemiology, 157*(5), 446–455.

Dreyfuss, M.L., Msamanga, G.I., Spiegelman, D., Hunter, D.J., Urassa, E.J.N., Hertzmark, E., et al. (2001). Determinants of low birth weight among HIV-infected pregnant women in Tanzania. *American Journal of Clinical Nutrition, 74,* 814–826.

Duncan, C. (2002). Smoking and pregnancy: An update. *Women and Reproductive Nutrition Report, 3*(2), 1–3.

Erikson, E.H. (1968). *Identity, youth, and crisis.* New York: Norton.

Flynn, L. (1999). The adolescent parenting program: Improving outcomes through mentorship. *Public Health Nursing, 16*(3), 182–189.

Garovic, V.D. (2000). Hypertension in pregnancy: Diagnosis and treatment. *Mayo Clinic Proceedings, 75,* 1071–1076.

Goldenberg, R.L., Iams, J.D., Mercer, B.M., Meis, P.J., Moawad, A.H., & Copper, R.L. (1998). The preterm prediction study: The value of new vs standard risk factors in predicting early and all spontaneous preterm births. *American Journal of Public Health, 88*(2), 233–238.

Hankin, J., McCaul, M. E., & Heussner, J. (2000). Pregnant, alcohol-abusing women. *Alcoholism: Clinical and Experimental Research, 24,* 1276–1286.

Health Connection. (1994). *The vegetarian food pyramid.* Hagerstown, MD: Author.

Howell, E.M., & Chasnoff, I.J. (1999). Perinatal substance abuse treatment: Findings from focus groups with clients and providers. *Journal of Substance Abuse Treatment, 17*(1–2), 139–148.

Jolly, M.C., Sebire, N., Harris, J., Robinson, S., & Regan, L. (2000). Obstetric risks of pregnancy in women less than 18 years old. *Obstetrics & Gynecology, 96*(6), 962–966.

Kaiser Permanente. (2000). *Healthwise Handbook: A self-care guide for you and your family.* Boise, ID: Healthwise Publications.

Kaskutas, L.A. (2000). Understanding drinking during pregnancy among urban American Indians and African Americans: Health messages, risk beliefs, and how we measure consumption. *Alcoholism: Clinical and Experimental Research, 24*(8), 1241–1250.

Koniack-Griffin, D., Anderson, N.L.R., Brecht, M.L, Verzemnieks, I., Lesser, J., & Kim, S. (2002). Public health nursing care for adolescent mothers: Impact on infant health and selected maternal outcomes at 1 year postbirth. *Journal of Adolescent Health, 30,* 44–54.

Koniack-Griffin, D., Anderson, N.L.R., Verzemnieks, I., & Brecht, M.L. (2000). A public health nursing early intervention program for adolescent mothers: Outcomes from pregnancy through 6 weeks postpartum. *Nursing Research, 49,* 130–138.

Koniack-Griffin, D., Verzemnieks, I.L., Anderson, N.L.R., Brecht, M.L., Lesser, J., Kim, S., et al. (2003). Nurse visitation for adolescent mothers: Two-year infant health and maternal outcomes. *Nursing Research, 52*(2), 127–136.

MacDorman, M.F., Minino, A.M., Strobino, D.M., & Guyer, B. (2002). Annual summary of vital statistics–2001. *Pediatrics, 110*(6), 1037–1052.

March of Dimes. (2003). Professionals and researchers quick reference and fact sheets. Retrieved January 10, 2004, from *http://www.marchofdimes.com/professionals/681_1169.asp*

McComish, J.F., Lawlor, L.A., & Laken, M.P. (1996). INREACH: Linking walk-ins and their infants to community-based care. *MCN: American Journal of Maternal Child Nursing, 21,* 132–136.

Minkoff, H. (2003). Human immunodeficiency virus infection in pregnancy. *Obstetrics and Gynecology, 101*(4), 797–810.

Mondestin, M.A.J., Ananth, C.V., Smulian, J.C., & Vintzileos, A.M. (2002). Birth weight and fetal death in the United States: The effect of maternal diabetes during pregnancy. *American Journal of Obstetrics and Gynecology, 187,* 922–926.

Olds, D.L., Henderson, C.R., Kitzman, H.J., Eckenrode, J.J., Cole, R.E., & Tatelbaum, R.C. (1999). Prenatal and infancy home visitation by nurses: Recent findings. *Future of Children, 9*(1), 44–65.

Olds, D., Hill, P., Robinson, J., Song, N., & Little, C. (2000). Update on home visiting for pregnant women and parents of young children. *Current Problems in Pediatrics, 30,* 109–141.

Piaget, J. (1950). *The psychology of intelligence.* London: Routledge & Kegan Paul.

Sherwen, L.N., Scoloveno, M.A., & Weingarten, C.T. (2001). *Media edition of maternity nursing: Care of the childbearing family* (3rd ed.). Upper Saddle River, NJ: Prentice–Hall.

Simonsen, S.M. (2001). *Telephone health assessment: Guidelines for practice.* Stamford, CT: Appleton Lange.

Singer, L.T., Arendt, R., Minnes, S., Salvator, A., Siegel, A.C., & Lewis, B.A. (2001). Developing language skills of cocaine-exposed infants. *Pediatrics, 107*(5), 1057–1064.

Southwick, K.L., Guidry, H.M., Weldon, M.M., Mert, K.J., Berman, S.M., & Levine, W.C. (1999). An epidemic of congenital syphilis in Jefferson County, Texas, 1994–1995: Inadequate prenatal syphilis testing after an outbreak in adults. *American Journal of Public Health, 89*(4), 557–560.

United States Census Bureau. (1999). *Statistical abstract of the United States, 1999* (119th ed.). Washington, DC: Author.

United States Department of Agriculture. (1992). *The food guide pyramid.* Washington, DC: Author.

United States Department of Health and Human Services. (2000). *Healthy people 2010* (Conference ed., Vols. 1 & 2). Washington, DC: U. S. Government Printing Office.

Venes, D., & Thomas, C.K. (Eds.). (2001). *Taber's cyclopedic medical dictionary* (19th ed.). Philadelphia: F.A. Davis.

Watkins, M.L., Rasmussen, S.A., Honein, M.A., Botto, L.D., & Moore, C.A. (2003). Maternal obesity and risk for birth defects. *Pediatrics, 111,* 1152–1158.

Weber, M.K., Floyd, R.L., Riley, E.P., & Snider, D.E. (2002, September 20). National task force on fetal alcohol syndrome and fetal alcohol effect: Defining the national agenda for fetal alcohol syndrome and other prenatal alcohol-related effects. *MMWR: Morbidity and Mortality Weekly Report, 51*(RR14), 9–12.

Wingood, G.M., & DiClemente, R.J. (2002). *Handbook of women's sexual and reproductive health.* Norwell, MA: Kluwer Plenum.

World Health Organization. (1998). *The world health report, 1998: Life in the 21st century—a vision for all.* Geneva: Author.

World Health Organization. (2000, December 5). Making pregnancy safer. EB107/26. Geneva: Author.

World Health Organization. (2001). Maternal mortality in 1995: Estimates developed by WHO, UNICEF, UNFPA. Retrieved January 10, 2004, from *http:/www.who.int/reproductive-health/publications/ Abstracts/maternal_mortality_1995.html*

SELECTED READINGS

Alexander, G.R., Kogan, M.D., & Nabukera, S. (2002). Racial differences in prenatal care use in the United States: Are disparities decreasing? *American Journal of Public Health, 92*(12), 1970–1975.

Beckwith, J.B. (2003). Defining the sudden infant death syndrome. *Archives of Pediatrics and Adolescent Medicine, 157*, 286–290.

Callister, L.C. (2001). Culturally competent care of women and newborns: Knowledge, attitude, and skills. *Journal of Obstetric, Gynecologic, and Neonatal Nursing, 30*(2), 209–215.

Dodgson, J.E., Duckett, L., Garwick, A., & Graham, B.L. (2002). An ecological perspective of breastfeeding in an indigenous community. *Journal of Nursing Scholarship, 34*, 235–241.

Ferrence, R., Pope, M., Room, R., & Slade, J. (Eds.). (2000). *Nicotine and public health.* Washington, DC: American Public Health Association.

Franko, D.L., Blais, M.A., Becker, A.E., Delinsky, S.S., Greenwood, D.N., Flores, A.T., et al. (2001). Pregnancy complications and neonatal outcomes in women with eating disorders. *American Journal of Psychiatry, 158*(9), 1461–1466.

Goodburn, E., & Campbell, O. (2001). Reducing maternal mortality in the developing world: Sector-wide approaches may be the key. *British Medical Journal, 322*, 917–920.

Haider, R., Ashworth, A., Kabir, I., & Huttly, S.R.A. (2000). Effect of community-based peer counselors on exclusive breastfeeding practices in Dhaka, Bangladesh: A randomized controlled trial, *The Lancet, 356*, 1643–1647.

Hall, R.T., Mercer, A.M., Teasley, S.L., McPereson, D.M., Simon, S.D., Santos, S.R., et al. (2002). A breast-feeding assessment score to evaluate the risk for cessation of breast-feeding by 7 to 10 days of age. *Journal of Pediatrics, 141*, 659–664.

Holditch-Davis, D., Miles, M.S., Burchinal, M., O'Donnell, K., McKinney, R., & Lim, W. (2001). Parental caregiving and developmental outcomes of infants of mothers with HIV. *Nursing Research, 50*(1), 5–14.

Lester, B.M., LaGasse, L., Seifer, R., Tronick, E.Z., Bauer, C.R., Shankaran, S., et al. (2003). The Maternal Lifestyle Study (MLS): Effects of prenatal cocaine and/or opiate exposure on auditory brain response at one month. *The Journal of Pediatrics, 142*, 279–285.

Li, R., Ogden, C., Ballew, C., Gillespie, C., & Grummer-Strawn, L. (2002). Prevalence of exclusive breastfeeding among U. S. infants: The third national health and nutrition examination survey (phase II, 1991–1994). *American Journal of Public Health, 92*(7), 1107–1110.

MacLean, L.M., Estable, A., Sims-Jones, N., & Edwards, N. (2002). Concurrent transitions in smoking status and maternal role. *Journal of Nursing Scholarship, 34*(1), 39–40.

Malloy, M.H. (2002). Trends in postneonatal aspiration deaths and reclassification of sudden infant death syndrome: Impact of the "Back to Sleep" program. *Pediatrics, 109*(4), 661–665.

McCormick, M.C., Deal, L., Devaney, B.L., Chu, D., Moreno, L., & Raykovich, K.T. (2001). The impact on clients of a community-based infant mortality reduction program: The national healthy start program survey of postpartum women. *American Journal of Public Health, 91*(12), 1975–1977.

Olds, D.L., Robinson, J., O'Brien, R., Luckey, W., Pettitt, L.M., Henderson, C.R., et al. (2002). Home visiting by paraprofessionals and by nurses: A randomized, controlled trial. *Pediatrics, 110*(3), 486–496.

Pollack, H., Lantz, M., & Frohna, J.G. (2000). Maternal smoking and adverse birth outcomes among singletons and twins. *American Journal of Public Health, 90*(3), 395–400.

Rasinski, K.A., Kuby, A., Bzdusek, S.A., Silvestri, J.M., & Weese-Mayer, D.S. (2003). Effect of a sudden infant death syndrome risk reduction education program on risk factor compliance and information sources in primarily black urban communities. *Pediatrics, 111*(4), e347–e354.

Ryan, A.S., Wenjun, Z., & Acosta, A. (2002). Breastfeeding continues to increase into the new millennium. *Pediatrics, 110*(6), 1103–1109.

Vintzileos, A.M., Ananth, C.V., Smulian, J.C., Scorza, W.E., & Knuppel, R.A. (2002), The impact of prenatal care in the United States on preterm births in the presence and absence of antenatal high-risk conditions. *American Journal of Obstetrics & Gynecology, 187*, 1254–1257.

Willinger, M., Ko, C.W., Hoffman, H.J., Kessler, R.C., & Corwin, M.J. (2003). Trends in infant bed sharing in the United States, 1993–2000: The National Infant Sleep Position Study. *Archives of Pediatrics and Adolescent Medicine, 157*, 43–49.

Internet Resources

Alcoholics Anonymous (AA): *http://www.aa.org*

Child Welfare League of America: *http://www.cwla.org*

National Council on Alcoholism and Drug Dependence: *http://www.ncadd.org*

National Institute on Alcohol Abuse and Alcoholism: *http://www.niaaa.nih.gov*

National Network for Child Care Health and Safety: *http://www.nncc.org/health/health.safe.page.html*

National Organization on Fetal Alcohol Syndrome: *http://www.nofas.org*

The National Healthy Mothers, Healthy Babies Coalition (HMHB): *http://www.hmhb.org*

27

Infants, Toddlers, and Preschoolers

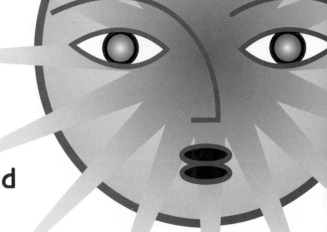

Learning Objectives

Upon mastery of this chapter, you should be able to:

- Identify the changing demographics found in the infant, toddler, and preschool populations.

- Identify major health problems and concerns for infant, toddler, and preschool populations globally and in the United States.

- Describe a variety of programs that promote and protect health and prevent illness and injury of infant, toddler, and preschool populations.

- State the recommended immunization schedule for infants and children, and give the rationale for the timing of each immunization.

- Give examples of methods the community health nurse might use in working with infants, toddlers, and preschool populations to help promote their health.

Healthy children are a vital resource to ensure the future well-being of a nation. They are the parents, workers, leaders, and decision makers of tomorrow, and their health and safety depend on today's decisions and actions. Their futures lie in the hands of those people responsible for their well-being, including the community health nurse.

The well-being of children has been a subject of great concern globally and in this country for many years. In the United States, its importance has been emphasized through development of numerous laws and services, yet the needs of millions of children continue to go unmet. Many young children often go to bed hungry. Some infants and toddlers do not receive even the most basic immunizations before they reach school age. Accidents and injuries are a leading cause of death. Preventable communicable diseases increase mortality among the very young. For a country that leads in many areas, including technology, business, agriculture, and education, the failure to protect and promote the health of its youngest citizens is a blemish that must not be ignored. In many other nations, infant health and well-being are in even greater jeopardy.

This chapter explores the global needs of and related services available for the youngest and most vulnerable of society's members. Health services that are commonly available in the United States for infants, toddlers, and the preschool population are examined, and the role of the community health nurse in providing those services is explored.

GLOBAL VIEW OF INFANT, TODDLER, AND PRESCHOOL HEALTH

The health of children in one country can affect that of children in other countries, including the United States. Infants and young children travel internationally with their parents. Refugees cross the borders of other countries in an attempt to escape intolerable political changes. Major natural disasters place whole populations at risk, especially the very young and the very old. Examples include the nationwide flooding in Mozambique during the winter and spring of 2000, earthquakes that occurred in Turkey in 2002, and the severe acute respiratory syndrome (SARS) epidemic in 2003. It behooves each country to consider these facts and do what is necessary to promote and protect the health of children worldwide. A review of changing demographics and the current health status of the world's infants, toddlers, and preschool-aged children provides a more complete picture of where we came from, where we are, and what we still need to accomplish.

Global History of Children's Health Care

Only recently in the history of the world have children been considered valuable assets, even in countries where there are now well-developed programs of infant health promotion and protection, infant and child day care services, and strict educational expectations for all children. In some countries today, however, female infants and children are not valued. They may be sold to another family or prevented from going to school to get an education. Some countries such as China limit population growth, and couples are allowed to raise only one child. Subsequent pregnancies are forbidden, and termination is encouraged. In some cultures, a child born with a congenital anomaly is not treated. Some birth, growth, and developmental rituals are harsh and would be considered illegal if judged by Western laws. Cultural practices that are fostered by political forces prevent many countries from improving the health of infants and young children.

In many developing countries, the health care system is one of superstition and faith, as was true in colonial America (Spector, 2000). In the United States, the system is presently "predicated on strong scientific beliefs; the epidemiological model of disease; highly developed technology; and strong values of individuality, competition, and free enterprise" (Spector, 2000, p. 51). Many other countries follow a similar pattern in their approach to health care.

Countries burdened with political unrest, poverty, and a lack or political misuse of natural resources have elevated numbers of low-birth-weight infants. Low birth weight is associated with an elevated risk of infant mortality, congenital malformations, and other physical and neurologic impairments (Cooke, 2003; Valanis, 1999). The most developed countries tend to have the lowest infant mortality rates, yet even in these countries, infants and young children are not always provided with the services they need (Display 27–1).

Demographics

Spectacular global improvements in infant and child health have occurred in the past 50 years and are likely to continue into the new millennium (World Health Organization [WHO], 2002). For example, in 1955, one in five children died before their fifth birthday—a total of 20.6 million deaths. By 1995, the death rate had fallen to less than half that rate, and it is projected to decline to 3.5 children per 100 by 2025 (WHO, 2002).

When tracking global morbidity and mortality trends of the infant-through-preschool population over the past 50 years, three dimensions of health development must be taken into account:

- Each country's epidemiologic patterns of disease and deficiencies
- Social, economic, and health infrastructure of the country
- Priority strategies and adequacy of the actions taken to address the preventable and treatable causes of death and illness in infants and children

Quality of family living conditions, prevalence and mode of transmission of infectious disease agents, and nutritional status of the child are among the strongest immediate determinants that affect mortality rates in children younger

DISPLAY 27-1

Countries With the Lowest Infant Mortality Rates, 2002	
Country	**Rate (per 1,000 live births)**
Iceland	2.3
Sweden	3.5
Norway	4.1
Finland	4.2
Luxembourg	4.2
Austria	4.8
Switzerland	4.8
France	5.0
Netherlands	5.1
Hong Kong	5.1
Denmark	5.2
Australia	5.3
Italy	5.5
Spain	5.5
Israel	5.8
United Kingdom	5.9
Belgium	6.0
Germany	6.0
Canada	6.1
Ireland	6.2
Greece	6.3
United States	7.1

(From Population Reference Bureau. [2002]. *World population data sheet*. Available at: *http://www.prb.org*.)

than 5 years of age. Significant improvement in at least one, but preferably all three, of these factors is required to produce a substantial overall decline in the rates. For example, the decline in deaths among the population younger than 5 years of age in developed countries since the late 1940s is largely attributable to improved sanitation, safe water supply, secure housing, adequate food supply and distribution, and general hygiene. Various childhood diseases such as diphtheria, scarlet fever, and rheumatic heart disease were in steady decline long before immunizations and antibiotics became widely available.

In most developing countries, general improvements in sanitation, water supplies, education, and access to preventive and curative health care have led to declines in childhood mortality similar to those seen in the Western industrialized countries 50 to 80 years ago. Progress in these countries has been comparatively more rapid, because of the lessons learned from the experience in other nations and improved technologies for disease prevention and treatment, nutrition, and fertility management.

Unfortunately, progress is not rapid in all countries. In the least developed countries, progress either has not been made or has not been sustained over the years. In a few re-gions, child mortality levels are as high as 15% of live births; examples include the western Sahara, where progress in child health is almost 50 years behind.

Health Status

In the poorest of countries, infants and young children are most vulnerable. They frequently die of diarrhea, acute lower respiratory tract infections, measles, tuberculosis, or pertussis. In the morbidity associated with these diseases, malnutrition is a significant factor. "Weight is a contributing factor in 60% of all child deaths in developing countries" (WHO, 2002). WHO estimates that approximately 27% of all children younger than 5 years of age are underweight, a condition that caused an estimated 3.4 million deaths in 2000 (WHO, 2002). Although childhood mortality rates have markedly decreased in most countries since the early 1900s, morbidity rates remain high (Fig. 27–1).

The most common types of acute conditions seen in the United States are respiratory illnesses (which account for the largest group), infectious and parasitic diseases, injuries, and digestive diseases (U. S. Department of Health and Human Services [USDHHS], 2000).

Other childhood health problems, less easy to detect and measure but often as debilitating, are those of emotional, behavioral, and intellectual development. Although these problems are not new, awareness and concern for them have increased as the rates of occurrence for infectious diseases such as measles, mumps, rubella, and polio have diminished. Emotional disorders are prevalent, and "it is estimated that 20% of children and adolescents may have a diagnosable mental, emotional, or behavioral problem that can lead to school failure, alcohol or other drug use, violence, or suicide" (Centers for Disease Control and Prevention [CDC], 2002). The roots of these problems are often traced to the toddler and preschool years. For example, studies have found an association between learning disorders in children and violent behavior in adolescents and adults (Barkley et al., 2002; Kendall et al., 2003).

Causes of learning disorders and emotional and behavioral problems appear to have genetic and environmental influences. Increased use of illicit drugs by pregnant women has produced a generation of children with developmental delays and learning disabilities (Butz et al., 1998). Childhood disabilities caused by parental drug use have surpassed those caused by lead poisoning, another major contributor to developmental problems in children.

In the United States, 21% of children live below the poverty level compared with 11% of adults (U. S. Census Bureau, 2000). Because many poor adults have more than two children, the total number of children who are poor is greater than the number of poor adults. Single parents also contribute to this number, as may cultural factors. For example, it is traditional in Southeast Asian, northern Laotian, and Hmong cultures for teenage girls to marry as young as 15 or 16 years of age to young men in their late teens. Fam-

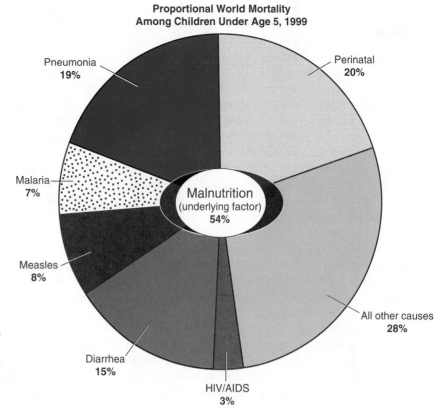

**Proportional World Mortality
Among Children Under Age 5, 1999**

Perinatal
20%

Pneumonia
19%

Malaria
7%

Malnutrition
(underlying factor)
54%

All other causes
28%

Measles
8%

Diarrhea
15%

HIV/AIDS
3%

FIGURE 27–1. Proportional world mortality among children under age 5. (World Health Organization. [2001]. Evidence and Information for Policy/WHO, Child and Adolescent Health and Development, 2001. Available: *www.who.int/child-adolescent-health/inegr.htm*)

ily planning measures are not widely practiced, and it is not unusual for the young couple to eventually have 6 to 10 children. Such early marriages and large families limit educational and employment opportunities and promote poverty. Additionally, there are millions of children worldwide in moderate-income families who have inadequate care, poor housing, limited health insurance, and limited access to higher education.

HEALTH PROBLEMS OF INFANTS, TODDLERS, AND PRESCHOOLERS

The **infant** (birth to 1 year), **toddler** (ages 1 and 2 years), and **preschooler** population (ages 3 and 4 years) has a low mortality rate in the United States, and it decreases every year. Currently, the infant mortality rate, often considered to be a fairly sensitive indicator of the general health status of a population, is 6.1 per 1000 live births (Martin, Park, & Sutton, 2002). There has been a steady decline since infant mortality rates were first recorded in 1915, when the rate was 99.9 per 1000 live births; by 1940, it had fallen to 47 per 1000 (Kovner & Jonas, 1999). This dramatic change can be credited to improved maternal health, the spacing of children, infant immunizations, and infant safety. The major causes of death among the birth-to-4-year-old population is unintentional injuries (motor vehicle accidents, falls, drownings,

fires, and burns), followed by malignant neoplasms, birth defects, and heart disease (CDC, 2003c).

Accidents and Injuries

Toddlers and preschoolers are vulnerable to many types of accidents and unintentional injuries, such as those caused by unsafe toys, falls, burns, drownings, automobile crashes, and poisonings. Injury from many sources may result in death.

The loss of children's lives resulting from all injuries combined adds up to a staggering number of years of productive life lost to society. Unintentional injuries are the leading cause of death for people aged 1 to 34 years and the fifth leading cause of death in the United States (USDHHS, 2000). Motor vehicle crashes account for approximately half the deaths from unintentional injuries. Greater efforts are being made to reduce play and recreational injuries to young children through better monitoring of toy safety and improved playground construction and maintenance. Product safety is monitored by the Federal Consumer Product Safety Commission.

Infants are at risk of falling when they are not supervised adequately. Falls from a bed or other furniture item that occur when a baby is not properly secured or supervised can cause permanent injury or death. Infants should never be left unattended when not in a crib or play yard. Even a safely made crib near a window with a dangling window blind cord presents the possibility for injury or possibly death. Many children are killed each year by entanglement in such cords.

As the infant grows and learns to walk, frequent falls are common and continuous supervision and "childproofing" of the home are essential. Young children are curious, and their explorations can lead to additional forms of injury, such as burns, drowning, and poisoning.

Injury from burns can happen to children of all ages. Child deaths and injuries from burns result primarily from house fires but also from electrical burns, cigarette lighters, matches, and scalds. Cigarette lighters and matches are fascinating to young children. Toddlers or preschoolers may be able to start a flame, injuring or killing themselves or others. Infants are often burned by touching a parent's cigarette or by reaching for a cup of hot coffee or the handle of a pot on the stove. Bath water that is too hot can cause a scalding injury. A crawling or toddling child can pull an iron cord, causing the iron to topple on him or her, resulting in a burn or injury. Electrocution can result from inserting a finger or toy into an electrical outlet.

Preventing all possible sources of injury or death from burns can be accomplished by eliminating opportunity and source. Through child supervision, safe storage of matches and lighters, and keeping children away from stoves and electrical outlets, burns can be prevented. Adults can protect children from burns by keeping pot handles turned toward the center of the stove, by not using stove burners or ovens to heat their homes, by reducing temperatures in water heater, by always testing bath water with an elbow before placing a child in the bath, and by keeping electrical outlets covered with inexpensive plastic inserts. Many local fire departments and public health programs offer safety education in this area; such programs emphasize the use of heat- and smoke-detecting systems, fire drills, home evacuation plans, use of less flammable structural materials, furnishings, and clothing; and careful smoking—or better yet—not smoking.

Young children are at risk for drowning wherever water occurs in depths exceeding a few inches such as in toilet bowls, bathtubs, buckets or cans filled with rainwater, puddles, ponds, and swimming pools. Infants, toddlers, and preschool-aged children are especially vulnerable because they are not aware of water dangers and explore unafraid. Parents need to provide a "drown-free" environment by

- Bathing young children in shallow water
- Never leaving young children unattended during a bath
- Keeping the lids down on toilets and bathroom doors closed—preferably secured with childproof safety handles
- Eliminating water collection sites around the home by turning over or removing empty buckets, containers, flower pots, and other items that can collect rainwater
- Fencing swimming pools and installing childproof locks or alarm devices that sound when the water is disturbed
- Promoting water safety measures, including teaching young children to swim
- Vigilantly observing young children at play to protect them from wandering off toward neighborhood water sources

Injuries and deaths from automobile crashes continue to be a major safety problem in the United States. Some families do not use infant restraint seats consistently even though they have been required by law for decades. Other families have them and use them regularly but do not install them properly, placing the child at as much risk as if there were no restraint. There is much opportunity in this area for the community health nurse to educate the public and ensure that parents have the information and skills to properly secure their children when traveling by car.

Poisoning is a constant safety concern for young children. Sources of poisoning include household plants, prescription medications, over-the-counter drugs, unintentional medication overdoses, household cleaning products, other chemicals stored within a child's reach, and lead.

Childproofing the home to eliminate major sources of poisoning is the best method of keeping children safe. This includes keeping plants out of a child's reach or eliminating them from the home until the child is older, locking up household chemicals and storing them out of a child's reach, using childproof medication containers, storing all medicines in a locked box with a key that is kept out of reach, and eliminating sources of lead.

A major cause of childhood poisoning is lead. The primary sources of lead exposure in preschool-aged children continue to be lead-based paint, lead-contaminated soil and dust, and drinking water from lead-soldered pipes (Cohen, 2001; Markowitz & Rosner, 2000). Children who live and play in substandard housing areas remain at risk for direct exposure to significant sources of lead. Community health nurses should promote opportunities for blood screening for lead levels if it is suspected that children in certain homes, apartments, or neighborhoods are at risk for lead poisoning.

Safety programs seek to protect children from the hazards of poisonings, ingestion of toxic substances, prescription medications, and over-the-counter drugs. Poison control centers in many localities offer information and emergency assistance. Toxic household substances, such as cleaning supplies, must be clearly labeled, and harmful drugs must be packaged with special seals and safety caps. Generally, the community health nurse can educate families to recognize potentially hazardous situations and encourage efforts to eliminate them.

Homicide is the most frequent cause of death for infants (8.3 per 100,000 in 1997). The 2010 target is 3.2 per 100,000 from a 1998 baseline of 6.2 (USDHHS, 2000). Homicides of children younger than 3 years of age most often result from family violence.

A child's culture influences the level of violence to which the child is exposed. Increased aggressive behavior among children has been attributed to violence in the child's home (spousal and child abuse) and in the community, as well as violent scenes on television and in movies.

Communicable Diseases

Toddlers and preschool-aged children experience a high frequency of acute illnesses, more than any other age group. Such illnesses account for a large number of days of restricted activity and disability requiring bed rest. Respiratory illnesses account for more than one half of acute conditions in toddlers and preschoolers (USDHHS, 2000). Morbidity from communicable diseases among young children is high. Respiratory illnesses, followed by infectious and parasitic diseases, injuries, and digestive conditions, are the most common. The incidences of measles, rubella (German measles), and infectious parotitis (mumps) have dropped considerably because of widespread immunization efforts, yet cases still occur. Some communicable diseases (eg, pertussis) have potentially serious complications. The *Healthy People 2000* goal for pertussis was 1000 cases, but the incidence has remained high, with 3417 cases in 1998 (USDHHS, 1998; 2000). The *Healthy People 2010* goal was revised to 2000 cases.

Vigorous campaigns have been undertaken by health departments to get children immunized. For example, routine infant hepatitis B vaccination was first recommended in 1991; within 5 years, the proportion of 19- to 35-month-old children who received three doses of the vaccine increased from less than 10% to 82% (USDHHS, 2000). After the introduction of *Haemophilus influenzae* type b (Hib) conjugate vaccine in 1990, the incidence of Hib meningitis among infants declined by 95% since 1993 (Zhou et al, 2002). A vaccine for mumps, measles, and rubella (MMR) has been available for several decades, and one for varicella (chickenpox) since 1995. In 1998, immunization coverage for children aged 19 to 35 months was at a record high level (CDC, 1999).

Guidelines for polio immunization have recently undergone change. Experts recommend giving most infants inactivated polio virus (IPV) for the first two doses, and the oral polio virus (OPV), which is made from live, attenuated virus, for the second two doses, rather than using just one or the other. This new schedule is intended to decrease the incidence of vaccine-associated paralytic polio. Approximately nine such cases occur each year after administration of OPV (Forshner & Garza, 1999).

The financing of immunizations for infants and children has significantly improved as a result of two major initiatives. The Vaccines for Children Program and the Child Health Insurance Program cover children on Medicaid, uninsured children, and American Indian and Alaska Native children. In addition, underinsured children who receive immunizations at federally qualified health centers and rural health clinics are covered. Additional state programs and funds help provide free vaccines for children who are not covered by the other programs. There are several ways for community health nurses to help all families obtain free immunizations.

Even if financial barriers are removed, there are other barriers. Transportation is a significant problem for some parents, especially in rural areas, and for families in urban areas who have several children and need to take public transportation. In spite of public health announcements in the media, there are mothers who are unaware of the disabling consequences of diseases such as polio and do not realize the importance of fully vaccinating their children (Fig. 27–2).

There are no immunizations against human immunodeficiency virus (HIV) infection, which causes acquired immunodeficiency syndrome (AIDS). In 1996, there were 830,000 HIV-positive children worldwide (CDC, 2003b). In 1999, more than 10,000 children in the United States were HIV positive. AIDS is the seventh leading cause of death among children between ages 1 and 4 in the United States. These children acquire the virus while in utero and are infected at birth. Pediatric AIDS is in decline due to the use of antiretroviral agents in HIV-positive pregnant women; there were 947 new cases in 1992 and 225 in 1998 (CDC, 2003b). The United Nations Programme on HIV/AIDS, as of 2002, estimated that 3.2 of the 42 million people thought to be living with HIV/AIDS are children younger than 15 years of age. AIDS caused the deaths of an estimated 610,000 children in 2002 (CDC, 2003b). Many young children become orphaned at an early age because their mothers die of AIDS. The children may enter foster care because of the mother's declining health or because other family members are reluctant or unable to care for an HIV-infected child. Because HIV-infected children are infrequently adopted, they often remain in foster care throughout their short lives.

Chronic Diseases

Many young children are afflicted with chronic diseases that affect quality of life. Asthma is the most common chronic illness among young people in the United States, affecting 4.8 million children and adolescents (Akinbami & Schoendorf, 2002; Diverte, 2002). Many begin to show signs and symptoms of asthma as infants and toddlers. It is a leading cause of hospitalization in children. Inner city, low-income, and minority children are affected disproportionately. **Head Start**, a federally funded program that provides early childhood education to low-income children between 3 and 5 years of age, is an ideal setting for community health nurses to address asthma awareness, education, and prevention.

The incidence of food allergies is increasing in the population. Fortunately, once allergies are diagnosed, they can be managed through dietary changes and by avoidance of allergy-producing foods. Food allergies can be identified early in an infant's life by offering one new food at a time, with a 3-day interval between new foods. This helps to determine which foods cause an allergic reaction. Parents need to be educated so that they can read food labels consistently and can alert family members to the child's allergy so inappropriate foods are not given.

Other chronic illnesses have a more profound effect on child and family. Muscular dystrophy (MD) and cystic fibrosis (CF) are two diseases that not only affect quality of life but also severely shorten the child's life. MD is a familial disease characterized by progressive atrophy and wasting of muscles. Onset usually occurs at an early age, and MD is more common in boys than in girls. The cause is thought to be a genetic defect in muscle metabolism. A child with MD is often confined to a wheelchair and needs assistance with activities of daily living, especially as the disease progresses.

CF usually begins in infancy and is characterized by chronic respiratory infection, pancreatic insufficiency, and increased electrolytes in sweat. It is the major cause of se-

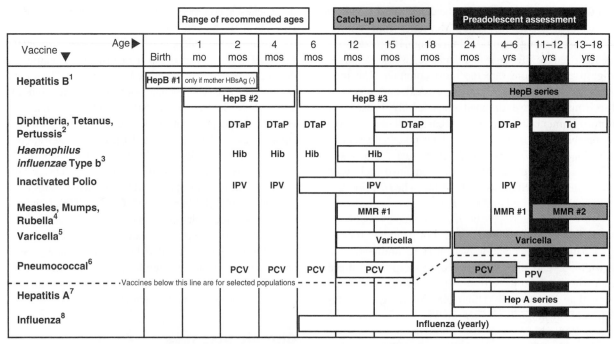

This schedule indicates the recommended ages for routine administration of currently licensed childhood vaccines, as of December 1, 2003, for children through age 18 years. Any dose not given at the recommended age should be given at any subsequent visit when indicated and feasible. ▓▓▓ Indicates age groups that warrant special effort to administer those vaccines not previously given. Additional vaccines may be licensed and recommended during the year. Licensed combination vaccines may be used whenever any components of the combination are indicated and the vaccines's other components are not contraindicated. Providers should consult the manufacturers' package inserts for detailed recommendations.

1. Hepatitis B vaccine (HepB). All infants should receive the first dose of HepB vaccine soon after birth and before hospital discharge; the first dose may also be given by age 2 months if the infant's mother is HBsAg-negative. Only monovalent HepB vaccine can be used for the birth dose. Monovalent or combination vaccine containing HepB may be used to complete the series. Four doses of vaccine may be administered when a birth dose is given. The second dose should be given at least 4 weeks after the first dose, except for combination vaccines which cannot be administered before age 6 weeks. The third dose should be given at least 16 weeks after the first dose and at least 8 weeks after the second dose. The last dose in the vaccination series (third or fourth dose) should not be administered before age 6 months.

   Infants born to HBsAg-positive mothers should receive HepB and 0.5 mL Hepatitis B immune globulin (HBIG) within 12 hours of birth at separate sites. The second dose is recommended at age 1–2 months. The last dose in the vaccination series should not be administered before age 6 months. These infants should be tested for HBsAg and anti-HBs at 9–15 months of age.

   Infants born to mothers whose HBsAg status is unknown should receive the first dose of the HepB vaccine series within 12 hours of birth. Maternal blood should be drawn as soon as possible to determine the mother's HBsAg status; if the HBsAg test is positive, the infant should receive HBIG as soon as possible (no later than age 1 week). The second dose is recommended at age 1–2 months. The last dose in the vaccination series should not be administered before age 6 months.

2. Diphtheria and tetanus toxoids and acellular pertussis vaccine (DTaP). The fourth dose of DTaP may be administered at age 12 months, provided that 6 months have elapsed since the third dose and the child is unlikely to return at age 15–18 months. Tetanus and diphtheria toxoids (Td) is recommended at age 11–12 years if at least 5 years have elapsed since the last dose of tetanus and diphtheria toxoid-containing vaccine. Subsequent routine Td boosters are recommended every 10 years.

3. *Haemophilus influenzae* type b (Hib) conjugate vaccine. Three Hib conjugate vaccines are licensed for infant use. If PRP-OMP (PedvaxHIB® or ComVax® [Merck]) is administered at age 2 and 4 months, a dose at age 6 months is not required. DTaP/Hib combination products should not be

used for primary immunization in infants at age 2, 4, or 6 months but can be used as boosters following any Hib vaccine.

4. Measles, mumps, and rubella vaccine (MMR). The second dose of MMR is recommended routinely at age 4–6 years but may be administered during any visit, provided that at least 4 weeks have elapsed since the first dose and that both doses are administered beginning at or after age 12 months. Those who have not previously received the second dose should complete the schedule by the age 11–12 year old visit.

5. Varicella vaccine. Varicella vaccine is recommended at any visit at or after age 12 months for susceptible children, i.e. those who lack a reliable history of chickenpox. Susceptible persons age ≥13 years should receive two doses given, at least 4 weeks apart.

6. Pneumococcal vaccine. The heptavalent pneumococcal conjugate vaccine (PCV) is recommended for all children aged 2–23 months . It is also recommended for certain children aged 24–59 months. Pneumococcal polysaccharide vaccine (PPV) is recommended in addition to PCV for certain high-risk groups. See *MMWR* 2000;49(No. RR-9):1–38.

7. Hepatitis A vaccine. Hepatitis A vaccine is recommended for children and adolescents in selected states and regions, and for certain high-risk groups; consult your local public health authority. Children and adolescents in these states, regions, and high-risk groups who have not been immunized against hepatitis A can begin the hepatitis A vaccination series during any visit. The two doses in the series should be administered at least 6 months apart. See *MMWR* 1999;48(No. RR-12):1–37.

8. Influenza vaccine. Influenza vaccine is recommended annually for children aged ≥6 months with certain risk factors (including but not limited to asthma, cardiac disease, sickle cell disease, HIV, diabetes, and household members of persons in groups at high risk (see *MMWR* 2002;51(RR-3): 1–31), and can be administered to all others wishing to obtain immunity. In addition, healthy children age 6–23 months are encouraged to receive influenza vaccine if feasible because children in this age group are at substantially increased risk for influenza-related hospitalizations. Children aged ≤12 years should receive vaccine in a dosage appropriated for their age (0.25mL if 6–35 months or 0.5 mL if ≥3 years). Children aged ≤8 years who are receiving influenza vaccine for the first time should receive two doses separated by at least 4 weeks.

F I G U R E   2 7 – 2 .   Recommended childhood and adolescent immunization schedule—United States, January–June 2004. (Centers for Disease Control and Prevention [2003]. General recommendations on immunizations: Recommendations of the Advisory Committee Practices [ACIP], American Academy of Pediatrics and American Academy of Family Physicians. *Morbidity and Mortality Weekly Report, 52,* Q1–4.)

vere chronic lung disease in children. CF occurs in 1 in 2000 white and 1 in 17,000 African-American live births. Parents must be taught positioning, clapping, and vibration followed by deep breathing and coughing as treatments to help mobilize secretions. Community health nurses reinforce these techniques and teach the family to avoid respiratory infections and to initiate prescribed antibiotic prophylaxis promptly. The young child should be involved in his or her own care, offered valid choices, and encouraged to participate in decision-making. The family needs emotional support as members work through feelings of anticipatory grief.

Behavior and Learning Problems

Behavioral disorders and developmental disabilities are first recognized in children in this age group and often become exacerbated when the child enters school. Their prevalence is difficult to measure epidemiologically, but as many as 20% of school-aged children have learning disabilities and behavioral problems that were first recognized in preschool years. The causes are multifaceted and often difficult to identify. The child's future mental health as an adult is influenced by how well emotional needs are met during the early childhood phase of development.

Attention deficit hyperactivity disorder (ADHD) is a cluster of problems related to hyperactivity and impulsivity. **Attention deficit disorder (without hyperactivity; ADD)** is a cluster of problems related mainly to inattention, poor motivation, and disorganization. Both are seen in children and adults. It is estimated that 3% to 17% of American children are affected, boys more commonly than girls (Kendall et al., 2003). These disorders are diagnosed with increasing frequency in children, adolescents, and adults; the signs are often recognized in the preschool years (Barkley et al., 2003). Descriptions of ADHD and ADD are displayed in

Table 27–1 (Aust, 1994; Marks, 1998). A detailed discussion of ADHD occurs in Chapter 28.

Oppositional defiant disorder (ODD) is a set of "externalizing" behavior problems that include noncompliance, temper tantrums, and other socially provocative behaviors first diagnosed in the preschool years (Speltz et al., 1999). ODD is often considered to be a "gateway" for diverse psychopathologies in later life, and preschool-aged children (predominantly boys) with confirmed diagnoses of ODD or ODD/ADHD have clear indicators for ongoing risk (Speltz et al., 1999). Children diagnosed with ODD have lower verbal IQ scores, higher probability of insecure attachments to parents, and conflicted family interactions (DeKlyen et al., 1998; Stormschak et al., 1997).

There is much controversy about the medications prescribed to modify and control behavior in these children. The use of mood-modifying drugs begins for some during the preschool years, and even more children are medicated by school age. Drugs used in combination with behavior modification practices can be tapered off after the symptoms improve, providing a productive approach to out-of-control behavior.

Developmental disabilities are severe, chronic disabilities that manifest before the person reaches 22 years of age. They share the following characteristics:
1. They are accompanied by a mental or physical impairment or a combination of mental and physical impairments.
2. They are likely to continue indefinitely.
3. Impairments result in substantial functional limitations in three or more of the following areas:
   a. Self-care
   b. Receptive and expressive language
   c. Learning
   d. Mobility
   e. Self-direction
   f. Capacity for independent living
   g. Economic sufficiency

TABLE 27–1

ADHD and ADD: The Differences

Attention Deficit Disorder With Hyperactivity (ADHD)	Attention Deficit Disorder Without Hyperactivity (ADD)
A child with this diagnosis often:	
Is impulsive	Has difficulty following through on instructions
Distracts easily	Has difficulty sustaining attention
Is inattentive when spoken to	Seems not to listen
Has difficulty waiting turn in group situations	Loses things necessary for tasks
Interrupts or intrudes on others	Fails to give close attention to details
Blurts out answers to questions	Is disorganized
Has difficulty playing quietly	Makes careless mistakes in schoolwork or work
Doesn't stay seated	Is forgetful
Runs about or climbs excessively	Daydreams when should be attending
Fidgets or squirms	Is unmotivated to complete tasks
Talks excessively	
Acts as if "driven by a motor" and cannot remain still	

Categories of causes for such developmental disability include birth defects, prematurity, birth trauma, injury from falls, auto crashes, poisonings, and near-drowning. Other disabling chronic conditions that limit activities and self-care include speech, hearing, and visual defects, seizure disorders, asthma, cancer, and AIDS. Disabilities affect approximately 12% of children through school age. The percentage is smaller among the infant, toddler, and preschool population because developmental and other chronic conditions may not occur until the child is older. Children with special needs affect family health and educational, and support services in communities, as well as the role of the community health nurse.

Poor Nutrition and Dental Hygiene

Other health problems found in this age group include nutritional problems (underfeeding or overfeeding, overeating, and inappropriate food choices) and poor dental health. Nutritional and dental health needs are great during this period of rapid growth. Many factors contribute to early nutritional and dental problems.

A healthy start is foundational to well-being later in life. Nutrition is basic in strengthening this foundation. Bonding between mother and infant and overall maternal health are predictors of infant weight gain. Both nutrition and bonding can be accomplished by breast feeding. Some of the benefits of breast feeding are as follows (Wiggins, 2001):

Convenience: Milk is always at the perfect temperature, and no preparation is needed.

Cost: Costs are limited to healthy diet for the mother, breast pads, nursing bras, and (possibly) a breast pump.

Nutrition: Breast milk is species specific; the proteins are easily digested, and fats are well absorbed

Anti-infective and anti-allergic properties: Breast milk contains immunoglobulins, enzymes, and leukocytes that protect against pathogens, and it decreases the incidence of allergy by eliminating exposure to potential antigens.

Overfeeding of an infant can lead to childhood obesity and becomes a risk factor for heart disease, hypertension, and diabetes. Eleven percent of school-age children are overweight, with the foundation begun in the preschool years (Hodges, 2003; USDHHS, 2000). The propensity for obesity begins as early as infancy and by childhood for most people. Obesity is a contributing factor to the worldwide increase in diabetes type 2 and has been reported to result in lower health-related quality of life (Kimm & Obarzanek, 2002; Schwimmer, Burwinkle, & Varni, 2003).

Young children's diets, often unreasonably high in sugar, increase the incidence of dental caries in this population group. The practice of allowing infants to bottle feed beyond 15 to 16 months, or to fall asleep with a bottle, can lead to "nursing bottle syndrome." This causes the decay of the front teeth and, eventually, the molars, requiring extraction of the affected teeth (American Academy of Pediatrics, 2003). Parents of infants older than 6 months of age should be instructed to rub the infant's gums with a damp, clean cloth and to be-

gin tooth brushing, using a soft pediatric toothbrush without toothpaste, after several teeth have erupted.

Liquid vitamins with added fluoride should be used if formula is premixed and not made from local fluoridated water supplies, or if local water is not fluoridated. As children reach the toddler years, they are able to brush their own teeth with enthusiasm. Toothpaste should be used sparingly, and tooth brushing should be supervised by an adult. Children of this age can get overzealous with the amount of toothpaste they use and it should not be ingested. At age 3 years or earlier, a first visit to a dentist should be planned and biannual visits should commence. American children begin a lifetime history of dental caries as preschoolers.

Dental caries is a preventable condition that, if left unaddressed, can lead to self-esteem issues and body image disorders when children live with teeth that are discolored, misshapen, or missing. Chronic health conditions such as heart disease and nutritional problems from bacteria forming in the rotted teeth or inability to masticate food properly can occur if teeth are missing. Dental caries increases with age and is more prevalent in Native-American populations (68% of children 2 to 4 years of age with dental decay go untreated), in groups underserved by dentists, and in areas where there is no fluoridated water (USDHHS, 2000).

The Effects of Poverty

Poverty steals childhood from more than one in five American children. It robs them of the resources needed to build a strong foundation for a healthy life. Urban and rural poverty affect greater numbers of children each year and are addressed in detail in Chapters 31 and 32.

Contributing to the growing numbers of children living in poverty is the increasing number of single-mother households. In addition, there are higher rates of mortality, morbidity, and disability in families with lower income, less education, lower occupational level, and racial or ethnic minority status.

The parents of children living in poverty tend not to seek preventive family care, underuse existing health care services, lack general or systematic communication with health professionals, and suffer from more acute and chronic health problems (Guasasco, Heur ,& Lausch 2002). These problems are exacerbated if the poverty is severe and the family is homeless (Averitt, 2003).

Homelessness brings additional problems that affect the health of young children. Exposure to the elements places children at risk for illness and injury. Sleeping in the street, parks, or occasional shelters interrupts a child's sleep patterns. The lack of a stable physical home environment can contribute to self-esteem, emotional, and mental health disturbances.

Community health nurses can make a big difference in the well-being of families with young children living in poverty. Helping the family apply for financial resources and locate permanent, low-cost, and safe housing are priorities. Helping the parents locate employment, health care, and educational resources promotes wellness and gives them the skills to help themselves and their children. Community health nurses can provide ongoing contact to teach preventive health practices and to provide anticipatory guidance for young families.

HEALTH SERVICES FOR INFANTS, TODDLERS, AND PRESCHOOLERS

There are many ways in which the health of a child can be influenced. The goal is for health to be influenced positively. A variety of programs now exist that directly or indirectly serve the health needs of children. Community health nurses play a major and vital role in delivering these services. In community health, programs fall into three categories, which approximate the three practice priorities of community health nursing practice: health prevention, protection, and promotion.

Preventive Health Programs

Neighborhood community centers found in urban and rural settings provide families with parenting education, health and safety education, immunizations, various screening programs, and family planning services. In some areas, nurse-run clinics are established at local schools to assist in outreach services to the community. Community health nurses, in collaboration with an interdisciplinary team, are usually the primary care providers in these programs. The major goals are to keep communities well by focusing on primary and secondary prevention services.

Two examples of preventive health programs for infants and young children are immunization programs and quality day care services. In addition, parenting classes and other parental support services yield long-term benefits to children.

Immunization Programs

Health departments and the private sector continue to offer immunizations against the major childhood infectious diseases—measles, mumps, rubella, chickenpox, polio, diphtheria, tetanus, pertussis, and *Haemophilus influenzae*—some of which can cause permanent disability and even death. Although the threat of these diseases has been substantially reduced, vigilance cannot be relaxed. Low immunization levels in many areas, particularly among the poor, and increased disease rates signal the need for constant surveillance, outreach programs, and educational efforts. Community health nurses are deeply involved in each of these preventive activities. Health departments and schools often work collaboratively to provide immunization services (see Fig. 27–2). A compulsory immunization law, varying in its application from state to state, has enabled public health personnel to carry out these preventive services.

Quality Day Care Programs

Quality child care provides a significant avenue for preventing illness and injury among young children. In 1975, 39% of

women with children younger than 6 years of age were in the labor force; by 1994, more than 60% were employed (Gormley, 1995). Today, those figures are even higher as a result of economic necessity, changes in family structure, or personal career and lifestyle choice, making the two-wage-earner family the single largest employee group in the United States (Carabin et al., 1999). Seventy-five percent of children younger than 5 years of age are in some form of child care on a regular basis (American Academy of Pediatrics, 2001). With these changes comes the demand for accessible and quality child care and, for some parents, the desire to provide children with educational experiences in preparation for school (Lucarelli, 2002).

Children in day care tend to contract a significantly higher number of illnesses than do children cared for at home. Carabin and colleagues (1999) found that there was an incidence rate of 6.1 upper respiratory tract infections (URTIs) per toddler in day care over a 6-month period, compared with 3.8 URTIs per child cared for at home, a figure established in an earlier study. An incidence rate difference of 2.3 episodes per child (a 38% increase) was observed among toddlers in day care. Many day care disease occurrences can be prevented through improved policies regarding sick children and adherence to those policies. Making sure that the requirements for immunization for all children and staff are met should be part of the community health nurse's role in services provided to community aggregates. Further preventive measures are needed to ensure cleanliness, good nutrition, proper ventilation, lighting, exercise, and a safe, emotionally secure environment (Lucarelli, 2002). Many children suffer injuries and even death due to lack of safe child care; one important preventive measure is to ensure lower child-to-caregiver ratios (Table 27–2).

The availability of affordable, quality, licensed day care facilities is recognized as one long-term solution for the prevention of child abuse. When their young children are safely

TABLE 27-2

The National Association for the Education of Young Children (NAEYC) Guidelines

Developed in 1984, the NAEYC criteria for accreditation were based on research and professional consensus. The criteria include guidelines for staff–child interactions, curriculum content, parental involvements, staff qualifications and training, administration, staffing patterns, physical environment, health and safety, and nutrition and food service. One example is the NAEYC standards for group size and adult–child ratio:

Age of Child	Number of Children per Group	Adult–Child Ratio
0 to 12 months	6 to 8	1:3 to 1:4
12 to 24 months	6 to 12	1:3 to 1:4
2 years	8 to 12	1:4 to 1:6
3 years	14 to 20	1:7 to 1:10
4 to 5 years	16 to 20	1:8 to 1:10

cared for, two parents or a single parent can work and provide more resources for the family, thereby decreasing the stress that often precipitates abuse. The quality of day care and preschool programs varies considerably. Licensing laws can regulate only minimum safety and health standards. In addition, numerous child care operations are too small to require licensing, which leaves their quality open to individual discretion. Community health nurses can influence the quality of day care and preschool programs through active educational efforts, monitoring of health and safety standards, and working to improve the state's role in passing stronger licensing laws.

Parental Support Services

Parental support services, available through many public and private agencies, including religious communities, have long-range effects on children's health. Emotionally healthy parents and stable families offer a healthful environment and support system for growing children. In most states, community health nurses provide teaching and counseling services to parents in their homes and in groups. Discussing parenting concerns and increasing parents' understanding of normal child growth and development allay fears and prevent problems. Through such efforts, family violence and abuse can be reduced or averted.

Health Protection Programs

Health protection programs for infants and young children are designed to protect them from illness and injury. Ultimately, these programs may even protect their lives.

Safety and Injury Protection

Accident and injury control programs serve a critical role in protecting the lives of children. Efforts to prevent motor vehicle crashes, a major cause of death, include driver education programs, better highway construction, improved motor vehicle design and safety features, and continuing research into the causes of various types of crashes. Injury prevention and reduction have been addressed through strategies such as state laws requiring the use of safety restraints, availability of front and side driver and passenger airbags, substitution of other modes of travel (air, rail, or bus), lower speed limits, stricter enforcement of drunk driving laws, safer automobile design, and helmets for motorcyclists, bicycle riders, and skaters.

For infants, toddlers, and preschool-aged children to be safe when traveling in vehicles, they must be restrained in an approved infant carrier, child restraint seat, or booster seat. These must be positioned and secured as described by the manufacturer; used at all times, even for the shortest distances; placed in the back seat, never in the front seat; and installed in the appropriate position (facing rear or front) based on the weight or age of the infant or toddler. Children younger than 12 years of age should never sit in the front seat. The force of a deploying airbag during a crash may be great enough to seriously injure or kill a small child.

Falls, a major killer of infants, toddlers, and preschool-

aged children and the cause of injury for millions of children each year, occur mostly in the home. Here, the community health nurse plays a major role in observing potential hazards, teaching safety measures, and reinforcing positive practices.

Preventive and protective measures may be achieved through simple and inexpensive changes in the home. These include installation of guards on windows and across stairways; removal, securing, or shortening of window blind cords; provision of safer walking surfaces; and elimination of sharp objects or modification of surfaces against which a child might fall. Clearly, close supervision of infants and young children is primary to their safety and survival.

Programs to reduce environmental hazards for all people, not just young children, begin at the federal level, where the government sets and enforces pollution standards and regulates environmental contamination. At the state and municipal government levels, enforcement of regulations occurs. Measures include monitoring air and drinking water safety; installing carbon monoxide detection devices in housing units; providing proper sewage disposal; controlling ionizing radiation; removing asbestos or lead; reducing radon contamination by installing barriers; enforcing auto safety and emission standards; and controlling use of agricultural chemicals and pesticides. Local protective measures include educational programs that warn against toxic agents in the environment, community surveillance, and enforcement of environmental health standards. At all levels, epidemiologic research probes the causes and seeks answers to provide better protection for the public. Community health nurses need to be alert to environmental hazards and to work collaboratively with other members of the public health team to report problems and educate parents so their children are safe. Improved environmental control protects today's children against disease and disability and tomorrow's children against birth defects and the long-range hazards of environmental contamination. Chapter 10 explores environmental health and safety.

Protection from Communicable Disease

It has been demonstrated in community health that infectious diseases can be controlled and, in some cases, eliminated. Witness the successful worldwide eradication of smallpox, the dramatic decline in paralytic polio, and the decreasing incidence of the other communicable diseases of childhood, especially measles and chickenpox. Control of infectious diseases comes largely through immunization programs, discussed earlier, and surveillance of communicable disease incidence.

Programs that protect children against infectious diseases encompass efforts such as closing swimming pools with unsafe bacteria counts, conducting immunization campaigns in conjunction with influenza or measles outbreaks, and working with hospital pediatric units to reduce the incidence and threat of iatrogenic disease.

Protection from Dental Caries

Dental caries is the single most common chronic disease of children in the United States, occurring five to eight times more frequently than asthma (USDHHS, 2000). Eighteen percent of children aged 2 to 4 years have been affected by dental caries. The average number of decayed and filled teeth among 2- to 4-year-olds has remained unchanged for the past 25 years. Children whose parents or caregivers have less than a high school education or whose parents and caregivers are Hispanic-Americans, American Indians, or Alaska Natives appear to be at markedly increased risk for development of early childhood caries (USDHHS, 2000).

Fluoridation of community water supplies is the single most effective, safe, and low-cost means of protecting the dental health of children and adults. Fluoride makes teeth less susceptible to decay by increasing resistance to bacterial acids in the mouth. Public acceptance of community water fluoridation has been slow, despite 40 years of research indicating its safety and effectiveness. In 1980, just 62% of persons served by community water systems in the United States received optimally fluoridated water (USDHHS, 2000). The goal for 2010 is to increase this figure to at least 75% of the population (USDHHS, 2000). For those without this passive protection, supplemental fluorides, both systemic and topical, are available. In addition to regular dental care, good nutrition, and proper oral hygiene, community health nurses can promote public water fluoridation as an important program for protecting children's dental health.

There remains the need to focus on good dental health care. Professional dental health care has not changed dramatically in recent years, yet there are new products such as fluoride-releasing sealants, antibacterial rinses, plaque- and tartar-control dentifrices, and slow-release, intraoral drug delivery systems. Nevertheless, none of these products or treatments takes the place of personal oral health care supplemented with regular professional care. *Healthy People 2010* has a goal of reducing the incidence of untreated cavities in the primary teeth to no more than 9% of children 2 to 4 years old, a reduction from the baseline of 16% in the period between1988 and 1994 (USDHHS, 2000).

Some barriers to children's dental health are more prevalent among minority populations and the poor. Financial barriers and lack of education lead to poor dental health values and adversely affect use of dentists and conscientious personal oral health care. Only about 40% of the population is covered by dental insurance, which accounts for 48% of dental reimbursement. The greater cost of dental care is assumed directly "out of pocket" by the consumer. Furthermore, dental insurance often provides limited coverage, requires high copayments, and is available only to children of employed parents or guardians with coverage (USDHHS, 2000). Medicaid pays for less than 4% of dental expenditures. The disparities in oral health care need to be reduced and, ideally, eliminated (Display 27–2).

Protection From Child Abuse and Neglect

Child abuse and neglect are major concerns for the United States. In 2000, an estimated 879,000 children in this country

---

DISPLAY 27–2

Disparities in Oral Health Care Among Young Children

Health Status
The level of untreated dental caries among members of racial and ethnic minority groups is greater than the national average.

Access
Poor children and members of racial and ethnic minority groups have less private dental insurance than the average for all children.
Poor children have 37% fewer dental visits than non-poor children.
Smaller proportions of members of racial and ethnic minority groups have dental insurance than the national average.
Smaller proportions of members of racial and ethnic minority groups had a dental visit in the preceding year.

Preventive Services
Smaller proportions of minority and poor children have dental sealants.

(From U. S. Department of Health and Human Services [2000]. *Healthy people 2010* [Conference ed., Vols 1 & 2]. Washington, DC: Author.)

---

were victims of neglect or abuse or were at risk. An estimated 1200 children died from such maltreatment (ACF, 2002). Child abuse is the maltreatment of children, which may include any or all of the following: physical abuse, emotional abuse, neglect (physical, medical, or educational), and sexual abuse (including sexual exploitation and child pornography) (Child Abuse, 2002). Exposure of infants to drugs while in utero is a form of abuse (see Research: Bridge to Practice).

It is believed that many more children also suffer from forms of abuse and neglect, but thousands of cases are not reported and not reflected in the statistics. The problem is often difficult to detect and is underreported. In recent years, there has been an increase in reported cases of physical and sexual abuse in day care centers, nursery schools, children's organizations, and churches. It is alarming to note that, regardless of race, culture, or socioeconomic origin, today's children run a high risk of suffering violence at the hands of their own caregivers.

Risk factors for abusive behavior include immaturity, stress, poverty, alcoholism, unstable employment, and physical and social isolation (English, 1998). Child abuse is seldom the result of any single factor, but rather a combination of stressful situations and parents who are unable to cope with problems and stress in a normal manner. Abusive adults, who often were abused, molested, or neglected as

RESEARCH: BRIDGE TO PRACTICE

Butz, A. M., Lears, M. K., O'Neil, S., & Lusk, P. (1998). Home intervention for in utero drug-exposed infants. *Public Health Nursing, 15*(5), 307–318.

Researchers from Johns Hopkins University conducted a study in 1997, which included 204 mother–infant dyads, to determine whether intensive early intervention, including home-based intervention, is an effective method to improve cognitive development, parent–child interaction, and health-related problems in high-risk children. There is a paucity of home intervention studies specifically examining in utero drug-exposed (IUDE) infants. This study was part of a larger clinical trial examining the effectiveness of home nurse interventions for the little-studied IUDE infants.

Each infant in this study received a total of 16 home visits during the first 18 months of life. Home visits were conducted by community health nurses who were adept in home visits to inner-city populations, who specialized in pediatrics, and who were trained in basic pediatric assessment for IUDE infants.

On each home visit, the nurse assessed for signs and symptoms of in utero drug exposure, developmental problems, and common infant conditions. At 3, 6, 12, and 18 months of age, each infant received the Denver Developmental Screening Test (DDST-II) in the home to screen for developmental delays. Parenting information was provided, and selected skills were taught to the mother/caregiver to enhance maternal-infant interaction. In addition,

role modeling was used by the community health nurse to promote positive maternal–infant interaction.

An analysis of home visit data for the first 20 enrolled mother–infant dyads was based on 229 visits to these 20 pairs of study participants. Health problems were encountered during approximately one third of the home visits and social problems during 80% of the visits. Basic parenting and personal skills were the primary educational information shared with the mother/caregiver. Basic parenting skills were important teaching topics in addition to well-child care. One third of the mothers continued drug use during the infant's first year of life. Infectious disease symptoms and preventable dermatologic problems were common, suggesting that basic personal hygiene is a necessary component of parent education before discharge of high-risk infants. Most mothers were unable to receive support from an identified support person and tended to be socially isolated, which can contribute to depression and continued drug use.

The implications for nursing practice indicate the need for vigilant monitoring through frequent home nurse visits for the first 12 months of life. These mothers experience a myriad of social, economic, and health problems during the first 12 months after birth. The authors suggested that home visiting should be incorporated into the discharge planning of any IUDE infant to monitor the safety of these infants and maintain them in the health care delivery system.

---

children themselves, carry low self-images into their adult lives and are unable to cope with the demands of parenting (see Chapter 25). Other characteristics of abusive parents include immaturity, dependency, inability to handle responsibility, and low self-esteem. They often believe in the value of physical punishment, misunderstand their children's abilities to comprehend and perform certain tasks, and frequently make unreasonable demands. During times of crisis, these parents often direct their anger and frustration at their children. Such negative life patterns can continue for generations if intervention does not occur (CDC, 2002).

Families at high risk for child abuse may be those that are either chronically troubled or temporarily stressed. Teenage mothers and parents with closely spaced children also may be more likely to engage in abusive behavior. Although poverty and lack of education are often linked with child abuse and neglect, no socioeconomic level is immune.

Services to protect children from abuse are not as well developed or effective as safety and injury prevention programs, an observation accounted for by a variety of factors.

Most child abuse occurs in the home, so only the most blatant situations become evident to outsiders. Community health nurses and physicians who see injured children may find parents' explanations plausible and may not suspect or want to believe that abuse might be responsible. Avoidance of legal involvement keeps others from reporting suspected cases. Fortunately, this attitude is changing among professionals who work with children and other community members.

For many years, states have had mandatory reporting laws. The first law was passed in 1963 and required mandatory reporting by physicians of cases suspicious for child abuse. By 1966, all states had a reporting law. Over the years, numerous amendments have expanded the definition of child abuse and the persons who are required to report. People mandated to report suspected child abuse include all those who work with children—day care providers, teachers, social workers, nurses, doctors, clergy, coaches, and so forth. In addition, animal humane workers and commercial photograph developers are mandated reporters. Procedures for reporting categories of child abuse have also been clarified. Today, professionals and the public are more aware of the problem, and there has been an increase in reporting. Nonetheless, it is estimated that fewer than 10% of cases are actually reported. In 1974, the National Center for Child Abuse and Neglect was established as a result of the Child Abuse Prevention and Treatment Act. The center collects and analyzes information on child abuse and neglect, serves as an information clearinghouse, publishes educational materials on the subject, offers technical assistance, and conducts research into the problem. In addition, this act spurred all of the states to pass mandatory reporting laws and set up procedures for investigating suspected cases of child abuse and neglect. The government entity known as Child Protective Services was also established (Child Abuse, 2002).

Most professionals adopt the "levels of prevention" model to define child abuse and neglect prevention efforts.

Primary Prevention

Primary prevention measures include establishing community education to enhance the general well-being of children and their families. Provide educational services designed to enrich the lives of families, to improve the skills of family functioning, and to prevent the stress and problems that might lead to dysfunction and abuse or neglect. Prevention should focus on parent preparation during the prenatal period; practices that encourage parent–child bonding during labor, delivery, the postpartum period, and early infancy; and provision of information regarding support services for families with newborns. Provide parents of children of all ages with information regarding child-rearing and community resources.

Secondary Prevention

Services are designed to identify and assist high-risk families to prevent abuse or neglect. **High-risk families** are those families who exhibit the symptoms of potentially abusive or neglectful behavior or who are under the types of stress associated with abuse or neglect.

Tertiary Prevention

Intervention and treatment services are designed to assist a family in which abuse or neglect has already occurred so that further abuse or neglect may be prevented. These measures range from "early" intervention, in the initial stages of abuse or neglect, to "late-stage" intervention, in severe cases or after services have failed to stop the abusive or neglectful behavior.

The community health nurse has a major role in primary prevention of child abuse. In addition, the nurse is in a unique position to detect early signs of neglect and abuse. The nurse must establish rapport with abusive parents, family members, or others and assist with appropriate interventions and referrals at the secondary and tertiary levels of prevention. An interdisciplinary approach with teachers, the department of social services, foster families, and other health care providers is necessary (Chernoff et al., 1994) (Display 27–3).

The effectiveness of local programs depends, in large measure, on the willingness of community health professionals to increase their awareness and work as a team to detect, report, and develop interventions for abusers and abused children. Ongoing education of health care providers is recommended to increase awareness of changing child abuse patterns, new reporting laws, and resources available to families.

Health Promotion Programs

Early childhood programs are designed to have positive effects on the outcomes of children's cognitive and social development. Some have considered children's physical health, and fewer have focused on parent–child interaction and parenting skills. All are considered health promotion programs.

Early Childhood Development Programs

Early childhood development programs serve an increasingly important function for the escalating number of children enrolled in day care centers and preschools. More than half of all children today have mothers who work, a figure that continues to rise. Economic pressures eat into family time together and often diminish the quality of children's physical and psychosocial nourishment. Childhood development programs such as Head Start provide physical, emotional, intellectual, and social stimulation during a critical period in children's growth, when impressions and patterns are formed that will influence the kind of adults these children will become.

Comprehensive preschool programs promote good physical health, proper nutrition, a positive self-concept, and development of cognitive and social skills. Many such programs exist, but more are needed.

In 1990, the President and the state governors set six national education goals to be reached by the year 2000. The first was "By the year 2000, all children in America will start school ready to learn" (U.S. Department of Education, 1990). That goal has not been achieved. Children are entering school without being ready to learn; for many children, major emotional, physical, financial, and social barriers still exist. A physically and emotionally healthy child is able to start school ready to learn. Where and how a child arrives at that healthy state is the challenge to society. The stresses some parents feel are compounded when affordable and accessible licensed child care is not available; stressed parents are more likely to abuse their children or to place their children at risk of abuse, neglect, or exploitation.

Nutritional Programs

Adequate nutrition must begin at birth. Some low-income children in the United States (8% in 1997) had retarded growth (USDHHS, 2000), which is defined as height-for-age below the 5th percentile. One of the most productive health outcome programs is the Special Supplemental Food Program for Women, Infants, and Children (WIC). In addition to supporting women and young children with nutritious

D I S P L A Y 27-3

Reports of an Emergency Foster Home

The following are examples of the various situations from which abused and neglected children come, as reported by a couple who had an emergency foster home for the county department of social services. The examples represent children placed with them over a 2-year period, during which they cared for 256 children.

- Two-week-old Jose was brought to their home because the parents (under the influence of drugs) were found swinging Jose upside down in circles in an infant carrier as they walked along a downtown street at 3 AM. After being returned to his parents, he was brought again to foster care 1 month later after being found abandoned in an infant carrier at the county fair.
- Andre, Otis, and Selma, ages 8, 5, and 4 years, were brought to the foster home after social services discovered they had been living with their father in an abandoned car for 2 years. They stayed for 3 weeks while the social worker found suitable housing for this family and counseling for the father.
- Victoria, 5 years old, a loving and passive child, arrived wearing a diaper and appeared developmentally delayed. She had a history of being physically and sexually abused. Her family was very dysfunctional, and it took the social worker several weeks to sort out relatives and their intentions before placing Victoria in a long-term foster home.
- Ronald and Randall, 6-year-old twin boys who were forced to "sexually please their mother" for several years, came to the emergency foster home before being placed with relatives while their mother underwent

psychiatric treatment. The boys began counseling during their stay in the emergency foster home.
- Antoinette, age 7 years, had severe asthma and was very withdrawn. She came to the emergency foster home because her mother (and the mother's boyfriend) refused to care for her. The child came with every photograph of herself and personal mementos because the mother wanted no reminders of the child. The social worker located a grandmother who would be the child's guardian.
- Thirteen-year-old Robert came home from school one day and found his mother and all their furniture gone. After he had lived a few weeks in the basement of the apartment building, someone alerted social services and Robert was placed in the emergency foster home for 2 months. His mother finally called social services after 6 weeks, saying Robert was too difficult for her to handle, but she might want to see him again someday. Robert was eventually placed in a group home for boys.
- Quyn, a 17-year-old Laotian girl, came into foster care after being referred by the school nurse because of wounds observed on her wrists and ankles. Quyn reported being strapped to a chair for 12 or more hours at a time by her father because she was not following the old ways and was shaming the family by being seen in public, unchaperoned, with a boy. Several meetings were held between the parents, a Southeast Asian community leader, and the social worker to resolve this situation so that Quyn could go home safely.

---

foods, WIC can make a difference between life and death for some children. Moss and Carver (1998) found that participation in the WIC program during pregnancy and infancy was associated with a reduced risk of infant death.

Nutrition and weight control programs form an additional important set of health-focused promotion services. Children need to learn sound dietary habits early in life, so that they can establish healthy lifelong patterns. Some preschool programs both teach and provide good nutrition and encourage eating patterns that prevent obesity and reinforce the importance of a healthy breakfast and lunch. Weight control programs are available for overweight young children through health departments, community health centers, health maintenance organizations, and private groups.

Parents have become more aware of the need to reduce consumption of saturated fat, salt, sugar, and overprocessed foods in order to feel and look better. They pass these beliefs along to their children. The community health nurse, through nutrition education and reinforcement of positive practices, plays a significant role in promoting the health of infants and young children (see Levels of Prevention Matrix).

Physical Fitness Programs

The value of developing a lifetime pattern of exercise and physical fitness has been recognized for some time. Organized groups, such as the YMCA, YWCA, Boy and Girl Scouts, and Campfire have offered sports and character development programs for many years. Good day care and preschool programs provide equipment and opportunities for large-muscle activity as well as fine-motor development. Schools, parks, and recreation centers encourage exercise through use of playground equipment and organized sports activities. In addition, many programs are available for the very youngest children and their mothers, through "Mommy and Me" programs. Such programs include simple play and exercises that mother and baby can participate in together. Another option is swimming classes for infants and toddlers, who are attended in the water by a parent. Despite these opportunities, many children do not exercise often enough or vigorously enough. Team sports such as soccer and baseball that begin for children as young as 4 or 5 years of age, keep players inactive much of the time and are not activities that most children continue into adulthood. Comprehensive

LEVELS OF PREVENTION MATRIX

SITUATION: Obesity in young children.

GOAL: Using the three levels of prevention, negative health conditions are avoided, or promptly diagnosed and treated, and the fullest possible potential is restored.

PRIMARY PREVENTION		SECONDARY PREVENTION		TERTIARY PREVENTION		
Health Promotion and Education	*Health Protection*	*Early Diagnosis*	*Prompt Treatment*	*Rehabilitation*	*Primary Prevention*	
					Health Promotion and Education	*Health Protection*
• Foster good eating habits from infancy • Introduce food types and amounts according to health care provider's recommendations • Reward good behavior with items or activities and not food • Family dietary practices should model the recommendations in the Food Guide Pyramid (see Chapter 1) • Encourage an active lifestyle, with physical activity being a more important and time-consuming part of early childhood than television and video games	• Reserve "empty calories" for special occasions only • Utilize regularly kept information in height/weight charts and the BMI index as a guide to appropriate weight management	• Establish that the child is overweight early—from height/weight charts and the BMI index	• Increase age-appropriate physical activity • Have fruits and vegetables available for snacks • Do not focus on the child's dieting—the entire family should eat appropriately—the child should not loose weight if the increased weight is mild to moderate, but weight should stabilize as the child grows	• Assist the family to recognize the need for the young child to lose weight • Get the child a physical examination by a health care provider before any major dietary changes are made • Initiate other actions according to those listed in primary and secondary prevention • If child is morbidly obese, additional medical intervention may be necessary, including family psychiatric interventions	• Same as in primary prevention	• Same as in primary prevention

physical education programs that encourage and focus on vigorous individual exercise and self-discipline as lifetime habits would better serve the health needs of even the youngest in this population. Community health nurses can promote development of and participation in such programs in their contacts with children of all ages.

Programs For Children With Special Needs

Many children have special needs. They may have a congenital or acquired developmental disability or a chronic emotional, mental, or physical disease. Infants, toddlers, and preschoolers may be diagnosed with asthma, diabetes, cerebral palsy, cystic fibrosis, muscular dystrophy, autism, ODD, ADHD, or ADD. Educational, health, and social or recreational services should be available for all children.

Public schools have been mandated by federal law since the 1970s to provide a full and equal educational program for all children, regardless of their ability level. Children as young as 3 months of age can receive infant stimulation services at home or in some schools especially designed to meet the needs of the very young. These programs are offered on a part-time basis for 1 to 2 hours, two to three times a week. By preschool age, children advance to half-day programs. Additional services are provided to assist the families in getting children to the programs. Door-to-door bus service in specially equipped small buses or vans safely transports young children who arrive at school in wheelchairs or with other assistive devices.

Head Start programs serve 3- to 5-year-olds from low-income families to give them a "head start" at being successful in school. Head Start programs seek to prepare children for the challenges of a structured school environment.

Availability of health services for children with special needs varies with the size of the community. In small rural communities, children and their parents may have to travel long distances to receive specialized services that the child needs. In inner-city neighborhoods, lack of money for transportation can make even nearby services equally inaccessible. Accessibility is also influenced by lack of knowledge, attitudes, and prejudices. Community health nurses must recognize the power of these immobilizing factors and be able to deal with them effectively in order to make positive changes.

Most communities offer additional social and recreational programs for children with special needs. Children as young as 3 to 4 years of age can participate in special camping programs, run by voluntary organizations, that usually are "disease specific." For example, American Lung Association affiliate offices sponsor camping programs for children with asthma or other lung diseases. Often, these are week-long sleep-away camps for school-aged children, but they may also be day camps with parents in attendance for preschoolers. Nationwide programs such as the Special Olympics offer recreational competition for children of all ages with special needs in a variety of sports, such as bowling, track and field, skiing, and swimming.

The community health nurse best serves families as a resource for such programs. Some parents are not aware of the rights or services available for their special needs children. Nurses can advocate for parents and help establish services in communities where needed services are lacking.

ROLE OF THE COMMUNITY HEALTH NURSE

Community health nurses face the challenge of continually assessing each population's current health problems, as well as determining available and needed services. Some gaps can be filled by nursing interventions. Others must be filled by referrals to various members of the community health team, with whom the nurse may sometimes collaboratively develop services.

Community health nursing interventions with infant, toddler, and preschool populations are focused on education, engineering, and enforcement. The nurse uses educational interventions when teaching family planning, nutrition and exercise, safety precautions, or child care skills. Such interventions involve providing information and encouraging client groups (parents and young children) to participate in their own health care. Engineering interventions are those strategies in which the nurse uses a greater degree of persuasion or positive manipulation, such as conducting voluntary immunization programs, encouraging enrollment in nutrition programs, preventing communicable diseases, and encouraging appropriate use of child safety devices such as car seats. Finally, the nurse uses enforcement interventions that coerce people into compliance with laws that require certain immunizations or mandate reporting of suspected child abuse and environmental health standards violations such as sanitation issues.

The community health nurse acts as an advocate and a resource for families of young children. The nurse is aware of federal, state, and local laws that preserve and protect the rights of children. Availability of educational, medical, social, and recreational services needed by young families is a necessity. The nurse helps to secure these services in the community she or he serves. Ensuring that families have the resources to provide a safe and healthy environment for their children can take many forms. The nurse may lobby to change existing laws, initiate the effort needed to establish programs and services in the community, and teach families infant safety or the importance of immunizations as part of a home visit (Table 27–3).

SUMMARY

Young children are an important population group to community health nurses, because their physical and emotional health is vital to the future of society and because the very youngest are unable to help themselves.

Mortality rates for children in the United States have decreased dramatically since the early 1900s, but morbidity rates among young children remain high. Children are still vulnerable to many illnesses and injuries, often as a result of a complex and stressful environment. In many other countries, child health has improved. However, in countries with long histories of political unrest and a lack of natural resources, the welfare of young children still remains bleak.

Worldwide, toddlers and preschoolers are at risk for accidents (falls, drowning, burns, and poisoning); acute illnesses, particularly respiratory illnesses; and nutritional, dental, and emotional ailments. Violence against children and deaths from homicide have alarming rates of occurrence in the United States. These problems create major challenges to the community health nurse who seeks to prevent illness and injury among children and promote their health.

Health services for children span three categories: preventive, health-protecting, and health-promoting. The community health nurse plays a vital role in each. Preventive services include quality child care, immunization programs, parental support services, and family planning programs.

T A B L E   27-3

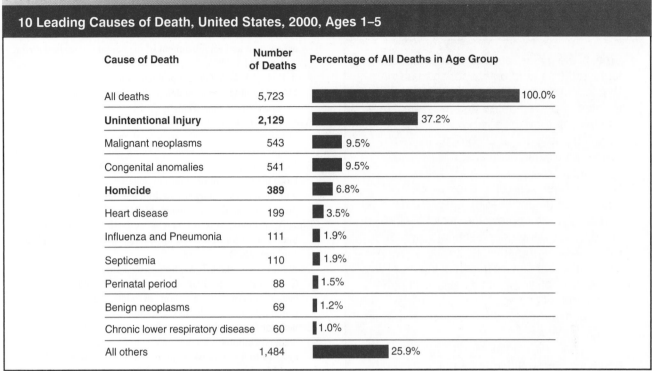

10 Leading Causes of Death, United States, 2000, Ages 1–5

Cause of Death	Number of Deaths	Percentage of All Deaths in Age Group
All deaths	5,723	100.0%
Unintentional Injury	**2,129**	37.2%
Malignant neoplasms	543	9.5%
Congenital anomalies	541	9.5%
Homicide	**389**	6.8%
Heart disease	199	3.5%
Influenza and Pneumonia	111	1.9%
Septicemia	110	1.9%
Perinatal period	88	1.5%
Benign neoplasms	69	1.2%
Chronic lower respiratory disease	60	1.0%
All others	1,484	25.9%

Health protection services include accident and injury control, programs to reduce environmental hazards, control of infectious diseases, services to protect children from child abuse, and fluoridation of community water supplies to protect children's dental health. Health promotion services include health outcome programs in early childhood development, nutrition and weight control, and exercise and physical fitness.

The role of community health nurses includes three basic interventions to serve young children's health needs. With educational interventions for the young child, such as nutrition teaching, nurses provide information and encourage parents to act responsibly on behalf of their children to assist in healthy habit formation for a lifetime. With engineering interventions, such as encouraging age-appropriate immunizations, nurses employ persuasive tactics to move clients toward more positive health behaviors. With enforcement interventions, such as reporting and intervening in child abuse, nurses practice some forms of coercion to protect children from threats to their health.

ACTIVITIES TO PROMOTE CRITICAL THINKING

1. What is the major cause of death among infants, toddlers, and preschool-aged children? What community-wide interventions could be initiated to prevent these deaths? Select one intervention for each age group, and describe how you and a group of community health professionals might develop this preventive measure.

2. Describe one health promotion program that you as a community health nurse could initiate and carry out to improve the health of children in a day care center or preschool program.

3. How can environmental health protection programs affect the future health of infants? Why is control of environmental hazards important for children of any age? List three things a nurse can do to protect children from environmental hazards.

4. A 1-year-old girl from a middle-class family and a 4-year-old girl from a poor family both come to the office you use when working with one preschool program in your community. The girls have similar symptoms that possibly indicate pediculosis capitis (head lice). Would your assessment and interventions be the same or different for the two girls? What are your values and attitudes toward people with "nuisance" diseases such as pediculosis capitis? Does social class, race, age, or sex make any difference in how you feel about them? What is one action the community health nurse can take to prevent such diseases in this population group?

5. Using the Internet, locate national Web sites that give you current information about progress toward meeting some of the *Healthy People 2010* goals with infants, toddlers, and preschool-aged children. Are we making progress? Will we meet the 2010 goal with these populations? What can a community health nurse do locally to promote the positive trend, if one exists, or to turn around a negative trend in the community? What needs to be done on the regional, state, or national level?

REFERENCES

Administration on Children, Youth and Families (ACF) (2002). *Child maltreatment 2000.* Washington, DC: U.S. Government Printing Office.

Akinbami, L.J., & Schoendorf, K.C. (2002). Trends in childhood asthma: Prevalence, health care utilization, and mortality. *Pediatrics, 110*(2), 315–322.

American Academy of Pediatrics. (2003). Oral health risk assessment and establishment of the dental home. *Pediatrics, 111*(5), 1113–1116.

Aust, P.H. (1994). When the problem is not the problem: Understanding attention deficit disorder with and without hyperactivity. *Child Welfare, 73*(3), 215–227.

Averitt, S.S. (2003). "Homelessness is not a choice!" The plight of homeless women with preschool children living in temporary shelters. *Journal of Family Nursing, 9*(1), 79–100.

Barkley, R.A., Fischer, M., Smallish, L., & Fletcher, K. (2003). Does the treatment of attention deficit/hyperactivity disorder with stimulants contribute to drug use/abuse? A 13-year prospective study. *Pediatrics, 111*(1), 107–109.

Butz, A.M, Lears, M.K., O'Neil, S., & Lusk, P. (1998). Home intervention for in-utero drug exposed infants. *Public Health Nursing, 15*(5), 307–318.

Carabin, H., Gyorkos, T.W., Soto, J.C., Penrod, J., Joseph, L., & Collet, J.P. (1999). Estimation of direct and indirect costs because of common infections in toddlers attending day care centers. *Pediatrics, 103*(3), 556–564.

Centers for Disease Control and Prevention. (1999). Notice to readers: National vaccination coverage levels among children aged 19 to 35 months—United States, 1998. *MMWR Morbidity and Mortality Weekly Report, 48*(32), 829–830.

Centers for Disease Control and Prevention. (2002). Child maltreatment facts. Retrieved April 2004 from *www.cdc.gov/ncipc/factsheets/cm_facts.htm*

Centers for Disease Control and Prevention. (2003a). General recommendations on immunizations: Recommendations of the Advisory Committee on Immunization Practices (ACIP), American Academy of Pediatrics and American Academy of Family Physicians. *MMWR Morbidity and Mortality Weekly Report, 52*(04), Q1–Q4.

Centers for Disease Control and Prevention. (2003b). HIV/AIDS surveillance report, year end 2001. Retrieved January 24, 2004, from *http://www.cdc.gov/hiv/stats/hasrlink.htm*

Centers for Disease Control and Prevention. (2003c). Web-Based Injury Statistics Query and Reporting System (WISQARS). Retrieved April 2004 from *www.cdc.gov/ncipc/wisqars*

Chernoff, R., Combs-Orme, T., Risley-Curtiss, C., & Heisler, A. (1994). Assessing the health status of children entering foster care. *Pediatrics, 93*(4), 594–601.

Child Abuse. (2002). Child Abuse Prevention and Treatment Act. Retrieved April 2004 from *http://www.uscode.house.gov/usc.htm*

Cohen, S.M. (2001). Lead poisoning: A summary of treatment and prevention. *Pediatric Nursing, 27*(2), 124–130.

Cooke, R.W., & Foulder-Hughes, L. (2003). Growth impairment in the very preterm and cognitive and motor performance at 7 years. *Archives of Disease in Childhood, 88,* 482–487.

DeKlyen, M., Speltz, M., & Greenberg, M. (1998). Attachment of disruptive preschool boys to their fathers. *Clinical Child and Family Psychology Review, 1,* 3–21.

Divertie, V. (2002). Strategies to promote medication adherence in children with asthma. *Maternal Child Nursing, 27*(1), 10–18.

English, D.J. (1998). The extent and consequences of child maltreatment. *The Future of Children, 8*(1), 39–53.

Forshner, L., & Garza, A. (1999). Childhood vaccines: An update. *RN, 62*(4), 32–37.

Gormley, W.T. (1995). *Everybody's children: Child care as a public problem*. Washington, D.C.: Brookings Institute.

Guasasco, C., Heur, L.J., & Lausch, C. (2002). Providing health care and education to migrant farm workers in nurse managed centers. *Nursing Education, 23*(4), 166–171.

Hodges, E.A. (2003). A primer on early childhood obesity and parental influence. *Pediatric Nursing, 29*(1), 12–22.

Kendall, J., Hatton, D., Beckett, A., & Leo, M. (2003). Children's accounts of attention-deficit/hyperactivity disorder. *Advances in Nursing Science, 26*(2), 114–130.

Kimm, S.Y., & Obarzanek, E. (2002). Childhood obesity: A new pandemic of the new millennium. *Pediatrics, 110*(5), 1003–1007.

Kovner, A.R., & Jonas, S. (Eds.). (1999). *Jonas and Kovner's health care delivery in the United States*. New York: Springer.

Lucarelli, P. (2002). Raising the bar for health and safety in child care. *Pediatric Nursing, 28*(3), 239–241.

Markowitz, G., & Rosner, D. (2000). "Cater to the children": The role of the lead industry in a public health tragedy, 1900–1955. *American Journal of Public Health, 90*(1), 36–46.

Marks, M.G. (1998). *Broadribb's introductory pediatric nursing* (5th ed.). Philadelphia: Lippincott-Raven.

Martin, J.A., Park, M.M., & Sutton, P.D. (2002). Births: Preliminary data for 2001. *National Vital Statistics Reports, 50*(10), 1–20.

Moss, M.E., & Carver, K. (1998). The effect of WIC and Medicaid on infant mortality in the United States. *American Journal of Public Health, 88*(9), 1354–1361.

Population Reference Bureau. (2002). World population data sheet. Retrieved January 24, 2004, from *http://www.prb.org*

Schwimmer, J.B., Burwinkle, T.M., & Varni, J.W. (2003). Health related quality of life of severely obese children and adolescents. *Journal of the American Medical Association, 289*(14), 1813–1819.

Spector, R.E. (2000). *Cultural diversity in health and illness* (5th ed.). Upper Saddle River, N.J.: Prentice-Hall Health.

Speltz, M.L., McClellan, J., DeKlyen, M., & Jones, K. (1999). Preschool boys with oppositional defiant disorder: Clinical presentation and diagnostic change. *Journal of the Academy of Child and Adolescent Psychiatry, 38*(7), 838–845.

Stormschak, E., Speltz, M., DeKlyen, M., & Greenberg, M. (1997). Family interactions during clinical intake: A comparison of families containing normal or disruptive boys. *Journal of Abnormal Child Psychology, 25,* 345–357.

United States Census Bureau. (2000). *Statistical abstract of the United States, 2000* (120th ed.). Washington, DC: Author.

United States Department of Education (1990). *America 2000: An education strategy sourcebook*. Washington, DC: Author.

United States Department of Health and Human Services. (1998). *Healthy People 2010 objectives: Draft for public comment*. Washington DC: Author.

United States Department of Health and Human Services. (2000). *Healthy People 2010* (Conference ed., Vols. 1 & 2). Washington, DC: U. S. Government Printing Office.

Valanis, B. (1999). *Epidemiology in health care* (3rd ed.). Stamford, CT: Appleton & Lange.

Wiggins, P.K. (2001). *Why should I nurse my baby?* Franklin, VA: L.A. Publishing.

World Health Organization. (2002). *The world health report, 2002: Reducing risks, promoting healthy life*. Geneva, Switzerland: Author.

Zhou, F., Bisgaed, K.M., Hussain, Y., Deuson, R.R., Bath, S.K., & Murphy, T.V. (2002). Impact of universal *Haemophilus influenzae* type b vaccination starting at 2 months of age in the United States: An economic analysis. *Pediatrics, 110*(4), 653–661.

SELECTED READINGS

Baker, A.J., Piotrkowski, C.S., & Brooks-Gunn, J. (1999). The home instruction program for preschool youngsters (HIPPY). *The Future of Children, 9*(1), 116–133.

Centers for Disease Control and Prevention. (1996). Progress toward elimination of *Haemophilus influenzae type b* disease among infants and children—United States, 1987–1995. *MMWR Morbidity and Mortality Weekly Report, 45,* 901–906.

Foley, H.A., Carlton, C.O., & Howell, R.J. (1996). The relationship of attention deficit hyperactivity disorder and conduct disorders to juvenile delinquency: Legal implications. *Bulletin of the Academy of Psychiatry Law, 24,* 333–345.

Kimmel, S.R. (2002). Vaccine adverse events: Separating myth from reality. *American Family Physician, 66*(11), 2113–2120.

McCarthy, M.J., Herbert, R., & Brimacombe, M. (2002). Empowering parents through asthma education. *Pediatric Nursing, 28*(5), 465–504.

McEvoy, M. (2003). Culture and spirituality as an integrated concept in pediatric care. *Maternal Child Nursing, 28*(1), 39–43.

28

School-Age Children and Adolescents

Learning Objectives

Upon mastery of this chapter, you should be able to:

- ● Identify major health problems and concerns for school-age and adolescent populations in the United States.
- ● Describe types of programs and services that promote health and prevent illness and injury of school-age and adolescent populations.
- ● State the recommended immunization schedule for school-age children and give the rationale for the timing of each immunization.
- ● Describe some common roles and functions of school nurses.
- ● Evaluate the potential benefits of school-based health centers, and discuss possible parental or community objections.

T here are projected to be approximately 48 million school-age children and adolescents in the United States by 2005 (U. S. Department of Education, 2003). Every school day, they attend more than 92,000 schools (National Center for Education Statistics [NCES], 2003a). These children are the parents, workers, leaders, and decision makers of tomorrow, and their future success depends in good measure on achievement of their educational goals today. Their school success in turn depends to some degree on the state of their health.

Think back to your own elementary and secondary schooling. Did you have access to a school nurse? If so, how did that person influence your health and the health of your peers? If you did not have a school nurse, how do you think a school nurse might have improved your school environment or educational experience? This chapter explores the health needs of school-age children and adolescents. Various services that address those needs are described, and the role of the school nurse as a key provider of these services is emphasized. This chapter should increase your understanding of the vital role of the school nurse in promoting the health of school-age and adolescent youngsters. It may also lead you to investigate a career in school nursing for yourself.

HEALTH PROBLEMS OF SCHOOL-AGE CHILDREN

The well-being of children has been a subject of great concern in this country for many years. International organizations, including the World Health Organization (WHO), the United Nations Children's Fund (formerly, United Nations International Children's Education Fund [UNICEF]), and U. S. governmental agencies, nonprofit groups, and charitable foundations have focused their resources on improving the health and well-being of children. Nonetheless, the needs of millions of children worldwide continue to go unmet. Even in the wealthiest nations, many children face complex and often chronic health problems that cause them to miss school days or participate only marginally in the classroom. The chronic health problems of children younger than 18 years of age are ranked in Display 28–1; many of these problems are explored in this chapter.

Problems Associated With Economic Status

Although the poverty rate for children living with family members has decreased from a 1993 high of 22%, it is still very much an issue for children and adolescents affected by a lack of resources (America's Children, 2002). Single-parent families (usually without an adult man present), welfare reform, and economic trends that keep less well-educated populations from entering all but the most menial jobs combine to produce a powerful synergistic effect for children and adolescents (Shields & Behrman, 2002). In 2000, more than

---

DISPLAY 28–1

Chronic Health Problems of School-Aged Children and Adolescents Younger Than 18 Years of Age (Ranked by Prevalence)

1. Hay fever or allergic rhinitis without asthma
2. Chronic sinusitis
3. Asthma
4. Chronic bronchitis
5. Dermatitis
6. Deformities/orthopedic impairments
7. Acne
8. Chronic disease of tonsils/adenoids
9. Heart disease
10. Deafness/hearing impairments/speech impairments

(From Collins, J. [1997]. *Prevalence of selected chronic conditions: United States, 1990–1992.* Washington, DC: National Center for Health Statistics.)

16% of children younger than 18 years of age lived in poverty, and three of every four poor children came from a home where someone worked full- or part-time for at least part of the year (Children's Defense Fund, 2003). Poverty has profound effects on children. Poor children and adolescents are more likely to experience poor health, score lower on standardized tests, be held back a grade, drop out of school, have out-of-wedlock births, experience violent crime, and end up as poor adults (Lewit, Terman, & Behrman, 1997). A longitudinal study in New Zealand by Poulton and colleagues (2002) found that childhood poverty can lead to health problems in adulthood (eg, poor cardiovascular health, periodontal disease) even if socioeconomic status later increases. According to the Children's Defense Fund (2002), 1 in 16 children lives in extreme poverty, and 1 in 3 children will experience poverty at sometime throughout childhood. Poor children are about twice as likely as children from higher-income families to have stunted growth, to be affected by lead poisoning, and to be held back in school. As the Children's Defense Fund (2002) stated, it is clearly in society's best interest to care for its children, because they will become the taxpayers of tomorrow.

Welfare reforms enacted in 1996 (ie, The Personal Responsibility and Work Opportunity Reconciliation Act) have been successful in moving many families from welfare to work. By 2000, the number of families receiving cash assistance fell to half the number served in 1996 (Shields & Behrman, 2002). Despite dire predictions of failure, some studies have shown that school-age children in families that participate in these programs do better in school and exhibit fewer behavior problems than those who do not participate. More negative outcomes, however, were found for adolescents, even though employment and income levels were increased (Morris, Huston, & Duncan, 2001). Some small but significant improvements in parenting practices of participating mothers were also noted (Chase-Lansdale & Pittman, 2002). There is a need for high-quality child care and after-school programs to support these families (Fuller et al., 2002). Some studies indicate that about half the families who leave welfare actually have fewer economic resources than they had while on welfare. A good number actually return to welfare rolls because of their inability to survive in the work world (Loprest, 2001).

The many needs of America's 11.7 million poor children are only part of the picture (Children's Defense Fund, 2003). There are millions more children in moderate-income families who have inadequate child care, limited health insurance, limited access to higher education, and poor housing. In fact, a classic study by Vissing and Diament (1997) surveyed more than 3600 high school students in New Hampshire and Maine and found that between 5% and 10% had been homeless during the past year. Almost 20% lived in distressing situations and were at risk of being homeless. Currently, more than 11.8% of children age 18 years or younger lack health insurance (Maternal and Child Health Bureau,

2002g). In some states, this figure is 21% or higher, even though more than 90% of uninsured children have one or more parents who work, and more than 66% have family incomes greater than the poverty level (see Research: Bridge to Practice).

There are specific physical health problems related to poverty (eg, lead poisoning, iron deficiency anemia, increased susceptibility to illness). Many school-age children suffer from the effects of poverty-related hunger. It is difficult to concentrate and to learn properly if meals are often skipped or if food consistently does not provide enough nourishment. Alaimo, Olson, and Frongillo (2001) found that younger school-age children were more likely to have had difficulty getting along with other children, to have seen a psychologist, and to have repeated a grade if they reported food insufficiency. Food-insufficient adolescents were more likely to have had problems getting along with other children, to have seen a psychologist, and to have been suspended from school. Food insufficiency was characterized by the child reporting that "his or her family sometimes or often did not get enough food to eat" (p. 44). According to a

---

RESEARCH: BRIDGE TO PRACTICE

Morris, R.I., & Butt, R.A. (2003). Parents' perspectives on homelessness and its effects on the educational development of their children. *Journal of School Nursing, 19*(1), 43–50.

Homelessness is an increasing problem—and families with children are the fastest growing segment of the homeless population. Poor children without a home more often report health and mental health problems, as well as hunger and barriers to school attendance. A retired nursing professor and a school nurse consultant examined parents' perceptions about how their homelessness affected the academic achievement and overall development of their children. They used a qualitative method of study, grounded theory, to determine the meaning homeless parents gave to their lifestyles. They conducted 1- to 2-hour interviews with 34 homeless families, using an interview guide to collect demographic data and open-ended questions to "explore the meaning of experiences" (p. 44). All families were currently residing in homeless emergency shelters, transitional housing, or motels/hotels and were composed of at least one adult and one child. Fewer than 15% were intact families; most were single-parent families.

Three major themes emerged from the data: (1) unstable relationships, (2) abdication of responsibility, and (3) perception of children's educational needs. Abuse, addiction, inadequate parenting models, and continuing crisis/conflict with family defined the theme of unstable

relationships. Parents often reported that school was "a place for their children to be cared for by others" (p. 46). Denial, blaming, and dependency were the hallmarks of the second theme, abdication of responsibility. Many parents either stated that they had noticed no behavior changes in their children since becoming homeless or, if they had been confronted by the school about problems, blamed the school as the source of the problem. The relationship between parents and the schools was a tenuous one—parents did not think absences were a significant problem, and they felt incapable of helping their children with homework. Frequent changes of residence and child embarrassment about the lack of a stable home were noted educational barriers. Parents perceived their children to be socially competent, and many children persevered despite hardships, demonstrating great resilience.

The researchers concluded that deprivation in security and parental attention contributes to poor academic achievement among homeless children. This study has implications for school nurses, because they frequently are the liaison between the school and the family. The researchers suggested development of interventions to empower homeless parents to assume more responsibility and become more proactive in working with schools to improve their childrens' educational outcomes. School nurse collaboration with interdisciplinary teams to design programs, policies, and parenting classes were also suggested as interventions.

2000 survey by the Food Research and Action Center (2003), 11.5% of all American households were food insecure, and 3.3 million people were classified as hungry. Weinreb and colleagues (2002) studied the effects of hunger on preschool and school-age children. They found that, even after controlling for variables such as housing status, mother's distress, child life events, and low birth weight, severe hunger was a predictor for adverse outcomes of both physical health (ie, chronic illness) and mental health (ie, anxiety, depression, internalizing behavior problems). In a U. S. Department of Agriculture survey (2001), only about half of food-insecure households reported use of any of the largest federal food assistance programs—food stamps, free or reduced school lunches, and Special Supplemental Food Program for Women, Infants, and Children (WIC). Children go hungry because many eligible families do not use these worthwhile services. In a survey of emergency food recipients, only 30% reported participation in the Food Stamp Program, even though almost 75% were eligible based on income; 34% stated that the program's application process was too difficult, and 7% cited social stigma as a reason for not participating. Those children who participate in school lunch and breakfast programs suffer fewer side effects of hunger that affect learning. However, not all schools participate in these programs (Food Research and Action Center, 2003).

Death From Injuries

The loss of children's lives that results from all injuries combined suggests a staggering number of years of productive life lost to society. Motor vehicle crashes are the leading cause of injury death for children ages 1 to 14 years—19% in children and 38% in adolescents (Maternal and Child Health Bureau, 2002h). For the 5- to 14-year-old age group, firearm-related deaths and drowning deaths follow motor vehicle crashes as the top three causes of injury death (Maternal and Child Health Bureau, 2002e). For this age group, 59% of firearm-related deaths were homicides and 35% were suicides, with the remainder classified as unintentional (Maternal and Child Health Bureau, 2002b). Childhood unintentional injury deaths in the United States have declined by more than 40% in the past 20 years (Centers for Disease Control and Prevention [CDC], 2003c) but are still much higher than in other developed countries (Deal et al., 2000). It is estimated that the cost of childhood unintentional injuries in 1996 alone resulted in $66 billion in present and future work losses, $14 billion in lifetime medical spending, and $1 billion in other resource costs (Miller, Romano, & Spicer, 2000).

Communicable Diseases

The mortality rates of school-age children (5 to 14 years old) are comparatively low and have decreased substantially over the last century (Arias & Smith, 2003). This reduction can be attributed to effective prevention and control of the acute infectious diseases of childhood.

Although mortality rates are low, morbidity among schoolchildren is high. Children of this age group are most often affected by respiratory illnesses, followed by infectious and parasitic diseases, injuries, and digestive conditions. Among schoolchildren, the incidence rates of measles, rubella (German measles), pertussis (whooping cough), infectious parotitis (mumps), and varicella (chickenpox) have dropped considerably because of widespread immunization efforts. Cases of these communicable diseases still occur, some with potentially serious complications, such as birth defects from rubella and nerve deafness from mumps. Although the number of cases of *Haemophilus influenzae* infection increased between 1999 and 2000, those of measles, rubella, mumps, hepatitis A and B, and pertussis decreased. Reported cases of pertussis usually occur in infants younger than 7 months of age who have not yet received all three doses of the vaccine (Maternal and Child Health Bureau, 2002i). Vigorous campaigns have been undertaken by health departments to get children immunized. An immunization for mumps, measles, and rubella (MMR) has been available for more than 20 years, and newer vaccines for *H. influenzae* type b (Hib), hepatitis A and B, and varicella have been developed and are now part of the childhood immunization schedule. As increasing numbers of school-age children must show proof of required vaccinations before they are allowed to enroll in school, the percentages of children in this age group who are immunized against specific diseases will continue to rise. However, some studies reveal that immunization compliance for adolescents is a continuing problem due to lack of sufficient insurance coverage and poor systems for tracking and recall (Schaffer et al., 2001).

Chronic Diseases

The number of school-age children afflicted with chronic diseases is rising. Commonly seen problems include hay fever, sinusitis, dermatitis, tonsillitis, asthma, diabetes, seizure disorders, and hearing difficulties. Stomachaches, headaches, colds, and flu are frequent complaints of school-age children. Asthma is the most common chronic disease of childhood. It is estimated that 12% of children younger than 18 years of age have at some time been diagnosed with asthma (CDC, 2002a). Non-Hispanic Blacks exhibit the highest asthma attack rates, and boys more often than girls reported an episode within the past year (CDC, 2001b).

Although reasons for the increased cases of asthma are somewhat unclear, experts speculate that better recognition and diagnosis of the disease; overcrowded conditions; and exposure to air pollution, allergens, and irritants in the environment are probable culprits (Daisey, Angell, & Apte, 2003; Ross et al., 2002; Shima et al., 2002). According to a study by Tortolero and colleagues (2002), children with asthma may have attacks triggered by exposure to cigarette smoke, stress, strenuous exercise, weather changes (eg, cold, windy, rainy weather), allergens, irritants, or air pollutants (indoor or outdoor). Many schools have high levels of allergens and irritants.

Treatment for asthma usually includes inhaled corticosteroids (Parameswaran, O'Byrne, & Sears, 2003). Parent and child education, along with adequate primary medical care, would help decrease the number of emergency room visits (Boudreaux et al., 2003; Lara et al., 2003).

School nurses often work with a student, the families, and the child's doctor to develop an asthma action plan to control, prevent, or minimize untoward effects of acute asthma episodes. Peak flowmeters can be used frequently to determine early signs of asthma problems. Monitoring asthma medications and teaching proper methods of inhaler use are also vital school nursing functions.

Diabetes is another common chronic illness in children, with the American Diabetes Association (2000) reporting that the incidence of diabetes among those younger than 20 years of age is 1.7 per 1000. Experts now conclude that both type 1 and type 2 diabetes mellitus are found in school-age children. Type 2 diabetes is rising almost exponentially in this age group, which has led some scientists to call this a major public health crisis, one caused largely by obesity, sedentary lifestyle, and the predisposition of certain ethnic groups (see Levels of Prevention).

Obesity-related hospital costs for the 6- to 17-year-old age group has reached $127 million a year (Goran, Ball, & Cruz, 2003). Identified risk factors for type 2 diabetes include insulin resistance syndrome, obesity (including increased body fat and abdominal fat), family history, diabetic gestation, and underweight or overweight for gestational age (Silverstein & Rosenbloom, 2001). During adolescent development, these risk factors may be most problematic.

LEVELS OF PREVENTION MATRIX

SITUATION: The School Nurse and Children with Type 2 Diabetes.

GOAL: Using the three levels of prevention, negative health conditions are avoided, or promptly diagnosed and treated, and the fullest possible potential is restored.

PRIMARY PREVENTION		SECONDARY PREVENTION		TERTIARY PREVENTION		
Health Promotion and Education	*Health Protection*	*Early Diagnosis*	*Prompt Treatment*	*Rehabilitation*	*Primary Prevention*	
					Health Promotion and Education	*Health Protection*
• Educate to promote good nutrition and a physically active lifestyle • Provide classroom contact in the early primary grades to encourage children to make good food choices • Limit passive activities and increase sports and physical activity • Teach older children how to make better food choices at fast food restaurants		• Teach older students to calculate their BMI • Monitor BMI scores • Yearly screenings for height and weight (calipers are useful) • Complete health histories on at-risk children	• Initiate referrals for health care provider follow-up in collaboration with parents on students at risk for type 2 diabetes • Initiate referrals to health care providers in collaboration with parents for students with signs and symptoms of type 2 diabetes	• Monitor the child's health • Work closely with the child, family, physician, and teacher to ensure proper follow-up • Be alert to monitor for any possible complications (e.g., medication side effects)	• Continue to promote a healthy lifestyle that includes appropriate food choices and daily physical activity within the limitations of diabetes type 2	• Educate the teachers on safety precautions for children in their classroom diagnosed with diabetes type 2 • Monitor children taking medications for diabetes type 2 (e.g., overdosage, under-dosage, adverse reactions)

Prevention of type 2 diabetes through education and improvement in exercise, nutrition, and lifestyle, can be one of the most important areas of focus for health professionals who work with the school-age population. Younger children with type 1 diabetes, especially those who use insulin pumps, may need careful monitoring, something that is not always possible for the school nurse who is assigned to several school sites and may not be present when problems arise. A multidisciplinary team approach is needed, with family and physician collaboration. Diabetic children and adolescents may be reluctant to comply with medical regimens, although strict adherence has been proven to reduce later microvascular complications (Tapper-Strawhacker, 2001). Testing blood sugar and taking insulin at school can be frustrating and can cause children to feel singled out or different from their peers. One study found that adolescents with type 1 diabetes have significantly higher rates of depression than those without diabetes (Kanner, Hamrin, & Grey, 2003). It is important for school nurses to understand each child's unique concerns and to alert teachers and school personnel to the signs and symptoms (as well as treatment) of hypoglycemia. In addition to the obvious emergency health-related concerns for diabetic children, a classic study showed that diabetes-related severe hypoglycemia can affect memory tasks (Hershey et al., 1999). Over time, memory deficits can affect learning and progress in school.

Juvenile rheumatoid arthritis is a painful autoimmune disorder characterized by persistent joint swelling and stiffness with periods of remission and flare-up. It is treated with nonsteroidal anti-inflammatory drugs (NSAIDs), disease-modifying antirheumatic drugs (DMARDs; eg, methotrexate) and sometimes corticosteroids or biologic agents (National Institute of Arthritis and Musculoskeletal and Skin Diseases, 2001; Wilkinson, Jackson, & Gardner-Medwin, 2003). Exercise is often an important component of therapy, and an adapted physical education program may be developed for these children. Long-term sequelae may result, and many adolescents with this disorder require additional support and counseling (Bowyer et al., 2003).

Seizure disorders are not uncommon in the school-age population. Epilepsy is a disorder of the brain in which neurons sometimes give abnormal signals. For almost 80% of those diagnosed, seizures can usually be controlled with medication or surgical treatment. Vagus nerve stimulators are now used in some cases after other treatments have failed (Buchhalter & Jarrar, 2003; National Institute of Neurological Disorders and Stroke, 2001). Treatment of epilepsy has been greatly enhanced by the use of newer antiepilepsy drugs (AEDs) specific to the pediatric population and, in some cases, by a diet rich in proteins and fats and low in carbohydrates—a ketogenic diet (Buchhalter & Jarrar, 2003; Kossoff et al., 2003). It is important to monitor medication compliance and teach school staff about first aid measures for seizure victims. Children and adolescents with seizure disorders may feel embarrassed or be the victims of teasing or bullying. They may exhibit signs of school avoidance. It is im-

portant for school nurses to work with these children and to teach all students about the disease process and the need for empathy and understanding.

The fourth leading cause of death in the 1- to 19-year-old age group is cancer (Gloeckler-Ries, Percy, & Bunin, 1999). Childhood cancers (eg, leukemia) now have better outcomes than ever before. More than 70% of childhood cancers are now considered curable, with survivors more concerned about the later complications of treatment rather than cancer recurrence (Wallace et al., 2001). Many children return to school after initial hospitalization and treatment. School nurses can help children make this transition by educating their classmates about cancer facts (eg, it is not contagious), helping them make necessary adjustments, and being vigilant in protecting any immunocompromised students from communicable diseases.

Behavioral Problems and Learning Disabilities

Other childhood health problems, less easy to detect and measure but often as debilitating, are those of emotional, behavioral, and intellectual development. Although these problems are not new, awareness and concern have increased as the rates of occurrence for other life-threatening childhood diseases have diminished. Emotional or behavior problems and learning disabilities are prevalent in childhood. In one survey, 6% of respondents reported having attention deficit hyperactivity disorder (ADHD) and 8% had some type of **learning disability** (CDC, 2002a). More boys than girls reported ADHD (9% versus 3%) or a learning disability (10% versus 5%). Children and adults with average or above-average intelligence who demonstrate significant difficulties in one or more areas of learning (eg, reading, writing, mathematics) may have a learning disability. Causes of learning disabilities and emotional behavioral problems appear to have genetic, environmental, and cultural influences. The number of children with learning disabilities in the lowest economic group is twice that in the highest group (CDC, 2002a). Children who were characterized as being in fair or poor health were more than four times as likely to have a learning disability and three times as likely to have ADHD as children with excellent, very good, or good health status (CDC, 2002a). High-risk families have a high incidence of child abuse (physical and sexual) and neglect. The number of children affected by parental drug use has surpassed that of children with disabilities caused by lead poisoning, another major contributor to developmental problems in children.

Behavioral and emotional problems of school-age children stem from many causes. The rate of divorce in the United States is double what it was in the 1950s. Over the last 30 years, the percentage of children living in two-parent families decreased from 85% to 69%; and more than 26% of children today live with one parent, usually their mother (Schor, 2003). Children of divorce are more likely to exhibit conduct problems. They often have lower academic achievement, more symptoms of psychological maladjustment, more social problems, a poorer self-concept, and a lower standard of living, compared with children raised in intact families. Those children who are products of highly contentious divorces are most at risk. The results of this maladjustment can also be observed in later adult life. School nurses can be alert to early symptoms and refer parents to marital counseling or suggest family therapists. Some schools are also now offering support groups for children of divorce.

Attention deficit hyperactivity disorder (ADHD) is a cluster of problems related to hyperactivity, impulsivity, and inattention (Display 28–2). It affects about 6% of school-age children (Lesene, Visser, & White, 2003), with estimates of prevalence ranging from 2% to 18% (Rowland, Lesesne, & Abramowitz, 2002). However, it is diagnosed with increasing frequency. One study found an increased rate of ADHD

diagnosis, from 0.9 per 100 children in 1987 to 3.4 per 100 in 1997, with the largest increase among low-income and poor children in the 12- to 18-year-old age group (Olfson et al., 2003). Although there were fewer treatment visits, an increase was noted in stimulant prescriptions during this same period. Another study found a positive association between stimulant treatment for ADHD and age, male gender, fewer child dependents, higher income, white communities, and living in the Midwest or South (Cox et al., 2003). Interestingly, girls are at increased risk for not receiving appropriate services because they often do not exhibit the hyperactivity component and are not diagnosed.

Some research has shown that prenatal exposure to nicotine and psychosocial adversity are associated with ADHD (Biederman & Farraone, 2002). There seem to be multiple reasons for ADHD, but new research focuses on inherited

D I S P L A Y 2 8 – 2

Diagnostic Characteristics of Attention-Deficit/Hyperactivity Disorder

A. Either (1) or (2):
   (1) six (or more) of the following symptoms of **inattention** have persisted for at least 6 months to a degree that is maladaptive and inconsistent with developmental level:

   Inattention
   (a) often fails to give close attention to details or makes careless mistakes in schoolwork, work, or other activities
   (b) often has difficulty sustaining attention in tasks or play activities
   (c) often does not seem to listen when spoken to directly
   (d) often does not follow through on instructions and fails to finish schoolwork, chores, or duties in the work-place (not due to oppositional behavior or failure to understand instructions)
   (e) often has difficulty organizing tasks and activities
   (f) often avoids, dislikes, or is reluctant to engage in tasks that require sustained mental effort (such as schoolwork or homework)
   (g) often loses things necessary for tasks or activities (e.g., toys, school assignments, pencils, books, or tools)
   (h) is often easily distracted by extraneous stimuli
   (i) is often forgetful in daily activities
   (2) six (or more) of the following symptoms of **hyperactivity-impulsivity** have persisted for at least 6 months to a degree that is maladaptive and inconsistent with developmental level:

   Hyperactivity
   (a) often fidgets with hands or feet or squirms in seat

   (b) often leaves seat in classroom or in other situations in which remaining seated is expected
   (c) often runs about or climbs excessively in situations in which it is inappropriate (in adolescents or adults, may be limited to subjective feelings of restlessness)
   (d) often has difficulty playing or engaging in leisure activities quietly
   (e) is often "on the go" or often acts as if "driven by a motor"
   (f) often talks excessively

   Impulsivity
   (g) often blurts out answers before questions have been completed
   (h) often has difficulty awaiting turn
   (i) often interrupts or intrudes on others (e.g., butts into conversations or games)

B. Some hyperactive-impulsive or inattentive symptoms that caused impairment were present before age 7 years.

C. Some impairment from the symptoms is present in two or more settings (e.g., at school [or work] and at home).

D. There must be clear evidence of clinically significant impairment in social, academic, or occupational functioning.

E. The symptoms do not occur exclusively during the course of a Pervasive Developmental Disorder, Schizophrenia, or other Psychotic Disorder and are not better accounted for by another mental disorder (e.g., Mood Disorder, Anxiety Disorder, Dissociative Disorder, or a Personality Disorder).

(From American Psychiatric Association. [2000]. *Diagnostic and statistical manual of mental disorders,* 4th ed., Text Revision. Washington, DC: Author.)

tendencies for problems with dopamine receptor and transporter genes, along with evidence of decreased blood flow in prefrontal regions of the brain. These findings support a neurobiologic basis for the condition. Some family and twin studies reveal a higher heritability factor (0.8) for ADHD than for other psychiatric disorders (Weiss & Murray, 2003). Although some health professionals believe that many of the symptoms found in people with ADHD are part of the spectrum of human behavior, others note that people with ADHD have functional impairment in academic, social, or occupational areas resulting from their problem behaviors. Noted differences have even been reported in the results of electroencephalograms (Swartwood et al., 2003). Nursing researchers have documented qualitative data from children and adolescents who described their difficulties. Corresponding similarities to psychological diagnostic criteria were noted (Kendall et al., 2003).

At each stage of development, those with ADHD are presented with distinct challenges. For example, children in elementary school often have conflict with peers and problems organizing tasks. They may be more accident prone and may have more school-related problems, such as grade retention and suspension or expulsion. They often have problems with grooming and with handwriting, and they exhibit difficulty sleeping. As adolescents, 80% still exhibit symptoms of inattentiveness, hyperactivity, and impulsiveness. Compared with non-ADHD teens, they may have more conflict with their parents, poorer social skills, and ongoing problems at school. In adulthood, they tend to have more marital and occupational problems. They often have fewer years of schooling, and poor social skills continue to be an issue (Barkley et al., 2002; Weiss & Murray, 2003).

ADHD is sometimes found with associated disorders, such as communication or language disorders and learning disabilities. Common comorbid conditions are bipolar, depressive, and anxiety disorders, as well as conduct disorders (Biederman & Faraone, 2002). An earlier age at onset of ADHD is associated with more parental reports of child aggressive behavior, and later age at onset with more anxious/depressive symptoms (Connor et al., 2003). For some children, ADHD might even be a precursor of a child-onset subtype of bipolar disorder (Masi et al., 2003).

There is a need for collaboration between the child's family, the school, and the child's physician to diagnose ADHD and to plan appropriate interventions and educational accommodations. Teacher confirmation of ADHD-related behaviors is very important. School nurses can assist parents in recognizing the symptoms of ADHD and obtaining appropriate treatment and follow-up (Subcommittee on Attention-Deficit/Hyperactivity Disorder, 2001). A multimodal treatment approach is recognized as most effective. This includes medication, usually methylphenidate (Ritalin or Concerta) or dextroamphetamine and amphetamine (Adderall); school accommodations for learning problems; and social skills training for the child with ADHD (Pelham et al., 1999). Family and individual counseling, parent support groups,

and training in behavior management techniques, as well as family education about the condition, are also essential features of this method of treatment. Not all children and adolescents respond to medication, and medication dosage must be carefully monitored and titrated. The main goal of medication for school-age children is academic improvement. If this does not occur, medication may need to be changed or discontinued. Parental depressive symptoms and severity of ADHD symptoms in children have been found to decrease the rate of response to medication and combined treatments (Owens et al., 2003). School nurses and community health nurses can work closely with school staff, parents, and physicians in determining the efficacy of treatment regimens.

Some families wish to pursue treatments other than stimulant medication. One study revealed that 54% of parents used some type of complementary and alternative medicine (eg, acupuncture, nutritional supplements, diet) and 11% did not discuss this fact with their child's physician (Chan, Rappaport, & Kemper, 2003). Promising results with neurofeedback were found in a German study (Fuchs et al., 2003). A new nonstimulant medication, Strattera (atomoxetine), is now being used for children. Parents often voice concern about giving their children a stimulant medication to treat ADHD. Resistance to treatment may stem from fears about later abuse of substances. As adolescents, those with ADHD may experiment with alcohol and other substances earlier than non-ADHD teens do; however, newer research indicates that treatment with medication for ADHD in childhood does not lead to an increased risk for substance use or abuse in adulthood (Barkley et al., 2003).

Children with disabilities account for more than 10% of the total school-age population. In the period from 1998 to 1999, 130 of every 1000 students were disabled. During that same period, 47% of those students with disabilities spent most of their time in the regular classroom—sometimes posing a challenge for teachers and school nurses who tried to meet their needs (NCES, 2003c). In descending order, the most common disabilities are learning disorders; speech or language impairment; mental retardation; serious emotional disturbances and other disabilities such as autism; deafblindness; orthopedic problems; traumatic brain injury; and other health impairments such as asthma, diabetes, and epilepsy. The prevalence of disability increased greatly over the past 30 years and was greater for Black than for White children (Newacheck et al., 2003).

Many children with perceived disabilities or problems are referred for assessment and possible placement in special education programs each year. In a classic evaluation of special education practices, Hocutt (1996) found that teachers and other school personnel refer 3% to 5% of the school-age population each year. Of the children referred, 92% are tested and 74% of those tested are ultimately placed in special education. However, most children receive special services in a regular classroom because of "full inclusion" or "mainstreaming" mandates; fewer children are segregated into special classes or separate schools.

Head Lice

Pediculosis (head lice) is a frustrating and common problem for many school-age children. It is estimated that 6 to 12 million children between the ages of 6 and 12 years get infested with head lice each year (Frankowski & Weiner, 2002). An infestation of *Pediculus humanus* var. *capitis,* the parasite that lives and feeds on the human scalp, can be an embarrassing nuisance to families of any socioeconomic level. These very tiny, wingless insects need blood to survive and can cause itching and skin irritation. They are most often found toward the nape of the neck, where hair is usually thickest, but their pearly white eggs (nits) are distributed all over the head. They are attached to the hair shaft with a glue-like substance and can be detected by careful examination of the scalp. Because nits hatch within 10 days and the immature louse can reach reproductive maturity within 8 to 9 days, recurring cycles of infestation are common. If no treatment is given, the cycle repeats every 3 weeks (Frankowski & Weiner, 2002). Complete eradication requires that all nits be removed along with lice.

Head lice are transmitted by direct contact or through shared items such as combs and brushes, hats, scarves, sheets, and towels (called fomites). Contrary to some popular myths, lice do not fly or jump and they cannot be contracted from animals. Many schools have recurring outbreaks of head lice that can be traced back to particular families who have failed to completely eradicate an infestation (Pollack, Kiszewski, & Spielman, 2000). Because of perceived social stigma, some families are defensive and unresponsive to attempts at education and intervention. Some schools resort to "no nit" policies and establish routine head lice examinations with a goal of early detection and treatment. However, the American Academy of Pediatrics and the National Association of School Nurses now discourage such policies because they have not been effective in curbing head lice infestations and they often result in significant lost school days and negative social impact (Williams et al., 2001).

Treatment of head lice commonly includes over-the-counter insecticide shampoos, such as pyrethrin-based RID or A200. A permethrin cream rinse (Nix) is currently the recommended choice for treatment (Frankowski & Weiner, 2002). Other treatments include Kwell (lindane), Ovide (malathion), oral agents such as Septra (an antibiotic) and Ivermectin (an anthelmintic agent—not yet approved by the U. S. Food and Drug Administration as a pediculicide), and occlusive agents such as petroleum jelly (Frankowski & Weiner, 2002; Jones & English, 2003). School nurses also need to educate families about reducing reinfestation by careful cleaning and treatment of any fomites (eg, combs, hats, towels, sheets, clothing, upholstered furniture) and scrupulous nit removal. In some larger cities, entrepreneurs have started nit removal businesses (eg, Nit Pickers) to assist parents with this tedious task.

Poor Nutrition and Dental Health

Other health problems found in this age group are nutritional problems (primarily overeating and inappropriate food choices) and poor dental health. Obesity often begins in childhood and becomes a risk factor for cardiovascular disease and diabetes later in life. Fifteen percent of children ages 6 to 19 years are characterized as being overweight (defined as a body mass index [BMI] at or above the 95th percentile). This represents a 4% increase over the previous survey (Ogden et al., 2002). Obese children are more likely to become obese adults. Results of a recent Youth Risk Behavior Survey indicated that 79% of those surveyed ate fewer than five servings of fruits and vegetables the day before, and 84% drank less than 3 glasses of milk per day in the previous week (CDC, 2001a).

The poor eating habits that develop during childhood are generally thought to persist into adulthood, contributing to the leading causes of death and disability—cardiovascular disease, cancer, and diabetes. In fact, evidence of early atherosclerosis and fatty streaks has been found in autopsy studies of children as young as 6 years of age (Harrell, Pearce, & Hayman, 2003). Aside from its relationship with inactivity, television viewing has been associated with higher intake of fats, sweet and salty snacks, and carbonated drinks, and lower intakes of fruits and vegetables (Coon & Tucker, 2002). Food is the most heavily advertised product on children's television, and highly sweetened products, as well as fast food, are the most frequently advertised foods. Going to bed late, decreased sleeping time (Sekine et al., 2002), and increased snacking (Jahns, Siega-Riz, & Popkin, 2001) have also been associated with childhood obesity. As children move from elementary to middle school, their food choices change dramatically. A study of 291 students by Lytle and colleagues (2000) illustrates this point. Consumption of breakfast, milk, fruits, and vegetables decreased and soft drink consumption increased between third and eighth grades. As children become older, families have less influence on food choices, and peers begin to have more influence. This is a time when school-based nutrition education programs can have an influence (Perez-Rodrigo & Aranceta, 2001) (see Using the Nursing Process).

Undernutrition can also have serious consequences, including effects on the cognitive development and academic performance of children (Cook, 2002; Hall et al., 2001). Irritability, lack of energy, and difficulty concentrating are only part of the problems that arise from skipped meals or consistently inadequate nutrition. Infection and illness that lead to loss of school days can affect academic progress and interfere with the acquisition of basic skills such as reading and mathematics. Undernutrition is frequently associated with poverty and hunger, but social pressure to be thin can also spark purposeful undernutrition. Because prepubertal children often exhibit a period of adiposity before a growth spurt, they are at risk for development of eating disorders (Dietz & Gortmaker, 2001). A Stanford University study of third

USING THE NURSING PROCESS

James Lopez is entering third grade. His teacher comes to you, the school nurse, because she is concerned about his poor performance in school. He frequently comes to school late and often puts his head on his desk and appears to be falling asleep. You notice that James has gained a significant amount of weight over the summer. His face is much fuller now than in his second grade picture.

ASSESSMENT (INITIAL VISITS)

You call James' mother and make an appointment for a home visit.

You do a health history, noting family history of diabetes, current eating, and activity and sleeping patterns for James and the family, and determine whether he has a regular physician and insurance or Medicaid.

You assess his vital signs, height and weight, hearing, and vision.

You talk more with his teacher about his activity on the playground and any signs of excessive thirst, hunger, or general fatigue.

NURSING DIAGNOSES

After a home visit, a meeting with James' teacher, and two observations/interviews with James, you decide on the following nursing diagnoses:
1. Nutrition: more than body requirements related to James' eating as a way of coping and his sedentary lifestyle.
2. Altered family process related to mother's recent change from being a stay-at-home single mom to attending truck driving school (necessitating absences of several days at a time, with James cared for by a married teenage sister and her husband).

FINDINGS, PLAN AND IMPLEMENTATION

James has been eating large quantities of snack food and fast food meals for the last 3 months, since his mother started her training. He has also quit participating in soccer and baseball, because his mother can no longer provide transportation. His bicycle was recently stolen, and he spends a lot of time playing video and computer games. James misses his mother when she is away and says that he "stays up late watching television" and has "trouble getting up for school" when he is at his sister's house.

You plan to work with the family to refer James to his physician to rule out diabetes. A family meeting is scheduled so that you can provide some health education on childhood obesity and inactivity. You discuss some possible interventions that the family can put into place:
- Decrease reliance on fast food meals.
- Have a regular evening meal time and encourage less snacking.
- Provide fresh fruit and vegetable snacks and decrease purchases of high-calorie, high-fat snack foods.
- Decrease sedentary activity (e.g., video and computer games, television viewing) and increase physical activity (e.g., team sports, walking, bicycling, active outdoor games).
- Establish a reasonable bedtime and consistently enforce it.
- Offer referral for family counseling so that James can discuss his feelings in a safe environment.
- With the family's input, seek ways for James and his mother to keep in better contact and for his sister to gain a greater understanding of good parenting practices.
- Meet with the teacher, the family, and James to discuss ways to help with his school performance.
- Continue to monitor James' progress with monthly height and weight checks, personal interviews, home visits, and teacher conferences.

EVALUATION

The physician reported that James does not have diabetes; however, if he continues to gain weight and remains inactive he is at a higher risk for type 2 diabetes. Evaluation of nursing diagnoses 1 and 2 includes the following goals:
- The family will report less reliance on fast food and more meals cooked at home.
- The family will report more purchases of fresh fruits and vegetables and fewer purchases of high-calorie, high-fat snacks.
- James will report more physical exercise (by the use of a calendar) and less hours spent in sedentary activity (corroborated by family).
- James will exhibit less tardiness and fewer signs of sleep deprivation at school, and his school performance will improve.
- James and his family will complete sessions with a family counselor.
- James' weight will remain stable or will decrease as his height increases over time.

through sixth grade students found that 50% "wanted to weigh less" and 16% had tried diet and exercise to lose weight (Schur, Sanders, & Steiner, 2000; p. 74).

Inactivity

An association between poor eating habits and physical inactivity has been found in studies of school-age children and adolescents (Chatrath et al., 2002; Trost et al., 2001). The Youth Risk Behavior Survey revealed that 48% of children surveyed were not enrolled in physical education classes, and 68% who were enrolled did not attend class on a daily basis. In addition, 31% of respondents stated that they did not participate in either vigorous or moderate physical activity (CDC, 2001a). Increased physical activity was shown to decrease BMI in a large study of overweight girls and boys (Berkey et al., 2003).

Dental Health

Dental caries affects more than half of school-age children and is the most common chronic disease for that age group. School days are lost to dental problems and dental visits, with poor children reporting almost 12 times more restricted-activity days due to dental-related illness than higher income children (CDC, 2003b). Although there has been a downturn in the rate of dental caries in school-age children over the past 2 decades (Brown, Wall, & Lazar, 2000), the prevalence of dental caries remains high in this country. The cost for dental services in 2003 was estimated to be $68 billion (CDC, 2003a). The peak incidence of dental caries is found among school-age children and adolescents, although the effects of decay are observed in adulthood as caries activity recurs or various restorations fracture or wear out and must be replaced. One study found that school-age dental decay could be predicted in toddlers by determining the frequency of brushing and other variables. This suggests the importance of regular brushing for young children (Clarke, Fraser-Lee, & Shimono, 2001).

Fluoridation of drinking water, school-based fluoride rinse or gel, and dental sealant programs are cost-effective, proven methods of reducing dental caries in school-age children (CDC, 2003b; Levy, 2003; Marinho et al., 2003; Task Force on Community Preventive Services, 2002). Between 11% and 72% of poor children have been found to have early childhood caries—an infectious disease thought to be caused by *Streptococcus mutans* and exacerbated by poor dietary practices. Topical antimicrobial therapies show some promise (Berkowitz, 2003). Some research has also shown an association between passive smoking and tooth decay (Aligne et al., 2003).

Barriers to dental care are more prevalent among the poor and those who are institutionalized. In a national survey, almost 10% of low-income children had a need for dental care, and more than 30% reported not seeing a dentist in the preceding year (Maternal and Child Health Bureau, 2002f). Financial barriers and lack of education lead to poor dental health values and adversely affect use of dental services and conscientious personal oral health care. Lack of dental insurance or access to a local dentist may deter people from seeking oral health care; however, only 19% of eligible children received preventive dental services under the Medicaid Early and Preventive Screening, Diagnosis, and Treatment (EPSDT) program in 1999 (Maternal and Child Health Bureau, 2002f).

HEALTH PROBLEMS OF ADOLESCENTS

A growing number of youth suffer from spiritual poverty and disengagement from home and school. Plagued with boredom, low self-esteem, and lack of motivation, children in wealthy homes are often insulated from challenge and risk. Many of the same problems exist for children of the rich as for those of the poor, with a number of young people turning to drugs, alcohol, and indiscriminate sexual activity. Although murder and robbery rates have declined over the last decade, the school shootings in the late 1990s attracted much public attention (Blumstein, 2002). Clearly, there is a need for improvement in the nation's efforts to prepare young people adequately for the future.

During the period that roughly encompasses the teen years, adolescents encounter many complex changes—physically, emotionally, cognitively, and socially. Rapid and major developmental adjustments create a variety of stresses with concomitant problems that have an impact on health. Mortality and morbidity rates for adolescents are low overall and demonstrate considerable improvement since the early 1900s. However, the proportion of deaths due to injury is much higher for 18-year-olds (81%) than for 10-year-olds (47%), and injuries are the most common cause of death in the 10- to 19-year–old age group (National Center for Health Statistics [NCHS], 2000). Injury death rate for adolescent males is 2.7 times higher than for females.

Unintentional injury, homicide, and suicide are the top three causes of death in the 15- to 19-year-old age group (Maternal and Child Health Bureau, 2002c). The death rate from motor vehicle-related injuries for this age group peaked during the 1970s and 1980s, and then declined throughout the 1990s to 25.9 deaths per 100,000—still the number one cause of injury mortality for this age group (Maternal and Child Health Bureau, 2002c). A gender difference is apparent, with the rate for males between 1.3 and 2.5 times greater than that for females (NCHS, 2000). The death rate from homicide was 9.4 per 100,000 for 15- to 19-year-olds, compared with the overall rate for all ages, 5.5 per 100,000 (Blumstein, 2002; NCHS, 2000). Death rates from firearm-related injuries have almost doubled since 1970 (NCHS, 1998).

Emotional Problems and Teenage Suicide

The adolescent years are a time of rapid growth and change. New research highlights changes to both the gray and white matter of the adolescent brain and shows marked differences in the frontal lobes of teens compared with young adults (National Institutes of Mental Health [NIMH], 2003). Hormonal influences may cause a teen to be emotional and unpredictable at times. Peer pressure becomes more important than parental concerns. Teens test family rules and generally search for their own identity and individuality apart from the family. Most parents and teens ride out this period with love and understanding and no long-term negative effects. For some children, however, a real or perceived lack of emotional support can lead to temporary or permanent emotional problems.

Depression, schizophrenia, and eating disorders may first appear during adolescence. Almost 21% of 9- to 17-year-olds were found to have a diagnosable mental illness or addictive disorder that caused some life impairment (NIMH, 2002a). Many adolescents are reluctant to seek help for emotional problems, or help may not be readily available to them. It is estimated that only 1 out of 5 of those who need treatment actually receive it. Common mental health disorders in adolescence include anxiety, depression, ADHD, eating disorders, bipolar disorder, and schizophrenia (NIMH, 2002a). Treatment for serious mental health problems may include hospitalization or placement in a group home. New intervention models, taking into account the importance of peers and family, have shown great promise in keeping troubled adolescents in the community and are more cost-effective (NIMH, 2001; 2002).

Suicide is the third leading cause of death in 13- to 20-year-olds (NCHS, 2000). As youth move toward adulthood, they become more likely to take their own lives. In 1999, 20% of all high-school students reported that they had seriously considered or had attempted suicide in the past year (NCHS, 2000). Girls attempt suicide more frequently than boys, but the actual suicide rate (those that actually kill themselves) is higher among boys (NCHS, 2000). The suicide rate among American Indians is highest, and the rate among African-Americans is lowest. A large study in Belgium by Vermeiren and colleagues (2003) found that male teens who have suicidal thoughts and exhibit violent behavior demonstrate higher levels of depression, overt and covert aggression, somatization, and risk-taking behavior than any of the other groups studied (ie, suicidal only, self-harming, violent only).

It is important to question a teen about his or her history of depression or feelings of hopelessness, as well as social support systems and intentions or availability of means to follow through on suicide threats (Van Heeringen, 2001). Suicide prevention programs and direct intervention by counselors or school nurses to determine an adolescent's suicide intentions are the most effective school-based approaches (Eggert et al., 2002). Hendin and colleagues (2001) noted that it is important for counselors to identify markers such as a precipitating event, intense affective state, suicide ideation or actions, deterioration in social or academic functioning, or increased substance abuse. Community health nurses and community mental health counselors may serve as consultants to schools in the development of sound prevention programs. Hallmarks of good prevention programs include school policies and inservice training on suicide prevention; collaboration between teachers, counselors, and nurses; student education on suicide prevention; peer assistance programs, school-family-community partnerships; activities that increase school connectedness; and crisis intervention teams (King, 2001).

Violence

Arrests for violent youth crimes peaked in the decade between 1983 and 1993 (Surgeon General of the United States, 2002). These high rates have dropped, but approximately 3.4 million adolescents are still victims of violent crimes each year, with boys 50% more often victims than girls (NCHS, 2000). Surveys have shown that between 15% and 40% of teens admit to having committing a serious violent offense by 17 years of age, and serious youth violence is part of a constellation of risk-taking behaviors that also includes precocious sex, drugs, and guns (Surgeon General of the United States, 2002). Children assault and kill other children at school and on the streets. More than 20,000 children and adolescents are killed or injured by firearms each year, and almost 85% of all firearm injuries treated in emergency rooms or hospitals are sustained by teens age 15 to 19 years. Only 1% of all firearm-related deaths for school-age children occur on school grounds (Fingerhut & Kaufer-Chrisoffel, 2002).

Gangs are often associated with teen violence. However, the proportion of schools reporting gang activity has dropped (Surgeon General of the United States, 2002). Incidents of high school shootings have raised concerns among parents and teachers. School violence has been linked to bullying (Nansel et al., 2003) and school environments. In a recent study of teachers' perceptions of school violence, 56% of teachers noted that violence or the threat of violence affected the quality of education that they provided (Fisher & Kettl, 2003). The researchers also found that elementary teachers were more likely to be the victims of physical assault by students and more likely to fear students' parents than other teachers. Another study by nurse researchers found that teachers cited probable causes of school violence as lack of knowledge and support along with inadequate safety measures (Johnson & Fisher, 2003). Comprehensive school safety plans are advised; grants and technical assistance are available to local school districts through the federal government.

Cultural and environmental influences include the violence to which children and adolescents are exposed. Increased aggressive behavior among children and teens has been attributed to violence in the environment, the home (spousal and child abuse), and the community, as well as what children see on television and in movies. A study of 9- to 15-year-olds who lived in public housing demonstrated that adolescents who witness violence (not as victims themselves) may suffer symptoms that victims of violence experience such as difficulty concentrating, vigilant/avoidant behavior, and intrusive thoughts and feelings (Howard et al., 2002). Violence is an increasing threat for teenagers. The percentage of young adolescents who do not feel safe at school is increasing dramatically. In the most recent Youth Risk Behavior Survey, 17% of adolescents reported carrying a weapon to school during the past month, and more than 35% were involved in physical fights in the last year (CDC, 2001a). Following the lead of the federal government with the implementation of the Safe and Drug-Free Schools and Communities Act, most schools have developed zero-tolerance policies to counteract and prevent violence (King, Wagner, & Hedrick, 2001). Many schools now have metal detectors and security guards, and some schools conduct random searches of students' lockers in an effort to prevent violence. More than half of violent acts involve someone who has taken drugs or alcohol (CDC, 2003d).

Substance Abuse

Substance abuse among young people was almost unknown before 1950 and rare before 1960. Now, adolescent drug experimentation and use pose serious physical and psychological threats. By the time they complete high school, 53% of teens report having tried an illicit drug, and 78% have consumed alcohol (Johnston, O'Malley, & Bachman, 2003). The Youth Risk Behavior Survey revealed that 24% of respondents had used marijuana in the past month and 9% had used cocaine at some time. Almost half drank alcohol, and 15% had sniffed or inhaled substances in the past month (CDC, 2001a).

Early drinkers more often reported academic problems, use of other substances, and delinquent behavior in middle and high school. By the time they were young adults, people with a history of early alcohol use had problems related to abuse of other substances, employment problems, and criminal and violent behavior (Ellickson, Tucker, & Klein, 2003). Almost 70% of high school students reported in 2001 that they had smoked a cigarette, and almost 14% stated that they were frequent smokers. More than 23% reported that they purchased their own cigarettes from a store or gas station (CDC, 2002b). Of those 10th grade students who were surveyed, 88% said that they could "fairly easily" or "very easily" get cigarettes if they wanted them, even though it is illegal in all 50 states to sell cigarettes to persons younger than 18 years of age. Comprehensive merchant education programs have reduced illegal sales to minors (Tobacco Information & Prevention Source, 2003).

Inhalant abuse is another very real problem. Approximately 9% of adolescents reported in 2001 that they had sniffed inhalants at least once (eg, glue, lighter fluid, spray paint) (National Clearinghouse for Alcohol and Drug Information [NCADI], 2003c). Inhalant abuse can result in severe nervous system damage. Control of such legal products as spray paint, lighter fluid, household solvents, gasoline, and glue is difficult, making the scope of this problem almost impossible to adequately monitor.

The illicit use of anabolic steroids is also difficult to monitor; however, more than one-half million 8th and 10th grade students reported using these synthetic compounds. High school seniors surveyed stated that they did not believe that anabolic steroids are dangerous, even though use of steroids has been proven to halt bone growth. This category of drugs is also associated with heart, kidney, and liver damage and increased levels of aggression known as "roid rage" (Zickler, 2000). Coaches have sometimes turned a blind eye to steroid abuse, and the National Institute on Drug Abuse has launched an educational campaign to fight the rising level of abuse in adolescents.

Other drugs that have become increasingly popular with adolescents and young adults include "club drugs" such as Ecstasy (MDMA, a synthetic drug with amphetamine and hallucinogenic properties), Rohypnol (the "date rape" drug that is often mixed with alcohol to produce sedative hypnotic effects), ketamine (a rapid-acting anesthetic), LSD (lysergic acid diethylamide, an hallucinogen originally popularized in the 1960s), and GHB (gamma hydroxybutyrate, a drug touted as a synthetic steroid in fitness clubs that has been associated with sexual assaults). Many of these drugs are part of the rave scene—all-night dance parties that originally began in England. Visits to the emergency department and some deaths have occurred from the use of these drugs (NCADI, 2003a; Wood & Synovitz, 2001).

Cocaine use has remained steady in recent years, peaking in 1980 for 12- to 17-year-olds and reaching a low point in 1991 (NCADI, 2003b). Heroin use among teenagers also was fairly steady in 2002 (at about 1%), down from a recent peak. Smoking or snorting of heroin, which is popular among adolescents and young adults because they mistakenly believe it precludes the strong physical addictiveness of this drug, frequently leads to intravenous abuse (Johnston, O'Malley, & Bachman, 2003). Methamphetamine use, reported at 2.2% for 8th graders and 3.6% for 12th graders, is a growing concern (Johnston, O'Malley, & Bachman, 2003). It may also be smoked, along with marijuana, or injected. "Meth labs" are a public health hazard and can often be found in rural areas.

Substance abuse problems and substance use disorders were associated with self-reports of psychiatric symptoms, especially mood and disruptive behavior disorders, in a large study of adolescents ages 14 to 18 years (Shrier et al., 2003). Both outpatient and inpatient treatment programs have shown some success in treating adolescent substance abusers. In 1998, some 100,322 adolescents participated in residential and outpatient treatment programs in the United States. Collaboration with families and schools is essential, because transitions back to school can be difficult (Wood et al., 2002).

Teenage Pregnancy

Teenage pregnancies, sexually transmitted diseases (STDs), and human immunodeficiency virus/acquired immunodeficiency syndrome (HIV/AIDS) are public health concerns associated with the sexual activity of adolescents. The United

States leads most developed nations in rates of teenage pregnancy, abortion, and child bearing. In the mid-1990s, rates for teen pregnancy in the United States were twice as high as in Canada, England, or Wales, and eight times as high as in Japan (NCHS, 2000). There was a 24% rise in births to teenage mothers between 1986 and 1991. More recently, however, the rate has declined, reaching a record low for the 15- to 19-year-old age group (Maternal and Child Health Bureau, 2002a). Between 1991 and 2001, teen birth rates for all ethnic groups combined declined by 26%. The rate in 2002 was 41.7 per 1000 adolescent girls for Whites, 73.1 for Blacks, and 92.4 for Hispanics (Maternal and Child Health Bureau, 2002a).

The fall in teen birth rates is encouraging because of the public health concerns related to teen pregnancy and birth. Young mothers are at high risk of bearing infants with low birth weight and are more likely to smoke. They are also less likely to receive adequate prenatal care or to gain the recommended weight during pregnancy. They are at risk for a greater number of physical, psychological, and social problems, including dropping out of high school, limited earning potential, social isolation, unstable relationships with child's father, and child abuse and neglect (NCHS, 2000). Those who choose to end their pregnancies by abortion may encounter other physical and psychosocial complications.

Primary care providers often miss opportunities to provide counseling on prevention of pregnancy, HIV, and STD (Burstein et al., 2003). It is important for community health nurses to provide education and health counseling on these subjects.

Sexually Transmitted Diseases

More than 20 diseases can be transmitted sexually; only the most common are reportable. Each year, about one quarter of new STD cases in the United States, other than HIV infection, occur among teens (Illinois Department of Public Health [IDPH], 2003). These diseases include syphilis, gonorrhea, chlamydia, human papillomavirus, and herpes simplex virus. It is estimated that prevalence rates for chlamydia in young women range from slightly less than 10% to 11.9%. The highest age-specific gonorrhea rate among women and the third-highest rate among men were in the 15- to 19-year-old age group (CDC, 2000). Compared with adults, adolescents (10 to 19 years) and young adults (20 to 24 years) are at increased risk for acquiring STDs (also called sexually transmitted infections, or STIs). Reasons for this may include a greater likelihood of multiple sex partners, unprotected intercourse, and selection of higher-risk partners. Adolescent girls also have a physiologically increased susceptibility to infection because of cervical ectopy (CDC, 2000). Serious complications from STDs include pelvic inflammatory disease (PID), sterility, increased risk of cancers of the reproductive system, and, with syphilis, blindness, mental illness, and death. There are also complications for unborn children of those infected with STDs (IDPH, 2003).

Even though death rates from HIV/AIDS have dramatically fallen, new HIV infections reported annually do not reflect the same steep decline. New medications are thought to be the cause of the declining death rate. As cohorts enter their late teens and early 20s, the rate of infection for HIV increases; an average of 2 young people are infected with HIV every hour (IDPH, 2003). In 2000, new cases of AIDS were reported in 1688 youths age 13 to 24 years, for a cumulative total of 31,293 cases in this age group (CDC, 2002c). Half of all new HIV infections are now thought to occur among people younger than 25 years of age, and most of these infections are traced to sexual transmission. Sixty-one percent of HIV-infected persons in the 13- to 19-year-old age group were female, and African-Americans were the largest racial/ethnic group (CDC, 2002c).

Effective methods of preventing STDs and HIV/AIDS include reduction of sexual activity among adolescents. This can be done by promoting abstinence or delaying sexual initiation, as well as by fostering safer sex messages that promote the use of condoms. Sex education is effective at both delaying the onset of sexual activity and decreasing sexual activity in adolescents who are already sexually active. It is also effective in increasing safer sex practices, knowledge of birth control method efficacy, and overall sexual knowledge (Aarons et al., 2000; Song et al., 2000). A comprehensive review of 73 studies of programs to reduce adolescent sexual risk taking, unintended pregnancy, and STDs revealed strong evidence that such programs can delay sex, increase condom or contraceptive use, and reduce teen pregnancies. The most effective programs included specific sex/HIV education curricula and certain intensive multimodal youth development programs (Kirby, 2002).

Acne

Between 79% and 95% of adolescents in Western societies have acne, leading some researchers to suspect environmental influences (Cordain et al. 2002). Acne is generally recognized as a genetic disease; three out of four children whose mother or father had acne as a teenager will also have it (National Institute of Arthritis and Musculoskeletal and Skin Diseases, 2003). Acne begins during puberty (10 to 12 years of age) with the increase in circulating male hormones that stimulate sebaceous glands in the skin. The excess sebum (oil) causes irritation in the pores and results in a buildup of cells, leading to whiteheads. Open pores are known as blackheads. A red and inflamed pustule can develop or, in serious cases of acne, cysts or nodules can form. This can lead to pitting and scarring if not treated.

It is now known that greasy foods and chocolate do not cause acne but may be aggravating factors (along with stress, environmental irritants, and certain cosmetics) in susceptible adolescents. Common treatment regimens include skin cleansers, peelers, and medications to decrease sebaceous gland activity. Girls are often prescribed oral contraceptives, which have been shown to be effective in treating acne

(Rosen, Breitkopf, & Nagamani, 2003). Benzoyl peroxide is used to kill bacteria on the skin and in the pores. It may be sold over-the-counter (OTC) or by prescription. Other OTC medications include salicylic acid, sulfur, and resorcinol. Retin A (a topical vitamin A ointment), glycolic acid, and a-hydroxy acids help to peel the impacted cells from the pores. Accutane (isotretinoin) reduces the size and activity of sebaceous glands but can cause liver or kidney dysfunction. Because of an extremely high risk of birth defects, female adolescents taking Accutane are prescribed oral contraceptives (National Institute of Arthritis and Musculoskeletal and Skin Diseases, 2003). Oral antibiotics may be prescribed, and corticosteroids may be injected directly into the comedones. Oral contraceptives are prescribed for some female adolescents to regulate their hormonally influenced acne.

The best preventive measures are keeping the skin clean, eating a balanced diet that includes fresh fruits and vegetables, drinking lots of water, and getting adequate sleep. It is important for male adolescents to shave carefully and for all teens with acne to avoid touching their faces or picking at their blemishes. Adolescents with severe acne may need to be referred to dermatologists who specialize in this skin disorder.

Poor Nutrition and Eating Disorders

Poor nutrition and obesity are not uncommon among adolescents, whose diets often consist of snacks with limited nutritional value interspersed among unhealthful meals. Increased fast food consumption has been tied to the increase in obesity in the United States (Brinkley, Eates, & Jekanowski, 2000). A national study found that adolescents and young adults got more of their energy intake from restaurants and fast food outlets than from home, with increased consumption of pizza, cheeseburgers, and salty snacks (Nielsen, Siega-Riz, & Popkin, 2002). Adolescent eating behavior is influenced by psychosocial factors, family and peers, availability of fast food, and mass media marketing (Story, Neumark-Sztainer, & French, 2002). Girls are more at risk for problems with nutrition for several reasons: they tend to diet inappropriately, to have more finicky eating habits, and to be less physically active than teenage boys. Boys typically eat large quantities of food, which increases the likelihood of obtaining adequate nutrients, and they also tend to be more physically active than girls. A large study of high school students found that "consumption of fruits and vegetables and a healthy breakfast and lunch related both to family and individual factors"; as family situations deteriorated, the percentage of adolescents who ate a healthy breakfast or lunch decreased (Young & Fors, 2001; p. 487).

Issues with body image and control are at the heart of anorexia nervosa and bulimia nervosa, common problems for adolescent girls. **Anorexia nervosa** is an eating disorder with an emotional etiology that is characterized by body image disturbance (ie, girls see themselves as fat although they may be extremely thin), an intense fear of becoming fat or gaining weight, and refusal to maintain adequate body weight (ie, BMI of 18 or greater). **Bulimia** is an eating disorder that is characterized by recurrent episodes of binge eating with repeated compensatory mechanisms to prevent weight gain, such as vomiting (purging type) and fasting or exercise (nonpurging type). **Binge eating**, which is also a recognized eating disorder, involves recurrent episodes of binge eating without fasting, self-induced vomiting, or other compensatory measures (Bulik, Sullivan, & Kendler, 2000). A woman's lifetime risk of developing a bulimic syndrome is estimated to be 8%; the estimated risk of developing an anorexic syndrome is 3% (Patton et al., 2000). These diseases have emotional causes that pose complex challenges to treatment. Nutrition education, psychological counseling, and cognitive-behavioral techniques that teach clients how to control stimuli, substitute alternative behaviors, and use positive visualization are all part of treatment; development of a support network is also important. Self-concept is often distorted and self-esteem is low; therefore, activities are initiated to improve the adolescents' feelings about themselves and to bolster their coping mechanisms. Medications (eg, antidepressants) have been helpful in treating some adolescents with eating disorders (Sharma, 2001). A study by Stock and colleagues (2002) found that female adolescents with eating disorders differed in their use and abuse of substances such as alcohol and marijuana. Those with a purging disorder were more likely to have rates of substance use similar to those of the general adolescent population. Their drug preferences included tobacco, alcohol, marijuana, hallucinogens, tranquilizers, stimulants, PCP (phencyclidine), cocaine, and Ecstasy. Those with restrictive eating disorders were less likely to use alcohol, tobacco, and marijuana than the general adolescent population. Both groups used caffeine and laxatives.

The key to prevention may be tied to education about the risks of dieting. One study indicated that adolescent girls who were severe dieters were 18 times more likely to develop an eating disorder than those who did not diet. Even moderate dieters were at risk; they were 5 times more likely to develop an eating disorder (Patton et al., 2000). Psychiatric morbidity was also a factor; it increased risk sevenfold. Exercise is seen as a more viable alternative than extreme dieting for adolescents who want to control their weight.

HEALTH SERVICES FOR SCHOOL-AGE CHILDREN AND ADOLESCENTS

A number of programs serve the health needs of school-age children and adolescents. Community health nurses play a major and vital role in delivering these services. Such programs fall into three categories that approximate the three practice priorities of community health nursing practice: illness prevention, health protection, and health promotion.

Preventive Health Programs

Immunizations

Low immunization levels in many areas, particularly among the poor, and increased disease rates signal the need for constant surveillance, outreach programs, and educational efforts. Community health nurses are deeply involved in each of these preventive activities. Health departments and schools often work collaboratively to provide immunization services (see Fig. 9-2 in Chapter 9). Compulsory immunization laws that vary from state to state have enabled public health personnel to carry out these preventive services. Most adolescents are now required to be immunized against hepatitis B. School nurses work with nurse volunteers and community health nurses to provide immunization clinics at elementary and middle schools, sites that are convenient for adolescents and their parents (Mark, Conklin & Wolfe, 2001). Although immunization clinics may improve rates of compliance, it is recommended that 11- to 12-year-olds be scheduled for routine visits to their physicians so that immunizations can be checked and updated (Schaffer et al., 2001). A second dose of MMR can be given at that time (if not already done), along with a tetanus-diphtheria booster. This booster should be repeated every 10 years, and children with chronic illnesses (eg, diabetes, asthma, sickle cell disease) may receive pneumococcal vaccine and an annual influenza vaccine (Maternal and Child Health Bureau, 2002d). Adolescents who have not had chickenpox and have not received prior vaccination should be given the varicella virus vaccine. In some areas, hepatitis A vaccine is also given to certain high-risk groups. Research studies have examined the feasibility of combining hepatitis A and B vaccines or administering a two-dose hepatitis B vaccine for adolescents in an effort to improve compliance in this age group (Levaux et al., 2001; Van Damme & Van der Wielen, 2001).

In addition to immunizations required for school entry, many states or local school districts now require tuberculosis (TB) skin tests for school-age children and adolescents. Children have a much higher risk of disease progression than adults do; annual testing is often recommended for children and adolescents from high-risk populations (CDC, 2001c). Children should be screened for TB if they meet any of the following criteria:

- Close contact with persons with known or suspected TB
- Foreign birth, foreign travel, or contact with a foreign visitor
- Medically underserved, low-income populations (especially Blacks, Hispanics, and Native Americans)
- Contact with HIV-infected persons or inmates
- Foster children (due to poor history)
- Medical risk factors (diabetes, asthma, HIV infection)
- Local epidemiology (health department recommendation)

Education and Social Services

Education of school-age children and adolescents includes a wide variety of approaches and can range from the basics of hand-washing for elementary school students (Guinan, McGuckin, & Ali, 2002; White et al., 2001) to hearing conservation for students who like to listen to loud music (Folmer, Griest, & Martin, 2002).

Parental support services are commonly available through many public and private agencies including churches. They can have long-range effects on the health of school-age children. Emotionally healthy parents and stable families offer a healthful environment and support system for children and can facilitate their progress in school. In most states, community health nurses provide teaching and counseling services to parents in their homes and in groups. School nurses, school mental health counselors, and school psychologists also organize parent support groups in local schools. This is particularly important during periods of transition (eg, from elementary to middle school, from middle to high school). Discussing parenting concerns and increasing parents' understanding of normal child growth and development help to allay fears and prevent problems. Through such efforts, family violence and abuse can be averted. Reduction in rates of divorce and the attendant consequences may also be a benefit of strengthening family resilience.

Family planning programs, often stationed strategically in inner cities, near schools, or in school-based clinics, provide birth control information and counseling to young people. In some communities, the school-based clinic dispenses condoms. Community health nurses, in collaboration with an interdisciplinary team, are usually the primary care providers in these programs. Their major goals are to prevent teenage pregnancy, educate teens about reproduction and contraception, and encourage responsible sexual behavior.

Providing STD services and HIV/AIDS education can be a daunting task. Young people with STDs are often afraid or embarrassed to seek help. Others who have been exposed to the HIV virus may not know that they are infected. Gay and bisexual young men are particularly at risk (CDC, 2002c). Furthermore, community health professionals receive very little training in these areas and may be uncomfortable and judgmental in their approaches. Quality services that are easily accessible, provide anonymity for clients, are age-appropriate or targeted to adolescents, and are staffed with health care providers who exhibit nonjudgmental attitudes are better able to attract young people who need help. Some argue that drastic changes in the provision of services to young people—working to ensure economic development, privatization of prevention activities, and employment of innovative models and strategies—are needed to effect change (Rotheram-Borus, 2000).

Vulnerable groups, particularly minority youths, inner-city residents, and homosexuals, are reached through STD clinics, HIV testing sites in clinics and health departments, family planning clinics, private health care providers, schools, and employers. Community health nurses are available in most of these settings and usually the professionals who deal most directly with these clients. Improved public awareness and education, screening of high-risk groups, appropriate treatment of infected people, and identification and treatment of sexual partners can reduce the threat of STDs.

Physicians are also concerned about the health risks common to adolescents. Pediatricians, especially, have instituted better history taking, more consistent monitoring, and anticipatory guidance for risks from unintentional and intentional injury, substance abuse, and sexual activity (Boekeloo et al., 2003; Pbert et al., 2003). Community health nurses need to work with local physicians and other community care providers to ensure that adequate education and social services are available to school-age children and adolescents.

Educational efforts to prevent risk-taking behaviors that can lead to adverse health conditions are effective. An examination of 44 studies that used interventions to reduce HIV in adolescents over a 15-year period revealed that reductions in sexual risk were greater for subjects who received HIV risk-reduction intervention than for those in comparison groups. The increased use of condoms, condom use negotiation skills, and sexual partner communication, along with delaying the onset of sexual activity and decreasing the number of sexual partners, were the outcomes of intensive behavioral interventions (Johnson et al., 2003). Peer educators are effective in HIV/STD prevention programs for adolescents (Ott et al., 2003; Ross & Williams, 2002).

The effectiveness of a universal drug abuse prevention program (eg, drug refusal skills, self-management, general social skills) was studied in 29 inner-city middle schools. About one fifth of the subjects were considered to be at high risk for use of substances. Participating high-risk youth reported less drinking, smoking, inhalant use, and polydrug use at the 1-year posttest than did high-risk youth in the control group (Griffin et al., 2003). In addition to school-based education, peer leadership, and parental education and involvement, and community-wide task forces have been developed to lobby for local legislation and strengthen community–school ties. One study from Chicago gathered information about billboard advertisements for alcohol and tobacco products. A disproportionate number were located in African-American and Hispanic neighborhoods close to schools, parks, and playgrounds. This information was used to lobby the city council for tougher ordinances controlling advertising content and zoning (Hackbarth et al., 2001).

Other intervention programs that rely on social influence have been successful in reducing cigarette and alcohol use (Elder et al., 2002; Komro & Toomey, 2002). Those with peer-led, interactive education were more effective than teacher-led, noninteractive programs in reducing use of alcohol, tobacco, and other drugs among adolescents. Enforcement of laws that restrict tobacco sales to minors are another highly effective method of prevention, as is consistent enforcement of school anti-tobacco policies (Tubman & Soza-Vento, 2001). Community health nurses often work in conjunction with law enforcement officials, school district administrators, and other community agencies to ensure compliance with local regulations and prevent or delay tobacco use.

Health Protection Programs

Safety and Injury Prevention

Accident and injury control programs serve a critical role in protecting the lives of school-age children and adolescents. Efforts to prevent motor vehicle accidents, a major cause of death, include driver education programs, better highway construction, improved motor vehicle design and safety features, and continuing research into the causes of various types of crashes. Injury prevention and reduction have been addressed through strategies such as state laws requiring the use of safety restraints, installation of driver and front passenger airbags, substitution of other modes of travel (air, rail, or bus), lower speed limits, stricter enforcement of drunk driving laws, safer automobile design, and helmets for motorcyclists, bicycle riders, and skaters. Students Against Drunk Driving (SADD) and Friday Night Live activities can promote more responsible driving habits among teens. Communities can also work with law enforcement officials to ensure compliance with mandatory seat belt laws and to promote safe speeds and appropriate driving behaviors near schools.

Child deaths and injuries from burns result primarily from house fires, but also from electrical burns, cigarette lighters, and scalds. Many local fire departments and public health programs offer safety education in this area. Emphasis is placed on the use of heat— and smoke—detecting systems, fire drills, and home evacuation plans; use of less flammable structural materials, furnishings, and clothing; and careful smoking or, better yet, no smoking.

Safety programs also seek to protect school-age children from the hazards of poisonings, ingestion of prescription or OTC drugs, product-related accidents (unsafe toys, bicycles, skateboards, skates, playground equipment, and furniture), and recreational accidents, including drownings and sports-related injuries. Safety services assume various forms. Poison control centers in many localities offer information and emergency assistance. Product safety is monitored by the Federal Consumer Product Safety Commission. Education programs in schools or through local fire or police departments teach school-age children about bicycle and water safety, fire dangers, and hazards related to poisoning.

Generally, the community health nurse can educate families to recognize potentially hazardous situations and encourage efforts to eliminate them. Working with school nurses and school district officials to reduce playground hazards can contribute to the reduction of school-related injuries.

Environmental hazards and other dangers await school-age children and adolescents in the workforce. It is estimated that more than 70 teenage workers die from work-related injuries each year, and more than 64,000 are seen in emergency departments. Between 15% and 45% of these nonfatal injuries are serious enough to lead to work restriction or permanent disability. Older, white, male adolescents are at greater risk (Runyan & Zakocs, 2002). The highest number of work-related injuries to youths younger than 18 years of age occurred in eating establishments and food stores (Mardis & Pratt, 2003). Deaths caused by exposure to toxic vapors, electrocution, and work-related motor vehicle accidents are not uncommon. Community health nurses can join with occupational health nurses and school nurses to teach parents and children about the dangers and risks inherent in the workplace, and they can work with local employers to ensure safe working conditions and reasonable hours of employment that do not interfere with school.

Infectious Diseases

Programs that protect school-age children and adolescents against infectious diseases encompass efforts such as closing swimming pools that have unsafe bacteria counts, conducting immunization campaigns in conjunction with influenza or measles outbreaks, and working with hospital pediatric units to reduce the incidence and threat of iatrogenic disease.

Child Protective Services

An estimated 879,000 children and adolescents were victims of abuse or neglect in 2000, and 79% of the abusers were parents (Maternal and Child Health Bureau, 2002j). Most victims suffered from neglect (63%), but almost 20% were physically abused, 10% were sexually abused, and 8% were psychologically abused (Maternal and Child Health Bureau, 2002j). Long-term costs of child maltreatment have been estimated at $94 billion per year. Consequences for affected children include lower self-esteem, depression, suicide, self-abuse, substance abuse, eating disorders, less empathy for others, antisocial behavior, delinquency, aggression, violence, low academic achievement, and sexual maladjustment (Dake, Price, & Murnan, 2003). Neglectful families often are characterized by high levels of adult problems, reports of stressful life events, and a higher incidence of maternal depression. One study found that those mothers who were more highly educated, had fewer stressful life events, and had more positive encounters with social services generally were better able to provide physically for their children (Casady & Lee, 2002).

Services to protect children from abuse are not as well developed or effective as safety and injury protection programs, for a variety of reasons. Most child abuse occurs in the home, so only the most blatant situations become evident to outsiders. Avoidance of legal involvement keeps others from reporting suspected cases, although this attitude is changing among professionals who work with children and other community members. Education, social and mental health services, and law enforcement personnel were the three highest reporters of child abuse in 2000, alleging abuse of approximately 3 million children and adolescents (Maternal and Child Health Bureau, 2002d). In some areas, community health nurses are working together with social workers, mental health workers, and substance abuse counselors as part of a team that provides services to families. Improved training of mandated reporters, such as teachers and physicians, has led to better reporting of abuse. Today, professionals and the public are more aware of the problem, and there is an increase in reporting. In 1974, the National Center for Child Abuse and Neglect was established as a result of the Child Abuse Prevention and Treatment Act. The center collects and analyzes information on child abuse and neglect, serves as an information clearinghouse, publishes educational materials on the subject, offers technical assistance, and conducts research into the problem.

Child abuse prevention education programs can be found in many school districts as a primary preventive intervention. Evaluation of one of these programs indicated a significant increase in knowledge regarding child abuse among the third graders surveyed (Dake, Price, & Murnan, 2003).

Oral Hygiene and Dental Care

School-based programs that provide fluoride rinses and dental sealants and promote toothbrushing and nutrition education for dental health can be found across the country.

Fluoridation of community water supplies is considered the most effective, safe, and low-cost means of protecting children's dental health (Gillcrist, Brumley, & Blackford, 2001; Griffin, Jones, & Tomar, 2001). Fluoride makes teeth less susceptible to decay by increasing resistance to the bacteria-produced acid in the mouth. Since 1945, public water supplies have been fluoridated at relatively low cost to communities. Water fluoridation has been ranked as one of the 10 greatest public health achievements of the 20th century, and children in communities with fluoridated water reportedly have 29% less dental caries. For every dollar spent on water fluoridation, between $7 and $42 in treatment costs are saved (CDC, 2003b).

Some individuals and groups oppose fluoridation because of possible adverse effects (including fluorosis, which can cause mottling of tooth enamel). Research results have been mixed, although most studies have supported the low risk of water fluoridation and the benefits of decreased caries. For instance, a British study examined the risk of hip fracture in adults older than 50 years of age who lived in areas with fluoridated water supplies. There was a very low risk of hip fracture with lifetime exposure to drinking water concentrations of fluoride at 1 ppm (Hillier, 2000). A longitudinal study found that adults (ages 18 to 45 years) who grew up with fluoridation and a greater emphasis on preventive dentistry had significantly reduced dental caries, compared with the previous cohort studied (Brown, Wall, & Lazar, 2002). In the United States, some researchers have concluded that because of children's potential for multiple exposures to fluoride through drinking water, processed foods and beverages, toothpaste, gels, and rinses, lower doses or no fluoride supplements are now required.

In addition to regular dental care, good nutrition, and proper oral hygiene, community health nurses can safely promote public water fluoridation as an important program for protecting children's dental health (CDC, 2003b). School nurses often conduct dental screenings at schools and make referrals to local dentists in an effort to promote better dental health for children and adolescents.

School Health Screening Programs

Most local school districts provide some type of health screening services, usually through the school nurse or local health care providers. A 2003 School Health Policies and Programs Study (SHPPS) noted that 73% of reporting school districts offered vision screening (CDC, 2003d). Routine vision screenings are done at periodic intervals for early detection of vision problems that can interfere with learning (eg, nearsightedness, farsightedness, strabismus, amblyopia). Lions Clubs may be involved in paying for local optometrists to assist or direct screenings or to provide follow-up care.

Hearing screenings were reported by 68% of districts (SHPPS, 2003). These mass screenings are done to detect any serious hearing deficits that may be related to recurrent ear infections or some type of sensorineural hearing loss. Height, weight, and sometimes blood pressure and cholesterol screenings are done on a regular basis to monitor normal growth and development and allow for early intervention with populations who are especially susceptible to hypertension and heart disease.

In some areas, scoliosis screening is also done, frequently during middle school years, to permit early detection and referral for medical intervention (eg, bracing, surgery). Some 52% of schools reported doing scoliosis screenings (SHPPS, 2003).

Dental screenings or clinics may be conducted to determine the incidence of dental caries, especially in elementary schoolchildren, and to encourage follow-up with local dentists for necessary restorations. Only 20% of schools reported doing some type of oral health screening (SHPPS, 2003).

The goal of all screening is to promote early intervention. Referral information is usually given to parents, and school nurses may contact parents to encourage follow-through. Children who are not present in school may not receive the benefits of these screenings. A growing number of children in this country are being homeschooled by their parents (approximately 1.7% of the total school-age population) and therefore also miss the socialization experiences that are part of school attendance. The number of homeschooled children more than doubled over the 5-year period ending in 1996, to an estimated 850,000 children in 1999 (NCES, 2003b).

Health Promotion Programs

Nutrition and Exercise Programs

Nutrition and weight control programs form another important set of health promotion services. Children need to learn sound dietary habits early in life to establish healthy lifelong patterns. Being overweight during childhood or adolescence may persist into adulthood and may increase the risk for some chronic diseases later in life. Some school programs teach and provide good nutrition and encourage eating patterns that prevent obesity (Baranowski et al., 2003). A number of weight control programs for overweight children and adolescents are available through schools, health departments, community health centers, health maintenance organizations (HMOs), and private groups.

Adolescents are particularly vulnerable to media and peer pressures with regard to their food choices. Because of increased rates of childhood obesity and greater awareness of the need for better nutrition in adolescence, legislative support to limit soft drink sales at public schools is growing (Fletcher, 2003). Fad diets can be harmful if they are not nutritionally balanced. Programs aimed at more nutritionally sound advertising are having a positive effect. Parents and children are becoming more aware of the need to cut down consumption of saturated fat, salt, sugar, and overprocessed foods in order to feel and look better. The U. S. Department of Agriculture's Food Guide Pyramid provides a sensible guide to daily food choices and eating that can assist people in limiting consumption of foods that may negatively affect health. The nurse, through nutrition education and reinforcement of positive practices, plays a significant role in promoting the health of children.

The value of exercise and physical fitness programs for young people has been recognized for some time. Organized groups such as the YMCA, YWCA, Boy Scouts, Girl Scouts, and Campfire have offered sports and character development programs for many years. Schools, parks, and recreation centers encourage exercise through use of playground equipment and organized sports activities. Despite these opportunities, many young people do not exercise often enough or vigorously enough. The greatest decline in physical activity occurs during adolescence (Lowry et al., 2001). Even team sports keep players inactive much of the time and are not activities that young people continue in their adult lives. More comprehensive physical education programs that encourage and focus on vigorous individual exercise and self-discipline as lifelong habits would better serve the health needs of this population group. Schmitz and colleagues (2002) found that levels of physical activity and sedentary leisure habits could be predicted in a large sample of seventh grade students. Caucasian students; students who perceived themselves as high achievers or had high academic expectations; girls who reported high measures on health, appearance, and achievement; and girls whose mothers used authoritative parenting styles all had greater levels of physical activity and lower levels of sedentary leisure activity. Students reporting more depressive symptomatology had higher levels of sedentary leisure activity. Community health nurses can promote such programs in the schools, as well as encouraging these activities in their contacts with students of all ages.

Education to Prevent Substance Abuse

The well-known hazards of cigarette smoking, inhalant use, and alcohol and drug abuse have prompted the development of substance abuse programs that target school-age children and adolescents. Health education efforts by school nurses, teachers, and counselors have influenced students to make responsible decisions about smoking, drinking, and other behaviors affecting their health (Distefan, Gilpin, & Pierce, 2000; Tingle, DeSimone, & Covington, 2003).

Health departments, community health nursing agencies, and private groups such as the American Cancer Society and the National Lung Association provide educational materials and promote antismoking and drug use prevention campaigns. The more successful programs emphasize how the human body works and how behaviors affect it. They also help young people resist social pressures to smoke and take drugs by pointing out that those who do are in the minority and by showing the deleterious effects of such practices. These groups can also work as advocates for change in the schools that permit broader health education (Leger & Nutbeam, 2000). Using students themselves as health educators is a positive use of peer pressure and can be a successful means of influencing attitudes.

Other groups, such as 4-H clubs, churches, the Catholic Youth Organization, and Boy Scouts, use peer counseling to influence young people to assume responsibility for healthy lifestyles. Decision-making skills that lead to healthy lifestyle choices in adolescence and through adulthood are the goals. The community health nurse participates in and supports existing programs in addition to counseling and referring young people who need help.

Counseling and Crisis Intervention

Stress control programs for children and adolescents do not exist in any great number, yet they are very much needed. Many of the health problems discussed in this chapter relate to the emotional health of young people. Reckless driving, suicide, homicide, unplanned pregnancy, smoking, alcoholism, illicit drug use, obesity, anorexia nervosa, and bulimia, as well as other problems, signal the presence of stress and the absence of coping skills sufficient to handle it. Social skills training is often needed by children and adolescents with behavioral or emotional disorders. Social skills deficits have been linked to poor peer relationships and a greater likelihood of abuse of tobacco, alcohol, or drugs (Evans, Axelrod, & Sapia, 2000).

Crisis intervention programs and services that treat a problem after it occurs are helpful and can prevent problems from worsening, but many children and adolescents need an emphasis on primary preventive mental health interventions. Social and emotional learning programs that focus on the student's awareness of self and others, positive values and attitudes, and responsible decision-making, as well as social skills training, are effective in enhancing the ability of students to recognize and manage emotions and deal with relevant developmental tasks (Payton et al., 2000). Programs that build coping skills early, including conflict resolution, self-help, peer counseling, peer intervention, and mutual support activities, are needed. Support groups for children of divorce or children with chronic health problems (eg, asthma, diabetes), groups that promote proper nutrition and weight man-

agement, and groups focused on preventing teenage pregnancies have been instituted in diverse areas with varying degrees of success. Many of these activities occur in the schools; however, they may be discontinued if grant funding ends or budget cuts must be made.

Programs offered in a group context have proved most effective. For the nurse, recognition of young people at risk, counseling, and early referral to sources of help can prevent crisis situations. Reduction of stresses in the family and community environments can further enhance health (Caccamo, 2000).

School-Based Health Clinics

Because of the complex and intertwined emotional, physical, and educational needs of school-age children and adolescents, a more comprehensive interdisciplinary approach to services is needed than the piecemeal approaches attempted previously. On a national level, experts are recognizing the link between learning and health and calling for an integrated, coordinated approach. The goal is to keep children and adolescents healthy and in school so they will have a greater chance of graduating and succeeding as citizens.

Adolescents are notorious for low utilization of health care services, lower rates of health insurance than other age groups, and participation in high-risk behaviors (CDC, 2001a). Emotional and physical problems frequently are entwined and can be discerned only by a well-trained, caring, and consistent practitioner. By 2020, school-age children are expected to comprise 24% of the U. S. population (America's Children, 2002). In addition, more parents are working and less available to take care of their children's health care needs during the day. Almost three fourths of women with school-age children are currently employed (Maternal and Child Health Bureau, 2002j). **School-based health centers (SBHC)** provide ready access to health care for large numbers of children and adolescents during school hours, making absences from school due to health care appointments unnecessary. SBHCs provide a variety of services in a user-friendly manner at a convenient location.

There are currently more than 1200 SBHCs in the United States, up from only 200 in 1990 (Brindis et al., 2003). Some clinics provide services only to schoolchildren, whereas others extend services to their families and to other families with preschool-age children in the neighborhood. Most centers are open full-time. Those located in middle or high schools may provide pregnancy testing and STD diagnosis and treatment as well as birth control. However, many SBHCs do not provide contraceptive services on the school site because of school district policy or state law (Santelli et al., 2003). Students who were younger, ethnically diverse, or from more rural areas were more likely to access available family planning and STD-related services from SBHCs, according to a national survey (Crosby & St. Lawrence, 2000).

The most commonly reported diagnoses are mental health/substance abuse (eg, crisis intervention, counseling) and health supervision/acute disease (eg, immunizations, physical examinations, risk behavior screenings). SBHCs are staffed by interdisciplinary teams of helping professionals, paraprofessionals, and staff. Many hospitals, HMOs, and health departments are sponsors of these school clinics, because it is a cost-effective way to decrease visits to the emergency department and promote health, especially to underserved groups such as adolescents. Third-party billing, especially to access Medicaid funding, is increasingly more common among SBHCs, and private foundations have also been instrumental in providing financial and technical support.

Evaluation research has demonstrated that SBHCs are effective in increasing student access to health care, especially for adolescent boys (Marcell et al., 2002); decreasing emergency department expenses, and improving use of preventive services for elementary schoolchildren (Adams & Johnson, 2000); and decreasing hospitalization while improving asthma morbidity in children from preschool through eighth grade (Lurie, Jones-Bauer, & Brady, 2001). Sexually active girls who received family planning services through onsite SBHCs began hormonal contraception sooner and were more consistent in its use (Zimmer-Gembeck, Doyle, & Daniels, 2001). Parents have cited the low cost (or no cost) of the SBHC, its close proximity, availability of appointments, ease of being seen without an appointment, and short waiting times as important benefits (Meerdink-Carpenter & Stanley-Mueller, 2001).

ROLE OF THE SCHOOL NURSE

Historical Background

At the end of the 19th century, immigrants flooded the northeastern cities of the United States, and mandatory education was instituted. Poor foreign-born children enrolled in schools, and, as early as 1870, New York City immunized children in public schools. Sanitation and identification of sources of contagion were the focus, and many children were excluded from school with no follow-up. Some schools reported that 10% to 20% of their students were absent. Lillian Wald sent one of her Henry Street Settlement visiting nurses to four schools with high numbers of exclusions in New York City, and the numbers of absentee children dropped significantly within 1 year, from 10,567 to 1101 (Hawkins, Hayes, & Corliss, 1994; Woodfill & Beyrer, 1991). Not only were medical inspections of schoolchildren conducted, but medical clinics were established in schools. Home visits and health education were also provided. Over the years, school health services dwindled and medical care was shifted to private practitioners, largely at the insistence of the American Medical Association. By the 1920s, school health services consisted mainly of health education and minimal health services (eg, emergency care, periodic health assessments, documentation of state or district health requirement compliance). During the 1960s and 1970s, federal legislation

providing Early Periodic Screening Diagnosis and Treatment (EPSDT) examinations for children and education for disabled students (Education for the Handicapped, Americans with Disabilities Act) expanded services to children and adolescents in public schools (Hawkins, Hayes, & Corliss, 1994; Woodfill & Beyrer, 1991). During this time, the first nurse practitioner programs began at the University of Colorado. Nurse practitioners continue to work in conjunction with school nurses, especially in SBHCs. The school nurse role in these clinics is one of triage, referral, and follow-up. A school nurse can be especially effective in the role of case manager for children and their families (National Association of School Nurses [NASN], 2001).

School nurses began working in public schools at the turn of the 20th century, and they continue as a specialty branch of professional nursing that serves the school-age population. It is estimated that there are more than 60,000 school nursing working in schools today (NASN, 2003). School nurses deliver services to students from birth through age 21 years. They also work with students' families and the school community in regular and special education schools, as well as other educational settings (eg, preschools, court/community schools). A school nurse, depending on the state of residence, is usually a registered nurse (frequently with additional education beyond the bachelor's degree in nursing, including a master's degree) who has primary responsibility for the health care of school-age children and school personnel in an educational setting. In some areas of the country, licensed practical nurses (LPNs) or licensed vocational nurses (LVNs) may be hired by school districts. The National Association of School Nurses (NASN) is a professional organization of school nurses that has been incorporated since 1979. There are chapters in each state, and members attend a national meeting every summer to address the professional needs of school nurses. It is the position of NASN (2002) that school nurses should, at minimum, possess a bachelor's degree (see Voices From the Community).

Responsibilities of the School Nurse

The primary responsibilities of the school nurse are to prevent illness and to promote and maintain the health of the school community (Display 28–3). The school nurse serves not only individuals, families, and groups within the context of school health but also the school as an organization and its membership (students and staff) as aggregates.

The school nurse identifies health-related barriers to learning, serves as a health advocate for children and families, and promotes health while preventing illness and disability (NASN, 1999). Further, the role of the school nurse includes that of care provider, change agent, teacher, manager, and educator. Health services include programs such as vision and hearing screening; scoliosis screening; monitoring of height, weight and blood pressure; oral health; TB screening; immunization assessment and monitoring; medication administration; care of children with specialized

vices (more than 70% rated them as important), not many understood the range of school health services or believed that their children had accessed them (Clark et al., 2002).

Functions of School Nursing Practice

Three main functions of school nursing practice are health services, health education, and promotion of a healthy school environment. Health services have been discussed. The health education function of school nursing practice involves planned and incidental teaching of health concepts; curriculum development, which includes classes in health science and healthful living; and use of educational media, library resources, and community facilities. These activities integrate health information with students' daily living experiences to build positive attitudes toward health and to establish sound health practices that will carry forward into adulthood.

The third function of school nursing practice is the promotion of healthful school living. Emphasis on a healthful physical environment includes proper selection, design, organization, operation, and maintenance of the physical plant. Consideration should be shown for areas such as adaptability to student needs; safety; visual, thermal, and acoustic factors; aesthetic values; sanitation; and safety of the school bus system and food services. Promotion of healthful school living also emphasizes planning a daily schedule that monitors healthful classroom experiences, extra class activities, school breakfasts and lunches, emotional climate, program of discipline, and teaching methods. It also includes reporting illegal drug use, suspected child abuse, and violations of environmental health standards. It seeks to promote the physical, mental, and emotional health of school personnel by being accessible as a resource to teachers and staff regarding their own health and safety.

Liaison With the Interdisciplinary School Health Team

School health, like all health programs in the community, requires an interdisciplinary team effort (NASN, 2001). The school nurse is part of a coordinated school health program that provides school health services, health education, and health promotion programs for faculty and staff. The nurse collaborates with counseling and psychological services as well as physical education and works to provide a healthy school environment with family and community involvement (NASN, 2002). Although the school nurse plays a central role, collaboration with many other individuals is important. The coordinated school health program includes eight components and involves a variety of professionals and other people ranging from teachers, administrators, and school staff to families. The components are

- School health services (preventive services, referral)
- Health education (kindergarten through 12th grade curricula)

VOICES FROM THE COMMUNITY

I have a new job that I love and have been shooting for since I graduated from nursing school. I now work for a school district as a school nurse. I have three year-round elementary schools in the central area of town, and it was exactly the assignment that I wanted because I wanted to expand my Spanish. It doesn't pay as much as I would get if I were still working at a hospital, but I have a life, good pay and benefits and, out of 365 days a year, I work 183 days. This job allows me to continue with other work interests and to do the traveling and mission work I've always wanted to do. I do love working with kids. I feel like I'm able to make a positive impact on the kids' health and their future. I have to admit that the job is very different than I had expected. Some people, especially other nurses, think that school nurses aren't "real nurses." Boy, they could not be more wrong. In the hospital, you have all these backups. If someone stops breathing, you call the code blue team. If a patient has some family problems, you call the social worker. If a patient's symptoms are puzzling, you grab another nurse or the doctor. As a school nurse, you are the code blue team, the other nurse, the social worker, and often, although you are not the doctor, you become a diagnostician (enough so that you send people to the emergency department or the doctor's office). You go from putting Band-Aids on knees, to running out to the playground hoping the kid on the ground is breathing and hasn't broken his neck (oh, yes, we've been there, done that one). Then, there is the paper work. You know the wave that can roll over us? This is more like a tsunami. I manage the cases of 3400 kids, give or take a hundred. They are actually being nice to the new school nurses. Most of us only have three schools. The more experienced nurses may have five or more schools. I have to admit, my boss is great to work for. She is very encouraging and gives us a lot of support, both in orientation and mentoring and in kindness. It is a very challenging job, and I love it. I head back to school in the fall to get my school nurse certification, and am also working toward my nurse practitioner license.

Kate, new school nurse, in a letter to a friend

health care needs; first aid; assessment of acute health problems; health examinations (especially for athletic participation or school entry); health education; and referrals. One study found that, although parents valued school health ser-

DISPLAY 28–3

Standards of School Nursing Practice (American Nurses Association and the National Association of School Nurses, 2001)

Standards of Care

I. **Assessment**—The school nurse collects client data
  The school nurse involves client, family, school staff, community, and other providers.
  Priority is determined by nursing diagnosis, client's immediate condition and needs.
  Pertinent individual and aggregate data are collected, using appropriate assessment techniques, and reviewed in light of supporting information.
  Data are documented in a retrievable form.

II. **Diagnosis**—The school nurse analyzes the assessment data in determining the nursing diagnoses.
  Nursing Diagnoses (Individual and Aggregate) are derived from evaluation of assessment data.
  Nursing Diagnoses (Individual and Aggregate) are validated with the student, family, school staff, community, and other providers if appropriate.
  Nursing Diagnoses (Individual and Aggregate) are documented in a manner that facilitates the determination of expected outcomes and plan of care or action.

III. **Outcome Identification**—The school nurse identifies expected outcomes individualized to the client.
  Outcomes are derived from nursing diagnoses.
  Outcomes are mutually formulated with student, family, school staff, community, and other providers.
  Outcomes are culturally appropriate and realistic in relationship to the client's present and potential capabilities.
  Outcomes are obtained in relation to necessary and attainable resources.
  Outcomes include a reasonable time line.
  Outcomes provide direction for continuity of care and the plan of care or action.
  Outcomes are documented as measurable goals.

IV. **Planning**—The school nurse develops a plan of care or action that specifies interventions to attain expected outcomes.
  The plan is individualized to student's nursing diagnoses.
  The plan is a component of the individual program for students with special health care needs.
  The plan is developed in compliance with local, state, and federal regulations, as needed.
  The plan is collaboratively developed with the student, family, school staff, community, and other providers, as appropriate.
  The plan reflects current standards of school nursing practice.

The plan provides for continuity of care and a plan of action to be taken.
  Priorities for care and action and a time line for interventions are established.
  The plan is documented in a retrievable form.

V. **Implementation**–The school nurse implements the interventions identified in plan of care/action.
  Interventions are consistent with the established plan of care/action.
  Interventions are implemented in a safe, timely, and appropriate manner.
  Interventions are documented in a retrievable form.
  Interventions reflect current standards of school nursing practice.

VI. **Evaluation**—The school nurse evaluates the client's progress toward attainment of outcomes.
  Evaluation is systematic, continuous, and criterion based.
  The student, family, school staff, community, and other providers are involved in the evaluation process, as appropriate.
  Ongoing assessment data, including incremental goal attainment in achieving the expected outcomes, are used to revise diagnoses and outcomes and the plan of care or action, as needed.
  Revisions in nursing diagnoses, outcomes, and the plan of care or action are documented in a retrievable form.
  Client's responses to interventions are documented in a retrievable form.
  Effectiveness of interventions is evaluated in relation to outcomes.

Standards of Professional Performance

Std I. **Quality of Care**—The school nurse systematically evaluates the quality and effectiveness of their school nursing practice.
  The school nurse participates in quality assurance activities as appropriate to position and practice environment (eg, identification of aspects of care necessary for quality monitoring; development of policies, procedures, and adoption of practice guidelines to improve quality of care; collection of data to monitor quality and effectiveness of nursing care; formulation of recommendations to improve school nursing practice or client outcomes; implementation of activities to enhance the quality of nursing practice; evaluation or research to test quality and effectiveness).
  The school nurse uses results of quality of care activities to initiate changes in school nursing practice, as appropriate.
  The school nurse continuously strives to improve the quality and effectiveness of school health services.

DISPLAY 28-3

Standards of School Nursing Practice (American Nurses Association and the National Association of School Nurses, 2001) (continued)

Std II. Performance Appraisal—The school nurse evaluates his/her own practice in relation to professional practice standards and relevant statutes, regulations, and policies.

The school nurse participates in regular performance appraisals, identifying areas of strength and weakness, as well as ways to refine professional development.

The school nurse seeks out and acts on constructive feedback regarding his/her own practice.

The school nurse takes action to achieve goals identified during performance appraisal.

The school nurse initiates and participates in peer review, as appropriate.

The school nurse's practice reflects knowledge of current professional practice standards, education, and health care laws, and regulations, and school policies.

Std III. Education—The school nurse acquires and maintains current knowledge and competency in school nursing practice.

The school nurse acquires knowledge and skills appropriate to the specialty practice of school nursing on a regular and ongoing basis.

The school nurse consistently participates in continuing education activities related to current clinical knowledge and professional issues.

The school nurse seeks experiences to maintain current clinical skills and competence.

Std IV. Collegiality—The school nurse interacts with and contributes to professional development of peers and school personnel as colleagues.

The school nurse shares knowledge and skills with nursing and interdisciplinary colleagues.

The school nurse provides peers with constructive feedback regarding their practice.

The school nurse interacts with nursing and interdisciplinary colleagues to enhance professional practice and health care of students.

The school nurse contributes to an environment that is conducive to clinical education of nursing students, other health care students, and other employees.

The school nurse contributes to a supportive and healthy work environment.

The school nurse participates in appropriate professional organizations in a membership and/or leadership capacity.

Std V. Ethics—School nurse's decisions and actions on behalf of clients are determined in an ethical manner.

The school nurse practice is guided by *The Code for Nurses.*

The school nurse maintains client confidentiality.

The school nurse acts as client advocate.

The school nurse delivers care in nonjudgmental and nondiscriminatory manner and is sensitive to client diversity.

The school nurse delivers care in a manner that preserves and protects client autonomy, dignity, and rights.

The school nurse seeks available resources to help formulate ethical decisions.

Std VI. Collaboration—The school nurse collaborates with the student, family, school staff, community, and other providers in providing client care.

The school nurse communicates verbally and in writing with the student, family, school staff, community, and other providers regarding client care and nursing's role in the provision of care.

The school nurse collaborates with the student, family, school staff, community and other providers in the formulation of overall goals, time lines, the plan of care, and decisions related to care and the delivery of services.

The school nurse assists individual students in developing appropriate skills to advocate for themselves based on age and developmental level.

The school nurse consults with and utilizes the expertise of other providers for client care, as needed.

The school nurse makes referrals, including provisions for continuity of care, as needed.

Std VII. Research—The school nurse promotes the use of research findings in school nursing practice.

The school nurse utilizes available research in developing the health programs and individual client plans of care and interventions.

The school nurse participates in research activities, as appropriate to his/her education, position, and practice environment (eg, identifying clinical problems suitable for research; participating in data collection; participating in unit, organization, or community research committee or program; interpreting research findings with others; conducting research; critiquing research for application to practice; using research findings in the development of policies and procedures for client care and program development).

The school nurse contributes to the nursing literature when and if possible.

Std VIII. Resource Utilization—The school nurse considers factors related to safety, effectiveness, and cost when planning and delivering care.

The school nurse evaluates factors related to safety, effectiveness, availability, and cost when choosing between two or more practice options that would result in the same expected client or program outcome.

(display continues on page 666)

DISPLAY 28-3

Standards of School Nursing Practice (American Nurses Association and the National Association of School Nurses, 2001) (continued)

The school nurse assists the student, family, school staff, and community in identifying and securing appropriate and available services and resources to address health-related needs.

The school nurse assigns tasks or delegates tasks as defined by the state nurse practice act and according to the knowledge and skills of the designated caregiver.

If the school nurse assigns or delegates tasks, it is based on the needs and condition of the client and potential for harm, the stability of the client's condition, the complexity of the task, and the predictability of the outcome.

The school nurse assists the student, family, school staff, and community in becoming informed consumers about the costs, risks, and benefits of health promotion, health education, school health services, and individualized health interventions for students.

Std IX. Communication—The school nurse uses effective written, verbal, and nonverbal communication skills.

The school nurse communicates effectively with the student, family, school staff, community, and other providers regarding student care and the role of the school nurse in the provision of care.

The school nurse employs counseling techniques and crisis-intervention strategies for individuals and groups.

The school nurse utilizes communication as a positive strategy to achieve nursing goals.

The school nurse demonstrates knowledge of the philosophy and mission of the school district, the kind and nature of its curricular and extracurricular activities, and its programs and special services.

The school nurse demonstrates knowledge of the roles of other school professionals and adjunct personnel and coordinates roles and responsibilities of the adjunct school health personnel within the school team.

Std X. Program Management—The school nurse manages school health services.

The school nurse manages school health services as appropriate to the nurse's education, position, and practice environment.

The school nurse conducts school health needs assessments to identify current health problems and identify the need for new programs.

The school nurse develops and implements needed health programs using a program planning process.

The school nurse demonstrates knowledge of existing school health programs and current health trends that may affect client care, the sources of funds for each, school policy related to each, and local, state, and federal laws governing each.

The school nurse develops and implements health policies and procedures in collaboration with the school administration, board of health, and the board of education.

The school nurse orients, provides training, documents competency, supervises, and evaluates health assistants, aides, and unlicensed assistive personnel as appropriate to the school setting.

The school nurse uses the results of school health and environmental needs assessment, analysis of evaluation data, and quality of care activities to initiate changes throughout the health care delivery system, as appropriate.

The school nurse participates in environmental safety and health activities (eg, indoor air quality, injury surveillance & prevention).

The school nurse adopts and utilizes available technology, as appropriate to the work setting.

Std XI. Health Education—The school nurse assists students, families, school staff, and community to achieve optimal levels of wellness through appropriately designed and delivered health education.

The school nurse participates in the assessment of needs for health education and health instruction for the school community.

The school nurse provides formal health instruction within the classroom based on sound learning theory, as appropriate to student developmental levels.

The school nurse provides individual and group health teaching and counseling for and with clients.

The school nurse participates in the design and development of health curricula.

The school nurse participates in the evaluation of health curricula, health instructional materials, and other health education activities.

The school nurse acts as a resource person to school staff regarding health education and health education materials.

The school nurse furthers the application of health promotion principles within all areas of school life (eg, food services, custodial).

(Adapted from *Scope and standards of professional school nursing practice.* [2001]. Washington, DC: American Nurses Publishing; used with permission.)

- Health promotion for faculty and staff (employee health)
- Counseling, psychological, and social services
- School nutrition services
- Physical education programs
- Healthy school environment
- Family and community involvement (partnership between school, families, community groups)

The school principal influences all phases of the school health program by promoting good school health through active support of the school's health services, participation in setting of policies, and tapping community resources. The principal can reinforce positive efforts within the school ranging from health teaching to cleaning activities of the custodian. Because of the principal's influential position, it is absolutely essential for the nurse and principal to maintain a positive and cooperative working relationship.

Teachers, whether they are involved in regular instruction, physical education, or special education classes, play a major role in school health. Because they spend so much time with students, their observations, health teaching, and personal health habits have a profound effect on student health and the quality of school health services. The school nurse and teachers must collaborate constantly.

Other health team members, such as health educators, health coordinators, psychologists, audiologists, speech therapists, occupational therapists, physical therapists, counselors, health care providers, dentists, dental hygienists, social workers, security personnel, health aides, and volunteers, may be present depending on the size and financial resources of the school. All team members, including students, parents, bus drivers, and custodians, have a specialized role complementary to that of the school nurse. Consultation and referral between team members are crucial to the successful implementation of the school health program.

If the school system desires such services, a physician may work part-time or on a consultation basis. This role focuses largely on advising and consulting in policy and medical–legal matters. A community physician may serve on a school advisory panel as a liaison with the community, other health agencies, and the school. The physician or a nurse practitioner may become involved in student health appraisals, rescreening, health problem intervention, sports physical examinations, or sporting events.

Special Training and Skills of the School Nurse

School nurses operate from one of two administrative bases, the school system or the health department. There is controversy over which system best serves the population's needs. In most localities, school nurses are hired by public or private school systems, and they maintain a specialized, school-based service. An advantage of this specialized role is that the nurse can concentrate time and effort on the school health program and develop specialized skills in school health assessment and intervention. Today, with emphasis on delivery of health care at community sites where clients spend most of their time (schools for children, the workplace for adults), the nurse who is specialized in school health care seems better prepared to meet the complex needs of the school-age population.

In contrast, the community health nurse who operates under the board of health's jurisdiction provides services to schools as one part of generalized services to the community. The community health nurse working through the health department devotes only a portion of the workday to the school; she or he has additional responsibilities such as clinic nursing and home visits. Many argue that such generalized school nurses are at a disadvantage because not enough time is spent on meeting school health needs. The advantage is that this broader base allows contact with preschoolers and their families, strengthened knowledge of the community and its resources, and integration of in-school and out-of-school care.

School nurse practitioners are registered nurses with advanced academic and clinical preparation (certification or a master's degree in nursing) and experience in physical assessment, diagnosis, and treatment, so that primary care can be provided to school-age children. Many school districts see the advantage of having a school nurse practitioner on staff rather than the limited services of a physician. Assessment, diagnosis, treatment, and referral of injuries, communicable diseases, or other health problems can be managed more efficiently by a nurse practitioner who is educationally prepared to work holistically with the school-age population and is part of the educational setting. If this is impractical, one school nurse practitioner who is available to school nurses for consultation or employed on a part-time basis can be the start of the development of more comprehensive school health services.

As the needs of school-age populations become increasingly complex, some states require even more specialized training for school nurses. In California, school nurses are expected to hold a school health services credential. This credential is obtained through a postbaccalaureate program that includes a minimum of 24 semester units of coursework in audiology, guidance and counseling, exceptional children, school health principles and practice, a practicum in school nursing, child psychology, and health curriculum development in addition to other courses.

As the population continues to become more diverse and the problems of children and families grow in complexity, the school nurse with specialized training in school health, the education system, case management, and advanced practice nursing (eg, nurse practitioner, clinical nurse specialist) becomes even more essential.

A review of school nursing research by Maughan (2003) found that school nurses are associated with improved school performance, decreased absenteeism, increased graduation rates, better chronic disease management, and identification of high-risk students. Health education by school nurses decreases smoking rates, increases prenatal care, and provides positive changes in chronic conditions (eg, headaches, asthma) (see What Do You Think?).

WHAT DO YOU THINK?

1. Hunger—America is the world's food basket, yet many children and families go hungry. This can affect a child's school performance. Do you think that schools should provide breakfast, lunch, and after-school snacks to all children?
2. Communicable Diseases—Most schools require that children entering school be fully immunized and screened for tuberculosis. What would happen if schools no longer had this requirement?
3. Attention Deficit Hyperactivity Disorder—Do you think that schools should require children with behavioral problems to be evaluated and put on medication? Should taking that medication be a condition of their continuing enrollment? Who should pay for that evaluation and medication?
4. Obesity—Should schools have vending machines with soda and high-fat, high-calorie snacks? What would happen if these things were banned on school property? Should student groups be allowed to sell candy bars, for instance, to pay for band uniforms?
5. Emotional Health—Do you think that emotional health affects students' academic achievement? Should schools be in the business of dealing with the social and emotional problems of their students?
6. School Health—What if there were no school nurses? How would the health of the students and the role of the teacher be changed?

SUMMARY

Children and adolescents are important population groups to community health nurses because their physical and emotional health is vital to the future of society and because they require guidance and direction.

Mortality rates for children and adolescents have decreased dramatically since the early 1900s, but morbidity rates remain high. Children and adolescents are vulnerable to many illnesses, injuries, and emotional problems, often as a result of a complex and stressful environment.

Violence against children and deaths due to homicide occur in the United States at alarming rates. Unintentional injuries, suicide, and homicide are the leading threats to life and health for adolescents. Other health problems include alcohol and drug abuse, unplanned pregnancies, STDs and HIV/AIDS, and poor nutrition. All of these problems create major challenges for the community health nurse who seeks to prevent illness and injury among children and adolescents and to promote their health. Chronic illnesses such as asthma and diabetes are important to monitor. Irritating, somewhat common problems, such as head lice and acne, can respond to treatment and education.

Health services for children and adolescents span three categories: prevention, health protection, and health promotion. The community health nurse plays a vital role in each. Preventive services include immunization programs, parental support services, family planning programs, services for those with STDs, and alcohol and drug abuse prevention programs. Health protection services include accident and injury control, programs to reduce environmental hazards, control of infectious diseases, and services to protect children and adolescents from child abuse and neglect. Health promotion services include programs in nutrition and weight control; exercise and physical fitness; smoking, alcohol, and drug abuse education; and stress control. School-based health centers provide a convenient place for the provision of primary health care as well as health education and mental health counseling.

The role of school nurses includes three basic interventions. With educational interventions such as nutrition teaching, nurses provide information and encourage clients to act responsibly on behalf of their own health. Nurses employ persuasive tactics to move clients toward more positive health behaviors by engineering interventions, such as encouraging consistent use of contraceptives by adolescents. With enforcement interventions, such as reporting and intervening in child abuse, nurses practice a form of coercion to protect children from threats to their health.

Nursing of the school-age population involves providing health services and health education and ensuring a healthful school environment. School nurses may provide these services as part of their roles within health departments, or they may be hired by the school district full-time. The increasingly complex needs of the school-age population and the collective accessibility for delivery of primary health care services to children in the school setting are prompting schools to hire nurses with advanced preparation as nurse practitioners and credentialed school nurses expand their services to this aggregate.

ACTIVITIES TO PROMOTE CRITICAL THINKING

1. You are a community health nurse assigned to work at a school. You learn that more than 20% of the students in this school district are being treated with Ritalin, Concerta, Adderall, or some other medication for ADHD. What things should you consider in determining whether these medications are being appropriately prescribed?

2. What is the major cause of death among school-age children? What community-wide interventions could be initiated to prevent these deaths? Select one intervention and describe how you and a group of community health professionals might develop this preventive measure.

3. A 14-year-old girl from a middle-class family and a 14-year-old girl from a poor family both come to the office where you work as a school nurse. The girls have similar symptoms that possibly indicate gonorrhea. Would your assessment and intervention be the same for the two girls? What are your values and attitudes toward people with diseases that are sexually transmitted? Does social class, race, age, or sex make any difference in how you feel about them? What is one action the community health nurse can take to prevent such diseases in this population group?

4. Discuss possible methods of doing nutritional assessments in school-age children. What programs could be instituted to encourage healthier diets and increased exercise? What other factors might need to be considered? How could you, as a community health nurse, work with schools and parents to increase physical activity and improve nutrition for school-age children and adolescents?

5. Describe possible benefits of school-based health centers (SBHCs). What are the most common misperceptions? What are common barriers to starting SBHCs? What steps can community health nurses take to promote community awareness and facilitate development of SBHCs in local schools?

6. A new elementary school to which you have been assigned has repeated outbreaks of head lice and very limited access to health care. Using the Internet, research causes for recurrent head lice infestations and effective OTC treatments. Are head lice most often found seasonally? Discuss possible education programs you might implement or other innovative methods of treatment and control you might be able to institute.

REFERENCES

Aarons, S., Jenkins, R., Raine, T., El-Khorazaty, M., Woodward, K., Williams, R., et al. (2000). Postponing sexual intercourse among junior high school students: A randomized controlled evaluation. *Journal of Adolescent Health, 27*(4), 236–247.

Adams, E., & Johnson, V. (2002). An elementary school-based clinic: Can it reduce Medicaid costs? *Pediatrics, 105*(4), 780–788.

Alaimo, K., Olson, C., & Frongillo, E. (2001). Food insufficiency and American school-aged children's cognitive, academic, and psychosocial development. *Pediatrics, 108*(1), 44–53.

Aligne, C.A., Moss, M.E., Auinger, P., & Weitzman, M. (2003). Association of pediatric dental caries with passive smoking. *Journal of the American Medical Association, 289*(10), 1258–1260.

American Diabetes Association. (2000). Clinical practice recommendations 2000. *Diabetes Care, 23*(Suppl. 1), S1–S116.

American Psychiatric Association. (2000). *Diagnostic and statistical manual of mental disorders,* 4th ed., Text Revision. Washington, DC: Author.

America's Children. (2002). *Highlights.* Retrieved January 24, 2004, from *http://childstats.gov/ac2002/highlight.asp*

Arias, E., & Smith, B. (2003). Deaths: Preliminary data for 2001. *National Vital Statistics Reports, 51*(5), 1–44.

Baranowski, T., Baranowski, J., Cullen, K., Thompson, D., Nicklas, T., Zakeri, I., et al. (2003). The fun, food, and fitness project (FFFP): The Baylor GEMS pilot study. *Ethnicity and Disease, 13*(Suppl. 1), S30–S39.

Barkley, R., Fischer, M., Smallish, L., & Fletcher, K. (2002). The persistence of attention-deficit/hyperactivity disorder into young adulthood as a function of reporting source and definition of disorder. *Journal of Abnormal Psychology, 111*(2), 279–289.

Barkley, R., Fischer, M., Smallish, L., & Fletcher, K. (2003). Does the treatment of attention-deficit/hyperactivity disorder with stimulants contribute to drug use/abuse? A 3-year prospective study. *Pediatrics, 111*(1), 97–109.

Berkey, C., Rockett, H., Gillman, M., & Colditz, G. (2003). One-year changes in activity and in inactivity among 10- to 15-year old boys and girls: Relationship to change in body mass index. *Pediatrics, 111*(4), 836–843.

Berkowitz, R.J. (2003). Causes, treatment, and prevention of early childhood caries: A microbiologic perspective. *Journal of the Canadian Dental Association, 69*(5), 304–307.

Biederman, J., & Faraone, S. (2002). Current concepts on the neurobiology of attention-deficit/hyperactivity disorder. *Journal of Attention Disorders, 6*(Suppl. 1), S7–S16.

Blumstein, A. (2002). Youth, guns, and violent crime. *The Future of Children, 12*(2), 39–54.

Boekeloo, B., Bobbi, M., Lee, W., Worrell, K., Hamburger, E., & Russek-Cohen, E. (2003). Effect of patient priming and primary care provider prompting on adolescent-provider communication about alcohol. *Archives of Pediatrics and Adolescent Medicine, 157*(5), 433–439.

Boudreaux, E., Emond, S., Clark, S., & Camargo, C. (2003). Race/ethnicity and asthma among children presenting to the emergency department: Differences in disease severity and management. *Pediatrics, 111*(5), e615–e621.

Bowyer, S., Roettcher, P., Higgins, G., Adams, B., Myers, L., Wallace, C., et al. (2003). Health status of patients with juvenile rheumatoid arthritis at 1 and 5 years after diagnosis. *Journal of Rheumatology, 30*(2), 394–400.

Brindis, C., Klein, J., Schlitt, J., Santelli, J., Juszczak, L., & Nystrom, R. (2003). School-based health centers: Accessibility and accountability. *Journal of Adolescent Health, 32*(6), 98–107.

Brinkley, J., Eales, J., & Jekanowski, M. (2000). The relation between dietary changes and rising U. S. obesity. *International Journal of Obesity and Related Metabolic Disorders, 24*(8), 1032–1039.

Brown, L., Wall, T., & Lazar, V. (2002). Trends in caries among adults 18 to 45 years old. *Journal of the American Dental Association, 133*(7), 827–834.

Brown, L., Wall, T., & Lazar, V. (2000). Trends in untreated caries in primary teeth of children 2 to 10 years old. *Journal of the American Dental Association, 131*(1), 93–100.

Buchalter, J.R., & Jarrar, R.G. (2003). Therapeutics in pediatric epilepsy, part 2: Epilepsy surgery and vagus nerve stimulation. *Mayo Clinic Proceedings, 78*(3), 371–378.

Bulik, C., Sullivan, P., & Kendler, K. (2000). An empirical study of the classification of eating disorders. *American Journal of Psychiatry, 157*(6), 886–895.

Burstein, G., Lowry, R., Klein, J., & Santelli, J. (2003). Missed opportunities for sexually transmitted diseases, human immunodeficiency virus, and pregnancy prevention services during adolescent health supervision visits. *Pediatrics, 111*(5), 996–1001.

Caccamo, J. (2000). Sharing the vision: Healthy, achieving students: What can schools do? *Journal of School Health, 70*(5), 216–218.

Casady, M.A., & Lee, R.E. (2002). Environments of physically neglected children. *Psychological Reports, 91*(3), 711–721.

Centers for Disease Control and Prevention. (2000). *STD Surveillance 2000: STDs in adolescents and young adults.* Retrieved January 25, 2004, from *http://www.cdc.gov/std/stats00/2000SFAdol&YAdults.htm*

Centers for Disease Control and Prevention. (2001a). *Adolescent and school health.* Youth Risk Behavior Survey: Summary results, 2001. Retrieved January 25, 2004, from *http://www.cdc.gov/nccdphp/dash/yrbs/2001/summary_results/usa.htm*

Centers for Disease Control and Prevention. (2001b). *New estimates for asthma tracked.* National Center for Health Statistics. Retrieved January 24, 2004, from *http://www.cdc.gov/nchs/releases/01facts/asthma.htm*

Centers for Disease Control and Prevention. (2001c). *Screening for tuberculosis and tuberculosis infection in high-risk populations: Recommendations of the Advisory Committee for Elimination of Tuberculosis.* Retrieved April 5, 2004 from *http://www.cdc.gov/mmwr/preview/mmwrthtml/00001642.htm*

Centers for Disease Control and Prevention. (2002a). *Summary health statistics for U. S. children: National health interview survey.* Vital and Health Statistics, Series 10, No. 208. Washington, DC: Author.

Centers for Disease Control and Prevention. (2002b). Trends in cigarette smoking among high school students—United States, 1991–2001. *MMWR Morbidity and Mortality Weekly Report.* Retrieved January 24, 2004, from *http://www.cdc.gov/mmwr/preview/mmwrhtml/mm5119a1.htm*

Centers for Disease Control and Prevention. (2002c). *Young people at risk: HIV/AIDS among America's youth.* Divisions of HIV/AIDS Prevention. Retrieved January 24, 2004, from *http://www.cdc.gov/hiv/pubs/facts/youth.htm*

Centers for Disease Control and Prevention. (2003a). *Improving oral health.* Retrieved January 29, 2004, from *http://www.cdc.gov/nccdphp/bb_oralhealth/index.htm*

Centers for Disease Control and Prevention. (2003b). *Fact sheet: Preventing dental caries.* National Center for Chronic Disease Prevention and Health Promotion. Retrieved January 24, 2004, from *http://www.cdc.gov/oralhealth/factsheets/dental_caries.htm*

Centers for Disease Control and Prevention. (2003b). *U. S. injury mortality statistics.* National Center for Injury Prevention and Control. Retrieved from *http://www.cdc.gov/nchs/data/ad/ad303.pdf*

Centers for Disease Control and Prevention. (2003c). *Youth violence prevention: Facts and myths about youth violence.* National Center for Injury Prevention and Control. Retrieved from January 24, 2004, from *http://www.cdc.gov/ncipc/dvp/youth/myths.htm*

Centers for Disease Control and Prevention. (2003d). *Fact sheet: School health policies and programs study.* National Center for Chronic Disease Prevention and Health Promotion. Retrieved December 30, 2003, from *http://www.cdc.gov/nccdphp/dash/shpps/index.htm*

Chan, E., Rappaport, L., & Kemper, K. (2003). Complementary and alternative therapies in childhood attention and hyperactivity problems. *Journal of Developmental and Behavioral Pediatrics, 24*(1), 4–8.

Chase-Lansdale, P.L., & Pittman, L.D. (2002). Welfare reform and parenting: Reasonable expectations. *The Future of Children, 12*(1), 167–186.

Chatrath, R., Shenoy, R., Serratto, M., & Thoele, D. (2002). Physical fitness of urban American children. *Pediatric Cardiology, 23*(6), 608–612.

Children's Defense Fund. (2002). *The state of children in America's union: A 2002 action guide to leave no child behind.* Washington, DC: Author.

Clark, D., Clasen, C., Stolfi, A., & Jaballas, E. (2002). Parent knowledge and opinions of school health services in an urban public school system. *Journal of School Health, 72*(1), 18–22.

Clarke, P., Fraser-Lee, N.J., & Shimono, T. (2001). Identifying risk factors for predicting caries in school-aged children using dental health information collected at preschool age. *Journal of Dentistry in Children, 68*(5), 373–378.

Collins, J. (1997). *Prevalence of selected chronic conditions: United States, 1990–1992.* Washington, DC: National Center for Health Statistics.

Connor, D., Edwards, G., Fletcher, K., Baird, J., Barkley, R., & Steingard, R. (2003). Correlates of comorbid psychopathology in children with ADHD. *Journal of the American Academic of Child and Adolescent Psychiatry, 42*(2), 193–200.

Cook, J.T. (2002). Clinical implications of household food security: Definitions, monitoring, and policy. *Nutrition in Clinical Care, 5*(4), 152–167.

Coon, K.A., & Tucker, K.L. (2002). Television and children's consumption patterns: A review of the literature. *Minerva Pediatrics, 54*(5), 423–436.

Cordain, L., Lindeberg, S., Hurtado, M., Hill, K., Eaton, S., & Brand-Miller, J. (2002). Acne vulgaris: A disease of Western civilization. *Archives of Dermatology, 138*(12), 1584–1590.

Cox, E., Motheral, B., Henderson, R., & Mager, D. (2003). Geographic variation in the prevalence of stimulant medication use among children 5 to 14 years old: Results from a commercially insured U. S. sample. *Pediatrics, 111*(2), 237–243.

Crosby, R., & St. Lawrence, J. (2000). Adolescents' use of school-based health clinics for reproductive health services: Data from the National Longitudinal Study of Adolescent Health. *Journal of School Health, 70*(1), 22–27.

Daisey, J., Angell, W., & Apte, M. (2003). Indoor air quality, ventilation, and health symptoms in schools: An analysis of existing information. *Indoor Air, 13*(1), 53–64.

Dake, J., Price, J., & Murnan, J. (2003). Evaluation of a child abuse prevention curriculum for third-grade students: Assessment of knowledge and efficacy expectations. *Journal of School Health, 73*(2), 76–82.

Deal, L., Gomby, D., Zippiroli, L., & Behrman, R. (2000). Unintentional injuries in childhood: Analysis and recommendations. *The Future of Children, 10*(1), 4–22.

Dietz, W.H., & Gortmaker, S.L. (2001). Preventing obesity in children and adolescents. *Annual Review of Public Health, 22,* 337–353.

Distefan, J., Gilpin, E., & Pierce, J. (2000). The effectiveness of tobacco control in California schools. *Journal of School Health, 70*(1), 28–30.

Eggert, L., Thompson, E., Randell, B., & Pike, K. (2002). Preliminary effects of brief school-based prevention approaches for reducing youth suicide risk behaviors, depression, and drug involvement. *Journal of Child and Adolescent Psychiatric Nursing, 15*(2), 48–64.

Elder, J.P., Litrownik, A.J., Slymen, D.J., Campbell, N.R., Parra-Medina, D., Choe, S., Lee, V., Ayala, G.X. (2002). Tobacco and alcohol use-prevention program for Hispanic migrant adolescents. *American Journal of Preventive Medicine, 23*(4), 269–275.

Ellickson, P., Tucker, J., & Klein, D. (2003). Ten-year prospective study of public health problem associated with early drinking. *Pediatrics, 111*(5), 949–955.

Evans, S., Axelrod, J., & Sapia, J. (2000). Effective school-based mental health interventions: Advising the social skills training paradigm. *Journal of School Health, 70*(5), 191–194.

Fingerhut, L., & Kaufer-Christoffel, K. (2002). Firearm-related death and injury among children and adolescents. *The Future of Children, 12*(2), 25–38.

Fisher, K., & Kettl, P. (2003). Teachers' perceptions of school violence. *Journal of Pediatric Health Care, 17*(2), 79–83.

Fletcher, E. (2003, May 30). *Senate votes to move the fizz off-campus.* The Sacramento Bee. Retrieved January 29, 2004, from *http://nl.newsbank.com/nl-search/we/Archives?p_ product=SB&p_theme=sb&p_action=search&p_maxdocs= 200&s_dispstring=allfields(Senate%20votes%20move% 20fizz%20off-campus)%20AND%20date()&p_field_advanced- 0=&p_text_advanced-0=("Senate%20votes%20move% 20fizz%20off-campus")&p_perpage=10&p_sort=YMD_date: D&xcal_useweights=no*

Folmer, R., Griest, S., & Martin, W. (2002). Hearing conservation education programs for children: A review. *Journal of School Health, 72*(2), 51–57.

Food Research and Action Center. (2003). *Hunger in the U. S.* Retrieved January 25, 2004, from *http://www.frac.org/html/ hunger_in_the_us/hunger_index.html*

Frankowski, B.L., Weiner, L.B.; Committee on School Health, Committee on Infectious Diseases. American Academy of Pediatrics. (2002). Head lice. *Pediatrics, 110*(3), 638–643.

Fuchs, T., Birbaumer, N., Lutzenberger, W., Gruzelier, J., & Kaiser, J. (2003). Neurofeedback treatment for attention-deficit/hyperactivity disorder in children: A comparison with methylphenidate. *Applications in Psychophysiological Biofeedback, 28*(1), 1–12.

Fuller, B., Kagan, S., Caspary, G., & Gauthier, C. (2002). Welfare reform and child care options for low-income families. *The Future of Children, 12*(1), 97–120.

Gillcrist, J., Brumley, D., & Blackford, J. (2001). Community fluoridation status and caries experience in children. *Journal of Public Health Dentistry, 61*(3), 168–171.

Gloeckler-Ries, L., Percy, C.L., & Bunin, G.R. (1999). Introduction. In L. Ries, M. Smith, J. Gurney, M. Linet, T. Tamra, J. Young, et al. (Eds.), *Cancer incidence and survival among children and adolescents: United States SEER program 1977–1995* (NIH Pub. No. 99-4649, p. 1). Bethesda, MD: National Institutes of Health.

Goran, M.I., Ball, G.D., & Cruz, M.L. (2003). Obesity and risk of type 2 diabetes and cardiovascular disease in children and adolescents. *Journal of Clinical Endocrinology and Metabolism, 88*(4), 1417–1427.

Griffin, S., Jones, K., & Tomar, S. (2001). An economic evaluation of community water fluoridation. *Journal of Public Health Dentistry, 61*(2), 78–86.

Guinan, M., McGuckin, M., & Ali, Y. (2002). The effect of a comprehensive handwashing program on absenteeism in elementary schools. *American Journal of Infection Control, 30*(4), 217–220.

Hackbarth, D., Schnopp-Wyatt, D., Katz, D., Williams, J., Silvestri, B., & Pfleger, M. (2001). Collaborative research and action to control the geographic placement of outdoor advertising of alcohol and tobacco products in Chicago. *Public Health Reports, 116*(6), 558–567.

Hall, A., Khanh, L., Son, T., Dung, N., Lansdown, R., Dar, D., et al. (2001). An association between chronic undernutrition and educational test scores in Vietnamese children. *European Journal of Clinical Nutrition, 55*(9), 801–804.

Harrell, J., Pearce, P., & Hayman, L. (2003). Fostering prevention in the pediatric population. *Journal of Cardiovascular Nursing, 18*(2), 144–149.

Hawkins, J., Hayes, E., & Corliss, C. (1994). School nursing in America—1902 to 1994: A return to public health nursing. *Public Health Nursing, 11*(6), 416–425.

Hendin, H., Maltsberger, J., Lipschitz, A., Haas, A., & Kyle, J. (2001). Recognizing and responding to a suicide crisis. *Suicide and Life Threatening Behaviors, 31*(2), 115–128.

Hershey, T., Bhargava, N., Sadler, M., White, N., & Craft, S. (1999). Conventional versus intensive diabetes therapy in children with type 1 diabetes: Effects on memory and motor speed. *Diabetes Care, 22*(8), 1318–1324.

Hillier, S. (2000). Fluoride in drinking water and risk of hip fracture in the UK: A case-control study. *Lancet, 355*(9200), 265–269.

Hocutt, A.M. (1996). Effectiveness of special education: Is placement the critical factor? *The Future of Children, 6*(1), 77–102.

Howard, D., Feigelman, S., Li, X., Cross, S., & Rachuba, L. (2002). The relationship among violence victimization, witnessing violence, and youth distress. *Journal of Adolescent Health, 31*(6), 455–462.

Illinois Department of Public Health. (2003). *Adolescents at risk: Statistics on HIV/AIDS, STDs and unintended pregnancies.* Retrieved January 25, 2004, from *http://www.idph.state.il.us/public/respect/hiv_fs.htm*

Jahns, L., Siega-Riz, A., & Popkin, B. (2001). The increasing prevalence of snacking among U. S. children from 1977 to 1996. *Journal of Pediatrics, 38*(4), 493–498.

Jarrar, R.G., & Buchhalter, J.R. (2003). Therapeutics in pediatric epilepsy, part 1: The new antiepileptic drugs and the ketogenic diet. *Mayo Clinic Proceedings, 78*(3), 359–370.

Johnson, B., Carey, M., Marsh, K., Levin, K., & Scott-Sheldon, O. (2003). Interventions to reduce sexual risk for the human-immunodeficiency virus in adolescents, 1985–2000: A research synthesis. *Archives of Pediatric and Adolescent Medicine, 157*(4), 381–388.

Johnson, S.A., & Fisher, K. (2003). School violence: An insider view. *American Journal of Maternal Child Nursing, 28*(2), 86–92.

Johnston, L., O'Malley, P., & Bachman, J. (2003). *Monitoring the future: National results on adolescent drug use. Overview of findings 2002.* (NIH Publication No. 03-5374). Bethesda, MD: National Institute on Drug Abuse.

Jones, K., & English, J. (2003). Review of common therapeutic options in the United States for the treatment of pediculosis capitis. *Clinical Infectious Diseases, 36*(11), 1355–1361.

Kanner, S., Hamrin, V., & Grey, M. (2003). Depression in adolescents with diabetes. J*ournal of Child and Adolescent Psychiatric Nursing, 16*(1), 15–24.

Kendall, J., Hatton, D., Beckett, A., & Leo, M. (2003). Children's accounts of attention-deficit/hyperactivity disorder. *Advances in Nursing Science, 26*(2), 114–130.

King, K. (2001). Developing a comprehensive school suicide prevention program. *Journal of School Health, 71*(4), 132–137.

King, K., Wagner, D., & Hedrick, B. (2001). Safe and drug-free school coordinators' perceived needs to improve violence and drug prevention programs. *Journal of School Health, 71*(6), 236–241.

Kirby, D. (2002). Effective approaches to reducing adolescent unprotected sex, pregnancy and childbearing. *Journal of Sexuality Research, 39*(1), 51–57.

Komro, K., & Toomey, T. (2002). Strategies to prevent underage drinking. *Alcohol Research and Health, 26*(1), 5–14.

Kossoff, E.H., Krauss, G.L., McGrogan, J.R., & Freeman, J.M. (2003). Efficacy of the Atkins diet as therapy for intractable epilepsy. *Neurology, 61*(12), 1789–1791.

Lara, M., Duan, N., Sherbourne, C., Halfon, N., Leibowitz, A., &

Brook, R. (2003). Children's use of emergency departments for asthma: Persistent barriers or acute need? *Journal of Asthma, 40*(3), 289–299.

Leger, L., & Nutbeam, D. (2000). A model for mapping linkages between health and education agencies to improve school health. *Journal of School Health, 70*(2), 45–50.

Lesesne, C., Visser, S., & White, C. (2003). Attention-deficit/hyperactivity disorder in school-aged children: Association with maternal mental health and use of health care resources. *Pediatrics, 111*(5), 1232–1237.

Levaux, H., Schonfeld, W., Pellissier, J., Cassidy, W., Sheriff, S., & Fitzsimon, C. (2001). Economic evaluation of a 2-dose hepatitis B vaccination regimen for adolescents. *Pediatrics, 108*(2), 317–325.

Levy, S.M. (2003). An update on fluorides and fluorosis. *Journal of the Canadian Dental Association, 69*(5), 286–291.

Lewit, E.M., Terman, D.L., & Behrman, R.E. (1997). Children and poverty: Analysis and recommendations. *The Future of Children, 7*(2), 4–24.

Loprest, P. (2001). *How are families that left welfare doing? A comparison of early and recent welfare leavers.* Assessing the New Federalism Policy Brief No. B-36. Washington, DC.

Lowry, R., Wechsler, H., Kann, L., & Collins, J. (2001). Recent trends in participation in physical education among U. S. high school students. *Journal of School Health, 71*(4), 145–152.

Lurie, N., Jones-Bauer, E., & Brady, C. (2001). Asthma outcomes in an inner-city school-based health center. *Journal of School Health, 71*(1), 9–16.

Lytle, L., Seifert, S., Greenstein, J., & McGovern, P. (2000). How do children's eating patterns and food choices change over time? Results from a cohort study. *American Journal of Health Promotion, 14*(4), 222–228.

Marcell, A., Klein, J., Fischer, J., Allan, M., & Kokotailo, P. (2002). Male adolescent use of health care services: Where are the boys? *Journal of Adolescent Health, 39*(1), 35–43.

Mardis, A., & Pratt, S. (2003). Nonfatal injuries to young workers in the retail trades and service industries in 1998. *Journal of Occupational and Environmental Medicine, 45*(3), 316–323.

Marinho, V., Higgins, J., Logan, S., & Sheiham, A. (2003). Systematic review of controlled trials on the effectiveness of fluoride gels for the prevention of dental caries in children. *Journal of Dental Education, 67*(4), 448–458.

Mark, H., Conklin, V., & Wolfe, M. (2001). Nurse volunteers in school-based hepatitis B immunization programs. *Journal of School Nursing, 17*(4), 185–188.

Masi, G., Toni, C., Perugi, G., Travierso, M., Millepiedi, S., Mucci, M., et al. (2003). Externalizing disorders in consecutively referred children and adolescents with bipolar disorder. *Comparative Psychiatry, 44*(3), 184–189.

Maternal and Child Health Bureau. (2002a). Adolescent childbearing. In *Child Health USA 2002.* U. S. Department of Health and Human Services, Health Resources and Services Administration. Retrieved January 25, 2004, from *http:www.mchb.hrsa.gov/chusa02/main_pages/page_35.htm*

Maternal and Child Health Bureau. (2002b). Adolescent deaths due to injury. In *Child Health USA 2002.* U. S. Department of Health and Human Services, Health Resources and Services Administration. Retrieved January 25, 2004, from *http://www.mchb.hrsa.gov/chusa02/main_pages/page_47.htm*

Maternal and Child Health Bureau. (2002c). Adolescent mortality. In *Child Health USA 2002.* U. S. Department of Health and

Human Services, Health Resources and Services Administration. Retrieved January 25, 2004, from *http://mchb.hrsa.gov/chusa02/main_pages/page_46.htm*

Maternal and Child Health Bureau. (2002d). Child abuse and neglect. In *Child Health USA 2002*. U. S. Department of Health and Human Services, Health Resources and Services Administration. Retrieved January 25, 2004, from *http:www.mchb.hrsa.gov/chusa02/main_pages/page_28.htm*

Maternal and Child Health Bureau. (2002e). Childhood deaths due to injury. In *Child Health USA 2002*. U. S. Department of Health and Human Services, Health Resources and Services Administration. Retrieved January 25, 2004, from *http://www.mchb.hrsa.gov/chusa02/main_pages/page_33.htm*

Maternal and Child Health Bureau. (2002f). Dental care. In *Child Health USA 2002*. U. S. Department of Health and Human Services, Health Resources and Services Administration. Retrieved January 25, 2004, from *http://mchb.hrsa.gov/chusa02/main_pages/page_52.htm*

Maternal and Child Health Bureau. (2002g). Health insurance status of children through age 18: 2000. In *Child Health USA 2002*. U. S. Department of Health and Human Services, Health Resources and Services Administration. Retrieved January 25, 2004, from *http://www.mchb.hrsa.gov/chusa02/main_pages/page_66.htm*

Maternal and Child Health Bureau. (2002h). Introduction. In *Child Health USA 2002*. U. S. Department of Health and Human Services, Health Resources and Services Administration. Retrieved January 25, 2004, from *http://www.mchb.hrsa.gov/chusa02/main_pages/page_06.htm*

Maternal and Child Health Bureau. (2002i). Vaccine-preventable diseases. In *Child Health USA 2002*. U. S. Department of Health and Human Services, Health Resources and Services Administration. Retrieved January 25, 2004, from *http://www.mchb.hrsa.gov/chusa02/main_pages/page_27.htm*

Maternal and Child Health Bureau. (2002j). Working mothers. In *Child Health USA 2002*. U. S. Department of Health and Human Services, Health Resources and Services Administration. Retrieved January 25, 2004, from *http:www.mchb.hrsa.gov/chusa02/main_pages/page_14.htm*

Maughan, E. (2003). The impact of school nursing on school performance: A research synthesis. *The Journal of School Nursing, 19*(3), 163–171.

Meerdink-Carpenter, L., & Stanley-Mueller, C. (2001). Evaluating health care seeking behaviors of parents using a school-based health clinic. *Journal of School Health, 71*(10), 497–499.

Miller, T., Romano, E., & Spicer, R. (2000). The cost of childhood unintentional injuries and the value of prevention. *The Future of Children 10*(1), 137–163.

Morris, P., Huston, S., & Duncan, G. (2001). *How welfare and work policies affect children: A synthesis of research*. New York: Manpower Demonstration Research Corporation.

Morris, R.I., & Butt, R.A. (2003). Parents' perspectives on homelessness and its effects on the educational development of their children. *Journal of School Nursing, 19*(1), 43–50.

Nansel, T., Overpeck, M., Haynie, D., Ruan, W., & Scheidt, P. (2003). Relationship between bullying and violence among U. S. youth. *Archives of Pediatric and Adolescent Medicine, 157*(4), 348–358.

National Association of School Nurses. (1999). *Definition of school nursing*. Retrieved January 25, 2004, from *http://www.nasn.org*

National Association of School Nurses. (2001, October). *The role of the school nurse in school-based health centers*. Position statement. Retrieved January 25, 2004, from *http://www.nasn.org/positions/schoolbasedjoint.htm*

National Association of School Nurses. (2002, October). *Education, licensure and certification of school nurses*. Position statement. Retrieved January 25, 2004, from *http://www.nasn.org/positions/education.htm*

National Association of School Nurses (NASN). (2003). *Coordinated school health program*. Position Statement. Retrieved January 25, 2004, from *http://www.nasn.org/positions/coordinated.htm*

National Center for Education Statistics. (2003a). Elementary and secondary education. In *Digest of education statistics, 2001* (Chap. 2). Retrieved January 25, 2004, from *http://www.nces.ed.gov/pubs2002/digest2001/ch2.asp*

National Center for Education Statistics. (2003b). *Homeschooling*. Retrieved January 29, 2004, from *http://nces.ed.gov/fastfacts/display.asp?id=91*

National Center for Education Statistics. (2003c). *Inclusion of students with disabilities*. Retrieved January 25, 2004, from *http://www.nces.ed.gov/fastfacts/display.asp?id=59*

National Center for Health Statistics. (1998). *Health, United States*. Washington, DC: Author.

National Center for Health Statistics. (2000). *Health, United States, 2000*. With adolescent health chartbook. Hyattsville, MD: Author.

National Clearinghouse for Alcohol and Drug Information. (2003a). *Club drugs*. U.S. Department of Health and Human Services. Retrieved January 25, 2004, from *http://store.health.org/catalog/results.aspx?h=drugs&topic=13*

National Clearinghouse for Alcohol and Drug Information. (2003b). *Cocaine*. U.S. Department of Health & Human Services. Retrieved January 25, 2004, from *http://store.health.org/catalog/facts.aspx?topic=41*

National Clearinghouse for Alcohol and Drug Information. (2003c). *Inhalants*. U.S. Department of Health and Human Services. Retrieved January 25, 2004, from *http://store.health.org/catalog/facts.aspx?topic=5*

National Institute of Arthritis and Musculoskeletal and Skin Diseases. (2001). *Questions and answers about juvenile rheumatoid arthritis*. National Institutes of Health. Retrieved January 25, 2004, from *http://www.niams.nih.gov/hi/topics/juvenile_arthritis/juvarthr.htm#2*

National Institute of Arthritis and Musculoskeletal and Skin Diseases. (2003). Questions and answers about acne. Retrieved January 29, 2004, from *http://my.webmd.com/content/article/5/1680_50116.htm?lastselectedguid={5FE84E90-BC77-4056-A91C-9531713CA348}*

National Institute of Mental Health. (2001). *Teens: The company they keep: Preventing destructive behavior by harnessing the power of peers* (NIH Publication No. 01-4588). Bethesda, MD: Author.

National Institute of Mental Health. (2002a, October 3). *Brief notes on the mental health of children and adolescents*. Bethesda, MD: Author.

National Institute of Mental Health. (2002b, October 3). *Youth in a difficult world* (NIH Publication No. 01-4587). Bethesda, MD: Author.

National Institute of Mental Health. (2003). *Teenage brain: A work in progress*. Retrieved January 25, 2004, from *http://nimh.nih.gov/publicat/childmenu.cfm*

National Institute of Neurological Disorders and Stroke. (2001). *NINDS epilepsy information page.* National Institutes of Health. Retrieved January 25, 2004, from *http://www.ninds.nih.gov/ health_and_medical/disorders/epilepsy.htm?format=printable*

Newacheck, P.W., Stein, R.E., Bauman, L., & Hung, Y.Y. (2003). Disparities in the prevalence of disability between black and white children. *Archives of Pediatric and Adolescent Medicine, 157*(3), 244–248.

Nielsen, S., Siega-Riz, A., & Popkin, B. (2002). Trends in food locations and sources among adolescents and young adults. *Preventive Medicine, 35*(2), 107–113.

Ogden, C., Flegal, K., Carrol, M., & Johnson, C. (2002). Prevalence and trends in overweight among U. S. children and adolescents, 1999–2000. *Journal of American Medical Association, 288,* 1728–1732.

Olfson, M., Gameroff, M., Marcus, S., & Jensen, P.S. (2003). National trends in the treatment of attention deficit hyperactivity disorder. *American Journal of Psychiatry, 160*(6), 1071–1077.

Ott, M., Evans, N., Halpern-Felscher, B., & Eyre, S. (2003). Differences in altruistic roles and HIV risk perception among staff, peer educators and students in an adolescent peer education program. *AIDS Education Prevention, 15*(2), 159–171.

Owens, E., Hinshaw, S., Kraemer, H., Arnold, L., Abikoff, H., Cantwell, D., et al. (2003). Which treatment for whom for ADHD? Moderators of treatment response in the MTA. *Journal of Consulting and Clinical Psychology, 71*(3), 540–552.

Parameswaran, K., O'Bryne, P., & Sears, M.R. (2003). Inhaled corticosteroids for asthma: Common clinical quandaries. *Journal of Asthma, 40*(2), 107–118.

Patton, G., Selzer, R., Coffey, C., Carlin, J., & Wolfe, R. (2000). Onset of adolescent eating disorders: Population based cohort study over 3 years. *British Medical Journal, 318*(20), 765–768.

Payton, J., Wardlaw, D., Graczyk, P., Bloodworth, M., Tompsett, C., & Weissberg, R. (2000). Social and emotional learning: A framework for promoting mental health and reducing risk behavior in children and youth. *Journal of School Health, 70*(5), 179–185.

Pbert, L., Moolchan, E., Muramoto, M., Winickoff, J., Curry, S., Lando, H., et al. (2003). The state of office-based interventions for youth tobacco use. *Pediatrics, 111*(6), e650–e660.

Pelham, W., Aronoff, H., & Midlam, J. (1999). A comparison of Ritalin and Adderall: Efficacy and time-course in children with attention-deficit hyperactivity disorder. *Pediatrics, 103*(4), 43.

Perez-Rodrigo, C., & Aranceta, J. (2001). School-based nutrition education: Lessons learned and new perspectives. *Public Health Nutrition, 4*(1A), 131–139.

Pollock, R., Kiszewski, A., & Spielman, A. (2000). Overdiagnosis and consequent mismanagement of head louse infestations in North America. *Pediatric Infectious Diseases, 19,* 689–693.

Poulton, R., Caspi, A., Milne, B.J., Thomson, W.M., Taylor, A., Sears, M.R., et al. (2002). Association between children's experience of socioeconomic disadvantage and adult health: A life-course study. *Lancet, 360*(9346), 1640–1645.

Rosen, M., Breitkopf, D., & Nagamani, M. (2003). A randomized controlled trial of second- versus third-generation oral contraceptives in the treatment of acne vulgaris. *American Journal of Obstetrics and Gynecology, 188*(5), 1158–1160.

Ross, M., Persky, V., Scheff, P., Chung, J., Curtis, L., Ramakrishnan, V., et al. (2002). Effect of ozone and aeroallergens on the respiratory health of asthmatics. *Archives of Environmental Health, 57*(6), 568–578.

Ross, M., & Williams, M. (2002). Effective targeted and community HIV/STD prevention programs. *Journal of Sexuality Research, 39*(1), 58–62.

Rotheram-Borus, M. (2000). Expanding the range of interventions to reduce HIV among adolescents. *AIDS, 14*(Suppl. l), S33–S40.

Rowland, A., Lesesne, C., & Abramowitz, A. (2002). The epidemiology of attention-deficit/hyperactivity disorder (ADHD): A public health view. *Mental Retardation and Developmental Disabilities Research Reviews, 8*(3), 162–170.

Runyan, C., & Zakocs, R. (2000). Epidemiology and prevention of injuries among adolescent workers in the United States. *Annual Review of Public Health, 21,* 247–269.

Santelli, J., Nystrom, R., Brindis, C., Juszczak, L., Klein, J., Bearss, N., et al. (2003). Reproductive health in school-based health centers: Findings from the 1998–1999 census of school-based health centers. *Journal of Adolescent Health, 32*(6), 443–451.

Schaffer, S., Humiston, S., Shone, L., Averhoff, F., & Szilagyi, P. (2001). Adolescent immunization practices: A national survey of U. S. physicians. *Archives of Pediatric and Adolescent Medicine, 155*(5), 566–571.

Schmitz, K., Lytle, L., Phillips, G., Murray, D., Birnbaum, A., & Kubik, M. (2002). Psychosocial correlates of physical activity and sedentary leisure habits in young adolescents: The Teens Eating for Energy and Nutrition at School study. *Preventive Medicine, 34*(2), 266–278.

Schor, E.L. (2003). Family pediatrics: Report of the task force on the family. *Pediatrics, 111*(6), 1541–1571.

Schur, E., Sanders, M., & Steiner, H. (2000). Body dissatisfaction and dieting in young children. *International Journal of Eating Disorders, 27*(1), 74–82.

Scope and standards of professional school nursing practice. (2001). Washington, DC: American Nurses Publishing.

Sekine, M., Yamagami, T., Handa, K., Saito, T., Nanri, S., Kawaminami, K., et al. (2002). A dose-response relationship between short sleeping hours and childhood obesity: Results of the Toyama birth cohort study. *Child: Care, Health, and Development, 28*(2), 163–170.

Shields, M.K., & Behrman, R.E. (2002). Children and welfare reform: Analysis and recommendations. *The Future of Children, 12*(1), 5–26.

Sharma, A. (2001). Anorexia nervosa and bulimia nervosa: An appraisal. *Drugs Today, 37*(4), 229–236.

Shima, M., Nitta, Y., Ando, M., & Adachi, M. (2002). Effects of air pollution on the prevalence and incidence of asthma in children. *Archives of Environmental Health, 57*(6), 529–535.

Shrier, L.A., Harris, S.K., Kurland, M., & Knight, J.R. (2003). Substance use problems and associated psychiatric symptoms among adolescents in primary care. *Pediatrics, 111*(6 Pt. 1), e699–705.

Silverstein, J.H., & Rosenbloom, A.L. (2001). Type 2 diabetes in children. *Current Diabetes Report, 1*(1), 19–27.

Song, E., Pruitt, B., McNamara, J., & Colwell, B. (2000). A meta-analysis examining effects of school sexuality education programs on adolescents' sexual knowledge, 1960–1997. *Journal of School Health, 70*(10), 413–416.

Stock, S.L., Goldberg, E., Corbett, S., & Katzman, D. (2002). Substance use in female adolescents with eating disorders. *Journal of Adolescent Health, 31*(2), 176–182.

Story, M., Neumark-Sztainer, D., & French, S. (2002). Individual and environmental influences on adolescent eating behaviors. *Journal of the American Dietetic Association, 102*(Suppl. 3), S40–S51.

Subcommittee on Attention-Deficit/Hyperactivity Disorder. (2001). Clinical practice guideline: Treatment of the school-aged child with attention-deficit/hyperactivity disorder. *Pediatrics, 108*(4), 1033–1041.

Surgeon General of the United States. (2002). *Youth violence: A report of the surgeon general.* Retrieved January 25, 2004, from *http://www.surgeongeneral.gov/library/youthviolence/toc.html*

Swartwood, J., Swartwood, M., Lubar, J., & Timmermann, D. (2003). EEG differences in ADHD-combined type during baseline and cognitive tasks. *Pediatric Neurology, 28*(3), 199–204.

Tapper-Strawhacker, M. (2001). Multidisciplinary teaming to promote effective management of type 1 diabetes for adolescents. *Journal of School Health, 71*(6), 213–217.

Task Force on Community Preventive Services. (2002, August 26). *Oral health recommendations.* National Center for Chronic Disease Prevention and Health Promotion. Oral Health Resources. [Press release.] Atlanta, GA: Centers for Disease Control and Prevention.

Tingle, L., DeSimone, M., & Covington, B. (2003). A meta-evaluation of 11 school-based smoking prevention programs. *Journal of School Health, 73*(2), 64–67.

Tobacco Information and Prevention Source. (2001). *Fact sheet: Minors' access to tobacco.* National Center for Chronic Disease Prevention and Health Promotion. Retrieved January 25, 2004, from *http://www.cdc.gov/tobacco/sgr/sgr_2000/factsheets/factsheet_minor.htm*

Tortolero, S., Bartholomew, K., Tyrrell, S., Abramson, S., Sockrider, M., Markham, C., et al. (2002). Environmental allergens and irritants in schools: A focus on asthma. *Journal of School Health, 72*(1), 33–38.

Trost, S.G., Kerr, L.M., Ward, D.S., & Pate, R.R. (2001). Physical activity and determinants of physical activity in obese and non-obese children. *International Journal of Obesity and Related Metabolic Disorders, 25*(6), 822–829.

Tubman, J., & Soza-Vento, R. (2001). Principal and teacher reports of strategies to enforce anti-tobacco policies in Florida middle and high schools. *Journal of School Health, 71*(6), 229–235.

United States Department of Agriculture. (2001). *Household food security in the United States, 2001.* Food Assistance and Nutrition Research Report, No. 39. Washington, DC.

United States Department of Education. (2003). *The condition of education, 2003.* Washington, DC: Author.

Van Damme, P., & Van der Wielen, M. (2001). Combining hepatitis A and B vaccination in children and adolescents. *Vaccine, 19*(17–19), 2407–2412.

Van Heeringen, C. (2001). Suicide in adolescents. *International Journal of Psychopharmacology, 16*(Suppl. 2), S1–S6.

Vermeiren, R., Schwab-Stone, M., Ruchkin, V., King, R., Van Heeringen, C., & Deboutte, D. (2003). Suicidal behavior and violence in male adolescents: A school-based study. *Journal of the American Academy of Child and Adolescent Psychiatry, 42*(1), 41–48.

Vissing, Y.M., & Daiment, J. (1997). Housing distress among high school students. *Social Work, 42*(1), 31–41.

Wallace, H., Blacklay, A., Eiser, C., Davies, H., Hawkins, M., Levitt, G., et al. (2001). Developing strategies for long term follow up of survivors of childhood cancer. *British Medical Journal, 323*(7307), 271–274.

Weinreb, L., Wehler, C., Perloff, J., Scott, R., Hosmer, D., Sagor, L., et al. (2002). Hunger: Its impact on children's health and mental health. *Pediatrics, 110*(4), e41.

Weiss, M., & Murray, C. (2003). Assessment and management of attention-deficit hyperactivity disorder in adults. *Canadian Medical Association Journal, 168*(6), 715–722.

White, C., Shinder, F., Shinder, A., & Dyer, D. (2001). Reduction of illness absenteeism in elementary schools using an alcohol-free instant hand sanitizer. *Journal of School Nursing, 17*(5), 258–265.

Wilkinson, N., Jackson, G., & Gardner-Medwin, J. (2003). Biologic therapies for juvenile arthritis. *Archives of Diseases in Childhood, 88*(3), 186–191.

Williams, L., Reichert, A., MacKenzie, W., Hightower, A., & Blake, P. (2001). Lice, nits, and school policy. *Pediatrics, 107*, 1011–1015.

Wood, R., Drolet, J., Fetro, J., Synovitz, L., & Wood, A. (2002). Residential adolescent substance abuse treatment: Recommendations for collaboration between school health and substance abuse treatment personnel. *Journal of School Health, 72*(9), 363–367.

Wood, R., & Synovitz, L. (2001). Addressing the threats of MDMA (Ecstasy): Implications for school health professionals, parents and community members. *Journal of School Health, 71*(1), 38–41.

Woodfill, M., & Beyrer, M. (1991). *The role of the nurse in the school setting: A historical perspective.* Kent, OH: American School Health Association.

Young, E.M., & Fors, S.W. (2001). Factors related to the eating habits of students in grades 9–12. *Journal of School Health, 71*(10), 483–488.

Zickler, P. (2000). NIDA initiative targets increasing teen use of anabolic steroids. *NIDA Notes, 15*(3). Retrieved January 25, 2004, from *http://165.112.78.61/NIDA_Notes/NNVol15N3/Initiative.html*

Zimmer-Gembeck, M., Doyle, L., & Daniels, J. (2001). Contraceptive dispensing and selection in school-based health centers. *Journal of Adolescent Health, 29*(3), 177–185.

SELECTED READINGS

Amschler, D. (2002). The alarming increase of type 2 diabetes in children. *Journal of School Health, 72*(1), 39–41.

Armbruster, P. (2002). The administration of school-based mental health services. *Child and Adolescent Psychiatric Clinics of North America, 11*(1), 23–41.

Arnold, E., Smith, T., Harrison, D., & Springer, D. (2000). Adolescents' knowledge and beliefs about pregnancy: The impact of "ENABL." *Adolescence, 35*(139), 485–498.

Baker, L., & Cavender, A. (2003). Promoting culturally competent care for gay youth. *The Journal of School Nursing, 19*(2), 65–72.

Boyer-Chuanroong, L., & Deaver, P. (2000). Meeting the preteen vaccine law: A pilot program in urban middle schools. *Journal of School Health, 70*(2), 39–44.

Bussing, R., Zima, B., Gary, F., & Garvan, C. (2003). Barriers to detection, help-seeking, and service use for children with

ADHD. *Journal of Behavioral, Health and Service Research, 30*(2), 176–189.

Dorman, S. (2001). Web-based health calculators. *Journal of School Health, 71*(10), 500–501.

Elder, J., Litrownik, A., Slymen, D., Campbell, N., Parra-Medina, D., Choe, S., et al. (2002). Tobacco and alcohol use-prevention program for Hispanic migrant adolescents. *American Journal of Preventive Medicine, 23*(4), 269–275.

Escobar-Chavez, S., Tortolero, S., Markham, C., Kelder, S., & Kapadia, A. (2002). Violent behavior among urban youth attending alternative schools. *Journal of School Health, 72*(9), 357–362.

Gall, G., Pagano, M., Desmond, S., Perrin, J., & Murphy, J.M. (2000). Utility of psychosocial screening at a school-based health center. *Journal of School Health, 70*(7), 292–298.

Geller, B., Bolhofner, K., Craney, J., Williams, M., DelBello, M., & Gundersen, K. (2000). Psychosocial functioning in a prepubertal and early adolescent bipolar disorder phenotype. *Journal of the American Academy of Child and Adolescent Psychiatry, 39*(12), 1543–1548.

Gerber-Zimmerman, P. (2003). Assessment of abdominal pain in school-age children. *The Journal of School Nursing, 19*(1), 4–11.

Hatmaker, G. (2003). Development of a skin cancer prevention program. *The Journal of School Nursing, 19*(2), 89–92.

Jackson, L.L. (2001). Non-fatal occupational injuries and illnesses treated in hospital emergency departments in the United States. *Injury Prevention, 7*(Suppl. 1), i21–i26.

Kirchofer, G., Price, J., & Telljohann, M. (2001). Primary grade teachers' knowledge and perceptions of head lice. *Journal of School Health, 71*(9), 448–452.

Klein, J., Sesselberg, T., Gawronski, B., Handwerker, L., Gesten, F., & Schettine, A. (2003). Improving adolescent preventive services through state, managed care, and community partnerships. *Journal of Adolescent Health, 32*(Suppl. 6), 91–97.

Levine, S., & Coupey, S. (2003). Adolescent substance use, sexual behavior and metropolitan status: Is "urban" a risk factor? *Journal of Adolescent Health, 32*(5), 350–355.

Lohse, J. (2003). A bicycle safety education program for parents of young children. *The Journal of School Nursing, 19*(2), 100–110.

McCabe, M., & Ricciardelli, L. (2003). Body image and strategies to lose weight and increase muscle among boys and girls. *Health Psychology, 22*(1), 39–46.

Mejdell-Awbrey, L., & Juarez, S. (2003). Developing a nursing protocol for over-the-counter medications in high school. *The Journal of School Nursing, 19*(1), 12–16.

National Association of School Nurses. (2002, June). *The role of unlicensed assistive personnel (UAPs) in the school setting.* Position Statement. Retrieved January 25, 2004, from *http://www.nasn.org*

National Association of School Nurses. (2003). *School nurse day proclamation.* Retrieved January 25, 2004, from *http://www.nasn.org*

O'Dea, J., & Maloney, D. (2000). Preventing eating and body image problems in children and adolescents using the health promoting schools framework. *Journal of School Health, 70*(1), 18–21.

O'Donnell, L., Myint-U, A., O'Donnell, C., & Stueve, A. (2003). Long-term influence of sexual norms and attitudes on timing of sexual initiation among urban minority youth. *Journal of School Health, 73*(2), 68–75.

Pesa, J. (1999). Psychosocial factors associated with dieting behaviors among female adolescents. *Journal of School Health, 69*(5), 196–201.

Plomin, R., & Walker, S. (2003). Genetics and educational psychology. *British Journal of Educational Psychology, 73*(1), 3–14.

Poijula, S., Wahlberg, K., & Dyregrov, A. (2001). Adolescent suicide and suicide contagion in three secondary schools. *International Journal of Emergency Mental Health, 3*(3), 163–168.

Roberts, T., & Ryan, S. (2002). Tattooing and high-risk behavior in adolescents. *Pediatrics, 110*(6), 1058–1063.

Shannon, C., Story, M., Fulkerson, J., & French, S. (2002). Factors in the school cafeteria influencing food choices by high school students. *Journal of School Health, 72*(6), 229–234.

Skoner, D., & Adelson, J. (1999). *New developments in corticosteroid therapy for children with asthma.* Presented at the American Academy of Pediatrics Annual Meeting. Retrieved January 29, 2004, from *http://www.medscape.com/viewarticle/423404*

Taylor, L. (2000). Achieving coordinated mental health programs in schools. *Journal of School Health, 70*(5), 169–190.

Vila, G., Nollet-Clemencon, C., Vera, M., Robert, J., deBlic, J., Jouvent, R., et al. (1999). Prevalence of DSM-IV disorders in children and adolescent with asthma vs diabetes. *Canadian Journal of Psychiatry, 44*(6), 562–569.

Weiler, R., Pigg, R., & McDermott, R. (2003). Evaluation of the Florida coordinated school health program pilot school project. *Journal of School Health, 73*(1), 3–8.

29

Adult Women, Men, and Occupational Health

Key Terms

- **Adult**
- **Anorexia nervosa**
- **Bisexual**
- **Bulimia nervosa**
- **Chronic fatigue and immune dysfunction syndrome (CFIDS)**
- **Come out (coming out)**
- **Disabling injury**
- **Employee assistance program**
- **Ergonomics**
- **Gay**
- **Homosexual**
- **Infertility**
- **Lesbian**
- **Life expectancy**
- **Menarche**
- **Menopause**
- **Morbidly obese**
- **Obesity**
- **Occupational disease**
- **Occupational health**
- **Occupational and environmental health nurse**
- **Tubal ligation**
- **Unintentional injury**
- **Unsafe condition**
- **Vasectomy**

Learning Objectives

Upon mastery of this chapter, you should be able to:

- Identify key national and global demographic characteristics of women and men throughout the adult life-span.

- Provide a health profile of adult women and men in the United States.

- Identify desirable primary, secondary, and tertiary health promotion activities designed to improve the health of women and men.

- Identify potential physical, chemical, biologic, ergonomic, and psychosocial stressors in a variety of work environments.

- Describe the history of state and federal legislation related to the health of women and men in the occupational setting.

- Discuss a variety of occupational health problems, including disorders related to ergonomics and workplace violence.

- Compare and contrast three main types of occupational health programs.

- Describe the role of the occupational health nurse and other members of the occupational health team in protecting and promoting workers' health and safety.

The term *adult* has many different meanings in society. To children, an adult is anyone in authority, including a 14-year-old babysitter. As people age, they tend to redefine the term upward. It is not unusual, for example, to hear an elderly person describe a couple in their mid-30s as "kids." The U. S. criminal justice system distinguishes between adults and juveniles for purposes of delimiting types of crimes and possibilities for punishment, and labor legislation provides different protections for children than for adult workers. Even hospitals and health care systems vary somewhat as to the ages at which they distinguish pediatric and geriatric clients from middle-aged adults.

How would you characterize an adult? Does your definition rest solely on age, or is it influenced by other factors, such as marital status, employment status, financial independence, amount of responsibility for self and others, and so on? For the purposes of this chapter, an **adult** is defined as anyone between the ages of 18 and 64 years. Obviously, within this range are tremendous differences in health profiles and health care needs. This chapter begins with a discussion of the characteristics of adult clients.

Adults are separated into female and male gender groups in this discussion. Throughout history, the health care needs of women and men have differed more often then they have been alike. Many health promotion and health protection programs are designed for women or for men specifically. Mammography screening programs and prenatal clinics are designed with a woman's health in mind. Testicular self-examination teaching and prostate cancer screening are health promotion programs for men. Programs in many areas, such as cardiac rehabilitation, stress management, and dating violence prevention, may have had one gender in mind at one time but are now established as programs for both sexes. Nevertheless, morbidity and mortality statistics, historical development of research foci, and workforce changes required that the health care needs of women and men be examined separately.

This chapter also examines adult clients as workers. **Occupational health** is a specialty health practice that focuses on the health and well-being of the working population, including both paid and unpaid laborers, and therefore covers most of the country's able adults. The environmental factors that affect workers' health and the evolution of the roles of occupational and environmental health nurses in meeting those needs are discussed.

WOMEN'S HEALTH

The health of women can be observed over time, and in most societies the story remains the same. Women were not the focus of medical progression throughout the centuries. Any benefits achieved by women were incidental to the findings that were achieved with men as the focus. Advances in women's health are very recent and primarily an advantage for women in Western countries where the women's or feminist movement beginning in the 1960s made major inroads. This section looks at the health concerns of women over the adult life-span and the major causes of acute and chronic illness and death; the issues, trends, and policies that have had an affect on women; and the primary, secondary, and tertiary methods the community health nurse can use to make a difference among women as individuals, in families, or as aggregates.

Historical Overview of Factors Affecting Women's Health

For the most part, women's health has been overlooked in all societies. It is still overlooked in much of the world, and only in the past few decades has women's health been a formidable issue in the United States and other Western countries—coming not so incidentally with the women's movement that began in the 1960s.

Because of cultural mores arriving with the first white settlers to the American colonies in the 1600s and lasting for the most part through the early 1900s, women did not receive the quality and intensity of medical care that men did. Lay women attended childbirths at home. What family planning methods existed were crude and ineffective and may have included induced abortion through the use of herbs or homemade probing devices that were risky and frequently deadly for the woman. If the rare advice of a physician was sought for any ailment, the information gathered (history and physical) was done verbally, with the female client fully clothed, and often through a third party, her husband (see What Do You Think? I).

At the beginning of formal human research (most of the 20th century), the investigations were concerned with the health of men; women were not a focus of medical research. A large and well-known study that still provides valuable information on men's health is the Framingham Heart Study. It was begun in the 1940s among a group of male physicians in New England. They have now been monitored for more than half a century, and the study has provided significant information on health habits, risks, and cardiac health of men. It has only been in very recent decades that researchers have designed major studies that focus on women. One of these is the Women's Health Study, in which more than 39,000 women older than 45 years of age are being studied for the place aspirin has in primary prevention of coronary heart disease (CHD). This is a longitudinal and experimental study that has been securely funded for more than 10 years to ensure that the research can achieve maximum results.

The significant feminist movement that is a hallmark of the 20th century also resulted in more fair representation of women in medical research. The 1960s and early 1970s brought more than miniskirts and go-go boots. It was the time of the very public escalation of the women's health movement. In this second wave of feminism, women again fought to gain control of their own reproductive rights, continuing the struggle for women's rights to birth control started by

ered, and that these needs vary with age. Knowing what the needs are is primary to knowing how to help women promote their health.

Teenaged Women (12–18 Years)

Usually, a 12- to 18-year-old female is not considered a woman. However, because physical changes occur among teenage girls that promote their bodies to the status of woman, this is where a woman begins. Full adult height, breast development, and the menstrual cycle begin well before the 18th birthday. **Menarche**, the beginning of a woman's menstrual cycle, usually occurs between the 9th and 17th year (Venes & Thomas, 2001). Therefore, long before "adulthood," a girl experiences the hormonal and physical changes that enable her to procreate. Along with the physical changes come emotional changes, which can test the patience of the strongest parents. Appearances are important. Risk-taking is not just for teenage boys, and the values of peers become the standard for girls' behavior.

In addition, there are growth and developmental tasks that girls in this age group work on if they are not distracted into adult role tasks before they are ready. According to Duvall (1977), a family developmental theorist, healthy families raise adolescents by focusing on balancing independence with responsibility and maintaining open communication. Near the end of adolescence, the teenage child is better able to compromise and set limits, develop vocational goals, and establish values and a personal identity. This teen prepares to disengage from the nuclear family and leave home (for college, work, military) to have her own living space separate from her parents.

Not all teens follow this pattern, and it is not unusual for the community health nurse to visit or provide services to a teen mother who has one, two, or three children before she reaches 18 years of age (Koniak-Griffin et al., 2000). This teen has chosen, either actively or passively, an adult role. She may or may not be prepared for the demands of this stage in the life cycle. These young mothers have difficulty meeting adult tasks, especially if they haven't successfully met the tasks of adolescence. Adolescence is a launching time that prepares a young woman for the challenges of adulthood. Becoming a successful adult is easier if a girl is successful at being a teen.

It is during the teen years that a young girl learns basic health promotion behaviors that she will carry into adulthood. Such issues as feminine hygiene, prevention of sexually transmitted diseases (STDs), and pregnancy prevention and family planning choices are discussed, contemplated, and frequently initiated before adulthood. Other important health promotion issues can have lasting effects on a young woman's health and safety. Healthy attitudes and practices that include regular exercise, mental health promotion, rest and sleep balance, nutrition, dental health, avoidance of smoking and secondhand smoke, and pedestrian and driving safety must be incorporated at early ages to have lasting positive benefits throughout a woman's life.

WHAT DO YOU THINK? I

A woman's dressing style that included a tightly laced corset was popular from the late 1700s throughout the late 1800s in Germany, England, and the United States. It was brought into question by an anatomist, S. T. von Sommerring, in 1793 (Fee et al., 2002). He identified compression of rib cages and internal organs as contributing to digestive problems, fainting, and shortness of breath. For the next century, dress reformers advocated looser lacing and clothes that allowed for a more natural movement. However, these reformers belonged to the "radical fringe" of the feminist movement and the tiniest waists, regardless of their impact on health, continued to be in vogue as the "hourglass" figure was sought by middle class and upper class women. More recently, hiatal hernias caused by overly tight girdles and corsets have been termed "Sommerring's syndrome" in tribute to the first physician to warn of the dangers, more than 200 years ago.

Margaret Sanger decades earlier. Women have been victims of "the paternalistic and condescending medical community" (Nichols, 2000, p. 56), and reclaiming power was a common goal among a diverse group of feminists at mid-century.

These feminists paved the way for women to have their voices heard on many health, social, and political issues. Women sought out higher education opportunities in greater numbers and entered workplaces once solely occupied by men, especially during and after World War II. With these positive changes that escalated women toward greater equality with men came the freedom and pressure for women to compete with men in their social and work settings. This resulted in more women smoking, drinking, and experiencing stress than ever before. Women began suffering from the diseases of men, such as lung cancer (Brunetta, 2002/2003) and heart disease (Arslanian-Engoren, 2002), in record numbers. These changes in women's health were discovered as a result of research that now includes women with more regularity. It was only in 1986 that the National Institutes of Health (NIH) adopted a policy requiring the inclusion of women in clinical research (Nichols, 2000).

Women's Health Promotion Across the Life-Span

What health care needs do women have that are different from those of men? Is there a need to look at health promotion throughout the life cycle of adult women? How is the health of an 18-year-old different from that of a 64-year-old woman? Most of us would have no trouble agreeing that women have different health care needs that must be consid-

Young Adult Women (18–35 Years)

Women in the younger years of adulthood have different tasks to accomplish and issues to deal with than do women in later adulthood. The tasks and issues of concern at this age include the following:

1. Attracting and choosing a significant other for the long-term and establish a home together. (Note that this task is phrased as such to include **lesbian** women—women who have sexual intercourse with other women. At times, women in this age group have not **come out**, or revealed to others that they are lesbian or **bisexual** and have sexual intercourse with people of both sexes; therefore, this is an area in which the community health nurse can provide counseling or guide the client to the appropriate community resources.)
2. Preparing for and choosing a life's work that is economically appropriate and personally satisfying based on individual interests.
3. Planning for children by using a variety of parenting models (childbirth, adoption, foster parenting); being **infertile** and unable to achieve a pregnancy after at least 1 year of unprotected intercourse; or choosing not to have children but enjoy children from a distance through the role of aunt, cousin, friend, or volunteer.
4. Maintaining health through positive health practices that protect reproductive and breast health, support the female skeleton through exercise and diet, and promote overall physical and mental health and safety.
5. Developing a life's philosophy that encompasses meaningful and comforting spiritual beliefs consistent with day-to-day living.

Based on these five areas, the community health nurse can plan an approach with female clients targeted to their lifestyles and life choices. Using a nursing care plan matrix that includes the five areas and possible interventions and teaching areas, a community health nurse can individualize contact with young adult women to best meet their needs (Display 29–1).

The Nursing Care Plan Matrix is complete enough to guide the community health nurse in most areas of health promotion encountered by the young adult female client. The challenge to the nurse is to be prepared to discuss all issues, backed up with knowledge of and access to the appropriate community resources to meet client needs encountered. Other chapters discuss the roles and settings of community health nurses (Chapter 3), teaching of clients (Chapter 12), and making home visits to clients (Chapter 24)—each chapter enhancing the nurses interaction with clients.

Adult Women (35–65 Years)

Women in the adult age group of 35 to 65 years have established themselves into patterns of living that have served them well or ill. It is in this period that the results of years of choices present themselves in the form of chronic illnesses. Nevertheless, many women in this age group have time to change their health habits to possibly reverse encroaching chronic illnesses. For other women, lifestyle choices and un-detected diseases have shortened their life-span, and in large numbers women are dying prematurely.

Menopause and Hormone Replacement Therapy

Women in this age group experience **menopause**, "the period that marks the permanent cessation of menstrual activity, usually occurring between the ages of 35 and 58" years (Venes & Thomas, 2001, p. 1329). Natural menopause occurs in 25% of women by age 47 years, in 50% by age 50, in 75% by age 52, and in 95% by age 55. Surgical removal of the ovaries, which produces menopause, occurs in 30% of U. S. women who are 50 years of age and older. Cigarette smoking causes menopause to occur 1 to 2 years prematurely (Venes & Thomas, 2001).

Symptoms of menopause vary among women and last from months to years; they range from hardly noticeable in some women to very severe in others. Symptoms include vasomotor instability, nervousness, hot flashes (flushes), chills, excitability, fatigue, apathy, mental depression, crying episodes, insomnia, palpitation, vertigo, headache, numbness, tingling, myalgia, urinary disturbances, and various disorders of the gastrointestinal system. The long-range effects of lower estrogen levels are osteoporosis and atherosclerosis (Venes & Thomas, 2001).

Recently there has been controversy over the benefits and side effects of hormone replacement therapy (HRT). In 2002, researchers found an unexpectedly high rate of invasive breast cancer, myocardial infarction (MI), and stroke among women in the Women's Health Initiative study who were taking estrogen combined with continuous progestin (Healy, 2002). An initial knee-jerk reaction to this information, including headlines in London such as "Millions in HRT danger: Biggest study ever abandoned amid massive health risks," preceded a more rational retrospective look at the findings. Researchers sorted through the state of hormone science, and the essential points remain: long-term HRT is not right for every woman, but it is for some. All HRT is not the same. The part of the study that was terminated involved women taking the estrogen and progestin combination; 11,000 estrogen-only participants remained in the study and had no problems. Estrogen alone was the hormone used by 8 million women in 2002. The decision to use HRT needs to be revisited regularly, and the "sometimes irrational exuberance for HRTs should not become an irrational backlash against it" (Healy, 2002, p. 53). However, many physicians in 2002 were taking women off of all HRT.

Heart Disease

Heart disease is the number one killer of women. In 1999, a total of 262,391 women in the United States died from CHD. Almost 3 million women older than 20 years of age have a history of MI, and approximately 439,000 women have an MI each year. Women most typically experience MI approximately 8 years later than men do, and they are twice as likely to die after an MI as men are (American Heart Association, 2002). Risk factors for heart disease and the types of symptoms women experience are presented in Table 29–1.

DISPLAY 29–1

Nursing Care Plan Matrix of Health Promotion for Young Adult Women (18–35 Years)

Community health nurses can use this matrix to individualize teaching, services, or care to young adult female clients. Use the questions to stimulate the development of an individualized approach that is client focused and client driven, with the community health nurse acting as the catalyst. In any or all of these areas, the community health nurse may (1) discuss the issues and commend the client for positive attitudes and behaviors (eg, making healthy decisions for her health and the health of her significant others), (2) discuss the issues and guide the client to resources that will enhance more positive behaviors and decisions (eg, flu shot clinic or a "Mommies and Me" program for mothers of toddlers), or (3) discuss the issues, inform the client that immediate changes must be made to protect the health of herself or others, and inform or utilize the appropriate resource as soon as possible (eg, children's protective service).

1. Life partner

   Ascertain whether the client is looking for a life partner or is choosing to live a single life. Discuss how the single life is satisfying for the client and ways to make it richer.

   Discuss settings where client can meet others (male or female based on sexual preference) with same interests, philosophy, and so on, such as work settings, school settings, faith communities, and recreational communities.

   Discuss what the client is looking for in a potential life partner; expectations for the relationship; what the client contributes; how the client compromises and resolves conflict, and similar issues. If the client is in a relationship, discuss what is good about it; what needs improving; and how to initiate.

2. Life's work

   How is client preparing for her life's work (education, formal training, on-the-job training)? Will this work provide the resources for the client's life plans? Will the work choice provide long-term satisfaction? Is the work choice a "stepping stone" to another work role? How will or does she handle work and having children? What needs changing or improvement in the

work/children arrangement? If working outside the home is not possible or desirable, how will or does she support herself?

3. Planning for children

   What is the client's family planning knowledge base? What methods fit best with her philosophy, religious beliefs, lifestyle? What are the long-term effects of the choices? What number of children is the client planning? Has she thought through all ramifications of this number? If choosing not to have (or unable to have) children, how will she deal with this situation? Does she want alternative suggestions for being a parent (adoption, foster parenting) or information about interacting with children (volunteering)?

4. Maintaining physical and mental health

   Explore all areas of health promotion for a woman's health in addition to general health and safety promotion: sexually transmitted disease prevention; reproductive health; primary prevention (diet) and secondary prevention (monthly self–breast-examination, regular mammograms based on age and present recommended guidelines) of breast cancer or of cervical cancer (regular Pap smear), uterine cancer, or ovarian cancer (alertness to subtle abdominal changes and regular health provider examinations); smoking (prevention or cessation and avoidance of secondhand smoke); nutrition for women (bone health/osteoporosis prevention, iron depletion); exercise (cardiac and bone health); safety (an all-inclusive overview of personal safety—stranger awareness, dating violence, pedestrian, driving, home safety, work, and recreational safety); general health maintenance (regularly scheduled health provider visits, yearly flu shots, tetanus shots every 10 years, regular use of sunscreen and avoidance of sunburn).

5. Developing a life's philosophy

   Discuss client's personal life satisfaction which may include religiosity and spirituality, living in congruence with cultural/ethnic/family beliefs and expectations, and coming to a comfortable level of satisfaction with life choices—having no regrets.

Except for family history and advancing age, women can make lifestyle changes to alter their risk factors. The remaining risk factors are areas the community health nurse can discuss with female clients in this age group.

Cancer

Cancer is the second leading cause of death for women, killing 169.9 of every 100,000 women in the United States each year, or 43,300 women in 1999. It kills women of color in fewer numbers, except for black women, for whom the rate is much higher. In all areas—cancer of the trachea, bronchus, lung,

colon, rectum, anus, and breast—black women die more frequently than white women, while all other women of color experience lower rates than black or white women (Table 29–2).

With statistics like these, it behooves the community health nurse to focus early screening programs and cancer prevention teaching in communities where black women have access to the services and information. In addition, transportation, child care, and other incentives may provide the motivation many women need. The statistics may represent disparity in the health care system rather than racial differences in susceptibility.

TABLE 29-1

Risks and Symptoms of Coronary Heart Disease in Women

Risks	Symptoms
Family history	Electrocardiographic changes:
Sedentary lifestyle	Non–Q wave
Excess body weight	Pain location:
Diabetes mellitus	Chest, neck
Hypertension	Epigastric, back
Hyperlipidemia	Treatment-seeking behaviors:
Race (highest in black women)	>6 hr after symptom onset
Cigarette smoking	Gastrointestinal symptoms:
	nausea and loss of appetite

(From American Heart Association [2002], *2001 heart and stroke statistical update.* Dallas, TX: Author.)

After skin cancer (which causes relatively few deaths), breast cancer is the most common cancer among women (more women *die* from lung cancer than from breast cancer). The sooner breast cancer is discovered, the more successfully it is treated. With routine breast self-examinations, regular mammograms, a diet low in fat and high in fruits and vegetables, breast feeding if possible, and avoiding prolonged use of estrogen replacement therapy, a woman is doing what she can to promote breast health. The community health nurse has many resources available to provide this information and to teach breast self-examination individually to women in their homes, or in small groups in clinic, work, or school settings (see Chapter 12).

Women should begin breast self-examinations by age 20 years, doing them monthly for the rest of their lives. Clinical breast examinations conducted by a health care provider are done as part of or with routine gynecologic examinations until menopause, every 1 to 2 years after menopause, and according to individual decision between the client and her

TABLE 29-2

Breast Cancer Death Rates Among All Women, 1999

Women	Rate per 100,000
All women	27.0
White	26.4
Black	35.6
Hispanic	15.4
American Indian/Alaskan Native	15.4
Asian/Pacific Islander	13.1

(From Centers for Disease Control and Prevention. [2002]. Deaths: Final data for 1999. *National Vital Statistics Reports, 49*[8], 119–122.)

health care provider after age 75 years (Kaiser Permanente, 2002). Mammography is not usually recommended for women younger than 40 years of age, but it is recommended every 1 to 2 years thereafter.

Cancer prevention diet teaching can occur during home, clinic, or school teaching sessions at the same time that breast self-examination is taught. The dietary influence on all cancers has been explored through more than 4500 studies and will grow in importance as more research is conducted in years to come (American Institute for Cancer Research, 1999).

Modern mammography, usually recommended for women older than 40 years of age, may not be the only or best method of early detection. There are other breast examination possibilities that in time may prove to be more effective than the standard mammography of today (Table 29–3).

Colorectal cancer is the third leading cause of cancer deaths among American women, claiming 28,800 women's lives in 1999. Many cases are preventable with regular screening (occult blood in stool, or detection of polyps that are considered precancerous on flexible sigmoidoscopy, or both); regular exercise; and a diet that is low in fat and high in fruits, vegetables, and whole-grain foods.

With the advent of the Papanicolaou (Pap) smear, early detection and prevention of cervical cancer have improved dramatically. Both the incidence and the death rate from this disease have declined by 40% since the early 1970s. However, many elderly, low-income, and rural women remain at high risk because they are not obtaining regular Pap screenings. Cigarette smoking and infection with certain types of the human papillomavirus (HPV) are major risk factors for cervical cancer. In 1999, 12,800 new cases of cervical cancer were diagnosed in the United States, and 4800 women died of the disease.

Smoking

Lung cancer killed approximately 65,700 women in the United States in 2002 (Women's Health Statistics, 2003). It kills more women than breast cancer and ovarian cancer combined. Almost 90% of lung cancer cases are smoking related. Other lung cancer deaths come from breast cancer that has metastasized. The disease is almost as preventable as it is deadly. A main problem is that teenagers begin smoking before they understand the health risks, and they become addicted (Brunetta, 2002).

Fifty years ago, lung cancer in women was rare. Since then, lung cancer mortality rates for women have jumped 600%. Lung cancer rate increases can be directly correlated with the increase in smoking among women that started in the 1940s, not long after tobacco companies began heavy cigarette marketing geared toward the female population. In 1968, Virginia Slims cigarettes capitalized on the changing role of women with its "You've Come a Long Way, Baby" ad campaign. The ads linked smoking with freedom and independence. By 1974, the number of 12-year-old girls who smoked had increased 110%, according to research published in the *Journal of the American Medical Association* (Brunetta, 2002). The risk of lung cancer and trends are un-

T A B L E   2 9 – 3

Cancer Detection Imaging Guide

Name	Description	Use	Limitations
Mammography	X-ray imaging of breasts requires compression and proper positioning.	Gold standard for early detection and diagnosis	Misses 15% of breast cancers; difficult to interpret in women with dense breasts
Digital mammography	Digital x-ray images displayed on monitor, can be enhanced to improve detection.	Screening and diagnosis, better visualization of dense breast tissue	Equipment is expensive; future may produce better results
Ultrasound	High-frequency sound waves produce images of breasts.	Differentiates between fluid-filled cyst or solid; useful for women with dense breasts	Time-consuming; needs a skilled operator; does not pick up small lesions
Magnetic resonance imaging	Radio waves and magnetic fields produce images, requires injection and contrast agent.	Not for screening; shows promise for evaluating lesions, for women with dense breasts; helps avoid unnecessary biopsies	Costly; limited availability; further study needed
Positive emission tomography	Radioactive tracers are used to identify areas of increased metabolic activity—common in cancer tissue.	Presently used to check cancer spread beyond the breast; may be useful in women with dense breasts, implants, or scar tissue	Expensive; not widely used; more studies needed; not good for lesion smaller than 1 cm

derrecognized by women. The community health nurse has much work to do in the area of smoking prevention, especially among teenaged girls and young women.

Chronic Health Conditions

There are several chronic health conditions affecting the overall health of women 35 to 65 years of age. Such conditions as substance abuse, anorexia, bulimia, obesity, chronic fatigue and immune dysfunction syndrome are chronic health conditions that have major effects on a woman's health.

Substance abuse may involve alcohol and other legal or illicit drugs. It is a serious and continuing problem among American women. This abuse costs society more than 235 billion dollars each year, in addition to approximately 120,000 deaths attributed to alcohol and drug use annually.

Almost 4.1 million women in this country currently use illicit drugs. More than 1.2 million misuse prescription drugs for nonmedical reasons (U. S. Department of Health and Human Services [USDHHS], 2001). Drug use often occurs among women with histories of mental illness. This issue is covered in greater detail in Chapter 35.

Uncontrolled alcohol consumption and cigarette smoking are behaviors that contribute to negative health states. Each habit (cause) alone has its effect, and in combination they are even more lethal. Negative health behaviors, if occurring together, exacerbate other health problems. Likewise, improvement in one area improves another.

Alcohol consumption in moderation (1 to 2 oz of liquor, 12 to 24 oz of beer, or 5 to 10 oz of wine per day) is not detrimental to a woman unless she is pregnant. No alcohol should be consumed during pregnancy, because the fetus can be permanently damaged (see Chapter 26). Women who drink can become impaired after consuming fewer ounces of liquor,

beer, or wine than their male counterparts. Women in general weigh less than men and have a greater percentage of body fat, so alcohol is absorbed faster, and smaller quantities are required for the same degree of impairment. Women may be less likely to be alcoholics than men, but the death rates among female alcoholics are 50% to 100% higher than those among men. In 1998, 2.1% of American women were heavy drinkers (USDHHS, 2001).

Problem drinking is of increasing concern among the population as a whole. The community health nurse may be the first health care provider to suspect that alcohol use is a problem or is out of control for a client visited at home. The nurse can use the list of questions in Display 29–2 to initiate a discussion with a female client about whom the nurse is concerned.

Anorexia nervosa is an eating disorder that is marked by weight loss, emaciation, a disturbance in body image, and a fear of weight gain. The clients lose weight either by excessive dieting or by purging themselves of calories they have ingested. This illness is typically found in industrialized nations and usually begins in the teen years. Young women are 10 to 20 times more likely than young men to suffer from the disorder. The young woman claims to feel fat even when she is emaciated, and refusal to maintain body weight can be life-threatening due to electrolyte disturbances, anemia, and secondary cardiac arrhythmias. The disease often resists therapy, but it is out of the realm of expertise for a community health nurse. If anorexia nervosa is suspected, the client must be referred to a health care practitioner for follow-up as soon as possible.

A related disorder, **bulimia nervosa**, is marked by recurrent episodes of binge eating, self-induced vomiting and diarrhea, excessive exercise, strict dieting or fasting, and an

DISPLAY 29-2

Do You Have a Problem with Alcohol? 20 Questions for Women

1. Do you get someone to buy liquor for you because you are ashamed to buy it yourself?
2. Do you buy liquor at different places so no one will know how much you purchase?
3. Do you hide the empty cans/bottles and dispose of them secretly?
4. Do you plan in advance to "reward" yourself with drinking after you've worked hard in the house?
5. Are you ever permissive with your children because you feel guilty about the way you behaved when you were drinking?
6. Do you have "blackout," periods about which you remember nothing?
7. Do you ever phone the hostess of a party the next day and ask if you hurt anyone's feeling or made a fool of yourself?
8. Do you find cigarette holes in your clothes or the furniture and can't remember when it happened?
9. Do you take an extra drink or two before leaving for a party to help you get in the party mood?
10. Do you ever wonder if anyone knows how much you drink?
11. Do you feel wittier or more charming when you are drinking?
12. Do you feel panicky when faced with nondrinking days, such as a visit to out-of-town relatives?
13. Do you invent social occasions for drinking, such as inviting friends for lunch, cocktails, or dinner?
14. Do you avoid reading articles or seeing television shows about women alcoholics when others are present but read and watch when no one is around?
15. Do you ever carry liquor in your purse?
16. Do you become defensive when someone mentions your drinking?
17. Do you become irritated when unexpected guests reduce your liquor supply?
18. Do you drink when under pressure or after an argument?
19. Do you try to cover up when you can't remember promises and feel ashamed when you misplace or lose things?
20. Do you drive even though you've been drinking, but feel certain you are in complete control?

ALL of these are problems with alcohol. If you are troubled by these questions, and especially if you answered "YES" to three or more, contact someone for help. Whatever your situation, you are not alone.

Adapted from *Do you have a problem with alcohol? 20 questions for women.* Los Angeles: Alcoholism Center for Women.

---

exaggerated concern about body shape and weight. In many ways, the two disorders are similar, except that women with anorexia nervosa rarely binge eat. A woman suspected of practicing bulimic behaviors should be referred to an appropriate health care provider by the community health nurse.

Females in careers in which low weight is required (eg, modeling), individuals who have been sexually abused or who come from families with a history of eating disorders, and individuals with low self-esteem and a history of not being "in control" or with communication and emotional difficulties are at greater risk for either disorder.

Obesity is becoming the nation's number one health problem. It is estimated that **obesity**, or the unhealthy accumulation of body fat—in lay terms, generally defined as being more than 50 and less than 100 lb overweight—is most prevalent among women, minorities, and the poor. Thirty-six percent of white women, 52.3% of African American women, and 50.1% of Mexican-American women are considered obese. Obese individuals have an increased risk of developing diabetes mellitus, hypertension, heart disease, stroke, and other illnesses. In addition, obese individuals may suffer psychologically and socially. Often the community health nurse can intervene by suggesting a method of weight reduction, providing the support needed, and assisting with weight loss monitoring. Nutrition teaching, coach-

ing, and motivation of obese clients are part of the counselor and teacher roles of the community health nurse.

For women who are **morbidly obese**, or more than 100 pounds overweight, the physical challenges of mobility and socializing are a daily struggle. For example, the morbidly obese woman may have difficulty walking to the corner bus stop, be painfully self-conscious when eating in a restaurant, or be unable to fit into theater seats. In addition, the morbidly obese individual is at greater risk for other chronic diseases or death. This woman needs to be referred to a health care provider for exploration of extreme options available to lose weight in order to save her life (eg, bariatric surgery). Morbid obesity becomes that choice—it is not a matter of appearance; it is a life-or-death condition that needs intervention.

Chronic fatigue and immune dysfunction syndrome (CFIDS) is characterized by persistent and debilitating fatigue and additional nonspecific symptoms such as sore throat, headache, tender muscles, joint pain, difficulty thinking, and loss of short-term memory. CFIDS affects as many as 500,000 persons in the United States, and 80% of those diagnosed with the syndrome are women between 25 and 45 years old. Rest does not relieve the fatigue. Symptoms may wax and wane and are difficult to validate objectively, but they are subjectively debilitating. Symptoms can last for months or years. Because the cause is unknown, there is no specific treatment and no prevention suggestions. Treatment is focused on supportive care for the associated pain, depression, and insomnia. The community health nurse can assess activity level and degree of fatigue, emotional response to the illness, and coping ability. Emotionally supportive family members and health care providers are helpful. Referring women to mental health or career counseling or to a local support group is helpful for many women and within the role description of the community health nurse.

A major chronic health condition is diabetes mellitus (DM). Many women in the 35- to 65-year-old age group develop DM type 2, the adult-onset type often called non–insulin-dependent diabetes. Diabetes is more prevalent among minority ethnic groups than in the white population. With this difference come additional disparities: higher numbers of women with the disease in minority populations, greater seriousness of the diabetes, inadequate access to proper diabetes prevention and control programs, and inadequate quality of care. Disparity in health care services is a major public health issue. Additionally, diabetes is a major public health concern, with 800,000 new cases diagnosed each year. More than 10.5 million people are currently diagnosed with diabetes, and an estimated 5.5 million more have the disease but are undiagnosed (USDHHS, 2000).

Factors that contribute to DM 2 include improper nutrition (especially a diet that is high in fat and processed foods), decreased physical activity, and obesity. Women are less likely to be physically active than men, especially women older than 40 years of age who are African-Americans or American Indians/Alaskan Natives (Brownson et al., 2000). These facts contribute to higher numbers of ethnic women with diabetes. The control of this disease is often affected by obesity or moderate excess weight. Increased weight, smoking, and poorly controlled diabetes contribute to hypertension. The combination of these factors increases the risk of heart disease and stroke. If weight and blood pressure are within healthy ranges, smoking ceased and diabetes controlled, heart disease and stroke can be avoided or at least postponed until mature adulthood or old age. Increasing the years of good health and compressing the years of morbidity is a goal of public health. It is one of the goals of *Healthy People 2010.*

Chronic lung disease can be attributed to a lifetime of negative health habits or environmental factors, or both. Emphysema or chronic obstructive pulmonary disease (COPD) in women who smoke can be the cause of death before a diagnosis of lung cancer occurs. A work history of exposure to fibers, dust, or toxic substances can make working women just as vulnerable to occupationally related diseases as men are. Asthma is becoming an alarming urban problem among people living in poverty and in some agricultural communities, especially among children.

Client teaching by the community health nurse is a major factor in the prevention and management of chronic diseases. What the nurse can accomplish can be quite dramatic in terms of reducing days in the hospital because of chronic disease control problems, improving quality of life for the chronically ill person at home, and preventing a combination of unhealthy habits from becoming causative factors in new cases of chronic disease.

Mature Adult Women (65–85 Years)

Women in this age group outnumber men about two to one, especially in the later years. This occurs because women are not risk takers to the extent that men are, and only in this age group do they die from accidents in higher numbers than men. Although men die more frequently in vehicular crashes at younger ages, women more often sustain life-threatening falls during the mature years of 65 to 85 because of osteoporosis and its debilitating effects. Chronic diseases begin in women later and they die approximately 6 years after men from CHD, stroke, lung diseases, diabetes, and cancers. People in these later years are on their way to being expert older adults.

In the age group of 65 to 85 years, women are meeting tasks and dealing with the following issues:

1. Learning to manage financially on a fixed income for a potentially long life, which may mean living in more affordable and physically manageable housing choices.
2. Managing to cope with loss: work (retirement), income, space (smaller housing decision), spouse, friends, peers, and at times adult children.
3. Finding meaning in life that may be different from the preceding decades in that the years remaining are much shorter than the years that have gone by.
4. Finding support and comfort from family, friends, and spiritual beliefs.
5. Feeling satisfied with the life lived and having few regrets.

Women have a greater propensity for meeting social and emotional needs. They reach out to others, are able to share feelings and needs and manage old age with a support system made up largely of other women.

Community health nurses, when working with women in this age group, focus on anticipatory guidance, problem solving health-related or medication administration issues, monitoring vital signs, and assisting clients with the decision-making process. This age group is often experiencing dramatic health changes and has many health-related and social/environmental decisions to make.

One woman beginning at age 65 lives 5 to 7 healthy and stable years and then falls and fractures a wrist. Managing with a cast may upset her balance, causing her to fall a few months later and break a hip. She is now in a long rehabilitation process and needs to make decisions about housing and living independently.

Another woman may be fairly healthy until age 75, after which she is diagnosed with Parkinson's disease that is progressing rapidly, needs to have a cystocele and rectocele repair, and is advised to have both knee joints replaced. This woman has many decisions to make, must cope with a progressive disease, and needs to weigh the ratio of benefits and costs (financially, emotionally, and physically) of moving ahead with proposed surgeries. Quality-of-life issues need to be explored, and the practical issues of caregiving must be addressed.

Then there is the physically active and healthy 84-year-old who volunteers, does water aerobics daily, walks twice a week, is active in her church, plays cards each week, and maintains her own home. She drives older (and younger) or less physically able friends to social activities, and she had planned well financially so that she has no financial constraints.

Each of these women has a different set of needs, would benefit in different ways from working with a community health nurse, and portrays an example of the issues and concerns of the mature adult woman.

The community health nurse can intervene and provide information on health and social resources; encourage health promotion activities; cut the "red tape" between the elder and various social agencies; and teach ways to promote physical and medication safety. The roles of counselor, teacher, and clinician are the nursing focus. The goal is to keep the older adult as healthy as possible within the constraints of ongoing disease processes. The health of older adults is more thoroughly explored in Chapter 30.

Expert Adult Women (85 Years and Older)

Women are survivors: Of all the people living beyond age 85, 71% are women. This elderly group is the fastest growing segment of the population (USDHHS, 2001). Because women survive beyond mature old age in such greater numbers than men, their age group category has been expanded into "expert adult women," those older than 85 years of age. These women have learned to survive the "slings and arrows" of life and have outlived many peers in their struggles with diseases that cause premature death.

The greatest concerns for women in this age group are safety, housing needs, and socialization. Personal safety in regard to medication administration, falls, and exploitation is especially important. Osteoporosis occurs in 50% of women older than 65 years of age, and it increases significantly in the expert older adult age group. Each year, osteoporosis causes 1.5 million fractures of the hip, wrist, vertebrae, and other bones. It accounts for 70% of all fractures that occur annually in people older than 45 years of age (USDHHS, 2001). Twenty percent of the women who sustain a hip fracture die within 1 year after that event. Osteoporosis is a major reason women enter long-term care settings and unwillingly give up the independence of other housing arrangements.

Many older women are trusting and gullible, which makes them vulnerable to become victims of family members, caretakers, or strangers who may bilk their social security checks or life savings. The community health nurse can be alert for signs of such happenings with expert elders while visiting them in their homes. If signs of exploitation are suspected, calling the Adult Protective Services (APS) in the community is an appropriate intervention while securing the safety of the elder until APS responds.

As people age, their senses decrease. Vision fades, and hearing is less acute. Short- and long-term memory may not be as sharp, even in elders without a diagnosis of Alzheimer disease (AD). The combination of these changes creates a dilemma for aged women as they attempt to administer their own medications. They may forget, take double doses, or take the wrong medications. The problems that mistaken medication administration can create are many and should be avoided if at all possible. Prolonged inappropriate drug administration can have irreparable consequences.

Women in this age group have most often outlived their spouses and are living alone, either in their home of many years or in a smaller apartment. Because debilitating chronic diseases, effects of falls, or sensory changes can occur together, a change in housing may be necessary for future safety and security. A variety of housing choices are available for older adults, from senior apartments to long-term care arrangements. The community health nurse can help the older client become aware of the services offered and the costs of various choices in addition to the challenges of staying in her present housing arrangement. The options are discussed in detail in Chapter 30.

Health changes and housing changes alter elders' interactions with their social groups. Involvement in a faith community may be curtailed because of mobility problems. Attending functions in the evening may have to be dropped because of failing night vision. Reduced reaction times and memory problems may make participating in card parties or volunteer activities impossible. The combination of the changes of advanced old age and a new housing option may cause the client to become immobilized in her decision-making ability. Community health nurses can serve these expert elders best by helping them to make decisions and to find fulfillment and dignity in their choices. Additional goals should include maintaining stable health while coping with chronic illnesses and remaining safe and secure in her surroundings

HEALTHY PEOPLE 2010 GOALS FOR WOMEN

As a nation, we have been focusing on improving the health of all citizens through the Healthy People initiatives. *Healthy People 2000* set a standard of change and improvement in objectives that were met or exceeded in some areas and were far from being reached in other areas. In that initiative, there were 14 areas in which the objectives focused specifically on women's health issues. In *Healthy People 2010,* the focus is still on improving the nation's health, but the objectives have been reevaluated. Objectives have been eliminated, broadened, expanded, or tailored to meet the changing needs of society. However, many still focus on the health of women (Display 29–3). As the community health nurse works with women at various stages in their lives, the objectives in *Healthy People 2010* can give structure to the program plan-

DISPLAY 29–3

Healthy People 2010 Objectives for Women (Including Eight Developmental Objectives)

1. Reduce the breast cancer death rate, from 27.7 deaths per 100,000 women to 22.2 deaths per 100,000.
2. Reduce the death rate from cancer of the uterine cervix, from 3.0 deaths per 100,000 to 2.0 deaths per 100,000 women.
3. Increase the proportion of women who receive a Pap test; from 92% to 97% for women older than 18 years of age who have ever received a Pap test, and from 79% to 90% for women who have received a Pap test within the preceding 3 years.
4. Increase the proportion of women aged 40 years and older who have received a mammogram within the preceding 2 years, from 68% to 70%.
5. (Developmental) Decrease the proportion of pregnant women with gestational diabetes.
6. Increase the proportion of pregnancies that are intended, from 51% to 70%.
7. Reduce the proportion of births occurring within 24 months after a previous birth, from 11% to 6%.
8. Increase the proportion of women at risk for unintended pregnancy (and their partners) who use contraception, from 93% to 100%.
9. Reduce the proportion of women experiencing pregnancy despite use of a reversible contraceptive method, from 13% to 7%.
10. Reduce pregnancies among female adolescents, from 72 pregnancies per 1000 girls aged 15–17 years to 46 pregnancies per 1000.
11. Reduce maternal deaths, from 8.4 maternal deaths per 100,000 live births in 1997 to 3.3 per 100,000 in 2010.
12. Reduce maternal illness and complications due to pregnancy, from 32.1 maternal complications per 100 deliveries during labor and delivery in 1997 to 20.0 in 2010.
13. (Developmental) Reduce ectopic pregnancies and postpartum complications, including postpartum depression.
14. Increase the proportion of pregnant women who receive early and adequate prenatal care, from 83% beginning in the first trimester of pregnancy to 90%, and increase early and adequate prenatal care, from 74% in 1997 to 90% in 2010.
15. (Developmental) Increase the proportion of pregnant women who attend a series of prepared childbirth classes.
16. Reduce cesarean deliveries among low-risk women (full-term, singleton, vertex presentation), from 17.8% to 15.5% among women with no prior cesarean delivery, and from 71% to 63% among women with prior cesarean delivery.
17. (Developmental) Increase the proportion of mothers who achieve a recommended weight gain during their pregnancies.
18. Increase abstinence from alcohol, cigarettes, and illicit drugs among pregnant women: alcohol, from 86% to 94%; binge drinking, from 99% to 100%; cigarette smoking, from 87% to 98%; and illicit drug use, from 98% to 100%.
19. Increase the proportion of mothers who breast feed their babies in the early postpartum period, from 64% to 75%; at 6 months, from 29% to 50%; at 1 year, from 16% to 25%.
20. Reduce anemia among low-income pregnant women in their third trimester, from 29% to 20%.
21. (Developmental) Reduce iron deficiency among pregnant females.
22. (Developmental) Reduce human immunodeficiency virus (HIV) infections associated with heterosexual contact in adolescent and young adult women aged 13 to 24 years.
23. (Developmental) Increase the proportion of sexually active women aged 25 years and younger who are screened annually for genital chlamydia infections.
24. (Developmental) Increase the proportion of pregnant women screened for STDs (including HIV infection and bacterial vaginosis) during prenatal health care visits, according to recognized standards.
25. Increase smoking cessation during pregnancy, from 12% smoking cessation during the first trimester of pregnancy to 30%.

(Adapted from U. S. Department of Health and Human Services. [2000]. *Healthy people 2010* [Conference ed., Vols. 1 & 2]. Washington, DC: U. S. Government Printing Office).

ning and services offered to women in the community at the primary, secondary, and tertiary levels of prevention.

ROLE OF THE COMMUNITY HEALTH NURSE

The community health nurse works with women in all age groups using the three levels of prevention—primary, secondary, and tertiary—as a guide. Interventions are conducted individually, in families, in small groups, and in aggregates

to assist the woman and to make progress toward *Healthy People 2010* objectives.

Primary Prevention

Primary prevention activities focus on education to promote a healthy lifestyle. Much of the community health nurse's time is spent in the educator role. During home visits to pregnant women, the nurse teaches nutrition, provides anticipatory guidance, emphasized the importance of staying drug and alcohol free, and teaches about bodily changes during pregnancy. With small groups of women in the work setting, the nurse can teach safety, illness prevention, use of safety devices, and balancing work and home responsibilities. Among aggregates, the community health nurse focuses on community needs in services and programs that will keep that aggregate healthy, such as providing flu clinics in assisted living centers that are 85% female or working with the community high schools and college health services in teaching sexual responsibility and prevention of STDs.

Women as an aggregate have health care teaching needs separate from those of men, and a significant amount of the community health nurse's time is focused on the primary level of prevention. The community health nurse may collaborate with community leaders and other stakeholders in designing programs, work with committees to secure funding, or approach the state legislature to lobby for needed changes to state laws and policies governing the health of women. At other times, the nurse works with small groups of women who could benefit from making healthy choices in diet, rest, and physical activity. Likewise, it is not unusual for the community health nurse to work with an individual woman in her home to promote her health.

Secondary Prevention

Secondary prevention focuses on screening and early diagnosis of disease or injury. A significant amount of the community health nurse's time is spent in assessing the need for, planning, implementing, or evaluating programs that focus on the early detection of diseases. This is followed with teaching to prevent further damage from the disease in progress or to prevent the spread of the disease if it is communicable. Examples of secondary prevention programs include establishing mammography clinics, teaching breast self-examination, administering tuberculosis skin tests to groups of women in their work setting or to residents of a long-term care center, conducting blood pressure screening booths at shopping malls or among groups of women when they come to a senior center for flu shots. Wherever women gather in groups is a good place to provide both primary and secondary health care services.

One community health nurse lives in a community where she is a member of a women's service club. At one monthly meeting a year, she is the program speaker; she brings lots of pamphlets on disease prevention and early disease detection and screens everyone who is interested for cholesterol level, blood pressure, height and weight, and occult blood in stool. If she speaks in the fall, she arranges to provide flu shots for a nominal fee. She is a community health nurse, whether employed or not, as long as she maintains her license.

Tertiary Prevention

The tertiary level of prevention focuses on rehabilitation and preventing further damage to an already compromised sys-

tem. Many of the women a community health nurse works with have chronic diseases, long-standing injuries with resulting disability, or conditions resulting from another disease. Examples include DM that is out of control because the client is 100 pounds overweight and broken bones resulting from falls in a woman with advanced osteoporosis.

Ideally, negative health conditions can be prevented. If not, the next best thing is for them to be diagnosed early, without damage to the woman's health. But if negative health conditions have not been treated or brought under control, then the woman is at a tertiary level of prevention when someone intervenes. At this level of prevention, the nurse focuses on quality of life and may even take a life-saving stance in the approach used.

For example, a 62-year-old woman who is 70 pounds overweight with out-of-control DM, symptoms of congestive heart failure, and difficulty walking more than 20 feet has much to accomplish in order to feel healthy. Can the nurse help the woman lose weight? Will weight loss bring her DM under control and alleviate congestive heart failure symptoms? With some weight reduction, will she be able to walk more easily? Or, will the woman feel better with physical therapy and a different medication regimen? Is that a quicker, safer, and better approach? On assessment, the nurse discovers that the woman has been as much as 80 pounds overweight for 40 years. Will this information alter the nurse's approach to helping this woman? What additional information does the nurse need?

Caring for people at the tertiary level of prevention can become quite complicated, because so many systems become involved. In addition, all people function within many social systems, which may include family expectations, roles people have within the family, expected behaviors, community system knowledge and involvement, personal expectations, motivation, and support. This is not to say that efforts are a waste of the nurse's time, but working at the tertiary level involves all of the nurse's skills in addition to community resources and a client who can be or wants to be motivated.

MEN'S HEALTH

Historical Overview of Factors Affecting Men's Health

Over the centuries, men have been the dominant gender. They left the caves and did the hunting while women stayed at the hearth and cared for the family. Things did not change much as we move forward in time. Women were sold or traded to men of different tribes or nations to promote status or political connections (a practice still going on in some countries today). In many societies, males have been the favored and anticipated offspring, with female newborns often being left to die. Throughout time and into the 1800s, women were controlled by fathers, brothers, and later, husbands. They were not permitted to work or even to leave the home without the consent of the man in charge. Decisions were made by the male head-of-household, inheritances were left to the sons, only the sons attended school, and a woman had to marry well (to a husband chosen for her) to have a fair chance at a decent life. It was only in the 1900s that women in Western countries began to be considered as equals, and this is still a challenge in many areas, such as equal pay for equal work. But the 20th century brought about many changes for women—greater changes than all the prior centuries combined.

Given this tradition, men have been the main focus of health-related research. Research generated statistics about men, and the resulting programs or approaches to health care services were male oriented. Therefore, more is known about the health of men than of women.

More males than females die at birth; men die earlier from chronic diseases; and greater numbers of men commit suicide or die in vehicular crashes. Some of the reasons are that men are risk takers; they have been exposed to toxic, stressful, and unsafe working conditions longer than women; they do not express their emotions as well or seek out support from peers as much as women do; and they have been smoking more and longer than women (until recently). Considering all of this, what are the health care needs of men at various stages, and how can the community health nurse best meet the needs of men throughout their life-span?

Men's Health Promotion Across the Life-span

Men's health begins in adolescence with the male teenager—an interesting bundle of hormones. Even the young adult male is not finished "growing" in the early years of that stage marked by the years 18 to 35. Adult men aged 35 to 65 years have reached maturity, the peak of their physical and intellectual development, and their greatest earning power. The mature adult male older than 65 years of age is an endangered species compared with women in the same age group. It is during this stage that men retire and must find new meaning in their lives if their focus was on work in prior years. Many men in this age group die prematurely.

What specific needs do men in these age groups have? Are their needs being met through services now provided, or are they thought of as having specific organs with problems and not looked at holistically?

Teenaged Men (12–18 Years)

Male teens have the same developmental needs as females in this age group. They are striving for independence, exploring the qualities in the opposite sex that one day will be sought in a mate, and making plans for their future by working or planning for education beyond high school. It is in these years that the teenage male goes through puberty, experiencing and learning about the hormonal and physical changes going on in his body.

Like female teenagers, teenaged men are physically able to procreate before they are emotionally or economically ready to support a family. The choices and decisions made by a young man at this age may affect him for a lifetime.

Some of the decisions a young man makes are whether to begin smoking, drinking alcohol, using drugs, or having sex. The young man learns to drive and chooses to be a responsible and safe driver or is influenced by peers and drives recklessly. It is a challenging period in his life, one that frequently creates many sleepless nights for his parents.

Teenaged boys usually begin puberty between ages 10 and 13 years. Prepubescent boys have a growth spurt in their feet that occurs a few years before pubic hair appears, genitals grow, and the voice deepens. These are awkward years for boys. Some may be maturing physically before others, so showering together at school can be embarrassing. The breaks in their changing voices can make public speaking in the classroom difficult. This will change as the boy completes puberty. At times, in boys who are a bit overweight, breast tissue grows, making it uncomfortable for them to wear tight shirts. This subsides as the boy matures and chest muscles develop.

In these years when young teens are developing a sense of self, body image becomes very important. Teenaged men may judge themselves by stereotypical images of masculinity seen on television and in magazines—men with "perfect" bodies and "six-pack" abdominal muscles. GI Joe dolls are so abnormally proportioned that their biceps could be achieved in a real body only through the use of steroids. Such role models as these can create body image problems in teen males. Females have similarly distorted role model images in Barbie dolls. Community health nurses can intervene through education and discussions on resisting media-driven images, being realistic, and eating for power. Access to young teens occurs at boys club meetings, scouting meetings, health or science classes, and team sports practice sessions (Display 29–4).

DISPLAY 29–4

Body Image Problems—Symptoms in Young Men

Young men with this disorder:
1. Believe they are "small" or "puny" despite being well above average in muscle development.
2. Work out excessively and follow strict diets, even if it means neglecting relationships and responsibilities.
3. Feel anxious if they go off their diet or miss a single day of exercising, even if they are ill or injured.
4. Stay away from social events or wear bulky, loose-fitting clothing to avoid exposing their bodies.
5. Are at increased risk for abuse of steroids and supplements.

(Adapted from Mueller, M. [2002]. *Men: You and your body.* Santa Cruz, CA: ETR Associates).

A concern for the young male is the risk for testicular cancer. Teaching testicular self-examination is an important role for the community health nurse. This can be done in small social, service, or sports groups of young men. The highest risk group is 15- to 30-year-old men and men with a family history of testicular cancer or a personal history of undescended testicles. It is a rare form of cancer, and it is not on the list of national objectives in *Healthy People 2010*. However, if detected early it is highly curable. It is worth it to the overall health of a young man to know how to do a testicular self-examination (Display 29–5).

Of greater concerns are sexual experimentation, drug and alcohol use, and driving safety. Teenage men are risk takers, believing they are invincible. They take risks without thought of the consequences. They respond to challenges such as drag racing, exceeding speed limits, binge drinking, or experimenting with drugs. Community health nurses make sure that school curricula contain content on these subjects early enough to reach teens before they begin experimenting. The nurse should suggest that the information be reinforced in other settings, especially the teenagers' homes.

Parents are very important during the teen years. They need to approach the subjects first with their children and provide open and continuous channels of communication with the family values and religious beliefs intertwined as facts are shared. It is imperative that parents know their teen's friends and preferably also the friend's parents. They need to know where their teen is going, when he'll return, and who he will be with. This is a good time for a teen to have access to a cell phone so that he and his parents can communicate when he is out alone or with friends.

Another issue with some teenaged men is the question of their sexuality. It is in these years that many gay men come to the realization that they are homosexual. **Gay** is the commonly accepted term for a **homosexual**—a person who has sexual interest in, or has sexual intercourse exclusively with, members of his or her own sex. The teen years are full of self-doubts and feelings of inadequacy that may contribute to some teens' having doubts about their sexuality. These feelings are infrequently shared with adults and may be discussed only with a close friend, leaving the teen with misinformation or continuing doubts.

Sexual experimentation, whether heterosexual or homosexual, can put the teen at risk for diseases that affect health for a long time or are life-threatening. The clear message that needs to reach teens is that being sexually active demands responsibility. The community health nurse has a plethora of resources available to assist sexually active teens. Many health departments have condoms that can be distributed and STD clinics that teens can access. Nurses can provide the address or a referral to a Planned Parenthood teen clinic. This organization focuses on sexual responsibility, with the teen couple attending together, and can prescribe a variety of birth control methods as well as answering questions and clearing up any misinformation. In addition, there is literature designed for any reading level, including comic book format, pamphlets, and books, that the community health nurse can acquire for the teen.

DISPLAY 29–5

Testicular Self-Examination

The best time to do the examination is after a warm bath or shower, when the scrotal skin is relaxed. You should do the examination monthly. You should also inspect your penis for any changes. Select a date that you will remember, such as the first day of each month or your birthdate.

1. Stand and place your right leg on an elevated surface. A tub side or toilet seat works fine.
2. Explore the surface of the right testicle by gently rolling it between the thumb and fingers of both hands. Feel for any hard lumps or nodules. The testicle should feel round and smooth, about the size of a large almond.
3. Notice any enlargement of the testicle or change in its consistency from previous months. It is normal for one testicle to be slightly larger than the other. Any major size difference should be reported to a health care professional.
4. Repeat, lifting the left leg and examining your left testicle.
   Report to your health care professional any of the following:
   • Unusual lumps or nodules in the testes
   • Unexplained pain or swelling in the testes or scrotum
   • Any penile discharge or sores on your penis

(From Kaiser Permanente. [2002], *Kaiser Permanente healthwise handbook,* Boise, ID: Healthwise.)

Young Adult Men (18–35 Years)

The young adult male goes through many changes in this age group that spans the first 17 years of adulthood. The awkward 18-year-old who does not know what to do with his future becomes the responsible spouse and father, possibly within a decade. There is much to accomplish in this stage: pursuing the training or education that leads to a personally and financially rewarding career; selecting a compatible mate and establishing a life together; finding comfort with and meaning to his existence through practicing and internalizing a belief and value system that works for him; actively planning for having (or not having) children; and participating in the betterment of the greater community, both actively (volunteering, committee work, leadership positions) and passively (voting, being a good citizen, obeying laws).

While this young adult male is achieving these developmental tasks, there are also health-related issues he needs to focus on. Choices made during these years to establish healthy eating, work, rest, and exercise habits will benefit him for a lifetime. He should eat for power and good health, following the recommended foods in the U. S. Agriculture Department's Food Guide Pyramid, considering his personal likes and dislikes. He and his family benefit if he is able to balance work and home, doing his best in both settings. Establishing a pattern of rest that allows his body to recover and refresh from a day full of meaningful activities will help him look forward to each day renewed. He should establish an exercise routine that meets his personal needs, fits with his skills and talents, and includes some physical activities that involve his family.

These choices provide him with the knowledge that he is doing all he can to keep himself healthy and to prevent the two major killers of men, heart disease and cancer. However, there are additional considerations. Monogamy between the spouses eliminates the chance of getting an STD, but many men may be single for all or most of this age span. In those single years, dating, using drugs or alcohol, and beginning smoking are all possibilities. If the young man establishes a sexual relationship during these years, he is at risk for STDs. Using condoms correctly and limiting the number of sexual partners he has will help to provide some protection.

Depending on his attitudes and practices before he entered this age group, he may or may not be enticed to experiment with or use drugs. Many young men (and women) are tempted to experiment with smoking, alcohol, and illicit drugs while on their own in college, in the military, or in their first full-time jobs in the early years of this stage. This is an important age group for the community health nurse to reach with health information, because the decisions made in the more formative years of this stage affect how these clients live the rest of their lives. The nurse can meet with young adult men in the occupational setting, on college campuses and in fraternities in collaboration with the college health nurse and other college health team members, in communities where there are military bases, at single-adult groups sponsored by religious communities, and even in health clubs and bars.

Late in this stage the man, if a husband and father, may participate in discussions with his wife regarding the choice of permanent birth control. The choices include **tubal ligation** for the woman and vasectomy for the man. Tubal ligation is done in one of two ways. In the more minimally invasive procedure, surgery is done through three 2-cm openings in the abdomen; a tube is inserted, and lasers are used to permanently sever the fallopian tubes. This is usually completed on an outpatient basis. The other approach involves traditional abdominal surgery; it is more invasive and may include overnight hospitalization. For the man, a **vasectomy** includes removal of all or a segment of the vas deferens; the procedure is almost always conducted on an outpatient bases and does not internally invade the client. These choices may be explored at this age and then postponed until the next stage, especially if the couple is not sure they have completed their family.

Typically, young adult clients have few interactions with health care providers in any given year. It is often as-sumed that young adult males in this age range are not at risk for physical or psychological disease. This is a nonproductive belief. It is important for people in this age group to have regular health checkups to assess for the early signs of disease.

Adult Men (35–65 Years)

Men in the developmental stage between 35 and 65 years of age face the issues of parents with children reaching maturity at the same time as their own parents and in-laws demand more attention. This puts physical, economic, and emotional demands on the family. The older adults may have extended care needs while, simultaneously, there are economic burdens of putting children through college. Meanwhile, the adults are adjusting to the reality that their career path is now set.

Men and women in this age group experience normal physical changes. Because body parts age at varying rates, a physical profile of middle-aged adults is organized by body system (Display 29–6).

The term of "midlife" is applied to the first half of this age group. It is a time to focus on reappraisal of values, priorities, and personal relationships, especially marriage. As the term "midlife crisis" implies, this is one of the more difficult stages and tends to challenge the adult's ability to solve problems. Successful navigation of this stage can be very fulfilling but may require enhanced coping skills. The community health nurse can provide anticipatory guidance to adults approaching this stage and help them with ways to more effectively manage the challenges.

The later years in this stage, age 50 to 64, involve preparation for retirement. In anticipation of retirement, these years are marked by expanded social relationships and pursuit of new hobbies to fill leisure time along with anticipating finishing of a career and accumulation of the best retirement benefits. The decisions made during these years will play out over the rest of the man's life and beyond. How his spouse lives out her years may be altered according to the retirement decisions made at this time.

Chronic health problems that were left undiagnosed when younger are now beginning to emerge. Peers may be suffering and succumbing to diseases, and the man begins to adjust to the potential loss of loved ones, particularly a spouse.

The community health nurse has much to do to help men move through this stage successfully. Most men are employed during these years, and the first nurse they interact with may be the occupational and environmental health nurse at their workplace. This nurse can conduct classes that keep clients safe at work, provide information about cardiac and cancer risks, screen for many forms of cancer, and monitor blood pressure or cholesterol levels. These activities can be scheduled so that the men do not have to miss work to reap health care benefits. In non-work settings, parish nurses, community health nurses at a health department clinic, or nurses making home visits may be resources for the adult male to access to meet health promotion needs.

D I S P L A Y   2 9 – 6

Physical Profile of Middle-Aged Adults by Body System

Body System	Physical Characteristic
Skeletal system	Intervertebral disks flatten over time
Integumentary system	Decreased secretions by sebaceous glands leads to drier skin
	Sweat glands diminish in size and number
	Skin loses elasticity and is more prone to wrinkles
	Hair bulbs lose melanin usually resulting in gray hair by age 50
Muscular system	Muscle fibers decrease by approximately 10%
	Lean body mass is replaced by adipose tissue
	Decreased grip strength occurs at this age
Endocrine and reproductive system	Menses stops
	Synthesis of estrogen decreases
	Tissues of the reproductive system (eg, cervix and uterus) gradually atrophy
	Uterine changes make pregnancy less likely
	Intercourse may be more painful due to diminishing natural lubrications
Neurologic system	Nerve impulses are conducted 5% slower
	Cognition is unaffected, although there is a gradual loss of neurons
	Eyesight is poorer due to loss of elasticity in the lens
	Auditory discrimination of certain tones and consonants gradually decreases
Cardiovascular system	By age 50, the heart's efficiency may be only 80%
	Elasticity of heart and blood vessels decreases
	Cardiac output decreases
Respiratory system	Elasticity of lungs decreases
	Breathing capacity decreases to 75% due to diminished strength of chest wall muscles
Urinary system	Decreased glomerular filtration rate appears in women
	Loss of bladder tone and tissue atrophy may lead to incontinence or possibly prolapse
	In men, an enlarged prostate may result in nocturia or dribbling

In addition to promoting cardiac health and living to prevent cancer, men in the later half of this stage should be aware of changes in their sexual response and their prostate health. Erection problems are common among men of all ages, but especially in men as they age. An erection problem is difficulty in raising or maintaining an erection capable of intercourse. Problems can often be solved with self-care remedies. The cause may be stress at work, tension in relationships, depression, fatigue, lack of privacy, physical injury, or side effects of medications (Kaiser Permanente, 2002). The self-care remedies the community health nurse can suggest include the following:

- Rule out medications. The nurse can check the medications the man is taking or have the man check with his pharmacist or health care provider for possible side effects involving sexual function.
- Avoid alcohol and smoking, which make erection problems worse.
- Cope with stress. Tension in the man's life can distract him and make erections difficult. Regular exercise and other stress-relieving activities may help ease tension.
- Try for more foreplay. Suggest that the man's partner focus more time on stroking the man to extend foreplay for him.
- Give himself time. If the man has experienced a recent loss or change in a relationship, he may not yet be emotionally ready for erections. Usually the stress will subside and the erection problem will disappear after a few weeks.

The man should find out whether he can have erections at other times. If he can achieve them with masturbation or has them on awakening, the problem is probably related to stress or an emotional problem.

If all of these measures have been tried, the drug sildenafil (Viagra) may help. There are some medical restrictions to the use of this drug, and the man's health care provider can decide with him whether the drug is recommended.

Prostate health is another concern that may occur later in this life stage. The prostate is a doughnut-shaped cluster of glands located at the bottom of the bladder, about halfway between the rectum and the base of the penis, that encircles the urethra. The walnut-sized gland produces most of the fluid in semen. Men can experience infection (prostatitis), prostate enlargement (benign prostatic hypertrophy), and prostate cancer.

The most serious is prostate cancer, which is a leading cause of cancer deaths in men. The American Cancer Society estimated that there were 180,400 cases of the disease and 31,900 deaths from prostate cancer in 2000 (Venes & Thomas, 2001). It usually occurs in men older than 65 years of age and does not shorten their lives. However, if the cancer is large or advanced, or appears at a younger age, it can be very serious. If it is detected early, before it has spread to other organs, the cancer may be curable. Screening of men should begin at age 50 years and should include a blood test to assess levels of prostate specific antigen (PSA), a digital rectal examination, or assessment of the gland with ultrasonography. A prostatectomy—excision of part or all of the prostate gland—is one treatment. If a nerve-sparing method is used, impotency will result in 20% to 30% of the patients, compared with up to 70% for other surgical methods. Incontinence, in 4% to 30%, also occurs (Venes & Thomas, 2001). A prostatectomy is considered a life-saving surgery, and the serious side effects mentioned need to be shared with the man before surgery and managed as effectively as possible afterward. A community health nurse can reinforce or clarify information shared with the man by his health care provider, discuss his options with him and his family, and provide the support they may need if cancer is the diagnosis.

Mature Adult Men (65 Years and Older)

This life stage is earmarked by retirement for most men, and by loss of health, income, status, and loved ones. These dramatic losses are somewhat offset by the benefits of increased leisure time, which provides time for travel, volunteering, hobbies, new relationships, and enjoying grandchildren and great grandchildren. Usually chronic diseases come about slowly, allowing feelings of wellness for many years and the ability to perform most chosen activities. If well planned for and happily anticipated, retirement can be a wonderful time. Avocations can be developed.

The developmental tasks for a man in this age group include coping with the various losses experienced, coming to terms with the decisions he has made in life, realizing that his life had meaning, and preparing for death.

The community health nurse can work with older adults on all of their developmental tasks. The nurse has information about resources in the community that encourage the older adult to spend his leisure time in meaningful activities. Volunteer opportunities abound. There are senior programs and centers with many social activities. There are travel groups for the "experienced traveler" and Elderhostel programs for men that want to continue learning without tests or papers to write. Other men may want to attend adult education or college classes. Most universities offer classes at very nominal fees for people older than 60 years of age—often as low as $5.00 per academic unit.

Regarding the man's health, the community health nurse can direct the client toward health promotion and maintenance programs in the community that provide free or low-cost immunizations (flu, pneumonia, tetanus) and screening services (tuberculosis, hypertension, cholesterol), to supplement the services covered by Medicare. This helps him to stretch his retirement income by keeping his health care costs down.

Some men become depressed from dealing with losses. The community health nurse can spend time helping the client reflect on the positive aspects of his life while assessing for signs of depression. The nurse can then guide the man to appropriate referrals in the community while continuing to provide supportive involvement in his holistic health care needs.

HEALTHY PEOPLE 2010 GOALS FOR MEN

Although *Healthy People 2010* has 25 health objectives specifically for women and just 5 for men, there are hundreds that apply to both women and men of all ages. The five men's objectives focus on prostate health, reproductive health, and disease prevention among gay men (Display 29–7).

ROLE OF THE COMMUNITY HEALTH NURSE

Many of the specific activities in which the community health nurse can become involved to promote the health of men throughout their life-span have been described previously. This section focuses on activities stratified into primary, secondary, and tertiary prevention strategies that the nurse can use.

Primary Prevention

Primary prevention strategies, such as providing health and safety education and encouraging men to keep their immunizations up to date, are a healthy start. In addition, men should be encouraged to learn moderate eating habits and to gradually increase their exercise if they have not established an active plan in their early adult years. Using safety guidelines to move oneself and to lift people or materials at work and in day-to-day activities is an important health promotion activity.

DISPLAY 29-7

Healthy People 2010 Objectives for Men

1. Reduce the prostate cancer death rate, from 31.9 prostate cancer deaths per 100,000 males to 28.7 deaths per 100,000.
2. (Developmental) Increase male involvement in pregnancy prevention and family planning efforts.
3. Reduce the number of new cases of acquired immunodeficiency syndrome (AIDS) among adolescent and adult men who have sex with men, from 17,847 new cases of AIDS in 1998 to 13,385 new cases in 2010.
4. Reduce the number of new AIDS cases among adolescent and adult men who have sex with men and inject drugs, from 2122 new cases of AIDS in 1998 to 1592 new cases in 2010.
5. Increase the proportion of sexually active persons who use condoms, from 23% to 50%.

(Adapted from U. S. Department of Health and Human Services. [2000]. *Healthy people 2010* [Conference ed., Vols. 1 & 2]. Washington, DC: U. S. Government Printing Office.)

Other measures that promote health include regular physical examinations, moderate drinking, no smoking, and learning relaxation techniques. Men often sacrifice their need for enjoyable leisure activity to their work schedule, but they need an emotional release to avoid frustration. If men do not have hobbies or favorite pastimes, encourage them to develop an avocation. Men who retire and enter old age often have trouble adjusting to the loss of what their jobs meant to them—status, income and a place to go each day—if they have not already built up other interests.

Secondary Prevention

Secondary prevention focuses on screening for early detection and prompt treatment of diseases. Throughout the lifespan there are screening tests that will help men catch disease early, at a point where it can be treated and cured. Many managed care organizations have their own schedule for routine screening, but for men in health care programs without such a schedule it is often the occupational and environmental health nurse who provides screening. At times the man may encounter other community health nurses in health department clinics, at flu clinics, or at health fairs. If the nurse asks the right questions at these times, the man will benefit from referrals to get low-cost or free health screening services. As with youth and teens, adult men gather in places where a community health nurse could reach them to provide information about screening services—at sporting events, sites of team activities (eg, bowling, soccer), bars, or work settings.

Tertiary Prevention

Tertiary prevention includes all activities taken after there has been an insult to the body. It often involves rehabilitation. Depending on the client's age, tertiary prevention can be simple or very complicated. A 19-year-old man who breaks his leg while skiing and lives with his parents needs information about using crutches safely, a reminder to eat protein foods for bone healing, and a reminder to return to his health care provider to get the cast taken off or if he experiences various symptoms. He needs no additional help from others. Tertiary prevention in this case is easy. On the other hand, if a 72-year-old man who lives alone breaks his leg slipping on ice on his sidewalk, his DM may begin to go out of control, his cardiac arrhythmia may exacerbate, his compromised mobility may affect his eating habits, and he may begin getting depressed. Providing appropriate intervention with this client becomes more complex; it requires a skilled community health nurse and involvement of community resources.

DEMOGRAPHICS OF ADULT CLIENTS—MALE AND FEMALE

It is difficult to identify the transition from wellness to poor health for both women and men. Therefore, mortality statistics are considered the most reliable indicator of the health status of a population. In addition, they can be used to calculate other important measures, such as life expectancy.

In the year 2000, a total of 2,404,598 people died in the United States. The crude death rate was 873.6 per 100,000 for all people. Causes of death vary by age, but the 15 leading causes of death among all people has shifted and now includes, in rank order, the following (National Center for Health Statistics, 2001):

1. Coronary heart disease (CHD)
2. Cancers
3. Stroke
4. Chronic obstructive pulmonary disease (COPD)
5. Unintentional injuries
6. Diabetes
7. Pneumonia and influenza
8. Alzheimer disease (AD)
9. Kidney disease
10. Septicemia
11. Suicide
12. Chronic liver disease
13. Essential hypertension
14. Aspiration pneumonia
15. Homicide

What has changed in this list is that AD and aspiration pneumonia, causes of death among the very oldest members of the population, are now among the leading causes of death overall. As people are living longer, there are more people in the over-75 age category, and they are the ones with AD and pneumonia deaths. Homicide has moved up to be the 15th item on the 2000 list. Some of the rates have changed, in that CHD is still number one but not as far away from cancer rates as it was in previous years.

The 20th century has seen a shift in the mortality statistics. At the turn of the century, communicable diseases such as tuberculosis and pneumonia were the leading causes of death. However, the impact of significant advances in biomedical research and public health have been such that noncommunicable diseases are now the leading causes of death. At present, 70% of all deaths in the United States are attributed to heart disease, cancer, cerebrovascular disease, or chronic lung disease.

LIFE EXPECTANCY

Life expectancy is another standard measurement that is used to compare the health status of various populations. **Life expectancy** is defined as the average number of years that an individual member of a specific cohort (usually a single birth year) is projected to live. Health statistics often report life expectancy figures for birth and 65 years of age (Table 29–4). In the United States, life expectancy has increased consistently over time, although U. S. life expectancy trails that of more than 20 other countries (Table 29–5). Japan reports the highest life expectancy figures. In all countries, there is a dif-

T A B L E 2 9 – 4

Life Expectancy (Years) at Birth and at 65 Years of Age According to Sex: United States, Selected Years, 1900–2000

Year	At Birth			At 65 Years		
	Both Sexes	Male	Female	Both Sexes	Male	Female
1900	47.3	46.3	48.3	11.9	11.5	12.2
1950	68.2	65.6	71.1	13.9	12.8	15.0
1960	69.7	66.6	73.1	14.3	12.8	15.8
1970	70.8	67.1	74.7	15.2	13.1	17.0
1980	73.7	70.7	77.4	16.4	14.1	18.3
1990	75.4	71.8	78.8	17.2	15.1	18.9
1995	75.8	72.5	78.9	17.4	15.6	18.9
2000	76.9	74.1	79.5	17.5	16.0	19.0

(Adapted from National Center for Health Statistics. [2000]. *Health, United States, 2002 with chartbook on trends in the health of Americans* [DHHS pub. no. 1232]. Hyattsville, MD: Public Health Service.)

ference between female and male life expectancy of as much as 8 years.

MAJOR HEALTH PROBLEMS OF ADULTS

Four selected major causes of death among adults are presented in this section. Heart disease and stroke are the first and third leading causes of death in adults and are discussed together. Cancer is the second leading cause of death, and unintentional injuries (accidents) have moved lower on the list, to fifth in 2000. Selected additional major causes of death are covered in detail in other chapters: suicide (Chapter 35), AD (Chapter 30), and homicide (Chapter 20).

T A B L E 2 9 – 5

Life Expectancy (Years) at Birth for Selected Countries by Sex

Country	Female	Male	Disparity
Japan	82.9	76.4	6.5
France	82.6	74.2	8.4
Switzerland	81.9	75.1	6.8
Spain	81.5	74.2	7.3
Canada	81.2	75.2	6.0
Australia	80.9	75.0	5.9
Greece	80.3	75.1	5.2
Germany	79.8	73.3	6.5
United States	79.5	74.1	5.4

(From U. S. Department of Health and Human Services. [2000].)

Coronary Heart Disease and Stroke

More than one fourth of all deaths of adults aged 25 to 64 years are due to cardiovascular diseases, primarily CHD and stroke or cerebral vascular accidents (CVAs). Heart disease has been the leading cause of death for men older than 40 years of age, and about 12 million Americans have CHD (USDHHS, 2000). Heart disease is also the largest contributor to permanent disability claims for workers before age 65, and it accounts for more days of hospitalization than any other single disorder. It is the principal cause of limited activity for some 5 to 6 million Americans younger than 65 years of age.

Risk factors contributing to coronary artery disease can be separated into three categories: personal, hereditary, and environmental. Personal risk factors include gender, age, race, cholesterol level (specifically the ratio of low-density to high-density lipoproteins), blood pressure, and cigarette smoking. The most preventable of these factors are cholesterol, high blood pressure, and cigarette smoking. Heredity obviously cannot be changed. The understanding of environmental risk factors, especially as they relate to occupational exposures, is limited. The likelihood of heart disease or CVA multiplies with the increasing number of risk factors present.

The disparities in heart disease have remained consistent. The incidence is higher in men than in women and higher in the African-American population than in the white population. In addition, over the last 30 years, the CHD death rate has declined differently by gender and race, at times favoring one sex or one race. The incidence of heart disease in women is only one third that in men until menopause, after which it increases. But men still have twice the incidence rate up to age 75 years. By age 85, the rates are almost the same.

Disparities also exist in treatment outcomes for clients who have a heart attack. Women, in general, have poorer outcomes after a heart attack than do men: 44% of women who have a heart attack die within 1 year, compared with 27% of men. At older ages, women who have heart attacks are twice as likely as men to die within a few weeks (USDHHS, 2000).

Approximately 600,000 Americans suffer strokes each year, resulting in 158,000 deaths (USDHHS, 2000). Between the ages of 25 and 64 years, African-Americans are almost twice as susceptible to stroke as whites, largely because of the high incidence of hypertension in the black population. In the southeastern United States (the so-called stroke belt), stroke death rates for both blacks and whites are higher than in any other part of the country.

Disparities also exist among people with strokes. Racial differences in the number of new cases of stroke and in the number of deaths due to stroke are even greater than those for CHD. Stroke deaths are highest in African-American women born before 1950 and in African-American men born after 1950.

Cancer

Chronic disease poses a significant threat to the health of American adults. Cancer is the major chronic illness in the United States. It affects more people older than 15 years of age than any other disease, and it remains the leading cause of death for these people. Overall, it is the second leading cause of death in the United States.

Major preventable risk factors that contribute to cancer include smoking, alcohol abuse, diet, exposure to radiation and sunlight, water pollution, and air pollution. There is a proven link between exposure to cigarette smoke and lung cancer, and, until legislation curtailed it, many workers were exposed to secondhand smoke in the workplace.

Chemicals and other potential cancer-causing materials are produced and used every year. In addition, known carcinogens, such as asbestos and vinyl chloride, continue to threaten the health of workers who, without adequate protection, develop malignancies not commonly found in the general population. In fact, mesothelioma, a lung cancer related to asbestos exposure, has been documented among people whose only known exposure was from the contaminants carried home on the shoes and clothing of a worker. Because asbestos was once a common construction material, it is being removed from older buildings to protect people from asbestos exposure. Asbestos removal experts are at risk of exposure and, therefore, must follow elaborate procedures to protect themselves.

Unintentional Injuries

Unintentional injuries, refers to any injury that results from unintended exposure to physical agents, including heat, mechanical energy, chemicals, or electricity. For example, a motor vehicle collision could result in unintentional injuries, as could exposure to pesticides. When we think about injuries, what usually comes to mind are mechanical injuries of the musculoskeletal system. However, chemical injuries

commonly affect the skin, eyes, lungs, and gastrointestinal organs, and both heat and electricity typically injure the skin.

In 1997, 149,691 Americans died of injuries from a variety of causes, such as motor vehicle crashes, firearms, poisonings, suffocation, falls, fires, and drownings. About 345 people older than 18 years of age die each day from unintentional injuries (USDHHS, 2000). It is estimated that 42,000 people die each year in motor vehicle crashes.

Although the greatest impact of injury is in human suffering and loss of life, the financial cost is staggering. By the late 1990s, injury costs were estimated at more than $224 billion annually, with an increase of 42% compared with the 1980s. As with other health problems, it costs far less to prevent injuries than to treat them. For example (USDHHS, 2000):

- Every child safety seat saves $85 in direct medical costs and an additional $1,275 in other costs.
- Every bicycle helmet saves $395 in direct medical costs and other costs.
- Every smoke detector saves $35 in direct medical costs and an additional $865 in other costs.
- Every dollar spent on poison control centers saves $6.50 in medical costs.

Disabling injuries occur disproportionately among the young and the elderly. Child safety seats, bicycle helmets, smoke detectors, and poison control centers save billions of dollars in direct and indirect medical costs. Primary prevention saves lives and money. A **disabling injury** is one that results in restriction of normal activities of daily living beyond the day on which the injury occurred.

An **unsafe condition** is any environmental factor, either social or physical, that increases the likelihood of an unintentional injury. An icy walkway is an example of an unsafe condition: although it poses a hazard, it does not cause an injury, but only makes it more likely that an injury will occur.

Injury prevention and *injury control* refer to any effort to prevent injuries or lessen their severity. These efforts often focus on assessment of the environment for unsafe conditions, such as loaded guns in the home or asbestos in school buildings and workplaces.

EVOLUTION OF OCCUPATIONAL HEALTH

Modern occupational health is an outgrowth of the 19th-century Industrial Revolution in England. Deplorable work conditions and worker exploitation created a growing public concern and spawned the development of many protective laws. This influence was felt in the United States, which was rapidly becoming an industrialized nation. Between 1890 and 1914, more than 16.5 million immigrants from all over the world poured into the United States. As industrial growth escalated, these new citizens worked in the plants, factories, railroads, and mines, creating a new market for manufactured goods. Workers—children as well as adults—commonly worked 12- to 14-hour shifts, 7 days a week, under unspeakable conditions of grime, dust, physical hazards, smoke, heat, cold, and noxious fumes. People accepted work-related illnesses and injuries as part of the job and lived shorter lives, frequently dying in their 40s and 50s, with workers in some trades dying in their 30s (Lee, 1978).

No connection was made between work conditions and health. Employers attributed employees' poor health and early deaths to their personal habits on the job or their living conditions at home. Physicians, uneducated in the relationship between work and health, blamed industrial-related diseases, such as silicosis, lead poisoning, and tuberculosis, on other causes.

Early Research in Occupational Health

Public awareness and understanding were necessary before changes could be made to improve working conditions. That understanding was based on continuing research into occupational health.

Bernardino Ramazzini (1633–1714), an Italian physician known as the "father of occupational medicine," conducted the earliest systematic and scholarly study of occupational disease. His treatise of 1700 was entitled *De Morbis Artificum Diatriba [Diseases of Workers]*. Ramazzini had the foresight, when attempting a diagnosis, to ask about his patient's occupation. He found that those who sat at their work, such as cobblers and tailors, became bent, hump-backed, and kept their heads held down like people looking for something on the ground. In addition, he felt they suffered from general ill health caused by their sedentary life. However, potters and weavers, for example, who exercised their arms and feet and in fact the whole body, were in better health. He studied bakers, carpenters, printers, porters, and other workers. Ramazzini realized that not all workers' diseases were attributed to chemical or physical agents in the environment, but that "a variety of common workers' diseases were caused by prolonged, violent, and irregular motions and prolonged postures. Such cumulative trauma and repetitive-motion injuries have recently been called the occupational epidemic of the 1990s" (Franco, 2001, p. 1382). Ramazzini suggested that all physicians ask their patients about the kind of work they did. Despite his influence, interest in and information concerning worker health evolved slowly.

It was not until the early 1900s that the Public Health Service conducted one of the first scientific studies on occupational hazards by investigating dust conditions in mining, cement manufacturing, and stone cutting. Other studies followed. Lead poisoning was as high as 22% among the pottery workers studied. A 1914 study of garment workers showed a high incidence of tuberculosis related to poor ventilation, overcrowding, and unsanitary work conditions. Other investigations revealed phosphorus poisoning among workers in the match industry (1912), radium poisoning among watchmakers (1920s), and mercury poisoning in

WHAT DO YOU THINK? II

In November of 2000, the U. S. Congress passed the nation's landmark ergonomics standard. However, a very few months later, in March 2001, with the support of President George W. Bush, the Congress voted to undo this standard of the Occupational Safety and Health Administration (OSHA). This standard was supported by public health and labor advocates and was the result of more than 10 years of work and 1 year of hearings and public comment.

This legislation would have required employers to create programs informing workers about musculoskeletal disorders and their symptoms, to encourage reporting, and to evaluate the workplace and take action to address risks. The standard was consistently under fire from business groups, who claimed that it would be too costly to enact. However current the battles over OSHA's ergonomic standard may be, these types of occupational hazards were recognized by astute public health and medical observers centuries ago, as documented by Ramazzini in 1700.

Yearly, more than 1.8 million US workers report musculoskeletal disorders such as carpal tunnel syndrome and back injuries. In 600,000 of these cases, the disorders are serious enough that workers take time off from work. These injuries costs industry an estimated $9 billion each year in sick days and decreased productivity.

those who manufactured felt hats (1930s) (Lee, 1978). The public was awakening to the effect of work conditions on people's health.

The birth of the labor movement increased the demand for healthful and safe working conditions. Workers' compensation laws provided for occupational injury and disease coverage, and other efforts were made to protect workers against health hazards in the workplace. Unfortunately, it took such disastrous events as the Triangle Shirtwaist Factory fire to create the impetus for further legislation. This notorious fire, which occurred in New York City in 1911, took the lives of 154 workers, most of whom were young women. Investigations after the incident revealed nonexistent fire escapes and locked exit doors. This tragic event resulted in establishment of the first serious safety laws to protect working people (Morris, 1976).

Current Legislation

Today, a growing body of legislation exists to protect the health and safety of workers. The following is a list of current laws that employers must follow to meet health and safety codes.

The Workmen's Compensation Act of 1910 was initially enacted in New Jersey before it became national law in 1948. This law requires employers to carry employee insurance that provides compensation for lost wages and medical and rehabilitative costs associated with work-related disease and injury. Application of the law varies from state to state. All states, however, emphasize early intervention and rehabilitation.

The Social Security Act of 1935 was enacted to provide financial resources to the "aged, blind, and disabled," as well as state and federal unemployment insurance programs. Amendments to the act in 1965 and 1972 created benefits for high-risk mothers and children and additional benefits for the elderly.

The Federal Coal Mine Health and Safety Act of 1967 is the only federal program that deals with a specific occupational disease. The act originally established health standards in coal mines and provided medical examinations for actively employed underground coal miners. Through the Social Security Administration, it also provided benefits for black lung disease (pneumoconiosis). Specifically, it required all exposed workers to have radiographic examinations and made available federal funds to compensate victims and their families. The subsequent *Federal Mine Safety and Health Amendments Act of 1977* retains most of the original provisions.

The Occupational Safety and Health Act of 1970 generally provides workers with protection against personal injury and illness resulting from hazardous working conditions. More specifically, its purpose and functions are "to ensure safe and healthful working conditions for working men and women by authorizing enforcement of the standards developed under the act; by assisting and encouraging the states in efforts to ensure safe and healthful working conditions; by providing for research, information, education, and training in the field of occupational safety and health; and for other purposes" (Lee, 1978, p. 50).

The 1970 Act created two federal agencies: the Occupational Safety and Health Administration (OSHA) and the National Institute for Occupational Safety and Health (NIOSH).

OSHA, housed in the Department of Labor, has been a controversial agency, criticized by detractors in the private sector and by legislators. Contributing to its controversy is that it is perceived solely as a regulatory agency. However, since its inception, OSHA has had a multifaceted mission to promote and protect worker safety and health through regulation, consultation, training, and outreach. All have been long-standing and well-subscribed programmatic activities offered by OSHA (McDiarmid, 2000). OSHA brought about several changes in the workplace. One of the most critical changes is that, for the first time, an employee may request an OSHA inspection for any suspected violation of work standards. And the employee may remain anonymous if he or she wishes to do so. In addition, OSHA provides grants to states to assist in compliance with the act, and some states OSHA regained local authority over occupational safety and health.

NIOSH is part of the Centers for Disease Control and Prevention (CDC), under the USDHHS, and is responsible for research. NIOSH responsibilities include the following adaptations (NIOSH, 2002):

* Enumerate hazards present in the workplace
* Investigate potential hazardous working conditions when requested by employers or employees
* Identify the causes of work-related diseases and injury
* Evaluate the hazards of new technology and work practices
* Create ways to control hazards
* Train safety and health professionals
* Sponsor research on psychological, motivational, and behavioral factors as they relate to occupational safety and health
* Make recommendations and disseminate information on preventing workplace disease, injury, and disability
* Recommend occupational, safety, and health standards

The Toxic Substances Control Act of 1976 ensures that the risk of using chemical substances in the workplace does not present an undue hardship for either the employee or the environment. The Act requires that certain chemical substances and mixtures be tested and their use restricted. It is also concerned with the manufacture, processing, commercial distribution, and disposal of such substances. The Environmental Protection Agency enforces this act.

The Hazard Communication Act of 1986, known as the worker right-to-know legislation, ensures that workers are adequately educated regarding hazards in their places of work through a hazards communication program. This is especially important because all hazards and toxic substances cannot be removed from workplaces, due to the nature of the product being developed or the service provided by the company. This standard was extended in 1988 to all employers covered by OSHA. One of the most frequently cited OSHA violations has been noncompliance with this standard.

The Americans with Disabilities Act (ADA) was passed by Congress in 1990 as a civil rights law to prevent discrimination against qualified workers with disabilities. For employers with 25 or more employees, the law went into effect in 1992. Employers with 15 to 24 employees were obligated to comply with its provisions by 1994. A *disabled person* is someone with a physical or mental impairment that substantially limits an aspect or aspects of daily living and work activity. Employees must identify themselves as disabled. The employer and employee then begin a process of defining the essential characteristics of the job and the accommodations that need to be made to allow the employee to work. This is usually done through a job description or a collective-bargaining contract.

The OSHA Blood-borne Pathogens Standard was enacted in 1992. Guidelines published since the early 1970s have addressed infection-control compliance for the protection of health care workers against the transmission of blood-borne diseases. This new standard requires employers to do two things: offer the hepatitis B vaccine free of charge to all employees and practice general infection control, as recommended by the CDC. The universal precautions recommended by the CDC instruct health care workers to consider any direct contact with blood or body fluids as potentially infectious and to provide guidelines on ways of handling such materials. This requires employers to provide such personal protective equipment as gloves, masks, gowns, and eye protectors and to establish education, training, and some form of record keeping.

Annual compliance costs to employers are considerable, and noncompliance with this new standard puts employers at risk for costly citations. However, the responsibility for adhering to universal precautions remains literally in the hands of the employees. With human immunodeficiency virus (HIV) infection the most significant ongoing public health crisis, compliance with standards for bloodborne pathogens becomes the responsibility of every health care employer and employee.

The Family and Medical Leave Act of 1993 was enacted as a labor standards act. It requires employers of 50 or more people to provide unpaid leave of up to 12 weeks to their employees to care for family members with serious health conditions, for their own serious medical condition, or for newborn or newly adopted children. The employer must also continue to provide medical benefits and must ensure that the employee can return to the same or comparable job.

ENVIRONMENTAL WORK FACTORS

Healthy employed women and men, in both urban or rural settings, have similar issues in their work environment. Five environmental factors are common to every work setting: (1) physical factors, (2) chemical factors, (3) biologic factors, (4) ergonomic factors, and (5) psychosocial factors.

Physical Factors

Physical factors are structural elements of the workplace that influence worker health and productivity. The various features that make up the physical work environment include work space, temperature, lighting, noise, vibration, color, radiation, pressure, and the soundness of the building and the equipment. The effects of such elements can influence worker health. Excessive noise, for example, may disrupt concentration, prevent verbal communication, impair job performance and safety, and, over time, cause hearing loss.

Exposure to the sun is another problem. Those who work outdoors, including migrant farm workers, construction workers, and groundskeepers, are especially at risk for skin cancer and for deleterious effects of dust, chemical pollutants, and so forth. These workers are also exposed to temperature extremes that put them at risk for frostbite in the winter and heatstroke in the summer.

Exposure to bloodborne pathogens, such as hepatitis B and C and HIV, can have serious or deadly effects on health

care workers. Extremes in pressure, such as those experienced by deep-sea divers or by persons working at high altitudes or in tunnels, can cause improper gas exchange and tissue damage affecting the ears, sinuses, and teeth.

Some employees work in confined spaces in mines, chemical plants, oil refineries, cargo ships, and airplanes. These workers typically breathe recycled air and may also suffer from insufficient exposure to sunlight. They may be exposed to additional hazards as a result of sudden events such as fires or explosions. Many physical factors in confined work areas can threaten safety, such as lack of protection against sparks from an acetylene torch, insufficient lighting, or weak scaffolding. Despite awareness of these hazards, incidences of occupational injury leading to death continue to remain high.

Each day, an average of 9000 workers suffer a disabling work-related injury, and 17 of them die from that injury, while 137 persons die from work-related diseases (USDHHS, 2000; NIOSH, 2002). There were 4.3 fatal injuries per 100,000 workers in 2000 among the total workforce, with motor vehicle–related fatalities at work accounting for the single largest percentage (23%) of deaths since 1980. Industries with the highest traumatic occupational fatality rates per 100,000 workers are mining, agriculture, forestry and fishing, and construction (USDHHS, 2000).

Chemical Factors

Chemical factors are the chemical agents present in the work environment that may threaten worker health and safety. Numerous chemicals are found in the raw materials, production processes, and daily operations of industries and businesses, including petroleum and chemical industries, dry cleaners, painters, food companies, photographers, automobile manufacturers, plastics factories, pharmaceutical companies, and hospitals. In addition, farming continues to introduce herbicides and insecticides into the environment at an alarming rate, with devastating consequences (Buranatrevedh & Roy, 2001). Although chemicals are frequently associated with gases, they are also present in solvents, mists, vapors, dusts, and solids.

Depending on their form and structure, chemicals can enter the human body through the lungs, gastrointestinal tract, or skin. Understanding the toxicology of chemicals is essential for identifying (1) the amount of chemical exposure that produces toxicity, (2) the routes by which chemicals enter the body, and (3) the appropriate personal protection for workers. For example, lead enters the body through all three routes—lungs, gastrointestinal tract, and skin. Workers exposed to toxic levels of lead must wear protective clothing, maintain good hand-washing practices, avoid eating or smoking on the job to prevent ingestion, and employ appropriate respiratory protection to prevent inhalation.

Many toxic chemicals, such as insecticides, are taken for granted in daily use, and their toxicity is frequently ignored. But careless handling and needless exposure can cause serious burns, poisoning, asphyxia, tissue damage, or even cancer. Some inert, nontoxic industrial materials, such as resins and polymers, may decompose and form toxic byproducts when heated. Workers need to be warned of and protected from the hazards associated with the materials they use on the job. With proper handling and protection, toxicity can be prevented. Ideally, all toxic substances should be eliminated through substitution of nontoxic agents, if such chemicals exist.

Inhalation of harmful substances is common in the workplace. The highest rate of inhalation-related deaths (from all substances) occur among miners, firefighters, farmers, and those in forestry and fishing occupations. Almost half of all inhalation victims are constructing, repairing, cleaning, inspecting, or painting when the injury occurs. Overall, carbon monoxide is the most frequently inhaled substance (33.5%), and the incidence of carbon monoxide poisoning is twice as high in the winter as in the summer (Valent et al., 2002).

Biologic Factors

Biologic factors are living organisms found in the work environment. These include bacteria, viruses, rickettsiae, molds, fungi, parasites of various types, insects, animals, and even toxic plants. Potential hazards, such as infectious or parasitic diseases, may derive from exposure to contaminated water or to insects. Other vehicles include improper waste or sewage disposal, unsanitary work environments, improper food handling, and unsanitary personal practices.

Workers in every setting have a unique set of potential biologic hazards. Agricultural workers, for instance, are subject to a condition called "farmer's lung," which comes from inhaling fungi-contaminated grain dust. Employees at an automobile brake manufacturing facility in Ohio who were routinely exposed to metalworking fluid became ill from exposure to aerosolized nontuberculous mycobacteria (NTM), which probably multiplied in the thousands of gallons of fluid they worked with on a regular basis ("Respiratory illness," 2002). Other employees were hospitalized with respiratory illness traced to *Staphylococcus aureus*, hepatitis B virus, HIV, and other infectious agents that threaten many health care workers. Brucellosis (undulant fever) and Q fever from infected cattle are threats to slaughterhouse workers. Outdoor workers, such as builders, forest rangers, and environmental specialists, face the hazards of insect and animal attack as well as exposure to toxic plants such as poison oak and poison ivy.

Ergonomic Factors

Ergonomic factors include all the interactions between the worker, the demands of the job, the work setting, and the overall environment. **Ergonomics** (sometimes called human engineering) has become a field of study in occupational health concerned with workplace, tool, and task design and how well they match the physiologic, anatomic, and psychological characteristics and capabilities of the worker.

For our purposes, ergonomic factors are the customs, laws, design, and expectations of the work itself, such as all the physiologic and psychological demands on the job as well as other workplace stressors that can cause anxiety. These include physical conditions in a work space (engineering stressors), such as the design of necessary tools, equipment, lighting, or ventilation; physical positions workers must assume; motions they must make to do the job; and bad habits associated with carrying out the work, such as improper lifting habits. Increasing diversity, technology, and task complexity underscore the need for changes in the work environment.

Migrant farm workers in some southwestern states as recently as 1984 were required to use short-handled hoes to speed production and maximize crop yield and were required to spend hours stooping over plants in this doubled-up position. This caused serious skeletal and internal injuries, some of which were permanent. Farm workers often suffer from a lack of toilet facilities or drinking water in the fields. Stooping or squatting for hours can cause bladder and uterine problems in females (Olmos, Ybarra, & Monterrey, 1999) (see Chapter 33).

There can be organizational stressors in the company or industry itself involving the chain of command, policies, or procedures. Sometimes, an employer's expectations or unrealistic job demands can provoke stress as well. In such situations, the organization becomes the target of treatment, not the individual. When these factors begin to have an impact on individuals' health, job stress results. Long periods of job stress, which is manifested in feelings of anxiety, frustration, and fatigue, can lead to job strain. Job strain can cause workers to lose interest in the job; it can also undermine the morale of others and may even be unsafe. Some extreme cases of job burnout result in former employees' using violence or sabotage against the company or its employees.

Psychosocial Factors

Psychosocial factors include the responses and behaviors that workers exhibit on the job. These behaviors come from the attitudes and values learned from their culture, life experiences, and worksite norms. They are the workers' responses to the work and the work milieu. Similar work conditions can evoke different responses. Within the same work setting, some people may seem fatigued, tense, bored, angry, depressed, or agitated, whereas others may seem enthusiastic and energized. Repetitive work bores some people, whereas others see it as an opportunity for reflection. Certain types of work may challenge some but threaten others.

The nature of the work, as much as the working conditions, can evoke certain responses. Work that is time sensitive or that conflicts with personal values can create tremendous stress for some employees. Ethical dilemmas, such as selling or promoting a product or service that might be injurious to the public (eg, unreliable used cars), can cause emotional conflict for people. Peer pressure can also add stress—for instance, when one employee is forced to agree with the majority, such as during strikes or labor disputes. Unrealistic personal expectations and unattainable aspirations can lead to chronic stress and fatigue. Psychological stress can result from personal problems such as a terminally ill spouse, a painful divorce or child custody battle, or other family difficulties or crises. Such problems can result in depression or even despair. These types of personal dilemmas influence the quality and quantity of work produced and, in many professions, can compromise worker safety if a worker is preoccupied and functioning inadequately. Furthermore, chronic work stress combined with marital dissolution increases the risk of mortality in men (Matthews & Gump, 2002).

Obviously, these five factors vary in their intensity and in their potential for threat to worker health, depending on the individual and the work environment. They present a core of critical data for occupational health assessment and planning (see Levels of Prevention Matrix). The nurse is required to assess not only the environment but also the workers' response to the factors discussed.

LEVELS OF PREVENTION MATRIX

SITUATION: Back Injuries Among Home Health Workers.

GOAL: Using the three levels of prevention, negative health conditions are avoided, or promptly diagnosed and treated, and the fullest possible potential is restored.

PRIMARY PREVENTION		SECONDARY PREVENTION		TERTIARY PREVENTION		
Health Promotion and Education	*Health Protection*	*Early Diagnosis*	*Prompt Treatment*	*Rehabilitation*	*Primary Prevention*	
					Health Promotion and Education	*Health Protection*
• Good body posture, movements, and lifting are necessary to prevent back injuries • Inservice training is required of all staff who provide direct client care: include positioning, transferring, and lifting clients • Appropriate safety techniques need to be used consistently with clients	• Health care workers should use the following appropriately: lifting devices, back supporters, and other working attire, such as wearing sturdy shoes	• A suspected injury needs prompt attention: report of the injury, discontinuing work (if needed), assistance to health care provider or emergency department, and prompt diagnosis	• Take appropriate actions, including rest, medical follow-up, drug therapy, exercise, heat, or hydrotherapy	• On return to work, the employee should gradually work up to full potential and use all safety precautions mentioned earlier • For long-term back injury, seek alternative treatment, including transcutaneous electric nerve stimulation (TENS) units, acupressure, acupuncture, biofeedback, surgery, or other treatment modalities offered at reputable pain clinics	• Maintain long-term back health by using all primary prevention techniques as a "way of life"	• If alternative treatments provide no relief, consider a change of occupation, part-time work, or, as a last resort, disability and the consequences of living on a limited income

WORK-RELATED HEALTH PROBLEMS

What are the health problems of the working population specifically? As previously mentioned, Americans are exposed to numerous safety and health hazards in the workplace. The goal of *Healthy People 2010* is to "promote the health and safety of people at work through prevention and early intervention." The objectives focus on the following 11 occupational health areas (USDHHS, 2000):

1. Reduce deaths from work-related injuries
2. Reduce work-related injuries resulting in medical treatment, lost time from work, or restricted work activity
3. Reduce the rate of injury and illness cases involving days away from work due to overexertion or repetitive motion
4. Reduce pneumoconiosis deaths
5. Reduce deaths from work-related homicides
6. Reduce work-related assault
7. Reduce the number of persons who have elevated blood lead level concentrations from work exposures
8. Reduce occupational skin diseases or disorders among full-time workers
9. Increase the proportion of worksites employing 50 or more persons that provide programs to prevent or reduce employee stress
10. Reduce occupational needlestick injuries among health care workers
11. Reduce new cases of work-related, noise-induced hearing loss

Occupational Disease

Occupational disease is any condition or disorder that results from an exposure related to employment. Collecting data on occupational diseases has been difficult because the lag time is so great between exposure, onset of the disease, and actual clinical evidence (Verma, Purdham, & Roels, 2002). Silicosis, for example, takes 15 years to develop. Some cases of mesothelioma have not become evident until 25 years after the worker was last exposed to asbestos. Lung disease in workers occurs gradually over time. Most often, exposures do not result in acute symptoms, and, once the symptoms do occur, little can be done. It is for this reason that respiratory disease prevention is so important. Many workers who have changed jobs or retired only later discover a disease that may be connected to previous employment. Documenting this connection poses problems. Nonetheless, more sophisticated epidemiologic methods and an improved database are enabling public health and industrial researchers to demonstrate linkages and make more accurate predictions.

Occupational settings give rise to a number of environmental health hazards. Workers who are exposed to heavy metals such as lead, mercury, and arsenic are likely to develop related diseases. Although miners are often exposed to high levels of radon, sawmill workers are at greater risk for lymphomas. Researchers have also demonstrated the relationship between cotton mill dust and byssinosis, a lung disease formerly thought not to exist in the United States.

Many rescue workers at the World Trade Center in 2001 were exposed to toxic materials in the burning rubble pile after the buildings' collapse. Exposures included asbestos from insulation and fireproofing materials; crystalline silica in the concrete; mercury from fluorescent lights; carbon monoxide from fires and engine exhaust; heavy metals from building materials; hydrogen sulfide from sewers, anaerobically decomposing bodies, and spoiled food; and many other toxic chemical compounds ("Occupational exposures," 2002).

Epidemiologists are also studying the connection between skin diseases and materials used on the job, a problem of considerable magnitude because dermatologic problems are among the most common occupational diseases.

It is estimated that 30 million workers are exposed to noise levels that can cause impaired hearing, and more than 9 million workers in the United States have some degree of noise-induced hearing loss. As many as 28% of all reported occupational conditions relate to noise-induced hearing loss. In a study of three construction trade group workers— roofers, laborers, and carpenters—it was determined that there are tasks or tools producing high levels of noise that had not been previously identified by trade representatives. Computer-based training programs provided construction workers with information on noise levels specific to their trades. The information presented allowed them to put their exposures into perspective and gave them knowledge and thus power over their decisions to wear hearing protection, ensuring better decision-making and, in the long term, greater likelihood of hearing loss prevention (Kerr, Brosseau, & Johnson, 2002). Occupational health and environmental nurses will be better equipped to design more effective protective and preventive measures as knowledge of occupational injuries and illnesses increases.

Health Problems Related to Ergonomics

Another set of health problems affecting workers stems from the ergonomic stressors. With increasing technology and changing work environments, new concerns about such factors as lack of natural light and air, poor lighting, loud noise, isolation, and temperature extremes have surfaced. Also, an increasing amount of research is being devoted to the study of video display terminal exposure, which may result in visual problems, and to musculoskeletal problems such as carpal tunnel syndrome, which may result from inappropriate positioning at workstations. Among hazardous waste workers in one study, the limited use of protective respiratory equipment was based on ineffective employee knowledge, beliefs, and attitudes; complaints of physical and psychological effects when using the equipment; and work-related conditions and the support of others (Salazar et al., 2001).

Work-Related Emotional Disturbances

There is evidence that "the number of employees experiencing psychologic problems related to occupational stress has increased rapidly in Western countries" (van der Klink et al., 2001). In Britain, it is estimated that 40 million workdays are lost each year related to mental and emotional problems. Pressures at work to increase productivity or a physically stressful work environment (eg, one with excessive noise, heat, or vibration), coupled with the perception of an inability to control the demands, can result in job stress and strain. Personal problems, such as those dealing with finances or relationships, can also adversely affect a worker's job performance. Either source of stress creates a vicious circle, perpetuating and escalating the problems in both settings with the potential for unsafe practices at work and harmful behaviors at home.

Workplace Violence

A related stressor is violence in the workplace stemming from "disgruntled employee syndrome" or from interpersonal relationship problems that escalate into violent acts against an employed spouse or significant other. Each year between 1992 and 1996, more than 2 million persons were victims of a violent crime while they were at work (USDHHS, 2000). Homicide is the second-leading cause of death at work. Workers in retail establishments, taxi drivers, and people working at night are the most vulnerable when robbery is the motive. Increasingly, individuals with relationship problems have sought out an ex-spouse or ex-lover at work and killed the person, at times also jeopardizing others in the work setting. More than three fourths of workplace homicides involve a firearm.

Prevention strategies for violence in the workplace fall into three categories: administrative controls, behavior strategies, and environmental designs. Administrative controls include procedures for handling money and for unlocking and opening up for business each day and staffing policies. Behavior strategies include training for all employees in conflict resolution and implementation of a nonviolence policy. Environmental designs may include such factors as lighting, security alarm systems, and protective equipment.

OCCUPATIONAL HEALTH PROGRAMS

Because the working population is primarily composed of healthy adults, the goal of occupational health is to maintain that healthy, productive workforce by providing a safe and healthy work environment and promoting healthful personal behavior. Occupational health programs therefore encompass the entire spectrum of health care, including the practice of disease prevention, health protection, and health promotion (Pender, Murdaugh, & Parsons, 2002).

Occupational health programs have grown tremendously since World War II. Many manufacturing plants, service organizations, and commercial establishments, including department stores, have instituted some kind of health program for employees. Some programs still concentrate on providing emergency care, but most are beginning to recognize the importance of prevention and health promotion. For example, in 1981, the Adolph Coors Company opened the nation's first comprehensive wellness facility. Mesa Petroleum estimated annual savings of $1.6 million in health care costs for its 650 employees as a result of its wellness program. Other major companies, such as General Electric Aircraft, Tenneco, AT&T Communications, and Johnson & Johnson, have lowered absenteeism and health care costs by initiating health promotion programs.

The variety of work in the United States, as well as the number and type of workers employed, creates a wide range of potential hazards and the need for various on-site health programs. For example, construction and mine workers are at high risk for certain types of injuries and illnesses. Workers require an aggressive surveillance program that focuses on prevention and personal protection. In contrast, professionals such as lawyers and accountants are generally at low risk for encountering hazardous physical conditions at work but may experience psychological stress. Therefore, they may benefit from a health promotion program that emphasizes stress management and physical fitness.

Disease Prevention Programs

To determine the priorities for intervention and the appropriate health goals and objectives for an aggregate of workers, it is essential to conduct an assessment of both workers and the workplace environment. Knowledge of workers' job classifications and the types of materials they handle and are exposed to provides clues to potential hazardous substances and working conditions. This information should be compiled, together with data on the characteristics of the aggregate in terms of age, gender, race, and existing health conditions. In addition, workers' compensation claims and occupational safety and health reports should be examined to identify subpopulations at risk for occupational illness and injury.

The practice of making prevention a priority holds primary importance in occupational health, because work-related injuries and illnesses are frequently irreversible. Development of a mesothelioma from asbestos exposure and loss of a limb are conditions for which there are no cures. Interventions, therefore, are aimed at eliminating the hazards by such methods as redesigning equipment to provide safeguards and substituting materials that are as effective but less toxic. *Healthy People 2000* (USDHHS, 1997) intended to promote health and disease prevention objectives in the area of occupational health and safety:

The reduction of leading work-related injuries and illnesses and the prevention of new problems require that accrediting bodies of all scientific disciplines understand the role of their professions in recognizing or preventing occupational and environmental problems. Progress in this area also depends greatly on improvements in surveillance to identify high-risk groups and to assist in developing appropriate prevention strategies.

The *Healthy People 2010* objectives add the goal of eliminating health disparities to the framework (USDHHS, 2000) (Fig. 29–1).

Once occupational hazards are identified, they can be controlled by substituting safer materials or safer practices, or both. In addition, manufacturing processes can be changed and hazardous materials can be isolated. Exhaust methods and other engineering techniques can be used to control the source of occupational hazards. Special clothing and other protective devices can and should be used. Efforts must be made to educate and motivate employees and employers to comply with safety procedures that focus on prevention (Salazar et al., 2001).

Health Protection Programs

Making protection a priority becomes essential when hazardous exposures cannot be eliminated. Construction workers, for example, wear hardhats and steel-toed safety shoes to pro-

tect themselves from falling objects. Health care workers who may be exposed to bodily fluids wear gloves, gowns, masks, and eye protectors. The protection of workers is frequently achieved through legislation and regulation. The Occupational Safety and Health Act of 1970 provided the impetus for worker protection. More recently, employee right-to-know legislation focused on safety training for employees who are working with potentially hazardous agents. Some of the changes made in the workplace environment include the use of international symbols to warn employees of potentially hazardous materials (eg, red on white background for electrical hazard, black on red background for biohazard, black on yellow background for radiation hazard). Other OSHA-prompted changes include the use of Material Safety Data Sheets (MSDS) and implementation of OSHA's standards regarding exposure to bloodborne pathogens. The enforcement of such regulations will continue to be the key intervention for ensuring that workers are adequately protected on their jobs.

Occupational safety programs are available in most industries, especially those employing larger numbers of workers. These programs include plant surveillance, safety violation reporting, and worker safety education. All have the goal of protecting the employee.

Health Promotion Programs

A health promotion program is designed to promote healthier lifestyles by encouraging necessary behavioral change.

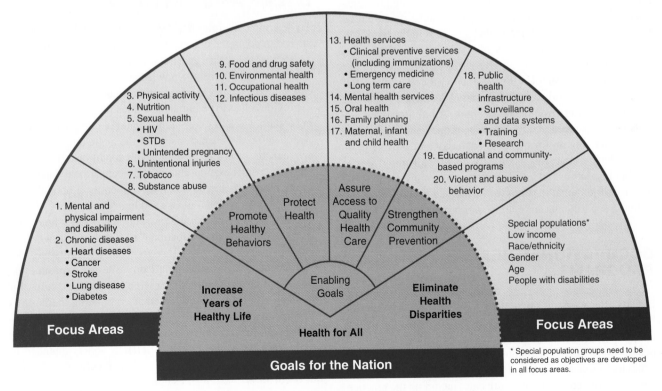

FIGURE 29–1.   Vision of 2010: Healthy people in healthy communities. (U. S. Department of Health and Human Services, Office of Disease Prevention and Health Promotion. [1997]. *Developing objectives for Healthy People 2010.* Washington, DC: U.S. Printing Office, p. 14.)

The practice of making health promotion a priority has appropriately received much attention and activity in the workplace over the past decade. The workplace is ideal for conducting health promotion efforts for two important reasons: (1) the majority of the healthy population can be reached at work, and (2) employers view wellness programs as legitimate, worthwhile employee benefits to promote and support.

Employee assistance programs are offered in federal and state governmental agencies and many private industries. These programs are cooperatively sponsored by employers and bargaining agencies. The intent is to promote the mental health of the employee by providing an outlet for employee concerns.

It is significant for community health that health promotion activities in the workplace can involve long-term interventions. This allows for the use of various educational and motivational strategies as well as a systematic plan for monitoring and evaluating the programs.

The work environment can serve as a model for a healthy community. Such health policies as creating a smoke-free environment, offering low-fat meals in the company cafeteria, discouraging alcohol abuse, and encouraging injury prevention (eg, using seat belts) establish health norms for company personnel. Many of these healthy behaviors can also have a positive impact on employees' homes and families (Pender, Murdaugh, & Parsons, 2002).

Typical health promotion programs include exercise, weight loss, smoking cessation, and nutrition education. There is growing evidence that wellness efforts are effective. Some research indicates that, as a result of wellness promotion, employees have increased self-esteem, improved job performance and job satisfaction, decreased absenteeism, and less use of company health services. The Health Action Plan is one attempt to promote health in corporations because it promotes the company name (Haughton et al., 2001) (see Research: Bridge to Practice).

Health promotion programs in the workplace have the potential to provide a significant contribution to adult health and to research and development in this new arena of wellness. Cost and production incentives increase employers' acceptance of methods that enhance employee wellness. More research is needed to demonstrate the correlation between healthy employees and increased productivity on the job. Health promotion will continue to be a vital area of emphasis for the working community in the 21st century.

Additional Workplace Health Services

Although employers are not presently required to provide treatment for nonoccupational injuries and illnesses (ie, injury or illness not incurred at work), many companies do provide such

---

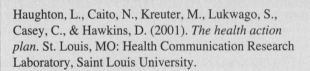

RESEARCH: BRIDGE TO PRACTICE

Haughton, L., Caito, N., Kreuter, M., Lukwago, S., Casey, C., & Hawkins, D. (2001). *The health action plan.* St. Louis, MO: Health Communication Research Laboratory, Saint Louis University.

In 2001, a team from the Health Communication Research Laboratory and a representative of the Missouri Department of Health worked on a project, "Worksite Wellness: An Environmental and Policy Approach."

Using statistical data in the areas of nutrition, physical activity, and tobacco, the team shared with various corporations the negative effects on their company name and the health of their employees if nutrition is compromised, physical activity is not encouraged, and tobacco is used. The researchers devised an assessment tool to assess the levels of corporate policies and follow-through in activities to promote wellness in the areas of nutrition, physical activity, and tobacco. They sought companies that, on being approached, invited them to conduct the assessment. A team assessed company policy and the worksite. A summary of the results was returned to company administration to use as they saw fit.

A "Health Action Plan" summary, utilizing a point system, was presented to each company in a spiral-bound report. It focused on the organizational climate, including characteristics and administrative support for worksite health promotion, tobacco policies and use, nutrition policies and the availability of healthy foods, and physical activity facilities, policies, and programs. In follow-up sections, the team rated how well the company name was doing in the area of cardiovascular health promotion, identified its current strengths, and described specific steps needed for the company to become a model for cardiovascular health promotion in the workplace. Tips were given to improve the company's total points and the number of points possible. Additional sections included local community resources and national resources for the three areas.

By using data from previous research studies, this health promotion plan focused on engaging a company to reflect on employee health, in policy and action, and enticed them into promoting employee health. The summary was designed to guide companies toward making positive policy changes and becoming model programs for employee cardiovascular health.

services. One reason is that it is difficult to determine where health problems such as muscle strain, influenza, and minor rashes are acquired. Therefore, it is simpler to provide care for the problem regardless of its source. The on-site treatment of minor acute injury and illness as well as employee counseling depends on the philosophy of the company, the employment of an occupational health nurse, and the company's prior experience with offering these services as an employee benefit.

From the nurse's perspective, the advantages of offering nonoccupational health services are the following:

1. The occupational health nurse develops rapport with employees and can detect health problems early.
2. Loss of employee productivity is minimized if treatment is given on site.
3. The occupational health nurse, through triage, can decide which cases require medical attention and which can safely be managed by the nurse.
4. The occupational health nurse can provide needed, ongoing, personal health education and counseling in the context of a more holistic view of the worker.
5. On-site chronic disease management (eg, hypertension monitoring) increases compliance, thereby saving costs of physician visits and complications associated with noncompliance.
6. The occupational health nurse provides employees with personal contact—a valued commodity in high-technology work environments.

A number of occupational health nurses have expressed concern that spending too much time on nonoccupational illnesses could keep them from pursuing an aggressive occupational health surveillance program. As occupational health nurses learn more about environmental factors that threaten workers' health, they will probably spend less time with illness management and move more aggressively toward primary prevention, protection, and health promotion efforts. The direction of health care programs in the future is covered later in this chapter.

ROLE OF THE OCCUPATIONAL AND ENVIRONMENTAL HEALTH NURSE

Community health nurses have a long history of involvement in occupational health. In 1895, the Vermont Marble Company hired the first industrial nurse in the United States to care for its employees and their families. At the time, it was an unusual demonstration of interest in employee welfare. The nursing service, which consisted mostly of home visiting and care of the sick, was free to employees and their families. Gradually that role changed. World War II showed a marked increase in employment of industrial public health nurses, who practiced illness prevention and health education among employees at work.

In addition to emergency care and nursing of ill employees, the activities of many industrial nurses involved safety education, hygiene, nutrition, and improvement of working conditions. Yet a significantly high number of industrial injuries and sick employees kept many nurses too busy to do anything but care for the ill. They might see more than 75 patients a day in the plant dispensary, where they provided first aid and medications. Employee health programs have improved as socioeconomic and political pressures have created improved safety and health standards for the work environment. Similarly, these developments have changed and expanded the nurse's role. The role of an **occupational and environmental health nurse** is to ensure that the workforce is healthy and productive, as evidenced by the nursing practice standards developed by the professional organization known as the Association of Occupational Health Nurses (Display 29–8).

Special Skills and Demands

The nurse's role in occupational health, as previously mentioned, has traditionally focused on illness and injury care. This directly resulted from the knowledge and skills obtained in basic nursing education. During the last decade, a number of nursing education programs (primarily on the graduate level) have developed a specialty focus in occupational and environmental health. In addition, many continuing education programs provide occupational and environmental health nurses with updated information and skill training for identifying and assisting in the management of the physical, chemical, biologic, ergonomic, and psychosocial factors in the work environment that can affect worker health and safety. As a result, the occupational health nurse's role is not universal; it depends on the type and philosophy of the company, type and number of workers, health professionals involved, exposures and potential hazards in the work environment, and knowledge and skills of the nurse.

Nurses who select the field of occupational health and safety encounter experiences that differ significantly from those found in an acute care setting. To make the adjustment, the nurse should be aware of the factors that make occupational health unique.

Unlike hospitals or ambulatory care centers, the workplace is a non–health care institution in which production or service (not health care) is the primary goal. The occupational and environmental health nurse participates in the organization's goals through activities that contribute to the productivity of the workforce.

An occupational and environmental health nurse in the organization is in a staff position, taking on the role of a consultant, educator, or role model in the workplace, but has no supervisory responsibilities or power to hire or fire workers. The nurse is generally responsible for management of the occupational health unit, serving the needs of employees and management personnel.

The occupational and environmental health nurse, especially in smaller organizations, may be the only nurse in the company. As a result, she or he has none of the on-site con-

DISPLAY 29-8

Standards of Occupational and Environmental Health Nursing Practice

Standards of Clinical Nursing Practice

Standard I. *Assessment:* The occupational and environmental health nurse systematically assesses the health status of the individual client or population and the environment.

Standard II. *Diagnosis:* The occupational and environmental health nurse analyzes assessed data to formulate diagnoses.

Standard III. *Outcome Identification:* The occupational and environmental health nurse identifies outcomes specific to the client.

Standard IV. *Planning:* The occupational and environmental health nurse develops a goal-directed plan that is comprehensive and formulates interventions to attain expected outcomes.

Standard V. *Implementation:* The occupational and environmental health nurse implements interventions to attain desired outcomes identified in the plan.

Standard VI. *Evaluation:* The occupational and environmental health nurse systematically and continuously evaluates responses to interventions and progress toward the achievement of desired outcomes.

Standard VII. *Resource Management:* The occupational and environmental health nurse secures and manages the resources that support an occupational health and safety program.

Standard VIII. *Professional Development:* The occupational and environmental health nurse assumes responsibility for professional development to enhance professional growth and maintain competency.

Standard IX. *Collaboration:* The occupational and environmental health nurse collaborates with employees, management, other health care providers, professionals and community representatives.

Standard X. *Research:* The occupational and environmental health nurse uses research findings in practice and contributes to the scientific base in occupational and environmental health nursing to improve practice and advance the profession.

(Adapted from American Association of Occupational Health Nurses. (2002). *Standards of occupational and environmental health nursing practice.* Retrieved on January 30, 2004, from www.aaohn.org/practice/standards.cfm)

There are various causes of job stress for the occupational and environmental health nurse, and there may be related personal, professional, and employer factors. The nurse may experience role ambiguity due to a lack of professional preparation or inadequate orientation and continuing education. The corporate culture and leadership may foster work overload, be nonsupportive, and have limited career opportunities for the nurse. Occupational and environmental health nurses need to apply strategies to reduce job stress and potential job strain by modeling health-affirming choices, networking with other nurses and professional organizations in the community, and setting appropriate occupational health standards.

The client base served in occupational health is a well-adult population with whom long-term contact is possible. Occupational and environmental health nurses, therefore, have the chance to know their clients well and have opportunities to work with them through various stages of personal as well as health service–related incidents. Such continuity of health care can challenge occupational health nurses to use all of the community health nursing model interventions—education, engineering, and enforcement.

Finally, the practice focus is oriented to the aggregate; the nurse serves a worker population. Environmental factors significantly influence the health and safety of workers. Therefore, occupational health nurses need to constantly monitor the work environment and assess the health needs of the entire worker population to identify those at risk, particularly workers in hazardous lines of work, and to develop prevention, promotion, and protection programs (Display 29–9).

Community-Based Occupational Health Nursing

Agencies external to business and industry also provide occupational and environmental health nursing services. Historically, public health nurses from visiting nurse associations made home visits to sick employees and their families. In subsequent years, public health agencies provided part-time nursing services to small companies. These services included supervising the work environment, conducting health examinations, keeping records, teaching about and counseling on health issues, providing first aid, giving immunizations, and referring workers to community resources. More recently, community health nursing services have offered health screening and health promotion programs. Furthermore, occupational and environmental health nurse consultants based in state departments of health provide consultation and continuing education programs to nurses employed in occupational health settings.

Hospital-based occupational health programs, large medical-industrial health clinics, and insurance companies also provide occupational and environmental health nursing services. These services may be in the form of direct care (rehabilitation of an injured worker) or indirect care (consultation on implementing regulations regarding record keeping or compiling health statistics).

sultation and direction that are needed for comfortable, competent, and independent decision-making. Nurses who use critical thinking skills to develop a framework for independent problem-solving enhance their efficiency. A nurse who works alone may feel isolated and need to collaborate with the occupational health and safety team members.

DISPLAY 29-9

Occupational and Environmental Health Nursing Care Plan

Evelyn Robbins has been the Occupational and Environmental Health Nurse at ABC Metals for 4 years. She works with management, the company physician (who works at ABC Metals 2 days a week), union representatives, unit foremen, individual employees, and representatives from the community businesses and neighborhoods surrounding the plant. The company employs 400 workers—380 in manufacturing, primarily an assembly line making telephone electrical boxes, and 20 management and administrative staff.

Recently, 12 employees came to the worksite clinic complaining of hand injuries that had not occurred before. Ms. Robbins treated the wounds, reported the occurrences to the foremen involved, and reported the incidents to management. In addition, she wanted to explore the cause of these injuries so that they could be interrupted. She used the nursing process in her exploration.

Assessment
- Tour the areas where the incidents occurred
- Inquire among the foremen to determine whether there was a change in routine, equipment, employee assignment, or product being manufactured
- Ask injured employees what they were doing when the injury occurred
- Reassess wounds for likenesses and differences; for example, was it the right or left hand and was it on the same part of the hand in each case?

Diagnoses
- Wounds occurred in factory areas where a new piece of equipment had been installed
- Injured employees did not receive orientation to the equipment

Plan
- Plan to work with foremen to provide an orientation for all employees who work with the new equipment
- Plan an orientation program (with foremen, union representative, and one employee from each unit in the factory) for all employees before working with new equipment in the future, to prevent further injuries

Implementation
- Implement the orientation for employees who work with the new equipment
- Initiate the orientation program as new equipment is introduced into the factory

Evaluation
- Have there been any new equipment-related injuries in the factory?
- Has there been any change in general safety in the factory related to the increased focus on safety with new equipment?

A continuing unmet need is attending to the health of workers in smaller companies. These companies have more hazards because equipment and controls are often inadequate. They seldom, if ever, have a health professional on site. Attempts have been made by some communities to provide needed health protection services, but no sustained efforts exist. Community health nurses are in a position to accept this challenge and develop a system that will ensure ongoing service to this high-risk population.

Members of the Occupational Health Team

Today, the two professionals who generally provide on-site occupational health services are the occupational and environmental health nurse and the safety engineer. Other members of the interprofessional team may include an industrial hygienist, epidemiologist, toxicologist, and occupational physician. However, these specialists usually are employed only by large corporations, or they provide only selected part-time services on a contractual basis. Therefore, the position of occupational and environmental health nurse in a large company or of the community health nurse who serves smaller companies is the cornerstone of occupational health.

Collaboration may take time, but it is worth the investment. The occupational health nurse must gain the respect and trust of management and establish open communication to influence company policies regarding the nature and scope of health programs.

Depending on the size of the company and its products or services, the occupational health nurse may also collaborate with any or all of the following people: insurance carriers, union representatives, employee assistance counselors, industrial hygienists, safety engineers, company or outside lawyers, toxicologists, human resources personnel, and the community. Any comprehensive assessment of employee health and safety problems, as well as any health promotion program, requires cooperation and assistance from many people working in various departments within the organization.

Finally, the occupational health team is not complete without the workers themselves. Employees can help identify problems and needs while contributing to decision-making about health programs. Their cooperation in implementing and evaluating programs is essential for an effective health protection and promotion effort.

Future Trends

A broad goal for occupational health is to promote and maintain the highest level of physical, social, and emotional health for all workers. In practice, this goal is only beginning to be realized in selected instances. Nevertheless, it is a worthy and, more importantly, an essential objective in the realization of an energized and productive working community.

However, the rapid and fundamental changes in U. S. businesses and the economy in the 1990s and early 2000s have added four critical issues that affect the practice of occupational and environmental health nursing. First, the downturn in the global economy, and in the economy of the United States specifically, has skeletonized many worksites, shut down companies, eliminated night or evening shifts, or moved companies to less expensive communities. In addition, several major scandals have eliminated employees within hours, such as with Enron and Worldcom corporations. Second, increasing worldwide competition requires businesses to remain competitive by reducing or controlling operating costs at the lowest level possible. Third, there has been an increase in technologic hazards that require a sophisticated approach as well as a knowledge of toxicology, epidemiology, ergonomics, and public health principles. Fourth, health care costs continue to escalate at faster rates than most company profits do (see The Global Community).

Current occupational and environmental health nurse practices will continue to evolve to meet future needs. The focus will shift from one-on-one health services to a new role involving broader environmental, business, and research skills.

Current occupational health nurse activities include the following:

1. Supervising care for emergencies and minor illnesses
2. Counseling employees about health risks
3. Following up with employees' workers' compensation claims
4. Performing periodic health assessments
5. Evaluating the health status of employees returning to work

Future occupational health nurse activities will involve the following:

1. Analyzing trends (health promotion, risk reduction, and health expenditures)
2. Developing programs suited to corporate needs
3. Recommending more efficient and cost-effective in-house health services
4. Determining cost-effective alternatives to health programs and services
5. Collaborating with others to identify problems and propose solutions

As we move further into the 21st century, occupational and environmental health nurses and management will share the goal of developing a healthy, productive, and profitable company. A healthy company consists of healthy and productive employees, and healthy employees mean lower health care costs. Lower costs result in an increased competitive edge and higher profits. Higher profits can make more

THE GLOBAL COMMUNITY

Shamian, J. (2000). On the heels of Florence Nightingale: Re-energizing hospital care. *Reflections on Nursing Leadership, 26*(1), 24–26.

IMPACT OF A NATIONAL HEALTH CARE SYSTEM ON CANADIAN NURSES

Health Canada's executive director of nursing, Dr. Judith Shamian, notes that Canada enjoys a first rate, publicly funded health care system. As a result, Canadian citizens view health as a right, not a privilege. Although most Canadian nurses share this perspective, they also acknowledge a dissonance between educational preparation of nurses and the demands that the current health care environment makes on their clinical practice. In 1998, Dr. Shamian was a co-investigator in a study of 8000 hospital nurses in Ontario, Canada. It was part of a comprehensive, multinational examination whose purpose was to determine which characteristics of the nurses are most likely to produce the best clinical outcomes and result in job satisfaction. Results from the Ontario study showed the following:

- When compared with other employee groups, nurses suffer greater emotional exhaustion.
- Nurses trust peers but are less trusting of their managers.
- The health condition of the nurse is described as being poor when compared with other employee groups.

Implications of the study are that nurses deserve greater respect for the important service they provide. Canadian nurses bear a tremendous social obligation to deliver health services in a system that does not appear to value them. Politicians and decision-makers need to be informed of nurses' contributions to both the physical and the economic well-being of a country. Health and nursing knowledge should address the impact of public policy. Continued research and resultant evidence-based practice have the potential to influence decisions regarding allocation of health care resources. The primary motivation for this paradigm shift is to enhance the health of the people served by any type of health care program.

resources available to support more programs and to improve employee health.

The occupational and environmental health nurse will particularly need skills in effective communication, leadership, change management, research, business acumen, and assertiveness. These tools will be crucial for effectively interpreting the occupational health nurse's role and promoting ideas. Success of programs developed by the occupational health nurse depends on establishment of positive working relationships with the other team members. Nurses involved in occupational health have a unique opportunity to help shape the health profile of the working population. The degree of that influence depends on how the nurse defines the occupational and environmental health nurse role. Also, the nurse must be able to overcome the many obstacles found in the occupational setting, including restrictive company policies, misunderstanding of the nurse's role, and lack of time for innovative program development. The nurse's role in occupational health, therefore, varies considerably. It ranges from providing only emergency care for on-the-job injuries or illness to establishing comprehensive policies and programs covering health promotion, accident and disease prevention, and innovative care for disease and disability.

Occupational and environmental health nursing demands a great deal from the nurse. Individual needs in the workplace always compete for the nurse's time and take attention away from aggregate needs, often to the detriment of the latter. To maintain a proper focus on aggregate needs requires discipline and commitment—commitment based on a different mindset and the realization that the health and productivity of workers are interrelated with the health of the community.

SUMMARY

The health care needs of adult women and men are of great concern. Many health care needs are the same among women and men, but there are significant differences that are addressed in this chapter.

Women have been neglected over the years in health research, and only in more recent years has there been a focus on women's health. Women have health care needs that change as they age from the teenage years to old age. Reproductive organ health concerns take a different focus after menopause. Diet and exercise, obesity, alcohol abuse, cancer, heart disease, and unintentional injuries remain issues that women must consider throughout their lives.

Men's health, like women's health, begins in the teen years. Decisions made as a teenager and young adult guide the man toward or away from health for the rest of his life. As risk takers, young men die from unintentional injuries more frequently than women do, and this relation is not reversed until old age. Young men should be concerned about testicular cancer, and many men are concerned with prostate health and erectile functioning as they age. However, heart disease and cancers remain important issues for men as well as women.

The 20th century has seen a shift in the leading causes of death, from communicable diseases to noncommunicable diseases. Currently, the five leading causes of death in adults are CHD, cancer, stroke, COPD, and unintentional injuries—none of them communicable diseases.

The working population in the United States, numbering 131 million, makes up the majority of the American people.

The profile of this aggregate is changing from an industrialized labor force to one of more white collar workers and professionals. The environment of the workplace is changing as well.

Five types of environmental factors, common to all work settings, can influence worker health or safety. Physical or structural elements include such things as temperature and noise extremes. Chemical factors refer to the presence of potentially hazardous chemical agents. Biologic organisms, such as viruses, bacteria, and fungi, may contaminate the work environment and cause disease. Ergonomic factors include the customs, design, and expectations of the job that influence the way people interact with their work environment. Psychosocial factors are the workers' feelings and behavior at work. Assessment of all of these factors is critical in determining appropriate occupational health interventions.

Historically, workers' health has been of little importance to the government. As a result, many have suffered unhealthy, dangerous working conditions and have contracted debilitating, often fatal, diseases and injuries. More recently, however, worker health has become a target for health intervention. Major legislation has been passed to ensure workers' rights to a safe and healthy work environment. Three of the most significant pieces of legislation are the Occupational Safety and Health Act of 1970, the Hazard Communication Act of 1986, and the Americans with Disabilities Act of 1990.

Leading work-related health problems include occupational lung diseases, injuries, and occupational cancers. New health concerns have arisen in this population that reflect the changing society, work patterns, and environment. They include job stress, ergonomic issues that relate to the computer age, emotional disturbances, and workplace violence.

The number and type of workplace injuries vary by place, time, and type of industry. Homicide is currently the second leading cause of deaths in the workplace. A variety of prevention strategies can be implemented to control workplace injuries.

Programs designed to serve the health needs of the working population should be based on an assessment of the unique needs of each setting. Occupational health services encompass the three public health practice priorities—prevention, protection, and health promotion. Preventive programs seek to eliminate potential hazards to worker health and safety. Protective services shield workers from remaining hazards. Health promotion or wellness programs seek to maintain and improve workers' health. Health services for workers may also cover nonoccupational illnesses.

Occupational and environmental health nursing applies the philosophy and skills of nursing, community, and environmental health to protecting and promoting the health of people in their workplaces. The occupational and environmental health nurse's role is evolving as business becomes more competitive and health care costs escalate at a frightening rate. That expanded role will include analyzing current trends, recommending more cost-effective and innovative in-house health services, and collaborating with other members of the multidisciplinary occupational health team, including management, to develop appropriate programs.

ACTIVITIES TO PROMOTE CRITICAL THINKING

1. Using a local newspaper, select three articles that relate to workplace violence. For each article, (a) summarize the content, (b) identify the likely cause of the violence, and (c) describe how the violence might have been prevented.
2. You are asked to offer a weight-control program for a local milk-processing plant that has 100 employees. What steps would you take to develop a successful program?
3. Using the Internet and the school library, research an injury and a disease often associated with your future profession. Write a two-page paper in which you identify the selected concerns and discuss both employee and employer responsibilities regarding management of these problems.
4. Survey your living quarters and make a room-by-room environmental assessment of potentially unsafe conditions. Describe a strategy for improving each condition.

REFERENCES

Alcoholism Center for Women. *Do you have a problem with alcohol? 20 questions for women.* Los Angeles: Author.

American Association of Occupational Health Nurses. (2002). *Standards of occupational and environmental health nursing practice.* Retrieved on January 30, 2004, from *http://www.aaohn.org/practice/standards.cfm*

American Institute for Cancer Research. (1999). *Food, nutrition and the prevention of cancer: A global perspective,* Washington, DC: Author.

American Heart Association. (2002). *2001 heart and stroke statistical update.* Dallas, TX: Author.

Arslanian-Engoren, C. (2002). Helping women seek treatment faster. *AWHONN Lifelines, 6*(2), 115–122.

Brownson, R.C., Eyler, A.A., King, A.C., Brown, D.R., Shyu, Y., & Sallis, J.F. (2000). Patterns and correlates of physical activity among US women 40 years and older. *American Journal of Public Health, 90*(2), 264–270.

Brunetta, P. (Fall 2002/Winter 2003). Lung cancer may strike women harder. *Breathe Easy* [American Lung Association of California], 3.

Buranatrevedh, S., & Roy, D. (2001). Occupational exposure to endocrine-disrupting pesticides and the potential for developing hormonal cancers. *Journal of Environmental Health, 64*(3), 17–28.

Centers for Disease Control and Prevention. (2001). Deaths: Final data for 1999. *National Vital Statistics Reports, 49*(8), 119–122.

Duvall, E.M. (1977). *Family development* (5th ed.). Philadelphia: J. B. Lippincott.

Fee, E., Brown, T.M., Lazarus, J., & Theerman, P. (2002). The effects of the corset. *American Journal of Public Health, 92*(7), 1085.

Franco, G. (2001). *De morbis artificum diatriba [Diseases of workers]*—Bernardino Ramazzini: The father of occupational medicine. *American Journal of Public Health, 91*(9), 1380–1382.

Haughton, L., Caito, N., Kreuter, M., Lukwago, S., Casey, C., & Hawkins, D. (2001). *The health action plan.* St. Louis, MO: Health Communication Research Laboratory, Saint Louis University.

Healy, B. (2002). Hormones of choice. *U. S. News & World Report, 133*(16), 53.

Kaiser Permanente. (2002). *Kaiser Permanente healthwise handbook.* Boise, ID: Healthwise.

Kerr, M.J., Brosseau, L., & Johnson, C.S. (2002). Noise levels of selected construction tasks. *AIHA Journal, 63*(3), 334–339.

Koniak-Griffin, D., Anderson, N.L.R., Verzemnieks, I., & Brecht, M. (2000). A public health nursing early intervention program for adolescent mothers: Outcomes from pregnancy through 6 weeks postpartum. *Nursing Research, 49*(3), 130–138.

Lee, J. (1978). *The new nurse in industry: A guide for the newly employed occupational health nurse* (DHEW [NIOSH] Pub. No. 78–143). Cincinnati, OH: U. S. Government Printing Office.

Matthews, K.A., & Gump, B.B. (2002). Chronic work stress and marital dissolution increase risk of posttrial mortality in men from the Multiple Risk Factor Intervention Trial. *Archives of Internal Medicine, 162*(3), 309–315.

McDiarmid, M.A. (2000). The Occupational Safety and Health Administration and the public health model. *American Journal of Public Health, 98*(2), 186–187.

Morris, R.B. (Ed.) (1976). *The United States Department of Labor bicentennial history of the American worker.* Washington, DC: U. S. Government Printing Office.

Mueller, M. (2002). *Men: You and your body.* Santa Cruz, CA: ETR Associates.

National Center for Health Statistics. (2000). *Health, United States, 2002 with chartbook on trends in the health of Americans* (DHHS Pub. No. 1232). Hyattsville, MD: Public Health Service.

National Institute for Occupational Safety and Health. (2002). *Mission and objectives statement.* Retrieved 4/9/04 from *http://www.cdc.gov/niosh/02-15658.html*

Nichols, F.H. (2000). History of the women's health movement in the 20th century. *Journal of Obstetric, Gynecologic, and Neonatal Nursing, 29*(1), 56–64.

Occupational exposures to air contaminants at the World Trade Center disaster site. (2002). *MMWR Morbidity and Mortality Weekly Report, 51*(21), 453–456.

Olmos, E., Ybarra, L., & Monterrey, M. (1999). *Americanos: Latino life in the United States.* Boston: Little, Brown.

Pender, N.J., Murdaugh, C., & Parsons, M.A. (2002). *Health promotion in nursing practice* (4th ed.). Upper Saddle River, NJ: Prentice-Hall Health.

Respiratory illness in workers exposed to metalworking fluid contaminated with nontuberculous mycobacteria—Ohio 2001. (2002). *MMWR Morbidity and Mortality Weekly Report, 51*(16), 349–352.

Salazar, M.K., Connon, C., Takaro, T.K., Beaudet, N., & Barnhart, S. (2001). An evaluation of factors affecting hazardous waste workers' use of respiratory protective equipment. *American Industrial Hygiene Association Journal, 62*, 236–245.

Shamian, J. (2000). On the heels of Florence Nightingale: Re-energizing hospital care. *Reflections on Nursing Leadership, 26*(1), 24–26.

U. S. Department of Health and Human Services. (2000). *Healthy people 2010* (Conference ed., Vols. 1 & 2). Washington, DC: U. S. Government Printing Office.

U. S. Department of Health and Human Services. (2001). *Womens's health issues: An overview.* Office on Women's Health, Washington, DC: U. S. Government Printing Office.

Valent, F., McGwin, G., Bovenzi, M., & Barbone, F. (2002). Fatal work-related inhalation of harmful substances in the United States. *Chest, 121*(3), 969–975.

van der Klink, J.J.L., Blonk, R.W.B., Schene, A.H., & van Dijk, F.J.H. (2001). The benefits of interventions for work-related stress. *American Journal of Public Health, 91*(2), 270–276.

Venes, D., & Thomas, C.L. (2001). *Taber's cyclopedic medical dictionary.* Philadelphia: F.A. Davis.

Verma, D.K., Purdham, J.T., & Roels, H.A. (2002). Translating evidence about occupational conditions into strategies. *Occupational Environmental Medicine, 59,* 205–214.

Women's Health Statistics. (2003). Cancer. Retrieved 4/8/04 from *http://www.womenshelp.com/information/women's_health_statistical_information/cancer.htm*

SELECTED READINGS

Abusabha, R., Peacock, J., & Achterberg, C. (1999). How to make nutrition education more meaningful through facilitated group discussions. *Journal of the American Dietetic Association, 99*(1), 72–76.

Agency for Toxic Substances and Disease Registry. *Living with asbestos-related illness: A self-care guide.* Atlanta, GA: U. S. Department of Health and Human Services.

Allen, J.D., Stoddard, A.M., Mays, J., & Sorensen, G. (2001). Promoting breast and cervical cancer screening at the workplace: Results from the woman to woman study. *American Journal of Public Health, 91*(4), 584–590.

Anderson, T. & Maslow, S. (2001). What do women want? *Path of Potential, 1*(3), 12–14.

Appel, S.J., Harrell, J.S., & Deng, S. (2002). Racial and socioeconomic differences in risk factors for cardiovascular disease among southern rural women. *Nursing Research, 51*(3), 140–147.

Banks-Wallace, J., & Conn, V. (2002). Interventions to promote physical activity among African American women. *Public Health Nursing, 19*(5), 321–335.

Brophy, M.O., Achimore, L., & Moore-Dawson, J. (2001). Reducing incidence of low-back injuries reduces cost. *AIHA Journal, 62,* 508–511.

Clark, S.P., Sloane, D.M., & Aiken, L.H. (2002). Effects of hospital staffing and organizational climate on needlestick injuries to nurses. *American Journal of Public Health, 92*(7), 1115–1119.

Cubbin, C., LeClere, F.B., & Smith, G. (2000). Socioeconomic status and the occurrence of fatal and nonfatal injury in the United States. *American Journal of Public Health, 90*(1), 70–77.

Ferrie, J.E., Shipley, M.J., Stansfeld, S.A., & Marmot, M.G. (2002). Effects of chronic job insecurity and change in job security on self reported health, minor psychiatric morbidity, physiological measures, and health related behaviors in British civil servants: The Whitehall II study. *Journal of Epidemiology and Community Health, 56*(6), 450–454.

Freedman, R.I., Krauss, M.W., & Seltzer, M.M. (1999). Patterns of respite use by aging mothers of adults with mental retardation. *Mental Retardation, 37*(2), 93–103.

Halm, M.A., & Penque, S. (1999). Heart disease in women. *American Journal of Nursing, 99*(4), 26–32.

Hull, J.B. (2002, November). Rip up your daily planner. *Working Mother, 24,* 26.

Kerr, M.J., Lusk, S.L., & Ronis, D.L. (2002). Explaining Mexican American workers' hearing protection use with the Health Promotion Model. *Nursing Research, 51*(2), 100–109.

Kim, Y., & Dunniway, D. (2001). Women's services: Without walls. *Nursing Management, 32*(5), 25–27.

Korrick, S.A., Hunter, D.J., Rotnitsky, A., Hu, H., & Speizer, F.E. (1999). Lead and hypertension in a sample of middle-aged women. *American Journal of Public Health, 89*(3), 330–335.

Lai, S.C., & Cohen, M. N. (1999). Promoting lifestyle change. *American Journal of Nursing, 99*(4), 63–67.

LaMontagne, A.D., Herrick, R.F., Van Dyke, M.V., Martyny, J.W., & Ruttenber, A.J. (2002). Exposure databases and exposure surveillance: Promise and practice. *AIHA Journal, 63,* 205–212.

Leigh, J.P., McCurdy, S.A., & Schenker, M.B. (2001). Costs of occupational injuries in agriculture. *Public Health Reports, 116*(3), 235–248.

Leigh, J.P., Romano, P.S., Schenker, M.B., & Kreiss, K. (2002). Costs of occupational COPD and asthma. *Chest, 121*(1), 264–272.

Linnan, L.A., Emmons, K.M., & Abrams, D.B. (2002). Beauty and the beast: Results of the Rhode Island smokefree shop initiative. *American Journal of Public Health, 92*(1), 27–28.

Loewenson, R. (2001). Globalization and occupational health: A perspective from southern Africa. *Bulletin of the World Health Organization, 79*(9), 863–865.

Miller, M., Azrael, D., & Hemenway, D. (2002). Firearm availability and suicide, homicide, and unintentional firearm deaths among women. *Journal of Urban Health: Bulletin of the New York Academy of Medicine, 79*(1), 26–38.

Rogers, B. (1998). Expanding horizons: Integrating environmental health in occupational health nursing. *AAOHN Journal, 46*(1), 9–13.

Strawbridge, W.J., Wallhagen, M.I., & Shema, S.J. (2000). New NHLBI clinical guidelines for obesity and overweight: Will they promote health? *American Journal of Public Health, 90*(3), 340–343.

Survey of Occupational Injuries and Illnesses. (2000). *Summary 02-01.* Washington, DC: U. S. Department of Labor, Bureau of Labor Statistics.

Internet Resources

Agency for Toxic Substances and Disease Registry (ATSDR): *http://www.atsdr.cdc.gov*

American Association of Occupational and Environmental Health Nurses: *http://www.aaohn.org*

American Lung Association of Washington: *http://www.alaw.org*

American Public Health Association (APHA): *http://www.apha.org*

American Red Cross: *http://www.redcross.org*

Bureau of Labor Statistics (BLS): *http://www.bls.gov*

Centers for Disease Control and Prevention (CDC): *http://www.cdc.gov*

Office of Radiation, Chemical, and Biological Safety, Michigan State University: *http://www.orcbs.msu.edu*

National Institute for Occupational Safety and Health (NIOSH): *http://www.cdc.gov/niosh/homepage.html*

National Institutes of Health: *http://www.nih.gov*

National Safety Council: *http://www.nsc.org*

U. S. Department of Health and Human Services: *http://dhhs.gov*

World Health Organization: *http://www.who.ch*

30

Older Adults: Aging in Place

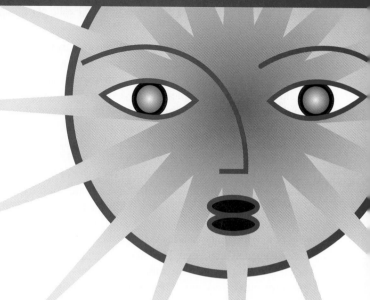

Learning Objectives

Upon mastery of this chapter, you should be able to:

- Describe the global and national health status of older adults.
- Identify and refute at least four common misconceptions about older adults.
- Describe characteristics of healthy older adults.
- Provide an example of primary, secondary, and tertiary prevention practices among the older population.
- Discuss four primary criteria for effective programs for older adults.
- Describe various living arrangements and care options as older adults age in place.
- Describe the future of an aging America and the role of the community health nurse.

Older Americans constitute a large and growing population group. You will be part of it in the future. Perhaps your parents and grandparents are in that group now. In fact, people age 65 years and older make up the fastest-growing segment of the American population (Eliopolous, 2001; Pan American Health Organization, 2002). This trend is expected to continue, with the most rapid increase expected between the years 2010 and 2030, when the "baby boom" generation reaches 65 years of age. Older adults make up a group whose health needs are not fully understood, and the nation has yet to offer the full complement of services they require and deserve.

For community health nursing, this population group poses a special challenge. The increasing number of seniors in the community increases the need for health-promoting and preventive services. These services help maximize an older person's ability to remain an independent, contributing member of society and to maintain a high quality of life. With this group's potential for longevity comes the myriad problems brought on by these extended numbers of years, including dwindling finances that may not be keeping up with inflation; increasing chronic disease and disability; diminishing functional capacity; and ongoing losses regarding work, home, family members, and other loved ones. Significant economic, environmental, and social changes create a demand for greater protective and preventive services for older adults in addition to requiring adjustments in health care provision patterns. The challenge is clear. Nursing must study the needs of this group and respond with appropriate, effective, and cost-effective interventions.

This chapter focuses on population-based nursing for the elderly. There are four fundamental requirements for effective nursing of any population:

1. Know the characteristics of the population.
2. Set aside stereotypes based on misconceptions about the population.
3. Know the health needs of the population as a basis for nursing intervention.
4. View the population from an aggregate, public health perspective that emphasizes health protection, health promotion, and disease prevention.

This chapter first examines the global challenge of an aging society and the characteristics of the aging population in the United States. Some myths and misconceptions about the elderly are described, and ageism is discussed. Next, the primary, secondary, and tertiary health needs of older adults are explored. Finally, population-based health services and nursing interventions applied to the health of the aging population are discussed in light of cost containment and comprehensive care at the beginning of the new millennium.

HEALTH STATUS OF OLDER ADULTS

Never before has the population of older adults been so large, and its numbers are on the increase. The progressive aging of populations is hailed as a triumph for the human species. People are living longer as a result of improved health care, eradication and control of many communicable diseases, use of antibiotics and other medicines, healthier dietary practices, safer global water supplies, regular exercise, and accessibility to a better quality of life. This is especially true for people in developed countries, and particularly for residents of the United States.

Global Demographics

It is estimated that more than 420 million people worldwide are older than 65 years of age. This is about 7% of the world's population. In the United States, more than 35 million people (12% of the population) are older than 65, and by 2050 that number is expected to increase to 20% of the population (National Center for Health Statistics, 2002). Between 1950 and 2000, the percentage of Americans younger than 18 years of age fell from 31% to 26%, and the percentage of elderly rose from 8% to 12% (Fig. 30–1).

Death rates have fallen steadily over the past 100 years. Life expectancy at birth in the United States increased from 51 to 80 years for women and from 48 to 74 years for men between 1900 and 2000 (Population Reference Bureau, 2003). Although there have been significant improvements in longevity, in 22 countries the percentage of the population older than 65 years of age is greater than in the United States. Countries with 16% or more of their population over age 65 years include Italy, Sweden, Norway, Greece, Belgium, Spain, Bulgaria, Japan, Germany, United Kingdom, and France. These high percentages are in part the result of actual

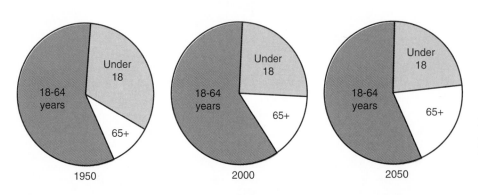

FIGURE 30–1.

Percentage of population in three age groups. (Source: U.S. Census Bureau, 1950 and 2000 decennial censuses and 2050 middle series population projections.)

increases in lifespan, but they also reflect the low birth rate in many countries. The fertility rate for the entire world population is now estimated to be 2.8 children per woman over the course of her lifetime. By 2050, it is projected to decline to 2.0 children per woman, slightly less than the level at which a population maintains its size over the long term. Already in 2003, China, Japan, almost all of Europe, and many parts of South and Southeast Asia have fertility rates lower than the replacement level. Presently the world population is at 6.3 billion people, but if fertility continues to decline at this rate, the world population in 2050 will be approximately 8.7 billion, not the 9.1 billion initially predicted by the United Nations (Population Reference Bureau, 2003).

Women outnumber men in the older population because they have an advantage in life expectancy that averages 6 years. In fact, older women outnumber older men in most countries, and more than half of the women in the United States older than 65 years of age are widowed (Eliopoulos, 2001). However, the advantage is partially offset by disability. There is no advantage to a longer life if the quality of that life is poor. In fact, extending the healthy years of life is a goal of the U. S. Department of Health and Human Services (USDHHS) *Healthy People 2010* objectives (USDHHS, 2000) and will be a focus of public health practices in the United States for the next decade. According to data from selected European countries, women in Switzerland can expect 15 disability-free years of life after age 65 and 5 years of disability, compared with a low of 8 disability-free years and 12 years of disability in the Netherlands. In the United States, the expectation is slightly more than 10 disability-free years after age 65, followed by 7 years of disability (National Institute on Aging, 2001).

National Demographics

As already stated, in 2000, the average life expectancy at birth for Americans was 80 years for women and 74 years for men. However, there are disparities in life expectancy among various subgroups in the population. Life expectancy is highest for white Americans and lowest for black Americans, who have the highest death rates of any of America's racial and ethnic groups (National Center for Health Statistics, 2002). Although life expectancies have been increasing for all Americans in general, a variety of factors has caused those figures to level off in recent years. These include unhealthy lifestyles; societal problems, such as deaths caused by firearms, substance abuse, and human immunodeficiency virus/acquired immunodeficiency syndrome (HIV/AIDS); and the rise of Alzheimer disease (AD) among the elderly.

Nevertheless, older people are healthier than ever before. Although statistics indicate that men in the United States who are 65 years old have an average of 14.8 years of life remaining, and women 19.5 years (National Institute on Aging, 2001). Increasing numbers of capable elderly people are living independently, and the **hearty elderly**—people older than 65 years of age who maintain a high level of wellness and activity, well above present expectations for that age—are increasing in number. Most people older than 65 years of age not only maintain independent living but continue to contribute to society. Many continue to work, and most stay involved in community programs and activities. Some have become valuable volunteers, helping others in such community activities as foster grandparents and literacy programs for adults, working in libraries and homeless shelters, or providing services such as Meals on Wheels.

Not only are more people living into old age, but also, once they get there, they are living longer. Specifically, the number of people living into "older" old age (75 years and older) is increasing. Forty percent of elderly people in the United States are among the "oldest old" (85 years and older)—4.2 million in the year 2000—and more than 200,000 are among the **elite-old**, or centenarians. Until the year 2030, the 85-and-older age group is projected to be the most rapidly growing segment of the entire U. S. population (Eliopoulos, 2001) and in the Americas (Pan American Health Organization, 2002). In 2011, the oldest of the large cohort (76 million) of **baby boomers**, those people born between 1946 and 1964, will turn age 65. This is a significantly sized population; by contrast, there were only 66 million births, in a larger U. S. population during the 19 years after the baby boom, which included the "baby bust" of the 1970s. Some 72 million people will be entering old age, significantly affecting health care resources, housing options for older adults, and national longevity statistics. As the number of "old-old" people increases, so, too, will the need for assistance with activities of daily living (ADLs) and other services. Many of these experts at aging will be among the **frail elderly**, those older than 85 years of age who need assistance in attending to ADLs such as dressing, eating, toileting, and bathing. Even now, about half of those 85 years old and older need some help with daily activities.

Other statistics on older adults may also help community health nurses anticipate the psychosocial needs of the older population. Most older men (76%) live out their years with their spouse and therefore have someone for companionship; in contrast, almost 60% of older women are widowed, single, or divorced (Eliopolous, 2001). In fact, there are five times as many widows (8 million) as widowers (1.5 million) in the United States, and the incidence of widowhood increases with advancing age. Community health nurses should anticipate the needs of many older adults (particularly women) who will face the loss of a spouse, helpmate, and companion and may experience loneliness, social isolation, and depression.

Only 6% of all older adults live in institutions; the overwhelming majority live in family settings (Ebersole & Hess, 2004). Two thirds (66%) of older adults live within 30 minutes of an adult child. Approximately 80% of older adults have seen one of their children within the previous week. These figures contradict the popular notion of abandoned elderly who have been forgotten or neglected by their families.

In the total U. S. population, almost twice as many women as men (16% versus 8%) live below the poverty level, and this trend continues into old age (Miller, 1999). More than one in eight older Americans (12.9%) are poor, and many live in profound poverty. They are unable to afford clothing, recreation, transportation, or other items that most people consider necessary for mental health, social status, and continued personal growth. The differences among various ethnic groups experiencing poverty in old age are broad. Among white older adults, approximately 10% live below the poverty level, whereas 30% of African-American elders and 23% of Hispanic elders live in poverty (Miller, 1999). In no other age group is there such a variance of assets, with 20% of the nation's elderly holding 50% of all assets held by this age group.

The education level of the older population is increasing. The percentage of older adults who have completed high school or a higher level of education is 66.7% among whites, 37% among African-Americans, and 30% among Hispanics (Miller, 1999). These figures are predicted to change as the United States witnesses a trend toward a more educated senior population because of the significant numbers of baby boomers who completed high school and entered college during and since the 1960s (see Voices from the Community I).

DISPELLING AGEISM

Stereotyping older adults and perpetuating false information and negative images and characteristics regarding older adults is called **ageism**. These stereotypes often arise from negative personal experience, myths shared throughout the ages, and a general lack of current information. Ageism can interfere with effective practice and prevent the kind of comprehensive and interdisciplinary service aging persons need and deserve.

Misconceptions About Older Adults

Community health nurses must guard against ageism in their practice by dispelling common misconceptions.

Misconception: Most Older Adults Cannot Live Independently

Ninety-four percent of elderly individuals live in the community, outside formal facilities or institutions. Some live alone or with friends, and others live in the homes of nonrelatives with room and board provided. In some homes, assistance with ADLs is provided. There are also alternative-housing arrangements—group-living situations for older adults in which many types of housing and care possibilities are offered. This concept is not new, but these centers are being built now in greater numbers to meet the needs of a growing segment of the older adult population. These situations are well suited to those who desire such comprehen-

VOICES FROM THE COMMUNITY I

"When did my parents get old? It seems it was only a couple of years ago that someone thought my mother was my sister. She was delighted, and gave an embarrassed laugh. My parents were strong, vibrant. Getting old was somewhere. . . . way out there. But suddenly, or so it seems, mom and dad are old. And vulnerable. I want to help, but how do I begin?"

Daniel, age 44

"The big issue is whether dad, 93, and mom, 83, can continue to live in their home. They're in a small town in South Dakota. Mom had a stroke 2 years ago, and dad has been taking care of her. Even though my brother lives in the same town and my sister is in Iowa, I'm a nurse, and they think I know more. It's also that I'm the eldest daughter. They turn to me for everything."

Ruth, age 57

"Mom just turned 79. She's determined to stay in her own home but wants me on call to help with everything, I'm doing the best I can because I'm all she has. But my job, my family, and everything else are suffering. She refuses to do laundry and go grocery shopping. I'm at my wits' end."

Eleanor, age 48

"Mom moved into a high-rise apartment building for the elderly after dad died. My sister, brother, and I have dinner at her apartment once a week. We bring the food. It makes her feel like she's still the hub of the family. My brother handles all medical appointments and prescriptions, my sister all the financial affairs, and I drive mom anywhere she wants to go. We're a close family and we're all helping."

Roger, age 42

sive living choices and have the financial means for the housing and care arrangements provided. The average age of older adults in residential care is getting older and is currently about 85 years—such facilities typically are not chosen by the hearty elderly or by totally independent young-elders (Hill et al., 2002).

Most elders who are vigorous and functioning independently live in their own homes. Only 6% live in institutions such as skilled nursing facilities, extended care facilities, supervised living facilities, and AD centers, and not all of these are permanent residents. Many are recovering from illnesses or undergoing rehabilitation after an injury or surgery and will return to their living situation in the community within weeks.

Misconception: Chronologic Age Determines Oldness

Older people are quite distinct from one another in the aging process, and they age at widely disparate rates. Some people at age 85 years still play golf, drive a car, and participate in social and community activities; others are frail and cannot move about well. Physical, social, and mental health parameters, life experiences, and genetic traits all combine to make aging an individualized process (see Levels of Prevention Matrix).

Misconception: Most Elderly Persons Have Diminished Intellectual Capacity or Are Senile

Studies show that intelligence, learning ability, and other intellectual and cognitive skills do not decline with age. Cognitive deficits are caused by certain risk factors. Nutritional status has been singled out as a physical health variable that influences cognitive functioning, particularly memory performance, regardless of a person's age. Anticholinergic ingredients that are present in many medications can interfere with memory and cognitive functioning. In healthy, mentally stimulated older adults, deficits are generally minimal and probably not even noticed. Speed of reaction tends to decrease with age, but basic intelligence does not. In fact, some abilities are viewed collectively as crystallized intelligence. Wisdom, judgment, vocabulary, creativity, common sense, coordination of facts and ideas, and breadth of knowledge and experience actually improve with age (Miller, 1999). Most older people are largely capable of making their own decisions; they want and need the freedom to make choices and to be as independent as their limitations will allow.

Senility, although not a legitimate medical diagnosis, is a term widely used by the lay public to denote deteriorating mental faculties associated with old age. Yet fewer than 1% of people aged 65 years, and only 18% of people older than 75 years, are affected by cognitive impairment, dementia, or AD (discussed later). Although most cases of cognitive impairment are not treatable, 10% to 20% of them are reversible. These include problems caused by drug toxicity, metabolic disorders, depression, or hyperthyroidism (Miller, 1999).

Certainly, AD and arteriosclerosis cause memory loss

LEVELS OF PREVENTION MATRIX

SITUATION: Making a healthy transition into a satisfying retirement.

GOAL: Using the three levels of prevention, negative health conditions are avoided, or promptly diagnosed and treated, and the fullest possible potential is restored.

PRIMARY PREVENTION		SECONDARY PREVENTION		TERTIARY PREVENTION		
Health Promotion and Education	*Health Protection*	*Early Diagnosis*	*Prompt Treatment*	*Rehabilitation*	*Primary Prevention*	
					Health Promotion and Education	*Health Protection*
• Early preparation—emotionally and financially • Avocation planning (preretirement workshops, support groups, financial planning)		• Plan or participate in a celebration activity • Reflect on past successes and contributions to the workforce	• Allow time for adaptation to this life transition • Organize new free time into satisfying and enriching activities	• Adapt to changed roles with spouse and significant others • Maintain health while assessing increasing dependency needs, including alternative housing, modifications in transportation, and changing health care needs	• Periodically review and update will, insurances, and other important documents as needed	• Keep beneficiaries or executors aware of changes in and location of documents and personal wishes regarding end-of-life care and funeral/burial arrangements

and altered behavior in the elderly, but many older adults have similar symptoms as a result of anxiety, loss, or grief, or simply from changes in their routine. These reactions need to be diagnosed by health care providers and differentiated from disease processes.

Misconception: All Older People Are Content and Serene

The picture of Grandma sitting serenely in her rocker with her hands folded in her lap is misleading. It is true that many older people have learned to accept rather than fight the hardships and vicissitudes of life. Yet, for most people, advancing age brings increasing physical, social, and financial problems to harass and worry them. Depression, which can be a problem among the elderly, is sometimes confused with dementia because of such symptoms as disorientation, failing memory, and eccentric behavior. However, one must not forget that, to attain the status of senior citizen (meaning one who has survived 65 years or more of living), one has had a great deal of strength, tenacity, and capacity for adaptation, as well as a sense of humor about many of the trials, tribulations, and absurdities in life. These people are survivors, and survivors do not always sit contentedly in a rocking chair on the sidelines of life.

Misconception: Older Adults Cannot Be Productive or Active

More than two thirds (between 65% and 68%) of the male work force retire before age 65 years. In contrast, the participation rate for women between 45 and 64 years of age is continually rising (Ginn, Street, & Arber, 2001; Rix, 2001). Some reasons for early retirement include health, availability of private pension benefits, social expectations, and long-held plans to do something else with their time (Menzey, 2001). These additional years give older adults time for travel, volunteering, and hobbies. This "third phase of life" is a gift of the 20th century that allows people to pursue these and other interests. Many older retired adults care for grandchildren, great-grandchildren, or even a very old surviving parent. Twenty-five percent of people aged 58 or 59 have at least one living parent; and 10% of older adults have at least one offspring who is older than 65 (Miller, 1999).

More than 4 million Americans older than 65 years of age work full- or part-time, and many others, who are not included in labor statistics, work but do not report their earnings. An example is the grandmother who chooses to give up full-time employment in an unsatisfying job to babysit for three preschool grandchildren and is paid in cash by her two children. The grandmother gets to spend time with growing grandchildren and not lose all her income potential; the parents feel comfortable that their children are being cared for by a loving family member; and the grandchildren are experiencing the joy of being with their grandparent. In another situation, active retired older adults assist with their two children's businesses. The mother types legal documents for the son's law practice

during busy times, and the father helps out on Saturdays in the daughter's pool supply store. Everyone wins in these situations.

Healthy older people usually do not disengage or withdraw and isolate themselves from society; rather, they are active and involved. Remaining active—through a daily routine, purposeful behavior, and a positive view of life—produces the best psychological climate.

Misconception: All Older Adults Are Resistant to Change

People at any age can learn new information and skills. Research indicates that older people can learn new skills and improve old ones, including how to use a computer. Learning occurs best in a self-paced, supportive environment (Morrell, Mayhorn, & Bennett, 2000). The elderly have spent a lifetime adapting to change, with varying measures of success. People older than 65 years grew up in an age when having an automobile was a luxury and many did not have a television, microwave oven, or VCR until they were in middle adulthood. Elders learned to adapt to these changes, and they are becoming increasingly computer literate today. The ability to change does not depend on age but rather on personality traits acquired throughout life or, sometimes, on socioeconomic difficulties. For example, elders living on fixed incomes may be faced with inflationary costs. This may cause them to vote against a school levy that would increase taxes, although they otherwise would support the schools.

Misconception: Social Security Will Not Be There When I Retire

The Social Security fund is healthy! Although the government has borrowed from it, the trust fund growth has been sufficient to keep Social Security solvent until 2041—which is 3 years longer than was projected in 2001 (American Association of Retired Persons, 2002). In addition, Medicare will stay financially healthy until 2030, also a 1-year gain over the 2001 estimate. Money still pours into the Social Security fund from payrolls, and not until 2019 will the administrators have to start tapping the trust fund to meet obligations. If there were no changes to the dispursement schedule of the fund for the next 35 years, the fund would become exhausted. Even with that worst-case scenario, however, payroll tax revenues would be enough to pay 75% of everyone's benefits for the next 75 years.

Even though the Social Security system is secure, most people who will reach retirement age in the next few decades have experienced a lifestyle well beyond what could be supported by the Social Security benefits they are scheduled to receive. This means that people must plan early and contribute to a retirement plan at work (or establish their own retirement fund if self-employed), invest, and save regularly. These multiple sources of income at the time of retirement will provide the resources necessary so that decisions about when to start or how to spend one's retirement can be based on personal preference rather than a restricted and fixed Social Security check.

Characteristics of Healthy Older Adults

No one knows conclusively all of the variables that influence healthy aging, but it is known that a lifetime of healthy habits and circumstances, a strong social support system, and a positive emotional outlook all significantly influence the resources people bring to their later years. Most people recognize a healthy older person when they meet one.

What is healthy old age? As was mentioned earlier, the vast majority (94%) of elderly individuals, even those with chronic diseases or other disabilities, are living outside institutions and are relatively independent. Their ability to function is a key indicator of health and wellness and is an important factor in understanding healthy aging. Good health in the elderly means maintaining the maximum possible degree of physical, mental, and social vigor. It means being able to adapt, to continue to handle stress, and to be active and involved in life and living. In short, healthy aging means being able to function, even when disabled, with a minimum of ordinary help from others (USDHHS, 1991, 2000).

Wellness among the older population varies considerably. It is influenced by many factors, including personality traits, life experiences, current physical health, and current societal supports. Some elderly people demonstrate maximum adaptability, resourcefulness, optimism, and activity (Display 30–1). Others, often those from whom we tend to draw our stereotypes, have disengaged and present a picture of dependence and resignation. Most of the elderly population fall somewhere in between those two extremes. Although the level of wellness varies among the elderly, that level can be raised. The challenge in community health nursing is to maximize the wellness potential of elderly clients. Nurses must analyze and capitalize on an older person's strengths rather than focus on the difficulties. The goal is to enable older people to thrive, not merely survive (Eliopoulos, 2001; Miller, 1999).

HEALTH NEEDS OF OLDER ADULTS

Effective nursing in any population requires familiarity with that group's health problems and needs. Aging in and of itself is not a health problem. Rather, aging is a normal, irreversible physiologic process. Its pace, however, can sometimes be delayed, as researchers are discovering, and many of the problems associated with aging can be prevented (Menzey, 2001). The aging process is subtle, gradual, and lifelong. One can see remarkable differences among individuals in the rate of aging. Even in a single individual, various systems of the body age differently (Eliopoulos, 2001).

DISPLAY 30–1

Profile of a Healthy Older Adult

Minerva Blackstone, affectionately called Minnie by her friends, is a lively 87-year-old woman who enjoys life. Every day, except in bad weather, she walks a half-mile to visit her granddaughter, Karen. There she works on the quilt, which is stretched on a frame, that she is making for Karen. In addition, twice a week Minnie takes the city bus to the senior citizens' center to join her friends in an exercise class. Although her eyesight has somewhat diminished, Minnie enjoys reading in the evening or crocheting while she watches television. Mysteries and comedies are her favorite kinds of stories.

She is not content, however, unless she is up on the latest political developments. She always has opinions on current events and expresses them with vigorous shakes of her curly white hair at her monthly group meeting on women and politics. She has a good appetite and generally sleeps well. Minor arthritis does not hamper her activities, nor does the hypertension that she controls by taking her medication with conscientious regularity. Minnie is enjoying a healthy, successful old age.

Therefore, chronologic age cannot serve as an indicator of health needs. However, the proportion of people with health problems increases with age, and as a group older adults are more likely than younger ones to suffer from multiple, chronic, and often disabling conditions.

The elderly, like any age group, have certain basic needs: physiologic and safety needs as well as the needs for love and belonging, self-esteem, and self-actualization. Their physical, emotional, and social needs are complex and interrelated. The following sections discuss these needs according to primary, secondary, and tertiary prevention activities.

Primary Prevention

As discussed previously in this text, primary prevention activities involve those actions that keep one healthy. Such primary prevention activities as health education, follow-through of sound personal health practices, and maintenance of an appropriate immunization schedule ensure that older adults are doing all that they can to maintain their health. The list in Display 30–2 includes strategies for successful aging. Taken from a variety of sources, it provides primary prevention activites the community health nurse can use when working with elders, either individually or in groups.

Nutrition Needs

People who have maintained sound dietary habits throughout life have little need to change in old age. Many have not established such habits but may wish to. It is generally believed

D I S P L A Y   3 0 – 2

Strategies for Successful Aging

1. Do at least 30 minutes of sustained, rhythmic, vigorous exercise four times a week.
2. Eat "like a bushman" (a healthy diet of fruits, whole grains, vegetables, and lean meat).
3. Get as much sleep and rest as needed.
4. Maintain a sense of humor and deflect anger.
5. Set goals and accept challenges that force you to be as alive and creative as possible.
6. Don't depend on anyone else for your well-being.
7. Be necessary and responsible; live outside yourself (give to others, become involved).
8. Don't slow down. Stick with the mainstream. Avoid the shadows. Stay together. Maintain energy flow in a purposeful direction; aging need not be characterized by losses. Maintain contacts with family and friends, and stay active through work, recreation, and community.
9. Get regular check-ups.
10. Don't smoke—it's never too late to quit.
11. Practice safety habits at home to prevent falls and fractures. Always wear seat belts when traveling by car.
12. Avoid overexposure to the sun and the cold.
13. If you drink, moderation is the key—when you drink, let someone else drive.
14. Keep personal and financial records in order to simplify budgeting and investing—plan long-term housing and financial needs.
15. Keep a positive attitude toward life—do things that make you happy.

VOICES FROM THE COMMUNITY II

"We want to stress that healthy ageing includes more than the mere absence of disease. Our goal is that everybody can enjoy a good quality of life and have a recognized role to play as full and useful members of society."

Dr. Gro Harlem Brundtland, Director-General,
World Health Organization

"The potential of older persons is a powerful basis for future development. This enables society to rely increasingly on the skills, experience, and wisdom of older persons, not only to take the lead in their own betterment but also to participate actively in that of society as a whole."

From the Political Declaration, Second World
Assembly on Ageing, Madrid, Spain, 2002

---

that older people need to maintain their optimal weight by eating a diet that is low in fats, moderate in carbohydrates, and high in proteins. Foods with "empty calories," such as salty snacks, candy, fatty foods, and alcohol, should be limited; they meet hunger needs by satisfying appetite only, while providing little nutrition (see Voices From the Community II).

Most people can keep their teeth for a lifetime with optimal personal, professional, and population-based preventive practices. Yet, in 1997, 26% of adults age 65 to 74 years had had all their teeth extracted. The *Healthy People 2010* target is to reduce this number to 20% (USDHHS, 2000). Since the 1960s, water supplies and toothpastes have been fluoridated, and regular dental care has become more accessible and acceptable to most people. These measures have helped prevent periodontal disease, a major component of tooth loss in adults. Oral health and hygiene needs do not decrease with age. Eating, chewing, and swallowing should be an uncomplicated and natural process. Frequently, older adults are taking medications that cause dry mouth, taste alterations, and loss of appetite that limit the desire for food. Eating should remain a pleasurable social experience, prefer-

ably taking place in the company of others. Community health nurses can assist older adults with meal management by following the suggestions outlined in Display 30–3.

In addition to maintaining a healthy diet, older adults should avoid the habitual use of laxatives, instead adding more fiber and bulk to their diet. Inadequate fluid intake often contributes to bowel and bladder problems. Consuming a diet that includes six to eight 8-oz glasses of fluid (water, juices, tea) each day assists the gastrointestinal and genitourinary system in their functions. Also, more exercise helps keep an older adult's bowel patterns regular.

Exercise Needs

Older adults need to exercise; in fact, they thrive when exercise is incorporated into their daily routine. Research shows that exercise can slow the loss of bone density and increase the size and strength of muscles, including the heart (Kressig & Echt, 2002; USDHHS, 2000). Aging does not and should not involve passivity; instead, physical activity and movement contribute to the quality of intellectual and physical performance in old age. Exercise, such as a daily walk, can keep muscles in good tone, enhance circulation, and promote mental health. Exercise may occur in connection with such activities as homemaking chores, gardening, hobbies, or recreation and sports. Often, such physical outlets are enjoyed in the company of other people, meeting social and emotional needs as well as physical ones. Preparing for exercise by warming up helps to keep muscles free from injury and to prevent falls (American Institute for Cancer Research, 2002). Even among the very old, an exercise routine that includes activities that improve strength, flexibility, and coordination may indirectly, but effectively, decrease the incidence of osteoporotic fractures by lessening the likelihood of falling (Burbank & Riebe,

D I S P L A Y   3 0 – 3

Meal Management Considerations

- Complete a safety check with the older adult to assess his or her ability to operate stoves and microwave ovens. Include the elder's ability to reach and to put things on and off stove burners.
- Arrange cupboards so that commonly used items can be reached from an easy standing level. Suggest use of turntables and long-handled "grabbers"; discourage use of stepstools or ladders.
- Assess the elder's typical meal for quality and availability. This can be accomplished for all meals by doing a 24 hour dietary recall—begin with the most recent meal and work backward.
- To ensure that elders eat an appropriate number of times a day, suggest that they "eat by the clock" or with a certain television show.
- Help older adults build support systems for sharing grocery shopping, cooking, and meals. Suggest that they bake once a week for an activity or shop with another elder.
- Suggest buying convenience foods, making sure they have nutritional value (eg, frozen vegetables or dinners).
- Consider community resources to assist with shopping, transportation, or meal preparation as needed. Keeping a continuous shopping list helps elders remember needed grocery items and provides a reference if someone offers to assist with shopping.
- Help elders consider increasing socialization by eating together with friends, rotating among three or four friends each week, or eating out with friends, selecting restaurants that are physically and financially accessible and that serve healthy food.

2002; Hill-Westmoreland, Soeken, & Spellbring, 2002) (see Research: Bridge to Practice).

Economic Security Needs

Economic security is another major need for older adults. Worrying about finances is often one of the most debilitating factors in old age. Fearing the potential costs of major illness and not wanting to be a burden on family or friends, many older people conserve their limited finances by establishing frugal eating patterns, using health resources sparingly, taking medications in partial doses, and spending little on themselves. Too often, the fear—let alone the reality—of financial difficulties prevents older adults from leading full and active lives.

For older adults today who have lived many years past retirement and perhaps had not planned for sufficient financial security to maintain them throughout these additional, unexpected years, the fears are not unfounded. Putting older people in touch with appropriate community resources can do much to relieve the source of that stress and anxiety. The community health nurse can also help younger, working adults plan for a physically and emotionally, as well as financially, vigorous old age.

Psychosocial Needs

All human beings have psychosocial needs that must be met for their lives to be rich and fulfilling. Without healthy relationships with other people, life can be very lonely and lacking in quality. With advancing age, the psychosocial issues are many. A major issue is coping with multiple losses. In addition, maintaining independence, social interaction, companionship, and purpose is necessary for a healthy old age. Older adults who have maintained good health and have developed a supportive system of family and friends have more fulfilled lives.

Coping With Multiple Losses

Elders experience multiple losses, including loss of income and prestige from a career once practiced or the economic stability of an enjoyable job; loss of space due to replacement of a larger residence by a much smaller home or apartment; and reductions in health and vitality that may result in limited movement or pain as a daily concern or necessitate another move to a more dependent setting. Repetitive losses occur as significant others, relatives, friends, and acquaintances die (Worden, 2002).

Inadequate coping with the compounding losses can make an older person believe that life holds no meaning. Depression may be a difficult problem for older adults. Social and emotional withdrawal can often occur, as can suicide. Although older populations have a much lower rate of suicide attempts than younger age groups do, the rate of completed suicide is high. It is highest among elderly men, who account for about 80% of suicides among those age 65 years and older. Moreover, elderly white men have a suicide rate six times the national average (USDHHS, 2000). Concern for the increased suicide rates among older white men led to a key health objective in *Healthy People 2000:* to reduce the suicide rate to 38.9 per 100,000 people, from the 1987 baseline of 46.1 per 100,000 (USDHHS, 1991). By 1997, for white men aged 65 years or older, the suicide rate was 35.5 per 100,000, exceeding the 2000 goal. Suicide continues to be of concern and is included in the *Healthy People 2010* objectives. Because most elderly persons who commit suicide have visited their primary care provider in the last month of their lives, recognition and treatment of depression in health care settings is a promising way to prevent suicide in this age group.

Mortality after bereavement is high and can be prevented through nursing intervention. Loss and the mourning process among elders have been examined in many studies. It has been found that the ability to mourn prior states of one's self and the past is crucial to successful aging. This can be liberating and can provide energy for current living, including planning for the future (Worden, 2002). Although men and women experience similar levels of depression dur-

RESEARCH: BRIDGE TO PRACTICE

Kressig, R.W., & Echt, K.V. (2002). Exercise prescribing: Computer application in older adults. *The Gerontologist, 42(2),* 273–277.

New approaches to health promotion are needed for all people, but can older adults find help from computer-generated educational tools that they would be required to operate? The purposes of this study were to determine whether adults older than 60 years of age are willing and capable to negotiate a computerized exercise promotion and to determine to what degree these older adults accept and use computer-generated exercise recommendations.

Thirty-four older adults who were cognitively alert, without chronic diseases that would limit exercise, and with some college or a college degree, volunteered to interact with a health promotion tool focused on exercise promotion. The men and women (equal numbers of each), ranged in age from 60 to 87 years. They rated the ease of use and acceptability of the computer-generated exercise recommendations.

The participants' average time to complete the items was 33 minutes. Each volunteer made three requests for assistance, of which 22% were mouse related. Age was directly related to the number of requests for assistance made and in particular to non–mouse-related requests. There was no significant relation between age and the time required to answer the items. Computer experience, not educational level or memory and concentration scores, was significantly related to shorter response times and requests for assistance.

The exercise prescription and the system's ease of use were rated as high, independently of prior computer experience.

The results of this study suggest that nurses, especially community health nurses, should consider encouraging computer literacy among community members and the dissemination of health promotion information found on the World Wide Web, especially for older adults. This study demonstrated that a highly educated, volunteer sample of older adults was able to obtain health-related information with minimal assistance, had few problems operating the mouse, and subjectively rated the computer program highly. Computer use by older adults for entertainment, educational information, travel opportunities, support and information on chronic health conditions, communication with friends and family, and health promotion information should be encouraged as community health nurses work holistically with elders in the community.

---

ing early bereavement, it is more difficult for widowers to seek and receive social support. Higher levels of perceived social support are associated with lower levels of depression in widows and widowers (Moore & Stratton, 2002). In addition, more men than women die soon after the death of their spouses. Women have stronger social support systems throughout their lives, and these help sustain them during losses in old age (Moore & Stratton, 2002).

In addition to preventing early deaths after the loss of a spouse, the greater goal for the nurse in promoting successful aging can be accomplished when the nurse recognizes the significance of accepting all the losses of aging. The loss of a spouse is much more frequent for women than for men (Eliopoulos, 2001). With this knowledge, a woman can age successfully by planning for the future through anticipatory guidance, with the help of a community health nurse. Many women can expect to live alone for up to 20 years at the end of their life, because of a longer life expectancy and the fact that women in most cultures marry men older than themselves. The nurse can help to make these years meaningful and as healthy as possible.

Maintaining Independence

Older people need independence, and those who stay independent are happier. As much as possible, the elderly need to make their own decisions and manage their own lives. Even those with activity limitations because of disability can still exercise decision-making options about many, if not most, aspects of their daily living. The need for autonomy—to be able to assert oneself as a separate individual—is great for all people. With life's restrictions ever increasing for the elderly person, this need is all the greater (Eliopoulos, 2001). Independence helps to meet the need for self-respect and dignity. The elderly need to have their ideas and suggestions heard and acted on and to be addressed by their preferred names in a respectful tone of voice. Respect for the older adult is not a strong value in American society, but it is highly valued in Asian, Italian, Hispanic, and Native American cultures. Older people represent a rich resource of wisdom, experience, and patience that is generally wasted in the United States.

Social Interaction, Companionship, and Purpose

Older people need companionship and social interaction, particularly if they live alone. The company of other people and the companionship of a household pet offer avenues for expression and response and add meaning to life. Many studies of mortality patterns demonstrate that older adults living together have a greater survival rate and retain their independence longer than do those who live alone (Miller, 1999).

The problem is of greatest significance for women, who outnumber men considerably in the later years and who live alone more frequently.

It is also important for older adults without companions to discover and develop a friendship with someone who can be considered a **confidant**, someone in whom the older adult can confide, reflect on the past, and trust. It could be a close friend, a sibling, a son or daughter, or an acquaintance. This person is usually seen daily or talked with on the telephone each week. In particular, mothers and daughters form confidant bonds. Many women consider a sibling a confidant, especially if that person lives close by; this is especially true for childless and single women.

Meaningful activity is another need of the elderly that adds purpose to life. Some kind of active role in community life is essential for mental health, satisfaction, and self-esteem. These activities can range from involvement in hobbies, such as gardening or crafts, to volunteer work or even full-time employment. Examples include the federally supported Foster Grandparents and Senior Companions programs, which engage the help of more than 20,000 seniors. These older adults work part-time offering companionship and guidance to handicapped children, the terminally ill, and other people in need. Senior Partners is another program that keeps older adults involved. Volunteers earn service credits by providing support services so that persons age 60 years or older can remain independent and active in their own homes. Each hour of volunteer service earns one service credit. Credits may be "spent" in several ways. They can be used to obtain services, should the volunteer need them, or they can be donated to another person in need or donated back to Senior Partners to help others.

Additional volunteering opportunities abound. Internationally, many older professionals join the Peace Corps, which was initiated in the early 1960s. In this program, people of all ages work for 2-year periods in global communities that are in need of services to improve personal health, education, environment, and the larger community. On the national level, the newer AmeriCorps*VISTA (Volunteers in Service to America) programs are similar, but with a 1-year commitment; the volunteer lives among and at the economic level of the low-income people in the United States served by its projects. Retired people can volunteer to help others, donating their skills at a time in their lives when they are in transition from employment to retirement or to fill active retirement years. The Retired and Senior Volunteer Program (RSVP) engages seniors in a bevy of activities designed to improve people's lives and the environment. Environmental Alliance for Senior Involvement (EASI) sponsors various environmentally focused programs, such as assisting the Hawk Mountain Sanctuary to protect birds of prey or monitoring streams and other waterways for cleanliness.

Many older adults choose not to engage in long-term volunteering, and other programs are more appropriate for them. Elderhostel, Inc., is a nonprofit organization with more than 25 years of experience providing high-quality, affordable, educational adventures for adults who are 55 years of age and older. It is the nation's first and the world's largest education and travel organization for adults age 55 and over, offering more than 10,000 learning adventures each year in more than 100 countries. Their theme-based, short-term (3 days to 3 weeks) educational programs are infused with a spirit of camaraderie and adventure (Elderhostel, 2002). In 2002, even when many others were limiting their travel, more than 175,000 adults took advantage of the unique experiences that Elderhostel has to offer. The success of this program is based on the fact that learning is a lifelong process that is rewarding at any age, and it is learning without testing or papers due! Elderhostel is inspired by the youth hostels and folk schools of Europe but guided by the needs and interests of older citizens.

Safety Needs

People of all ages have safety needs, and this concept has been threaded throughout the five chapters in this unit on developmental needs of clients. Likewise, safety issues are a major concern for older adults and the community health nurses who work with them. Several areas of safety focus are discussed here: personal health and safety, home safety, and community safety.

Personal health and safety include three major areas: immunizations, prevention of falls, and drug safety. Immunizations are not just for children. Older adults are at risk for not only contracting influenza or pneumonia but dying from them. Pneumococcal disease, influenza, and hepatitis B account for more than 45,000 deaths annually, mostly among older adults. Ninety percent of influenza-related deaths occur in people age 65 years and older (USDHHS, 2000). Although the overall influenza immunization rate among elders has increased, from 33% in 1989 to 63% in 1997, and pneumonococcal vaccine coverage rates have increased from 15% to 43%, improvement is still needed. Despite the increases, coverage rates for certain racial and ethnic groups remain substantially below that of the general population. For example, the influenza vaccination rate for whites was 66% in 1997, whereas for African-Americans it was 45% and for Hispanics it was 53%. In September of 1997, the USDHHS approved an agency-wide plan to improve adult immunization rates and reduce disparities among racial and ethnic minorities through their "Put Prevention Into Practice" program, a national campaign to improve delivery of clinical preventive services (USDHHS, 2000). Attempts to improve immunization coverage involve changing provider knowledge, attitudes, and behavior through reminders and standing orders so that "missed opportunities" when seeing clients are prevented. Additional opportunities for vaccinating people exist beyond the primary care setting, as community health nurses are well aware. People can be reached during emergency department visits, at neighborhood and senior centers, at religious facilities, and in other innovative settings where elders may gather. Regardless of the site, a method for tracking and communicating vaccinations is needed so that vaccination information may be documented and shared with the elder's primary care provider. Immunizations protect more than the at-risk population—they protect society as a whole. People of any age with a chronic illness, such as heart disease, diabetes, or chronic respiratory disease, and people older than 65 years of age should be encouraged to receive the flu vaccine each year and the pneumonia vaccine every 5 years.

Each year, approximately one third of people older than 65 years of age who are independent and living on their own experience a fall; for those individuals residing in long-term care settings, the percentage is 50% (Hill-Westmoreland, Soeken, & Spellbring, 2002). Every year in the United States, 300,000 people are treated for hip fractures, 90% of which are caused by falls (Jech, 2000). Causative factors involve both environmental hazards and host issues. Fall prevention, which involves education, strengthening and balance exercises, medication evaluation, and environmental improvements, is an important part of the role of the community health nurse. Use of a home safety checklist can give the nurse a baseline of information from which to begin teaching (Display 30–4).

A significant safety issue for the older adult arises from adverse drug effects. Older people may need to take several medications to control the effects of chronic conditions, and their bodies may react differently than those of younger people (on whom most new drugs are tested). It is not unusual for older people to be taking four to six medications daily and filling 13 prescriptions each year. It is estimated that 25% of all older people who live independently receive prescriptions for inappropriate medications (Jech, 2000). Elders receive multiple prescriptions from multiple providers and are in danger of receiving double doses of the same or similar medications. Multiple medications or complicated drug regimens for many older people can lead to unexpected and dangerous drug interactions. The use of more than four prescribed medications is related to an increased risk of falling (Jech, 2000). Elderly clients need education about the drugs they take and their possible effects. They also need proper supervision of their overall medication intake. This is an area in which the community health nurse can intervene very effectively and with much success.

Safety in the community is an additional concern. Safety involves pedestrian and driving issues, crime and fear of crime against elders, and environmental factors such as sun exposure, pollution, heat, and cold.

Because of age-related changes in vision, hearing, mobility, and the effects of polypharmacy, elders are at risk in the community as pedestrians and as drivers. Automobile crashes and pedestrian injuries can be life-threatening events when elders are involved. As pedestrians, elders must be increasingly vigilant to traffic patterns, sidewalk irregularities, and the possibility of being a victim of street crime. Often out of necessity and pride, elders drive longer than their abilities permit. In 1998, 23.7 of every 100,000 older adults died of motor vehicle-related injuries. Only the 15- to 24-year-old population had a higher rate (National Center for Health Statistics, 2002). All traffic and pedestrian fatality rates are higher in this age

group. On the basis of estimated annual travel, the fatality rate for drivers age 85 years and older is 9 times as high as the rate for drivers 25 through 69 years of age, with a 31.5 deaths per 100,000 people (U. S. Department of Transportation, 1998). To stop driving is usually a difficult and painful decision for the elder to make. At times, the car keys may have to be taken from the elder, for his or her own safety and that of others. This may be necessary especially with elders who have dementia, AD, uncorrectable vision problems, or stroke-related physical or cognitive after-effects.

Actual crime against elders in the community is as much as 50% lower than among other segments of the population. However, the fear of crime among elders is perceived as a major issue by the general public, and about 25% of elders consider the fear of crime a major concern. Display 30–5 lists client-centered nursing interventions designed to reduce fear among older adults and empower them to feel safer in their communities.

Environmental factors can have an effect on the health and safety of elders when they are outside. Sun exposure, pollution, and exposure to heat and cold can have negative effects on older adults. They are just as vulnerable as infants and children to climatic changes and should take a variety of preventive measures, including using sun block when gardening, reading, or walking outside for longer than 10 minutes, even on days with an overcast sky; staying indoors on days when the air quality is poor or there is an air safety alert; drinking additional fluids, wearing protective covering, and limiting outdoor activities and exposure on days with elevated temperatures; and, conversely, limiting outdoor exposure and wearing appropriate winter clothing, especially layers of clothes, on cold, snowy, or icy days. Teaching geographically and seasonally appropriate safety precautions is the responsibility of the community health nurse providing services to groups of elders in the community.

Spirituality, Advance Directives, and Preparing for Death

A final need of the elderly, and one that is receiving increasing attention, is that of preparing for a dignified death. Elisabeth Kübler-Ross (1975) described death as the final stage of growth and one that deserves the same measure of quality as other stages of life. Many older people fear death as an experience of pain, humiliation, discomfort, or financial concern for their loved ones. Planning for a dignified death is an important issue for many older people. For most, this includes choosing, if possible, where and under what circumstances death will occur; being free of financial worries; knowing that their affairs and their family members are taken care of; having the opportunity to receive spiritual counseling; and dying in peaceful surroundings, preferably at home with the support of loved ones (Cicirelli, 2002; O'Brien, 2003).

Some elders make arrangements with a funeral home of their choice, selecting interment or cremation, a memorial service or a celebration of life gathering, music to be played, and other personal details rather than leaving these choices

DISPLAY 30-4

Guidelines for Assessing the Safety of the Environment

Illumination and Color Contrast
- Is the lighting adequate but not glare-producing?
- Are the light switches easy to reach and manipulate?
- Can lights be turned on before entering rooms?
- Are nightlights used in appropriate places?
- Is color contrast adequate between objects such as a chair and the floor?

Hazards
- Are there throw rugs, highly polished floors, or other hazardous floor coverings?
- If area rugs are used, do they have a nonslip backing and are the edges tacked to the floor?
- Are there cords, clutter, or other obstacles in pathways?
- Is there a pet that is likely to be running underfoot?

Furniture
- Are chairs the right height and depth for the person?
- Do the chairs have arm rests?
- Are tables stable and of the appropriate height?
- Is small furniture placed well away from pathways?

Stairways
- Is lighting adequate?
- Are there light switches at the top and bottom of the stairs?
- Are there securely fastened handrails on both sides of the stairway?
- Are all the steps even?
- Are the treads nonskid?
- Should colored tape be used to mark the edges of the steps, particularly the top and bottom steps?

Bathroom
- Are grab bars placed appropriately for the tub and toilet?
- Does the tub have skidproof strips or a rubber mat in the bottom?
- Has the person considered using a tub seat?
- Is the height of the toilet seat appropriate?
- Has the person considered using an elevated toilet seat?
- Does the color of the toilet seat contrast with surrounding colors?
- Is toilet paper within easy reach?

Temperature
- Is the temperature of the rooms comfortable?
- Can the person read the markings on the thermostat and adjust it appropriately?
- During cold months, is the room temperature high enough to prevent hypothermia?
- During hot weather, is the room temperature cool enough to prevent hyperthermia?

Overall Safety
- How does the person obtain objects from hard-to-reach places?
- How does the person change overhead light bulbs?

- Are doorways wide enough to accommodate assistive devices?
- Do door thresholds create hazardous conditions?
- Are telephones accessible, especially for emergency calls?
- Would it be helpful to use a cordless portable phone?
- Would it be helpful to have some emergency call system available?
- Does the person wear sturdy shoes with nonskid soles?
- Are smoke alarms present and operational?
- Is there a carbon monoxide detector (if the house has gas appliances)?
- Does the person keep a list of emergency numbers by the telephone?
- Does the person have an emergency exit plan in the event of fire?

Bedroom
- Is the height of the bed appropriate?
- Is the mattress firm at the edges to provide enough support for sitting?
- If the bed has wheels, are they locked securely?
- Would side rails be a help or a hazard?
- When side rails are in the down position, are they completely out of the way?
- Is the pathway between the bedroom and bathroom clear of objects and adequately illuminated, particularly at night?
- Would a bedside commode be useful, especially at night?
- Does the person have sufficient physical and cognitive ability to turn on a light before getting out of bed?
- Is furniture positioned to allow safe use of assistive devices for ambulation?
- Is a telephone situated near the bed?

Kitchen
- Are storage areas used to the best advantage (eg, are objects that are frequently used in the most accessible places)?
- Are appliance cords kept out of the way?
- Are nonslip mats used in front of the sink?
- Are the markings on stoves and other appliances clearly visible?
- Does the person know how to use the microwave oven safely?

Assistive Devices
- Is a call light available, and does the person know how to use it?
- What assistive devices are used?
- Would the person benefit from any assistive devices that are not being used?
- Are assistive devices being used safely and properly, or do they present additional hazards?

(Adapted from Miller, C.A. [1999]. *Nursing care of older adults: Theory and practice* [3rd ed.]. Philadelphia: Lippincott Williams & Wilkins.)

D I S P L A Y   3 0 – 5

Reducing the Fear of Crime

1. Allow elder adults time to discuss their fears of crime.
2. Facilitate a realistic self-assessment of their ability to avoid crime and to defend themselves.
3. Teach basic safety and security techniques.
4. Correct the elder's sensory losses if possible, such as by getting a hearing aid or glasses.
5. Correct a physical disability if possible, such as by treating the pain of arthritis or obtaining physical therapy.
6. Facilitate access to safe, reliable, and affordable transportation.
7. Identify family members, friends, neighbors, or caregivers who can support efforts to leave the home on a more regular basis.
8. Encourage an elder to make a daily telephone or e-mail contact with at least one supportive person.
9. Encourage the elder to get to know his or her neighbors.
10. Encourage elders to travel and conduct community activities and errands together.
11. Encourage participation in local senior centers and other community-based programs.
12. Refer to alternative housing options available for older adults.
13. Provide information on local services that assist and support crime victims.

to their families. Others place less emphasis on the rituals, as was demonstrated by one elder who left these choices to her children by telling them, "Surprise me!"

Living wills and medical directives are legal documents whose purpose is to give people legal power over the medical treatment they would want if they became incapacitated or terminally ill. Living wills are legal in all states and the District of Columbia (Miller, 1999). Having such documents prepared and made known to significant others can ensure that the older adult's wishes will be honored.

Secondary Prevention

Secondary prevention focuses on early detection of disease and prompt intervention (see Chapter 1). Much of the community health nurse's time is spent in encouraging individuals to obtain routine screening for diseases such as hypertension or cancer, which, if identified early, can be treated successfully. Many nurses are in positions to establish screening programs based on the desires and demographics of the community and agency focus, making them accessible to the population being served.

Older adults need to be encouraged to follow the routine health screening schedule prescribed by their clinic or health care provider. The health screening schedule described in Table 30–1 is based on the recommendations of Kaiser Permanente (2000), an HMO serving millions of clients, and is presented here as a guide. A more comprehensive view of interventions and recommendations for the periodic health examination of people older than 65 years of age was proposed by the United States Preventive Services Task Force

T A B L E   3 0 – 1

Recommended Health Screenings and Immunizations—Older Adults

Test	Age 50–64 Yr	Age ≥65 Yr	Comments
Men and Women			
Blood pressure	Every 1–3 yr	Yearly	More often if elevated
Total cholesterol	Every 5 yr	Every 5 yr	More often if elevated
Flexible sigmoidoscopy	Every 10 yr	Every 10 yr	—
Vision	Every 4 yr	Every 2 yr	—
Hearing	Not recommended	Once	Evaluate at regular health care practitioner visits
Pneumonia vaccine	Not recommended	Once	—
Influenza vaccine	Yearly	Yearly	—
Tetanus and diptheria	Every 10 yr	Every 10 yr	After a closed/dirty wound if it has been >5 yr
Women			
Breast self-examination	Monthly	Monthly	—
Pap test	Every 2 yr after age 40 yr	Every 2 yr after age 40 yr	After a hysterectomy by health care practitioner evaluation
Clinical breast examination	Every 1–2 yr	Every 1–2 yr	—
Mammogram	Every 1–2 yr	Every 1–2 yr	Frequency decided on an individual basis

(Adapted from Kaiser Permanente. [2000]. *Kaiser Permanente healthwise handbook.* [14th ed.]. Boise: Kaiser).

DISPLAY 30-6

Health Maintenance Programs and Services for Older Adults

Resources for Community Health Nurses to Utilize With Clients

- Communication services (phones, emergency access to health care)
- Dental care services
- Dietary guidance and food services (such as Meals on Wheels, commodity programs, or group meal services)
- Escort and protective services
- Exercise and fitness programs
- Financial aid and counseling
- Friendly visiting and companions
- Health education
- Hearing tests and hearing-aid assistance
- Home health services (including skilled nursing and home health aide services)
- Home maintenance assistance (housekeeping, chores, and repairs)
- Legal aid and counseling
- Library services (including tapes and large-print books)
- Medical supplies or equipment
- Medication supervision
- Podiatry services
- Recreational and education programs (community centers, Elderhostel)
- Routine care from selected health care practitioners
- Safe, affordable, and ability-appropriate housing
- Senior citizens' discounts (food, drugs, transportation, banks, retail stores, and recreation)
- Social assistance services offered in conjunction with health maintenance
- Speech or physical therapy
- Spiritual ministries
- Transportation services
- Vision care (prescribing and providing eye glasses; diagnosis and treatment of glaucoma and cataracts)
- Volunteer and employment opportunities (Vista, RSVP)

(Adapted from U. S. Preventive Services Task Force. [2000–2003]. *Guide to clinical preventive services* [3rd ed.]. Retrieved January 30, 2004, from *http://www.uspstf.gov*)

(USPSTF). They identified age-specific, evidenced-based preventive services guidelines that are outlined in Display 30–6 (U. S. Preventive Services Task Force, 2000–2003).

Tertiary Prevention

Tertiary prevention involves follow-up and rehabilitation after a disease or condition has occurred or been diagnosed and initial treatment has begun. Chronic diseases that are common among older adults, such as congestive heart failure, emphysema, and arthritis, often cannot be prevented but frequently can be postponed into the later years of life through a lifetime of healthy living. However, when they occur, the debilitating symptoms and damaging effects can be controlled through healthy choices encouraged by the community health nurse and recommended by the primary care practitioner.

Although most older adults are healthy, 80% have at least one chronic condition, causing almost half of the elderly population to experience some kind of limitations in activity (Miller, 1999). A small proportion suffer more disabling forms of disease, such as chronic obstructive pulmonary disease (COPD), cerebral vascular accidents (CVAs), cancer, or diabetes mellitus (DM), the latter two requiring more extensive care. The most common health problems of older people in the community are arthritis, reduced vision, hearing loss, heart disease, peripheral vascular disease, and hypertension. In those older than 65 years of age, 40% have blood pressure recordings that are high enough to be considered hypertensive. Chapter 34 expands on clients with disabilites and chronic illnesses and the role of the community health nurse working with these populations in the community.

Alzheimer Disease

Alzheimer disease has been recognized in the medical literature since it was first described by Dr. Alois Alzheimer in a German medical journal in 1907. It is the same illness that produces the majority of cases of progressive dementia in the elderly today. At age 65 years, one's risk is about 5% for development of AD; by 75 years, it has increased to about 20%; and by age 85, the risk is substantial and may be as high as 50% (Vellas & Fitten, 2001). AD is the fourth leading cause of death among the very old in the United States. This disease robs its victims of everything learned in life, so that they are unable to fall back on preserved intelligence.

There is a simple way to describe the difference between the normal forgetfulness of aging and AD. With advancing age or increased stress, an individual may say, "Where are my keys? Where did I place them? I can't find them anywhere"; after several stressful moments, the keys are usually found and the event is over. However, if a person with AD is handed a set of keys, he or she looks at them blankly, handles them awkwardly, and has no idea what they are for or what to do with them.

Onset is gradual, and verbal memory is often affected first. Early in the disease process, clients may remember the details of a vacation in 1952 but cannot remember whether they took their medication 5 minutes earlier. Eventually AD clients lose judgment and reasoning, and safety becomes an issue as the disease process continues. Victims of AD may wander away from home and cannot tell anyone exactly where they live, or they may forget that a stove can get hot and burn themselves while trying to cook. They neglect their health and are even unaware of whether they are experiencing major health problems (Mace & Rabins, 2001).

Probable causes of AD are many. Promising leads involve the role of neurotransmitters, proteins, metabolism, environmental toxins, and genes. Discovering the cause and a means of preventing the disease will be a significant achievement that it is hoped may be realized early in this century. Currently 16 different agents are under study, compared with 90 for cardiovascular disease. The medical community is not putting the same amount of effort into research for AD as it does for other diseases. This lack of research interest today affects what will be available for those in need tomorrow.

How does this disease affect the role of the community health nurse? Often, the person is cared for at home until very late in the disease course. The intense caregiving these clients require drains the reserves of their families. The client demonstrates depression, agitation, sleeplessness, and anxiety, which upset the family's normal routine. In many situations, the main caregiver is an aged spouse. The stress of caregiving puts the caregiver's health at risk as well. The intensity of caregiving was aptly described in a book written for AD family members, called *The 36 Hour Day* (Mace & Rabins, 2001). Medications may be prescribed, but many are largely experimental, some having promise (Fillit & O'Connell, 2002). At best, available medications "turn back the clock somewhat," with the disease worsening at a slower rate, or the drugs control some of the client's behaviors that jeopardize safety, thereby promoting caregiver management.

The community health nurse is in a position to assess the levels of stress on family members, provide them with methods and means to cope and adapt as needed, and make referrals if appropriate. Most communities have resources for clients and their families. They may provide family and caregiver support groups, respite care (discussed later), counseling, and legal or financial consultation. These services are available through local agencies, but there are also government-sponsored national resources that offer information, referral services, and educational materials, all of which can be accessed by the community health nurse or the families in need. The nurse needs to know that resources are available in order to guide families to them (see What Do You Think? I and Using the Nursing Process).

Arthritis

Osteoarthritis is the deterioration and abrasion of joint cartilage. It is increasingly seen with advanced age and affects women more than men. Classic symptoms include aching, stiffness, and limited motion of the involved joint. Discomfort increases with overuse and during damp weather. It is the leading cause of physical disability in older adults (Eliopoulos, 2001). Acetaminophen is the first drug of choice; however, clients often find a combination of medications and daily routines that helps them the most. The nurse can best help these clients by assessing the safety of a particular regimen and suggesting treatment changes as they are developed, including new medications, surgical options for joint replacement, and dietary changes (eg, vitamins, foods high in essential fatty acids).

WHAT DO YOU THINK? I

Have you heard of the *Best Friends* approach to Alzheimer's care? The approach has changed the caregiving approach to Alzheimer's disease and is changing the lives of caregivers, families, and clients. It improves the quality of life not only for clients with Alzheimer disease (AD) but also for those providing care. *Best Friends* is a groundbreaking and upliftng method for the care of people with AD. It builds on the essential elements of friendship: respect, empathy, support, trust, and humor. These are the building blocks of a care model that is both effective and flexible enough to adapt to each person's remaining strengths and abilities. The *Best Friends* approach does not just prevent catastrophic episodes; it makes every day consistently reassuring, enjoyable, and secure.

From Bell, V., & Troxel, D. (2001). *The Best Friends staff: Building a culture of care in Alzheimer's programs*. Baltimore: Health Professions Press, and Bell, V., & Troxel, D. (1997). *The Best Friends approach to Alzheimer's care*. Baltimore: Health Professions Press. (*Best Friends* is a trademark of Health Professions Press, Inc.)

Rheumatoid arthritis (RA) begins in young adulthood and becomes disabling as the disease continues, causing systemic damage in the later years. This form of arthritis is an autoimmune disease that causes inflammation, deformity, and crippling. RA arthritis is treated with anti-inflammatory agents, corticosteroids, antimalarial agents, gold salts, and immunosuppressive drugs. Joint discomfort is often relieved by gentle massage, heat, and range-of-motion exercises.

The community health nurse must be aware of the major differences between these two prevalent forms of arthritis. Recommended treatments, including physical therapy, diet, and medications, change as more is discovered about arthritis. The community health nurse must keep up-to-date on treatments, because these conditions are treated in the community and affect a large portion of the midlife and older populations.

Cancer

Cancers, which are characterized by the uncontrolled growth and spread of abnormal cells, steadily increase in incidence in aging adults (Ebersole & Hess, 2004). One popular theory is that as the body ages the immune system deteriorates, losing its ability to serve as a buffer against abnormal cancer cells that have been forming in the body throughout life.

It is particularly important for the community health nurse to be aware of the increased incidence of cancer in older clients, because older people often underreport symptoms that

USING THE NURSING PROCESS

ASSESSMENT

Mr. and Mrs. Boxwell are in their late 70s and have lived modestly on a fixed income since Mr. Boxwell's retirement. However, their budget has been strained this year because they must pay $300 to $400 each month in out-of-pocket expenses for prescription medications. Mrs. Boxwell confessed to you, the community health nurse visiting them after receiving a referral from the coordinator of the senior center they attend, that in some months they skip medication doses to make "ends meet." They both take drugs for high blood pressure; Mrs. Boxwell is diabetic, and Mr. Boxwell has congestive heart failure. They live in a small, older home. Their 8-year-old car is seldom driven, because they report that "the traffic is getting worse" and they have come close to having an automobile crash twice while they were driving in the past 3 months. They are receptive to your suggestions and are trying to stay healthy and independent.

NURSING DIAGNOSES

1. The clients are at risk for an alteration in their health status due to insufficient finances to purchase needed medications for chronic diseases.
2. The clients are at risk for altered safety when driving related to chronic health problems, diminished driving skills, and a history of narrowly avoided automobile crashes.

PLAN/IMPLEMENTATION

Diagnosis 1.

The community health nurse will explore the clients' eligibility for Medicaid. It is possible that these clients are eligible yet unaware of this program.

The community health nurse will consult with the clients' primary health care provider and suggest that

their prescriptions be changed to generic from brand names and to have some medications ordered in larger doses (ie, ones that come in scored tablets). They are less expensive and the client can break them in half safely. For example, atenolol, the generic for Tenormin, is prescribed 25 mg qd—it comes in 50-mg scored tablets and costs just 20% more than the 25-mg tablets.

Mrs. Boxwell will check with her present distributor of diabetic supplies for larger quantities and generic brands of syringes, alcohol pads, and so on.

Diagnosis 2.

Mr. Boxwell will look into selling their car, exploring the bus schedule, and cost of taking a taxi to the doctor and the grocery store. Mr. and Mrs. Boxwell's daughter spends a day each month with them and takes them wherever they want to go, as long as it is "a fun outing."

EVALUATION

The couple is eligible for Medicaid, which will defray the out-of-pocket costs for medications. They have reduced medication costs as much as possible and report not missing any prescribed medications.

They sold their car and are negotiating the bus in good weather. They use a taxi in the winter or when it is raining. They figured that they save $1000 per year in auto insurance, auto maintenance, and gasoline, whereas the bus and taxi cost them about $22 per month.

Because the couple is receptive to the help you have provided, you initiate a discussion regarding their long-term plans for housing needs as they get older. They are not opposed to a senior housing option and have been talking about it with their daughter. They are going to talk with a realtor about selling their home, explore some senior apartments with their daughter on her monthly visits, and review their budget.

---

may be early signs of cancer. Thorough assessments in clinics, on home visits, or during participation in screening programs and encouraging reporting of untoward symptoms promote early detection, which gives clients their best chance of survival. Adherence to the health care practitioner's recommended schedule for health screening (see Table 30–1) should be encouraged. In addition, being aware of and educating clients about the American Cancer Society's seven warning signals of cancer can possibly save their lives (Display 30–7).

Depression

Depression in older adults is a major problem. It is frequently related to the experience of major multiple losses, such as

losses related to retirement, a health change, or the death of a significant other. Depression is reported to be more common in women than in men (Ebersole & Hess, 2004). However, as mentioned earlier in this chapter, depression in men is more severe, resulting in suicide at a higher rate than among women. Higher levels of perceived social support are related to lower instances of depression among all people, especially the elderly, and women seem to make these supportive connections throughout life more effectively than men do. The nurturance, reassurance, and support women get from intimate relationships with other women are not highly developed in men, and for this reason, men display more symptoms of depression after a loss.

D I S P L A Y   3 0 – 7

CAUTION

The seven warning signals of cancer can be remembered through the use of the mnemonic device, *CAUTION*, as follows:
1. **C**hange in bowel or bladder habits
2. **A** sore throat that does not heal
3. **U**nusual bleeding or discharge
4. **T**hickening or lump in breast or elsewhere
5. **I**ndigestion or difficulty in swallowing
6. **O**bvious change in wart or mole
7. **N**agging cough or hoarseness

Community health nurses can help elders prevent the overwhelming signs and symptoms of depression related to losses by working with aggregates of elders in the community. Through senior centers, adult housing units, senior day care centers, or men's and women's groups at religious centers, the community health nurse can meet with groups of seniors to offer support, teach ways to improve the quality and quantity of support systems, invite mental health speakers on the topic of depression prevention, and generally assess the holistic health status of the elders in that setting. The increased years added to life in the advances of the past century should be healthy and happy ones, filled with activities that bring joy and contentment. Years lost to depression are a wasted resource that could be prevented through early intervention.

Diabetes

DM is a chronic disease affecting 16 million people, or 5.9% of the population, in the United States. Each year, an additional 800,000 people are diagnosed with diabetes. The number of people with DM has increased sixfold since 1958, and 95% have type 2 diabetes (Holtrop et al., 2002). The incidence in people older than 65 years of age is now 18.4%, or almost one in five older adults (Oxendine, 1999). About 50% of all elders have some problems with glucose intolerance (Eliopoulos, 2001). More Americans than ever suffer from various forms of DM, and the resulting rates of death and serious complications, such as adult blindness, kidney disease, and foot or leg amputations, are especially high for elders and racial and ethnic minority populations (West, 1999). In the past, DM was not always managed effectively; fear and misinformation about the disease may hinder today's elders from getting an early diagnosis or from participating in an effective teaching–learning process if diagnosed with DM.

Being diagnosed with DM can cause depression or anger, and the community health nurse must tailor educational programs to meet individual client needs. The plan should be thorough, with special emphasis placed on the areas in which each client needs information. For example, a spouse may be concerned about preparing meals that meet her husband's needs, whereas the husband may be more concerned with how the disease will affect his long days on the

golf course; in contrast, a single older woman may worry whether she can see well enough to draw up her insulin and whether she can afford to pay for diabetic supplies and special foods. All newly diagnosed diabetics need a comprehensive overview of the disease process followed by an individualized approach.

Community health nurses are ideally situated to meet group and individual needs. They have the resources and skills to plan and implement diabetic education classes for groups of elders, in addition to making home visits to individual clients based on their specific concerns. The group setting allows elders to share their experiences, learn from each other, and benefit from the support of the group. Home visits permit the nurse to focus on an assessment of the client, home, family support, diabetic supplies and technique, and overall health management.

Cardiovascular Disease

Hypertension increases with age and affects men more frequently than women. It appears at an earlier age and is more severe, with higher rates of morbidity and mortality, in African-Americans than in whites (Miller, 1999). Older adults, however, do need to have a blood pressure that is high enough to provide sufficient cerebral circulation to avoid lightheadedness and dizziness. Therefore, slightly higher blood pressure readings for older adults than for younger people are within the normal range. Elders have difficulty managing ADLs if antihypertension medications lower their blood pressure too dramatically. Hypotension leads to problems of safety, including a higher risk of falling. This point is mentioned to alert the community health nurse to the negative effects of a blood pressure that is too low. Both hypertension and hypotension can have significant detrimental effects on the health of older adults.

Osteoporosis

Osteoporosis, the "silent disease," is characterized by low bone mass and microarchitectural deterioration of bone tissue that leads to increased susceptibility to fractures of hip, wrist, or vertebra (McKeon, 2002). It starts long before old age, making recognition essential for preventing its progression. Osteoporosis is a generalized, persistent, and disabling disease that can influence every facet of a person's life. It causes acute and chronic pain, subsequent fractures, decreased physical activity, changes in body image, role changes, a reduction in the ADLs, and chronic depression. It has become an increasingly prevalent problem that will only grow in magnitude as society ages. In fact, "a woman's lifetime risk for developing a hip fracture is greater than her combined risk for developing breast, uterine and ovarian cancer" (McKeon, 2002, p. 26). Eighty percent of the 1.5 million osteoporotic fractures that occur each year are in women.

Community health nurses can focus their teaching on primary prevention and ensure that people eat diets that are rich in calcium and include calcium supplements as needed. People should be encouraged to engage in weight-bearing activities, such as walking and weight lifting. Also, people should not smoke; women who smoke have a higher incidence of osteoporosis. The value of hormone replacement therapy (HRT) in women—its benefits and possible long-term side effects—must be considered on the advice of the primary care provider, whose judgment is based on the latest research findings along with the individual woman's needs.

APPROACHES TO OLDER ADULT CARE

In general, nursing service to seniors can be divided into two approaches: geriatrics and gerontology. In addition, healthy older adults can be effectively cared for in the community through case management approaches.

Geriatrics and Gerontology

Geriatrics is the medical specialty that deals with the physiology of aging and with the diagnosis and treatment of diseases affecting the aged. Geriatrics focuses on abnormal conditions and the treatment of those conditions, and geriatric nursing in the past has focused primarily on the sick aged.

Gerontology refers to the study of all aspects of the aging process, including economic, social, clinical, and psychological factors, and their effects on the older adult and on society. Gerontology is a broad, multidisciplinary practice, and gerontologic nursing concentrates on promoting the health and maximum functioning of older adults (Eliopoulos, 2001).

Community health nurses work with many older people. In one instance, the nurse works to promote and maintain the health of a vigorous 80-year-old man who lives alone in his home. As another example, the nurse gives postsurgical care at home to a 69-year-old woman, teaches her husband how to care for her, and helps them contact community resources for shopping, meals, housekeeping, and transportation services. Perhaps nursing intervention focuses on teaching nutrition and maintaining a healthful lifestyle in an extended family that includes a 73-year-old grandmother. The nurse may also lead a bereavement support group for senior citizens whose spouses have recently died.

A community health nurse works with older adults at the individual, family, and group levels. However, a community health perspective must also concern itself with the aggregate of older adults. There are many groups composed of seniors, such as those who attend an adult day care center, belong to a retirement community, live in a nursing home, or use Meals on Wheels. Other groups include residents of a senior citizens' apartment building, retired business and professional women, older postcataract-surgery patients at risk for glaucoma, the older poor, AD sufferers, and the homeless elderly.

Case Management and Needs Assessment

The **case management** concept involves assessing needs, planning and organizing services, and monitoring responses to care throughout the length of the caregiving process, condition, or illness. This concept, which has been practiced by community health nurses for many years, focuses primarily on the health needs of clients. Social workers use case management to address their clients' social needs, including their financial problems. Some HMOs provide a coordinated system of services for their enrolled clients. However, many communities provide no such advocate for their older residents, and a more comprehensive, community-wide system is needed to serve the entire older population. Such a system might be based on an agency specifically designed to serve as case manager or "agent," to assess clients' needs and assemble existing agencies and services to meet those needs.

Various techniques or tools are available to assess the needs of older adults:

- The Older Americans Resources and Services Information System (OARS), developed by Duke University, has two tools—Mental Health Screening Questions and the OARS Social Resource Scale. They establish baseline data on clients' well-being, available economic and social resources, physical and mental health status, and capacity for self-care.
- Clients' capacity for self-care is assessed by the Capacity for Self-Care Index, which ascertains clients' ability to go outdoors, climb stairs, move about their homes, bathe, dress, and cut their toenails.
- The Barthel Index assesses functional independence.
- The Katz Index of Activities of Daily Living is based on an evaluation of the functional independence or dependence of clients with respect to bathing, dressing, toileting, and related tasks.
- The Instrumental Activities of Daily Living Scale looks at an older adult's ability to perform such activities as using the telephone, shopping, doing laundry, and handling finances.
- Other techniques, such as the Ability to Perform Work-Related Activities survey, determine an elderly person's physical, psychological, and social needs.

A frequently overlooked area of assessment is an elderly client's spiritual needs (Moberg, 2001). Religious dedication and spiritual concern often increase in later years. Limited ability or lack of transportation may prevent older people from attending religious services or engaging in spiritually enhancing activities. Self-health ratings, including clients' reports on their spiritual needs, provide another useful assessment technique. A tool to assess a client's self-care practices is included in Chapter 23, Fig. 23-8.

HEALTH SERVICES FOR OLDER ADULT POPULATIONS

How well are the needs of older adults being met? To answer this question, other questions must be raised. Do health programs for the elderly encompass the full range of needed services? Are programs both physically and financially accessible? Do they encourage elderly clients to function independently? Do they treat senior citizens with respect and preserve their dignity? Do they recognize older adults' needs for companionship, economic security, and social status? If appropriate, do they promote meaningful activities instead of overworked games or activities such as bingo, shuffleboard, and ceramics? Games can be useful diversions, but they must be balanced with opportunities for creative outlets, continued learning, and community service through volunteerism (see What Do You Think? II).

WHAT DO YOU THINK? II

Services designed specifically for older homeless people are not widespread for three reasons: (1) there is little awareness of the circumstances and unmet needs of older homeless people, (2) the age group is not a high priority for policy makers—young homeless people are, and (3) there are few formal evaluations or published reports of successful experimental schemes and outcomes, so good practice is rarely disseminated.

Since the mid-1980s, services specifically for older homeless people have been initiated mainly in the larger cities of the United States, the United Kingdom, and Australia. The few services for older adults include drop-in and day centers, temporary housing with rehabilitation and resettlement programs, and various long-term housing options such as shared, supported, and high-care housing.

These services demonstrate that older homeless people can be helped by intensive work and specialized facilities, and can be rehoused in conventional accommodations. When offered these services instead of temporary drop-in night shelters, older men become more self-confident and sociable, drink less, eat better, and take care of their personal appearance and rooms.

Helping people soon after they become homeless is key to successful resettlement. Older homeless people must be encouraged to remain in contact with services and support staff long enough to benefit from help. In addition, more needs to be understood about effective ways of helping those with an alcohol problem; heavy drinking reduces the clients' ability to be rehoused and to live independently, increasing their chances of returning to the streets with compounded health problems, depression, and pessimism.

From Warnes, A.M., & Crane, M.A. (2002). The achievements of a multiservice project for older homeless people, *The Gerontologist, 40*(5), 618–626.

Criteria for Effective Service

Several criteria help to define the characteristics of an effective community health service delivery system for the elderly. Four, in particular, deserve attention.

For the delivery system of a community health service to be effective, it should be *comprehensive*. Many communities provide some programs, such as limited health screening or selected activities, but do not offer a full range of services to more adequately meet the needs of their senior citizens. Gaps and duplication in programs most often result from poor or nonexistent community-wide planning. Furthermore, such planning should be based on thorough assessment of elderly people's needs in that community. A comprehensive set of services should provide the following:

- Adequate financial support
- Adult day care programs
- Health care services (prevention, early diagnosis and treatment, rehabilitation)
- Health education (including preparation for retirement)
- In-home services
- Recreation and activity programs
- Specialized transportation services

A second criterion for a community service delivery system is *coordination*. Often, older people go from one agency to the next. After visiting one place for food stamps, they go to another for answers to Medicaid questions, another for congregate dining, and still another for health screening. Such a potpourri of services reflects a system organized for the convenience of providers rather than consumers. It encourages misuse and discourages use. Instead, there should be coordinated, community-wide assessment and planning. Communities must consider alternatives, such as multiservice agencies, that can meet many needs in one location.

A coordinated information and referral system provides another link. Most communities need this type of information network, which contains a directory of all resources and services for the elderly and includes the name and telephone number of a contact person with each listing. Such a network is available in some communities and should be developed in those without one. A simplified information and referral system that includes one number, such as an 800 number, to call to find out what resources and services are available and how to get them is particularly helpful to older people.

In most communities, coordination is not present, or it is not done with any regularity or thoroughness. Many agencies in a given community do not coordinate services, but instead deliver their own services to the elderly in a patchwork and uncoordinated fashion. Collaboration among those who provide services to seniors can provide vital information for planning and implementing needed programs. This was documented in a seven-county area in central California through the services of the San Joaquin Valley Health Consortium, a nonprofit community organization that focuses on identifying health care needs in central California and providing a center for health-related grant writing and grant administration.

A third criterion is *accessibility*. Too often, services for the elderly are not conveniently located or are prohibitively expensive. Some communities are considering multiservice community centers to bring programs and services for the elderly closer to home. More convenient and perhaps specialized transportation services and more in-home services, such as home health aides, homemakers, and Meals on Wheels, may further solve accessibility problems for many older adults. Federal, state, and private funding sources can be tapped to ease the burden on the economically pressured elderly population.

Finally, an effective community service system for older people should *promote quality programs*. This means services that truly address the needs and concerns of a community's senior citizens. Evaluation of the quality of a community's services for the elderly is closely tied to their assessed needs. What are the needs of this specific population group in terms of nutrition, exercise, economic security, independence, social interaction, meaningful activities, and preparation for death? Planning for quality community services depends on having adequate, accurate, and current data. Periodic needs assessment is a necessity to ensure updated information and to initiate and promote quality services.

Services for Healthy Older Adults

Maintaining functional independence should be the primary goal of services for the older population. Assessment of needs and the ability to function and use of techniques such as OARS, the Instrumental Activities of Daily Living Scale, or other previously mentioned tools form the basis for determining appropriate services. Although many of the well elderly can assess their own health status, some are reluctant to seek needed help. Therefore, outreach programs serve an important function in many communities. They locate elderly people in need of health or social assistance and refer them to appropriate resources.

Health screening is another important program for early detection and treatment of health problems among older adults. Conditions to screen for include hypertension, glaucoma, hearing disorders, cancers, diabetes, anemias, depression, and nutritional deficiencies (Eliopoulos, 2001). At the same time, assessment of elderly clients' socialization, housing, and economic needs, along with proper referrals, can prevent further problems from developing that would compromise their health status.

Health maintenance programs may be offered through a single agency, such as an HMO, or they may be coordinated by a case management agency with referrals to other providers. These programs should cover a wide range of services needed by the elderly, such as those listed in Display 30–6.

Living Arrangements and Care Options

Three types of living arrangements and care options are available for elders. Some living arrangements are based on

levels of care—from independent to skilled nursing care, and all levels of assistance in between. At times, seniors who remain in their own homes or apartments need home care services brought to them. Other seniors live with family members and go to an adult day care center during the day. The third category of living arrangements is those that are short term. It may be for respite care, which gives the usual caregiver a much-needed rest from 24-hour-a-day caregiving and helps prevent "burnout." Families of terminally ill clients cared for at home often use respite services. Finally, hospices provide comfort-focused care in a homelike atmosphere for people who have less than 6 months to live.

To meet the multiple housing and caregiving needs of today's elders and in anticipation of the larger numbers to come, many options are becoming available. A range of housing types, from luxurious retirement communities with all amenities for the active and healthier senior to secure and more modestly priced or low-income apartments for independent senior living, are being built in most communities.

Day Care and Home Care Services

Most older adults want to remain in their own homes for the remainder of their lives and be as independent and in control of their lives as possible. Some struggle to appear to be doing well in maintaining their independence. Often, they fear that their children or others will make decisions for them that include leaving their homes. Home, whatever form it takes, is where these people believe they are the happiest.

There is increased emphasis on providing needed services for elders at home. This trend started several years ago when it became evident that people improved more quickly and at lower cost when they were cared for as outpatients in their own homes. Today's heightened emphasis on health care cost control gives added support for providing services at home. Given the increase in longevity, the potential for cost savings appears great if dependent older people can be maintained at home. Doing so encourages functional independence as well as emotional well-being.

Home care provides services such as skilled nursing care, psychiatric nursing, physical and speech therapies, homemaker services, social work services, and dietetic counseling (see Chapter 37). Day care services offer a place where older adults can go during the day for social activities, nutrition, nursing care, and physical and speech therapies. Both services are useful for families who are caring for an elderly person if the caregivers work and no one is at home or available during the day. One disadvantage to those remaining at home is that services for the dependent elderly in the community are often fragmented, inadequate, and inaccessible, and at times they operate with little or no maintenance of standards or quality control.

The dependent elderly need someone in the community to assess their particular needs; assemble, coordinate, and monitor the appropriate resources and services; and serve as their advocate. Such case management roles are most appropriately filled by the community health nurse. This case management approach tailors services to the long-term needs of clients and enables them to function longer outside of institutions (Fast & Chapin, 2000).

Living Arrangements Based on Levels of Care

Although only 6% of the elderly population live in **skilled nursing facilities**, such organizations remain the most visible type of health service for older adults. These facilities provide skilled nursing care along with personal care that is considered nonskilled or **custodial care**, such as bathing, dressing, feeding, and assisting with mobility and recreation. Currently, approximately 2 million elderly people are receiving nursing home care.

Long-term care services "include all those services designed to provide care for people at different stages of dependence for an extended period of time" (Miller, 1999, p. 662). New choices are now available and provide housing for larger numbers of elders than nursing homes.

Nursing home reform was promoted in 1987 with passage of the Omnibus Budget Reconciliation Act (OBRA), which put increased demands on facilities to provide competent resident assessment, timely care plans, quality improvement, and protection of resident rights starting in 1990 (Miller, 1999). This increased complexity of services has resulted in increased costs in these facilities. Staffing needs increase as care becomes more complex and the resident population grows. Licensed personnel must be knowledgeable decision-makers, managers of unskilled staff, staff educators and role models, and efficient and effective administrators in an essentially autonomous practice setting.

In the past, nursing homes had stigmas attached to them. Many people saw them as places that enforced dehumanizing and impersonal regulations, such as segregation of sexes, strict social policies, and sometimes overuse of chemical and physical restraints. Media attention to such conditions, together with current licensing regulations, should make these types of practices the rare exception. Gradually, the fear and despair associated with such facilities will begin to dissipate. In addition, as competition comes from facilities offering lower levels of care (eg, assisted living centers), residents in nursing homes who are receiving more minimal care may be attracted to move to other types of housing.

Even in institutions in which the quality of care is outstanding, costs are so high that family resources are soon depleted if not planned for long in advance of the need. Although Medicaid pays for skilled nursing costs if the client meets low income and asset requirements, and Medicare pays for a limited period, clients and families pay more than half of the total costs (Eliopoulos, 2001). Life savings that older parents had hoped to leave to their children may be quickly consumed, forcing them into indigence. In 2004, it was not unusual for a skilled nursing facility to cost $4000 to $6000 per month based on level of caregiving needed and amenities offered.

Intermediate care facilities are less costly and still provide health care, but the amount and types of skilled care given are less than that provided in skilled nursing facilities. Frequently, older adults need **assisted living**. According to the mission statement of the Assisted Living Federation of America, "ALFA's primary mission is to promote the interests of the assisted living and senior housing industry and to enhance the quality of life for the population it serves" (Assisted Living Federation of America, 2004). This is a less intense level of care than intermediate care units or facilities provide. Medicare generally pays only for care in skilled nursing facilities. Medicaid pays for care in intermediate care facilities, but only after the client meets income and asset tests that leave them essentially indigent. Costs in 2003 for assisted living choices averaged $4000 a month.

Personal care homes offer basic custodial care, such as bathing, grooming, and social support, but provide no skilled nursing services. Payment may also come from private funds, Title XIX or XX (Social Security Act) funds, or Supplemental Security Income (aid to the aged, disabled, and blind). Boarding homes, board and care homes, and residential care facilities house elderly people who need only meals and housekeeping and can manage most of their own personal care. Government funds are not available to support these institutions. Costs averaged $2400 a month for a shared room in 2004. **Group homes** are an alternative for specific elderly populations, such as the mentally ill, alcoholics, or developmentally disabled individuals. They are often subsidized by concerned community organizations. Homes focusing on the care of people with AD are physically designed with clients safety and individual needs considered and are staffed with paraprofessionals trained to meet each person's needs.

The concept of **continuing care centers** (sometimes called total life centers), in which all levels of living are possible, from total independence to the most dependent, are designed to meet the continuous living needs of older aging adults (Display 30–8). This choice is usually expensive; however, it is a very attractive alternative for wealthier segments of the aging population. Others may choose to remain in their own home because they do not desire consolidated living arrangements in which only older adults reside or because they cannot afford such an arrangement. Nevertheless, demand is increasing for this type of housing option. Adults nearing retirement today are investigating this concept as a viable choice as they actively plan for a long old age. Many of these centers have a 5- to 10-year waiting list, so older adults need to seek them out long before they intend to live there.

Hospice and Respite Care Services

Respite care is a service that is receiving increasing attention. It is aimed primarily at caregivers' needs. Many older people at home are cared for by a spouse or other family member. The demands of such care can be exhausting unless

DISPLAY 30-8

Continuing Care Centers—Wave of the Future?

The Otterbein-Lebanon Retirement Community, a model continuing care center, is one of five Otterbein Homes located in Ohio. With housing options for more than 800 residents on a 1500-acre campus in rural southeastern Ohio, older adults can choose among freestanding two- or three-bedroom homes, one-bedroom cottages, or apartment-style one- or two-bedroom units or one-room studio units, where they live independently.

The 311 licensed beds include assisted living options from one-room studio apartments (with limited facilities for meal preparation) to semiprivate rooms in which nurses oversee administration of medications and staff members are available to assist with personal care. If caregiving needs become greater, additional services are available. Both skilled nursing services and a freestanding 30-bed Alzheimer's living unit exist for the frailest older adults.

Regardless of the living arrangement, the residents are free to come and go as they wish, and all have access to congregate dining in the large and attractive restaurant-style dining room.

The retirement community is expanding: 110 patio homes were built in 1999–2000, with additional expansions planned. The goal is to house 1200 residents by the year 2006.

The Otterbein-Lebanon Retirement Community also provides home health care services, adult day care, and the other usual services found in a community—a bank, a post office, an ice cream parlor, a small convenience store, a hairdresser, a library, a church (with a 70-member choir, a bell choir, and men's and women's clubs), a thrift shop, and an arts and craft shop open to the public. Because of the popularity of this community, there is a waiting list of 1 to 4 years for some independent living areas.

Many of the assisted living and skilled nursing beds are occupied by residents who moved into the independent living areas 10 to 15 years ago, while they were in their 70s or 80s. Their ages now range from the late 80s to older than 100, and caregiving needs have increased. In this type of setting, frail elderly people do not have to leave their community to get the care they need, and long-time friends are nearby to care for them or for companionship. It is not unusual to see many of the independent seniors volunteering to help feed frail elderly in the skilled nursing care units. In fact, residents volunteer more than 85,000 hours per year to the Otterbein-Lebanon Retirement Community. They know that when they need the care, a senior friend will be there for them.

(Otterbein-Lebanon Retirement Community Admissions Director, personal communication, April 4, 2003)

the caregiver gets some relief, or respite—thus the name of this service (see Chapter 37). Respite care may be available through an agency that provides volunteers to relieve caregivers, giving them time off regularly or permitting a periodic vacation. Some skilled nursing facilities or **board and care homes** provide an extra room to give temporary institutional housing for the elderly while caregivers take a break. Elderly clients may also need a change from the constant interaction with their caregivers.

Hospice care may be offered through an institution, such as a hospital or home health agency, or it may be a freestanding facility existing solely as an inpatient hospice. Hospices and other agencies providing hospice care offer services that enable dying people to stay at home with the support and services they need. The purpose of **hospice care** is to make the dying process as dignified, free from discomfort, and emotionally, spiritually, and socially supportive as possible. Some community health nursing agencies offer hospice programs staffed by their nurses. It is a service that has been well received by elders, meets important needs, and is growing in use. Hospice and respite care are two services most needed and used by the families of clients with AD.

THE COMMUNITY HEALTH NURSE IN AN AGING AMERICA

Community health nurses can make a significant contribution to the health of older adults. Because these nurses are in the community and already have contact with many seniors, they are in a prime position to begin needs assessments and mutual planning for the health of this group. Case management is often a critical aspect of the nurse's role, because the community health nurse must know what resources are available and when and how to make referrals for these older clients.

The health care scene in terms of availability of services for the elderly is changing dramatically. The numbers and types of home care services, for example, are mushrooming. Many entrepreneurs, including nurses, who recognize the potential of this growing market have begun offering goods and services targeted to older adults. Community health nurses must keep abreast of new developments, programs, regulations, and social and economic forces and their potential impacts on the provision of health services.

More importantly, community health nurses need to be proactive, designing interventions that maximize nursing's resources and provide the greatest benefit to elderly clients. For example, community health nurses might develop a case management program for older adults as a community-wide assessment, information, and referral service. Such a program might contract with existing agencies to serve as a clearinghouse for the elderly and to channel clients to appropriate services. Financing of such a program might be based on tax dollars (if it is a public agency), grants, or some innovative fee-for-service reimbursement system.

Many of the older population's health problems can be prevented and their health promoted. Changing to a healthier lifestyle is one of the most important preventive measures the nurse can emphasize.

The role of the community health nurse as a teacher is an important one. Educating the elderly about their health conditions, safety, and use of medications is another important way to prevent problems. Influenza and pneumonia can be prevented through regular health maintenance, which includes immunizations. Other problems associated with environmental conditions and the aging process, such as arthritis, diabetes, and some cancers, can be diagnosed and treated early, thereby minimizing their effect on functional independence.

Many types of accidents that frequently happen to older adults are 100% preventable. Community health nurses can make a difference through their work with individuals, families, and aggregates in teaching safety measures to avoid such accidents. As discussed earlier, falls are a leading cause of injury and death and result from a combination of internal factors (eg, diseases, effects of medicines) and external factors (eg, lighting, scatter rugs) that are preventable or controllable. Nurses can make a difference in the lives of older clients by using available materials and their own resources when teaching safety.

Community health nurses face a serious challenge in addressing the needs of the growing and aging elderly population. At the same time, nursing can be in the forefront of the development of innovative health services for that group, rising to meet the opportunity and the challenge.

SUMMARY

The number of older adults (age 65 years and older) is increasing, and they are becoming a larger percentage of the overall population. Women commonly outlive men by many years, making women a larger part of this older population. With improved medicines and medical technology, many people are now living into their 80s and 90s in relatively good health. They are able to enjoy these later years and still make contributions to their families and society. This extended life expectancy is, of course, good news; however, it has also created a myriad of new health needs and concerns, not only for the older population, but also for health care facilities and professionals who deliver services to older adults.

Healthy longevity is the goal for the aging population and is a focus of *Healthy People 2010*. That means being able to function as independently as possible; maintaining as much physical, mental and social vigor as possible; and adapting to life's changes and coping with the stresses and losses while still being able to engage in meaningful activity.

The most common health problems of older adults are chronic and often progressive conditions such as arthritis, vision and hearing loss, heart conditions, hypertension, and diabetes, all of which can become disabling conditions. Other major causes of death or disability are cancer, cerebral vascular accidents, AD, and accidents and injuries resulting from falls, fires, or automobile crashes. Older adults also often suffer adverse side effects from taking multiple medications prescribed for various chronic conditions. Many of these health problems associated with old age are preventable to some extent, and early diagnosis and treatment of some conditions can minimize their adverse effects. Many accidents and injuries that render older adults unable to live independently are preventable.

Too frequently, older adults suffer from the emotional side effects of aging, such as feelings of distress and anxiety regarding their future, loneliness and social isolation when loved ones or friends die, and even depression—feeling that life is over and they have no purpose or meaningful function in life. But older people can also enter this phase of life determined to keep physically and mentally healthy, interacting with others and making viable contributions to others and society.

To promote and maintain health and prevent illness, older people need to be educated about their own health care needs. In particular, they should understand the potential hazards of drug interactions if they are taking multiple medications. They also need good nutrition and adequate exercise; they need to be as independent and self-reliant as possible; they need coping skills to face the possibility of financial insecurity and the loss of a spouse or other loved ones; they need social interaction, companionship, and meaningful activities; and they need to resolve anxieties regarding their own impending death.

Many programs are available to older adults, both for those who are healthy, hearty, and active and for those who need some level of dependent or semidependent care. Programs for hearty older people include health maintenance programs that cover a wide range of health services, wellness programs, health screening, outreach programs, social assistance programs, and information about volunteering and educational opportunities in the community. A variety of living arrangements and care options are available from which to choose, according to the older person's desires and needs. These include the newest concepts of continuing care centers, which offer a full range of living arrangements, from totally independent living to skilled nursing services, all within one community. There are also facilities that provide skilled nursing and custodial care, home care, day care, respite care, and hospice care.

The community health perspective includes a case management approach that offers a centralized system for assessing the needs of older people and then matching those needs with the appropriate services. The community health nurse should also seek to serve the entire older population by assessing the needs of the population, examining the available services, and analyzing their effectiveness. The effectiveness of programs can be measured according to four important criteria—comprehensiveness, effective coordination, accessibility, and quality (targeted to the specific needs of the population).

The community health nurse can make significant contributions to the health of the older population as a whole by being aware of new developments and programs that become available, new regulations, and new social and economic forces and their impacts on the provision of health services. More importantly, the community health nurse can design interventions that maximize nursing resources and provide the greatest benefit to the older adult population.

ACTIVITIES TO PROMOTE CRITICAL THINKING

1. Picture an elderly person whom you know well or know a great deal about. Make a list of characteristics that describe this person. How many of these characteristics fit your picture of most senior citizens? What are your biases (ageisms) about the elderly?

2. If you were Minnie Blackstone's community health nurse (see Display 30–1), what interventions would you consider using to maintain and promote her health? Why?

3. As part of your regular community health nursing workload, you visit a senior day care center one afternoon each week. You take the blood pressures of several people who are taking antihypertensive medications and do some nutrition counseling. The center accommodates 60 senior clients, and you would like to serve the health needs of the aggregate population. What are some potential health needs of this group? What actions might you consider taking at an aggregate level? With whom would you consult as you plan programs at the center?

4. Assume that you have been asked by your local health department to determine the needs of the elderly population in your community. How would you begin conducting such a needs assessment? What data might you want to collect? How would you find out what services are already being offered and whether they are adequate?

5. Visit a continuing care center in your community. Assess the housing options, services, and health care provisions. Would you live here when you are older? How would you feel about a family member living here? What would you change if you could?

6. Using the Internet, locate innovative programs for elders in the community at the primary, secondary, and tertiary levels of care. Determine whether such programs could work in your community.

REFERENCES

American Association of Retired Persons. (2002). Social security finances improve despite recession. *AARP Bulletin, 43(5)*, 4.

Alzheimer, A. (1907). A unique illness involving the cerebral cortex. In D.A. Rottenberg & F. H. Hochberg (Eds.), *Neurological classics in modern translation*. New York: Hafner Press.

Assisted Living Federation of America. (2003). Mission statement. Retrieved April 9, 2004, from *http://www.alfa.org*

American Institute for Cancer Research, (2002). Smarter, safer exercise. *AICR Newsletter, 76,* 12.

Bell, V., & Troxel, D. (1997). *The Best Friends approach to Alzheimer's care*. Baltimore: Health Professions Press.

Bell, V., & Troxel, D. (2001). *The Best Friends staff: Building a culture of care in Alzheimer's programs*. Baltimore: Health Professions Press.

Burbank, P.M. & Riebe, D. (2002). *Promoting exercise and behavior change in older adults: Interventions with the transtheoretical model*. New York: Springer.

Cicirelli, V.G. (2002). *Older adults' views on death*. New York: Springer.

Ebersole, P., & Hess, P. (2004). *Toward healthy aging* (6th ed.). St. Louis: Mosby.

Elderhostel, Inc. (2002, June). *Elderhostel U. S. and Canada catalog: Fall 2002*. Issue 3. Boston, MA: Author.

Eliopoulos, C. (2001). *Gerontological nursing* (5th ed.). Philadelphia: Lippincott Williams & Wilkins.

Fast, B., & Chapin, R. (2000). *Strengths-based care management for older adults*. Baltimore: Health Professions Press.

Fillit, H., & O'Connell, A. (2002). *Drug discovery and development for Alzheimer's disease, 2000*. New York: Springer.

Ginn, J., Street, D., & Arber, S. (Eds.). (2001). *Women, work and pensions: International issues and prospects*. Philadelphia: Open University Press.

Hill, R.D., Thorn, B.L., Bowling, J., & Morrison, A. (2002). *Geriatric residential care*. Mahwah, NJ: Lawrence Erlbaum Associates.

Hill-Westmoreland, E.E., Soeken, K., & Spellbring, A.M. (2002). A meta-analysis of fall prevention programs for the elderly. How effective are they? *Nursing Research, 51(1)*, 1–8.

Holtrop, J.S., Hickner, J., Dosh, S., Noel, N., & Ettenhofer, T.L. (2002). "Sticking to it—Diabetes mellitus": A pilot study of an innovative behavior change program for women with type 2 diabetes. *American Journal of Health Education 33(3)*, 161–166.

Jech, A.O. (2000). A health crisis for the elderly: Taking a tumble. *Nurseweek, 13*(13), 20–21.

Kaiser Permanente healthwise handbook (14th ed.). (2000, revised). Boise, ID: Healthwise.

Kressig, R.W., & Echt, K.V. (2002). Exercise prescribing: Computer application in older adults, *The Gerontologist, 42(2)*, 273–277.

Kübler-Ross, E. (1975). *Death: The final stage of growth*. Englewood Cliffs, NJ: Prentice-Hall.

Mace, N.L., & Rabins, P.V. (2001). *The 36-hour day* (3rd Ed.—Large Print). Baltimore: Johns Hopkins University Press.

McKeon, V.A. (2002, February/March). Exploring HRT. *AWHONN Lifelines*, 24–31.

Menzey, M.K. (Ed.). (2001). *The encyclopedia of elder care: The comprehensive resource on geriatric and social care*. New York: Springer.

Miller, C.A. (1999). *Nursing care of older adults: Theory and practice* (3rd Ed.). Philadelphia: Lippincott Williams & Wilkins.

Moberg, D.O. (Ed.). (2001). *Aging and spirituality: Spiritual dimensions of aging theory, research, practice, and policy.* Binghamton, NY: Haworth Press.

Moore, A.J., & Stratton, D.C. (2002). *Resilient widowers: Older men speak for themselves.* New York: Springer.

Morrell, R.W., Mayhorn, C.B., & Bennett, J. (2000). A survey of World Wide Web use in middle-age and older adults. *Human Factors, 41*(2), 175–182.

National Center for Health Statistics. (2002). *Health, United States, 2002, with chartbook on trends in the health of Americans.* Hyattsville, MD: Author.

National Institute on Aging. (2001). Retrieved April 16, 2004, from *http://www.nia.nih.gov/news/2001guide.pdf*

O'Brien, M.E. (2003). *Spirituality in nursing: Standing on holy ground* (2nd Ed.). Sudbury, MA: Jones and Bartlett.

Oxendine, J. (1999, February/March). Who has diabetes? *Closing the Gap* [a newsletter of the Office of Minority Health, U. S. Department of Health and Human Services], 5.

Pan American Health Organization. (2002). *Health in the Americas—The Americas: A growing, urban, aging popluation. PAHO reports.* Washington, DC: Author.

Population Reference Bureau. (2003). *World population data sheets.* Retrieved April 16, 2004, from *http://www.prb.org/pdf/worldpopulationDS03_Eng.pdf*

Rix, S.E. (2001). The role of older workers in caring for older people in the future. *Generations, 25*(1), 29–34.

U. S. Department of Health and Human Services. (1991). *Healthy people 2000: National health promotion and disease prevention objectives* (S/N 017-001-00474-0). Washington, DC: U. S. Government Printing Office.

U. S. Department of Health and Human Services. (2000). *Healthy people 2010* (Conference ed., Vols. 1 & 2). Washington, DC: U. S. Government Printing Office.

U. S. Department of Transportation. (1998). *Traffic safety facts 1997—Older population.* Washington, DC: National Center for Statistics and Analysis, Research and Development.

U. S. Preventive Services Task Force. (2000–2003). *Guide to clinical preventive services* (3rd ed.). Retrieved January 29, 2004, from *http://www.uspstf.gov*

Vellas, B.J., & Fitten, L.J. (Eds.). (2001). *Research and practice in Alzheimer's disease* (Vol. 5). New York: Springer.

Warnes, A.M., & Crane, M.A. (2000). The achievements of a multiservice project for older homeless people. *The Gerontologist, 40*(5), 618–626.

West, J. (1999, February/March). National diabetes education program. *Closing the Gap* [a newsletter of the Office of Minority Health, U.S. Department of Health and Human Services], 1–3.

Worden, J.W. (2002). *Grief counseling and grief therapy: A handbook for the mental health practitioner* (3rd Ed.). New York: Springer.

SELECTED READINGS

Adler, P., Good, M., Roberts, B., & Snyder, S. (2000). The effects of Tai Chi on older adults with chronic arthritis pain. *Journal of Nursing Scholarship, 32*(4), 377.

Beckerman, A.G., & Tappen, R.M. (2000). *It takes more than*

love: A practical guide to taking care of an aging adult. Baltimore: Health Professions Press.

Blando, J.A. (2001). Twice hidden: Older gay and lesbian couples, friends, and intimacy. *Generations, 25*(2), 87–89.

Cantley, C. (2001). *A handbook of dementia care.* Philadelphia: Open University Press.

Estes, C.L. (2001). *Social policy and aging: A critical perspective.* Thousand Oaks, CA.: Sage.

Foote, C., & Stanners, C. (2002). *An integrated system of care for older people: New care for old.* Philadelphia: Jessica Kingsley.

Fulmer, T., Flaherty, E., & Medley, L. (2001). Geriatric nurse practitioners: Vital to the future of healthcare for elders. *Generations, 25*(1), 72–75.

Gray-Vickrey, P. (2001). Protecting the older adult. *Nursing Management, 32*(10), 36–40.

Gueldner, S.H., Burke, M.S., & Smiciklas-Wright, H. (2000). *Preventing and managing osteoporosis.* New York: Springer.

Heywood, F., Oldman, C., & Means, R. (2002). *Housing and home in later life.* Philadelphia: Open University Press.

Huyck, M.H. (2001). Romantic relationships in later life. *Generations, 25*(2), 9–17.

Ingersoll-Dayton, B., & Campbell, R. (2001). *The delicate balance: Case studies in counseling and care management for older adults.* Baltimore: Health Professions Press.

Kane, R.L., & Kane, R.A. (2000*). Assessing older persons: Measures, meaning, and practical applications.* New York: Oxford University Press.

Kimmel, D.C., & Martin, D.L. (2002). *Midlife and aging in gay America: Proceedings of the SAGE conference 2000.* Binghamton, NY: Haworth Press.

Klesges, L.M., Pahor, M., Shorr, R.I., Wan, J.Y., Williamson, J.D., & Guralnik, J.M. (2001). Financial difficulty in acquiring food among elderly disabled women: Results from the Women's Health and Aging Study. *American Journal of Public Health, 91*(1), 68–75.

Laditka, S.B. (Ed.). (2003). *Health expectations for older women: International perspectives.* Binghamton, NY: Haworth Press.

Lockett, D., Aminzadeh, F., & Edwards, N. (2002). Development and evaluation of an instrument to measure seniors' attitudes toward the use of bathroom grab bars. *Public Health Nursing, 19*(5), 390–397.

Montgomery, R.J.V. (2003). *A new look at community based respite programs: Utilization, satisfaction, and development.* Binghamton, NY: Haworth Press.

Moody, H.R. (2002). *Aging: Concepts and controversies* (4th ed.). Thousand Oaks, CA: Sage.

Post, S.G. (2000). *The moral challenge of Alzheimer disease: Ethical issues from diagnosis to dying* (2nd Ed.). Baltimore: Johns Hopkins University Press.

Ronch, J.L., & Goldfield, J. (2003). *Mental wellness in aging: Strengths-based approaches.* Baltimore: Health Professions Press.

Rowe, M.A., Straneva, J.A., Colling, K.B., & Grabo, T. (2000). Behavioral problems in community-dwelling people with dementia. *Journal of Nursing Scholarship, 32*(1), 55–56.

Savishinsky, J. (2001). Images of retirement: Finding the purpose and the passion. *Generations, 25*(3), 52–56.

Swanson, E.A., Tripp-Reimer, T., & Buckwalter, K. (2001). *Health promotion and disease prevention in the older adult: Interventions and recommendations.* New York: Springer.

Taira, E.D., & Carlson, J.L. (2000). *Aging in place: Designing, adapting, and enhancing the home environment.* Binghamton, NY: Haworth Press.

Tideiksaar, R., (2002). *Falls in older people: Prevention and management* (3rd Ed.). Baltimore: Health Professions Press.

Tucker, K.L., Bermudez, O.I., Castaneda, C. (2000). Type 2 diabetes is prevalent and poorly controlled among Hispanic elders of Caribbean origin. *American Journal of Public Health, 90*(7), 1288–1293.

Webster, J.D., & Haight, B.K. (2002). *Critical advances in reminiscence work: From theory to application.* New York: Springer.

World Health Organization. (2002). *Keep fit for life: Meeting the nutritional needs of older persons.* Geneva: Author.

Internet Resources

Administration on Aging: *http://www.aoa.dhhs.gov*

Alzheimer's Disease Education and Referral Center: *http://www.alzheimers.org*

American Association of Retired Persons: *http://www.aarp.org*

Andrus Foundation: *http://www.andrus.org*

Assisted Living Foundation of America: *http://www.alfa.org*

Association of Late Deafened Adults: *http://www.alda.org*

Elderhostel: *http://www.elderhostel.org*

Generations United: *http://www.gu.org*

Gerontological Society of America: *http://www.org*

GriefNet: *http://www.rivendell.org*

National Aging Information Center: *http://www.aoa.dhhs.gov/naic*

National Institute on Aging: *http://www.nih.gov/nia*

National Parkinson Foundation: *http://www.Parkinson.org*

SPRY Foundation: *http://www.spry.org*

Statistical Abstract of United States: *http://www.census.gov/statab/www/*

The Geezer Brigade: *http://www.thegeezerbrigade.com*

Promoting and Protecting the Health of Vulnerable Aggregates

31
Rural Health Care

Learning Objectives

Upon mastery of this chapter, you should be able to:

- Define the term *rural*.
- Discuss population characteristics of rural residents.
- Identify at-risk populations of rural residents.
- Describe five barriers to health care access for rural clients.
- Discuss how the terms *out-migration* and *in-migration* relate to the population trends associated with rural communities in recent decades.
- Relate the broad objectives of *Healthy People 2010* to the concept of "social justice" in rural communities.
- Discuss activities to assist in the orientation of a new community health nurse to a rural community.
- Compare and contrast the *"circle of formal support"* and the *"circle of informal support"* themes apparent in rural communities.
- Discuss the challenges and opportunities related to rural community health nursing practice.

Think about the last time you were in a rural community. What do you recall about it? Was there a hospital, nursing home, clinic, or public health department in the community? Were there schools and playgrounds? What types of small businesses lined the main street? What eating establishments were there? How many traffic signals were present? How would you describe the population living in the area in terms of age, income, occupations, faith, culture, and ethnicity? If you live in the rural community you describe, these questions are probably easy to answer, and you may have at least considered a career in rural nursing. If you live in an urban community, you probably have little familiarity with rural communities and have never considered this specialty practice.

Rural nursing practice offers many opportunities. Nurses are respected community members—their judgment and opinions count. Rural nurses are key members of the health care team. They can make a difference in the lives of their neighbors, friends, and community. The challenges are many, and the rewards are great! This chapter addresses the special health needs and concerns of rural clients and the ways in which a community health nurse can address those needs. After reading the chapter, you may come to appreciate the many advantages that rural nurses enjoy and consider rural nursing as a practice choice.

DEFINITIONS AND DEMOGRAPHICS

Definitions of Rural

There are various definitions of the term *rural*. The community health nurse needs to be aware of the precise meaning of the term as it is used in a particular agency, community, or piece of legislation, because differences in semantics can affect public policy regarding rural communities. For example, federal dollars are often distributed to communities based on rural or urban status.

The U. S. government provides several definitions of rural. The U. S. Census Bureau (2000a) identifies "urban" as all territory, population, and housing units within **urbanized areas (UAs)** and **urban clusters (UCs)**. A UA consists of densely settled territory that contains 50,000 or more people. A UC consists of a densely settled territory that has at least 2500 people but fewer than 50,000. Both UAs and UCs have a cluster of one or more block groups that have a population density of at least 1000 people per square mile. The U. S. Census definition of "rural" is all territory, population, and housing units located outside UAs and UCs.

The U. S. Office of Management and Budget (OMB) recently reclassified the United States into metropolitan and micropolitan statistical areas ("Standards for Defining," 2000). This new nomenclature identifies a **metropolitan statistical area** as a core-based statistical area associated with at least one urbanized area that has a minimum population of 50,000. **Micropolitan statistical areas** are core-based sta-

tistical areas associated with at least one urban cluster of no less than 10,000 and no more than 50,000 people. Both metropolitan and micropolitan statistical areas comprise the central county or counties containing the core; also included are adjacent outlying counties that have a high degree of social and economic integration with the central county (based on the number of people who commute). With such a broad definition, micropolitan statistical areas can include both rural and urban areas. Before 2003, the OMB defined urban and rural in terms of metropolitan and nonmetropolitan counties. Those terms are still used by the U. S. Department of Agriculture (USDA).

The USDA's rural-urban continuum codes break down the former OMB definition of metropolitan counties into four codes; nonmetropolitan counties are divided into six codes based on population density and proximity to metropolitan areas (Butler & Beale, 1994) (Display 31–1). Areas coded 8 (Adjacent to Metropolitan Area) or 9 (Not Adjacent to Metropolitan Area) have fewer than 2500 residents and are classified as "completely rural."

For the purposes of this chapter, **rural** is defined as communities with fewer than 10,000 residents and a county pop-

DISPLAY 31–1

U. S. Department of Agriculture Economic Research Service Rural–Urban Continuum Codes

Code	Metropolitan Counties
0	Central counties of metropolitan areas of 1 million population or more
1	Fringe counties of metropolitan areas of 1 million population or more
2	Counties in metropolitan areas of 250,000–1 million population
3	Counties in metropolitan areas of less than 250,000 population

Code	Nonmetropolitan Counties
4	Urban population of 20,000 or more, adjacent to a metropolitan area
5	Urban population of 20,000 or more, not adjacent to a metropolitan area
6	Urban population of 2,500 to 19,999, adjacent to a metropolitan area
7	Urban population of 2,500 to 19,999, not adjacent to a metropolitan area
8	Completely rural or less than 2,500 urban population, adjacent to metro area
9	Completely rural or less than 2,500 urban population, not adjacent to metro area

(From Butler, M. A., & Beale, C. A. [1994]. *Rural-urban continuum codes for metropolitan counties,* 1993. Washington, DC: Agriculture and Rural Economy Division, Economic Research Service, U.S. Department of Agriculture.)

T A B L E   3 1 – 1

Definitions of Rural

Source	Nomenclature	Definitions
U. S. Bureau of the Census	Rural	All territory, population, and housing units located outside of urbanized areas (UAs) and urbanized clusters (UCs)
U. S. Office of Management and Budget	Micropolitan statistical area	A core-based statistical area associated with at least one urban cluster of at least 10,000 but <50,000 people.
U. S. Department of Agriculture Rural-Urban Continuum Codes	Completely rural	<2500 urban population either adjacent to or not adjacent to metropolitan area.
U. S. Government	Frontier area	<6 people per square mile
Author	Rural	Communities with <10,000 residents and county population <1000 people per square mile.

ulation density of less than 1000 persons per square mile (Table 31–1). This definition of rural is arbitrary because rural clients do not just consider population density or community size when defining their "ruralness." They have a multitude of reasons for defining their community as rural, such as distance from a large city, major occupations in the area, or numbers of students in the local schools. If you have access to a small community, ask some of the residents why they consider their community to be urban or rural.

The term **frontier area** is used to designate sparsely populated places with six or fewer persons per square mile (Congdon, 2001; U. S. Department of Health and Human Services [USDHHS], 1998). Health issues of concern to rural areas may be of even greater concern to frontier areas. Another term critical to rural health is **health professional shortage areas (HPSAs)**, which are urban or rural geographic areas, population groups, or facilities with shortages of health professionals (National Advisory Committee on Rural Health, 2002). Current HPSA designations relate only to primary medical care, mental health, or dental care. The USDHHS determines which areas are HPSAs, thereby making them eligible for a variety of governmental assistance programs. Hundreds of counties in the United States have been designated as HPSAs (Fig. 31–1).

Population Statistics

The number of persons living in rural areas of the United States has tripled since the mid-1800s, to 59,367,367 in 2000 (U. S. Census Bureau, 2000b). During the same period, the proportion of persons living in rural communities decreased from about 85% of the U. S. population to 21% (Ricketts et al., 1999). The highest proportion of the rural population is located in the South (35%). The Midwest and West both have approximately 23% rural residents, and the Northeast has the smallest percentage (19%) (Eberhardt et al., 2001).

Of the poorest counties in America, 244 are rural (Congressional Rural Caucus, 2001). Poverty is common among rural Americans. Rural workers are more likely than urban workers to earn the minimum wage (12% versus 7%, respectively). Twenty-one percent of the nation's welfare population is rural (Congressional Rural Caucus, 2001). These

people are generally older than their urban counterparts, a fact that has health implications. It is also important to note the concentration of the rural population between 25 and 44 years of age, because this group is responsible for most of the child bearing in rural communities. Growth in population related to births is called "natural increase."

Changing Patterns of Migration

Population changes in rural areas are usually related to natural increase through births or through **out-migration**, the process of residents moving out of rural communities and into urban places (Ricketts et al., 1999). Johnson and Beale (cited in Ricketts et al., 1999) noted that during the 1800s there was more natural increase than out-migration in the United States, which caused growth in the rural population.

In the first half of the 1900s immigration was high and industrialization increased, causing cities to grow while rural areas remained essentially unchanged. This changed in the 1970s; the proportion of births decreased, but many people moved into rural communities, resulting in an increase in population. During the 1980s, the population trends shifted as most rural areas lost population to out-migration, and any gains were due to increased births. During the 1990s, the population trend in rural communities changed to **in-migration**, an increase in residents moving into rural communities from urban places. An additional 2.2 million Americans moved into rural communities (Congressional Rural Caucus, 2001). During this period, 70% of rural communities grew in population and 61% experienced more in- than out-migration. Since 1995, however, the growth rate in many rural communities has decreased. Population trends have many implications for the health services needed by rural people. The patterns of rural migration appear to be "shifting sand," which adds to the challenge of planning resources for rural communities.

POPULATION CHARACTERISTICS

The following information is meant to describe, not stereotype, rural clients. Each rural community is unique as are its resi-

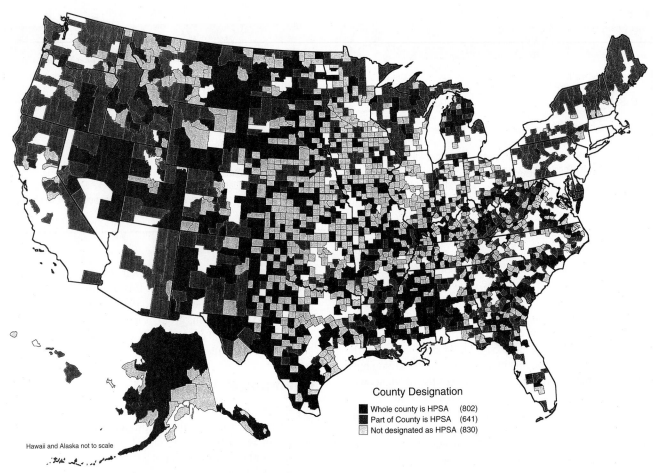

Note: Metropolitan counties are aggregated into white areas on the map.
Source: Division of Shortage Designation, BPHC, HRSA, DHHS, 1997.
Produced by: North Carolina Rural Health Research and Policy Analysis Center, Cecil G. Sheps Center for Health Services Research,
University of North Carolina at Chapel Hill, with support from the Federal Office of Rural Health Policy, HRSA, US DHHS.

FIGURE 31–1.   Primary care health professional shortage areas (HPSAs), 1997.
(Ricketts, T. [Ed.] [1998]. *Mapping rural health: The geography of health care in rural America* [p.
17]. Bethesda, MD: Office of Rural Health Policy, Health Resources, and Services Administration.)

dents. The community health nurse must determine whether the population characteristics discussed "fit" a specific rural community. Keep in mind that many rural clients reside in countries outside the United States. The nursing student who plans to practice in the international arena will need to seek out relevant information about the rural population to be served.

Age and Gender

Elderly persons, those 65 years of age and older, are the fastest growing population in the United States in every location, including rural America. Older women outnumber men by more than 1 million. The elderly use more health care resources than other age groups do. In 1998, Medicare was the payment source for almost one third of all health care expenditures (Eberhardt et al., 2001).

Population estimates in 1998 noted that 6.5% of the non-metropolitan population were younger than 5 years of age,

19.7% were 5 to 17, 59.2% were 18 to 64, and 14.6% were older than 65 years of age.

Population trends have a direct relationship to the kinds of health services that are needed in rural communities. Growing families with young children need maternity, pediatric, and family health medical services. They also can benefit from health promotion and disease prevention services. The elderly, on the other hand, need health care to manage increased numbers of chronic health conditions. Rural communities need to provide access to nursing homes and rehabilitative services, as well as to hospitals, clinics, and health promotion programs that serve the elderly and the entire community.

Race and Ethnicity

Rural areas have less racial diversity than urban areas do. In 1998, the U. S. Census Bureau estimated that 83.3% of nonmetropolitan (rural) residents were Caucasian, 9.1% were African-American, 4.8% were Hispanic, 1.8% were American Indian or Alaskan Native, and 1% were Asian or Pacific Islander (Eberhardt et al., 2001). Racial and ethnic subgroups tend to be more concentrated in certain areas of the country. These patterns influence geographic patterns of health status.

Rural Hispanics generally live in the western states and the state of Texas, whereas the majority of rural Asian-Americans live in Hawaii. Seventy percent of nonmetropolitan Native Americans live in the western United States or in Oklahoma. Most African-American rural residents live in the southern states.

Education

Rural clients in the United States generally have lower educational attainment than urban clients do. In 1998, 15% of adults (25 years of age and older) in nonmetropolitan areas had college degrees, compared with 27% of urban adults. Twenty percent of rural adults do not have a high school diploma, compared with 15% for urban adults. According to the Congressional Rural Caucus (2001), a disproportionate share of rural poor parents lack a high school education; 44.2% of adults in two-parent rural families, and 71.6% of those in single-parent families, are not high school graduates. Rural clients have little access to higher educational facilities such as community colleges or universities close to home. Travel to urban areas for educational pursuits adds to the burden of obtaining additional education beyond high school.

Income and Occupations

There are rural communities with some very wealthy residents. On the average, however, the income of people in rural communities is lower than that of persons living in urban communities. This is reflected in higher unemployment and lower per capita income (Hummel, 2001).

There are a number of economic advantages to living in a rural area. The cost of land is lower than in urban areas; therefore, housing costs are also lower. Taxes are usually less, and restrictions on land use are not as stringent. Less expensive land is advantageous to businesses such as manufacturing, which may need large parcels of land.

Although many people equate farming with rural life, only 1.9% to 2.4% of the total U. S. population were rural farmers as of 1990 (USDHHS, 1998). The United States is unique in that it feeds its population with a small proportion of workers committed to food production and still exports food products to the rest of the world.

When compared with urban areas, rural communities typically offer fewer job options. Types of rural work such as mining and forestry vary by locale. Rural areas have manufacturing, business, education, and service occupations just as urban communities do. Moreover, the use of the telephone and Internet for commerce is now common in rural areas.

RURAL POPULATIONS AT RISK

Homeless Families

The homeless are a population at risk in many rural communities. Although fewer in number, rural homeless families are similar to their urban counterparts. The heads of household are often female. They have frequently suffered a series of personal crises such as illness, loss of work, loss of housing, or other misfortunes that have led to their homelessness. Finally, although such families usually consider themselves to have few major health needs, studies frequently report heavy smoking, alcohol use, and illegal drug use of some members in this population (Cox et al., 2001). Homeless children are at risk for developmental delays, nutritional deficits, and other health problems.

In rural settings, the problems of homelessness may be compounded by lack of transportation, inadequate shelter, few employment opportunities, limited access to health and social services, and a lack of inexpensive housing. Community health nurses must try to address the multiple needs of this population. They should (1) seek out homeless families, (2) assess their health needs, (3) connect the families with available resources (eg, health, financial, housing), and (4) remain connected with the families until they have stabilized (see Research: Bridge to Practice).

Perinatal Clients

Historically, the best outcomes for obstetric clients have been observed for white urban women (Lishner et al., 1999). The question is whether rural women have adequate access to prenatal care to ensure the births of healthy infants. Perinatal clients are pregnant women in the last half of pregnancy and their newborn infants until 1 month of age.

Local access to obstetric care is basic to positive birth outcomes. The Council on Medical Education (cited in Lishner et al., 1999) stated that 20% of the U. S. population lives in rural areas, yet only 9% of physicians practice in these communities. Many pregnant women must either receive obstetric care from a primary care physician in their own community or travel to an urban center for care by an obstetrician. Babies born to these women enter the rural system of health care as soon as they are born.

It is important to consider the role of midlevel practitioners in perinatal care. Nurse practitioners (NPs), physician assistants (PAs), and certified nurse midwives (CNMs) provide innovative approaches to the delivery of prenatal and obstetric care in rural areas (Acosta, 2001). NPs and PAs are able to provide prenatal care and assist with some hospital "call" responsibilities when working with a family physician. They also can provide health care to newborns and well-child care. CNMs are able to assist rural physicians by providing care for low-risk clients, including prenatal care, delivery, and postpartum follow-up.

RESEARCH: BRIDGE TO PRACTICE

Craft-Rosenberg, M., Powell, S.R., & Culp, K. (2000). Health status and resources of rural homeless women and children. *Western Journal of Nursing Research, 22,* 863–878.

Nurses need to assess the health status of rural residents and understand their specific health needs in order to participate in the development of needed health services and resources. Often rural clients have different needs than urban residents do. Distance to health services and lack of health care providers are two common rural problems.

The purpose of this descriptive research study was to "describe the health status and health resources for homeless women and children in a midwestern rural community." Additionally, the following research questions were asked:

- What is the health status of rural women housed in a shelter for homeless women in a midwestern state including the dental status, substance use, mental health, and adverse life events?
- What is the health status of the children of rural homeless women?
- What are the health resources for health promotion and illness management for rural homeless women?

Several interview instruments were used to collect data from the 31 shelter guests—The Rural Homeless Interview Instrument, The Michigan Alcohol Screening Test, and the Beck Depression Inventory. The researchers did pilot testing to refine the process and instrument use. Questions were added about dental status after the pilot study was completed.

The study sample of 31 rural homeless women was collected at a single homeless shelter. Women were invited to participate, and all those signing up completed the 1-hour interview, physical assessment, and dental assessment. A graduate student in community health nursing conducted the interviews and assessments.

Selected findings from the study include the following:

- **Demographics**—The age of the participants ranged from 18 to 60+ years. Most were Caucasian; 4 were married, and 23 had not completed high school. Most were unemployed, and about half had incomes of $400 or less per month.
- **Children**—Six mothers reported having one child, and two mothers reported having two children. The mothers were not aware of the health status of their children because the children were adopted out, in foster care, or cared for by others. It was interesting that these women also reported a total of 69 pregnancies and 29 miscarriages, stillbirths, or abortions; obviously, the data on children are incomplete.
- **Health Status**—The 31 women reported 122 health problems, almost four per woman. They included 78 chronic issues such as asthma, diabetes, and high blood pressure. The women reported 44 acute health problems such as bronchitis, pneumonia, and colds.
- **Dental Status**—Dental screening identified 12 of the 31 women as having at least two missing teeth. Other reported dental problems included 10 women with bleeding gums and smaller numbers of women with dental odor or drainage. Seven of the participants reported dental pain.
- **Substance Use and Abuse**—Approximately one third of the participants reported a history of alcohol abuse. Five women reported current illegal drug use, and 22 of the 31 smoked tobacco.
- **Mental Health**—The women reported a wide variety of mental health issues, ranging from hallucinations to panic disorders, bipolar disease, and obsessive-compulsive disorder. Additional mental health-related symptoms were frequent; 13 of the 31 women had depression ranging from mild to severe. There were no data reported about recent or current treatment for these conditions.
- **Health of Children**—The data reported by the women in this category (20 children) did not match the data reported earlier (10 children). The women stated that their children had coughs and colds, sore throats, ear infections, and allergies as well as other health conditions.
- **Adverse Life Events**—The women described many losses, including loss of personal possessions (16), death of family members (15), and job loss (14).
- **Health Promotion/Illness Detection Measure**—Preventive care measures were practiced by many of the women. Eighteen reported having had a pap smear in the previous year, and 23 reported a breast examination conducted by a health professional within the last 2 years. Most women used contraception or were not sexually active. The women were informed about the need for dental self-care, and almost all reporting daily toothbrushing. The range of time since their last professional dental examination was 1 month to 10 years, with 15 of the women reporting a dental visit within the last year.
- **Resources: Health and Personal**—Some of the women reported limited income from part-time employment, disability insurance, welfare, or child support. Most received health care at a public clinic. The women shared that they would most likely seek help from a family member or friend rather than a professional or agency.

The findings from this research study have potential implications for community health nurses working with rural homeless women and children. Nurses should attempt to assess the medical, dental, and mental health needs of this special population and minimize the barriers for homeless women and children to receive needed health services. Community health nurses can also seek ways to inform homeless rural women about the health and prevention-related community resources available to them and their children.

An Iowa study (Hulme & Blegen, 1999) looked at the caesarean section birth outcomes of three different residential groups: urban women, rural women, and rural adjacent women (defined as women living in "counties adjacent to urban counties with at least 5% commuting to urban areas and a population base between 2500 to 50,000 people") (Hulme & Blegen, 1999, p. 178). Caesarean birth outcomes were best for rural adjacent women, the youngest and least educated group. Rural women had the worst birth outcomes and had to travel the farthest for obstetric care. In this study, both rural and rural adjacent women frequently lacked private health insurance and started prenatal care later than urban women did. The initiation of early prenatal care is an issue of concern for community health nurses seeking to optimize birth outcomes in their communities. High-risk infants born in rural hospitals are at risk for many potential complications. More research needs to be done to identify the needs of rural perinatal clients and to provide appropriate interventions.

The Elderly

The elderly are a population of special concern for rural community health nurses. Some elderly individuals are well and live independently throughout their lives. As an aggregate, however, the elderly have increased chronic disease, disability, and functional impairment. In The National Health Interview Survey (1990 to 1994), 35% of rural elders between 65 and 69 years of age rated their own health status as poor (Coburn et al., 1999).

Elders rarely have close access to the sophisticated health care that they need. Oncologists, cardiologists, neurologists, and other specialists do not typically practice in rural communities. Extended travel to these specialists can be a severe barrier to obtaining needed care.

Even when ill, older adults tend to stay in their own homes. They do not want to move to a dependent living situation. Rural elders in poor health often have limited options for alternative housing when they can no longer live by themselves. Many of the community services required to maintain ill elders in their homes are not available in rural communities. They may need to move to nursing homes if in-home or assisted living placements are not available.

A major ethnographic study of the rural elderly was conducted by a team of nurse researchers in 13 rural counties of Colorado (Magilvy et al., 2000). Over 4 years, the researchers explored the transitions that older adults experienced as they moved through various types and levels of health care. After being introduced to the residents by local community health nurses or home health nurses, the team interviewed 175 older adults in a variety of settings. A major theme from the study was "the crisis nature of health care transitions experienced by the rural older adults and their families and observed by rural nurses and other providers" (Magilvy et al., 2000, p. 339). In other words, the older adults had not anticipated the chronic and acute health conditions that they experienced. Additional findings of the research included the following:

- Crisis was compounded by surprise
- Limited knowledge of local resources exacerbated crisis
- Inconsistent discharge planning disrupted transitions
- Changing family support necessitated admission to nursing homes
- Continuity of care in nursing home discharges lessened transition crisis
- Rural home health care was identified as a strength

Because of these findings and their previous studies, the researchers recommended that nurses working with rural older adults develop resources for their clients within two "circles of care": the circle of formal support and the circle of informal support. The **circle of formal support** includes health services (eg, hospital, nursing homes, clinics), and professionals (eg, nurses, physicians, pharmacists). The **circle of informal support** includes family and other persons from the community who support the patient.

The Mentally Ill

Rural residents experience mental illness as do people in urban communities. The mental health resources available to rural residents, however, may be limited to primary care physicians, community mental health centers (CHMC), state hospitals, and clergy. CHMCs may be restricted to treating only individuals with severe mental illness. Less severely ill people may be placed on long waiting lists and never receive needed services. These individuals may lack health insurance that could enable them to seek private mental health services.

In a research study identifying the health care access needs of residents in 10 rural Washington counties, 17% to 35% of 391 rural households reported having at least one of six specific mental health care needs for a member or members of the household (Bayne et al., 2002). The mental health needs for these households were often met to a low degree—domestic violence (92%), drug abuse (90%), alcohol counseling (89%), crisis counseling (86%), chronic mental illness (82%), and anxiety/depression (71%). Many households reported multiple mental health needs (see Chap. 35).

There is a stigma associated with mental illness. Rural residents may be unwilling to use the services of mental health specialists because of concerns about confidentiality. Rural practitioners need to consider ways to reduce the stigma of mental illness, ensure confidentiality, and connect rural residents with the mental health services they need.

Ideally, there should be an integration of primary care and mental health care services so that people who need the latter services receive them. Primary care providers may be in the best position to make these connections. Physicians, PAs, and NPs should be alert to the signs and symptoms of depression and other mental health disorders. They need to be aware that depression in women may be an indicator of domestic violence. All women should be questioned about violence in their lives and offered services if they are living in a violent situation.

The elderly with mental health problems comprise another overlooked group in rural communities. Outpatient services for elders with mental illness may not be available. These elders may be unable to care for themselves without intensive home health and other support services, which may be limited or nonexistent in their areas. Rural residents may be admitted to nursing homes for long-term custodial care.

Community health nurses need to be aware of the mental health resources available in the rural community and assist rural residents in obtaining those services. Rural community health nurses can work with other professionals to "get the word out" about mental health and illness to churches, service clubs, businesses, and the community at large. Only then can the stigma of mental illness be lessened so that rural residents receive the mental health services they may need.

Native Americans

Almost 2 million Native Americans live in rural America, most of them on or near tribal reservations in 28 states (Joho & Ormsby, 2000) (Fig. 31–2).

A unique feature of a federally recognized tribe is that the tribe has a signed treaty with the U. S. government providing eligibility of the tribe to participate in federal programs such as the Indian Health Service (IHS) while at the same time placing the land once occupied by the American Indian in trust to the U. S. government; thus the term reservation (Joho & Ormsby, 2000, p. 210).

Native Americans may move back and forth between their rural homes and nearby cities because of unemployment and poverty. Native Americans who leave the reservation may be ineligible for health care services by IHS. This can be problematic because Native Americans are at risk for numerous health problems.

American Indians have an infant mortality rate twice that of whites. They also have some of the highest rates of diabetes, alcoholism, and smoking (USDHHS, 2000). Stubben (cited in Hartley, Bird, & Dempsey, 1999) stated that Native

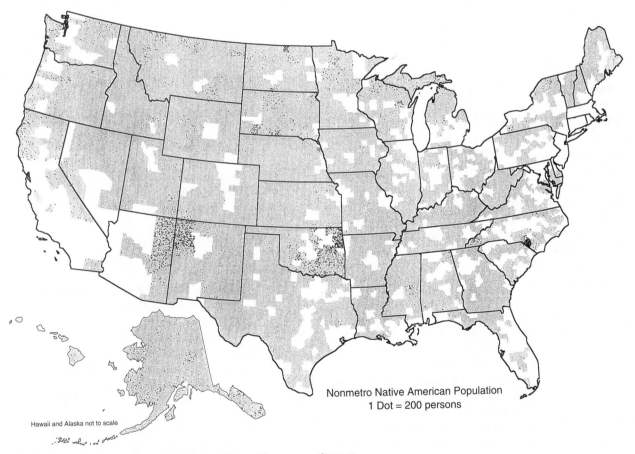

Nonmetro Native American Population
1 Dot = 200 persons

Hawaii and Alaska not to scale

Note: Metropolitan counties are aggregated into white areas on the map.
Source: US Bureau of the Census, 1990.
Produced by: North Carolina Rural Health Research and Policy Analysis Center, Cecil G. Sheps Center for Health Services Research, University of North Carolina at Chapel Hill, with support from the Federal Office of Rural Health Policy, HRSA, US DHHS.

FIGURE 31–2.   Distribution of nonmetropolitan Native American population, 1990. (Ricketts, T. [Ed.] [1998]. *Mapping rural health: The geography of health care in rural America* [p. 10]. Bethesda, MD: Office of Rural Health Policy, Health Resources, and Services Administration.)

American adolescents drink more alcohol and have higher suicide rates than other American adolescents do.

Nurses and other professionals working with Native Americans should attempt to identify the traditions and beliefs of their patients. They can ask their Native American clients about traditions related to healing and attempt to incorporate those into the health services delivered. Nurses who work with this population should encourage health promotion activities such as exercise, smoking elimination, and reduced alcohol consumption to minimize health consequences related to these behaviors.

Farm Workers

Agricultural workers operating family farms are another population at risk. There are many potential health and safety issues associated with farming. Agricultural workers are exposed to hazards every day, yet they usually receive little injury prevention education. For example, farming today is a high-technology industry with much potentially hazardous equipment. Heavy machinery such as tractors, forklifts, and combine harvesters can cause serious injuries, especially if operated by unskilled workers. Toxic pesticides and other chemicals are commonplace on farms. Power tools, ladders, and discarded farm equipment account for many electrical shocks, falls, and other injuries (see Chap. 33).

Farms are also places where people live and play. Farm families are exposed to potential dangers daily. Often, children do the work of adults and older adults continue to participate in the heavy labor associated with the farm. These groups are at special risk for serious or fatal injuries and acute or chronic illnesses (Bushy, 2000). Many farm children are injured each year from falls, drowning, electrical shock, suffocation, and other causes.

The community health nurse can intervene with farm workers by using tools that identify farm hazards. A walk-through of a farm can assist the nurse in the process. Farm safety checklists and a risk-mapping tool are available through the National Institute for Occupational Safety and Health (NIOSH), and additional assessment tools can be obtained through the local USDA extension agent. Community health nurses can include injury prevention in all interactions with farm workers and their families. A multifaceted approach works best with this population.

RURAL HEALTH ISSUES

Self, Home, and Community Care

Historically, self-management of health care problems has been the most common way for rural people to cope with illness. This may be a strength. Rural clients are resourceful and often have a supportive network to get their health needs met. Because cost, travel, weather, and distance are barriers to obtaining health services from formal health care providers, rural clients may employ a variety of folk treatments and home remedies before consulting a nurse or a physician; such clients tend to visit providers at a much later stage than people in urban areas.

Home health care (HHC) allows people to stay at home, supports their hardiness, and compensates for the long distance between home and formal health care. Adams and colleagues (2001) conducted a study to determine whether health status differed between rural and urban HHC patients and whether place of residence was a predictor of HHC direct care time. The study collected data from more than 2500 episodes of patient care using items from the Outcome Assessment and Information Set (OASIS). Home health nurse time in the home was also measured. The study results showed significant differences in rural versus urban health status, with urban patients being healthier. Rural HHC clients were more ill and received more home health nurse time. This study demonstrated need for higher Medicare reimbursement for rural patients and supported the importance of the availability of HHC for patients who need this service.

Major Health Problems

Cardiovascular Disease

"It is possible that geography is more powerful than any risk factor yet to be discovered" (Taylor et al., 2002, p. 550). Geographic concentrations of cardiovascular disease and other diseases vary from one rural location to the next, possibly related to inadequate health care, distance from care, environmental exposures, infectious disease in the area, and other factors. These multidimensional elements interact in such a way to cause cardiovascular mortality statistics to vary among regions and ethnic groups.

Cardiovascular disease is a leading cause of death in the United States, with ischemic heart disease accounting for more than 60% of deaths (Eberhardt et al., 2001). There are clear differences in cardiovascular mortality rates between urban and rural residents. The rates of cardiovascular death from ischemic heart disease for men 20 years of age and older are highest in the most rural counties. In the South, both men and women are more likely to die from ischemic heart disease than in other parts of the country. In the West, rural adults have less heart disease than urban residents do.

There are many reasons for these data. Cardiovascular disease, like some other chronic diseases, is characterized by a long latency period. Residence of diagnosis is of less interest than residence 10 to 30 years prior to diagnosis (Dennis & Pallotta, 2001). Rural residents may ignore early cardiovascular symptoms and give little heed to preventive interventions such as exercise and low-fat diets. Other risk factors such as smoking and poverty affect cardiovascular health. Adults in rural counties are most likely to smoke. This may be related to "delayed access to medical and media resources that help change unhealthy behaviors, and lower educational attainment, which is strongly associated with smoking" (Eberhardt et al., 2001, p. 34). In addition, rural areas usually have less high-tech health care equipment available, which may affect outcomes for patients with cardiovascular emergencies.

Human Immunodeficiency Virus Infection

Human immunodeficiency virus (HIV), the virus that causes acquired immunodeficiency syndrome (AIDS), was first identified among the urban U. S. population in the early 1980s. The Center for Disease Control and Prevention (CDC) estimates that more than 850,000 U. S. residents are living with AIDS, 25% of whom are unaware of their positive HIV status (National Institutes of Health, National Institute of Allergy and Infectious Diseases, 2002). Bushy (2000) reported that 36% of all HIV/AIDS cases are from nonmetropolitan areas of the country and that the number of HIV/AIDS cases is increasing especially in the rural South among young people, African-Americans, Hispanics, and women (see Chap. 9).

Early diagnosis and treatment of HIV/AIDS are issues that must be faced by all rural communities. Physicians, nurses, and other health practitioners need to be educated about the changing face of the disease. Because there are relatively few cases of HIV/AIDS in any one rural community, it can be a challenge to stay up to date with the newest treatment protocols. Each state health department has resource persons that can provide information to health professionals in rural communities about the HIV/AIDS epidemic.

It may be difficult for a person to seek diagnosis or treatment from a rural health practitioner. Confidentiality is an issue of concern, as is lack of anonymity. People with HIV/AIDS may fear for their jobs or their "place in the community" if their diagnosis is learned. Instead, rural people may choose to seek out HIV/AIDS testing through an urban health care facility where they know no one. Returning to the community can be devastating because of the lack of needed support services and the fear of sharing their diagnosis with others.

Another issue that has become common is that of urban residents with "rural roots" who return to their home communities as their illness worsens. These people seek family support and can overwhelm their caregivers, especially if the caregivers do not seek support for themselves. Community health nurses are in a good position to assist families with any health issues and can offer to facilitate connections to other social, spiritual, financial, and health care providers.

The impact of HIV/AIDS on other rural areas of the world is devastating. The disease is engulfing large populations of countries in Africa and elsewhere. The "face of HIV/AIDS" is changing: 50% of adults living with HIV/AIDS worldwide are now women (UNAIDS, 2002). Often, people with HIV/AIDS have no access to treatment modalities and little understanding about the epidemiology of the disease. Certainly, the key to this disease lies in its prevention. Nurses worldwide are in a position to provide education and advocate for policies that provide for humane treatment for people with HIV/AIDS (see What Do You Think? I).

WHAT DO YOU THINK? I

A rural resident friend shares that her 23-year-old son has AIDS and is coming home because he is getting more ill. Few people know about her son's condition. What might you recommend to your friend so that she can resolve this issue and get the support that she needs?

Access to Health Care

Insurance and Managed Care

Health insurance in today's market is costly, especially for individual purchasers. Some people, therefore, forego health insurance for themselves and their families. Depending on their income, these people may or may not be eligible for Medicaid. Even people who are eligible for government health assistance may not apply because of their belief that it is a sign of weakness to "accept a handout."

Historically, a traditional fee-for-service model delivered health care in rural and urban communities. However, it is challenging for rural providers to deliver the cost-effective, complex health care that rural persons need via solo or small group practices. The managed care model, which attempts to control costs and improve health care delivery, has diffused into rural communities slowly. One reason is that rural practitioners are reluctant to become part of organizations whose "governance, values, and objectives rest in the hands of people who no longer live in the local community" (Rosenblatt, 2001, p. 9).

Building provider networks in rural communities is time- and effort-intensive because rural providers are often inexperienced with managed care organizations (MCOs). Amundson (cited in "How Do We Make Managed Care Work For Us?," 1998) suggested three major choices for rural communities with respect to MCOs. Community providers can join an existing health maintenance organization (HMO), they can form a local or regional network for managed care, or they can operate their own health plans with their inherent costs. Amundson believed that rural communities should explore the formation of community health plans (CHPs). The CHPs are composed of local or regional organizations that pull together the providers and a financing system, often an existing MCO. This model supports local providers, maintains local control, and attempts to retain local dollars. However, the costs of MCOs are high, and their future development in rural areas is uncertain (see Bridging Financial Gaps).

Barriers to Access

Access to health care for rural clients has numerous barriers. The physical distance between place of residence and location of health care services can be considerable. Rural clients may be referred to a distant urban medical center for cancer therapy

BRIDGING FINANCIAL GAPS

Rural community health nurses often serve as school nurses for the local schools. One fall day, a 15-year-old student was referred to the nurse because he did not have the required physical examination form signed by a physician so that he might play basketball. The nurse met with the student, John, that day and inquired about the needed physical examination. John explained that his father had recently lost his job and now the family had no health insurance. He would have to wait until he could earn the money to pay for the examination. John said that he understood that he would not be able to start the basketball season with his classmates. Mrs. J., the community health nurse, asked if she could meet with John's parents; he agreed.

The next afternoon, Mrs. J. visited John's parents at their home and confirmed that John had their permission to play basketball. They discussed the family's loss of health insurance and limited income to purchase private insurance. Mrs. J. told the family that she would attempt to help John get a free or low-cost physical examination, if that was acceptable to them.

Mrs. J. made a few telephone calls that afternoon and was able to get John an appointment to see Dr. Z., the team doctor, at his office the next afternoon. Dr Z. was pleased to give John the necessary examination. Mrs. J. also let John and his parents know about the appointment; they were pleased. Mrs. J. then shared that she had an application for a new state-subsidized health insurance plan for families that was available at minimal cost. She encouraged John's parents to apply for the reduced-premium insurance.

Weeks later, at a basketball game, John's mother approached Mrs. J. and thanked her for helping their family to get enrolled in the subsidized insurance plan. The family now had added the basic health insurance to their family's health care, and John was enjoying playing basketball on the school team.

or other sophisticated care. Members of the population may be frustrated if they travel to a faraway site for care and do not have their problem solved. Rural clients need to be advised before they travel "into town" to make sure that the health care provider is not behind schedule or unable to see them.

Transportation can also be an issue, especially for people who do not drive or who lack dependable transportation. Unpredictable weather adds to potential barriers for rural clients. Snow, ice, wind, and rain can make travel dangerous, even for short distances. Parents may decide not to risk driving on poorly maintained roads to get their children immu-

nized or to have their own hypertension evaluated. Travel in emergency situations can be life-threatening, not only because of the emergency situation itself, but also because of the distance involved to get the ill or injured person to the nearest health care facility.

Limited choice of health care providers is a barrier for some rural residents. There are fewer physicians, nurses, dentists, and other providers in rural areas. Sometimes concerns about confidentiality or provider expertise cause clients to seek care from even more distant providers.

New Approaches to Improve Access

The *Healthy People 2010* objectives (2000) mandate improvements in health education, health screening, immunizations, and disease morbidity for the United States. Creative ways of delivering these and other services to rural clients need to be explored. Access to care is a social justice issue: clients who live in rural areas should receive quality health care. Their choice of a place to live should not be a "sentence" to less than ideal health options.

One approach that has been successful in numerous rural areas is the use of mobile clinics. These clinics bring health care providers to remote places for health screenings, immunizations, and other services. Mobile health clinics are frequently staffed by NPs and can improve access to health care for low-income residents.

School-based clinics are another approach that improves access. These clinics provide available, community-based, affordable, and culturally acceptable care to well and sick children. Often grant-supported, school-based clinics facilitate the receipt of health education and primary care by children who are otherwise without easy access to health services.

Telehealth is a new approach for increasing access to care. **Telehealth** provides electronically transmitted clinician consultation between the client and the health care provider. This option is especially useful for connecting home health nurses with their patients who need close monitoring at home. Patients and providers are "connected" via two-way audiovisual transmission over telephone lines without the need for patients to leave their residences. Clients can also be assessed quickly by interactive communication from physician offices and other sites. Telehealth technology may decrease visits to emergency departments and hospitalizations. The USDHHS provides Medicare reimbursement to health care providers for Telehealth services in designated HPSAs.

Healthy People 2010 Goals

The two broad objectives of *Healthy People 2010* are (1) to increase quality and years of healthy life and (2) to eliminate health disparities. The report noted that injury-related death rates are 40% higher in rural communities and that 20% of the rural population is uninsured compared with 16% of urban residents (USDHHS, 2000). Model standards are written by communities with community-specific objectives to reduce morbidity and mortality and to determine which preventive services to emphasize in their locale. It may be useful for rural communities to consider focusing on the following health indicators:

- Access to health care
- Mental health
- Tobacco use
- Injury and violence
- Overweight and obesity
- Environmental health

Rural community health nurses need to consider the *Healthy People 2010* objectives as guides for improving the health status of rural communities throughout the decade (see Using the Nursing Process).

USING THE NURSING PROCESS

You are a community health nurse working in a small town of 5000 residents in rural Idaho. One weekend at church, an elderly woman, Mrs. Richey, approaches you and asks for some help. It seems that Mr. Richey, her 78-year-old husband, a retired farmer, is becoming more confused and difficult to care for at home. Mrs. Richey explains that Mr. Richey was diagnosed with Alzheimer disease 2 years ago. He also has diabetes and problems walking without assistance. Mrs. Richey says that her grown children live out of the area and aren't able to help her much. They think that their Mom should consider placing their father in a nursing home. You agree to stop by and visit with the Richeys the following day.

ASSESSMENT—INITIAL CONTACT

These are some of the areas from your assessment done on your first two visits with Mr. and Mrs. Richey:

1. Introduce yourself and your agency's services to Mr. and Mrs. Richey.
2. Spend some time talking with the couple. Attempt to assess the couple's interactions, relationship, and needs.
3. Assess the home environment for safety hazards.
4. Spend some time talking with Mr. Richey about how he feels and what his health concerns are; assess his level of confusion.
5. Observe Mr. Richey as he ambulates.
6. Assess Mr. Richey's vital signs and his activities of daily living.
7. Assess the medications being taken by Mr. Richey. Assess the management of his diabetes.
8. Inquire about Mr. Richey's health care. Who are his providers? When was he last seen? When is his next appointment?
9. Ask Mrs. Richey about any support persons available for the couple. Whom do they call when they need assistance?
10. Assess Mrs. Richey about how she spends a typical day. How often does she get out of the house? Who cares for Mr. Richey when she is gone?

NURSING DIAGNOSES

After two home visits to the Richeys, you have determined that the following nursing diagnoses are appropriate:

1. Caregiver role strain related to the long hours that Mrs. Richey must put in caring for her husband and lack of respite and support.
2. Decisional conflict about the best options for Mr. Richey, related to Mrs. Richey's strong belief that she should care for her husband and not place him in a nursing home.
3. Impaired physical mobility, related to Mr. Richey's cognitive impairment, joint stiffness, and decreased strength and endurance.
4. Chronic confusion of Mr. Richey related to Alzheimer's disease.

PLANNING

After your assessment, you determine that Mr. Richey needs more assistance than his wife can provide safely. She is not sleeping well because she feels like she always needs to be alert, and she looks physically "drained." You contact Mr. Richey's physician to share your concerns about how the couple is doing. You suggest that Mr. Richey is in an unsafe setting at home, especially with his wife so exhausted. You advise that Mrs. Richey should contact their church about providing some respite temporarily. You decide to offer some intermittent home health aid assistance to the family until they can make other arrangements for more long-term care for Mr. Richey. You talk with Mr. Richey about the help that you think he needs. You offer to talk with the couple's children if they have questions.

IMPLEMENTATION (RELATED TO NURSING DIAGNOSIS 1)

1. Mrs. Richey will contact her pastor about her need for respite help with her husband for the next couple of weeks, at least three or four times each week.
2. Mrs. Richey will talk with her children about the family situation related to their father's health status within the next few days.

USING THE NURSING PROCESS

(continued)

3. Mrs. Richey will rest when the home health aide visits to assist with care for Mr. Richey.
4. You will encourage Mrs. Richey to ask one of the couple's children to visit them soon to assist her with planning for the care of Mr. Richey.
5. You will call Mrs. Richey to check on availability of respite care through the church.
6. You will gather information about nursing home placement options to share with Mrs. Richey at your next home visit.

EVALUATION (RELATED TO NURSING DIAGNOSIS 1)

1. Mrs. Richey has contacted her pastor, and respite support is available to the family for 3 hours, three times a week.

2. Mrs. Richey talked with her children and reports that her children are supportive of her. They continue to think that their Dad needs a nursing home placement.
3. Mrs. Richey reports that she has "put her feet up" when the home health aide has visited and states she is feeling a little better.
4. Mrs. Richey reports that her oldest son will be arriving Friday and will be able to stay for 1 week.
5. You call and verify that the respite care is in place.
6. You gather information about the nursing home options available locally and up to 50 miles away. You plan to share this information with Mrs. Richey and her son at your next home visit.

RURAL COMMUNITY HEALTH NURSING

Working in a Rural Community

Rural community health nurses are most often women who either grew up in rural areas or lived for a time in small communities. They frequently have extended family there (Bushy, 2000). Rural nurses are active members of their community and are highly respected professionals.

Display 31–2 lists the characteristics of a rural nurse (American Nurses Association [ANA] Rural/Frontier Health Care Task Force, 1996). The ANA stated in its "Statement on Rural Nursing" (1990) that the organization is concerned about the availability and quality of rural health services. The ANA recommends recruitment of rural residents into nursing and rural nurses into leadership roles.

Rural community health nurses use the levels of primary, secondary, and tertiary prevention in their practices (see The Global Community). Primary prevention is used when the community health nurse provides immunizations to children at a well-child clinic or influenza vaccine to elders at the local community center. The nurse may engage in secondary prevention while doing blood pressure checks with adults or screening schoolchildren for scoliosis. Rural community health nurses have opportunities to practice tertiary prevention as they work with children who have special health care needs or visit recently hospitalized rural residents who need home health care. It is important for rural community health nurses to emphasize each of the levels of prevention (see What Do You Think? II).

How does one learn about a rural community? If you are going to have a rural clinical experience in community health nursing, these simple steps are for you (Display 31–3). Your community assessment skills (see Chapter 18) will come in handy. It is helpful to (1) approach the community without preconceived ideas and (2) observe and describe the people, places, and activities of the community at different times of day. You should (3) use your senses—your eyes, ears, and nose—to learn about the neighborhoods and (4) identify key informants and talk with them about their community. **Key informants** are people who know much about their communities and are willing to share that information. You need to (5) review the demographic, morbidity, and mortality data that are available for the locale and (6) determine potential strengths and problems of the community. Lastly, you must (7) verify your impressions with community members, in-

D I S P L A Y   3 1 – 2

Rural Nurse Characteristics

- They have close community ties.
- They are expected to be all things to all people.
- Confidentiality is a concern because of blurring of social and professional roles.
- Autonomy is important in retaining and satisfying rural nurses.
- Rural nursing staffs are generally cohesive; there is less burnout than urban nurses.
- Rural nurses are seen as positive assets to their community.

(Adapted from American Nurses Association [ANA] Rural/ Frontier Health Care Task Force [1996]. *Rural/frontier nursing: The challenge to grow.* Washington, DC: American Nurses Publishing.)

THE GLOBAL COMMUNITY

Cox, H., Cash, P., Hanna, B., D'Arcy-Tehan, F., & Adams, C. (2001). Risky business: Stories from the field of rural community nurses' work in domestic violence. *Australian Journal of Public Health, 9*, 280–285.

Family violence is a major health concern in Australia, where it is estimated that about 500,000 women experience domestic violence yearly. This descriptive study conducted in various regions of rural Victoria, Australia, sought to "understand" domestic violence from the perspective of 24 community (health) nurses working there.

After instituted ethical approval was obtained, focus groups were held with the 24 community nurses to identify issues related to domestic violence. Each focus group met once for about 2 hours. The sessions were audiotaped with participant permission and later transcribed to identify major themes from the discussions.

Results from the study included the fact that the nurses preferred to call the issue "family violence" rather than domestic violence. They further defined family violence to be "any type of abuse toward someone who is known to them, be it physical, sexual, financial, emotional, or verbal." In rural Victoria, victims of family violence live in isolated geographic areas, and many lack the transportation to leave their abuser. Additionally, the abused individuals are often unable to share their situation with others in their small communities. Some felt that they would not be believed because their abusers were well respected in the community.

The four themes derived from the community nurse focus groups are as follows:

- **Picking up the cues**—Community nurses can easily "pick up the cues" of bruising or other physical injuries. Subtle cues, including nonverbal ones, are more difficult for the nurse to identify.
- **Helping and helplessness**—Community nurses often feel unable to manage the complexities of family violence. The nurses shared that sometimes they were able to help victims of family violence because others viewed them as coming to the home to learn about the infant or child of the family and not the mother.

Other nurses shared that they were approached by victims at sporting or other events. These discussions could be more discreet when held in a very public place.

- **Holding secrets**—Community nurses often know information about family violence in various families. They sometimes need to "hold secrets" while supporting individuals to seek help or leave the abusive situation. Community nurses also need to share information with professional colleagues sometimes, to ensure the safety of their clients and themselves.
- **Quiet resistance**—The rural community nurses reported that they "often undertook a supportive and counseling role, but this may not be evident in their records." Instead, the nurses might record a "baby visit" because some feared that recording the real information might cause harm to the victim or the nurse.

All four themes can be summarized by the overriding theme of "Risky Business." Community nurses working with families in rural areas experiencing family violence are doing "risky business" on a daily basis. Confidentiality of community nurse records is another risky issue, when those records are shared inappropriately. The authors recommended that further research is needed about family violence in rural Australia. Further efforts must be made to address the issue of family violence there. They also recommended "further exploration into the professional and bureaucratic barriers" that make it so challenging for community nurses to work with families experiencing family violence.

There are implications from this research for community health nurse practicing in the rural areas of the United States. Rural community health nurses need to be aware that working with families who are experiencing family violence can be "risky business." Nurses need to seek support for themselves as they attempt to work with these families. They also need to determine whether the four themes related to family violence as described by rural Australian community nurses are applicable to their clients in the United States.

WHAT DO YOU THINK? II

There have been two serious car wrecks in your rural county recently involving adolescents driving under the influence of alcohol. What might you be able to do to address this problem through your consultation with the local high school?

cluding the health providers you will be working with, and (8) enjoy your learning experience!

Roles of the Nurse

There are many roles for the rural community health nurse:

1. *Advocate:* assists rural clients and families in obtaining the best possible care
2. *Coordinator/Case Manager:* connects rural clients with needed health and social services

DISPLAY 31-3

Working as a Community Health Nurse in a Rural Community

- Approach the community without preconceived ideas.
- Observe/describe the people, places, and activities.
- Use all of your senses.
- Talk with key informants.
- Review available demographic, morbidity, and mortality data.
- Determine potential community strengths and problems.
- Verify your impressions.
- Enjoy your learning!

3. *Health Teacher:* provides education to individuals, families, or groups on health promotion or other health-related topics (eg, prepared childbirth, parenting)
4. *Referral Agent:* makes appropriate connections between rural clients and urban service providers
5. *Mentor:* helps new community health nurses, nursing students, and other nurses new to the rural community
6. *Change Agent/Researcher:* suggests new approaches to solving patient care or community health problems based on research, professional literature, and community assessment
7. *Collaborator:* seeks ways to work with other health and social service professionals to maximize outcomes for individual clients and the community at large
8. *Activist:* takes appropriate risks to improve the community's health

It may be helpful to see how all these roles come into play during a typical day for a rural community health nurse. Carol M. arrives at the Stevens County Public Health Department in rural America. She reviews her caseload for the day and begins her work. First, she telephones the principal of the local high school to let him know that she is able to speak next week to the Parent-Teacher Association about raising healthy adolescents (*health teacher*). Then, Carol calls the family of a hospitalized patient (*coordinator/case manager*) to plan the discharge of their family member. At 10:00 AM, Carol makes a home visit to the Wesley family. The family members explain that they have been unable to enroll for needed food stamps because they do not understand the process. Carol encourages the family to contact the appropriate agency (*referral agent*) and even calls her neighbor who works at the office to inform her of the need for special attention for the family (*advocate*). At lunch, Carol runs into a social worker colleague and they discuss their concerns about the hospitalized individual with whom Carol spoke earlier in the day (*collaborator*). Both question whether the family will be able to manage the care needed for the family member without much outside support. After

lunch, Carol returns to her office for a staff meeting and discusses a new charting system that she is recommending (*change agent/researcher*) for implementation by the department. At the same meeting, she is asked and agrees to work with a visiting community health nursing student during his rural practicum (*mentor*). That evening, Carol, as a concerned citizen, participates in a meeting at the town hall about concerns related to local water quality. She addresses the group (*activist*) and volunteers to lead others who are concerned about the issue. It is obvious that community health nurses like Carol M. often play many roles during the day. As a nursing student working in a rural community, you may have the opportunity to "try on" many of these roles (see Voices from the Community).

Challenges and Opportunities

Autonomy

Rural community health nurses have the opportunity to use autonomy in daily practice. Nurses must rapidly assume independent and interdependent decision-making roles because of the small workforce and large workload. Rural community health nurses learn to prioritize tasks quickly and work efficiently with others to "get the job done." Referrals to other rural providers are facilitated because providers frequently know one another. The rural community health nurse has an advantage over urban nurses in that the rural health care system is smaller and easier to influence and change.

"Always a Nurse"

Anonymity is not easy for the rural community health nurse, who is always "on duty." A trip to the grocery store on a Saturday morning may include interactions with rural clients and their families about their pressing health concerns. Rural community health nurses may have confidentiality and personal/professional boundary issues that need to be addressed. However, rural community health nurses are often respected, known, and trusted by the populations they serve.

Funding Your Education

Some of the educational loans available to you at the undergraduate and graduate levels may be reduced or forgiven if you practice in a rural community after graduation. You should inquire through your nursing program about that possibility. It is also possible to contact a specific rural community as to whether they can offer some monetary support in return for a pledge to return to the host community to work for several years.

Isolation

Rural community health nurses may experience the challenge of physical isolation from personal and professional opportunities associated with urban areas. Travel to cities for basic and continuing education can be a barrier. Rural nurses may also feel isolated in their clinical practices because of the scarcity of professional colleagues. Many rural community

VOICES FROM THE COMMUNITY

I knew where this road would end. After a mile or so, I would have to stop, open, drive through, and then close the cattle gate before arriving at a complex of old buildings. There would be two houses, a trailer home, plus all the other assorted ranch buildings. The end house was the home of an elderly lady that I had visited monthly for an injection. She was the mother of the two men who ran this rural ranch, and the visits that accompanied the treatment to the elderly lady were delightful. As a rural public health nurse, I now had been called to visit the home of the hired man. His wife had given birth to a new baby the month before. The new mom, Ellen, invited me into her cluttered kitchen. She was somewhat quiet and only 17 years old. She stated that her delivery had gone well, and that this was her first baby. Her husband had three other children living with his first wife. He was quite a bit older than Ellen and was not particularly interested in another child. Ellen's family was in another state, and I got the indication that marriage was a good reason for her to leave home. When I asked to see the baby, I was led into another small room in the trailer. The 1-month-old infant was lying on his back, awake, staring at the ceiling. Ellen stated that her son was a good baby, who rarely cried and spent most of his time in the crib. She made no effort to talk with him or pick him up. I told her what a beautiful baby he was, and that I would like to visit her several times to help answer her questions about child care, or any other matters. Before I left that day, she began asking questions about mixing formula and feeding her infant, and I felt that she truly wanted to be a good mom. As I drove back to town, I contemplated where to start with my next visit. Basic infant care needed to be addressed, as well as how Ellen and her son would get to their medical appointments, when her husband and the beat-up pickup truck were her only means of transportation. The ranch owners were neighborly but did not appear interested in supporting Ellen in the mothering of her son. Isolation certainly was a potential problem for Ellen. I also was very concerned about the brain development of an infant with such little stimulation. Unfortunately, before I could put any more interventions into place, I learned that the family had moved without leaving a forwarding address. To this day, I still wonder about the life of that child, and whether Ellen was able to find the resources to parent effectively.

health nurses overcome these barriers and learn to appreciate the benefits of clinical practice in a rural setting by discussing their concerns with peers and seeking ways to combat isolation.

Dollars and "Sense"

The rural community health nurse often receives a salary that is lower than that of urban nurses in comparable positions. However, there are benefits to rural nursing. Housing costs are usually less than in larger cities, and long commutes to and from work on congested highways are avoided. Rural communities are great places to live and raise a family. The slower pace of life, open spaces, clean air, and friendly atmosphere may make more "sense."

Many Possibilities

The smaller system of health care in a rural community can be an advantage to the community health nurse. It may be easier to "understand the system" and initiate planned change. For example, if a rural nurse wants to continue his or her education, a college of nursing could be contacted to offer the needed classes. There are many possibilities to enhance rural nursing practice, including continuing education by satellite or Internet, partnerships with larger medical centers, and invitations to clinical experts to provide on-site workshops. Grants can be written to facilitate these endeavors.

SUMMARY

Rural clients are a unique aggregate. Community health nurses are key to ensuring the delivery of appropriate health services to this population. There are numerous definitions of the term *rural*. In this chapter, rural is defined as communities with fewer than 10,000 residents and a county population density of fewer than 1000 people per square mile. The number of people living in rural communities has increased over the last century. Since 1995, however, the growth rate in many rural communities has decreased. The elderly are a rapidly growing population in rural communities. Rural areas have less diversity than urban places, and rural clients generally have lower educational levels than urban clients, due in part to less access to higher education. Income levels and housing costs are frequently lower than in larger cities.

Healthy People 2010 identifies national goals applicable to rural communities. There are many at-risk populations in these communities. Homeless families often face inadequate shelter, few employment opportunities, lack of inexpensive housing, and limited access to health and social services. Rural elders may have limited alternatives for housing if they can no longer live alone. Perinatal clients may not have the health services they need close to home. Mental health services are limited, even though the need may be great. Health care providers need to ensure confidentiality and attempt to reduce the stigma of mental illness for these clients. There are numerous risks associated with farming. The community health nurse must help this population identify hazards and practice injury prevention. Native American clients are at great risk for diabetes, obesity, alcoholism, and smoking.

A community health nurse needs to engage in community assessment of the rural area as a part of orientation. It is helpful to identify the strengths of the community. Rural clients are frequently resourceful and have a supportive network of people to meet their needs.

Access to health care is an important issue in rural communities. Health insurance is expensive, and some rural residents choose not to purchase it. Others may be too proud to apply for government assistance. Managed care organizations are diffusing into rural communities, and their long-term impact is uncertain. Barriers to access include distance, weather, transportation, and limited choice of providers. Some ways to improve access in these communities are school-based clinics, mobile health vans, and use of the latest technology. University-sponsored nursing centers that could serve rural populations should be explored.

Rural community health nurses are key members of the professional community. Their roles include advocate, coordinator/case manager, health teacher, referral agent, mentor, change agent/researcher, collaborator, and activist. Community health nurses have challenges and opportunities related to their clinical practices. There may be confidentiality and personal/professional boundary issues. Salaries for rural nurses may be lower than for nurses in urban areas. Rural community health nurses are highly respected individuals who make a difference for the communities they serve. Maybe you should consider a career as a rural community health nurse.

ACTIVITIES TO PROMOTE CRITICAL THINKING

1. Interview a peer who grew up in a rural community about his or her family and school life. What were his or her best experiences growing up? Compare the peer's best experiences with your own.
2. Complete a community assessment of a rural community with a small group of peers. Compare your assessment findings with an assessment done in an urban neighborhood. Discuss the similarities and differences of the community assessments with your peers.
3. Assume you are a community health nurse in a rural community. Describe your approach to solve the problem of overuse of the emergency room for minor childhood illnesses by community residents.
4. Go on the Internet to locate rural health programs in various states. In addition, see whether the Internet has rural job opportunities for community health nurses.
5. Suggest to your faculty that the class debate whether rural residents should have access to sophisticated care, such as intensive care units for adults and children, medical specialists (oncologists, cardiologists), and emergency care equal to what can be found in an urban area.

REFERENCES

Acosta, D.A. (2001). Obstetric care. In J.P. Geyman, T.E. Norris, & L.G. Hart (Eds.), *Textbook of rural medicine* (pp. 15–26). New York: McGraw-Hill.

Adams, C.E., Michel, Y., DeFrates, D., & Corbett, C. F. (2001). Effect of locale on health status and direct care time of rural versus urban home health patients. *Journal of Nursing Administration, 31,* 244–251.

American Nurses Association. (1990). Statement on rural nursing. *The Kansas Nurse, 65*(5), 6–7.

American Nurses Association Rural/Frontier Health Care Task Force. (1996). *Rural/frontier nursing: The challenge to grow.* Washington, DC: American Nurses Publishing.

Bayne, T., Higgs, Z., Gruber, E., & Bendel, B. (2002, July). *Eastern Washington access to health care consumer study.* Spokane, WA: Tina Bayne (Intercollegiate College of Nursing, 2917 W Fort George Wright Dr., Spokane, WA 99223.)

Bushy, A. (2000). *Orientation to nursing in the rural community.* Thousand Oaks, CA: Sage.

Butler, M.A. & Beale, C.A. (1994). *Rural-urban continuum for metropolitan counties, 1993.* Washington, DC: Agriculture and Rural Economy Division, Economics Research Service, U. S. Department of Agriculture.

Coburn, A.F., & Bolda, E.J. (1999). Rural elderly and long-term care. In T.C. Ricketts (Ed.), *Rural health in the United States* (pp.179–189). New York: Oxford University Press.

Congdon, J.G., & Magilvy, J.K. (2001). Themes of rural health and aging from a program of research. *Geriatric Nursing, 22,* 234–238.

Congressional Rural Caucus, United States House of Representatives. (2001, October 1). *Frequently asked questions—Fast facts: Why rural matters.* Retrieved February 3, 2004, from *http://www.house.gov/emerson/crc/overview/faq.html*

Cox, H., Cash, P., Hanna, B., D'Arcy-Tehan, F., & Adams, C. (2001). Risky business: Stories from the field of rural community nurses' work in domestic violence. *Australian Journal of Rural Health, 9,* 280–285.

Craft-Rosenberg, M., Powell, S.R., & Culp, K. (2000). Health status and resources of rural homeless women and children. *Western Journal of Nursing Research, 22,* 863–878.

Dennis, L.K., & Pallotta, S.L. (2001). Chronic disease in rural health. In S. Loue & B.E. Quill (Eds.), *Handbook of rural health* (pp. 189–207). New York: Kluwer Academic/Plenum.

Eberhardt, M.S., Ingram, D.D., Makuc, D.M., & Harper, S.B., et al. (2001). *Urban and rural health chartbook: Health, United States, 2001.* Hyattsville, MD: National Center for Health Statistics.

Hartley, D., Bird, D., & Dempsey, P. (1999). Rural mental health and substance abuse. In T.C. Ricketts (Ed.), *Rural health in the United States* (pp. 38–51). New York: Oxford University Press.

How do we make managed care work for us? (1998, Fall). *State Rural Health Watch, 5*(1), 2–3, 8–10.

Hulme, P.A., & Blegen, M.A. (1999, June). Residential status and birth outcomes: Is the rural/urban distinction adequate? *Public Health Nursing, 16,* 176–181.

Hummel, J. (2001). Population-based medicine: Links to public health. In J.P. Geyman, T.E. Norris, & L.G. Hart (Eds.), *Textbook of rural medicine,* (pp. 55–72). New York: McGraw-Hill.

Joho, K.A., & Ormsby, A. (2000). A walk in beauty: Strategies for providing culturally competent care to Native Americans. In M.L. Kelley & V.M. Fitzsimons (Eds.), *Understanding cultural diversity: Culture, curriculum, and community in nursing* (pp. 209–218). Sudbury, MA: Jones & Bartlett.

Lishner, D.M., Larson, E.H., Roisenblatt, R.A., & Clark, S.J. (1999). In T.C. Ricketts (Ed.), *Rural health in the United States* (pp. 134–149). New York: Oxford University Press.

Magilvy, J.K., & Congdon, J.G. (2002). The crisis nature of healthcare transitions for rural older adults. *Public Health Nursing, 17,* 336–345.

National Advisory Committee on Rural Health. (2002). *A targeted look at the rural health care safety net: A report to the Secretary, U. S. Department of Health and Human Services.* Washington, DC: U. S. Department of Health and Human Services.

National Institutes of Health, National Institute of Allergy and Infectious Diseases. (2002, December). *Fact sheet: HIV/AIDS statistics.* Retrieved February 3, 2004, from *http://www.niaid.nih.gov/factsheets/aidsstat.htm*

Rickets, T.C. (Ed.). (1999). *Rural health in the United States.* New York: Oxford University Press.

Ricketts, T.C. (2001). The rural patient. In J.P. Geyman, T.E. Norris, & L.G. Hart (Eds.), *Textbook of rural medicine* (pp. 15–26). New York: McGraw-Hill.

Rural and urban health care needs: Hearing before the Subcommittee on the Judiciary, United States Senate. 107th Cong., 26 (2002).

Rosenblatt, R.A. (2001). The health of rural people and the communities and environments in which they live. In J.P. Geyman, T.E. Norris, & L.G. Hart (Eds.), *Textbook of rural medicine* (pp. 3–14). New York: McGraw-Hill.

Standards for defining metropolitan and micropolitan statistical areas. (2000, December 27). *Notice,* 65 Fed. Reg. 82,238.

Taylor, H.A., Hughes, G.D., & Garrison, R.J. (2002, April). Cardiovascular disease among women residing in rural America: Epidemiology, explanations, and challenges. *American Journal of Public Health, 92,* 548–551.

UNAIDS (Joint United Nations Programme on HIV/AIDS). (2002, December) *AID epidemic update.*

United States Census Bureau. (2000a). *Appendix A: Census 2000 geographic terms and concepts.* Retrieved February 3, 2004, from *http://www.census.gov/geo/www/tiger/glossary2.pdf*

United States Census Bureau. (2000b). *Detailed tables: Urban and rural-universe Total population.* Retrieved February 3, 2004, from *http://factfinder.census.gov*

United States Department of Health and Human Services, Office of Rural Health Policy. (1998). *Definitions of rural: A handbook for health policy makers and researchers.* Technical Issues Paper. Bethesda, MD: Equal Three Communications.

United States Department of Health and Human Services. (2000, January). *Healthy people 2010* (Conference ed., Vols. 1 & 2). Washington, DC: U. S. Government Printing Office.

SELECTED READINGS

Ander, K. L., Uscian, M. & Robertson, J. F. (1999). Improving client outcomes through differentiated practice: A rural nursing center model. *Public Health Nursing, 16*(3), 168–175.

Fisher, K. & Shumaker, L. (2004). Assessment of depression and cognitive impairment among elders in rural housing facilities. *Journal of the American Psychiatric Nurses Association, 10*(2), 67–72.

Kenny, A. & Duckett, S. (2003). Educating for rural nursing practice. *Journal of Advanced Nursing, 44*(6), 613–622.

Leight, S. B. (2003). The application of a vulnerable populations conceptual model to rural health. *Public Health Nursing, 20*(8), 440–448.

Sullivan, T., Weinert, C., & Cudney, S. (2003). Management of chronic illness: Voices of rural women. *Journal of Advanced Nursing, 44*(6), 566–574.

Wilkinson, D. & Blue, I. (2002). *The new rural health.* New York: Oxford University Press.

Internet Resources

National Rural Health Association: *www.nrharural.org*

The National Rural Recruitment and Retention Network: *www.3rnet.org/index.asp*

Rural Health Research: *http://www.nrharural.org/pagefile/rh.html*

Rural Health Webguide: *http://www.scdhec.net/elsa/elsarurh.html*

Rural Nurse Organization: *www.rno.org/index.htm*

Rural Policy Research Institute: *http://www.rupri.org/*

32

Urban Health Care, Poverty, and Homelessness

Key Terms

- Disenfranchised
- Distributive justice
- Feminization of poverty
- Ghettos
- Health disparity
- Homelessness
- Indigent
- Marginalized
- Poverty threshold
- Social justice
- Social status
- Social support
- Temporary Aid to Needy Families (TANF)

Learning Objectives

Upon mastery of this chapter, you should be able to:

- Discuss health and safety factors experienced by people living in urban areas.
- Discuss the concepts of ethics and social justice surrounding urban health issues.
- Identify common characteristics of people living in poverty.
- Analyze political and ethical dimensions of American poverty.
- Identify common health effects of poverty.
- Analyze causes of homelessness and its effects on health.
- Explain the forces determining global poverty and strategies for its elimination.
- Propose intervention strategies at the community, agency, and individual level to reduce or eliminate poverty.
- Assess your own attitude toward poverty and homelessness, and identify self-caring strategies to use when working with impoverished people.

Have you ever lived in, driven through, or provided nursing care to an urban neighborhood? Perhaps you are one of many people who drive by such neighborhoods very quickly, never looking right or left. Your only experience with urban areas may be watching the nightly news on television and seeing apartment fires, the results of gang shootouts on the street, or a homeless shelter that has closed down because of lack of financial support. This chapter describes some of the major sociopolitical and health care issues of people living in urban areas, those living in poverty, and the homeless. To provide a clearer focus on each of these three issues, they are discussed separately in this chapter.

It is important to be aware that poverty is a national dilemma and is found in all communities—urban, suburban, and rural. There are homeless people in small towns and in very rural areas, although the largest numbers of homeless people are congregated in urban areas. In addition, urban health care issues affect all of society in clear and subtle ways: higher health care costs, less income for the urban area because consumers avoid spending money there, increased crime by substance users that occurs in the urban area and spreads to surrounding areas, and disease transmission to others from urban inhabitants with lifestyle-related diseases. Those of low income are directly affected, but many of the negative aspects about living in urban areas are of concern to all inhabitants, rich or poor.

HISTORY OF URBAN HEALTH CARE ISSUES

Urban living has a long and "checkered" history in the United States. Arriving immigrants increased the population density especially of the large eastern and midwestern cities. Millions of immigrants arrived in the United States between the mid-1800s and the early 1900s. Most had some family or distant relative who had arrived here earlier and made their ways to where these people lived, hoping to receive temporary shelter while work was sought. Many came with large families and roomed with other large European and Eastern European families. Others came alone or as a family without close ties to others already here. Nonetheless, they gathered in **ghettos**, thickly populated sections of cities inhabited predominantly by members of the same minority group, so that they could be with people from their homeland—people who knew the same language and the same ways. In one poignant photograph from 1910, a mother and small child sit in a crowded kitchen with wash hung to dry over the stove and a large wash basin on a paper-strewn table. Information about the photo reveals,

The mother and child in the photograph are identified as part of a Hungarian Jewish family with 10 children. The entire family occupied three crowded rooms, including the kitchen, shown here. Nine of the children slept in a single windowless bedroom. The father, who spoke little English, made his living in the winter by carrying advertising signs for a clothing store; in the summer, he sold ice-cream sodas from a stall in front of the tenement (Fee, Brown & Theerman, 2001, p. 1764).

This situation was not atypical for large cities, such as New York City, Pittsburgh, and Chicago at the turn of the 20th century.

As time went on, many families left ghetto communities and found housing in smaller towns or in the beginnings of suburbs. For instance, the Irish left New York City in the early years of the 20th century; then blacks, coming from the south, moved in. Many black families later left for outlying city areas, and Puerto Rican families moved in. Today, Haitian and Middle Eastern families inhabit the same neighborhoods. After 100 years, many of the same buildings continue to provide inadequate shelter for a new group of immigrants. Ghetto living provides a sense of belonging, but for many it is temporary because it has more negatives than positives. Children and grandchildren of the original immigrants seek out a different life for themselves, away from the urban area riddled with crime, unsafe housing, and disease. Others, because of poverty, drugs, or being near-homeless, remain in urban slum areas.

URBAN HEALTH DISPARITY

Today, the declining urban situation is not confined to a few large cities. More than one fourth of the U. S. population still live in central cities. To achieve the vision of "healthy people in healthy communities," as discussed throughout the *Healthy People 2010* document, more must be done to promote health and prevent disease in urban areas. Although some significant improvements have been made in the last decade, no more than 15% of the goals identified in *Healthy People 2000* have been achieved (Freudenberg, 2000). The reason for this is primarily **health disparity**, the disproportionate burden of certain health problems in urban areas. Overcrowding and poor-quality housing have a direct relation to poor mental health, developmental delay, and even short stature (Bashir, 2002). Problems such as human immunodeficiency virus (HIV) infection, asthma, cirrhosis, diabetes, violence (including homicide), unintentional injury, substance abuse, preterm delivery, infant mortality, heart disease, cancer, and stroke affect the poor and people of color more than other groups, and they are increasingly concentrated in cities. As an illustration, in 1998 the age-adjusted death rate for heart disease among non-Hispanic black people was 40% higher than the rate for non-Hispanic whites (Phillips & Grady, 2002). Throughout this text, each of these diseases or conditions as it relates to the health of individuals and the entire population has been discussed individually, along with the roles of the community health nurse as advocate, researcher, clinician, educator, and leader.

T A B L E 3 2 - 1

Top 10 Metropolitan Growth Areas, 1990–2000

Location	Year 2000	% Increase
1. Las Vegas, NV/AZ	1,563,000	83.3
2. Naples, FL	251,000	65.3
3. Yuma, AZ	160,000	49.7
4. McAllen-Edenburg-Mission, TX	569,000	48.5
5. Austin-San Marcos, TX	1,250,000	47.7
6. Fayetteville-Springdale-Rogers, AR	311,000	47.5
7. Boise, ID	432,000	46.1
8. Phoenix-Mesa, AZ	3,252,000	45.3
9. Laredo, TX	193,000	44.9
10. Provo-Orem, UT	369,000	39.8

Although it is clearly recognized that health disparities concentrate in the cities, there is no national urban political agenda for improving social conditions. More than 80% of the population in America lives in metropolitan areas, including the cities and their surrounding suburbs (Table 32–1). Over the past 25 years, cities and their suburbs have become more similar, and the demographic and health profiles that were previously uniquely urban are now shared by "edge cities" and suburbs populated by poor and minority families. Political power has shifted to more affluent suburban areas, where the tax base and spending practices are greater, at the expense of the cities. Monies that once came to cities to support new resources have also declined. While these changes were occurring, the national government lost power to the states and multinational corporations, which invested tax dollars and incentives in the growing suburbs. In the 20 years between 1970 and 1990, the number of people living in poor inner-city neighborhoods doubled (Freudenberg, 2000). These are the people who live a marginal existence—substance abusers, poor elderly, undocumented immigrants, the very ill, and the disabled. They are economically trapped where they are, as the inner city declines around them.

SOCIAL JUSTICE AND THE COMMUNITY HEALTH NURSE

What is happening to people in decaying urban areas is an example of social injustice. **Social justice** is demonstrated by a society that sees that the health needs and health care issues of all people have economic and social ramifications and can be met only by treating people fairly, regardless of where they live or who they are. Community health nurses who practice social justice have broad and holistic views of health; they have strong convictions that health care is a basic human right, and that improving the health of communities is a social justice issue (Couto, 2000). Community health nurses must have a heightened sense of the value of cultural, racial, and socioeconomic differences and an awareness that these differences are often turned into discrimination in health care services and policies. They need to be determined to "extend the bonds of community to give everyone a firm place to stand as equally entitled to services from a health care system with a single high standard" (Couto, 2000. p. 4).

The Community Environmental Health Resource Center (CEHRC) in Washington, D.C., works with grassroots organizations engaged in the fight for social justice in low-income communities (Bashir, 2002). Their primary focus is empowering residents and increasing economic opportunities to address the environmental health hazards posed by substandard housing. Children and other vulnerable persons in low-income urban communities are at greatest risk. CEHRC addresses the major negative health outcomes of childhood asthma and lead poisoning along with increased risk for depression and poor mental health among people living in substandard housing in urban areas (see Research: Bridge to Practice).

WHO ARE THE POOR?

Do you have experience with poverty or the poor? Have you or your family lived in poverty? Do you give money to charities for the poor? What are your opinions of the needs of impoverished people? Poverty is of great concern to nurses because of the resulting human hardship and association with poor emotional and physical health.

This section provides some general characteristics of the poor in America. It then examines the politics and ethics of poverty, the health effects of poverty, and homelessness in America, and looks briefly at global poverty. Finally, the role of the community health nurse in caring for clients living in urban or rural poverty is explored.

Poverty Defined

To be poor is to have few or no material possessions as well as inadequate access to family and community resources. Low socioeconomic position in society is determined by social and economic deprivation that includes poor income, no accumulated assets, no access to power, poor education, and low-status occupation. People are said to be **indigent** when they are impoverished and deprived of basic comforts.

The U. S. government has an official poverty line or **poverty threshold**; people living below this income line are defined as poor. In 2003, the poverty threshold for a reference family of two adults and two related children (excluding the states of Alaska and Hawaii) was a cash income of $18,660; for a single adult under 65, it was $9,573 (U. S. Census Bureau, 2004). This number is updated every year with changes in the federal consumer price index. Many government programs, such as Medicaid, Head Start, food stamps, the national school lunch program, low-income

RESEARCH: BRIDGE TO PRACTICE

Freeman, N.C. G., Schneider, D., & McGarvey, P. (2002). School-based screening for asthma in third-grade urban children: The Passaic asthma reduction effort survey. *American Journal of Public Health, 92(1)*, 45–46.

The researchers in this study targeted 1052 third grade children in public and private schools in Passaic, New Jersey in the 1998–1999 school year. Parents (78%) and children (93%) completed questionnaires about their perceptions of asthma diagnosis or asthma-like symptoms. Spirometry readings from 615 children were obtained. The population distribution by race/ethnicity of the children with abnormal spirometry readings reflected the population of Passaic. Questionnaires from parents and children and spirometry readings were completed on 455 children and results were as follows:

RACE/ ETHNICITY	% POPULATION DISTRIBUTION	% WITH ABNORMAL SPIROMETRY
Dominican	22.6	28.2
Mexican	19.8	10.0
Puerto Rican	19.3	8.0
Black	11.2	38.2
Mixed other Hispanic	9.7	4.5
Peruvian	4.0	11.1
White	4.0	27.8
Asian	3.7	47.1
Mixed non-Hispanic	3.1	14.3
Columbian	2.6	8.3

Parents indicated that 21% of the children had diagnoses of asthma, yet only 11% of the chidren were reported to be taking medications. Almost 19% of the participating children had forced vital capacity values lower than 75%. Significant differences in abnormal evaluations were found by race/ethnicty, with Blacks and Asians showing more abnormal evaluations and Dominicans having more than other Hispanic groups in the community. Environmental tobacco smoke in the home showed a dose response to impaired spirometry, and children from homes with no tobacco smoke had fewer abnormal readings.

The outcomes of this study seem not to tell the entire picture of asthma-related symptoms in so many children. This urban community has a large minority population. How does the poverty level of these children compare with that of other children in the country? What is the condition of housing in this community? What other health problems do these children have? Do other family members have symptoms or diagnoses of ill health (38% of the parents reported asthma in other family members)? It appears that this population is at risk for many health-related disparities and should be studied further.

home energy assistance programs, and the Childrens' Health Insurance Program (CHIP) determine eligibility based on the poverty threshold.

How is the poverty threshold determined? It is assumed that a family spends one third of its budget on food. Therefore, subsistence living costs are calculated by taking a meager food budget and multiplying by three, then identifying the lowest amount of income needed for all other expenditures, such as utilities, clothing, and shelter. This method of defining poverty is under government evaluation because it does not take into account many factors. It may underestimate poverty by not considering escalating housing costs, medical expenses, or day care costs. Likewise, it may overestimate poverty by ignoring noncash government benefits such as housing assistance and food stamps.

Absolute poverty is defined as not having enough money for shelter, clothing, and food. However, many more people live in relative poverty, meaning that they cannot afford goods and services that most would consider necessities. These people are isolated from consumer America and must "make do" without safe child care or health care, reliable transportation, heat, telephone service, or electricity for months or years at a time. They survive by trading, bartering, and sharing among friends and relatives (see What Do You Think? I).

Demographics

The demographics of poverty can be examined in terms of how many people are poor in any given year and how many people experience poverty during their lifetime. About 34 million Americans, or 12.1% of the population, were poor in 2002. This number is based on a U. S. Bureau of the Census population survey in 2002 and does not include people who are homeless and living in shelters (U. S. Bureau of the Census, 2003).

WHAT DO YOU THINK? I

How would your family live with a cash income at the poverty line?

The number of extreme poor—those trying to survive on less than half of the official poverty threshold—is increasing. In 1997, 14.6 million Americans were classified as extremely poor.

Most impoverished Americans are white. However, compared with their numbers in the population, a disproportionate number of people of color are poor. For example, 22.1% of blacks are poor, as are 21.2% of Hispanics and 10.8% of the Asian-American population, in contrast to 9.4% of non-Hispanic whites (U. S. Bureau of the Census, 2000).

Approximately 13.5 million or 12% of American children live in poverty. Fifty-nine percent of children younger than 6 years of age who lived with single mothers heading the household were poor in 1997 (U. S. Bureau of the Census, 1998). Poverty also affects the aged; 10% of people older than 65 years of age live below the poverty threshold. In addition, 17% of elders are considered "near poor," with incomes less than 125% of the poverty line.

Poverty also has its own geographics. Sixteen percent of people in rural areas are poor, as are 19% of those in central cities. New Mexico and Washington, D.C., have the highest rates of poverty in the nation (see Chap. 31).

Chronic illness and disability increase the chances of living in poverty. One third of adults with disabilities live in households with annual incomes less than $15,000 (Kilborn, 1999). Growing numbers of disabled people live without income, health insurance, or family support (see Chap. 34).

More striking than the actual proportion of people who are poor at any given time is the likelihood of living in poverty sometime during one's lifetime. It is projected that by 40 years of age, slightly more than one third of all Americans will have lived in poverty (Rank & Hirschl, 1999). By age 75, more than one half of adult Americans will have experienced poverty. This includes 91% of African-Americans and 53% of European-Americans. When viewed across the lifespan, poverty is a prevalent experience of mainstream Americans, not one afflicting a small marginal population! The typical spell of poverty is relatively brief; it often occurs when people living just above the poverty threshold lose employment income or a couple separates. Long-standing poverty, lasting longer than 10 years, affects approximately 15% of the poor. Because poverty is so prevalent, many students of nursing have been touched personally by its hardships.

Social Characteristics

The wealthiest Americans have vast resources at their disposal. The average income of the top 20% of the population in 1998 was $127,529 per year, and for the bottom 20% it was $9,225—lower than the poverty threshold (AmeriStat, 2000). This discrepancy is deeply troubling to those who believe in equal opportunity for all. Most impoverished Americans have few resources with which to escape from poverty or to live with dignity despite extreme poverty. In particular, the marginalization of the poor, their social status, social support, and neighborhood resources all influence their ability to escape persistent poverty (O'Toole et al., 2002).

Marginalization

Despite their numbers, the poor in America remain invisible, easily denied by mainstream America. This is, in part, because the poor are often **marginalized**, meaning that they live on the margins, or edges, of society rather than in the mainstream. Another term used is **disenfranchised**; enfranchisement refers to having full privileges and rights as a citizen. People who live in persistent poverty are especially likely to be isolated in inner-city neighborhoods through which the middle-class person never travels. The most vulnerable—the elderly, the disabled, and the young—seldom leave their own neighborhoods (Display 32–1).

D I S P L A Y   3 2 – 1

The Human Face of Poverty: Tommy

Four generations of Cora's impoverished African-American family live in the shadows of Chicago's loop surrounded by outstanding medical centers. The family narrative by Laurie Abraham (1993) reveals the failure of the health care system. Cora is 69 years old and suffers from diabetes and hypertension. She lives with her granddaughter, Jackie, who is caring for Cora, Jackie's three children, and Jackie's husband Robert, whose kidneys failed when he was 27 years old. Tommy is Cora's son and Jackie's father; he lives with his girlfriend, who works full time. Tommy had a stroke at age 48, when he was employed as a bartender. He has been hardened by a lifetime on the rough inner-city streets and does not trust outsiders. Tommy believes that his high blood pressure was caused by stress, and he suspects that his stroke was caused by a relative's curse; he believes he was vulnerable because he had not led a virtuous life. Before the stroke, he was a drinker and smoker; he stopped taking his antihypertensive medication because it made him impotent. Now, his left arm remains partially paralyzed; he has trouble with most activities of daily living. He has stopped drinking but continues to smoke and eat a high-fat diet; he rarely exercises. Tommy leaves home primarily to cash his disability check, buy lottery tickets, and visit the doctor. He worries that he is losing strength, but he has no insurance coverage for physical therapy. Counseled by his physician to walk regularly, Tommy responds, "I do not want to be no prey" (p. 140). He is afraid of being assaulted in his crime-ridden neighborhood. Likewise, dietary advice is hard to follow, with the ingredients of a healthy diet too expensive and not available at neighborhood convenience stores. Tommy appears to agree when his doctor lectures him on smoking, but he continues his habit. The doctor concludes that Tommy is morally responsible for his persistent unhealthy choices; he is the cause of his own suffering. What do you think about Tommy's choices?

Rural poverty is also "off the beaten path." Diminished opportunities to earn a decent living in mining, farming, and forestry have left many rural people living in grinding poverty. They reside in picturesque regions that mainstream America hurries through on the way to tourist destinations.

Both the inner-city poor and the rural poor are politically invisible. They are less likely to vote, and they are seldom organized to have a voice. They are not property owners. They are not represented by policy makers (Williams & Collins, 2001).

The poor are also rendered invisible by the difficulty of others, even in health care professions, in understanding and identifying with them. Perhaps they lack the language skills and education to explain their circumstances, or to provide an adequate health history (Display 32–2). Perhaps their social circumstances are so different that the health care worker has trouble identifying with the clients' problems. Unable to empathize with their circumstances, they may fail to see poor clients as persons.

Social Status

Social status is a person's rank or standing in society. Social status is affected by gender, age, and race. In the United States, women have a lower social status than men. Children and the elderly also have low social status, as do people of color. Therefore, a very young or very old woman of a minority race has the lowest status and least opportunity in American society. Middle-aged Caucasian men have the highest status. It is not surprising, then, that rates of poverty are highest among women of color and lowest among white men (Fergerson, 2001).

Social Support

Social support involves the quality of interpersonal ties between individuals; the strength and extent of these personal ties determine the individual's abilities to cope with adversity. A single, adolescent mother living apart from family and friends has little social support and is, therefore, most vulnerable to an array of social, physical, and emotional problems.

Neighborhood Resources

Neighborhood resources can be valuable in helping people reach their potential. Such community assets include religious organizations, safe housing, crime-watch programs, good schools, libraries, safe and affordable day care centers, recreational facilities, public health care clinics, and other social services.

Consider the likelihood of persistent poverty for a Native American woman living with paraplegia. She lives on a reservation, marginalized from mainstream society. She is of low social status as a disabled woman of color. The quality of her life and health and the opportunity to move beyond poverty are, therefore, determined by the strength of social support available from her family and friends and by the resources available in her community. If vocational rehabilitation, wheelchair-accessible housing, transportation, and employment opportunities are lacking, she is unlikely to escape poverty.

Gender and Age

Almost two out of three poor adults in the United States are women (U. S. Bureau of the Census, 2000). In a process that has been called the **feminization of poverty**, growing numbers of women have fallen into poverty due to weakening of the nuclear family, women heading households alone, low-wage jobs for unskilled work, and the dismantling of social programs for women. Society expects women to care for others. Women's lives are woven into a web of caring for children, the elderly, grandchildren, men, and other relatives and friends. They are also responsible for managing households by cooking, cleaning, and organizing. How can women in poverty sustain these roles and survive economically?

As mentioned earlier, 12% of American children are poor. Indeed, among Western industrialized nations, the United States has the highest rate of child poverty. This means children are going to school hungry and, therefore, are unable to learn. Lacking preventive dentistry, they suffer from dental caries. Sometimes they are poisoned by lead from the old lead-based paint peeling off the wall of deteriorating housing. Perhaps they cannot breathe because of asthma caused by roach droppings in their infested housing.

DISPLAY 32–2

The Human Face of Poverty: Mary

Mary is a poor mother in a foreign country she cannot understand. She is Haitian-American, pregnant with an infant on her arm, hungry, and living on the streets of a small agricultural community in central Florida. The public health nurse received a referral from the obstetric clinic nurse, asking her to call on this woman because she was considered "peculiar in the head." Mary lost her welfare benefits and, therefore, her single room because the baby's father was living with her. The father was HIV positive and took any money she had. She had a single room, but the father had taken over the entire space with stored items he planned to sell overseas. There was no room to sleep. People tell the public health nurse just to leave this crazy woman alone. She does appear to have a personality disorder, but most of the difficulty is that she cannot articulate what is going on in her life because she speaks Creole and little English. Her mental illness estranges her from the local Haitian community, and she does not know how to access community resources in the broader community. Mary lives apart from mainstream society, and it will be the nurse's role to connect her to the community. What nursing priorities are evident in this situation?

Because of poor access to preventive health care, they have more, and more severe, health problems.

Employment Status

In 1998, 42% of Americans classified as poor were employed. However, only 10% had full-time jobs year round. Some had part-time employment, often in low-paying retail service industries. Others worked seasonally as migrant farmworkers or sporadically as "temps" or day laborers. Much American poverty is a consequence of work that has disappeared or no longer pays a living wage.

America has shifted from an industrial economy to a postindustrial economy based on service industries such as retail trade, banking, and health care. Manufacturing plants have closed or moved overseas. The remaining manufacturing industries are becoming more and more technologically oriented, with jobs that require advanced training. These jobs are typically located in the suburbs, where they are inaccessible to inner-city and rural residents. Whereas low-skilled fathers in the past were able to work in manufacturing trades, low-skilled sons today can get only the lowest-paid part-time retail or service jobs. Similarly, undereducated women are likely to be working in low-wage, dead-end positions.

Consider just some of the challenges of obtaining and maintaining a higher wage position: completing high school and vocational training, money for the bus or to maintain a car, child care, and money for presentable clothing. These factors often have forced poor Americans—especially single mothers—to rely on public assistance at least until their children reach school age.

Persistent joblessness perpetuates self-doubt and feelings of hopelessness and powerlessness that can infect whole neighborhoods. The lack of economic opportunities for millions of American men can consign them to a lifetime at the bottom of the class structure and to estrangement from community and family commitments. They become resigned to their inability to play the traditional "breadwinner" role and may walk away from fatherhood.

Even for those who are employed full-time year round, low wages perpetuate poverty. In 2002, the minimum wage in California was $6.75 per hour; in other states, it was lower. At the California minimum wage, a full-time worker grosses just over $14,000 a year—above the poverty for a single person, but below the poverty rate for a family of three or four. This does not permit a decent standard of living. Factors conspiring to keep the minimum wage down include the increased political power of American industry, decline of union representation of workers, exporting of manufacturing operations overseas, and increased reliance on part-time and temporary workers.

Lifestyle

In 1959, anthropologist Oscar Lewis first described common beliefs and coping mechanisms held by people living in persistent poverty (Carney, 1992). These patterns are seen when wage earners are continuously unemployed or employed with low wages in unskilled work. Cash is chronically short. Possessions are pawned and money is borrowed at inflated interest rates. Food is purchased in small amounts daily. Living quarters are crowded, with no privacy. Attitudes and behaviors can include fatalism, cynicism about government, marginal connection to mainstream organizations, present-time orientation with little postponement of immediate gratification, early sexual initiation, abandonment of women and children, high frequency of alcoholism, and violence toward women and children. The external environment may be hostile, crowded, polluted, and violent. Over time, the chronically poor have "internalized their poverty. . . . Many simply do not believe that they can influence the course of their lives" (Hilfiker, 1994, p. 158).

A public health nurse explains the attitude of sexually active, drug-using teen women whose families live in persistent poverty with no economic opportunities in their local community:

Over the years, it took me a while to figure out why the drugs and the sex and the babies. They're so poor, and the older men will come along and say, "I'm going to show you a better life. Be with me and be my girlfriend and I'll give you all the stuff you never had." Now, delayed gratification is not in their mind. They can't envision 5 years from now. I tell them, "Five years from now, you finish high school, go to vocational school or community college, and you'll be able to buy as many pairs of shoes once you're working." Instead, they can't see beyond 6 months of high living with him. It's the poverty and hopelessness causing them to take all of these risks. Then comes the babies and the HIV.

Communication patterns can be very different from those used within the middle class. Verbalization may be minimal; silence might be valued over exploring feelings or ideas. Indirect communication of feelings is likely. Poor people are often skilled at picking up nonverbal communication of acceptance or apparent rejection. If the nurse shares some details of her or his own personal life, the disclosure is more likely to break down social barriers, which then encourages client disclosure of self.

POLITICS AND ETHICS OF POVERTY

The existence and alleviation of poverty in America are best understood in the context of American political and ethical forces.

Tensions Between Community and Self-Interest

Mainstream American values emphasize materialism and the work ethic. Individualism, focusing on individual self-interest and self-determination, has fashioned our social conscience. As a society, we believe that people do well by having strong wills and working hard. When people fall into hard times, the dominant assumption is that they are weak and failed to work hard enough. In other words, we blame the poor for their impoverished state.

Because American social conscience denies that society is responsible to help the poor, we resist paying taxes to support community services. In contrast, Canada and Western Europe have emphasized sustenance rights for the population, ensuring basic social protections such as food, housing, and health care for all. European programs include housing subsidies, medical care, child care, and unemployment insurance that benefit all levels of society. The European public believes in the social origins of poverty and that society as a whole benefits when poverty is prevented or relieved.

Cycles of Government Involvement

English and American history reveal cycles of political focus on the poor (Carney, 1992). The English Poor Law of 1601 first established government responsibility for relieving poverty. In the American colonies, the first Poor Law was established in Plymouth in 1642. Helping people in their own homes was neglected in favor of removing them to workhouses, almshouses, and indentured servitude. The Protestant ethic emphasized individual hard work and explained poverty as individual failure. In the 1800s, counties took responsibility for public assistance, primarily in the form of almshouses. Orphanages were established; most of the children had living parents who were too poor to care for them. Not until the early 1900s was there public support for aiding needy families and reversing the policy of taking children from their own homes.

In the United States, as a consequence of the Great Depression, President Franklin Roosevelt enacted the New Deal in 1935. It included Social Security and Aid to Dependent Children, which added a grant for the mother's expenses and was renamed Aid to Families with Dependent Children (AFDC) in 1950. Receiving AFDC came to be equated with "receiving welfare." AFDC was administered at the state level with federal grants; payments provided varied dramatically from state to state. The cash benefit was supposed to be enough to provide basic needs for food, clothing, shelter, and essential necessities.

In 1964, a War on Poverty was declared, ushering in Medicare and Medicaid and the Equal Opportunity Employment Act. Then, in the 1980s, many programs to assist the poor were cut in the belief that such assistance was fostering irresponsibility. The American dream continued to be that anyone can make it to the middle class through hard work. The sentiment against the poor became so strong that, in 1996, the United States abolished welfare as it had been known. In contrast, most of the industrialized, developed world continues to support women and men in their dual responsibilities as workers and parents. Cash benefits are given to supplement wages that are considered inadequate to nurture children. Mothers receive maternity leave and leave to care for sick children; day care is government sponsored.

Temporary Aid to Needy Families

In 1996, the Personal Responsibility and Work Opportunity Reconciliation Act restructured AFDC into **Temporary Aid to Needy Families (TANF)**. Financing is through federal funding to individual states, which have great latitude in setting up programs. The government limits the duration of family support to 5 years; this is a lifetime limit. Most states have reduced the eligibility duration even further. TANF also mandates that states require that the recipient find work within 2 years. Secondary school or postsecondary education does not postpone the work requirement, although it is well known that education is a significant factor predicting whether welfare recipients work and eventually can earn enough to escape poverty. Federal law does not require child care provisions, although it is also known that subsidizing child care enables about one third of families living in poverty to eventually escape. Individual states impose requirements for keeping benefits, such as up-to-date immunizations, limits on child absenteeism from school, or identification of fathers and requiring their child support cooperation (Chavkin, 1999). Mothers are required to work outside the home and be highly responsible for their children, but they are given little assistance to accomplish these ends.

After this work-based welfare reform was enacted in 1997, the U. S. Census Bureau reported in 2002 that there had been a dramatic reduction in the number of welfare recipients, to 1.5 million women (from 8.2% to 3.9%), making the program appear effective. However, many women are forced to rely on extended family or friends to subsidize household costs, and with a less than robust economy in 2001–2002 entry level jobs were being cut, directly affecting many of the newly employed women (Wesphal, 2002). In addition, President George W. Bush proposed a plan in 2002 that would require 70% of welfare recipients to work at least 40 hours a week by 2007. Time will tell whether this plan is enacted and, if so, what additional problems it may create, rather than helping women and children as intended.

Income eligibility requirements are now stricter than Medicaid requirements, which causes administrative complications by creating two separate sets of criteria. The Act also cut back Medicaid benefits for mentally impaired children and for many noncitizen immigrants. Today, many immigrants have no recourse except the emergency department; they wait until their conditions become life-threatening, or they use emergency services inappropriately for minor problems, without having a personal health care provider for consultation. As had been feared by health advocates, many people have lost Medicaid coverage and become uninsured as a result of the TANF reforms (Pear, 1999). Even for those who have found employment, their low-wage jobs usually do not have any health benefits.

The effects of welfare-to-work programs are continuing to be evaluated. A key element of their success will be the strength of accompanying health insurance and child care provisions. Tough long-range issues will be the lack of employment opportunities, low wages, and unaffordable housing. Other challenges to maintaining steady employment include mental health issues, drug or alcohol abuse, jealous or violent male partners, unreliable babysitters, sick children, nonoperating cars, and neighborhood dangers. For the most emotionally and socially impoverished, the cutoff of welfare benefits mandated by the Welfare Reform Act of 1996 could result in an enlarged group of people living in extreme hardship with no financial safety net.

TANF has been called successful because it has dramatically reduced the number of people receiving assistance (a 50% drop in the 1990s) (Westphal, 2002). However, true success will be measured by a long-standing reduction of the number of families living in poverty. Low-wage jobs typically allow no paid leave or flexibility to meet children's health needs. Current policy forces mothers to choose between meeting their children's basic health needs and keeping a job to ensure family survival (Heymann & Earle, 1999). Many children are left alone to care for even younger children, sick and well. Whom will we blame for the resulting tragedies? In contrast, interventions that support work success include education and skill development, child care, work flexibility and family leave, and programs to respond to domestic violence and chronic disabilities, particularly those related to substance abuse (Antai-Otong, 2002).

Human Service Programs

Contrary to the myth that nothing can be done and that helping the poor only weakens them, many human service programs have proved their effectiveness in alleviating hardship and improving well-being of impoverished people. Effective programs are interdisciplinary and comprehensive; they combine intensive social, educational, and health interventions. They consider people in the context of family and community, not in isolation. Successful programs include professionals who establish trusting relationships and respond to the needs of people they serve rather than the demands of bureaucracies. Such programs deliberately reduce barriers of access, money, and fragmented services. They do not wait for people to make it through the overwhelming service maze. They go where people live and work and go to school, often at nontraditional hours. Pregnancy prevention and prenatal care programs that meet these criteria have excellent outcomes. Perinatal nurse home visiting with these characteristics has been demonstrated to have dramatic effects to reduce maternal smoking, newborn low birth weight, emergency department visits, and child abuse and to improve mothers' return to school and work and

postponement of further pregnancies (Olds, Henderson, Kitzman, et al., 1999) (see Levels of Prevention Matrix).

There is strong evidence that federally funded public assistance programs intended to alleviate the effects of poverty on children and families are effective. Food stamps provide nationwide food assistance to all households based on financial need. They are considered central to the food assistance safety net for children. The Special Supplemental Food Program for Women, Infants, and Children (WIC) has increased intake of essential nutrients for pregnant mothers and children. School nutrition programs offer free or low-cost breakfasts and lunches to qualifying children. Head Start is a model of comprehensive services that was launched in 1965 as a preschool educational program for the disadvantaged, providing educational, social, health, and nutritional interventions. Short-term benefits include improved physical, social, and cognitive development. The Low Income Home Energy Assistance Program cuts monthly utility bills for people within predetermined income ranges. And finally, the Childrens' Health Insurance Program (CHIP) provides physical examinations, immunizations, and other health care needs for children up to 18 years of age, free of charge and separate from parent's eligibility for Medicaid or other assistance.

Distributive Justice

Justice is concerned with treating people fairly. **Distributive justice** refers to the justified distribution of burdens and benefits throughout society. Just distribution means challenging when resources are considered scarce; the paradox of growing American wealth is that resources are hoarded rather than distributed. Philosophies of economic justice are contradictory. Some believe that resources should be distributed according to merit, determined by factors such as social status and work contribution. Whom does this leave out? Some believe that resources should be distributed to ensure that basic human needs (food, shelter, education, health) are met (see What Do You Think? II).

In the United States, the distribution of goods and services is largely determined by the marketplace. Although equality is claimed as a social ideal, dramatic inequities are accepted as being determined by the law of the marketplace. In contrast, community health nursing is grounded in commitment to a just distribution of primary goods for all members of society. The founder of American public health nursing, Lillian Wald, was in the forefront of social reform movements emphasizing just allocation of resources for the immigrant and poor laborer (Wald, 1971). Public health nurses inherit her legacy in the beginning of the 21st century.

HEALTH EFFECTS OF POVERTY

Increased Morbidity and Mortality

Public health professionals are committed to reducing the greater risk of illness and death that is caused by poverty.

LEVELS OF PREVENTION MATRIX

SITUATION: Preventing illness and diminishing poverty among poor single mothers and their children while effectively detecting and treating health problems of marginalized young families.

GOAL: Using the three levels of prevention, negative health conditions are avoided, or promptly diagnosed and treated, and the fullest possible potential is restored.

PRIMARY PREVENTION		SECONDARY PREVENTION		TERTIARY PREVENTION		
Health Promotion and Education	*Health Protection*	*Early Diagnosis*	*Prompt Treatment*	*Rehabilitation*	*Primary Prevention*	
					Health Promotion and Education	*Health Protection*
• Support social policy that fosters income-earning opportunities so that women can make enough to move out of poverty • Encourage opportunities for women to achieve a secondary education and jobs that pay living wages with benefits and child care • Eliminate racial and gender discrimination • Develop accessible health education programs with priorities on compelling issues such as family planning, strengthening parental bonds, violence prevention, smoking prevention, drug and alcohol abuse, mental health, and injury prevention	• Ensure availability of client-friendly preventive measures such as nutrition supplementation and counseling and immunization administration • Advocate for those whose personal and social circumstances prevent employment for a living wage • Encourage support systems	• Develop comprehensive, humanized health services focusing on women's health and well-child screening • Develop outreach screening programs in the neighborhoods, schools, and workplaces • Develop trusting partnerships with women to diagnose health problems	• Encourage local community development to strengthen the capacity of women to help one another • Develop trusting partnerships with women to manage health problems	• Ensure effective case management of chronic conditions • Work with agencies and individuals to support women living with domestic violence and alcohol and substance abuse • Advocate for expansion of counseling and rehabilitative services in the community	• Continue with primary prevention activities	• Continue with primary prevention activities

WHAT DO YOU THINK? II

Do you believe that there are some human beings so unworthy that they do not get to eat or to have a roof over their head?

Complex mechanisms related to socioeconomic disadvantage result in disadvantaged health status. As socioeconomic position improves, health improves. Just how causal variables relate to each other and result in poor health requires further investigation; however, it is clear that poverty and race are entwined as determinants of health (Levine et al., 2001; Satcher, 2000). The greater relative risks for racial minorities are particularly striking in the rates of infant and maternal mortality, cardiovascular disease, diabetes, HIV infection, cancer, and immunization. African-Americans have a shorter life expectancy, and twice as many African-American newborns die in the first month of life as European-American newborns. Even if adequately insured, members of minority groups are less likely to receive advanced therapies. Institutional racism is a major reason. One study presented 720 physicians with videotaped actors posing in identical clothing with identical occupations, health insurance, and health histories (Schulman et al., 1999). The physicians chose to refer significantly fewer women and African-Americans for cardiac catheterization. Earlier studies also identified gender and race as factors affecting how aggressively heart disease is managed.

Other variables known to interact with poverty in promoting poor health include lack of education, low occupational status, jobs with high demands and low control, selected cultural health beliefs, social isolation, poor nutrition, and poor housing (Bashir, 2002; House et al., 2000). Inadequate housing may lack heat or cooling, proper ventilation, access to bathing, adequate refrigeration and cooking facilities, and security from violence. Houses with deteriorating lead paint are home to 1.8 million children, and 42 million dwellings in the United States contain lead paint (Potula, Hegarty-Steck, & Hu, 2001). Inadequate housing may also be plagued with rats, fleas, roaches, and other vermin. Environmental hazards outside the home include toxic wastes in the neighborhood and toxic materials at work.

The chronic stressors of poverty, including racism, classism, self-doubt, and learned helplessness, contribute to poor health. Similarly, morbidity and mortality are greater where social bonds and the level of social trust have eroded (Williams & Collins, 2001). Residents in high-trust neighborhoods are more willing to help one another and share resources; they are healthier, despite poverty. Any intervention that strengthens human connections within a community can be predicted to improve individual health (Pittman et al., 2000).

Individual health behaviors such as inactivity, tobacco and alcohol abuse, and obesity are clearly correlated with poor health and must be understood in their social context. Persons with the least education and the lowest income are more likely to be smokers, overweight, and physically inactive (Ganz, 2000; Lantz et al., 1998). However, it is unwise to focus public health policies solely on reduction of individual risk behaviors, because they explain only some of the health disadvantage.

Reduced Access to Health Care

Low-income people are less likely to have access to preventive and therapeutic health services. In addition to lack of transportation and inability to leave low-wage jobs to keep medical appointments, access to care is impeded by lack of health insurance and inability to pay out-of-pocket charges. Places where the poor have traditionally received care have been called "safety net providers." Lacking an insurance card

in their pocket or purse, they have, in the past, been able to receive care in emergency departments, public health departments, community free clinics, public and teaching hospitals, some not-for-profit hospitals, and from physicians and practitioners who have voluntarily provided uncompensated care. Now, although the demands for uncompensated care are increasing, with 44.3 million uninsured Americans in 1998 and more than 70 million people lacking insurance for at least 1 month each year, subsidies for indigent care have been cut at all levels of government (Smith-Campbell, 2000). As managed care aggressively seeks to control costs, there is no longer a way to subsidize care for the indigent ("Managed Care Cost Pressures," 1999).

Those who receive Medicaid often receive unequal care. For instance, mothers covered by Medicaid in some south Florida hospitals must pay $500 or more out of their pockets if they want epidural anesthesia during childbirth; they must pay anesthesiologists up front before labor begins or endure the pain. Many Medicaid recipients are unable to access medical specialists because these physicians consider Medicaid reimbursement to be inadequate.

When they do access care, impoverished clients of the health care system are unlikely to receive health-promoting advice and unlikely to have their chronic conditions carefully managed. Instead, they are likely to be treated for the most obvious symptoms of a single illness episode. This situation may often be attributed to the negative attitudes of agencies and care providers. Often, agencies founded to serve the poor have developed so many regulations and obstacles for clients that they are essentially inaccessible. For instance, a nurse practitioner not long ago sought to immunize a population of 300 adolescents in a dropout prevention program against hepatitis B and measles, but the nursing supervisor interpreted the regulations of the local health department to preclude both delivery of the vaccine to the practitioner and authorization of transportation of the youth to the department. Additionally, the resources of institutions mandated to serve the poor may be stretched so thin that essentially no adequate services are provided. Finally, service providers may be so numbed or "burned out" by their exposures to human hardship that they decide clients are beyond help. It is often in the institutions charged with providing for the poor that one can find the highest proportion of workers who are no longer responsive to the real needs of clients.

Lack of access to services for prevention and treatment of alcohol and drug dependency is an immense burden on the poor (Antai-Otong, 2002; Wells et al., 2001). The national failure to ensure access to substance abuse treatment has been estimated to cost the nation up to $276 billion annually. The cost of untreated chemical abuse includes law enforcement, motor vehicle crashes, lost work productivity, medical expenses, and incarceration (Amaro, 1999). Treatment has been proven to be more effective than law enforcement and incarceration in reducing demand, yet the federal government spends almost double the amount on reducing supply (interdiction) than on prevention and treatment. Every dollar spent on treatment generates $7 in future costs saved. Publicly funded treatment is demonstrated to save money over time and is essential, along with expansion of private insurance benefits, to provide comprehensive and effective treatment.

HOMELESSNESS IN AMERICA

Poverty results in **homelessness** when limited resources make housing unaffordable. Homeless people lack a regular address. In a major study on national homelessness, Link and colleagues (1995) estimated that 14% of Americans become homeless at some point during their lifetime. Finding, interviewing, and counting the homeless are challenging to officials; their numbers are always likely to be underestimated. If they have not yet exhausted the resources and good will of friends or relatives, people without their own home stay overnight in other people's homes. This condition, called "doubling-up" with family and friends, may exist for up to 4 years before the "near-homeless" become literally homeless (Bolland & McCallum, 2002). When they become unable to continue to double-up, the most deprived homeless people sleep in parks, in abandoned buildings, in cars, on benches in bus stations, on roofs, under viaducts, or in homeless shelters.

For most people, being homeless is temporary or cyclic as they struggle to keep a roof over their heads. Homeless people on the doorsteps and streets of America have become familiar sights since the 1980s. We have come to accept and even to ignore this profound hardship, although being without a home was once common only in impoverished nations, not in the United States.

Why Are People Homeless?

The absence of low-cost housing is a tremendous burden on the poor, who must pay an expanding percentage of their paycheck for housing. Over the last 25 years, 2.2 million low-rent apartments have disappeared quietly due to urban renewal; the process of upgrading urban housing has created what the National Coalition for the Homeless defines as a high-rent burden: rents that absorb a high proportion of income (Strehlow & Amos-Jones, 1999). At the same time, the federal government has reduced its commitment to build and maintain inexpensive housing. The resultant widening gap between affordable housing units and people needing them has created a housing crisis. Many impoverished people are forced to live in overcrowded and substandard housing. The most severe housing needs are among the elderly, families with children, and low-income disabled people. Government housing assistance programs are unable to keep up with the demand. Waiting lists are 3 to 4 years long for government programs such as Section 8 housing.

In addition to poverty and the unavailability of affordable housing, several other factors can lead to homelessness in America. Battered women without resources are often forced to choose between enduring abuse at home and becoming homeless. In addition, many uninsured or underinsured people who suffer severe physical or emotional illness eventually become homeless (Rosenheck, 2000). Approximately one fourth of the adult homeless population is mentally ill. The lack of community mental health support services (eg, case management, treatment, supportive housing options) often forces patients onto the streets, under the bridges, or into the woods. Likewise, people who are poor and addicted to drugs or alcohol are at high risk of becoming homeless. Uninsured homeless people face long waits to get into treatment programs, and then they are likely to be discharged after treatment back onto the streets or into shelters. In 1996, new federal legislation denied Social Security Income and Social Security Disability Insurance, including Medicaid, to people whose disability resulted from addictions. As a result, many chemically dependent people are unable to afford even the worst sort of housing (Strehlow & Amos-Jones, 1999).

Living as a Homeless Person

The poor are continually faced with multiple stressors. Mothers living in shelters report minimal social support and alienation from human relationships (Caton et al., 2000). One third suffered physical abuse as children, and one fourth were battered in adult relationships. Having no place of their own makes mothers feel angry, controlled by rules they did not make. They dislike the absence of privacy and the lack of an address and telephone number, which are needed to seek health care for Medicaid or other third-party payers and to manage eligibility requirements. They are surrounded by the hardships of others. In a life involving frequent moves, mothers worry about where they will sleep next. They are concerned that their children's schooling is interrupted and inferior. Children suffer emotionally and psychologically. They feel imprisoned, miss school, do not like their new schools, and perform significantly lower than housed children in tests of academic performance. Relationships are impaired by shelter rules that prohibit visitors. Living so publicly causes tensions between everyone. Homeless people yearn for a stable family life, and their children dream of houses (Craft-Rosenberg, Powell, & Culp, 2000).

Health of the Homeless

Consider how the living environment contributes to health. Living outside results in exposure to assault and the weather. Hypothermia or the effects of sun and heat are constantly threatening. Trauma and impaired skin integrity are common. Living in shelters results in exposure to violence and communicable diseases ranging from scabies to tuberculosis, readily transmitted due to overcrowding. What basic activities of daily living would be difficult if you were homeless? You would face sleep deprivation, fear, hunger and thirst, inadequate bathing and oral hygiene, inadequate laundry facilities, nowhere to store medicines, no privacy, no control, and perhaps no hope. If you or your children were persistently hungry, would you consider begging, stealing, selling drugs, or engaging in prostitution? A whole new set of problems would result (see Clinical Corner).

Homelessness and health are interrelated in three ways: homelessness precipitates ill health, homelessness complicates the treatment of ill health, and ill health causes homelessness (Amarasingham, Spalding, & Anderson, 2001; Synoground & Bruya, 2000). Infant mortality and low birth weight are disproportionately high among infants born to homeless women. Homeless children experience chronic physical disorders at double the rate of the general population. Most common are malnutrition, anemia, and asthma. Acute illnesses such as upper respiratory tract infections, ear infections, gastrointestinal problems, and skin disorders are especially frequent. Children's mental health is profoundly affected, with half of preschool children experiencing developmental delays and half of school-aged children manifesting anxiety and depression, including suicidal ideation. Posttraumatic stress disorder is commonly diagnosed in children (Caton et al., 2000).

Homeless adults suffer disproportionately from most physical and mental illnesses. Tuberculosis and acquired immunodeficiency syndrome (AIDS) can be prevalent, depending on the region. Residents of homeless shelters in New York City die at an extraordinary four times the rate of the general population of the same age (Barrow et al, 1999). Homeless adults suffer disproportionately from permanent physical disabilities and have a life expectancy 20 years less than that of middle-class adults.

Programs to Help the Homeless

The Interagency Council on the Homeless coordinates federal homeless resources and is made up of the leaders of 16 federal agencies that have programs for the homeless. However, health care programs for the homeless are limited and fragmented.

Like most people living in poverty, homeless people tend to receive their health care in emergency departments after their health problems have reached crisis proportions. Typically, there is no plan for continuity of care. Some homeless people receive health care in community clinics, often experiencing long waits and insensitive care from health care providers who find them noncompliant with medical regimens.

Frequent barriers to health care for the homeless include the following: lack of health insurance, insensitivity of health care providers, stereotyping on the part of providers, cultural barriers regarding health beliefs and behavior, the homeless person's first priority of food and shelter instead of health, breakdown in communication between client and provider and among providers, bureaucratic paperwork to obtain services, transportation to those services, and homeless people's fear of "the system" (Strehlow & Amos-Jones, 1999).

The best services for the homeless provide social, educational, and health interventions. For instance, the Henry

CLINICAL CORNER

NUISANCE DISEASES IN A HOMELESS SHELTER

Scenario
As a public health nurse working for the Capitol City health department, you are assigned to rotate through three homeless shelters once each week. Your role is assessment of physical and mental health issues, health education, basic first aid, and appropriate referrals. In recent weeks, you have noticed that individuals staying in a particular homeless shelter have complained of an increased incidence of pediculosis capitis and pubis.

The shelter is operated by an interfaith religious organization. Twelve religious groups are members of this organization, including churches, synagogues, and mosques. Each agency assumes responsibility for operating the shelter three to four times per month. The hours of operation for the shelter are from 5:00 PM until 10:00 AM. Clients are provided an evening meal, a cot and blankets, and a morning meal. Hot showers are available in the morning, with clients rotating through the two showers in the shelter.

Funding and oversight of this program are provided by a volunteer organization working with officials in city government.

Available assessment data related to the problems include the following:

- Inclement weather has led to an increase in clients requesting shelter.
- Many of these clients would otherwise camp in the woods or sleep on the streets.

Questions
1. Discuss additional assessment data needed to address the issue of pediculosis in the shelter. How will you go about gathering these data?
2. Based on data presented in this scenario, present host, agent, and environmental factors that may be contributing to the problems.
3. Discuss interventions your program will perform at the primary, secondary, and tertiary levels of prevention.
4. Analyze issues related to social justice for this aggregate.

Street Settlement in New York City, originally established by the founder of American public health nursing, Lillian Wald, has offered model supportive services. Mental health and children's school involvement improve markedly with a safe shelter, around-the-clock staff, day care, tutoring after school, job training, help with obtaining government assistance, and help locating homes. It is fruitless to treat symptoms in the absence of broad-based interventions that address underlying problems.

Primary prevention of homelessness requires affirmation of shelter as a basic human right. Primary prevention involves changes in social policy, including affordable housing, accessible education and job training, work at a living wage, accessible child care, timely drug treatment, health education that includes pregnancy prevention, and public assistance that guarantees shelter for all.

GLOBAL POVERTY: THE DEVELOPING NATIONS

The right to a life free from poverty is proclaimed by the United Nations Charter. Internationally, poverty thresholds are defined in terms of the cost of a basic diet. One common definition of poverty is daily subsistence on $1 or less in the U. S.; one third of people in developing countries meet this definition. For example, one third of India's 1 billion people live on less than $1 a day (Crossette, 1999).

The concept of human poverty goes beyond income to identify deprivations such as lack of political freedom, lack of personal security, and inability to participate in the life of the community (United Nations Development Programmes, 1998). The Human Poverty Index measures illiteracy, child malnutrition, early death, poor health care, and inadequate access to safe water (see The Global Community). It reveals environmental and population characteristics that lead to health risks that are strikingly similar across the globe. Poverty, overpopulation, urbanization, and environmental deterioration are strongly interrelated.

Overpopulation

Poverty leads to population growth, and population growth leads to poverty. High child mortality leads parents to have more children. Lack of resources increases the need for children to help in home and field and to ensure help during infirmity and aging. Poverty engenders helplessness and hopelessness, which does not lead to planning ahead to limit children. Likewise, low education and low status of women means less knowledge of family planning and less personal power over fertility.

Migration and Urbanization

As the population expands, growing numbers of people are exhausting the soil and then moving to cultivate environmentally vulnerable areas, where they denude the hillsides

---

THE GLOBAL COMMUNITY

Cancun, Mexico, is famous as a luxury destination resort. However, 15 minutes away is a community of 110,000 people, many of whom are Mayan Indians. For several years, Jackie Adames, a nurse, who attended Florida Atlantic University's nursing program, visited these people as a member of a medical mission team. Her community assessment, presented in class, provided the information that follows regarding the environment, the people, and their health risks.

There are significant environmental hazards. The climate is persistently warm and humid. The air is thick with dust; most streets are not paved. Pesticides are used weekly to prevent yellow fever and dengue fever transmission by mosquitoes. Air is polluted from the exhaust of numerous buses and cabs. There is constant migration to and from the area. Although some houses are sturdy, others are made of cardboard or bamboo with thatched roofs and dirt floors. There are no child labor laws and no mandatory school laws. The cost of living has more than doubled in the past few years. Health services are available for employed people.

There are 110,000 people living in this community, which has been experiencing a 21% annual population growth. Most are younger than 45 years of age; they live in extended families with many children. They speak Spanish and Mayan at home. Most are impoverished, with no employment or low-wage employment. The diet is tortillas, pork, rice, cheese, animal fat, and few vegetables. Newborn babies are not named for 3 months to reduce attachment if they die. Prenatal care is inadequate. Mothers work, and children babysit younger children. Water is available from an outside pipeline at set times of the day. Electricity is inconsistent. Development of neighborhood infrastructure and government services cannot keep up with the explosive community growth.

Health risks are extensive, with a particularly high incidence of respiratory infections, asthma, gastroenteritis, and premature or low-birth-weight infants. Infectious diseases and diseases of malnutrition are of great concern. Dental problems include gum disease and tooth decay. Physical injuries from manual labor and domestic violence are prevalent.

and deforest the tropics. Short-term survival takes precedence over preservation of natural resources. When rural life becomes unsustainable, the poor migrate into cities and towns. Almost half of the world's people now live in cities, creating an unprecedented density of people. Their concentrated numbers have resulted in dramatic environmental degradation and urban sprawl that makes water a scarce commodity and causes immense problems with waste disposal. Increased motorization results in gridlock and air pollution. Public spending cannot keep up with the needs for food, transportation, water, sewer, garbage collection, public health protection, communication, and education. Urban crowding is strongly linked to respiratory infections. Dirty air and water are causing serious health problems worldwide. Seventy percent of the health problems in Ghana, on the southern coast of West Africa, are environmentally related diseases. Whether poor people are urban or rural dwellers, the immediacy of making a living overshadows preservation of the forest, land, water, or air. Poverty is destroying the ecosystem, and environmental degradation disproportionately affects the lives of the poor.

Underemployment and Industrialization

The poor are often underemployed in the "informal sector," in activities such as domestic service or street vending. Those who are formally employed often have temporary work and are underpaid. Industries in the underdeveloped world are under great pressure to be competitive internationally. They push production costs down by keeping wages down and hiring part-time, temporary workers. Increasingly, children, the elderly, and women are pressed into manufacturing, with all the attendant occupational hazards and none of the safety requirements enforced in the United States. The greed of the commercial interests in the developed world is felt in the everyday struggles of the working poor in developing countries.

Eradicating Global Poverty

The poorest countries are so heavily burdened with debt to industrialized nations that they are falling behind in meeting the basic needs of their people (Display 32–3). Eradication of poverty requires honest central governments working in partnerships with local governments and the private sector. Vital to antipoverty programs are the organization and activation of impoverished communities themselves. Because poverty causes illness and illness causes poverty, community development is central to international public health nursing.

ROLE OF THE COMMUNITY HEALTH NURSE

There are many points at which the community health nurse can make a difference in the lives of people. Nurses provide

DISPLAY 32–3

Eradicating Global Poverty

Six policies are proposed by the United Nations to eradicate extreme poverty in the underdeveloped global community:
1. Empowerment of women
2. Programs to promote economic growth of developing countries where growth has been failing
3. Fair trade policies that allow poor countries to enter the world market
4. Support for poor communities to organize and act collectively
5. Promotion of accountable, open governments with active citizen participation
6. Debt reduction and peace-building for nations in particularly difficult circumstances

(From United Nations Development Programmes, 1998.)

services in deteriorating urban areas, with those living in poverty wherever they live, and among the homeless. Nurses need, first, to assess themselves for their attitudes and preconceptions. All low-income people in urban areas can have access to care improved, and some mostly need an advocate. The urban communities, and poor or homeless people living in them, need strenghtening and interventions that can be initiated by community health nurses using the nursing process as a guide (see Using the Nursing Process).

Self-Assessment

Confronting poverty and caring for people who are poor require reflective assessment of one's own assumptions and beliefs. Because poverty is prevalent over a lifetime, many students of nursing have personal or family experience of living in poverty. However, because the stigma is so great and fault finding is so pervasive in our society, acknowledging and reflecting on this experience may well be painful. In contrast, because poverty is so hidden and frequently denied, many students of nursing have lived apart from any knowledge of the human experience of poverty. They may have come to believe many of the negative stereotypes about poor people. How have your judgments been shaped? How can you open yourself to caring for those from whom most of society turns away?

We learn from one another's stories. First, learn from your classmates, friends, and neighbors who are courageous enough to tell you their own experiences of living with poverty. Ask them and listen well. Then let your patients teach you. One honor we have as nurses is the opportunity to work with people from all walks of life. You are particularly likely in clinical experiences in community health to meet impoverished individuals and families living outside the

USING THE NURSING PROCESS

When "Nursing on the Streets"......

David Morton, a community health nurse, noticed that there were many homeless people sitting, sleeping, and wandering around in two vacant lots near the health department where he worked. He wanted them to know about and use the clinics in the health department but had not as yet made any contact with them. Often thinking "outside of the box," David thought he would bring a few card tables and folding chairs to one of the lots and set up a "mobile" clinic. He convinced two other nurses to spend a morning with him and do case-finding on the street. The first day they brought free hand-out items (condoms, vitamin samples, Band-aids, liquid hand wash, and so on) that they had in the department. David brought some juices and cookies from home to have available. In addition, they brought equipment to check blood pressure and blood sugar and informational material about the services of the health department and allowed time to chat with the people and answer any questions they might have.

ASSESSMENT

As people began to gather around, the nurses introduced themselves and described the services of the health department.

The nurses "assessed" 15 people on the first morning and got a better understanding of the needs of those who dropped by, including immediate needs, presenting health problems, and suggestions of services the nurses could provide if they set up weekly for 2 hours, (the amount of time the nurses could spare), including the best day and time.

NURSING DIAGNOSIS

After the first day, the nurses determined that the following nursing diagnoses were the most pressing and began working on #1 immediately (which would also help #3 and #4, and solve problem #5):
1. Sleep pattern disturbances
2. Altered nutrition at risk for less than body requirements
3. Impaired skin integrity
4. At risk for injury
5. At risk for hypothermia
6. Ineffective community coping

PLAN

After assessment and diagnoses development the nurses developed a plan based on presented needs and observations. Most presented problems were related to a lack of food and shelter. Diagnosis #1 was focused on first, because it had a major effect on the other items.

IMPLEMENTATION

The community health nurse will contact nearby family shelters for housing of two mothers with five children; care at a Veterans' Hospital for two elderly men with stasis leg ulcers, and temporary overnight shelter for the remaining six men.

The cohort of homeless mothers, children and elderly agreed to the arrangements and working with the staff to have other needs met, such as school for two children, health care maintenance, long-range counseling, housing, education, and work training and preparation for the adults as needed.

The nurses agreed to work with the six men temporarily housed to find long-term solutions or provide supportive services for those choosing to live on the street.

The nurses agreed to return to the vacant lots weekly to keep in touch with those who may return there and to work with others who would hear about the nurses' services.

EVALUATION

The two elderly mens' leg ulcers healed after 2 months, and through social services at the Veterans' Hospital low-income, subsidized housing was secured.

One woman with three children went to Alcoholics Anonymous meetings at the family shelter, found work in her son's new school, and found low-income housing through the supportive services of the family shelter. She stayed there for 6 months while becoming sober, receiving counseling, and preparing for a job.

The second woman stayed at the family shelter for 2 months and then moved to a nearby city to live with her sister. The nurses made referrals to the health department in that city to provide follow-up as needed.

Among the six homeless men, two find shelter housing on most nights. The others stay in the vacant lots, but they now know where to get food more regularly, and they use the health department clinic for illness or injury. They frequently refer others to seek out the nurses who "come to help us, rain or shine."

mainstream. Many years ago, a nursing faculty member had a one-to-one postclinical conference with a student at a small Roman Catholic college. The student had made many visits to an African-American teen mother of two thriving children. The young mother lived in a dangerous housing project, and, although she locked him out of her second-floor apartment, her abusive boyfriend had been known to climb up the drainage pipe and over the porch roof. Sometimes, he forced open a window and beat her. The mother worked every day at a fast food establishment; her grandmother took care of the children. After a couple of months of weekly visits, the student exclaimed, "When I read her chart, I saw her as a immoral girl—a slut—and I expected her to be a loser. Now I can't believe what I've learned about how strong she is. She just keeps fighting for herself and the kids to survive! She's a great mom and I told her so!"

Another faculty member who taught community health nursing in a midwestern school of nursing was having an informal discussion with a student who related her experience trying to get comfortable making home visits with low-income young women. She was making brave attempts at home visits to a pregnant woman about her age who lived in the deteriorating outskirts of a major city. She thought she had established rapport and was making progress with the client. One day the client asked the student, with concern in her voice, if she had "broken off her engagement?" The student then had difficulty explaining the absence of her engagement ring, which she had never mentioned but the client had noticed. During the previous week, she had suddenly realized she was wearing this special ring in marginal neighborhoods and thought it best to leave it at home. Of course she had to fabricate another reason to tell the client, but she felt badly for being so judgmental when the client was identifying with the student and felt they had something in common (see Voices from the Community).

VOICES FROM THE COMMUNITY

A nurse who has practiced with many disenfranchised patients living with mental illness or infected with the human immunodeficiency virus (HIV) describes *breaking the fear* as essential to caring:

"All of us at some level have a fear of the disenfranchised, whether it's because we could be in that place or because there may be potential harm to us. But I seek to break that fear and see someone as human. The more I work with her, the more I see her as human."

(Zerwekh, J.V. [2000]. Caring on the ragged edge: Nursing persons who are disenfranchised. *Advances in Nursing Science, 22*[4], 47–61.)

Improving Access

Even when government-sponsored health insurance and services are available, as we have seen, extensive barriers prevent poor people from accessing services. The community health nurse serves as an advocate and bridge for families who need to gain access. Barriers to access associated with the clients themselves include reluctance to seek coverage because of feelings of pride or independence or mistrust; feeling powerless; being unaware that such services exist or are worthwhile; lacking resources such as a telephone, transportation, or fare for children who need to go along because no babysitter is available; being illiterate; and preoccupation with meeting survival needs and competing life priorities instead of health needs (Bamberger et al., 2000). Barriers associated with applying for health insurance include a system that is unfriendly and complicated. Paperwork is overwhelming and may be returned for correction; presentation of paid utility bills or other statements not saved may be required. Informative materials may be too difficult to understand; programs may seek to restrict enrollments by restricting information. The process may require a car, a telephone, and appointments at inconvenient times. The nurse can intervene as a coach and guide, interpreting the system to the client and the client to the system. Likewise, the nurse can act as change agent to improve the system whenever possible.

Strengthening Communities

We are all connected. All of us as citizens have a stake in preventing the adverse hardships of poverty. All of society pays to support community members who do not contribute, to house those who are incarcerated, and to ignore the homeless. This weakens us. We fear crime in our homes, schools, businesses, and communities in general. Our society is impaired by adults who are incapable of providing nurturing environments for their children. And the alienation of many groups in society erodes our sense of community as a nation.

The common good is enhanced by strengthening community resources, including investing in people of historically low status, developing and strengthening ties within families and among people involved in neighborhood mutual support, and redeveloping neighborhood resources. Recognizing that the foundational causes of poverty are economic, the community health nurse realizes that the alleviation of poverty can come only with major changes in American economic and social policy. Whenever possible, the nurse voices support of economic redevelopment of neighborhoods to enhance schools, housing, and employment. The community health nurse can also work to promote subsidized carpools, school-to-work transition programs, universal health insurance, and inner-city economic development programs.

Many caution well-intentioned professionals to beware of seeking solutions to poverty in service programs alone. First of all, a whole population of people can become defined in terms of their problems instead of their strengths. In addition, citizens acting to help themselves within their community can be weakened when they are seen as "clients" requiring professional services. Finally, there is a disabling effect of being dependent on multiple human services, which reduces self-worth and leads to feelings of powerlessness. If you doubt this, go sit in the waiting room of your nearest public clinic. Notice how people are addressed as they wait, are processed through various clerks, and are finally seen. If you are really courageous, try seeking help for one of your own health problems in such an environment, so often dehumanized and even designed to discourage people from seeking help. Because human service interventions can have negative as well as positive effects, it is important to consider whether more community agencies are the answer to resolving community hardship. Community health planning should take seriously an organizing process that builds community, focusing on developing neighborhood competence to problem-solve and create solutions for itself (see the discussion of community development in Chapters 18 and 19).

Strengthening Individuals

Poverty nursing requires careful attention to how medical regimens can be made workable despite poverty (Display 32–4). The nurse needs to ask many questions to translate mainstream health care to what is feasible, given the person's living circumstances. For every treatment prescribed, the

DISPLAY 32–4

Strengthening Individuals

When working with the poor, it is imperative for the community health nurse to follow these guidelines:

- Create trust.
- Show respect and concern.
- Modify assessments and interventions as needed.
- Make no assumptions regarding underlying need.
- Remember the basics, such as food, shelter, and survival.
- Accept that appointments will be missed—surviving is a more pressing priority, drop-in, stop-by contacts may be more feasable.
- Collaborate with community agencies to form a network of services for referrals.
- Advocate for accessible health services.
- Focus on prevention, yet provide for health promotion and maintenance.
- Know when to take initiative on behalf of the client and when to back off and let the client take it—this allows "ownership" of the problem.
- Develop a support network for oneself.

(From Synoground & Bruya, 2000; Rew, Chambers & Kulkarni, 2002.)

nurse must question how it will be accomplished. Can the client afford medications? Can the client obtain the dressings? Is it possible for the client to rest or exercise or eat as prescribed? Are caregivers available among family and friends? What compromises are necessary? What is practical? What agencies or services can be mobilized to help, and for how long?

Seven nurses who were well respected for their compassionate work with disenfranchised people were interviewed. Their clients are people from whom many others withdraw and walk away. These exemplary nurses described their clients as fellow human beings who frighten many of us and are themselves afraid. Their poverty, accompanied by mental illness, HIV infection, end-stage illness, alcoholism, or status as an unwanted immigrant, has "pushed them out of the human family." They are disconnected and fearful. It seems as if there is a wall between them and the rest of the community (see Voices From the Community). The abandonment of the poor results in tragic "trickle-down" consequences. The abandonment is internalized by the adults and children who had not been adequately loved see themselves as unlovable. Being pushed down so many times, they see failure as inevitable. The nurses interviewed said that compassionate caring for patients who are disenfranchised and apart from the mainstream requires a different kind of nursing. Analysis of their reflections and stories reveals three practice categories: the Human Connection, the Community Connection, and Making Self-Care Possible (Zerwekh, 2000).

The Human Connection involves deliberately honoring the human dignity of the poor, coming to know them well, and sharing one's own humanity rather than maintaining professional distance. The nurses remind other professionals who have forgotten about their clients' humanity. Clients know they are held in regard. One nurse explained, "They call me because I respect them." They are proud of knowing the clients well, drawing them out through authentic listening and paying attention. They discover their past. With discretion, they share their own life struggles and stories and insist that other nurses should do the same. One expert asserts, "They have to perceive you as real."

The Community Connection involves connecting the disconnected to other community members and services, mediating between clients and services, and persisting with the case. The nurse has to find a way around the wall that separates clients from community. One nurse said this might require "tunneling through the wall. There's always another way around."

In many cases, this means making exceptions to bureaucratic rules. Although others get tired and give up, expert nurses keep trying to pull in and coordinate resources. One nurse calls this kind of persistence "haunting the case." They seek to develop rapport with each person, developing and maintaining a trusting connection. In addition, the nurses establish and maintain a provider network to get the client into the health delivery system. This requires excellent working relationships and personal influence. Finally, they actively link the homeless person to the health care system. The goal is continuity of care that addresses underlying problems, instead of a Band-Aid approach.

Making Self-Care Possible has to do with strengthening people to care for themselves. Nurses listen at length. They "help them get the anger out" and do not take it personally. One nurse explains, "I help them get through the rough spots." They teach understanding of body and emotions. Another nurse tells her clients, "You should know more about the illness than I do. You have to walk it, wash it, live it, breathe it." Another nurse who works with indigent mentally ill clients teaches them how to separate from "the voices that tell them all day long that they are no good and ugly." Nurses encourage impoverished clients to take control of their lives, and they develop practical health care plans with clients in charge. "Always, always let them know that they are in control." And, as we have seen, poverty nursing—whether urban, suburban, small town, or rural—involves working at the community level to pull the entire wall down and help change underlying circumstances.

Care for Oneself as Caregiver

Sustained work with the poor requires significant self-awareness and deliberate self-caring. Work with the truly broken, people who are physically unappealing, odorous and unclean, disturbed and possibly violent (to self and others), abusive, confused, unreachable, often visibly "ungrateful," and frequently seen as people who "use the system" and do "nothing" to help themselves, can exhaust the emotional and spiritual reservoirs of even the most highly motivated caregivers. Some clients are deeply damaged and degraded by poverty and feel powerless. When they fail to make the changes that we as professionals repeatedly recommend, our caring intentions can become fault finding and blaming and can turn to indifference if we do not care for ourselves.

As we experience inevitable frustration and failure, self-protection results in growing detachment and less willingness to feel the pain, anger, and cynicism. We retreat behind the wall. In contrast, sustained engagement requires ongoing, conscious exploration of one's own motivations and behaviors. Sustained caring requires continuous, conscious care of self: nurturing through spiritual practices, rest, retreat, celebration, friendship, art, music, exercise, therapy, self-reflection, and group support with colleagues.

Many community health nurses find meaning in working with the disenfranchised through a sense of personal calling: "These are the people I am meant to help." To work effectively with the poor, nurses hold a strong conviction of their common humanity and right to sustenance and respect. Many nurses are invigorated by the ongoing challenges of helping the neediest of the needy: "They are the sickest people, and I am putting an end to them falling through the cracks." Might this be your mission also?

SUMMARY

To integrate and apply your understanding of urban health care needs, the poor and homeless, and the role of the community health nurse in caring for these clients, consider the information from this chapter.

Urban health issues have existed for hundreds of years in the United States, and they continue today. Deteriorating inner-city neighborhoods and marginal suburbs on the outskirts of large cities evoke feelings of despair and fear for most people not living in these communities. These areas are plagued with crime, violence, disease, injury, unemployment and underemployment, and, above all, poverty. For many disenfranchised and minority groups, inner cities are called home. In some "downtown" areas, upper middle-class people are renovating old buildings and returning to the city, in the process moving out the poor literally to the streets.

Poverty is a disease; it handicaps and disables as surely as an illness. Some people are in such a cycle of poverty that they spin down to homelessness. These clients are in the depths of despair, hopelessness, and helplessness.

Caring for people who are living in poverty takes the most skilled of community health nurses. Nurses should follow these guidelines for practice:

1. Vote for candidates and laws that diminish poverty and diminish suffering of the poor.
2. Advocate for the poor in all community groups of which you are a member.
3. Listen and keep listening to people living in poverty.
4. Consciously develop trusting, respectful relationships with poor people.
5. Based on your search to understand their life circumstances, develop preventive and treatment approaches that are workable.
6. Link poor people with each other and with helping resources.
7. Translate medical and psychiatric information in practical ways that assist the poor to understand themselves and to take charge of their lives.
8. Maintain your own hope and well-being through deliberate self-care.
9. Always consider how you could contribute to community-level or organizational changes that diminish poverty or its hardships.
10. Find meaning that sustains your compassion and nursing effectiveness with every impoverished person you encounter.

ACTIVITIES TO PROMOTE CRITICAL THINKING

1. Check the World Wide Web for the latest U. S. Census Bureau poverty threshold (*http//www.census.gov/hhes/www/poverty.html*). Now, check the costs in your community for the simplest nutritional diet, shelter, clothing, and basic necessities. Create a budget for a subsistence living in your community, and compare it with the most recent poverty threshold established by the government.

2. What is your own family history of poverty? Because poverty is so stigmatized, such a background in your own family may be difficult to acknowledge. Family encounters with poverty may be family secrets.

3. Drive through your own community. Are there places where the tourist books advise visitors never to venture? Are there neighborhoods with unpaved streets and homes slowly falling down on top of the residents, who live in escalating fear of the drug selling of youths on the street? How many children grow up in these places? How many finish high school? How many find work that pays a living wage?

4. Drive through two local communities, one affluent and one impoverished, to evaluate local resources.

5. What do you believe about the worth of individual human beings?

6. Are the poor to blame for their poverty?

7. See Display 32–1. What sorts of social, educational, and economic assistance programs would make it possible for Tommy to become employed at a living wage? Are there limits to his potential for self-sufficiency? What is society's responsibility?

8. Why do you think our nation emphasizes policing and punishment of drug trafficking instead of prevention and treatment of drug use? What do you believe, and how does this affect your nursing care?

9. Do you believe that shelter and food are basic human rights?

10. Go sit in the waiting room of your nearest public clinic. Notice how people are addressed as they wait, are processed through various clerks, and are finally seen. Try seeking help for one of your own health problems in such an environment. What have you learned?

11. You may have come to believe many of the negative stereotypes about poor people. How have your judgments been shaped? How can you open yourself to caring for those from whom most of society turns away?

REFERENCES

Amarasingham, R., Spalding, S.H., & Anderson, R.J. (2001). Disease conditions most frequently evaluated among the homeless in Dallas. *Journal of Health Care for the Poor and Underserved, 12*(2), 162–176.

Amaro, H. (1999). An expensive policy: The impact of inadequate funding for substance abuse treatment. *American Journal of Public Health, 89*(5), 657–659.

AmeriStat. (2000, February). *The rich, the poor, and the in-between.* Retrieved February 12, 2004, from *http://www.ameristat.org/*

Antai-Otong, D. (2002). Culturally sensitive treatment of African Americans with substance-related disorders. *Journal of Psychosocial Nursing and Mental Health Services, 40*(7), 14–21.

Bamberger, J.D., Unick, J., Klein, P., Fraser, M., Chesney, M., & Katz, M.H. (2000). Helping the urban poor stay with antiretroviral HIV drug therapy. *American Journal of Public Health, 90*(5), 699–701.

Barrow, S., Herman, D., Cordova, P., & Struening, E. (1999). Mortality among homeless shelter residents in New York City. *American Journal of Public Health, 89*(4), 529–533.

Bashir, S.A. (2002). Home is where the harm is: Inadequate housing as a public health crisis. *American Journal of Public Health, 92*(5), 733–738.

Bolland, J.M., & McCallum, D.M. (2002). Touched by homelessness: An examination of hospitality for the down and out. *American Journal of Public Health, 92*(1), 116–118.

Carney, P. (1992). The concept of poverty. *Public Health Nursing, 9*(2), 74–80.

Caton, C.L.M., Hasin, D., Shrout, P.E., Opler, L.A., Hirshfield, S., Dominguez, B., et al. (2000). Risk factors for homelessness among indigent urban adults with no history of psychotic illness: A case-control study. *American Journal of Public Health, 90*(2), 258–263.

Chavkin, W. (1999). What's a mother to do? Welfare, work, and family. *American Journal of Public Health, 89*(4), 477–478.

Couto, R. A. (2000). Community health as social justice: Lessons on leadership. *Family and Community Health, 23*(1), 1–17.

Craft-Rosenberg, M., Powell, S.R., & Culp, K. (2000). Health status and resources of rural homeless women and children. *Western Journal of Nursing Research, 22*(8), 863–878.

Crossette, B. (1999, August 5). In days, India, chasing China, will have a billion people. *New York Times,* p. A10.

Fee, E., Brown, T.M., Lazarus, J., & Theerman, P. (2001).

Immigrant mother and child: Chicago, 1910. *American Journal of Public Health, 91*(11), 1764.

Fergerson, G. (2001). Culture, class, and service delivery: The politics of welfare reform and an urban bioethics agenda. *Journal of Urban Health: Bulletin of the New York Academy of Medicine, 78*(1), 81–87.

Freudenberg. N. (2000). Time for a national agenda to improve the health of urban populations. *American Journal of Public Health, 90*(6), 837–840.

Ganz, M.L. (2000). The relationship between external threats and smoking in Central Harlem. *American Journal of Public Health, 90*(3), 367–371.

Heymann, S., & Earle, A. (1999). The impact of welfare reform on parents' ablity to care for their children's health. *American Journal of Public Health, 89*(4), 502–505.

Hilfiker, D. (1994). *Not all of us are saints: A doctor's journey with the poor*. New York: Ballantine Books.

House, J.S., Lepkowski, J.M, Williams, D.R., Mero, R.P., Lantz, P.M., Robert, S. A., et al. (2000). Excess mortality among urban residents: How much, for whom, and why? *American Journal of Public Health, 90*(12), 1898–1904.

Kilborn, P. (1999, May 31). Disabled spouses increasingly face a life alone and loss of income. N*ew York Times,* p. A8.

Lantz, P., House, J., Lepkowski, J., Williams, D., Mero, R., & Chen, J. (1998). Socioeconomic factors, health behaviors, and mortality. *Journal of the American Medical Association, 279*(21), 1703–1708.

Levine, R.S., Foster, J.E., Fullilove, R.E., Fullilove, M.T., Briggs, N.C., Hull, P.C., et al. (2001). Black-white inequalities in mortality and life expectancy, 1933–1999: Implications for *Healthy People 2010*. *Public Health Reports, 116*(5), 474–483.

Link, B., Phelan, J., Bresnahnm, M., Steuve, A., Moore, R., & Susser, E. (1995). Lifetime and five-year prevalence of homelessness in the United States: New evidence on an old debate. *American Journal of Orthopsychiatry, 65*, 347–354.

Managed care cost pressures threaten access for the uninsured. (1999, March). *Findings from Health System Change, 19,* 1–6.

Olds, D.L., Henderson, C.R. Jr., Kitzman, H.J., et al. (1999). Prenatal and infancy home visitation by nurses: Recent findings. *The Future of Children, 9*(1), 44–65.

O'Toole, T.P., Gibbon, J.L., Seltzer, D., Hanusa, B.H., & Fine, J. (2002). Urban homelessness and poverty during economic prosperity and welfare reform: Changes in self-reported comorbidities, insurance, and sources for usual care, 1995–1997. *Journal of Urban Health: Bulletin of the New York Academy of Medicine 79*(2), 200–210.

Pear, R. (1999, May 14). Study links Medicaid drop to welfare changes. *New York Times,* p. A18.

Phillips, J. & Grady, P.A. (2002). Reducing health disparities in the twenty-first century: Opportunities for nursing research. *Nursing Outlook, 50*(3), 117–120.

Pittman, K.P., Wold, J.L., Wilson, A., Huff, C., & Williams, S. (2000). Community connections: Promoting family health. *Family and Community Health, 23*(2), 72–78.

Potula, V., Hegarty-Steck, M., & Hu, H. (2001). Blood lead levels in relation to paint and dust lead levels: The lead-safe Cambridge Program. *American Journal of Public Health, 91*(12), 1973–1974.

Rank, M., & Hirschl, T. (1999). The likelihood of poverty across the American adult life span. *Social Work, 44*(3), 201–214.

Rew, L., Chambers, K.B., & Kulkarni, S. (2002). Planning a sexual health promotion intervention with homeless adolescents. *Nursing Research, 51*(3), 168–174.

Rosenheck, R. (2000). Cost-effetiveness of services for mentally ill homeless people: The application of research to policy and practice. *American Journal of Psychiatry, 157*(10), 1563–1570.

Satcher, D. (2000). Eliminating racial and ethnic disparities in health: The role of the ten leading health indicators. *Journal of the National Medical Association, 92*(6), 315–318.

Schulman, K., Berlin, J., Harless, W., Kerner, J., Sistrunk, S., Gersh, B., et al. (1999). The effect of race and sex on physicians' recommendations for cardiac catheterization. *The New England Journal of Medicine, 340*(8), 618–626.

Smith-Campbell, B. (2000). Access to health care: Effects of public funding on the uninsured. *Journal of Nursing Scholarship, 32*(3), 295–300.

Strehlow, A.J., & Amos-Jones, T. (1999). The homeless as a vulnerable population. *Nursing Clinics of North America, 34*(2), 261–274.

Synoground, G., & Bruya, M.A. (2000). Meeting the health needs of homeless or low-income persons: Role of the nurse practitioner. *Clinical Excellence for Nurse Practitioners, 4*(3), 138–144.

United Nations Development Programmes. (1998). *UNDP poverty report 1998: Overcoming human poverty*. New York: United Nations.

United States Bureau of the Census. (1998). *Current population reports: Poverty in the United States*—1997 (Series P60–201). Washington, DC: U. S. Government Printing Office.

United States Bureau of the Census. (2003). Retrieved on 4/7/04 from *http://www.census.gov/hhes/www/income.html*

United States Bureau of the Census. (2004). Poverty guidelines and poverty thresholds. Retrieved on 4/7/04 from *http://www.ssc.wisc.edu/irp/faqs/faql.htm*

Wald, L. (1971/1915). *The house on Henry Street*. New York: Dover Publications. (Originally published by Henry Hold and Co., New York).

Wells, K., Klap, R., Koike, A., & Sherbourne, C. (2001). Ethnic disparities in unmet need for alcoholism, drug abuse, and mental health care. *American Journal of Psychiatry, 158,* 2027–2032.

Westphal, D. (2002, June 6). Moms on welfare drops 50% in 1990s. *The Fresno Bee,* p. A2.

Williams, D.R., & Collins, C. (2001). Racial residential segregation: A fundamental cause of racial disparities in health. *Public Health Reports, 116*(5), 404–416.

Zerwekh, J.V. (2000). Caring on the ragged edge: Nursing persons who are disenfranchised. *Advances in Nursing Science, 22*(4), 47–61.

SELECTED READINGS

Abernathy, T.J., Webster, G., & Vermeulen, M. (2002). Relationship between poverty and health among adolescents. *Adolescence, 37*(145), 55–67.

Abraham, L.K. (1993). *Mama might be better off dead: The failure of health care in urban America*. Chicago: University of Chicago.

Anderson, J.A. (2001). Understanding homeless adults by testing the theory of self-care. *Nursing Science Quarterly, 14*(1), 59–67.

Andrulis, D.P. (2000). Community, service, and policy strategies to improve health care access in the changing urban environment. *American Journal of Public Health, 90*(6), 858–862.

Beech, B.M., Myers, L., & Beech, D.J. (2002). Hepatitis B and C infections among homeless adolescents. *Family Community Health, 25*(2), 28–36.

Beiser, M., Hou, F., Hyman, I, & Tousignant, M. (2002). Poverty, family process, and the mental health of immigrant children in Canada. *American Journal of Public Health, 92*(2), 220–227.

Bustos, P., Amigo, H., Munoz, S.R., & Martorell, R. (2001). Growth in indigenous and nonindigenous Chilean schoolchildren from three poverty strata. *American Journal of Public Health, 91*(10), 1645–1649.

Greenspan, B. (2001). Health disparities and the US health care system. *Public Health Reports, 116*(5), 417–418.

Harrington, M. (1962). *The other America: Poverty in the United States.* Baltimore: Penguin.

Hunter, J.K., Ventura, M.R., & Kearns, P.A. (1999). Cost analysis of a nursing center for the homeless. *Nursing Economics, 17*(1), 20–28.

Kushel, M.B., Vittinghoff, E., & Haas, J.S. (2001). Factors associated with the health care utilization of homeless persons. *Journal of the American Medical Association, 285*(2), 200–206.

Leviton, L.C., Snell, E., & McGinnis, M. (2000). Urban issues in health promotion strategies. *American Journal of Public Health, 90*(6), 863–866.

Marks, S.M., Taylor, Z., Burrows, N.R., Qayad, M.G., & Miller, B. (2000). Hospitalization of homeless persons with tuberculosis in the United States. *American Journal of Public Health, 90*(3), 435–438.

Merzel, C. (2000). Gender differences in health care access indicators in an urban, low-income community. *American Journal of Public Health, 90*(6), 909–916.

Pratt, C.N.U., Paone, D., Carter, R.J., & Layton, M.C. (2002). Hepatitis C screening and management practices: A survey of drug treatment and syringe exchange programs in New York City. *American Journal of Pubilc Health, 92*(8), 1254–1256.

Skinner, C.S., Arfken, C.L., & Waterman, B. (2000). Outcomes of the learn, share & live breast cancer education program for older urban women. *American Journal of Public Health, 90*(8), 1229–1234.

Warnes, A.M., & Crane, M.A. (2000). The achievements of a multiservice project for older homeless people. *The Gerontologist, 40*(5), 618–626.

Zabos, G.P., Northridge, M.W., Ro, M.J., Trinh, C., Vaughan, R., Howard, J.M., et al. (2002). Lack of oral health care for adults in Harlem: A hidden crisis. *American Journal of Public Health, 92*(1), 49–52.

Internet Resources

Environmental Protection Agency Information Center: *http://www.epa.gov*

National Public Health Information Coalition: *http://www.nphic.org*

National Center for Health Statistics (NCHS): *http://www.cdc.gov/nchs/*

National Clearinghouse on Families and Youth (NCFY): *http://www.ncfy.com*

Office of Minority Health Resource Center: *http://www.omhrc.gov*

Office of National Drug Control Policy Clearinghouse on Drugs and Crime: *http://www.whitehousedrugpolicy.gov*

The Community Environmental Health Resource Center (CEHRC): *http://www.cehrc.org*

U. S. Population Information (Population Reference Bureau): *http://www.ameristat.org*

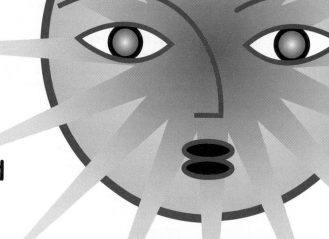

33

Migrant Families and Seasonal Workers

Key Terms

- Camp health aide
- Crew leader
- Cultural brokering
- Curanderas
- Familialism
- Homebase
- Lay workers
- Machismo
- Migrant farmworker
- Migrant health program
- Migrant streams
- Outreach
- Patterns of migration
- Personalismo
- Seasonal farmworker
- Simpatica

Learning Objectives

Upon mastery of this chapter, you should be able to:

- Discuss the historical background of migrant workers including their demographics and patterns.
- Describe the migrant lifestyle.
- Explain how hazardous living and working conditions contribute to migrant workers' increased risk for health problems.
- Identify at least three health problems common to migrant workers and their families.
- Describe social issues resulting from the migrant lifestyle.
- Discuss barriers and challenges to migrant health care.
- Identify methods for effective health care delivery to migrant populations.
- Discuss goals and implications for effective health care delivery to migrant populations.

Y ou may never have seen migrant workers, yet you are a direct beneficiary of their labor. Have you ever thought about the people who harvest the fruits and vegetables that you eat? Have you ever thought about exactly who these people are, where they come from, where they live, or what their health is like? This chapter addresses these questions, but you will probably come away with many new questions and concerns as you explore migrant health issues in community health nursing.

Migrant farmworkers are an integral part of the farming community in the United States. The agricultural industry relies heavily on migrant workers to harvest the almost endless array of fresh, frozen, and canned fruits and vegetables that mark the United States as a country of plentiful harvests. Almost 5 million migrant farmworkers are employed in the United States, and they harvest more than half of the produce in many communities.

Despite their importance to American agriculture, migrant workers are rarely visible beyond the fringes of the camps and farms to which they travel to pursue their livelihood. Most come to the United States from Mexico and other underdeveloped countries with the hope of improving their impoverished lives. Some are legal residents, whereas others are undocumented and live in fear of deportation. All endure backbreaking, menial labor for low wages and are often deprived of basic rights to safe working conditions, adequate sanitation, decent housing, quality education for their childre, and health care.

Because they are concerned with the health needs of underserved populations at risk, community health nurses are the prime implementers of health care to migrant workers and their families. Primarily, nurses who work with migrant communities try to simultaneously reduce their high incidence of disease and increase their low access to health care. By creating options for this vulnerable aggregate and helping them reach beyond their often abysmal conditions, community health nurses also promote social justice.

MIGRANT FARMWORKERS: PROFILE OF A NOMADIC AGGREGATE

Maintaining a low public profile, migrant workers are, for the most part, marginalized from mainstream society. They remain unseen, unheard, poorly understood, and excluded from many programs that provide health care assistance for low-income people. The migrant worker is a kind of disenfranchised citizen, for whom no one wants to take responsibility. Yet the needs of these workers are great. They are plagued with different, more complex, and more frequent health problems than the general population (McCarthy, 2000). Their demographics, socioeconomic conditions, and lifestyle resemble those of a Third World country despite the fact that they live and work in one of the most prosperous countries on earth. Some of their most common problems are

poverty, malnutrition, infectious and parasitic diseases, limited education, hazardous working conditions, and unsafe housing. Although migrant families are in dire need of health resources, economic, cultural, and language barriers prevent this aggregate from accessing available health services. According to the National Advisory Council on Migrant Health, fewer than 20% of migrant farmworkers use available health services (Hawkins, 2001). This astounding fact makes it essential to understand the history, demographics, environment, culture, and health care needs of the migrant worker.

Historical Background

Both historically and internationally, farmers have rarely been able to employ permanently the large workforces needed to harvest their crops. Through the 19th century, however, the small, family-owned farms typical in the United States got through the harvest by using schoolchildren, neighbors, and local day laborers. However, during the Great Depression many of these small, independently run farms went bankrupt. Within a few years, the outbreak of World War II caused an increased need for food production. To keep abreast of the demand for produce, the surviving, larger farms turned to migrant labor for help. The Bracero Agreement of 1942 enabled Mexicans to enter the United States for up to 6 months to provide agricultural assistance to farmers. The goals of the Bracero Agreement were to contract for Mexicans who would leave as soon as the harvesting season was over, to prevent Mexican workers from displacing American workers, and to provide for transportation and living expenses. Between 1951 and 1964, more than 400,000 Mexicans were brought to the United States annually. The Bracero Agreement lasted more than 20 years and established a large core of Mexican migrant workers. Despite the Bracero Agreement, however, many employers, wanting to save time and expenses, started importing immigrants across the border illegally. Living apart from society, the plight of migrant farmworkers was largely ignored until exposure on a television documentary created a national outcry. This led to the passage of the Migrant Health Act of 1962, which addressed the health needs of migrant workers for the first time in U. S. history.

The Migrant Health Act authorized delivery of primary and supplementary health services to migrant farmworkers. Federally funded migrant health clinics serve areas in the United States where there are significant numbers of migrant farmworkers. Staffing usually includes doctors, nurses, outreach workers, social workers, and health educators. An important source of health care for migrant workers, the federally funded clinics also receive monetary help from more than 100 organizations. They provide health care services throughout more than 400 clinic sites (Fig. 33–1). However, funding is often insufficient, and many clinics are not sufficiently staffed or operated to meet the health needs of migrant farmworkers and their dependents. Additionally, although these clinics exist throughout the United States, there

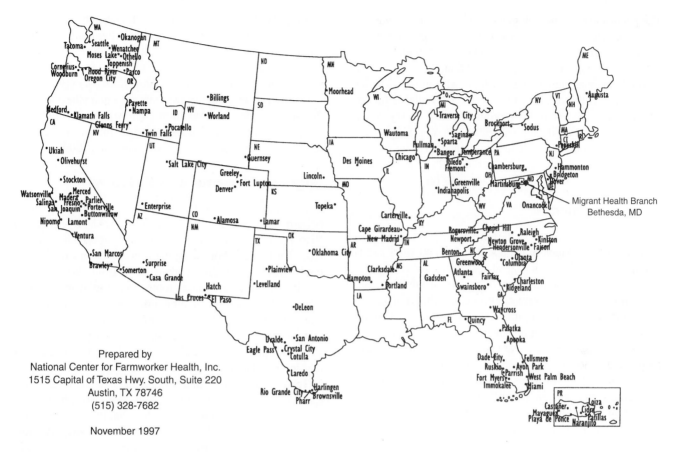

FIGURE 33-1.   Health centers serving migrant and seasonal farmworkers.

are large geographic regions that are not being served well or at all. Migrant workers in these areas must rely on local health departments and emergency departments or go without health care at all. These facts may explain why migrant health clinics have struggled to provide care for more than 40 years. A law passed in 1997 under the Clinton administration, the Children's Health Insurance Program (CHIP), Title XXI of the Social Security Act, insures the nation's 10.6 million uninsured children. Hopefully, CHIP will improve health care access for the almost 1 million migrant children who move from field to field and state to state with their parents to harvest the crops (Health Resources and Services Administration [HRSA], 1998).

Migrant Hero

An outstanding migrant hero, Cesar Chavez, was born near Yuma, Arizona, on March 31, 1927 and died on April 23, 1993. Chavez founded the National Farm Workers Association (NFWA)—whose name was later changed to United Farm Workers (UFW)—the first union in agricultural labor history to successfully organize migrant farmworkers. He spent his life fighting for social justice, "La Causa," and his tireless commitment inspired people to join the movement for social change. He traveled with his family to harvest crops, but they rarely had enough food to eat and lived in shacks. Work was often scarce, wages were low, and labor contractors cheated the family out of the money they earned. Moving to California during the Great Depression, the family became part of the migrant community. Chavez attended as many as 65 different schools, and after completing eighth grade, he dropped out of school to help support his family by working full-time in the fields. As a young man he served in the Navy during World War II, married in 1948, and continued migrant work. His experiences as a migrant worker deeply affected him and later motivated him to devote his life to organizing farmworkers.

In early 1972, Chavez successfully organized the UFW, whose membership now numbers 100,000, to campaign against antilabor legislation in California, Oregon, Arizona, and Florida. In 1975, the Agricultural Labor Relations Act was passed, guaranteeing farmworkers secret ballots in union elections. Chavez organized many successful strikes and boycotts, the most famous one being the boycott of California grapes against the indiscriminate use of pesticides by growers, which lasted for longer than 5 years. In 1968 and again in 1988, he fasted as a protest against the use of agricultural pesticides. His efforts united people who, as individuals, had no significance in the power structure. His legacy is an example of how people build power together.

The persistent commitment that Chavez had for the cause of social change serves as an example to all people. He never owned a home or a car and never made more than $6000 a year (Sahlman & Strandberg, 2003). Throughout his life, he ignored personal hardships to struggle with union victories and losses. As he so eloquently expressed, "Fighting for social justice . . . is one of the profoundest ways to say yes to human dignity." California recognizes Chavez with a state holiday each March 31st. Schoolchildren learn of his efforts, and in several central California communities streets have been renamed for Chavez. His legacy lives on.

Demographics

Comprehensive, national studies on the migrant population need to be done. Much of the research from 40 years ago is out of date, and there is a general agreement that census figures are not reliable indicators of the actual numbers. Because migrant farmworkers constitute a mobile population with shifting composition, it is difficult to know their numbers precisely or to determine their origins. Estimates of the number of migrant workers vary also because of the influx of illegal and undocumented workers. Most of the estimated 5 million migrant farmworkers tend to be either newly arrived immigrants with few connections or established legal residents with limited opportunities and skills who rely on farm labor for survival. The majority of migrant and seasonal farmworkers (70%) were born outside the United States, mostly in Mexico (90%) and central America, and many speak little English (Alderete et al., 2000; Coughlin & Wilson, 2002). Most of the migrant workers are young. Two-thirds are younger than 35 years of age; 7% of farmworkers are adolescents, and some are even younger. In addition, many mothers bring infants and young children to work with them, and the children spend their days strapped to their mother or playing among the pesticide-laden fields (Alderete et al., 2000; McCauley et al., 2002). Some are U. S. citizens; although they are predominantly Hispanic Mexicans, many are African-American, Haitian, Creole, Native American, or Asian. The pool of farmworkers is increasingly diverse in California, with people coming from Latin American and Asia, such as the Hmong from Southeast Asia, the Mixtec and Zapotec from Mexico, and the Maya from Guatemala (Alderete et al., 2000). No one can accurately count immigrants who cross the Mexican border every day, yet as many as one fourth of the migrant population may be unauthorized to work in the United States.

Farmworkers are defined as having income derived primarily from work in the agricultural industry. **Seasonal farmworkers** live in one geographic location and labor in the fields of that particular area, whereas **migrant farmworkers** travel to find agricultural work throughout the year, usually from state to state. Some live apart from their families, forming groups of single men; others travel with their entire families. The average migrant farmworker spends from June to September doing seasonal harvesting, with about 8 weeks on the road traveling from farm to farm for work, and is then un-

employed unless nonagricultural work such as hauling or canning is found (Sandhaus, 1998). Agricultural labor requirements vary greatly in the various phases of planting, cultivating, harvesting, and processing. This labor is crucial to the production of a large variety of crops in almost every state of our nation, yet migrant farmworkers are among the poorest of the working poor. Income for migrant workers is well below the poverty line. The median personal income is between $2500 and $5000 in the U. S. (Alderete et al., 2000).

Migrant Streams and Patterns

Migrant farmworkers usually have their permanent residence, or **homebase**, in California, Texas, Florida, Mexico, or Puerto Rico. From their homebase, they mobilize as each new crop is ready for harvest. Following the harvest seasons of agricultural crops, migrant farmworkers move from place to place, usually along predetermined routes called **migrant streams** (Fig. 33–2). Most migrant farmworkers are multigenerational; that is, their families have been farmworkers for several generations, traveling the same streams for many years.

Three principal streams formulate the agricultural routes that migrant laborers follow. The *eastern stream* originates in Texas, Puerto Rico, and Florida and extends up the East Coast to states east of the Mississippi as far as northern New York. Although predominantly Mexican, this stream is ethnically diverse, including African-Americans, Anglos, Haitians, and Jamaicans. The *midwestern stream* begins in Texas and reaches across the southwestern and midwestern states, going north to the states bordering Canada and both east and west of the Mississippi. The *western stream*, the largest of the three, originates in California and Arizona and moves up the West Coast to all western states. Mexicans, Native Americans, and Southeast Asians follow the midwestern and western streams.

Weather conditions and employment opportunities affect movement and patterns of migration. Because of the unpredictable nature of farm work, the three streams are not clearly delineated, pointing to more complex patterns of movement. In addition to the migrant streams, **patterns of migration** exist, with varying lengths of stay. In a *restricted circuit,* many people travel throughout a season within a small geographic area. *Point-to-point migration* entails leaving a homebase for part of the year to travel to the same place or series of places along a route during the agricultural season. *Nomadic* migrant workers travel away from home for several years, working from farm to farm and crop to crop, relying on word of mouth about job opportunities. Some of these workers eventually settle in the areas to which they have migrated, whereas others return to their homebase. A given ethnic group usually follows its own particular stream and pattern of migration.

Migrant Lifestyle

To understand the health needs of migrant farmworkers and their families, it is important to understand their lifestyle. Mi-

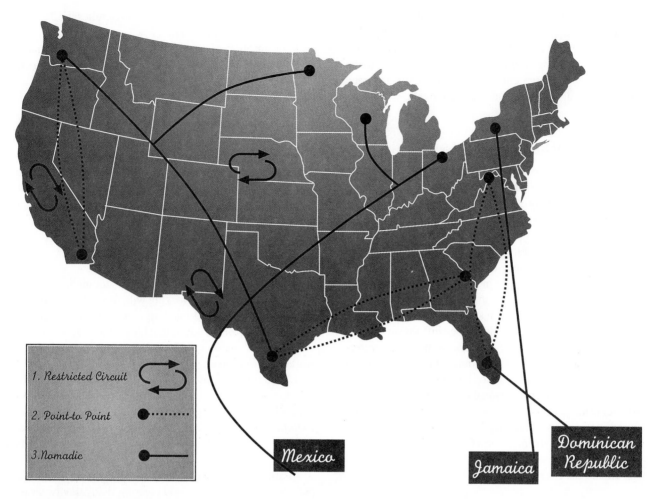

FIGURE 33–2.   Migrant patterns. (From the Migrant Clinicians Network Monograph Series. [1998]. The TB Net System.)

grant workers and their families endure a transient and uncertain life, with long hours, stressful working conditions, low wages, and poor health care. Substandard housing, unsafe working conditions, and language difficulties make life even more difficult.

Migrant workers must confront the vagaries of an unpredictable world. Migrants typically remain in an area for only 6 to 8 weeks, working the fields 6 days a week from sunrise to sunset. Depending on weather and crop conditions, work may be plentiful one week and virtually gone the next. Because yearly income must be earned during the harvest season, all family members contribute to harvesting. Children are essential to the core group's economy and must help in the fields and at home. Migrant laborers learn about employment opportunities from recruiters and crew leaders and from other migrants. Interestingly, there are towns in Mexico where the majority of the people migrate each year. Migrant laborers who travel in crews, or groups, use a **crew leader**, who acts as the mediator between themselves and the farmer. The farmer usually pays the crew leader, who, in turn, pays the workers. An unscrupulous crew leader could withhold payment and keep the migrant workers in constant debt.

Entry into the migrant camps is contingent on the approval of the farmer and crew leader. Crew leaders often organize their crews at the beginning of a season and then transport them throughout the stream. Usually, crew leaders and crews remain the same year after year. It is not uncommon for an entire crew to be composed of a family of uncles, aunts, cousins, and siblings traveling together.

Migrant workers often drive night and day as they move from crop to crop. Typically, they travel with their children and only their most essential possessions, in aging cars, vans, and trucks. Occasionally, van loads of "solos," or single men, migrate together. Their status is even more precarious, because they lack family support systems.

Depending on the economy and the crop, a migrant farmworker may earn as little as 40 cents per 5-gallon bushel of harvested crops. At that rate, a worker can earn up to $100 on a good day, but rain, poor harvest, injury, and disease make the average earnings only $30 to $60, causing annual income to fall below the poverty level (National Center for Farmworker Health [NCFH], 2003). Men, women, and older children all work in the fields. Because inexpensive child care is often unavailable, mothers often leave very young children alone playing in fields exposed to sun, chemicals, and dangerous machinery. Sometimes children are brought to the fields and left in cars or in cardboard boxes. Often a teenage girl or the mother of an infant remains in the camps to babysit all the children; she is usually stranded there, because all available cars are used to take workers to the fields.

Recent Population Changes

Although there is little evidence to suggests that the total number of migrant farmworkers has changed significantly in recent years, two important changes have occurred in this population. The first major change is the declining number of migrant workers traveling independently in organized work crews. Instead, family units now predominate. As a result, the number of women, young children, and infants exposed to the stress of migrant life has increased.

A second major change is in the increased number of Hispanics, particularly Mexicans, in the midwestern and western states. This change reflects the shift toward family working units, with Mexican farmworkers showing a preference for traveling in family units. Migrant farmworkers from Mexico typically have low rates of literacy and often accept employment regardless of personal cost to health. Although most Mexicans tend to resettle in the Southwest, many are now settling in areas where they were not found in previous years, such as Pennsylvania, North Carolina, and Minnesota. Work crews composed mostly of African-Americans still dominate the eastern stream.

HEALTH RISKS OF MIGRANT WORKERS AND THEIR FAMILIES

A community with varied and profound health needs complicated by disease and social isolation, migrant farmworkers and their families are at risk. Because seasonal earnings must last the entire year, the migrant farmworker avoids or delays seeking health care until illness becomes debilitating. When work is primary, health is eclipsed (Sandhaus, 1998). Migrant farmworkers and their families suffer illnesses caused by poor nutrition, lack of resources to seek care early in the disease process, and infectious diseases resulting from overcrowding and poor sanitation. Keep in mind these shocking health statistics (NCFH, 2003):

- The life expectancy of a migrant worker is 49 years, compared with 73 years for the general population.
- The migrant infant mortality rate is 125% higher than the national average.
- The death rate from flu and pneumonia is 20% higher than the national average.
- The rate of parasitic infection is estimated to be 11 to 59 times higher than that of the general population.
- The death rate from tuberculosis (TB) and other communicable diseases is 25 times higher than the national average.

- The hospitalization rate of migrant families is 50% higher than the national average.
- Poor nutrition often results in infant deaths, anemia, extreme dental problems, vision problems, and poor mental and physical development of children.

Occupational Hazards

The hazards of agricultural employment, coupled with limited legal protection, jeopardize the health of the migrant farmworker. Agricultural work surpasses mining and construction as the most hazardous occupation in the United States, with more deaths occurring among agricultural workers than in other occupations (Table 33–1) (U. S. Department of Health and Human Services, 2000). Frequent falls, cuts, muscle strains, and repetitive motion injuries (eg, carpal tunnel syndrome) afflict migrant laborers.

Agricultural work often requires stooping, long hours working in wet clothes, working with the soil, climbing, carrying heavy loads, and touching plants. Failure to perform these activities on a rigid timetable dictated by seasons and weather can result in crop loss. This urgency compels farmworkers to work in all weather conditions, including extreme heat, cold, rain, bright sun, and damp. Some plants, such as tobacco and strawberries, emit toxic chemicals that cause severe allergic reactions (See Research: Bridge to Practice). Extreme cold causes frostbite; overexposure to the sun creates heat stroke, which occurs almost four times as often among farmworkers as in the general population.

Farmworkers spend much of their time on their feet, picking crops, irrigating, and clearing fields. Footwear usually is not adequate, and foot problems are often ignored until walking becomes painful, because the migrant worker cannot afford the time off from work or the treatment expenses. Minor injuries usually receive superficial treatment in the field, from coworkers or from the crew chief. Non-emergencies and chronic health conditions merit minimal attention. Leaving work means loss of pay, because farmers are not required to pay health insurance or Workers' Com-

TABLE 33–1

Deaths from Work-Related Injury—*Healthy People 2010* (Deaths per 100,000 Workers Aged 16 Years and Older)

Work Area	Baseline	2010 Target
All industry	4.5	3.2
Agriculture, forestry, and fishing	24.1	16.9
Mining	23.6	16.5
Construction	14.6	10.2
Transportation	11.8	8.3

From U. S. Department of Health and Human Services. (2000). *Healthy People 2010)* (Conference ed., Vols. 1 & 2. Washington, DC. Author.

RESEARCH: BRIDGE TO PRACTICE

Quandt, R.P., & Arcury, T.A. (2002). Hispanic farm-worker interpretations of green tobacco sickness. *Journal of Rural Health, 18*(4), 503–511.

In this study, the researchers explored green tobacco sickness (GTS) in migrant and seasonal farmworkers in North Carolina. The workers use an explanatory model, which is compared with the research-based biobehavioral model. GTS is a form of acute nicotine poisoning that affects those who work in wet tobacco fields. This condition is characterized by anorexia, nausea, vomiting, headache, dizziness, and insomnia. There are no standard diagnostic criteria for GTS; clinicians base the diagnosis on a combination of symptoms and exposure risk. GTS resembles pesticide poisoning, but the treatment is quite different.

Many farmworkers today are Spanish-speaking immigrants from Mexico with limited experience in tobacco fields. This study involved in-depth interviews with 23

Hispanic farmworkers in central North Carolina, whose understanding of the problem of GTS was explored.

The workers generally attributed the symptoms to other aspects of working in tobacco, such as pesticides or heat, rather than nicotine. They cited many of the same risk factors identified in the biobehavioral model, such as wet working conditions and inexperience with the work required in tobacco fields.

Prevention and treatment include a combination of exposure avoidance and common medications. The symptoms of most importance to the farmworkers were insomnia and anorexia, both of which impaired the ability to work, jeopardizing their income as well as their work security.

Community health nurses and other health care workers can benefit by understanding the explanatory model held by farmworkers. They can be more effective in managing (teaching, diagnosing, and treating) GTS. The goal is to prevent future episodes.

pensation, although migrant workers are entitled to these benefits (NCFH, 2003).

Few states impose the minimum age of 16 years for field labor outside of school hours. Because migrant workers are paid on a piecework basis, the contribution of each member, including young children, is significant income. Taken out of school to work in the fields, children are at great risk for accidents and pesticide and sun exposure (McCauley et al., 2002). Beyond physical injury, children are at risk for school failure that is compounded by mobility and poverty.

Pesticide Exposure

Migrant farmworkers are at greater risk for pesticide poisoning when fields are sprayed or at initial reentry into the field. Many migrant camps are located within large open fields or on the periphery. Overhead pesticide sprayings then endanger not only those at work in the fields but also those in the camp. One study of migrant children found that 48% worked in fields still wet with pesticides, 36% were sprayed with chemicals directly or indirectly, and 34% were sprayed in the process of spraying nearby fields (HRSA, 2004).

Pesticide exposure produces higher rates of miscarriages, birth defects, upper respiratory tract infections, visual problems, excessive thirst, sweating, and tremors. Skin reactions include rashes, welts, excoriations on the arms, facial swelling, and intense itching. Severe cases can result in blindness or death. Pesticide burns and rashes often go untreated because of lack of education about the dangers of pesticides and lack of available services. Migrant workers are often unaware of the hazards of pesticides. A study among

adolescent Latino farmworkers found that 64.7% were traveling and working in the United States independent of their parents, and few reported having received pesticide training; however, 21.6% of the sample reported that their current work involved mixing or applying agricultural chemicals (McCauley et al., 2002). Farmers do not always comply with the law to post Environmental Protection Agency (EPA) warnings of pesticide safety and dangers in the migrant camps and in the fields. Gloves and long-sleeved shirts are not always supplied or used. The Department of Labor cannot keep up with the reports of violations of safety standards. If a farm is reported, it often is closed down only for a few days; although large fines may be assessed, they are seldom collected (see Clinical Corner).

Contaminated water sources in the field enhance the absorption and spread of pesticides. EPA standards that bar entry to a field for at least 24 hours after a spraying are often ignored. Pesticides can drift from the fields to contaminate food or children playing nearby. Children are at greater risk for pesticide-induced illnesses because of their higher metabolism rate, greater surface absorption, and chronic long-term exposure. The EPA estimates that 300,000 farmworkers suffer pesticide poisoning each year (EPA, 2004). Many cases are unreported because the workers do not seek treatment. In addition, pesticide poisoning is often misdiagnosed, because the symptoms can mimic those of viral infections.

Although the impact of acute pesticide poisoning is widely recognized, little is understood about the long-term effects of the repeated low-level exposures to which migrant farmworkers are constantly subjected. Some farmworkers report long-term allergies and colds that last 2 or 3 years. Al-

CLINICAL CORNER

MIGRANT AND SEASONAL FARMWORKERS

As you looked at your reflection in the mirror this morning, you said to yourself, "It's finally here . . . the day I've been waiting for the past 6 years." You are now a public health nurse working with migrant farmworkers in the maternal–child program of the county health department! You are excited but somewhat anxious. You can hardly believe this moment has arrived. The years of Spanish courses, along with your already challenging nursing coursework, 2 years working on the medical–surgical unit of your local hospital, then resumes, interviews, . . . You've finally made it!

After a brief orientation to your new workplace and introductions to new colleagues, your supervisor hands you a chart. "This is the first client we'll be seeing today," she tells you. "I'd like you to review the record and tell me what you think we ought to do during our home visit today." Okay, here goes!

The record indicates a referral from the family planning clinic after a positive pregnancy test. Your client is Angelica, a 23-year-old, monolingual Spanish-speaking woman who came to this country 5 years ago from El Salvador. Angelica is married to Hector, a 38-year-old migrant farmworker from the same village in El Salvador. They have a 4-year-old daughter, Esperanza.

As you read through Angelica's chart, you note the following significant information:

- Angelica had gestational diabetes with her previous pregnancy. She sought prenatal care at 7 months' gestation after presenting in the emergency room with complaints of dizziness. Esperanza weighed 11 lb 13 oz at birth.
- The family has expressed concerns about the fact that they are "undocumented." They are concerned about deportation, and, although they seem to trust the health department staff, they seem reluctant to use other available services.
- Angelica is at approximately 16 weeks' gestation.

Questions

1. What issues have you identified as priorities for your visit this morning? How do you plan on addressing those issues with the client?

    Your supervisor advises you that the Spanish-speaking community health worker contacted the family yesterday and told them you would be visiting this morning.

    You feel excited and confident as you drive to the family's home.

    The home is a two-room shack in a complex for migrant field workers. After entering the home, you greet Angelica. She advises you that Hector has gone to work but hopes to come home early from working in the field so he may participate in the visit as well. You see Esperanza watching a small television, drinking a bottle of chocolate milk. Angelica invites you to sit on the couch and asks if you'd like a soda.

2. What will you do in the first few minutes of your visit to develop rapport with your client?

    Angelica tells you, "I am glad to have you as my nurse, and I am happy that you came to my home. I don't like going to that doctor's office. They always tell me I weigh too much and that I have to stop eating the food that is good for my baby."

    After several minutes, Hector comes in from working in the fields and says, "Let me wash my hands. I've been spraying 'chemicos' (chemicals) in the field all morning."

3. Considering the information you garnered from the chart, along with the information obtained thus far during the home visit, discuss your plan for the remainder of today's visit. Present ways in which you will implement your plan.

4. What issues will you identify on subsequent visits? How have you prioritized those issues?

5. What issues does this situation elicit for you regarding the following:
    - Fears and anxiety in dealing with this family
    - Lack of immediate resources (supervisor)
    - Building partnerships with families, communities, and area resources

though there are no studies on the long-term effects of pesticide poisoning, some studies reveal multigenerational effects of pesticide exposure among farmworkers and their families. Of significance are the clusters of cancer and birth defects that have been documented in areas of California. Figure 33–3 is an assessment tool, the Assessment of Farmworker Pesticide Exposure form, developed by the Migrant Clinicians Network. It is useful for community health nurses working with migrant and seasonal workers who may be exposed to pesticides.

An arm of the EPA is the Association of Farmworker Opportunity Programs (AFOP), whose goal is to improve the quality of life for migrant and seasonal farmworkers and their families by providing information, education, support, advocacy, and representation at the national level (EPA, 2003). In addition, there are two innovative programs sponsored by the EPA.

The Serving America's Farmworkers Everywhere (SAFE) program enlists bilingual young adults who are dy-

PATIENT ID	Name: _____ DOB: _____ SS#: _____
	Farm: _____ Address: _____
EXPOSURE INFORMATION	Date of exposure: _____ Last time field sprayed: _____
	Name of pesticide: _____ Crop: _____
	Method of pesticide application: ☐ Aerial ☐ Hand spray ☐ Spray rig
	Type of work: ☐ Mixing ☐ Loading ☐ Picking/thinning/pruning crops
	Exposure: ☐ Aerial ☐ Hand spray ☐ Spray rig ☐ Sprayed directly ☐ Drift
	Other workers involved? ☐ Yes ☐ No ☐ Who? _____
	_____
	Had patient received training under the Worker Protection Standard? ☐ Yes ☐ No
SYMPTOMS	☐ Weakness ☐ Drooling ☐ Blurred vision ☐ Chest pain
	☐ Skin rash ☐ Tiredness ☐ Excessive sweating ☐ Red eyes
	☐ Headaches ☐ Nausea ☐ Loss of consciousness ☐ Convulsions
	☐ Shortness of breath ☐ Dizziness ☐ Vomiting ☐ Abdominal pain
	☐ Muscle twitches ☐ Productive cough ☐ Confusion ☐ Other: _____
	How long after exposure did symptoms occur? _____
	Other workers exposed who developed symptoms? ☐ Yes ☐ No
PHYSICAL SIGNS	☐ Hypotension ☐ Bradycardia ☐ Dermatitis ☐ ↓ DTRs
	☐ Confusion ☐ Convulsions ☐ Ataxia ☐ Muscle weakness
	☐ Paralysis ☐ Fasciculations ☐ Constricted pupils ☐ Other: _____
	☐ ↓ Visual accommodation ☐ Sweating ☐ Drooling _____
	☐ Bronchospasm ☐ Bronchial exudation ☐ Red eyes _____
	Cholinesterase testing: Date: _____ Results: _____
	Follow-up test ordered: ☐ Yes ☐ No Date: _____ Results: _____
TREATMENT	Atropine? ☐ Yes ☐ No Dose: _____ Response: _____
	2-PAM? ☐ Yes ☐ No Dose: _____ Response: _____
PROVIDER ID	Provider Signature: _____ Date: _____
	Address: _____ Phone: _____
ABOUT THIS REPORT	The original "Evaluation of Farmworker Pesticide Exposure" was developed by Mark Lyons, MPH, PAC, for the New Jersey Department of Health. This form was adapted by the Migrant Clinicians Network for use in a migrant health center setting and used with permission. This form may be duplicated as needed. For more information, contact MCN at 2512 South IH35, Suite 220, Austin, TX 78704, (512) 447-0770.

FIGURE 33–3. Migrant Clinicians Network evaluation of farmworker pesticide exposure.

namic, creative, and committed to working with migrant workers. They assist farmworkers and their families, teach about pesticide safety, and support the farmworker community. The program operates in coordination with the national AmeriCorps Programs, and the young people make a committment of 3 to 12 months. For this they receive a living allowance and an educational award to be used for college.

The second program is AFOP's Children in the Field Campaign, which is designed to end exploitation of children in agriculture. It has three foci. The government focus is on improving labor laws, regulations, standards, and conditions. It seeks to strengthen enforcement of protections for children working in the fields and to spur EPA-sponsored research to assess agricultural risks to children posed by use of pesticides, farm machinery, and so on. The consumer focus is designed to promote awareness of children working in the fields and its negative impact on their education, health, and safety. The consumer awareness arm of this campaign focuses on having consumers not buy foods for which children are employed in growing and harvesting. The industry focus is on providing incentives to eliminate child labor. Such steps might include providing farmworkers with day care for younger children, and accessible transportation to schools for school-age children, or encouraging farm owners to not hire minors in their fields (EPA, 2004).

Substandard Housing and Poor Sanitation

Agricultural fields are usually located in isolated areas on the outskirts of rural communities. While in these isolated fields, migrant workers often are not provided with sanitation facilities or fresh drinking water. The Occupational Safety and Health Administration (OSHA) mandates field sanitation (1 toilet) and fresh drinking water for farms with 11 workers or more working together within a quarter-mile stretch of field (EPA, 2003). Large corporate farms can, however, simply space workers out and legally avoid this regulation. Furthermore, one in six migrant or seasonal workers works on farms hiring 10 or fewer workers, where toilets and drinking water do not have to be provided.

When housing is available, several families live in one structure. Often 15 or more people share one or two rooms. Typical living quarters include dilapidated housing units, overcrowded barracks, trailers, buses, and sheds. Most have inadequate or absent heating and cooling, poor plumbing, and little privacy. Trailers used as living quarters are often in disrepair, lacking doors, screens, and even windowpanes (Perilla et al., 1998). Numerous pests such as roaches, fleas, snakes, rats, and scorpions invade the trailers and pose health threats to the workers and their families. Moreover, broken beer bottles, cans, intravenous drug needles and paraphernalia, and other trash often litter the living and outdoor spaces. Babies cannot be put down for fear of pests, toddlers are at risk as they explore their environments, and young children are at risk if they play outside (Perilla et al., 1998).

When housing is unavailable, workers and their families live in boxes, cars, garages, or in the fields and orchards where they work. Some migrant workers live at least temporarily without any shelter at all. For example, southern Arizona is a first stop for Mexicans coming into the United States. While looking for work or awaiting transportation to another state, many single men and families live under trees in orange groves. They sleep outside on the ground with no protection from cold, heat, or rain. They drink water from irrigation canals in the field and depend on food that is provided by charitable organizations. Lacking stoves, they often cook meals outside over open fires. Without proper refrigeration, their food spoils quickly.

Available housing often does not meet even minimal standards of adequacy. Many migrant quarters have neither sinks nor toilets. In one migrant camp in Alabama several years ago, workers were living in a converted chicken house (Cole & Crawford, 1991). An upper portion of the wall had been removed for ventilation, creating easy access for insects and birds. A dirt floor, a single light bulb, and two portable toilets located a distance away were some of the other features. Two sinks in a common living area provided the only water for the almost 60 people who lived in the chicken house. Many did not have mattresses, and because the workers were harvesting potatoes, potato baskets conveniently served as the only furniture. Such living situations still exist today.

Licensed and unlicensed field housing is especially likely to have a polluted water source contaminated by pesticides, chemical fertilizers, and organic wastes. Bathing or drinking in this water exposes the migrant worker to harmful chemicals and parasites. Migrant workers are sometimes ignorant of their hazardous conditions, but often they are fearful that if they complain to farmers they will lose their jobs.

COMMON HEALTH PROBLEMS

Health problems among migrant families are largely correlated with poverty, mobility, poor nutrition, neglect, crowded housing, and occupational hazards. Migrant community life is threatened by common denominators that threaten health, such as inaccessibility to medical care, lack of basic hygiene, and ignorance of exposure to environmental hazards. Furthermore, problems with drugs, alcohol, and prostitution erode health and family values. The growing numbers of women and children with different and specific health care needs pose even greater health challenges for community health nurses. The migrant lifestyle also places families at risk for chronic and communicable diseases. Surveys conducted in migrant camps reveal that the health problems most often encountered are nutritional deficiencies, urinary tract infections, diabetes, dental caries, skin infections, and head lice.

The hazards of agricultural work and the crowded, unsanitary living conditions, with frequent migration to new camps, expose migrant farmworkers and their families to many sources of infection and create the opportunity for diseases to spread rapidly. The stressors of living a life in which work is sporadic, with no guarantee of income, affect the entire migrant family. Life is physically and emotionally demanding, often causing high levels of anxiety and depression (Hovey & Magana, 2002). The lack of access to health care services results in a high incidence of preventable diseases, as well as diseases that are almost unheard of in the general population.

Migrant Family Health

Inadequate nutrition affects the health of the entire family. Because migrant farmworkers often cannot afford the fruits and vegetables that they harvest, they buy foods that are cheaper but higher in fat, salt, and processed sugar. These foods exacerbate the hypertension and diabetes already prevalent in Mexican groups. Poor nutrition results in anemia, greater infant mortality and morbidity, and poor physical and mental development in children. In one study, infants were given micronutrient supplements during the first year of life and had greater length gains (8.2 mm) than did the placebo group (Rivera et al., 2001).

Preschool children from Hispanic farmworker families represent a nutritionally vulnerable subset of the pediatric population. Health care providers must be aware of the nutritional risks these children face and the fact that many are not participating in public health supplemental food programs because of the family's migratory status and program funding limitations. Up to one half of migrant preschoolers show clinical signs of vitamin A deficiency, largely attributed to a diet lacking in fruits and vegetables. Vitamin A is essential for normal growth and for maintaining the integrity of the gastrointestinal, pulmonary, immune, and integumentary systems. Deficiencies can lead to conjunctival dryness, blindness, and increased susceptibility to infection (Venes & Thomas, 2001). Unhealthy diets also cause other vitamin deficiencies and obesity in migrant children. Obesity is particularly harmful for the Mexican migrant children who are susceptible to developing hypertension and diabetes. In addition, anemia and upper respiratory tract congestion resulting from a largely milk-based diet are common in migrant children. Sometimes, infants get only milk well beyond the age when solids should be given. Many migrant infants with milk allergies have chronic diarrhea and congestion because medical interventions are not sought and allergies are not recognized.

Because of frequent moves, children of migrant farmworkers receive only fragmented health care. Minor health problems of migrant children are similar to those seen in the general population and include rashes, sprains, upper respiratory tract infections, earaches, diarrhea, urinary tract infections, anemia, headaches, and dizziness (HRSA, 1998). Lack of awareness that a minor symptom such as diarrhea or fever may indicate a more serious underlying problem can cause delays in seeking medical attention. An earache is mi-

nor, but it can lead to a major problem, such as deafness, if left untreated. Deafness is a frequently mentioned major health problem in the migrant population (Kerr, Lusk, & Ronis, 2002).

Although parents of migrant families may seek help for a child's acute viral or bacterial infection, they may stop giving prescribed antibiotics after the child appears to be better, or they may have siblings share the medicine. As a result, infections often recur or develop into chronic, subacute conditions. Because head lice is not considered a serious health threat among migrant families, spending money on treatment is deferred. Both of these situations are seen in many families visited by community health nurses, not just migrant families.

Mexican women tend to marry young and to bear children in their teens. They have higher birth rates and need health care and teaching in the areas of family planning and preconception, prenatal, and pediatric health care—all of which is sorely lacking at this time. Hispanic women are more likely to have several children but are less likely to receive prenatal and postnatal care. Often anemic and with little or no prenatal care because of the constant moving, young mothers bear babies who are also anemic and often underweight. In addition, exposure to pesticides causes birth defects and contamination of breast milk.

Women report frequent urinary tract infections, at a rate almost two to three times higher than the national average, because of the demanding work conditions, dehydration from working in the hot sun, and lack of toilet facilities in the fields. Running water and working toilets are sparsely located in the fields. The toilets are often broken, and repairs are delayed (Perilla et al., 1998). Because migrant farmworkers are paid by the amount of produce harvested, they do not take out time to walk the distances to usable bathrooms. Workers, especially women, either reduce their water intake or wait up to 14 hours before using a toilet (Perilla et al., 1998). Frequent complaints of bladder and kidney problems are the consequence. Overcrowding in the migrant camps further hinders personal hygiene and access to toilets.

Money for treating chronic diseases is limited, and migrant families lack knowledge of and access to helpful health measures. In addition to the poor diets, high levels of stressful living and difficult working conditions exacerbate chronic diseases such as diabetes and hypertension that are common among Hispanic populations. Upper respiratory tract infections, eye problems, depression, anemia, and arthritis are commonly reported illnesses. Knowledge of appropriate skin and foot care is minimal. Spending much of their time on their feet with inadequate shoes picking crops, irrigating, and clearing fields, farmworkers develop painful foot problems. Although suffering skin rashes from exposure to pesticides and plants, migrant workers spend such limited time in one state that it becomes difficult for health care providers to identify the relationship between dermatitis and working conditions. Long-term effects of eye irritations and systemic pesticide poisoning include cancer and neuropsychological problems (see What Do You Think?)

WHAT DO YOU THINK?

On a per person basis, farming contributes roughly 30% more than the national average to occupational injury costs. Direct costs are estimated to be $1.66 billion and indirect costs, $2.93 billion. The costs of farm injuries are on a par with the costs of hepatitis C. This high cost is in sharp contrast to the limited public attention and economic resources devoted to prevention and amelioration of farm injuries. Agricultural occupational injuries are an under appreciated contributor to the overall national burden of health and medical costs.

Leigh, J.P., McCurdy, S.A., & Schenker, M.B. (2001). Costs of occupational injuries in agriculture. *Public Health Reports, 116*(3), 235.

Dental Problems

Dental problems are epidemic in the migrant population, yet dental care has very low priority among migrant families. Dental problems often are not assessed or treated. Obtaining oral health care is very difficult in migrant clinics, with waiting periods of up to 6 months for an appointment. Many migrant children are never screened for dental problems. Studies cite dental caries as the most common chronic disease of childhood (U. S. Department of Health and Human Services, 2000). Many adult migrant and seasonal workers have missing and decayed teeth and gingivitis. Migrant families seek to have teeth extracted when they become painful; little consideration is given to dental repair or restoration.

"Baby-bottle" syndrome, in which toddlers' teeth are rotted to the gum lines, frequently occurs when they are allowed to sleep with sweetened liquids in their bottles. Although refined sugars and soft drinks are not part of the traditional Mexican diet, migrant families frequently resort to low in nutritional value, convenience foods in the migratory lifestyle.

Many migrant families do not even own a toothbrush, and most have limited knowledge of dental care. Specifically, they have a poor understanding of the relationship between a sweet diet and caries, the connection between oral hygiene and periodontal health, and the role of fluoride in caries prevention. Oral health problems are caused by lack of early professional treatment, inadequate fluoride intake, and poor diets that, when combined with inadequate oral hygiene, lead to tooth decay.

Infectious Diseases

Although many diseases in migrant aggregates are also common in the general population, it is not unusual to find diseases that would be seen once in a lifetime, if ever, in other groups in the United States. Migrants not only live in Third World conditions but also suffer from Third World diseases. To understand why infectious diseases are so prevalent among migrant workers, one must consider their extreme poverty, need to travel great distances to find work, overcrowded living conditions, lack of proper sanitation, and limited access to health care. Diseases that have been almost eradicated in the United States are sometimes seen among migrant workers. These include typhus, encephalitis, yellow fever, malaria, and leprosy. The largest outbreak of typhoid in recent history occurred in a Florida migrant laborers' camp and was traced to contaminated water (Sandhaus, 1998). Many of the cases of polio in the United States in recent times have occurred in the migrant farmworker population. A significant percentage of migrant farmworkers come from Mexico, Central America, Haiti, and the Dominican Republic, where malaria is endemic. Migrant workers frequently travel back to these countries, placing themselves at risk of acquiring and spreading malaria (Barat, 1999). Discussing the concern for TB, one epidemiologist said, "A Mexican farmworker with tuberculosis who begins treatment in New Mexico might travel during the summer all the way to Canada after the harvests, and, even if successfully treated, may well go home to Mexico in the winter, only to be reinfected by an untreated family member" (McCarthy, 2000, p. 1021).

Cold and damp living quarters produce ear and respiratory tract infections that occur more frequently in the migrant population than in the general population. Toilets located in sleeping areas are associated with a higher incidence of anorexia and gastrointestinal diseases. Parasitic diseases, hepatitis, and gastroenteritis spread rapidly in the crowded living conditions, with no indoor plumbing or sewage disposal and open barrels used for garbage. For example, *Giardia lamblia,* the most commonly found parasite infection in the United States, had a 34% prevalence among migrant children, compared with a national incidence of 4% (Gwyther & Jenkins, 1998). Parasite infestation is rampant among migrant communities, as mentioned earlier in this chapter. (See Voices from the Community I.)

Tuberculosis and Acquired Immunodeficiency Syndrome

TB is again emerging as a serious public health problem, and the deplorable conditions of migrant life favor the spread of TB among migrant farmworkers. It has been estimated that the migrant farm population is six times more likely to develop TB than the general population (NCLR, 1998). With unsanitary, cramped, and poorly ventilated living conditions, respiratory infections and the transmission of TB become inevitable. Migrant farmworkers living in migrant camps report a great number of coworkers with coughs, weakness, and trouble breathing who refuse to go to a clinic because they would lose work hours, money, and possibly jobs. Although TB screening reveals a high prevalence of the disease, essential follow-up procedures are lacking. As many as

VOICES FROM THE COMMUNITY I

"I am the product of undocumented parents who dared to swim across the Rio Grande so that they could find a better opportunity for themselves and their children. My mother had no prenatal care, and none was available to her. I lived in tents. I picked fruit so I could get through school along with my other family members. I have had to deal with not wanting to be Hispanic because of the language and cultural barriers and what it did to women.

"I am the oldest of five children and became my parents' advocate because they could not speak English. . . . Being an advocate at the age of 7, when I learned English as a second language, I encountered a system that was not very sensitive to people who had a different culture and different language. And so, as I picked grapes and I was on my knees spreading those grapes for raisins, I decided that some day I would hope to work in the system. That I would try to change it so that it would be sensitive and poor people would get care with love, dignity, and respect for their cultural barriers.

"I think that it is incumbent on all of us to remember where we came from and turn our face around to the injustices. And that together we make a difference."

A. V., Nashville, Tennessee

"What we have to do is reeducate our people and let them know that we have many rights to live and work and to educate and to have health care. And without health care, we cannot have the other three."

Unidentified male farmworker, California

"We're used to working. We don't want to be given things. We just want to be respected and to be paid the salaries."

T. S., California

"The pesticides we live in day and night. . . . You go to the fields and you think that it's a foggy day because it's so pretty and it's white, but actually it's the chemicals that have been sprayed."

A. R., California

40% of migrant farmworkers have positive TB tests. Inaccessibility to a mobile chest x-ray van delays the confirmation of active TB cases, and financial constraints further preclude treatment. Those with positive tuberculin skin tests often relocate before treatment can be initiated. Some farmworkers with positive skin tests are given a 1-month supply of medication and never return for subsequent months of medicine. Although court-ordered compliance is required for active TB cases, the migratory lifestyle, absence of a nationwide tracking system, and large state financial burdens render this impossible.

AIDS is a growing problem in the migrant community. The incidence of prostitution and intravenous drug use, both risk factors for AIDS, is especially high in the eastern stream, where single migrant workers interact with day workers from large cities in which drug use is frequent. Not surprisingly, research points to increases in HIV infection in the East Coast migrant community that far exceed that in the general population. Migrant families are particularly at risk for both transmission of the virus and development of AIDS because of their lack of access to counseling, prevention, and treatment. In addition, many farmworkers traveling alone become infected in the United States and then return home to infect their wives (Hirsch et al., 2002). Studies reveal that migrant families do not know about the transmission of HIV and that, before going to a doctor, migrant workers often attempt to self-treat with herbal compounds and other folk remedies (Perilla et al., 1998). As a result, HIV infection may not be diagnosed until AIDS-related symptoms are manifested, and HIV may be spread unknowingly.

Immunization

Because of the nomadic life of this community, absence of adequate medical tracking and continuity of care are problems. Poor medical record keeping makes tracking of immunizations difficult, yet many of the diseases prevalent in the migrant population are preventable through proper immunization. Probably no other population in the United States has simultaneous high incidences of both overimmunization and underimmunization of children. Many migrant children are immunized four or five times in the same season because of poor tracking records, whereas others are missed completely for the same reason. The vast majority of migrant adults also do not have available or up-to-date health or immunization records. Acknowledgment of immunization is another problem. When immunizations are offered free of charge to migrant workers, some refuse because they do not want to risk a sore arm that would interfere with crop harvesting.

Risks to Communities

Limited information is available concerning which illnesses migrant farmworkers and their families have when they enter a state or which illnesses they take along with them when they leave. It is known that the migrant lifestyle leads to the creation and perpetuation of disease and illness, which then becomes a community health issue; examples are the HIV/AIDS and TB issues explored by McCarthy (2000) and Hirch et al. (2002), mentioned earlier. Migrant workers live in close quarters with others and may send their children to local schools for brief periods of time. They and their children may remain untreated for the duration of the time they spend in a community. Therefore, they may act as vehicles for disease transmission and incubators for diseases that develop into drug-resistant strains.

Many migrant workers eventually settle in the predominantly rural areas where they work. Then the need for decent health care and housing becomes more pressing, not only for their safety and comfort, but also for the good of the community at large. Host communities faced with people markedly different from themselves and with threatening health problems may become polarized and hostile to the migrant workers.

Social Issues

Migrant workers work and live in places and ways apart from the mainstream population. In Georgia, for example, more than 100,000 migrant workers and their families harvest approximately 90% of the crops, generating more than $300 million in sales for the farmers. Yet it is not rare to meet native Georgians who have never met a migrant farmworker or do not even know of their existence (Perilla et al., 1998). Living apart from established local communities, migrant workers are especially vulnerable to isolation and neglect. Fear of deportation, poverty, and limited education intensify social isolation, which sometimes results in chronic emotional problems such as depression. Display 33–1 lists some stressors in the Hispanic Stress Inventory evaluation tool.

Lack of recreational facilities and the stressors associated with migrancy also contribute to increased rates of substance abuse. Leisure time in the camps is sometimes spent drinking, smoking marijuana, or injecting illegal drugs. In one study, women in a Georgia migrant camp cited drug and alcohol abuse as the most significant health problem in their community (Perilla et al., 1998).

The children of these workers suffer homelessness, hunger, long hours of work, exposure to toxins, lack of friends, frequent relocation, poverty, and school interruption, all of which pose psychosocial, developmental, and health risks. Studies conducted by Rivera (2001), McCauley (2002) and Flores (2002) and their colleagues, as well as others, have documented the negative effects on children of being Latino (90% of migrant workers are Latino) in the United States or of living a migrant lifestyle. Many children are forced to leave school to work in the fields and have little more than a sixth-grade education. This limits their opportunities and forces them to repeat the life cycle of their parents. In addition, bilingual children often become negotiators for their parents. This stressful role requires skills well beyond their years. One community health nurse had to carefully approach the 9-year-old daughter of migrant parents to translate for her family, because her mother and father suffered from several health problems that needed immediate attention. This skilled nurse was able to gather important information without revealing facts that the parents would not have wanted their child to be aware of until a bilingual adult family member became available. Finally, adult roles are forced on migrant children early. Girls are viewed as adults when they are capable of taking care of the household and can bear children, and boys are considered men as soon as they start earning as much as their fathers.

Living in cramped, dirty, and unsanitary quarters often leads to domestic violence. Physical and sexual abuse of

DISPLAY 33-1

Hispanic Stress Inventory—Brief Version

Item	Yes	No
My spouse and I disagree about who controls the money.	❏	❏
My spouse expects me to be more traditional in relationships.	❏	❏
My spouse and I disagree on how to bring up our children.	❏	❏
I've questioned the idea that "marriage is forever."	❏	❏
There have been cultural conflicts in my marriage.	❏	❏
I've felt my spouse and I haven't communicated.	❏	❏
My spouse and I disagree on the language spoken at home.	❏	❏
Both my spouse and I have had to work.	❏	❏
My spouse hasn't adapted to American life.	❏	❏
I watch my work quality so others don't think I'm lazy.	❏	❏
My income is insufficient to support my family or myself.	❏	❏
Since I'm Latino I'm expected to work harder.	❏	❏
Since I'm Latino it's hard to get promotions/raises.	❏	❏
I've been criticized about my work.	❏	❏
I think my children used illegal drugs.	❏	❏
My children have been drinking alcohol.	❏	❏
My children received bad school reports/grades.	❏	❏
My children haven't respected my authority as they should.	❏	❏
My children's ideas about sexuality are too liberal.	❏	❏
My children have talked about leaving home.	❏	❏
There's been physical violence among my family members.	❏	❏
My personal goals conflict with family goals.	❏	❏
I've had serious arguments with family members.	❏	❏
Since I'm Latino it is difficult to find the work I want.	❏	❏
I thought I could be deported if I went to a social/government agency.	❏	❏
Due to poor English, people treat me bad.	❏	❏
Due to poor English, it's hard dealing with daily situations.	❏	❏

(From Garcia, D. [1997]. Assessing stress among migrant and seasonal farmworkers. *Streamline: The Migrant Health News Source, 3* [5], 1–5.)

LEVELS OF PREVENTION MATRIX

SITUATION: DOMESTIC VIOLENCE IN THE MIGRANT POPULATION.

Research is scant, but informal discussions occur among women and health care providers. Outreach workers sometimes possess lists of men who are abusive and their victims. Although the migrant lifestyle and experience is difficult for the entire family, women and children suffer most from family violence the migrant way of life promotes. Isolation and subjugation to a patriarchal system usually prohibit migrant women from seeking help if they are abused. Fear of consequences and difficulty expressing negative views about husbands prevent women from speaking out.
(Artemis, 1996; Rodriguez, 1993)

GOAL: Using the three levels of prevention, negative health conditions are avoided, promptly diagnosed and treated, and the fullest possible potential is restored.

PRIMARY PREVENTION		SECONDARY PREVENTION		TERTIARY PREVENTION		
Health Promotion and Education	*Health Protection*	*Early Diagnosis*	*Prompt Treatment*	*Rehabilitation*	*Primary Prevention*	
					Health Promotion and Education	*Health Protection*
• Create awareness of the harsh living conditions that migrant families endure • Advocate for improved and safe living conditions on state and national levels • Provide adequate housing that eliminates overcrowding and offers privacy	• Train bilingual and bicultural lay migrant women on the issues of wife abuse and help them form support groups • Provide opportunities for women and men to improve self-esteem, which will change attitudes toward each other	• Promptly identify an abused woman and remove her from the dangerous situation—self-identification or by other family members or professionals • Keep communication lines open, be culturally sensitive, examine for injuries	• Secure the victim in a safe battered women's shelter • Assist women to regain lost self-esteem	• Promote family rehabilitation—with or without abuser in the home • Encourage ways to eliminate or reduce social and geographic isolation among vulnerable women	• Alleviate stressors of the migrant lifestyle, such as over-crowding and substandard living conditions • Provide emotional support and educate on what constitutes abuse • Promote self-esteem to the point where a woman can take control of her situation	• Encourage women to contact health care providers as she migrates • Encourage women to find appropriate lay community outreach workers for support • Encourage migrant women to unite and create an environment that allows them to speak up and out while supporting one another against abuse

*Secondary Prevention is difficult because of lack of financial resources, transportation, nearby friends or relatives for support, English speaking capability, and safe battered women's shelters in rural areas.

women and children occurs, and migrant women are more susceptible to domestic and intimate partner violence than women in the general population. Lacking access to health services and fearing deportation and isolation, these women often have no choice but to endure the violence. One migrant woman related that while sharing one room with her husband, infant, and five single men, her husband became increasingly violent and unpredictable. He began to beat her and the baby, and she was unable to predict what would initiate a violent attack. She finally fled when one of the men living with them

also began beating her. She attributed the aggressive behavior to the powerlessness felt by the men. The Violence Against Women Act of 1994 affords protection for undocumented battered women and children by allowing them to seek legal immigration status without the help of their abusers (Camacho, 1998) (see Levels of Prevention Matrix).

Deterioration of family values is a concern of some migrant workers who see their children becoming acculturated into mainstream values and becoming less family oriented. Conflicts sometimes erupt when children start to identify with mainstream lifestyles despite parental enforcement of traditional values. Yet, despite concerns that the very fabric of their culture may be threatened by problems with drugs and alcohol, domestic violence, prostitution, and deterioration of family values, the migrant community remains extremely resilient and proud. Families place high premiums on work and self-sufficiency. Family and family structure are highly valued, and migrant families form cohesive units based on language, food, music, religion, social interaction, and beneficial folk health practices.

BARRIERS TO HEALTH CARE

When you get sick, you expect to go to a doctor and use your insurance to cover medical expenses. You expect your illness to be understood, and you expect to be treated as a person in need of medical attention. This is not the case with migrant workers. Migrant health clinics often fail to serve migrants by imposing legal, financial, and physical impediments. Many clinics do not account for cultural differences, and some have staff that are unable to speak the clients' language. Understanding why less than 20% of migrant workers use primary care health services is essential in providing better health care to this aggregate. Barriers to primary health care access include isolation, powerlessness, economic barriers, limited health resources, language difficulties, and cultural differences.

Isolation and Powerlessness

The rural communities in which migrant workers live generally lack primary care providers, and migrant workers lack the transportation necessary to get to clinics that may be far away from migrant camps. Lack of adequate child care facilities is also a hindrance for working mothers. Because migrant workers will not miss a day's work until their illnesses become dire, migrant clinics are not helpful unless they offer weekend and evening hours. Normal office hours are hours that migrant farmworkers spend in the fields (see Voices in the Community II).

Nomadic lifestyle and poverty render migrant workers politically powerless. Furthermore, they do not stay in their communities long enough to affect local decision-making processes that could improve their working and living conditions. Many state and federal agencies are too understaffed to adequately enforce health regulations and labor laws.

Migrant workers tend to be clannish and suspicious of strangers, and they mistrust outsiders for fear of deportation and job loss. They are even fearful of reporting minor injuries, because health care providers may be viewed as having policing power. The Immigration Law of 1986, which was designed to open up more jobs for American citizens by limiting the hiring of illegal immigrants, increased discrimination against Hispanics, even those who are citizens. Racism and discrimination abuses are pervasive among migrant farmworkers and their families. Suffering discrimina-

VOICES FROM THE COMMUNITY II

"Going out into the migrant camps, one of the migrant workers said, 'We expect one of us to die.' I thought, 'Why do you expect that to happen?' They shouldn't have this mentality when they go traveling state to state—that it's a part of life."

"They [women] also need child care. What happens with the children? Go out in the fields. They lay under the trees and there is a residue falling on the children. They are picking grapes, what happens? The sprayers are there with the residue falling on the children."

I.A., health promoter, La Clinica del Carino,
Hood River, Oregon

"They [farmworkers] don't demand to go to the doctor [for medical treatment after injuries] nor do they file any complaints. They feel that if they do not come back to work the next day, they will lose their job. The foremen do not help because they do not want people that will not produce for them."

"Now there are a lot of people who are making a living in the same way but are unable to find adequate housing, consequently having to live under the trees. What's even worse, the foremen even charged them for sleeping under the trees."

T. V., Migrant Health Center Board Member,
California

"I have seen people that work in the fields stay wherever, outside on the edge of their fields, and in their cars and vans. And we have the whole family, they come in their vans and they stay there. Those people just ask for permission to take a bath in some cabin or some field, to be able to take a bath or drink some water and that's all. And that's the way they spend their lives."

E. S., Board member, La Clinica del Carino,
Hood River, Oregon

tion due to their ethnicity and migrant status, many migrant men and women encounter prejudice and racism in medical facilities, grocery stores, shopping centers, restaurants, schools, and even churches (Perilla et al., 1998).

Economic Barriers and Limited Health Resources

Inability to obtain Medicaid, coupled with lack of health insurance, severely handicaps migrant farmworkers' ability to access health care. Because they are low-wage earners, migrant workers often cannot afford to pay for health care and are not willing to take time off from work when pay depends on each bushel picked (Gwyther & Jenkins, 1998). Migrant farmworkers usually are not covered by health insurance, because farm owners, especially those who own smaller farms, cannot afford to provide health insurance for their workers. Mobility disqualifies migrant families from Medicaid–managed care systems because of the inability to maintain a single primary care provider (Gwyther & Jenkins, 1998). Primary and secondary prevention are almost nonexistent because funds for these services are not available.

Migrant workers are unable to qualify for basic health and disability benefits such as Workers' Compensation, Social Security, occupational rehabilitation, and disability compensation because of loopholes in the legal system (NCFH, 2003). Although they are eligible for public programs such as Medicaid, food stamps, and WIC, migrant farmworkers as a whole do not participate. They may fear immigration penalties or be totally unaware of the available benefits. Although many have worked in this country for several years, they often are not U. S. citizens and may be in the country illegally. Some are eligible for Social Security benefits but do not possess the ability to process their claim (NCFH, 2003). Although undocumented immigrants are not eligible for public assistance, they do have protected rights to decent wages, health, and safety.

Medicaid was enacted to protect and increase health care for vulnerable populations such as the migrant community. However, as a group migrant farmworkers have more difficulty accessing Medicaid than any other population. Medicaid benefits have little value in the face of constant mobility, because they are not transferable from state to state. On one hand, although the low income of migrant workers meets the guidelines for state medical assistance, few families remain in one state long enough for the 30-day residency requirement. On the other hand, farmworker families may not qualify for Medicaid because, during certain months of the year, they earn more than the state's poverty limits. Ironically, migrant workers suffer from preventable and treatable diseases covered under Medicaid but are unable to obtain treatment.

In a New York migrant camp, a group of nurses made obtaining Medicaid a priority and worked to facilitate the Medicaid application process by assisting with the completion of the form, scheduling interviews, gathering appropriate documents, and interpreting as necessary. Although assisting with the Medicaid application was extremely time-consuming and labor intensive, it was an important strategy for expediting health care access. This strategy was helpful only if the applications were started as soon as the farmworkers arrived in the area; otherwise, they would be gone before Medicaid benefits started. Also, if the farmworkers began earning salaries before completing their application, they would make too much money to qualify for Medicaid benefits, because income guidelines are based on recent paychecks and not yearly earnings.

Often, the emergency department is the most accessible health care option for migrant families, yet it is the most expensive health care choice for all populations. Migrant families even hesitate to use this option, because hospitals are viewed with anxiety and mistrust and as a place to die.

Cultural and Language Barriers

Because many migrant workers do not speak or read English, they must overcome a language barrier to navigate difficult communication processes such as negotiating appointments, applying for insurance, or adhering to medical treatment. Many families do not comprehend the language in which application forms are written. Increasing the number of bilingual personnel and nurses at migrant centers is crucial for increasing health care access.

Many migrant families are unable to effectively communicate health care needs, and many health care providers lack sensitivity to understand the needs of this culturally diverse population. To become effective health care providers, community health nurses must embrace the notion of *cultural sensitivity,* the awareness of different values, beliefs, and behaviors of others. To become effective health care providers, nurses must work on developing the capacity to appreciate differences and value diversity and must assess their own reactions to different cultures (see Chapter 4).

In a New York state migrant camp, cultural sensitizing took place on several occasions. Nurses and staff discussed their cultural values and opinions about what was right and good in caring for migrant farmworkers. The sharing of this information sensitized staff members and nurses to migrant value systems and to the injustices these workers endure as migrants and also as members of an ethnic group. To learn about migrant family values, nurses observed behaviors and asked questions, especially about health care behaviors. They also visited migrant camps and interacted socially. Cultural sensitivity enabled the nurses to anticipate culturally based problems that could arise during health care encounters. In a similar situation, community health nursing students were taken to migrant camps as part of a summer course requirement. Forced to confront migrant culture, the working conditions, and unique health problems, the students soon learned that although economic, social, and racial issues may divide communities, the basic elements of wanting a better environment and enhancing self-worth transcend all differences.

Culture affects health beliefs. For example, folklore medicine and rituals are a strong component of Hispanic culture and are commonly practiced by many migrant workers. Because of limited access to health care and a tendency to distrust mainstream medical personnel, many migrant workers seek health care first from healers in their own communities (Perilla et al., 1998). Herbal medicines are common, as is seeking advice from **curanderas** (folk healers). If these means are unsuccessful, migrant workers will then seek out medical interventions. In rural areas of Mexico, strong beliefs in folk illnesses, such as the evil eye, require traditional folk remedies. Many Hispanics believe in hot and cold theories of illness. Mexican women refuse fruits and vegetables during the "hot" postpartum state because these foods are considered "cold" (Spector, 2000). Many recent Mexican immigrants use needles and syringes to give themselves vitamins, medications, and contraceptives purchased in Mexico. The needles are a threat to health because they may be shared for these injections, exposing the users to possible infection, including HIV.

The Mexican culture is patriarchal, with "machismo" men playing the dominant role in decision-making while women carry out the decisions (Spector, 2000). Treating disease involves use of remedies approved by the male head of the household and implemented by the female members of the household. Hispanics also appreciate the qualities of **simpatica** (positive interpersonal relationships) and **personalismo** (pleasant conversation). Although diseases are often viewed with fatalistic acceptance, migrant families expect health care providers to relieve their disease symptoms. Many nurses do not possess an adequate understanding of the impact of the migrant family's cultural beliefs and expectations of the nurse (Spector, 2000). Migrant families expect to have symptoms relieved quickly and effectively, with nurses using a personal, warm approach. The migrant worker must also be considered in the context of family, because family is an important source of emotional and physical support for members who become ill. Community health nurses who are sensitive to cultural beliefs can and do increase the effectiveness of treatment (Gwyther & Jenkins, 1998).

THE ROLE OF COMMUNITY HEALTH NURSES IN CARING FOR A MOBILE WORKFORCE

Beyond barriers to health care such as lack of health services, language and cultural impediments, inadequate to nonexistent transportation, financial strains, underinsurance, and questionable residency status, which are by themselves formidable obstacles, the migrant lifestyle is fraught with challenges. Because of the insecurity and instability inherent in a mobile lifestyle, long-term health goals are difficult to establish and long-term follow-up of any chronic illness is doubtful. Nonetheless, community health nurses provide much-needed services using community resources, innovative thinking, tenacity, and sensitivity.

Trenchant strategies for improving the health status and resource use of migrant workers and their families can be accomplished by

- Improving existing services
- Advocating and networking
- Practicing cultural sensitivity
- Using lay personnel for community outreach
- Utilizing unique methods of health care delivery
- Employing information tracking systems

Community health nurses are the major providers of migrant health services and have a crucial role in the development and management of interventions. In response to the growing need for available, accessible, and affordable health care for farmworker families, nurses are called on not only to understand the migrant lifestyle but also to help migrant families overcome the barriers to health care (see Voices from the Community III).

Evaluating and Improving Health Services

No clearly defined leadership to develop policies for migrant workers exists. Because the farmers themselves, under financial constraints, are not traditionally consulted regarding migrant health issues, health care for this population becomes fragmented in the federal domain. Federal appropriations for migrant workers are low, and most existing services exclude them because of residency requirements. The government's funding structure provides incentives for agencies that treat a greater number of clients rather than stressing quality, disease prevention, and continuity of care (Sandhaus, 1998). In addition, an effective tracking system to maximize services is desperately needed.

The National Advisory Council on Migrant Health recommends universal health coverage for migrant families, with Medicaid coverage transferable from state to state. It suggests that migrant health centers provide culturally sensitive health care to the diverse and underserved migrant populations that includes transportation, translation services, and case management. Currently, most translators at health care sites are clerical support staff. Untrained personnel can impede health care delivery if they are unable to translate accurately, and they may be perceived as threats to confidentiality by the clients.

Investigations to improve the health care of migrant workers are needed. Laws regulating safety, wages, sanitation, and employment must be better enforced. All migrant health centers should be funded to provide oral health care. Migrant workers should be included in mental health and substance abuse health services. The Office of Substance Abuse Prevention recommends increased appropriations for migrant-specific health issues. Assessment, intervention, and evaluation of health care delivery, areas in which community health nurses excel, are needed, as are increased numbers of culturally and linguistically competent nurses. To develop outreach and primary care services, increased federal funding for migrant health projects is essential. Regulations that limit reimbursement, especially for dental and eye examinations, hypertension and diabetes screening, mammograms, and preventive health care, should be reevaluated. Improving public health services, such as providing drinkable water, ensuring sanitation services in the fields, guarding against pesticide exposure, and addressing substandard housing, is crucial to disease prevention.

Advocacy, Networking, and Cultural Brokering

Advocating for the migrant population is an important strategy in facilitating health care. As advocates, community health nurses can effectively intervene when a treatment plan is incongruent with the migrant lifestyle. For example, if a doctor were to prescribe bed rest for a migrant farmworker who injured his leg, that protocol would most likely not be followed, because missing a day's work means missing a

"First of all, a nurse should expect the unexpected. Because of the migratory way of life . . . they do not always know where they will be next week or next month. Therefore we must understand that they do not always have their medical records, immunization records, or income records. Hours are very irregular, depending on what time the workers get in from the fields and what time the shifts are. Because of the distances we travel, we work anywhere from 8 to 12 hours a day. The most rewarding part of the job is bringing health services to the underserved and uninsured. The people are so gracious and appreciative of whatever services we provide."

J. S., RN, Michigan

"Since farmworkers come to our area for only 4 months of the year, it is rare that I care for a migrant woman through her entire pregnancy. I may diagnose her pregnancy, I may see her for three or four prenatal visits, or I may meet her only once before she goes into labor and delivers her baby. I struggle with the desire to make a difference in a short period of time and with the disappointment of not being able to follow-through."

C. K., CNM, RN, Pennsylvania

"Encourage clinicians to trust old diagnostic skills of palpation, auscultation, and careful listening. Exhaustive laboratory work or radiology studies are not likely to be welcomed by farm workers who seek relief of symptoms so that they may return to work. Be warm and interested in the whole family. If you do not speak Spanish or Creole, work with translators who under-

stand how you work. Use translators as . . . vehicles to get the information out and in. Eye contact and touch are crucial. Learning to be clinically relevant as well as competently utilizing a translator is an art, and takes time and experience to hone. Learning some phrases or some of the most frequently asked questions in the language of the farm worker should be encouraged. Even the attempt to speak the patients' language will build trust and confidence. These harvesters of the nation's food are very bright and resourceful people who travel great distances and undergo severe deprivation in order to work. The nobility of this pursuit is getting short shrift in the press and legislative bodies today, but the sheer enormity of the service [that] this group of oppressed people do for the rest of us needs to be acknowledged and honored by the clinicians who will provide primary health care to them and theirs."

W. H., RN, Michigan

"I'm dealing right now with Hispanic women, migrant workers, who do not have any access to prenatal care, none whatsoever. What I'm doing is creative financing, a lot of begging, a lot of pleading, a lot of being nice to people I don't even want to be nice to because it means that much to me for them to get help. So I find myself in situations that are sometimes uncomfortable, but nonetheless I do it because I feel that as a nurse that's my job. Having been a farmworker myself, I would want someone to do that for my mother, and they did."

Unidentified female nurse, Idaho Falls, Idaho

day's pay. An alternative plan, one more consistent with the migrant lifestyle, would be for the migrant farmworker to stay off the injured leg in the evening when he is not working. In advocating on the behalf of the injured worker, the community health nurse would have to ensure that the leg was elevated and that appropriate pharmaceutical treatments were applied. Although healing would probably take longer, this plan is more realistic.

When community health nursing students in an experimental learning program spent a summer in the fields working within a migrant community, they came across a migrant worker suffering from dehydration and nausea. Through an interpreter, he told the students that the crew leader would not allow the men to interrupt work to go to the bathroom. He also said that the crew leader was withholding his pay. A visit to the worker's trailer revealed that 16 other workers were living in one trailer and that they shared a bathroom with two other families. After advocating to both the crew chief and local officials to collect the wages that were due, the students helped relocate the worker to another camp so that he would not suffer recriminations for reporting the

squalid conditions to the authorities. In addition, the students contacted several state and federal agencies to report the unsanitary living conditions and attended a rural outreach forum to discuss health, labor, and migrant issues.

Community health nurses can obtain health care services for migrant workers through **cultural brokering**, whereby nurses intervene to assist in acquiring needed health care. Cultural brokering involves facilitating health care for migrant workers who are unable to overcome the barriers that exist. This includes negotiating, mediating, and innovating on behalf of migrant workers. Essential to this role are sensitivity to patient needs, knowledge of the barriers that impede health care, and commitment to facilitate health care for those who do not have the power to access health care on their own.

Cultural Sensitivity

Community health nurses who have consistent and frequent contact with the migrant community will become aware of migrant families' social and culturally based needs. Interventions with culturally diverse clients and communities must reflect cultural sensitivity, such as viewing culture as an enabler to pursue health care rather than a resistant force. Culturally sensitive assessments and interventions must include health, education, income, degree of acculturation, level of participation in traditional culture, and length of time in the United States (Spector, 2000). Incorporating cultural beliefs in plans of care that stress **familialism**, the act of taking time for pleasant conversation with Hispanic clients, for example, requires knowing about their culture, customs, beliefs, and language. Dialogues between the community health nurse and migrant workers should not be patronizing or one-sided but open, with an opportunity to learn and to teach. Each time migrant families are helped, they become encouraged and empowered for the common good of the entire community.

Because the traditional mainstream ideal of professionalism may be construed as cold and distant, a warm, accepting attitude and pleasant conversation are cornerstones of effective health care relationships (see Chapter 24). Successful intervention strategies include nonjudgmental communication and the ability to convey respect and genuine affection for the family. This may take time to nurture and develop, but in the end it very much enhances communication with migrant clients. For example, a migrant worker did not finish his prescribed antibiotic. By being less formal, warm, and showing concern and by avoiding criticism and confrontation, the nurse was able to explain the importance of finishing the antibiotic. This resulted in the client's becoming more receptive to care and even referring family members to the nurse.

Family is the most important source of support for those who become ill. Decision-making about health matters is a family function. Having family members present during assessment and teaching enhances client satisfaction and compliance. For example, when dealing with drug addiction in a migrant family, the entire family should be included. Fear of being isolated from family may prevent the drug-addicted member from seeking treatment. **Machismo**, or male qualities of dominance, has been described as a cultural reason why Hispanic men attempt to prove their masculinity through substance abuse and use of prostitutes, which carry high risks for HIV infection and AIDS (Hirsch et al., 2002).True machismo, however, translates into pride, honor, and dignity when men must take responsibility for their families and protect them from harm. By incorporating machismo and familialism into health education programs and stressing that the men are responsible for and capable of protecting their household, the community health nurse will have better success. Love of family and children is so strong that Mexican-Americans have shown themselves to be more likely than non-Hispanic whites to quit smoking if they perceive it to be a threat to their children.

Being nonjudgmental and nonthreatening provides a framework for communication. Inquiries about folk remedies, for example, should never be broached by direct questioning; rather, a third-person inquiry approach should be used. One should not attempt to dissuade migrant families from their folk remedies if they are harmless but should instead educate them on the importance of medical therapy (see Chapter 4). Combining folk and medical therapies may help increase compliance because it places medicine within the context of the culture and lifestyle. If a Hispanic mother wishes to give her child a harmless folk potion for asthma or massage the abdomen of a child with viral gastroenteritis as is culturally prescribed, no harm will be done if these remedies are continued along with prescribed medical treatments (Spector, 2000). Even Spanish-speaking Hispanics have a difficult time in getting migrant women to open up about domestic violence. If assessment questions are tried and fail, a new approach should be attempted. Ask the migrant women what a nurse should tell a woman who might come to her as a result of physical abuse by her partner. This third-person approach often meets with success, and women who had previously denied being physically abused offer information about their handling of abusive situations. It is a form of reverse role play discussed in Chapter 12, and it is an effective teaching method that assists people to open themselves up to discuss an issue (see Using the Nursing Process).

Lay Personnel for Community Outreach

Lay outreach personnel can overcome the language and cultural barriers as well as isolation. Use of migrant lay community **outreach** workers who have received basic training in health care and resources is a method of reaching and improving health care. Recognizing the value of family, friends, and the sharing of cultural values, migrant lay personnel are readily accepted within the migrant community, overcoming cultural and language barriers. Despite the stereotypic portrayal of Hispanic women as passive, they are, in fact, a source of strength for family members because they maintain and nurture strong family ties and loyalty (Olmos, Ybarra & Monterrey, 1999). Many Hispanic women become involved outside the family sphere in education and community activities as lay workers. **Lay workers** in migrant communities are typically trained and supervised by community health nurses (Gwyther & Jenkins, 1998). Already familiar with life in the migrant community, lay migrant outreach workers create formal and informal links with one another to promote health and provide continuity of care. Perhaps one of the most trenchant advantages of using lay personnel is the sense of empowerment engendered when these clients believe they can take control in caring for one another.

One successful program using lay migrant women is the North Carolina Maternal and Child Health Migrant Project. This program overcame stringent barriers to health care such as limited transportation, communication difficulties, and lack of child care. Volunteer women in the migrant camps were trained to become lay health advisors, providing health education, prescription instruction, and first aid. Bilingual staff also streamlined follow-ups, referrals, and appointments and acted as interpreters. The program used a bus and

USING THE NURSING PROCESS

When Working with Migrant Families

BACKGROUND DATA AND ASSESSMENT

Elena Vasquez is a community health nurse in rural Central California. She had two migrant camps in her service area and realized that during her normal working hours she was missing the adults in the camps. She met with several farmworker families one evening and brainstormed with them. They discussed their health needs and what type of services they needed most. A similar meeting was held at the other camp. At both camps, the families were willing to work with the nurse to enhance needed health care services. The information gathered helped Elena formulate nursing diagnoses which led to innovative planning and implementation.

NURSING DIAGNOSES

1. Alteration in family health status related to hazardous working conditions, poverty, and mobility.
2. At risk for occupational and situational injury, illness, and stress due to poverty-level working and living conditions.
3. Inadequate and inaccessible health care services related to poverty, work hours, and mobility.

PLAN AND IMPLEMENTATION

Elena enthusiastically approached the health department administration with the innovative ideas she was formulating. The administrator agreed to try the plan Elena proposed for 3 months if Elena could find the personnel she needed and the results were positive.

She enlisted four other community health nurses, two social workers and several bilingual students from the local university's community health nursing class, which used the agency as a clinical site. Each team of nurses, a social worker, and three students drove to a camp once a week on a Tuesday or Thursday evening from 5 to 9 PM (The professionals started their day at 1

PM on that day). They completed a family assessment for each family; established a health record for each person; conducted health appraisals; administered immunizations; enrolled families in the Women, Infants, and Children Supplemental Food Program (WIC); made early-evening dentist and doctor appointments and arranged transportation if needed; and held brief teaching sessions on safety, infant and child care, family planning, and any topic the people requested or Elena and her colleagues felt the families needed.

The students became as innovative as Elena. They gathered used clothing and household items from their fellow nursing students for distribution and got valuable practice teaching and delivering health care services. The volunteers' enthusiasm overflowed to the farmworkers. Some of the women planned an informal "day care" program after receiving child care classes from the nursing students. Some of the men organized a baseball team to play against the other camp on Sunday afternoons. Additional donations were solicited—toys and books for the day care program and bats and gloves for the ball teams.

EVALUATION

The interventions were so successful that the program became a permanent service of the health department. In the following months, a nurse practitioner was added, along with a preschool teacher and students from the early elementary education program at the university. The two camps became popular with migrant workers, who stayed healthier and were more productive. In addition, the camp managers found the grounds being kept cleaner and had fewer complaints and less abuse of the cabins and shower areas. With improved health and productivity, several families were motivated to establish a permanent home in the community and not continue the migrant lifestyle.

---

volunteer drivers to transport clients to appointments. Several years ago, when 40 migrant women trained as lay health advisors were evaluated in two migrant health centers in North Carolina, they were found to have interacted with 50% to 82% of the 470 migrant women and infants within the year-long study. Mothers who had contact with the lay advisors were more likely to visit health care providers when their children were sick. Furthermore, they had more knowledge about health than did the mothers without contacts to the lay advisors (Watkins et al., 1994).

Another intervention strategy using lay leaders is the camp health aide program. **Camp health aides**, who are bilingual and bicultural, are recruited to overcome language restrictions and negative stereotyping that prevent migrant workers from getting proper health care. Camp health aides, usually women and themselves workers, help reinforce positive health values and create a sense of self-esteem and empowerment (Sandhaus, 1998). Recruited in the same manner as lay health advisors, camp health aides are trained to teach their peers on topics such as hygiene, spread of disease, preventive health care measures, nutrition, prenatal care, pesticides, and availability of health services. Migrant women trained in this manner are able to provide on-site care, which decreases the amount of time lost from work and reduces the complications from inattention to health problems.

The Camp Health Aide Program in Monroe, Michigan, recruits lay workers to teach about nutrition, first aid, prenatal care, well-child care, environmental protection, diabetes, hypertension, sexually transmitted diseases, HIV/AIDS, and mental health. Gaining better access to health care, migrant farmworkers benefit by having illnesses diagnosed and treated sooner and in a more cost-effective manner (HRSA, 1998).

Unique Methods of Health Care Delivery

Because migrant health centers do not adequately meet the health needs of the migrant community, several innovative methods of health care delivery have been developed and implemented by community health nurses. Although changes are often minor and slow to occur in the migrant population, even minute changes are a milestone, because the migrant lifestyle does not support any type of health stability. Any progress made must be welcomed with recognition and support.

Mobile health vans staffed with bilingual community health nurses and lay workers can travel directly to migrant camps and are an effective strategy for outreach health screening and education (HRSA, 1998). By going to migrant camps and delivering care where the clients live and work, especially during nonwork hours such as evenings and weekends, community health nurses increase health access and overcome barriers of culture and lack of child care. Although migrant families receive only fragmented acute care, a nurses' outreach team can succeed by encouraging migrant farmworkers to prevent illness with immunizations, good nutrition, and healthy lifestyles. A viable alternative to traditional medical clinics, the mobile nursing clinic provides primary care to an underserved population through health promotion, disease prevention, and early treatment.

Other migrant services may include migrant ministries—ecumenical organizations formed to assist migrant workers with government and state grants as well as donations. For example, a ministry in Florida, supported by local donations, distributes sacks of food staples such as rice, beans, flour, and vegetables, as well as gas for cooking, to needy migrant families. Classes in English, basic parenting skills, banking needs, and understanding medicine labels are offered in the evenings (Jorn & Ros, 2004). The ministry has also developed vocational training programs and has goals of developing a day care center for children and educational programs that focus on gang violence and substance abuse prevention.

To streamline enrollment in Medicaid, Wisconsin operates a model Medicaid reciprocity system in which migrant farmworker families with valid medical assistance cards from other states automatically qualify for Medicaid without having to reestablish eligibility. Wisconsin also uses average annual income rather than monthly earnings to qualify families for Medicaid, because migrant farmworker earnings vary considerably from month to month, and a single higher-income month could disqualify the worker from Medicaid eligibility (HRSA, 1998). To help access primary care, vouchers can be implemented in areas that do not make separate services economically feasible. For example, in Colorado, voucher programs have evolved into migrant health programs that are trenchant strategies to meet health needs.

Whereas migrant health care centers provide direct service, **migrant health programs** depend on referrals and vouchers to address gaps in health care services (Castro, 1999). A migrant health program in Colorado maintains formal agreements with medical, dental, and pharmacy providers that accept reduced fees. With an identification card, migrant workers can directly access primary medical services themselves. Responding to the needs of the migrant workers, evening hours are maintained with bilingual community health nurses who also advocate for migrant workers to ensure that services are accessible and appropriate. A model worthy of replication, the Colorado migrant health program promotes health care advocacy, empowerment, continuity of care, improvement of living and working environments, and accountability to the community.

Resources

Community health nurses involved with migrant families benefit from using federally funded resources such as the National Advisory Council on Migrant Health, Midwest Migrant Health Information Office, Farmworker Health Services, Farmworker Justice Fund, and HRSA Bureau of Primary Care. Promoting health, social services, education, and employment, these agencies also are important networking sources.

Information Tracking Systems

Mobility impedes continuity of care, and the inadequate system of medical record keeping for the migrant population is particularly frustrating (Weinman, 1999). Data information systems are vital components for monitoring the health status of individual farmworkers as they migrate. Furthermore, these data are essential for generating research and follow-up care as well as long-range health planning. They also help justify appropriation of monies to migrant health agencies (Gwyther & Jenkins, 1998). Many proposals for data tracking systems have required the implementation of expensive and complicated computer systems that present almost insurmountable barriers to their widespread use. The HEART FAX, a simple and secure system for retrieving medical records using only telephones and fax machines, was initially developed to track cardiac patients who are part-time residents of Florida. HEART FAX functions as a medical database clearinghouse with continuous service via a toll-free telephone number. All instructions for accessing records are provided in both English and Spanish. Such a data retrieval system would improve continuity of care, especially for pregnant women and children who are most in need (Weinman, 1999).

Migrant children are susceptible to medical "feast or famine" and may be either overtreated or undertreated simply because their medical histories are unknown to current providers. One method for tracking the health status of migrant school-age children is through the Migrant Student Record Transfer System (MSRTS), a computerized system that collects and maintains health and academic records for migrant children. Records of more than one-half million migrant children collected by school nurses include data on personal and family history; immunization status; visual, auditory, and dental problems; nutritional status; and general physical condition. Although this tracking system does serve to enhance the health of migrant children, many do not attend school or do so only on a sporadic basis. The ability to track these children in the migratory lifestyle from work location to work location is often minimal. Early intervention for migrating children is unlikely, although it has been proven to greatly improve outcomes. The creation of a national database for information on the health status of migrant workers, paralleling the information included in the MSRTS, has also been suggested.

Health Goals

The challenge of providing a uniform strategy of care for a highly mobile population prompted the development of a compilation of goals by the National Migrant Resource Program and Migrant Clinicians Network. These goals include the promotion of better health, fewer risk factors, increased awareness, and improved services. Objectives are to improve nutrition, immunization, occupational safety, prenatal care, dental health, preventive services, and medical records and to reduce drug and alcohol abuse, violent behavior, mental illness, adolescent pregnancy, and HIV transmission (Display 33–2). These objectives both complement and enhance the health objectives for the nation for the year 2010 to increase years of healthy life and eliminate health disparities (U. S. Department of Health and Human Services, 2000).

The transience of the migrant workforce also makes it difficult to ascertain its numbers. A specific goal for the immediate future is to improve research data on migrant workers. Toward this end, community health nurses can gather information concerning changes in family relationships and acculturation to mainstream values to be used in designing health programs. Because few researchers have studied migrant health needs, status, and behavior, this information would ensure that health services closely match the needs of specific migrant cultures. Continued efforts must be made to conduct research assessing risks and hazards, especially those of pesticide exposure. Many government publications document the despair and isolation of migrant workers, yet very little has been done to address the living and working environments that contribute to diminished health. Although migrant workers are difficult to study as a mobile population,

---

DISPLAY 33–2

Migrant-Specific Health Objectives

1. Reduce alcohol and other drug abuse.
2. Improve nutrition.
3. Improve mental health and prevent mental illness.
4. Reduce environmental health hazards.
5. Improve occupational safety and health.
6. Prevent and control unintentional injuries.
7. Reduce violent and abusive behavior.
8. Prevent and control HIV infection and AIDS.
9. Immunize against and control infectious diseases.
10. Improve maternal and infant health.
11. Improve oral health.
12. Reduce adolescent pregnancy and improve reproductive health.
13. Prevent, detect, and control chronic diseases and other health disorders.
14. Improve health education and access to preventive health services.
15. Improve surveillance and data systems.

(From National Migrant Resource Program and Migrant Clinicians Network [1996]. *Migrant and seasonal farmworker health objectives for the year 2000.* Austin, TX: U. S. Department of Health and Human Services, National Center for Farmworker Health, Inc.)

---

they are important as an integral part of our economy and because infectious disease in their sector increases health risks for all (Hirsch et al., 2002).

Community health nurses can become involved in politics and educate the public on the importance of migrant workers to the American economy and their compromised health and living conditions. Community health nurses can influence and implement improvements in public health policy, especially increased funding to provide greater insurance coverage and better health care to migrant farmworkers. Health interventions, however, must reflect cultural sensitivity and language differences as well as environmental risks. Adequate follow-up and referrals and transferable medical records are crucial for continuity of care. To affect migrant health issues, community health nurses must advocate for funding to train lay health advisors, promote law enforcement to ensure safe environments, and educate community leaders regarding the special needs of migrant farmworkers.

SUMMARY

An aggregate at risk, migrant workers suffer higher frequency of illness, more complications, and more long-term debilitating effects. Diseases, often resembling those of a Third World country, are caused by poor nutrition, neglect and inadequate treatment, and occupational hazards and conditions arising from poverty and migration. Exacerbated by a magnitude of environmental and work stressors, the health of migrant families is also compromised by limited access to health care, mobility, language and cultural barriers, low educational levels, and few economic and political resources. Because migrant health needs are largely manageable within community settings, community health nurses are ideal health providers. Implementing health education at migrant camps, training lay health workers, and providing clinic hours to accommodate late workdays are successful interventions. Learning the language of the migrant workers and their unique cultures is also helpful in reaching this population. Community health nurses must advocate for the health of migrant workers, who have very little economic or political power, and also guide them through the complexities of a changing health care system. Although many resources and programs exist to help migrant families, the needs are still overwhelming. By aligning with the goals of *Healthy People 2010* to improve the health of one of our most underserved populations, the community health nurse will also be improving the health of the nation as a whole.

The abysmal conditions and health needs of migrant workers have changed little in the past 40 years. However, new needs are arising in the migrant community. In the past, migrant workers traveled primarily in organized crews; they are now traveling in family units with women and children. Added attention must be given to family members exposed to the hazards of the migrant lifestyle. Even as many migrant workers settle into communities, the cycle of poverty continues as others arrive from impoverished countries. With a paucity of health resources, the community health nurse is sometimes the only health provider who is able and willing to care for this population. Providing care for migrant workers presents a challenge to be innovative and to go beyond the boundaries of traditional health services.

Community health nurses are charged with the challenge of breaking the cycle of poverty by providing a voice for those who are not seen or heard. Migrant workers and their families, vital contributors to the American economy, can barely afford the produce that their grueling, underpaid labor provides. Awareness of this plight drives community health nurses to ensure that migrant worker families come to enjoy the harvest of bounty along with improved health and living conditions.

ACTIVITIES TO PROMOTE CRITICAL THINKING

1. In March 1999, on the Web site of the National Center for Farmworker Health, the following quotation from Paula Diperna appeared: "Justice in the fields slips through the fingers like a handful of soil." Considering what you have read in this chapter about social justice and migrant workers and undocumented immigrants, explain how these words express the inequities this aggregate endures regarding working and living conditions and health.

2. Download patient education materials for migrant workers from the NCFH Web site at *http://www.ncfh.org/00_ns_rc_pateduc.shtml.* Explain why the topics, which include diabetes, healthy eating, alcohol, teen sex, work injuries, family planning, high blood pressure, skin emergencies, care of teeth, and tips to reduce stress, are appropriate for this population. All of these teaching materials can be downloaded in Spanish or in English. Considering language barriers and lack of health care knowledge, discuss the need for using simplicity and pictures in teaching these topics to migrant families. Perhaps, if you live near a migrant camp, you could organize a project with groups of students to implement much-needed teaching strategies using this educational material.

3. The Hispanic Stress Inventory—Brief Version tool presented in Display 33–1 lists migrant-specific stressor items. How are these items unique to the migrant lifestyle? How are they different from yours?

4. Changes in the structure of health care and social services greatly affect farmworkers' access to care. Many states are choosing to limit the access of both legal and undocumented immigrants to social and health services. For example, federal food stamps were discontinued for hundreds of thousands of legal immigrants in Texas without plans for alternatives. Many migrant farmworkers return to Texas after 6 months of working in the northern states but cannot find work in the off-season. During this time, they rely on food stamps. Without food stamps, many migrant families will go hungry in the winter. Suggest ways to advocate for this group, and discuss implementing methods to ensure that health and nutritional needs can be met.

5. Compare and contrast health, living, and working concerns between migrant workers and recent immigrants. Discuss how many recent immigrants from places such as Asia, Kosovo, or Iraq experience the same hardships as migrant workers do. How does nomadic lifestyle affect and differentiate the needs of migrant workers and recent immigrants?

REFERENCES

Alderete, E., Vega, W.A., Kolody, B., & Aguilar-Gaxiola, D. (2000). Lifetime prevalence of and risk factors for psychiatric disorders among Mexican migrant farmworkers in California. *American Journal of Public Health, 90*(4),608–614.

Artemis, L. (1996). Migrant health care: Creativity in primary care. *Advanced Practice Nursing Quarterly, 2*(2), 45–49.

Barat, L. (1999). Management of the febrile migrant farmworker. *Streamline: The Migrant Health News Source, 4*(6), 1–4.

Camacho, L. (1998). Battered women and U. S. immigration policy: The Violence Against Women Act. *Streamline: The Migrant Health News Source, 4*(1), 2–3.

Castro, J. (1999). Migrant health programs: Essential component in health care [online]. *Migrant Health Newsline, 16*(l). Retrieved February 12, 2004, from *http://www.ncfh.org/newsline/99-01.htm#article2*

Cole, A., & Crawford, L. (1991). Implementation and evaluation of the health resource program for migrant women in the Americus, Georgia area. In A. Bushy (Ed.), *Rural nursing* (Vol. 1, pp. 364–374). Newbury Park: Sage.

Coughlin, S.S., & Wilson, K.M. (2002). Breast and cervical cancer screening among migrant and seasonal farmworkers: A review. *Cancer Detection and Prevention, 26(3),* 203–206.

Environmental Protection Agency. (2004). Citizen's guide to pest control and pesticide safety. Retrieved 4/10/04 from *http://www.epa.gov/oppfeadl/publications/cit_guide/cityvide.pdf*

Flores, G., Fuentes-Afflick, E., Barbot, O., Carter-Pokras, O., Claudio, L., Lara, M., et al. (2002). The health of Latino children: Urgent priorities, unanswered questions, and a research agenda. *Journal of the American Medical Association, 288*(1), 82–90.

Garcia, D. (1997). Assessing stress among migrant and seasonal farmworkers. *Streamline: The Migrant Health News Source, 3*(5), 1–5.

Gwyther, M., & Jenkins, M. (1998). Migrant farmworker children: Health status, barriers to care, and nursing innovations in health care delivery. *Journal of Pediatric Health, 12*(2), 60–66.

Hawkins, D. (2001). Migrant health issues—Introduction. National Center for Farmworkers Health, Inc. Retrieved 4/10/04 from *http://www.ncfh.org/docs/00%20-%20intro.pdf*

Health Resources and Services Administration. (2004). A plan of action for improving the health of migrant and seasonal farm workers [online]. Retrieved 4/10/04 from *http://www.hrsa.gov/migrant/migrant.html*

Hirsch, J.S., Higgins, J., Bentley, M.E., & Nathanson, C.A. (2002). The social constructions of sexuality: Marital infidelity and sexually transmitted disease—HIV risk in a Mexican migrant community. *American Journal of Public Health, 92*(8), 1227–1237.

Hovey, J.S., & Magana, C.G. (2002). Exploring the mental health of Mexican migrant farm workers in the Midwest: Psychosocial predictors of psychological distress and suggestions for prevention and treatment. *Journal of Psychology, 136*(5), 493–513.

Jorn, E., & Ros, R. (2004). Beth-El mission serves farmworkers in Florida [online]. Retrieved 4/10/04 from *http://beth-el.info*

Kerr, M.J., Lusk, S.L., & Ronis, D.L. (2002). Explaining Mexican American workers' hearing protection use with the health promotion model. *Nursing Research, 51*(2), 100–109.

Leigh, J.P., McCurdy, S.A., & Schenker, M.B. (2001). Costs of occupational injuries in agriculture, *Public Health Reports, 116*(3), 235–248.

McCarthy, M. (2000). Fighting for public health along the USA-Mexico border. *The Lancet, 356,* 1020–1022.

McCauley, L.A., Sticker, D., Bryan, C., Lasarev, M.R., & Scherer, J.A. (2002). *Journal of Agricultural Safety & Health, 8*(4), 397–409.

National Center for Farmworker Health. (2003). *Quick facts.* Retrieved February 12, 2004, from *http://www.ncfh.org/factsheets.shtml*

National Council of La Raza. (1998). *Tuberculosis update: Fact sheet.* Washington, DC: NCLR.

National Migrant Resource Program and Migrant Clinicians Network. (1996). *Migrant and seasonal farmworker health objectives for the year 2000.* Austin, TX: U. S. Department of Health and Human Services and National Center for Farmworker Health, Inc.

Olmos, E., Ybarra, L., & Monterrey, M. (1999). *Americanos: Latino life in the United States.* Boston: Little, Brown.

Perilla, J., Wilson, A., Wold, J., & Spencer, L. (1998). Listening to migrant voices: Focus groups on health issues in South Georgia. *Journal of Community Health Nursing, 15*(4), 251–263.

Quandt, R.P., & Arcury, T.A. (2002). Hispanic farmworker interpretations of green tobacco sickness. *Journal of Rural Health, 18*(4), 503–511.

Rivera, J.A., Gonzalez-Cossio, T., Flores, M., Romero, M., Rivera, M, Tellez-Rojo, M.M., et al. (2001). Multiple micronutrient supplementation increases the growth of Mexican infants. *American Journal of Clinical Nutrition, 74,* 657–663.

Rodriguez, R. (1993). Violence in transience: Nursing care of battered women. *AWHONN's Clinical Issues, 4,* 437–440.

Sahlman, R., & Strandberg, D. (2003). *Cesar Chavez.* Retrieved 4/10/04 from *http://www.incwell.com./biographies/chavez.html*

Sandhaus, S. (1998). Migrant health: A harvest of poverty. *American Journal of Nursing, 98*(9), 52–54.

Spector, R.E. (2000). *Cultural diversity in health and illness* (5th ed.) Stamford, CT: Appleton & Lange.

U. S. Department of Health and Human Services. (2000). *Healthy People 2010* (Conference ed., in Vols. 1 & 2). Washington, DC: U. S. Government Printing Office.

Venes, D., & Thomas, C.L. (2001). *Taber's cyclopedic medical dictionary* (19th ed.). Philadelphia: F.A. Davis.

Watkins, E., Harlan, C., Eng, E., Gansky, S., Gehan, D., & Larson, K. (1994). Assessing the effectiveness of lay health advisors with migrant farmworkers. *Family and Community Health, 16,* 72–78.

Weinman, S. (1999). Heart Fax makes migrant patient records available worldwide [online]. *Migrant Health Newsline, 15*(3). Retrieved February 12, 2004, from *http://www.ncfh.org/newsline/99-05.htm#article1*

SELECTED READINGS

Berkowitz, B., & Wolff, T., (2000). *The spirit of the coalition.* Washington, DC: American Public Health Association.

Clendon, J., & White, G., (2001). The feasibility of a nurse practitioner-led primary health care clinic in a school setting: A community needs analysis. *Journal of Advanced Nursing 34*(2), 171–178.

Estill, C.F., Baron, S., & Steege, A.L. (2002). Research and dissemination needs for ergonomics in agriculture. *Public Health Reports, 117*(5), 440–445.

Flaskerud, J.H., Lesser, J., Dixon, E., Anderson, N., Conde, F., Kim, S., et al. (2002). Health disparities among vulnerable populations. *Nursing Research, 51*(2), 74–85.

Frates, J., Diringer, J., & Hoganm L. (2003). Models and momentum for insuring low-income, undocumented immigrant children in California. *Health Affairs, 22*(1), 259–263.

Hanson, V.D. (2003). *Mexifornia: A state of becoming.* San Francisco: Encounter Books.

Kelaher, M., & Jessop, D.J. (2002). Differences in low-birthweight among documented and undocumented foreign-born and US-born Latinas. *Social Science and Medicine, 55*(12), 2171–2175.

Liller, K.D., Noland, V., Rigal, P., Pesce, K., & Gonzalez, R. (2002). Development and evaluation of the Kids Count farm safety lesson. *Journal of Agricultural Safety and Health, 8*(4), 411–421.

McGregor, A. (compiler). (2001). *Remembering Cesar: The legacy of Cesar Chavez.* Fresno, CA: Quill Driver Books.

National Alliance for Hispanic Health. (2002, March 19). *Policy brief.* Healthy People 2010: *Hispanic concerns go unanswered.* Washington, DC: Author.

Porterfield, D.S., & Kinsinger, L. (2002). Quality of care for uninsured patients with diabetes in a rural area. *Diabetes Care, 25*(2), 319–323.

Rothenberg, D. (2001). *With these hands: The hidden world of migrant farmworkers today.* Berkeley: University of California Press.

Schneider, D.L., Steiner, R., & Romaine, J. (2003). Human cargo: Health conditions of Chinese migrants interdicted offshore by U. S. authorities. *Journal of Community Health, 28*(1), 19–39.

Shaokang, Z., Zhenweim S., & Blas, E. (2002). Economic transition and maternal health care for internal migrants in Shanghai, China. *Health Policy Planning, 17*(Suppl.), 47–55.

Steinbeck, J. (2002/1939) *The grapes of wrath* (John Steinbeck Centennial Edition, 1902–2002). New York: Penguin USA.

Zambrana, R.E., & Carter-Pokras, O.D. (2001). Health data issues for Hispanics. *Journal of Health Care of the Poor and Underserved, 12,* 20–34.

Zambrana, R.E., & Logie, L.A. (2000). Latino child health: Need for inclusion in the U. S. national discourse. *American Journal of Public Health, 90*(12), 1827–1833.

Internet Resources

Association of Occupational and Environmental Clinics: *http://www.aoec.org*

Migrant Clinicians Network: *http://www.migrantclinician.org*

National Alliance for Hispanic Health: *http://www.hispanichealth.org*

National Center for Farmworker Health, Inc.: *http://www.ncfh.org*

34

Clients With Disabilities and Chronic Illnesses

Learning Objectives

Upon mastery of this chapter, you should be able to:

- Discuss the national and global implications of disability and chronic illness.

- Describe the economic, social, and political factors affecting the well-being of individuals with disabilities and chronic illness.

- Provide an example of primary, secondary, and tertiary prevention practices for disabled individuals.

- Describe the Americans with Disabilities Act.

At some point in our lives, most of us will be diagnosed with a chronic illness or develop some type of disability. We may be lucky enough to get early diagnosis and treatment of our health conditions so that they can be easily managed. We might find ourselves temporarily incapacitated, unable to manage our daily lives, and needing assistance from others. We can hope our ability to resume more normal activities will return swiftly. An estimated 54 million Americans (almost 20% of the population) live with some ongoing level of disability (United States Department of Health and Human Services [USDHHS], 2001). The human costs associated with disabilities aside, the cost of direct medical care and indirect annual costs related to disability have reached almost $300 million in the United States alone.

The *Final Review of Healthy People 2000* (USDHHS, 2001) indicated that, although rates of some disabling conditions such as significant hearing and vision impairments decreased between 1991 and 2000, the rates of many other conditions either remained stable or increased. For instance, arthritis is currently the leading cause of disability in the United States. It affects approximately 43 million individuals and more than 20% of the adult population. Asthma, a growing national health concern, is responsible for approximately 500,000 hospitalizations, 5000 deaths, and 134 million restricted-activity days each year. Since 1991, the number of people with diabetes who have developed end-stage renal disease has almost tripled. For persons younger than 45 years of age, chronic back pain now ranks as the most frequent cause of limitations in activity, the second leading cause of physician visits, and the third most common cause of surgery (USDHHS, 2001). The need to address health issues of disability and chronic illness is vital to the well-being of affected individuals and families and crucial to the financial health of the country.

Health promotion and preventive efforts at every level are necessary and are discussed in this chapter. Although treatment of chronic conditions has long been a mainstay of health care in the United States and globally, little attention has been paid to the additional health promotion required to maintain and improve overall well-being of individuals with chronic conditions. Nor has enough attention been directed

---

RESEARCH: BRIDGE TO PRACTICE

HEALTH PROMOTION CLASSES FOR INDIVIDUALS WITH INTELLECTUAL DISABILITIES

Marshall, D., McConkey, R., & Moore, G. (2003). Obesity in people with intellectual disabilities: The impact of nurse-led health screenings and health promotion activities. *Journal of Advanced Nursing, 41,* 147–153.

The high rates of obesity in people with intellectual disabilities prompted this study of the impact of health promotion classes on weight loss. Physical health and well-being of individuals with intellectual disabilities has received much less attention than those of nondisabled populations. This two-part study focused on the impact of health screening versus health promotion classes directed at weight control, which discussed healthy eating and exercise. The initial sample included 464 individuals from Northern Ireland, 10 years of age and older, who were attending a special school or day center or living in a residential facility; 73% were assessed as fully mobile, 15% required assistance with walking, and 12% were wheelchair users.

Individuals were assessed for body mass index (BMI), hypertension, cholesterol, smoking, multiple risks, and referrals (to their general practitioner or provided with health promotion advice). Of those assessed, 64% of the adults were overweight or obese, an increase from 52% for this population 6 years previously. This sample received only health screening, and only one third of those identified as needing to lose weight took action, weight reduction was achieved only in three cases.

Conversely, a smaller sample (*n* = 25) was recruited to participate in health promotion sessions (six to eight 2-hour sessions), which focused on healthy eating and exercise. At initial evaluation, 20% were normal or underweight, 36% were overweight, 12% were obese, and 32% were very obese. After the intervention, 2 people who had been underweight were normal weight, 1 moved from the obese to the overweight category, and 3 very obese people were classified as obese.

The study's findings suggested that implementing a proactive approach with intellectually disabled persons can have positive results in weight reduction even over as short a period as 6 weeks. Identifying weight loss needs and high-risk status alone had very limited impact on those individuals in terms of normalizing weight. Overall, the study supports other research showing that people with intellectual disabilities suffer from higher levels of obesity than nondisabled persons do. Moreover, health screenings alone have a limited impact on improving obesity levels in this population. Taking an active role in providing health promotion education, even over a short period, appears much more effective in achieving the health goal of normalizing weight for intellectually disabled persons. The authors argue that suitable exercise and healthy eating activities are vital for improving the health and well-being of this population and should be encouraged.

to those same needs for people with physical or psychological disabilities (see Research: Bridge to Practice). This chapter begins with an overview of disabilities and chronic illnesses, and thereafter discusses the current national and global trends in addressing these issues. The various organizations that focus on improving the well-being of those affected, the impact on families, and the role of the community health nurse in addressing the health care needs of individuals, families, and aggregates are also discussed.

PERSPECTIVES ON DISABILITY, CHRONIC ILLNESS, AND HEALTH

What does the word *disabled* mean to you? What thoughts come to mind when you think about the word as it applies to an individual? It is defined in one dictionary as "the incapacity to do something because of a handicap—physical, mental, etc." (Morehead & Morehead, 1995). It is linked with *inability*, which is defined as "the lack of ability to do something, whatever the reason, but usually through incompetence, weakness, lack of training, etc." (Morehead & Morehead, 1995). **Handicap** is explained in the same volume as "any encumbrance or disadvantage". Each of these definitions provides a decidedly negative connotation, similar in nature to the typical societal view faced daily by people with disabilities.

Challenges differ from one individual to the next and require different degrees of accommodation. Fortunately, long-held negative views of disabled persons and their conditions are being replaced with new and more positive approaches that view individuals and their challenges from a more holistic standpoint.

International Classification of Functioning, Disability, and Health

One such change in thinking about disability and chronic illness was expressed in *International Classification of Functioning, Disability, and Health* (ICF), published by the World Health Organization (WHO) in 2001. This document, the result of 5 years of work, replaces *International Classification of Impairments, Disabilities, and Handicaps* (ICIDH) (WHO, 1980). Even the change in terminology in the title shows the dramatic shift in thinking by the World Health Assembly; both *impairments* and *handicaps* were removed. In the revised document, **disability** serves as a broad term for impairments, activity limitations, or participation restrictions. It is linked with **functioning**, a term that encompasses all body functions, activities, and participation.

The ICF is an attempt to provide a universal classification system with standardized language and a way to view the domains of health from a holistic vantage point. It takes into account (1) body functions and structures, (2) activities and participation, (3) environmental factors, and (4) personal factors. This allows a multidimensional evaluation of an individual's circumstances in terms of functioning, disability, and health. Melding the "medical model" of health and health care for disabled persons with the "social model," the ICF provides a biopsychosocial approach for assessing people with disabilities; emphasis is placed on the observation that no two people with the same disease or disability have the same level of functioning (see The Global Community).

The purpose of the ICF reaches far beyond simply categorizing the health status of people with disabilities. Specific aims of the document are stated as follows (WHO, 2001, p. 5):

• Provide a scientific basis for understanding and studying health and health-related states, outcomes, and determinations

THE GLOBAL COMMUNITY

MEASURING QUALITY OF LIFE IN CHRONICALLY ILL CHINESE PEOPLE

Hwu, Y., Coates, V.E., Boore, J.R.P., & Bunting, B.P. (2002). The Concept of Health Scale. Developed for Chinese people with chronic illness. *Nursing Research, 51*, 292–301.

Recognizing the paucity of information regarding the concept of health in Chinese people with chronic illness, a scale was developed to help measure this concept. Utilizing a two-stage process, the tool was initially developed and tested with 80 Taiwanese individuals who were older than 20 years of age, spoke Mandarin, and had been diagnosed with a chronic illness for a minimum of 1 year. The resulting 34-item self-report questionnaire was then tested with a convenience sample of 372 individuals meeting the same criteria.

The overall study findings were as follows. The concept of health for this population was identified in structural terms as a construct with three dimensions: physical, psychological, and spiritual. From a cultural aspect, health was related to the specific first-order factors of (1) independence, (2) physical functioning, (3) contentment in social interaction, (4) zest for life, (5) serenity, and (6) meaning. Viewing the concept of health in this population from a cultural perspective, the meaning of health was a comprehensive term that referred to a broad range of quality-of-life factors. This holistic approach is consistent with a belief that harmony is achieved through the interaction of the individual, the society, and the natural universe. The researchers suggested further testing of the scale to determine whether quality of life measures are higher for patients with a positive concept of health than for patients with a more negative concept, as well as testing with different cultural groups.

- Establish a common language for describing health and health-related states in order to improve communication between different users such as health care workers, researchers, policy makers, and the public, including people with disabilities
- Permit comparison of data across countries, health care disciplines, services, and time
- Provide a systematic coding scheme for health information systems

The document provides a roadmap for using the ICF, based on experience with the ICIDH for more than 20 years. Table 34–1 shows the current and potential uses of the document by various entities ranging from insurance companies and health care providers to policy makers and educators.

In addition to the definitions of disability and functioning discussed previously, the following definitions serve to explain the ICF in terms of health (WHO, 2001, p. 10):

- **Body functions** are the physiologic functions of body systems and include psychological functions.
- **Body structures** are anatomic parts of the body such as organs, limbs, and their components.
- **Impairments** are problems in body function or structure, such as a significant deviation or loss.
- **Activity** is the execution of a task or action by an individual.
- **Participation** is involvement in a life situation, including personal and interpersonal roles and activities.
- **Activity limitations** are difficulties an individual may have in executing activities.
- **Participation restrictions** are problems an individual may experience when involved in life situations.
- **Environmental factors** make up the physical, social, and attitudinal environments in which people live and conduct their lives.
- **Personal factors** are the features of an individual's background, life, and living that are not part of a health condition or health status, such as gender, race, age, other health

TABLE 34–1

Applications of the International Classification of Functioning, Disability, and Health

Statistical Tool	Collection and recording of data: • Population studies & surveys • Management information systems
Research Tool	Measure: • Outcomes • Quality of life • Environmental factors
Clinical Tool	• Needs assessment • Matching treatments with specific conditions • Vocational assessment • Rehabilitation • Outcome evaluation
Social Policy Tool	• Social security planning • Compensation systems • Policy design and implementation
Educational Tool	• Curriculum design • Raising awareness • Undertaking social action

(From World Health Organization. [2001]. *International classification of functioning, disability and health.* Geneva, Switzerland: Author.)

conditions, fitness, lifestyle habits, upbringing, coping styles, social background, education, profession, past and current experience, overall behavior pattern and character style, individual psychological assets, and other characteristics—all or any of which may play a role in disability at any level.

For the community health nurse, the ICF facilitates assessment of an individual client based on a wide range of factors. The disability or disease is just one factor to be considered in planning and implementing a care plan for clients in

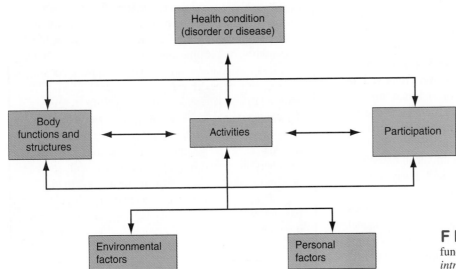

FIGURE 34–1. Model of functioning and disability. (WHO. [2001]. *ICF introduction.* Geneva, Switzerland: Author.)

the community. Two individuals may have the same disability, such as a below-the-knee amputation, but their health and well-being can be quite different. One may have a more positive or a more cynical outlook, one may have more social support than the other, or one may suffer more than the other from additional health issues that impede rehabilitation. What the community health nurse must always consider is the totality of the situation, including the biologic, psychological, sociocultural, and environmental realms. Diseases and disabilities are conditions, yet a client may often be referred to as "the paraplegic" or "the amputee" and not by his or her name. This type of designation should be avoided: a disease or disability is something one has, not something one is. Figure 34–1 depicts the interactions among the various components addressed by the ICF in evaluation and assessment of clients with disabilities. It can serve as a useful model for community health nursing practice in the overall assessment of people with disabilities.

The World Health Report

The 2002 release of the annual report by WHO (*The World Health Report 2002: Reducing Risks, Promoting Healthy Life*) set a new standard for addressing global health. It challenges the world community to focus more attention on unhealthy behaviors that lead ultimately to chronic disease, disability, and early mortality. The report stresses that although infectious diseases and malnutrition require ongoing vigilance because they continue to plague many parts of the world, they are not the only threat. It is increasingly clear that lifestyle choices play a major role in morbidity and mortality levels in affluent and poor countries alike, and intervention at all levels (local, national and international) is a high priority. With this new reality in mind, this document has a twofold purpose: (1) to quantify the most important risks to health and (2) to assess the cost-effectiveness of interventions designed to reduce those risks. The overall goal is "to help governments of all countries lower these risks and raise the healthy life expectancy of their populations" (WHO, 2002, p. 7).

No longer can health care providers across the globe continue to address acute illness by itself; lifestyle and behavior must be considered because of the impact they have on healthy years of life. The risks to health that the WHO report focused on include some that are the direct result of poverty, but many can be more aptly linked to excesses, notably in the more affluent countries. The 10 leading health risks are (1) underweight, (2) unsafe sex, (3) high blood pressure, (4) tobacco consumption, (5) alcohol consumption, (6) unsafe water, sanitation, and hygiene, (7) iron deficiency, (8) indoor smoke from solid fuels, (9) high cholesterol, and (10) obesity. Globally, these 10 health risks are responsible for more than 33% of all deaths and untold disability. Half of these risks—tobacco and alcohol consumption, high blood pressure, high cholesterol, and obesity—can be directly related to lifestyle and behavioral choices.

Nutrition is vital to health; nutritional imbalances can lead to severe chronic illness, disability, and premature death. Of the leading 10 health risks, 5 are directly related to consumption: underweight, hypertension, iron deficiency, high cholesterol, and obesity. The prevalence of obesity worldwide is estimated at more than 1 billion adults, with some 300 million who can be classified as clinically obese. In stark contrast, there are 170 million underweight children in poor countries, more than 3 million of whom will die each year from malnutrition. Being overweight increases the risk of coronary heart disease, stroke, diabetes, and some types of cancer. Malnutrition and the lack of important nutrients can lead to a wide array of preventable disabilities. For instance, the leading cause of acquired blindness in children is vitamin A deficiency, and the leading cause of mental retardation and brain damage is iodine deficiency (WHO, 2002).

The significance of the WHO report lies in its simplicity. If countries can make even minimal strides in improving the health of their citizens, a dramatic improvement in health outlook can occur within those countries and worldwide. What is required is for governments to take a proactive role in addressing the preventive health care needs of their citizens (Display 34–1). A shift in focus from the most high-risk individuals to the general population is essential. Primary and secondary prevention as the main focus is the approach that public health care professionals have stressed for decades. As difficult as it has been in the United States to im-

---

D I S P L A Y   3 4 – 1

WHO Recommendations to Improve Global Health

- Government/health ministry support for scientific research, improved surveillance systems, and better access to global information
- Development of effective, committed policies for the prevention of health risks such as tobacco consumption, unsafe sex associated with HIV/AIDS, and unhealthy diet and obesity
- Implementation of cost-effectiveness analysis to identify the most cost-effective and affordable interventions to reduce priority health risks
- Collaborative efforts (intersectoral and international) to reduce major extraneous risk to health caused by unsafe water, poor sanitation, or lack of education
- Supportive and balanced approach in addressing these major health risks that includes government, community, and individual action
- Empowerment and encouragement of individuals to make positive, life-enhancing health decisions (such as eliminating tobacco use, excessive alcohol consumption, unhealthy diet, and unsafe sex)

Adapted from World Health Organization. (2002). *The world health report 2002: Reducing risks, promoting healthy life.* Geneva, Switzerland: Author.

plement a shift in emphasis to health promotion efforts, it will be interesting to see if this "call to action" by WHO will result in less emphasis on tertiary prevention. The old adage, "An ounce of prevention is worth a pound of cure," is most appropriate for the years ahead.

Taken together, the ICF and the 2002 WHO report set a standard for health care in the 21st century. Chronic disease and disability prevention are vital to world health. The cost of health care treatment is high, but the cost in terms of lost productivity and decreased quality of life is even higher. Without control of preventable disability and chronic disease, these conditions could very well become the "new plagues" of the coming decades.

Healthy People 2010

The most influential document addressing health in the United States is *Healthy People 2010* (USDHHS, 2000), which defines areas of health and well-being that are most in need of attention. With its clearly delineated and measurable objectives, *Healthy People 2010* has far-reaching influence on national and state health initiatives, health care policy, research priorities, and funding. In terms of disability and chronic illness, *Healthy People 2010* has placed added emphasis on conditions expected to take a toll on the nation's health in the coming years. It also reflects a growing realization by health care providers, insurance companies, public health agencies, and health care facilities of the need to act proactively to avoid the economic toll that lack of attention can produce (see Bridging Financial Gaps).

It is difficult to discuss *Healthy People 2010* (USDHHS, 2000) without some mention of *Healthy People 2000* (USDHHS, 1991). A comparison of the two documents reveals some striking differences regarding disabilities and chronic conditions. Increased attention has been given to the growing national need to reduce the incidence of disability and chronic disease and improve the health of people affected by them. In *Healthy People 2000,* only one priority area was devoted to disability and chronic illness. Priority Area 17, "Diabetes and Chronic Disabling Conditions," emphasized diabetes with only limited attention to the broader range of other disabilities (asthma, chronic kidney disease, arthritis, deformities or orthopedic impairments, mental retardation, peptic ulcer disease, visual and hearing impairments, and overweight). In contrast, almost half of the *Healthy People 2010* focus areas directly address chronic illness and disability, and almost all of the focus areas can be related to these issues in some manner. Moreover, the section on "Disability and Secondary Conditions" is devoted exclusively to issues most relevant to people with disabilities.

The definition of **disability** in *Healthy People 2010* is somewhat different and more explicit than that used in the ICF (WHO, 2001); it is stated as "the general term used to represent the interactions between individuals with a health condition and barriers in their environment" (USDHHS, 2000, p. 25). Moreover, **people with disabilities** are "identified as having an activity limitation or who use assistance or

BRIDGING FINANCIAL GAPS

MANAGING CHRONIC ILLNESS TO IMPROVE HEALTH AND CONTROL COSTS

Rapaport, L. (2003, June 22). CalPERS seeks proof of payoff from prevention. *The Valley Times*, p. A5.

The California Public Employees' Retirement System (CalPERS) is planning to make disease management the centerpiece of its health program beginning in 2004. In an effort to improve the health of its workers and reduce insurance expenditures, all identified chronically ill patients enrolled in the system will be tracked in an effort to keep them from getting sicker. The two health maintenance organizations (HMOs) now contracted by CalPERS (Kaiser and Blue Shield) will be required to provide programs for asthma, diabetes, cardiovascular disease, and depression. Profit margins for those HMOs will now be directly tied to their ability to both treat and track those members enrolled in select disease management programs, with the added caveat that the data show improvement in the health of those patients. The benefit to the two HMOs was that they were now the sole health care options available to the enrollees, as opposed to more than a dozen companies available just a few years ago. CalPERS is also planning to spend $12 million on a new data warehouse to track every doctor visit, hospitalization, and prescription to determine whether the new effort is providing real benefits. The question remains: Will disease management provide cost savings to the system? The overriding goal of improved quality of life for the CalPERS members and cost control for the system are clearly at issue. The results will undoubtedly provide a clearer path to managing chronic illnesses in the coming years and will influence chronic disease management all over the country, not just in California.

who perceive themselves as having a disability" (USDHHS, 2000, p. 6–25).

This change in emphasis between the two documents was noted in *Healthy People 2010* (USDHHS, 2000), which cited lack of parity between disabled and nondisabled populations in terms of several selected objectives: leisure-time activity, use of community support programs, and receipt of clinical preventive services. One such example was the finding that the percentage of people with disabilities who reported some type of leisure-time activity was the lowest of any of the groups identified (including those older than 65 years of age and low-income persons). On the positive side, the percentage of people with disabilities who reported no leisure-time physical activity actually declined from the

T A B L E   3 4 – 2

Healthy People 2010: Disability and Secondary Conditions—Objectives

- Include in the core of all relevant Healthy People 2010 surveillance instruments a standardized set of questions that identify "people with disabilities"
- Reduce the proportion of children and adolescents with disabilities who are reported to be sad, unhappy, or depressed
- Reduce the proportion of adults with disabilities who report feelings such as sadness, unhappiness, or depression that prevent them from being active
- Increase the proportion of adults with disabilities who participate in social activities
- Increase the proportion of adults with disabilities reporting sufficient emotional support
- Increase the proportion of adults with disabilities reporting satisfaction with life
- Reduce the number of people with disabilities in congregate care facilities, consistent with permanency planning principles
- Eliminate disparities in employment rates between working-age adults with and without disabilities
- Increase the proportion of children and youth with disabilities who spend at least 80% of their time in regular education programs
- Increase the proportion of health and wellness and treatment programs and facilities that provide full access for people with disabilities
- Reduce the proportion of people with disabilities who report not having the assistive devices and technology needed
- Reduce the proportion of people with disabilities reporting barriers to participation in home, school, work, or community activities
- Increase the number of Tribes, States, and the District of Columbia that have public health surveillance and health promotion programs for people with disabilities and caregivers

(From U. S. Department of Health and Human Services. [2000]. *Healthy people 2010: Understanding and improving health.* Washington, DC: U.S. Government Printing Office.)

1985 level of 35% to 29% in 1995, although it was still far short of the 2000 target of 20%. Additional disparities noted for people with disabilities included increased likelihood of being overweight, adverse effects from stress, and reduced rates of preventive services (eg, tetanus boosters, Pap tests, breast examinations, and mammograms). Recognition that the health needs of disabled persons were not receiving needed attention resulted in placement of high priority on improvement of the health of people with disabilities.

Improving the health of the nation requires a multifaceted approach to improve parity among all individuals. *Healthy People 2010* states that "every person in every community across the nation deserves equal access to comprehensive, culturally competent, community-based health care systems that are committed to serving the needs of the individual and promoting community health" (USDHHS, 2000, p. 16). The goal of *Healthy People 2010* specific to disabled persons is to "promote the health of people with disabilities, prevent secondary conditions, and eliminate disparities between people with and without disabilities in the U. S. pop-

ulation" (USDHHS, 2000, p. 6-8). Thirteen individual objectives have been selected to measure progress toward this goal (Table 34–2). What is most significant about the changes in the *Healthy People 2010* objectives specific to disabled persons is the emphasis on healthy life-years and improved quality of life, similar to the recommendations by WHO (2002). Although the issues of function stressed in the ICF (WHO, 2001) were not as explicit in *Healthy People 2010*, the 13 objectives indicate a growing emphasis on a holistic approach that recognizes that life satisfaction is just as important to health and well-being as preventive services. It also indicates a growing realization that healthy life-years for persons with disabilities equate to decreased health costs at local, state, and national levels, just as they do for persons without disabilities.

CIVIL RIGHTS LEGISLATION

Policies such as *Healthy People 2010* are important features of an overall plan to address the health of people with disabilities and chronic diseases in the United States. Although it has a great deal of influence on the direction and type of programs initiated, policy alone cannot assure individuals with disabilities that the needed services and accommodations are or will be available. As has often been the case, an act of legislation is vital to ensure that every individual's rights are protected and that legal recourse is available if such protection is denied. The struggle for civil rights for disabled persons in this country is still in its infancy, but it has begun to gain the level of attention that racial and gender equality receive. As is true for other issues of equality, legislation is only the first of many steps that must be taken.

The **Americans with Disabilities Act** (ADA) was signed into law in 1990 to protect the civil liberties of the many Americans living with disabilities (see Chapters 15 and 29). This legislation was the result of a long and difficult struggle. Individuals with disabilities and their advocates made their voices heard by repeatedly demanding an end to inferior treatment and lack of equal protection under the law that impeded their daily lives. The ADA set the standard for a number of subsequent laws that, together with pre-ADA legislation, offer a broad spectrum of protections for disabled persons. These additional laws are listed in Table 34–3 and cover a variety of issues, including telecommunications, architectural barriers, and voter registration.

The ADA essentially "prohibits discrimination on the basis of disability in employment, state and local government, public accommodations, commercial facilities, transportation, and telecommunications [and] also applies to the United States Congress" (United States Department of Justice [USDOJ], 2002, p. 3). For an individual to be protected under the ADA, he or she must have a disability or some type of relationship or association with an individual who has a disability. The definition of a disabled person used in the application of the ADA is "a person who has a physical or mental impairment that substantially limits one or more major life activities, a person who has a history or record of such an impairment, or a person who is perceived by others as having such an impairment" (USDOJ, 2002, p. 2). A listing of the specific impairments covered under the law is notably absent, leaving open a broad range of interpretations and legal challenges with respect to who is actually covered.

T A B L E   3 4 – 3

Disability Rights Laws

Law	Summary	Contact
Telecommunications Act of 1996	Equipment and services are accessible	Federal Communications Commission (FCC)
Fair Housing Act (amended 1988)	Prohibits housing discrimination	U. S. Department of Housing and Urban Development (HUD)
Air Carrier Access Act	Prohibits discrimination in air transportation by domestic and foreign carriers	U. S. Department of Transportation
Voting Accessibility for the Elderly and Handicapped Act of 1984	Requires polling places to be physically accessible for federal elections	U. S. Department of Justice—Civil Rights Division
National Voter Registration Act of 1993	"Motor Voter Act"— makes it easier to vote by increasing low registration rates by minorities and persons with disabilities	U. S. Department of Justice—Civil Rights Division
Individuals with Disabilities Education Act	Make available free public education in the least restrictive environment for all children with disabilities	U. S. Department of Education—Office of Special Education Programs
Rehabilitation Act	Prohibits discrimination in all federal programs or programs receiving federal financial assistance	Agency's Equal Employment Opportunity Office U. S. Department of Labor—Office of Federal Contract Compliance Programs U. S. Department of Justice
Architectural Barriers Act	Buildings constructed or altered with federal funds must meet federal accessibility standards	U. S. Architectural and Transportation Barriers Compliance Board

(From U. S. Department of Justice. [2002]. *A guide to disability rights laws.* Available at: *http://www.usdoj.gov/crt.ada.cguide.htm*)

Although there is ongoing debate as to who is actually protected by the ADA, there is an equal amount of confusion as to who is actually required to comply with the provisions of the act and what specific actions are necessary. The following is a short summary of the ADA. All employers, including religious organizations with 15 or more employees, are subject to the act, as are all activities of state and local governments irrespective of size. Before 1994, the act applied only to employers with 25 or more employees. Public transportation, businesses that provide public accommodation, and telecommunications entities are all required to provide access for individuals with disabilities. It is important to note that the ADA does not override federal and state health and safety laws. However, successful legal challenges to those statutes have been made when they were clearly outdated or when it could be argued that the public safety was not actually at risk in a specific situation. There are considerable gray areas within the ADA, leaving open the prospect of challenges by those who are subject to the law and those who are protected by it.

Individuals who believe that their legal rights under the ADA have been violated may seek remedy by filing a lawsuit or submitting a complaint to one of four federal offices, depending on the specific type of alleged violation: (1) the U. S. Department of Justice—Civil Rights Division, (2) any U. S. Equal Employment Opportunity Commission field office, (3) the Office of Civil Rights—Federal Transit Administration, or (4) the Federal Communications Commission. The process for filing a complaint is not a simple task, and many seek the assistance of attorneys, legal aid societies, or various private organizations, some of which are discussed later in this chapter (see What Do You Think?).

WHAT DO YOU THINK?

The responsibility of the U. S. Department of Justice, Office of Civil Rights (OCR), is to investigate complaints of alleged violations of the Americans with Disabilities Act (ADA). An example of one of those complaints involved a 22-year-old Connecticut woman with cerebral palsy. She had been placed in a nursing home because of changes in her living situation and health care status and wanted to move back into the community. The OCR intervened to ensure that the woman secured appropriate housing and that counseling and intensive case management services were in place when she moved back into the community. Without the protection afforded under the ADA, the outcome could have been much different.

(From U. S. Department of Health and Human Services. [2003, May]. *Delivering on the promise: OCR's compliance activities promote community integration.* Available at: *http://www.hhs.gov/ocr/comlianceactiv.html*)

In a report on the enforcement history of the ADA between its inception and 1999, the National Council on Disability (NCD) noted that many of the federal agencies charged with protecting the civil rights of disabled persons suffered from insufficient funding and lack of a coherent and unifying national strategy (NCD, 2000). NCD recommendations included clarification of specific elements that provide a basis for evaluating agency performance and thereby serve to improve the full expression of the law as it was intended. These 11 elements or criteria are (1) proactive and reactive strategies, (2) communication with consumers and complainants, (3) policy and subregulatory guidance, (4) enforcement actions, (5) strategic litigation, (6) timely resolution of complaints, (7) competent and credible investigative processes, (8) technical assistance for protected persons and covered entities, (9) adequate agency resources, (10) interagency collaboration and coordination, and (11) outreach and consultation with the community.

It is important to those with disabilities and the professionals that serve them that a structure is in place to provide protection under the law, but this does not preclude discrimination, nor does the existence of such a structure suggest that immediate remedies will be available. Laws aside, the most difficult aspect of change comes when attempts are made to alter the perceptions and misunderstandings of others about people with disabilities. Voices from the Community offers one such example.

ORGANIZATIONS SERVING THE NEEDS OF THE DISABLED AND CHRONICALLY ILL

Although the impact of civil rights legislation cannot be underestimated, it did not come about without demands for change from the chorus of voices of all those who deal on a daily basis with the issue of disability (the individuals themselves, their families, coworkers, employers, and advocates). Without the hard work of those individuals and groups, it is unlikely that the efforts envisioned and accomplished by legislation would have occurred. Much of the credit for the legislative focus belongs to advocacy groups. The following section provides an overview of some of the groups that advocate for the disabled and chronically ill and their families. In serving those specific populations, they offer others an opportunity to learn more about the lives and struggles of disabled persons. Each of the organizations listed offers a wide range of information, some of which can be accessed via the Internet. For community health nurses, these organizations provide a starting point for exploring specific topics pertinent to practice. They also can be a source of valuable information for clients and families to access on their own. Families that cannot afford Internet service or computers can use them at public libraries, most of which now offer this service. Many Internet sites are not reliable or accurate, so it is important for the nurse to prescreen any specific sites that are recommended to clients and their families.

VOICES FROM THE COMMUNITY

I was always such an active and healthy person, so when I was diagnosed with multiple sclerosis it hit me like a ton of bricks. Here I was with two small children and I was only 30 years old; it just wasn't fair. Some days are good and some days are just awful. I finally broke down and applied for one of those disabled parking stickers. The doctor had to approve it, and he said it was a good thing to help me save my energy for the important things, like taking care of my family. I hated to use it, but I was just getting so tired. What is so awful are the looks on people's faces when I park in the special areas near the door. I know I don't look like I'm sick. I just hate those looks—I can hear them saying under their breath, "She can't be sick . . . I'll bet that sticker is for a family member and she's just abusing it—how lazy!" If I wasn't so tired I'd park in the regular parking places.

Pat N., Tampa, Florida

Government

The *National Council on Disability* (NCD) is an independent federal agency that is tasked with making recommendations to the President and to Congress about issues that face Americans with disabilities. The NCD has 15 Presidential appointees (all confirmed by the U. S. Senate), whose charge is to promote "policies, programs, practices, and procedures that guarantee equal opportunity for all individuals with disabilities, regardless of the nature or severity of the disability, and to empower individuals with disabilities to achieve economic self-sufficiency, independent living, and inclusion and integration into all aspects of society" (NCD, 2003, p. 1). In its 1986 report, *Toward Independence,* the NCD proposed that Congress should enact a civil rights law for people with disabilities; the result was the 1990 ADA.

Private

Many private organizations—local, national, and international—deal with a variety of disabilities and chronic diseases. Many of the better-known organizations such as the American Heart Association and the American Cancer Association are discussed in other chapters of this book and therefore are not covered here. Instead, examples of groups that deal most directly with disability and chronic illness are described. The reader is encouraged to search the Internet or other print resources for additional entities that deal with specific disabilities or chronic illnesses.

The **National Association of the Deaf** (NAD), headquartered in Washington, D. C., is a private, nonprofit organization that was established in 1880. As the oldest U. S. organization serving this population, it has the stated purpose of "safeguarding the accessibility and civil rights of 28 million deaf and hard-of-hearing Americans in education, employment, health care, and telecommunications" (NAD, 2003, p. 1). Specific programs and activities that NAD is involved with include advocacy, captioned media, certification of **American Sign Language** (ASL) professionals and interpreters, legal assistance, and policy development and research (NAD, 2003). Two goals of the 1993 *NAD Position Paper on ASL and Bilingual Education* (NAD, 1993) are the official recognition of ASL as an indigenous language and the implementation of bilingual education (ASL and English) for deaf children in the nation's schools. ASL uses "handshapes" to communicate ideas and concepts; it is used primarily in America and Canada by the deaf community (Grayson, 2003). Display 34–2 offers a brief summary of sign languages.

The *National Organization on Disability* (NOD), headquartered in Washington, D.C., has as its mission statement "to expand the participation and contribution of America's 54 million men, women, and children with disabilities in all aspects of life" (NOD, 2002a, p.1). An important contribution of NOD is the *2000 NOD/Harris Survey of Americans with Disabilities,* which sought to quantify the gaps between people with and without disabilities in terms of employment, income, education, health care, access to transportation, entertainment or going out, socializing, attending religious services, political participation/voter registration, life satisfaction, and trends (NOD, 2002b). One of the most notable findings of the study was that improvements in education and employment have been made for people with disabilities over that last decade (1990–2000). Nonetheless, people with disabilities are more likely than nondisabled persons to have low incomes. The NOD Web site connects visitors to a rich variety of sources on community involvement, economic/employment topics, and access issues (*http://www.nod.org*).

The *American Council of the Blind* (ACB) was founded in 1961 and states as its purpose, "to improve the well-being of all blind and visually impaired people" (ACB, 2003, p.1). Services advertised by the organization include information and referral, scholarship assistance, public education, and industry consultation, as well as governmental monitoring, consultation, and advocacy. Some of the major issues that are currently being pursued by the organization include improved education and rehabilitation for the blind and increased production and use of reading materials for the blind and visually impaired.

Guide Dogs for the Blind is a nonprofit charitable organization established to train and make available guide dogs for the visually impaired (Guide Dogs for the Blind, 2003). The dogs and services are free, and the organization relies on donations. It currently has two training sites, one in California and one in Oregon, with puppy raisers located throughout the Western states. The organization can be reached through its Web site at *http://www.guidedogs.com*.

Another organization dealing with issues affecting the blind and visually impaired is the *National Federation of the Blind* (NFB). Founded in 1940, it seeks to help "blind persons achieve self-confidence and self-respect and to act as a vehicle for collective self-expression by the blind" (NFB, 2003a, p.1). Citing the need for assistance to the more than 1.1 million people in the United States who are blind, the organization fulfills its mission by providing public education, information and referral, and support for increased availability of materials in **Braille** (Display 34–3).

The oldest organization devoted to eliminating barriers for the blind and visually impaired is the *American Foundation for the Blind* (AFB), which was founded in 1921. The AFB advocates for the visually impaired through increased

DISPLAY 34–2

Sign Languages in Brief

- Sign languages are not universal
- Sign language is the use of "handshapes" and gestures to communicate ideas or concepts
- American Sign Language is a unique language with its own rules of grammar and syntax
- American Sign Language is primarily used in America and Canada and is the natural language of the deaf community
- International Sign Language (Gestuno) is composed of vocabulary signs from various sign languages for use at international events or meetings to aid communication
- Systems of Manually Coded English (ie, Signed English, Signing Exact English) are not natural languages but systems designed to represent the translation of spoken language word for word

(From Grayson, G. [2003]. *Talking with your hands, listening with your eyes. A complete photographic guide to American Sign Language.* Garden City Park, NY: Square One Publishers.)

DISPLAY 34–3

What is Braille?

Braille takes its name from Louise Braille, an 18-year-old blind Frenchman who created a system of raised dots for reading and writing by modifying a system used on board sailing ships for night reading. Persons experienced in Braille can read at speeds of 200 to 400 words per minute, comparable to print readers. Braille consists of arrangements of dots to form symbols. The text can be written either by hand with a slate and stylus, with a Braille writing machine, or with the use of specialized computer software and a Braille embossing device attached to the printer.

(From National Federation of the Blind. [2003b]. *What is Braille and what does it mean to the blind?* Available at: *http://www.nfb.org/books/book1/ifbnd03.htm*)

funding at the federal and state levels in areas such as rehabilitation research for older, visually impaired persons; improved literacy for the visually impaired, including use of Braille and assistive technology; improved employment opportunities; and increased accessibility of technology. In addition, AFB houses the Helen Keller Archives, which contain her correspondence, photographs, and various personal items and documents (AFB, 2002).

The *American Obesity Association* (AOA) sees as its goal, "to address obesity as a public health concern and to remove the barriers to treatment through vigorous advocacy and education" (AOA, 2002). The organization addresses such issues as the need for attention to the impact of obesity on death and disability and for increased research, improved insurance coverage, and elimination of discrimination and mistreatment of people with obesity. The organization's Web site (*http://www.obesity.org*) offers informational literature covering topics that range from the global problem of obesity to Social Security benefits for obesity-related disability.

HEALTH PROMOTION AND PREVENTION NEEDS OF THE DISABLED AND CHRONICALLY ILL

Misconceptions Impede Improvement

Earlier, the influence of *Healthy People 2010* as it relates to people with disabilities was discussed. One of the most influential aspects of the document is its emphasis on a change in thinking within the health care community about the health promotion needs of people with disabilities. This shift is needed because the lack of health promotion and disease prevention activities for this population leads to an increase in the number and extent of **secondary conditions**, defined as "medical, social, emotional, mental, family, or community problems that a person with a disabling condition likely experiences" (USDHHS, 2000, p. 6–25). Approaching the health needs of disabled persons from the traditional standpoint of asking what medical, rehabilitative, or long-term care is needed has failed to reduce illness or improve the overall well-being of the disabled or chronically ill. Moreover, a number of misconceptions have resulted that impede progress in this area: (1) that all people with disabilities have poor health, (2) that public health activities need to focus only on preventing disability, (3) that there is no need for a clear definition of "disability" or "people with disabilities" in public health practice, and (4) that environment does not play a significant role in the disability process. Increased national attention to the needs of the disabled (those needs specific to disabled persons as well as needs that are universal to all) should greatly improve the outlook. This change of focus is clearly evident in the definition of **health promotion** used in *Healthy People 2010:* "efforts to create healthy lifestyles and

a healthy environment to prevent medical and other secondary conditions, such as teaching people how to address their health care needs and increasing opportunities to participate in usual life activities" (USDHHS, 2000, p. 6–25).

Missed Opportunities by Health Care Providers or Missed Opportunities to Affect Quality of Life

In this age of rapid growth in technology, it is easy to forget that clean water is a far more important commodity than having the latest prescription drug or surgical procedure. All of us, whether healthy, disabled, or chronically ill, require some basic elements to maintain health. Those elements are the same all over the world and include clean air and water, a safe place to live, sunshine, exercise, nutritious food, socialization, and the opportunity to be successful in life's pursuits. As self-evident as these health promoting elements may seem, for the millions of persons who deal with disability, chronic disease, or both, such basic needs seem too often to take second place to other issues. It is equally problematic that preventive measures, most notably at the primary and secondary levels, are often nonexistent or lacking.

The issue of missed opportunities in health promotion and prevention is depicted in Figure 34–2. The focus of the health care delivery system is increasingly skewed toward secondary and tertiary prevention efforts, and limited emphasis is placed on the health promotion and primary prevention needs of the population. Although this is a concern for all persons, it is of particular importance for persons with disabilities and chronic illnesses, because they are more likely to have these needs ignored altogether. As Figure 34–2 shows, an entire area of issues may be addressed with a basically healthy person but not with a disabled or chronically ill individual. There may be areas of secondary and tertiary prevention unique to persons with disabilities or chronic illnesses that are completely ignored. It is the nonreceipt of

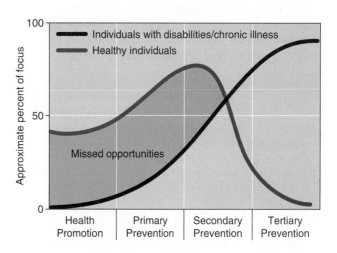

FIGURE 34–2. Difference in client focus between individuals with and without a chronic illness or disability.

health promoting or preventive education or actions vital to the health and well-being of those with disabilities or chronic illnesses that is of most concern. For example, issues such as sexuality are often not explored with the disabled or chronically ill. This skewed view of the lifestyles, behaviors, and needs of the disabled as "different" from those of the "able-bodied" is a clear example of lack of understanding by health professionals and the public alike.

It is likely that disability or chronic illness serves as the initial reason for an individual's encounter with the health care community, including the community health nurse. As a result, the disability or illness often drives the selection of prevention efforts, to the possible exclusion of other, equally important health issues. For example, for an individual with a primary diagnosis of type 1 diabetes, secondary prevention efforts often center on that disease (eg, screening for diabetic retinopathy). The need to refer the client for a Pap test or a baseline mammogram may be overlooked. Likewise, the treatment plan may include a consultation with a dietitian but

fail to address the basic needs for leisure-time activities, regular physical activity, a varied and interesting diet, fresh air and sunshine, and socialization—all of which may help prevent the development of depression, a common result of chronic illness. Display 34–4 offers several examples of missed opportunities in the areas of primary and secondary prevention. It is of particular concern to the practice of community health nursing that the broad range of health promotion and prevention needs of all clients be addressed.

Health Care Disparities and Discrimination

It is a growing concern to those who are disabled, and to their families and advocates, that the type and quality of the health-related services, referrals, and care that they receive may not be appropriate to their circumstances. This results in increased illness and disability and potentially decreased quality or length of life.

D I S P L A Y   3 4 – 4

Missed Opportunities

Example 1
A 60-year-old woman, blind since birth, self-sufficient and active all of her life, has developed severe arthritis. She encounters a health care system that far too often focuses on her "disabilities" and not her "abilities." The focus is placed squarely on her tertiary health promotion needs, often at the expense of health-promoting or lifestyle-enhancing needs. The result is a failure to recognize that the "disability" of arthritis is likely no less and no more an issue for her than for a sighted person. She receives the same medication therapy as a sighted person but may not be offered a physical therapy program due to her disability. Her need for physical therapy is no less important, but locating an appropriate, safe, and easily accessible program requires some additional work on the part of her provider. At issue is that options potentially discussed with a sighted person are more apt to be omitted completely, which may negatively affect the client's overall health and well-being.

Example 2
A 20-year-old man with learning disabilities, who is employed at a local factory, receives a regularly scheduled physical examination with a new provider. He lives in a **congregate care facility,** which is an out-of-home facility that provides housing for people with disabilities in which rotating staff members provide care for 16 or more adults or any number of children/youth younger than 21 years of age. It excludes foster care, adoptive homes, residential schools, correctional facilities, and nursing facilities (USDHHS, 2000). The major finding of the examination is that he is due for a tetanus booster and should also begin the series for hepatitis A, because he lives in a high-risk

area of the western United States. He takes the referral slip and leaves the office. One year later, at his regularly scheduled visit, it becomes clear that he never received his immunizations. Apparently, he didn't know what he was supposed to do with the paper, because he has difficulty reading, and he had no idea where to go to get his "shots." The primary prevention elements were provided, but clearly not in a manner appropriate for this individual. With additional explanation and follow-up, perhaps the outcome would have been quite different.

Example 3
A 34-year-old woman who has been severely obese since the birth of her last child (4 years ago) has not had a gynecologic examination since that birth. She is aware of the need to have regular examinations, yet she cannot bring herself to make an appointment. The reason is that she knows she will have to be weighed, and this terrifies her, especially because it is done in an open area where others can see. She finally gets the courage to call for an appointment and tells the clerk that she does not want to be weighed. The clerk's response is less than helpful and she is essentially told that it is "policy." She makes the appointment but does not keep it. This situation could have been handled in a compassionate manner, recognizing the painful experience that weighing is for many individuals and suggesting alternatives, one of which could have been simply to bypass the scales until after the interview and examination. At that point, the woman may have been more amenable to the measurement and a more discrete area could have been offered. In this case, the opportunities to provide primary, secondary, and tertiary prevention were lost.

The issue of health care access was one of a number of elements explored in a study involving 932 independently living Massachusetts adults with a major disability (Wilber et al., 2002). The purpose of the study was to determine whether factors such as having a consistent primary care provider, access to health promotion or disease prevention programs, and accessible transportation were related to the number and severity of secondary conditions experienced. The findings suggested that the more independent the individual and the fewer obstacles faced, the fewer secondary conditions were reported. The study used the definition of secondary conditions in *Healthy People 2010*; the most notable findings were the high prevalence rates of fatigue, depression, spasms, and chronic pain.

Additional disparities may exist in services received by those with chronic illness and disabilities. Racial and ethnic differences in immunization rates were found in a study analyzing data from the National Health Interview Survey of almost 2000 individuals with diabetes (Egede & Zheng, 2003). Even after controlling for access, health care coverage, and socioeconomic status, the rates of influenza and pneumococcal immunization were lower for certain racial/ethnic groups, primarily Blacks. What is not known from these results is whether the depressed immunization rates resulted from client acceptance issues, from differential provider recommendations, or from some combination of these factors.

A qualitative in-depth survey by Becker and Newsom (2003) that examined the issue of disparities found that economic status also appeared to affect dissatisfaction with health care among chronically ill African-Americans. In this study, low-income-status individuals were less satisfied with both the quality and the quantity of their care than were middle-income respondents. The potential impact of low satisfaction for selected groups is of real concern in addressing the ongoing needs of those individuals. Although neither study was confirmatory, it is nevertheless an issue that needs to be explored further.

It is discriminatory practice when an individual receives unequal, inappropriate, or limited services compared with those offered to others. Although the difference in treatment is often due to lack of understanding of the needs of disabled persons, it is nonetheless discriminatory. Such bias may not be intentional, but it can dramatically affect the health of clients and must be changed.

The good news is that the incidence of unequal and inappropriate practices can be reduced with education and training of health care providers, agency staff, and insurance carriers. A crucial aspect of community health practice is to ensure that those individuals with disabilities or chronic illnesses are afforded the best possible care, treatment options, and opportunities to improve their health—the same options that are provided for nondisabled persons and those who do not suffer from chronic illness.

Health promotion and primary, secondary, and tertiary prevention activities are essential aspects of quality care for all persons. Those with disabilities require specialized attention to needs resulting from or related to their disabilities, yet they also require the same attention to health and well-being as the rest of the population. Community health nurses are in a prime position to advocate needed changes for those with disabilities and chronic illnesses. Such changes can include increased attention to health promotion and disease prevention needs, accessible and appropriate delivery of those services, and specialized treatment plans that incorporate the latest knowledge of a specific illness or disability.

FAMILIES WITH A DISABLED OR CHRONICALLY ILL MEMBER

The Family's Role in Advocacy

Families that have a member with a chronic illness or disability face many challenges. They are required to navigate a health care system that they know little about and with which they often feel at odds. They serve as advocates for their member in need (whether child, spouse, or parent) and often feel tired and frustrated from their efforts, especially if they have been less than successful in meeting their goals. Many are forced to ask for or demand assistance from health care agencies, social services, or transportation sources to achieve the level of care needed by the family member. Many are required to open their home to others (eg, community health nurses, social workers) to access the services. Families may have little understanding of what services they are entitled to because of language barriers, difficult agency policies, or disjointed service delivery.

The community health nurse is usually not the first health care professional that the family encounters. They may already have been through a lengthy struggle to receive assistance. In these circumstances, the nurse often is confronted by a frustrated family that distrusts yet another "professional." The nurse must gain the trust and confidence of the family by practicing consistency, following through with promised actions, and always being truthful. Not all problems that the family faces can be remedied, and even for problems that do have solutions, time and effort may be needed to obtain the desired result.

The Impact on Families

A literature review of the needs of parents with chronically ill children reported a number of common themes in the studies surveyed: (1) the need for normalcy and certainty, (2) the need for information, and (3) the need for partnership (Fisher, 2001). Although these needs were associated with the presence of a chronically ill child in the family, the same needs are likely to occur in other families. These are certainly areas that can be addressed by the community health nurse in a practical way.

One major obstacle for families with a disabled or chronically ill member may be obtaining needed **assistive**

devices and technology. These are defined in *Healthy People 2010* as "any item, piece of equipment, or product system, whether acquired commercially, modified, or customized, that is used to increase, maintain, or improve the functional capabilities of individuals with disabilities" (US-DHHS, 2000, p. 6-25). With constant changes in available equipment, financing, and technology, it is little wonder that families struggle to find the best alternatives. Just because the technology exists does not mean that it can be obtained. Often the insurance carrier, whether private or governmental, sets limits on which products can be obtained or which brands are acceptable. The overriding issue of financing is no small hurdle. It is often left up to the family to learn about options and legal rights through a process of trial and error.

Intervention by the community health nurse can greatly reduce the burden on the family. With so many product lines available on the Internet, the nurse can assist families in this area, especially those without access to or understanding of computer technology. It is equally helpful for the nurse to intervene with insurance providers if coverage of equipment is not easily obtained or to find sources of funding for the equipment from private agencies if possible. Referring families to community groups or organizations that provide specific assistance can be very helpful. Other families who share similar struggles can provide a vital link to needed services and can be contacted through self-help groups or other sources. This is where the community health nurse can provide expertise on available community resources.

USING THE NURSING PROCESS

ASSESSMENT

Anna Lopez is a mother of three children aged 2 to 9 years old. The eldest, Ernesto, was diagnosed with severe Down syndrome at birth. He is confined to a wheelchair, requires total care, and remains at home with his mother and younger siblings, who are not yet in school. Anna's husband works long hours as a computer repairman for a large company. They have health insurance, but it does not cover additional expenses, such as day care for Ernesto. The family has done very well in providing for Ernesto's needs, and they receive periodic visits from you, the community health nurse, to evaluate his condition and check on the feeding tube used for his nourishment. Physically, Ernesto is stable, but you notice that Anna has been increasingly withdrawn at the visits, rarely offering information, but responding to questions appropriately. She seems less engaged with her other children as well, only occasionally smiling at them.

NURSING DIAGNOSES

1. At risk for depression related to ongoing caregiver demands and lack of respite care
2. At risk for altered health status due to limited focus on self-care needs

PLAN/IMPLEMENTATION

Diagnosis 1. The community health nurse will discuss with the client the need for a thorough physical assessment, including an evaluation for depression. The community health nurse will contact the insurance provider to discuss day care/respite options for Ernesto. If unavailable, local community organizations will be contacted for appropriate referrals. In addition, the need for

more frequent visits to the family will be discussed with the insurance carrier to address the needs of the mother as caregiver.

Diagnosis 2. The community health nurse will discuss with the client her concerns about her overall physical and mental health and discuss some self-care options that may improve her well-being: improved nutrition, physical activity, leisure time options, and adjustment of family schedule to accommodate more free time for self-care.

EVALUATION

The client was at first very reticent to make an appointment for an evaluation, but after thinking it over for a week and discussing it with her husband, she did so. Her husband was relieved that she had suggested the appointment, because he was growing increasingly concerned over her withdrawal but did not know how to bring up the subject. The family physician referred Anna to a psychologist for evaluation of the depression. The insurance carrier agreed to increase home visits on a short-term basis but did not have a respite care option available for Ernesto. Fortunately, a local faith-based community group was able to provide limited assistance to the family. They identified several members who had raised children with similar disabilities and were willing to stay with Ernesto and the other children once a week for 4 hours. This allowed Anna some free time to make appointments with her psychologist, shop, or visit friends. After several months, Anna has begun to smile more and seems much more relaxed at the home visits. The children are all doing fine, and the respite care is expected to continue for at least the next 6 months. The need for ongoing attention to her own self-care needs is emphasized with Anna by the community health nurse.

Respite care is another area of great importance for families of the disabled and the chronically ill. It can be emotionally draining to meet the daily needs of a member who cannot perform self-care. This often leads to caregiver fatigue and increased stress. It is also important to recognize the effect of the situation on non-caregivers in the family, particularly nondisabled siblings of a disabled child. With focus placed on the needs of one member, children may feel that their own needs are not as important. This can lead to behavioral and health-related problems. Respite care offers some needed relief to the family and allows for uninterrupted attention to the nondisabled children. This service can occur within the home or at an outside facility. Respite care may be provided by a private organization at little or no cost to the family, or it may be quite expensive and require financing by the insurance company or by the family itself. Whatever the source, some type of respite care is often vital to the family's health and should be a priority in the overall treatment plan of the family (see Using the Nursing Process).

With the enactment of the 1996 welfare reform legislation (the Personal Responsibility and Work Opportunity Reconciliation Act), a number of significant changes were implemented that potentially affect families with a chronically ill child, especially those living in poverty. Changes included the stipulation of a 5-year lifetime limit on receipt of benefits, institution of work requirements, and elimination of entitlement to cash benefits. The impact of these changes is of growing concern within the public health community. Smith, Wise, and Wampler (2002) explored this issue in a study of knowledge of welfare reform among families with a chronically ill child. They found that respondents often had incomplete knowledge of work requirements, even if they were entitled to exemptions because their children received Supplemental Security Income. In those cases, 37% of the respondents were unaware that they qualified for work exemptions, and 70% had not applied for the exemptions. This indicates that eligible families might not be receiving the exemptions to which they are entitled, adding additional and unnecessary burdens to families already at risk.

Another study explored the relationship between welfare status, health insurance status, and the health and medical care received by children with asthma (Wood et al., 2002). The most significant findings were (1) children of parents who had been denied Temporary Assistance for Needy Families (TANF) experienced more severe asthma symptoms and had more acute care visits than children in families that did not access the welfare system, (2) children of recent TANF applicants were more likely to be uninsured or transiently insured than those who had not applied, and (3) recent TANF applicants had the poorest mental health scores. The significance of this study is that it demonstrated the high-risk status of those families with a chronically ill child and the need to provide access to health insurance and health services.

Even for families that are ineligible for public assistance, the issue of employment is generally of great significance. Employment options may be quite limited when a family has a member with special needs. The family may have to remain in a particular location to access needed health and social services, reducing the possibility of increased earning potential at a different location or in another field of employment. The working family members may choose less favorable employment options because the position is convenient or has more flexible hours. For instance, a person may take a part-time position at a local convenience store that does not pay particularly well in preference to a higher-paying, full-time factory position because the store is close to home and allows for frequent adjustments in schedule.

Having a chronically ill family member often means that working individuals must take time off from work. Although some legal protections are provided under the Family and Medical Leave Act of 1993 (see Chapter 29), the Act does not apply in all situations. More importantly, it allows only for time off; it does not mandate payment during those periods. The choice becomes an issue of taking unpaid time off or continuing to work and dealing with the needs of the family member as best one can. Some individuals choose to work part-time or not to work at all so that they can care for family members. At a time when many families have two earners to help meet financial commitments, these families may have to rely on only one income. Limitations in income are particularly difficult when one considers the myriad needs of the disabled and chronically ill, many of which may not be covered by insurance.

Caregiver health needs and mental health status are yet another area of concern for families who must provide for a disabled or chronically ill member. One of the largest longitudinal studies in the United States, the Nurses Health Study, provided the data for an investigation of the impact of informal caregiving on the mental health status of caregivers (Cannuscio et al., 2002). Using data collected over a 4-year period (1992–1996), the study found that women who provided 36 or more hours per week of care for a disabled spouse were six times more likely than noncaregivers to report depressive or anxious symptoms. The frequency of symptoms was elevated but less dramatic if the women cared for a disabled or ill parent as opposed to a spouse. The findings support the necessity of attention to the needs of caregivers, the majority of whom are women. Poor health outcomes, both physical and mental, are of growing concern as the population ages and the need for family caregiving rises. Recognizing that caregivers within a family are at increased risk for poor health outcomes, the community health nurse must select appropriate interventions to address the health needs of the other family members.

Families of individuals with a disability or chronic illness are at increased risk for a number of negative consequences. Although families do not all have the same level of risk or disruption, the community health nurse should recognize the potential impact of the dependent member's needs on the entire family. Families may suffer from financial difficulties, poor physical or mental health, and a variety of other challenges. They are often ill prepared to deal with the complicated systems that must be accessed to obtain needed care. The community health nurse is in an optimal position to interpret those systems to the families and to advocate for the needed care, services, and equipment. The nurse must view the family holistically, recognizing additional needs that may develop as a result of the situation they currently face.

THE ROLE OF THE COMMUNITY HEALTH NURSE

This chapter has discussed a number of areas in which the community health nurse plays a key role. It is important to review those roles in the context of the individual, the family, and the community as prime areas for nursing intervention. Chapter 3 first examined the broad spectrum of roles that the professional nurse takes on within the community. It is helpful to review those roles and think about their application to disabled and chronically ill clients, their families, and the communities in which they live.

Table 34–4 provides a grid on which to record specific examples of the roles that community health nurses assume in relation to disabilities and chronic illnesses. Take note of each role that you participate in or observe while completing your clinical experience. If you cannot find examples of the various roles at each level, perhaps you can interview a community health nurse during your clinical experience and find examples of how he or she performs activities in each of

those roles. You will probably find that, while addressing a single issue with a client, the community health nurse serves in a variety of roles and at different levels.

Consider as an example of the variety of roles and multilevel practice that the community health nurse assumes with respect to a 55-year-old female client who uses a wheelchair. The client has difficulty obtaining a gynecologic examination because of the lack of accessible examination tables at the local clinic; as a result, she has not had an examination for more than 20 years. Recognizing the need for a complete examination, the community health nurse arranges with the clinic to find appropriate alternatives that will aid the client in receiving the needed examination, possibly by ensuring that additional personnel are provided (Advocate Role—Individual Level).

Because this solution is temporary and less than optimal, the nurse contacts a number of clinics in neighboring communities and finds one that has appropriate equipment for people who have difficulty transferring to a standard examination table. Unfortunately, this clinic is 1 hour away. The nurse then contacts a number of other community health nurses and discovers that they also have a significant number of women clients with this problem who have not received a gynecologic examination in many years (Research Role—Community Level).

Through a coordinated effort with a local transportation company and the clinic, the nurse is able to arrange a twice-yearly gynecologic screening program for the women in the

T A B L E   3 4 – 4

Roles of the Community Health Nurse

Role	Individual	Family	Community
Clinician			
Educator			
Advocate			
Manager			
Collaborator			
Leaders			
Researcher			

community who require special accommodations (Advocate and Coordinator Roles—Community Level). Information sheets that discuss the need for annual gynecologic examinations and advertise the program are distributed to area public health nurses, employers, and health clinics (Educator Role—Community Level). Data collection on examinations provided over the next few years shows a 65% increase in the number of women with special needs who have received a gynecologic examination within the past year (Research Role—Community Level).

This is not an uncommon scenario in the practice of community health nursing. Often, the needs of an individual open the door to areas of concern for many in a community and provide a basis for intervention that can benefit a larger population.

Like nursing practice in general, the role of the community health nurse with respect to disabilities and chronic illness requires broad and holistic practice. The complexity of issues surrounding these conditions requires creativity, tenacity, honesty, and, most of all, knowledge. Community health nurses who are informed about the issues that affect the disabled and chronically ill at local, state, and national levels are prepared to offer assistance to their clients and to their communities. Knowledge of civil rights for these individuals is crucial in serving as advocates.

The issues facing individuals and families with disabilities require strong and sustained efforts to achieve results. Although successes at the individual level are laudable, the extent to which the health and well-being of those affected is improved must be the ultimate goal. Community health nursing is in a prime position to initiate and support efforts to improve the health status of those populations. We can either leave the issues to other professionals or use our expertise and long history of caring for those less fortunate to make major and lasting changes. It is up to us.

SUMMARY

The issue of disability and chronic illness is of growing importance in community health, both nationally and internationally. Through the efforts of WHO, the international community has been challenged to provide increased attention to health promotion and disease prevention. Even in less developed countries, behavioral patterns linked to excesses in consumption (overweight and tobacco/alcohol use) have an impact on the quality and quantity of healthy years of life. The ICF provides a universal classification system that standardizes language and takes into account the biopsychosocial realms in health assessment and well-being of disabled persons. Along with the *World Health Report 2002*, this document now places the emphasis squarely on prevention of disease and disability. This means, of course, that the health promotion and disease prevention needs of the disabled and chronically ill must be given the same emphasis as the needs of those who are not disabled or ill.

The aging of the U. S. population and the rise in lifestyle-related illnesses such as diabetes and obesity are often linked with increasing rates of disability. Prevention of disability and disease is emphasized in *Healthy People 2010,* which serves as a wake-up call to Americans about the need to give serious attention to health promoting and disease prevention activities. What is unique about this current edition of *Healthy People* is the emphasis placed on health promotion and disease prevention needs of those with disabilities and chronic illness. It is no longer acceptable that these individuals be treated solely for tertiary health needs. Research has shown that when health promoting (lifestyle) issues are addressed with these clients, the rates of secondary conditions are reduced, including medical, social, emotional, mental, family, and community problems. Like the ICF, *Healthy People 2010* takes the position that disability and chronic conditions are not universally debilitating and that the overall well-being and health of these individuals must be a priority.

Legislation is but one step toward equality for those affected by disabilities and chronic illnesses. The ADA has provided for many improvements in accessibility and specific legal protections for the disabled, but it is only the beginning. Discrimination can occur at many levels; some is hurtful and intentional, but most results from misunderstanding of the needs and desires of disabled persons and their families. This may even occur in relation to the provision of health care because of lack of education. Improvement can be found only with increased community education programs for professionals and the public that target the myths and misunderstandings about those with disabilities and chronic illnesses.

Community health nurses are in a prime position to advocate for the health needs of the disabled and chronically ill. With a long history of serving those who are most vulnerable, community health nurses can help make needed changes at the individual, family, and community levels. Although it is often easier to focus on the needs of the individual, those needs are most often shared by many others. Nurses have long recognized the need to collaborate with other professionals in reaching the goal of improved health care for their clients; this continues to be an important aspect of successful efforts on behalf of the disabled and the chronically ill. It will take the concerted efforts of many to implement changes necessary to improve the lives of those most affected, their families, and the communities in which they live.

The next time you have difficulty opening a door that is unusually heavy or struggle to open the lid of a jar or feel that you were treated differently than someone else in the receipt of services, take that moment to think. Think about the challenges, struggles, and pain that face so many citizens. Although many argue against improving accessibility of city streets and sidewalks because of the expense, those same people may one day find that they, too, are faced with trying to master a curb that is just a bit too high.

ACTIVITIES TO PROMOTE CRITICAL THINKING

1. Arrange to interview an individual with a disability (eg, hearing, vision, mobility) about the challenges that they have faced in interactions with nondisabled persons.
2. Visit some of the nongovernmental sites listed under Internet Resources and read some of the personal stories that are included.
3. Take an inventory of your house or apartment and make a list of modifications you would need to make if you were suddenly confined to a wheelchair. Would you even be able to stay in your current residence?
4. As part of your regular clinical assignment in community health nursing, look at those clients and families who are dealing with either a disability or chronic illness and assess how often you or other community health nurses have addressed health promotion activities (eg, healthy eating, physical activity, leisure-time activities) with those clients.
5. Review your family history for chronic health conditions. Are you at risk? If so, what have you done to reduce your risk over the past 12 months?

REFERENCES

American Council of the Blind. (2003). *Organizational profile.* Retrieved February 9, 2004, from *http://www.acb.org/profile.html*

American Foundation for the Blind. (2002). *About us.* Retrieved February 9, 2004, from *http://www.afb.org*

American Obesity Association. (2002). *Disability due to obesity: Are you disabled?* Retrieved February 9, 2004, from *http://www.obesity.org*

Becker, G., & Newsom, E. (2003). Socioeconomic status and dissatisfaction with health care among chronically ill African Americans. *American Journal of Public Health, 93,* 742–748.

Cannuscio, C.C., Jones, C., Kawachi, I., Colditz, G.A., Berkman, L., & Rimm, E. (2002). Reverberations of family illness: A longitudinal assessment of informal caregiving and mental health status in the Nurses' Health Study. *American Journal of Public Health, 92,* 1305–1311.

Egede, L.E., & Zheng, D. (2003). Racial/ethnic differences in adult vaccination among individuals with diabetes. *American Journal of Public Health, 93,* 324–329.

Fisher, H.R. (2001). The needs of parents with chronically sick children: A literature review. *Journal of Advanced Nursing, 36,* 600–607.

Grayson, G. (2003). *Talking with your hands, listening with your eyes. A complete photographic guide to American Sign Language.* Garden City Park, NY: Square One.

Guide Dogs for the Blind. (2003). *Welcome to guidedogs.com!* Retrieved February 9, 2004, from *http://www.guidedogs.com*

Hwu, Y., Coates, V.E., Boore, J.R., & Bunting, B.P. (2002). The concept of health scale. Developed for Chinese people with chronic illness. *Nursing Research, 51,* 292–301.

Marshall, D., McConkey, R., & Moore, G. (2003). Obesity in people with intellectual disabilities: The impact of nurse-led health screenings and health promotion activities. *Journal of Advanced Nursing, 41,* 147–153.

Morehead, P., & Morehead, A. (Eds.). (1995). *The new American Webster handy college dictionary.* New York: Penguin Books.

National Association of the Deaf. (1993). *The NAD position paper on ASL and bilingual education.* Retrieved February 9, 2004, from *http://www.nad.org*

National Association of the Deaf. (2003). *About NAD.* Retrieved February 9, 2004, from *http://www.nad.org/about/index.html*

National Council on Disability. (1986). Toward independence: An assessment of Federal laws and programs affecting persons with disabilities—with legislative recommendations. Retrieved June 16, 2003, from *http://www.ncd.gov*

National Council on Disability. (2000). *Promises to keep: A decade of Federal enforcement of the Americans with Disabilities Act.* Retrieved February 14, 2004, from *http://www.ncd.gov/newsroom/publications/promises_1.html*

National Council on Disability. (2003). What's new. Retrieved June 16, 2003, from *http://www.ncd.gov*

National Federation of the Blind. (2003a). *About the NFB.* Retrieved February 9, 2004, from *http://www.nfb.org/aboutnfb.htm*

National Federation of the Blind. (2003b). *What is Braille and what does it mean to the blind?* Retrieved XXXX from *http://www.nfb.org/books/books1/ifblnd03.htm*

National Organization on Disability. (2002a). *About us.* Retrieved February 9, 2004, from *http://www.nod/org*

National Organization on Disability. (2002b). *Key findings: 2000 NOD/Harris Survey of Americans with disabilities.* Retrieved February 9, 2004, from *http://www.nod/org*

Rapaport, L. (2003, June 22). CalPERS seeks proof of payoff from prevention. *The Valley Times,* A5.

Smith, L.A., Wise, P.H., & Wampler, N.S. (2002). Knowledge of welfare reform program provisions among families of children with chronic conditions. *American Journal of Public Health, 92,* 228–230.

United States Department of Justice. (2002). *A guide to disability rights laws.* Retrieved February 9, 2004, from *http://www.usdoj.gov/crt/ada/cguide.htm*

United States Department of Health and Human Services. (1991). *Healthy People 2000: National health promotion and disease prevention objectives* (S/N 017-001-00474-0). Washington, DC: U.S. Government Printing Office.

United States Department of Health and Human Services. (2000). *Healthy People 2010: Understanding and improving health.* Washington, DC: Government Printing Office. Retrieved February 9, 2004, from *http://www.health.gov/healthypeople/Document/*

United States Department of Health and Human Services. (2001). *Healthy People 2000 final review.* Retrieved February 14, 2004, from *http://www.cdc.gov/nchs/products/pub/pubd/hp2k/review/highlightshp2000.htm*

United States Department of Health and Human Services. (2003, May). *Delivering on the promise: OCR's compliance activities promote community integration*. Retrieved February 9, 2004, from *http://www.hhs.gov/ocr/complianceactiv.html*

Wilber, N., Mitra, M., Walker, D.K., Allen, D., Meyers, A.R., & Tupper, P. (2002). Disabilities as a public health issue: Findings and reflections from the Massachusetts Survey of Secondary Conditions. *The Milbank Quarterly, 80,* 393–419.

Wood, P.R., Smith, L.A., Romero, D., Bradshaw, P., Wise, P.H., & Chavkin, W. (2002). Relationships between welfare status, health insurance status, and health and medical care among children with asthma. *American Journal of Public Health, 92,* 1446–1452.

World Health Organization. (1980). *International classification of impairments, disabilities, and handicaps.* Geneva: Author.

World Health Organization. (2001). *International classification of functioning, disability and health.* Geneva: Author.

World Health Organization. (2002). *The World Health Report 2002: Reducing risks, promoting healthy life.* Geneva: Author.

SELECTED READINGS

Damush, T.M., Stump, T.E., & Clark, D.O. (2002). Body-mass index and 4-year change in health-related quality of life. *Journal of Aging and Health, 14,* 195–210.

DiBenedetto, D.V. (2003). Finding disability-related information on the Web. *AAOHN Journal: Official Journal of the American Association of Occupational Health Nurses, 51,* 10–12.

Loeb, S.J., Penrod, J., Falkenstern, S., Gueldner, S.H., & Poon, L.W. (2003). Supporting older adults living with multiple chronic conditions. *Western Journal of Nursing Research, 25,* 8–23.

Lutz, B.J., & Bowers, B.J. (2003). Understanding how disability is defined and conceptualized in the literature. *Rehabilitation Nursing, 28,* 74–78.

Minder, C.E., Muller, T., Gillmann, G., Beck, J.C., & Stuck, A.E. (2002). Subgroups of refusers in a disability prevention trial in older adults: Baseline and follow-up analysis. *American Journal of Public Health, 92,* 445–450.

Nosek, M.A., Howland, C.A., Rintala, D.H., Young, M.E., & Chanpong, G.F. (1997). *National study of women with physical disabilities: Final report.* Houston, TX: Center for Research on Women with Disabilities.

Nunez, D.E., Armbruster, C., Phillips, W.T., & Gale, B.J. (2003). Community-based senior health promotion program using a collaborative practice model: The Escalante Health Partnerships. *Public Health Nursing, 20,* 25–32.

Resnick, B. (2003). Health promotion practices of older adults: Testing an individual approach. *Journal of Clinical Nursing, 12,* 46–55.

Spero, D. (2002). *The art of getting well. A five-step plan for maximizing health when you have a chronic illness.* Alameda, CA: Hunter House.

Thomsett, K., & Nickerson, E. (1993). *Missing words. The family handbook on adult hearing loss.* Washington, DC: Gallaudet University Press.

Tolson, D., Swan, I., & Knussen, C. (2002). Hearing disability: A source of distress for older people and careers. *British Journal of Nursing, 11,* 1021–1025.

Internet Resources

American Council of the Blind: *http://www.acb.org*
American Diabetes Association: *http://diabetes.org*
American Foundation for the Blind: *http://afb.org*
American Heart Association: *http://www.americanheart.org*
American Obesity Association: *http://www.obesity.org*
Guide Dogs for the Blind: *http://www.guidedogs.com*
National Association to Advance Fat Acceptance: *http://naafa.org*
National Association of the Deaf: *http://www.nad.org*
National Center for Health Statistics: *http://www.cdc.gov/nchswww*
National Council on Disability: *http://www.ncd.gov*
National Federation of the Blind: *http://www.nfb.org*
National Institute of Diabetes & Digestive & Kidney Diseases: *http://www.niddk.nih.gov*
National Organization on Disability: *http://www.nod.org*
Office of Minority Health Resource Center: *http://www.omhrc.gov*
Robert Wood Johnson Foundation: *http://www.rwjf.org*
U. S. Department of Justice (Americans with Disabilities Act Home Page): *http://www.usdoj.gov/crt/ada/adahom1.htm*
U. S. Department of Health and Human Services, Office for Civil Rights: *http://www.hhs.gov/ocr*
Women with Disabilities (The National Health Information Center): *http://www.4woman.gov/wwd*

35

Clients With Mental Health Issues and Addictions

Learning Objectives

Upon mastery of this chapter, you should be able to:

- Discuss the historical evolution of mental health care.

- Explain the obstacle of stigma in community mental health.

- Discuss the incidence and prevalence of mental illness and addictions in the United States.

- Compare and contrast various theories on the etiology of addiction.

- Discuss the needs of and treatment approaches for the mentally ill and those with addictions.

- Identify and describe community mental health and addiction resources.

- Define terms commonly used to describe addiction and addictive behaviors.

- Identify the *Healthy People 2010* objectives for reducing addiction and addressing mental health needs in the United States.

- Clarify your own assumptions and beliefs regarding clients living with mental illness and addictions.

- Discuss health-promoting interventions for community mental health.

- Describe the role of the nurse in caring for clients, families, and communities struggling with addiction or mental illness.

his might not be an easy chapter to read. It may stir thoughts of a loved one who is struggling with an addiction or challenge you to rethink your assumptions about people with mental illnesses. Nonetheless, the worldwide importance of addressing mental health issues can not be understated. Whether dealing with the psychological aftermath of tradegies such as the September 11, 2001, attack on the World Trade Center, the global problem of narcotic trafficking, the untreated mental illness of the homeless, or the lack of mental health treatment options for so many citizens, the issue of mental health is critical at all levels of health provision from the local to the international arena.

Mental illnesses are probably the least understood group of illnesses, and the most likely to go untreated, affecting the quality of life for many. Although not separate from the wider body of mental health issues, addictions and substance abuse are of particular concern to community health practice. Addiction is a devastating personal trauma, whether it is the result of self-medication for existing mental illness or the aftermath of out-of-control "recreational" substance abuse. In this chapter, addictions and substance abuse are addressed in depth as a distinct but not separate issue.

This chapter describes how epidemiologic information about the vulnerable population of clients with mental health issues becomes a roadmap to guide community mental health nursing practice in community health services, mental illness prevention, and mental health promotion. It also describes some of the most common addictions and the preventive measures that are most often used in approaching clients with addictions. The term *community mental health nurse* is used frequently throughout this chapter to denote individuals whose practice is centered on the mental health needs of the populations served. The information discussed is applicable to general community health nursing practice in a variety of settings. Community health nurses frequently have clients with mental health issues in addition to diagnoses such as pregnancy, chronic cardiac problems, and communicable diseases. Recognition of the link between mental and physical health is a vital component in developing effective interventions for many individuals served by community health nurses.

The following questions should be kept in mind while reading about the issues surrounding mental illness and addictions: In what sense do they threaten the health of communities? What are the global implications? Is there anything a community health nurse can do to help individuals, families, and communities cope with addictions and mental health issues?

COMMUNITY MENTAL HEALTH IN PERSPECTIVE

In the past century, research and public health innovations in the United States and worldwide contributed to significant improvements in health and treatment of disease. Once-dreaded diseases, such as cancer and human immunodeficiency virus/ acquired immunodeficiency syndrome (HIV/AIDS), are in-

creasingly survivable and even curable. The average American's lifespan has almost doubled, and the physical health of Americans overall has never been better. However, the picture has been different for mental health, which has remained a low national priority, and for mental illness, which has been mostly feared and misunderstood.

Only recently has mental health begun to receive the attention it needs and deserves. Speaking of the overall health and well-being of our nation, Tommy Thompson, Secretary of Health and Human Services, commented, "We have only begun to come to terms with the reality and impact of mental illnesses on the health and well being of the American people" (Substance Abuse and Mental Health Services Administration [SAMHSA], 2001). It is now recognized that, worldwide, 4 of the 10 leading causes of disability for persons 5 years of age and older are mental disorders (World Health Organization [WHO], 1999). Furthermore, depression is the leading cause of disability in all developed nations, including the United States. Mental disorders also tragically often lead to death, with suicide one of the main preventable causes of death in the United States and globally. Mental health is among the top 10 leading indicators of health, as identified in *Healthy People 2010* (U. S. Department of Health and Human Services [USDHHS], 2000a). Addressing these concerns, much research was conducted in the 1990s, declared the "Decade of the Brain" by the U. S. Congress, to gain understanding of mental functioning and mental illness (SAMHSA, 1999). The Surgeon General's report on Mental Health underscored the concept that mind and body are inseparable and that "mental health is fundamental health" (SAMHSA, 1999, p. 2). The supplement to this report, published in 2001, furthered the issue of disparities in mental health services for racial and ethnic minorities, a problem that affects the overall health and productivity of this population (SAMSHA, 2001).

Mental health, as defined in *Healthy People 2010,* is "a state of successful mental functioning, resulting in productive activities, fulfilling relationships, and the ability to adapt to change and cope with adversity" (USDHHS, 2000a, p. 37). Mental health, although a somewhat elusive and value-driven concept, clearly undergirds successful performance in life. On the other hand, **mental illness** "refers collectively to all diagnosable mental disorders [which] are health conditions that are characterized by alterations in thinking, mood, or behavior (or some combination thereof) associated with distress and/or impaired functioning" (SAMHSA, 1999, p. 8). Mental illness and mental health are not polar opposites; rather, they can be viewed as points along a health continuum. Mental disorders vary in severity and are manifested through specific, distinguishing characteristics. They may arise without regard to age, gender, or ethnicity, as a product of genetic, biologic, environmental, social, physical, or behavioral factors acting alone or in combination.

Serious mental illness (SMI) refers to any mental illness that has compromised both the client's level of function and his or her quality of life. **Serious and persistent mental**

illness (SPMI) is the preferred term for serious mental illness of a chronic nature. For example, schizophrenia is usually classified as an SPMI.

Neurosis is a general term commonly used to describe any of a variety of mental or emotional disorders involving anxiety, phobia, or other abnormal behavioral symptoms. It is considered less severe than psychosis, which is a mental disorder characterized by partial or complete withdrawal from reality.

Finally, the word insanity is a legal term reserved for mental impairment that may relieve a person from the legal consequences of his or her actions. Tests for insanity are usually conducted by psychiatrists who try to determine whether the accused individual can distinguish right from wrong, or whether his or her reason was overpowered by irresistible impulses when committing the criminal act (see Voices in the Community).

Evolution of Community Mental Health

The ways in which mental health and illness were viewed through the ages dictated how people with mental disorders were treated. It is helpful for the community mental health nurse to understand how those views have changed and how this history influences the field today. The following sections examine the historical evolution of mental health services up to the present time.

Mental Illness in Ancient Civilizations

The common term *lunacy* (from the Latin *luna*, "moon") has its basis in the ancient belief that the moon has the power to

drive people insane; people were once supposed to have become insane by being exposed to the full moon. Many ancient civilizations believed that mental illness was caused by possession, by either an evil spirit or a divine power. In some ancient societies, the mentally ill were believed to possess special powers of divination and healing and were supported and revered by the community.

In ancient Greece, Hippocrates (460–377 BC), called the Father of Medicine, was the first to attempt to explain diseases on the basis of natural causes (Simon, 1978). He combined bedside observations with the speculations of the philosphers of medicine. He was the first to recognize the brain as the most important human organ, although he believed that if the brain were plagued by heat, cold, or excessive moisture, madness would ensue. Hippocratic physicians first classified mental illness and described the symptoms of melancholia, which we call depression, believing that such conditions were caused by an accumulation of black bile.

Mental illness was considered nonexistent in ancient Chinese culture. The Chinese family was traditionally very large and hierarchical in structure, and individuals had little chance to express themselves. The family system along with the teachings of Confucius interfered with an individualistic concept of life. Much later, in the 20th century, the influence of Mao and Marxism redefined any sign of mental illness as reflections of guilt toward socialism and society. Depression, mania, and neurosis were viewed as expressions of guilt rather than symptoms of mental illness (Ng, 1990; Lee & Kleinman, 1997).

Egyptian beliefs in ancient times were influenced both by Oriental mysticism and by African views of nature. In 525 BC, Imhotep was named a god of medicine, and his temple at Memphis became a medical school and hospital. Here the Aesculapian priests developed a form of psychotherapy using incubation sleep. Patients were encouraged to occupy themselves with recreational activities such as painting, drawing, or concerts, which were believed to have therapeutic value. Egyptian medicine influenced Moses as well as Hippocrates. Egyptian physicians were as knowledgeable in their observations as they were magical in their explanations and esoteric in their teachings (Hurry, 1978).

Influence of the Church Through the Middle Ages

Medieval European society was dominated by the church. In this religious society, madness or any deviant behavior was viewed as demonic possession and the work of Satan (Rosen, 1968). Such beliefs existed before the 13th century and led to extensive witch hunts during the Inquisition. Deviants, or witches, were believed to be heretical agents of Satan from whom people needed protection. The protector was the inquisitor. Furthermore, the Church regarded women, especially midwives, as evil, so that women were persecuted as members of an inferior, sinful, and dangerous class of individuals. Physicians and priests were both involved in witch hunts. They used various methods to distinguish between those who were witches and those who were truly ill.

VOICES FROM THE COMMUNITY

I've always prided myself as being a "fair minded" person. Every year I make it a point to send in a check to the Salvation Army and the Red Cross—they do so much to help all those poor people in our community. But this is just too much; they want to convert one of those nice old homes in our neighborhood to house some mentally ill teenagers. The thought of them running around the neighborhood just scares me to death. Who knows what's wrong with them . . . for all I know they could be child abusers or drug addicts. I have two grandchildren who come over to see me all the time—I can't watch them every second. A few of my neighbors are sponsoring a meeting this evening to see how we can stop this. I feel guilty about not wanting to help out these kids but I know there are other places that would be better suited for this type of thing.

Mrs. Taylor, age 63 years

Witches, like involuntary mental patients, were cast into a degraded and deviant role against their will, subjected to certain diagnostic procedures, and finally deprived of their liberty or their lives, supposedly for their own benefit.

Emergence of the Scientific View

Toward the end of the Middle Ages, a pattern of hospital care for the insane began to emerge. The famous English hospital of Saint Mary of Bethlehem, commonly called "Bedlam," was founded in 1450 as an institution for those who had "fallen out of their wit and their health." However, the mentally ill were more likely to be housed in jails or poorhouses than hospitals. Almost 200 years would pass before a foundation was constructed for a scientific interpretation of insanity that would come to replace supernatural and religious interpretations (Rosen, 1968).

In the mid-17th century, the work of natural scientists such as Sir Francis Bacon and Sir Isaac Newton placed science at the forefront of human achievement. The universe was thought to be a complex mechanism, similar to a clock, whose structure and function could be examined, categorized, and understood. This approach influenced investigations of the human body and was buoyed by English physician William Harvey's demonstration of the function of the heart and circulatory system. Also at this time, the French philosopher Descartes proclaimed the preeminence of rational thinking as proof of existence, and the physician Thomas Willis, who is considered the father of neuroanatomy, placed the brain at the center of human action and disease.

By the early 18th century, the English physicians Thomas Wright and Robert Burton stressed the psychological causes and cures of insanity. In the "Age of Reason," madness stood out as a dark challenge. During this century, physicians discovered that the insane were amenable to medical intervention. Modern psychiatry began in 1775 when the French physician Philippe Pinel, chief physician at an asylum for women in Toulouse, removed the chains from the inmates. In a famous essay published in 1809, he advocated humane treatment of the mentally ill and a more empiric study of mental disease. By recognizing categories of mental illness and promoting symptom identification, Pinel revolutionized psychiatric medicine (Kiple, 1995).

Advances in the Nineteenth Century

In the first half of the 19th century, the treatment of mental illness was marked by asylum building (Grob, 1991). Originally, asylums were designed as centers for "moral treatment" of the mentally ill—places where troublesome persons would be subjected to occupational therapy and moral persuasion. Chains were replaced by admonitions, physical tasks, and distractions; however, treatment was still coercive and primitive (Gamwell & Tomes, 1973).

As the 19th century progressed, medical professionals turned increased attention on mental illness and the brain, some claiming care of the mentally ill as their special domain. With the formal development of the human sciences within and across disciplines, significant attention was devoted to the study of the human brain and human behavior. Not only physicians but also nurses, social reformers, and spiritual leaders became increasingly interested in humane treatment of the mentally ill. Dorothea Lynde Dix worked ceaselessly for humane treatment, health care, and social services for the mentally ill, and by the close of the century many of her reforms had been implemented in the United States and Europe.

The Twentieth Century and the Impact of Managed Care

During the early decades of the 20th century, the modern profession of psychiatry was born. Medical schools began to offer instruction in the medical treatment of insanity, and the Freudian model of psychoanalysis became increasingly popular. Psychiatric hospitals and long-term care facilities were constructed, and individuals with severe disorders were increasingly institutionalized, removed from their families and communities. Although institutionalization was intended to produce humane and effective treatment and care of the mentally ill, in reality conditions were often inhumane. Overcrowding, overmedication, sporadic or inexpert care, physical restraint, and even beatings were reported in many institutions. Once admitted, most patients remained in the institution for the rest of their lives, in part because the inadequate and even callous care did not effect an improvement in their conditions, and in part because the community had no resources for assisting recovery from mental illness.

In approximately the 1950s, the reform movement began. The quality and efficacy of institutional care came under attack, and new policies were implemented that sought to provide more humane treatment for the mentally ill (Grob, 1994). It was thought that people with mental disorders would fare better living in the community. In response to this movement, Congress enacted the 1963 Community Mental Health Centers Act (P.L. 88-164) to provide for community-based mental health services. This act was revised in 1991 to also authorize partial hospitalization services under Medicare Part B (USDHHS, 2002). With federal and state reimbursement in place, the promotion of community-based services further reduced the need for state-owned mental institutions, and many closed over the following decades.

The process of transferring the mentally ill from public institutions to community-based care settings was called **deinstitutionalization**. In the years after the end of the Vietnam War (1973) and during the Reagan Administration (1981–1989), the effects of deinstitutionalization were most evident. Many mentally ill individuals, who formerly would have been institutionalized in a secure and ordered residential setting, often had difficulty accessing services in the communities. The result was that many were left to wander the streets, unable to sustain employment or function adequately in a stressful and confusing world. Their feelings of abandonment, loneliness, and fear only exacerbated their mental disability. Stigmatization further jeopardized the health of these populations. Misperceptions and fears of the general public caused the mentally ill to become even more socially isolated and cut off from needed support. Added to this societal problem related to the chronically mentally ill were the significant numbers of Vietnam military combat veterans suffering from **posttraumatic stress disorder (PTSD)**, alcohol and drug abuse, and related mental illnesses, who were also in dire need of accessible community services. PTSD is described in the *Diagnostic and Statistical Manual of Mental Disorders,* 4th edition, Text Revision (known as DSM-IV-TR) as "the development of characteristic symptoms following exposure to an extreme traumatic stressor" (American Psychiatric Association, 2000, p. 463). It is estimated that as many as 30% of Vietnam veterans experienced this disorder at some point after the war (National Institute of Mental Health [NIMH], 2001). Both deinstitutionalization and the emerging mental health needs of the war veterans increased the demand for appropriate mental health services in the community; often beyond the ability of existing programs to meet that need.

In the late 20th century, the advent of managed care again altered treatment approaches for mental illness. Initially, managed care was heralded as a solution to spiraling health care costs, but disadvantages have also become evident. In order to control costs, most managed care plans severely restrict treatment for mental illness. These restrictions include limitations on length of treatment and choices of medications that can be prescribed. In addition, certain hospitals or clinics that are the sole designated providers of mental health care may be geographically inaccessible to the populations most in need of services. Finally, more funding is often allocated for inpatient care than for outpatient care, a policy that promotes crisis care as the preferred vehicle of treatment.

Community Mental Health Today

As is evident from this historical view, the understanding of mental illness and mental health has come a long way, yet many challenges remain. The treatment of mental illness re-

mains controversial. Whereas some see mental illness as primarily a physiologic disorder and advocate pharmacologic therapy, others see it as a crisis of meaning, development, or cognition that requires primarily "talk therapy" with a skilled psychotherapist, and still others view mental illness as a spiritual crisis requiring spiritual guidance, meditation, prayer, and a supportive community. All of these views have been prominent in different societies at different historical periods, and all still have some validity today.

Traditionally, mental health services have focused primarily on treatment of the mentally ill. However, in an era of greater enlightenment, the significance of prevention and health promotion are influencing community mental health workers to start expanding the range of services. Today, **community mental health** is a field of practice that seeks to address the needs of the mentally ill, prevent mental illness, and promote the mental health of the community. With a new national commitment for mental health, advances in research, and improved treatment modalities, the future for promotion of mental health and treatment of mental disorders looks promising.

The Obstacle of Stigma

Despite increased attention to the challenges faced by the mentally ill, the Surgeon General's report emphasizes that "a formidable obstacle to future progress" remains, and "that obstacle is stigma" (SAMHSA, 1999, p. 5). **Stigma** is an unjustified mark of shame and discredit attached to mental illness. It is the result of myths and misunderstandings that have been perpetuated down through the ages as illnesses of the mind remained a mystery and a threat. Stigma toward mental illness is largely attributable to ignorance and misconceptions. Until recently, society lacked knowledge about the mind, how it works, why mental illness occurs, and how to successfully recover from it. In addition, most people have experienced some form of mental health problem that is similar to the symptoms of mental illness and assume that anyone can get over it. They greatly underestimate the difficulty of dealing with a painful, disabling SMI. Stigma is also attributable to fear—fear that is spawned by ignorance. Consequently, it is easy to label these illness behaviors as shameful and to shun and discredit those who are the victims. Persistence of stigma and fear is a destructive force that prevents this client population from receiving the health services it needs.

Nevertheless, as discussed earlier, the tide is turning. The White House Conference on Mental Health in 1999 promoted a national anti-stigma campaign, and mental health has become a higher priority nationally, as evidenced in *Healthy People 2010* and in the Surgeon General's 2001 supplemental report calling national attention to ethnic and racial disparities in mental health care (SAMHSA, 2001). Finally, the Global Burden of Disease study (WHO, 1999) showed that mental illness is surprisingly significant in its contribution to the world's burden of disease. As these efforts spawn new information, expanded research, and more effective policies

WHAT DO YOU THINK?

For decades one of the world's largest mental hospitals existed in Long Island, New York. Pilgrim State Hospital housed 15,000 mentally ill patients; one building housed patients with mental illness and tuberculosis. This facility closed its doors in the early 1980s, because psychotropic drugs were helping patients control symptoms. In a matter of a few short years, thousands of clients were released, literally to the streets, because community mental health programs were in their infancy.

and programs, there will be increasing opportunities, particularly for community mental health nurses, to educate the public and start eradicating the obstacle of stigma.

EPIDEMIOLOGY OF MENTAL DISORDERS

Epidemiologic information about mental illness, which describes its occurrence and distribution in the community, provides a road map that guides community mental health nursing practice. Such information helps the nurse determine what, where, and for whom services are needed. However, in the past, it was not easy to epidemiologically measure the incidence and prevalence of mental illness in the community. Because mental illness has not been a reportable condition by law, only those individuals who were housed in mental hospitals or asylums could be accurately counted. An even larger number of persons, either receiving treatment through mental health centers and private practices or untreated and living in the community, were unknown to public health policy makers and program planners. Then, in 1952, the American Psychiatric Association first published its *Diagnostic and Statistical Manual: Mental Disorders* (DSM-I), in order to provide an official manual of mental disorders with a focus on clinical utility. The DSM became a source of diagnostic information for clinical practice, research, and education, in addition to providing a language for communicating about mental illness with other service providers and policy makers. For epidemiologic purposes, the DSM made it possible to more consistently define mental disorders and to estimate their occurrence in the community. The latest version of this manual, DSM-IV-TR, updates the 1994 publication of DSM-IV (American Psychiatric Association, 2000). With publication of DSM-V not expected until approximately 2006, the Text Revision was designed as an intermediary source to bridge the gap between major DSM publications. DSM-IV-TR reviews the following axis 1 clinical disorders:

- Disorders usually first diagnosed in infancy, childhood, or adolescence
- Delirium, dementia, and amnestic and other cognitive disorders
- Mental disorders due to a general medical condition
- Substance-related disorders
- Schizophrenia and other psychotic disorders
- Mood disorders
- Anxiety disorders
- Somatoform disorders
- Factitious disorders
- Dissociative disorders
- Sexual and gender identity disorders
- Eating disorders
- Sleep disorders
- Impulse-control disorders not elsewhere classified
- Adjustment disorders
- Other conditions that may be a focus of clinical attention

Incidence and Prevalence of Mental Disorders

Every year, one out of five Americans, or more than 51 million people, experience a diagnosable mental disorder. Of this group, more than 6.5 million, including 4 million children and adolescents, are disabled by an SMI (SAMHSA, 1999). More than 19 million Americans older than 18 years of age will suffer from a depressive illness at some time during their lives, and many of these individuals will be incapacitated for significant lengths of time by their illness. Over two thirds of suicides in the United States each year are caused by major depression, which is also the leading cause of disability. More than 2 million Americans 18 years of age and older, about 1% of the population, suffer from bipolar disorder, and an almost equal number of adults suffer from schizophrenia. Indeed, almost all people who kill themselves have a diagnosable mental disorder (NIMH, 2001).

Studies focusing on the prevalence of mental illness are limited and sometimes inconclusive; however, the poor, the poorly educated, and the unemployed typically experience higher rates of mental illness than the general population. A large portion of the mentally ill population, many of whom are homeless, remain untreated in the community. The poor, disproportionately representative of racial and ethnic minorities, are even more vulnerable due to lack of access to care and questionable quality of the care that is received (SAMHSA, 2001).

Age influences the patterns of mental illness in the community. Each year about one of every five children and adolescents has the signs and symptoms of a DSM-IV disorder. The most commonly occurring conditions among American children ages 9 to 17 years are anxiety disorders, disruptive disorders, mood disorders, and substance use disorders. Attention-deficit/hyperactivity disorder (ADHD) affects approximately 4% of U. S. school-age children, with boys two to three times more likely to be affected than girls. Autism, a developmental disorder, has a prevalence among children of 1 to 2 per 1000 people and is four times more common in boys than in girls (NIMH, 2001) (see Chapter 28). For American adults, the most prevalent mental disorders are anxiety disorders, followed by mood disorders, especially major depression and bipolar disorder. Anxiety, depression, and schizophrenia present special problems for this age group—anxiety and depression because they contribute to such high rates of suicide, and schizophrenia because it is so persistently disabling. For the growing number of older adults, there is increased incidence of Alzheimer disease, major depression, substance abuse, anxiety, and other disabling mental disorders. Particular problems arise with dementia, which causes significant dependency and results in costly long-term care; with depression, which contributes to the high suicide rates among men in this age group; and with the disabling effects of schizophrenia (SAMHSA, 1999).

Gender differences also arise in the prevalence of certain mental disorders. Anxiety disorders and mood disorders, including major depression, occur twice as frequently in women as in men. Women of color, women on welfare, poor women, and uneducated women are more likely to experience depression than women in the general population. The three main types of eating disorders (anorexia, bulimia nervosa, and binge eating) also affect more women than men (NIMH, 2001). Women attempt suicide more frequently than men, but completed suicides are more common among men. Analysis of national suicide data from 1991 to 1996 suggested that White and African-American widowed men younger than 50 years of age were at particular risk to commit suicide, compared with the general population of married men, and young African-American men were most at risk (Luoma & Pearson, 2002). Vital statistics data from 2000 indicated that White men older than 85 years of age had the highest suicide rate for any group in the United States (Minino et al., 2002).

Adding to the heavy toll that mental illness exacts is the financial burden it creates. Costs associated with treatment of mental disorders, poor productivity, lost work time, and disability payments are astronomical. The direct and indirect costs of mental illness and addictive disorders in the United States. are greater than $400 billion annually (USDHHS, 2000a). Furthermore, the cost to society when treatment is *not* provided for these illnesses has been estimated to be three to seven times the cost of direct treatment. Certainly, these facts have policy implications and suggest the need for greater preventive and mental health promoting efforts.

Risk Factors Influencing the Mentally Ill Population

As a community health nurse concerned about the mentally ill, you have examined some of the epidemiologic information about this population. What are some of the causative factors contributing to the at-risk status of the mentally ill? Using a vulnerability model, it is helpful to consider four categories of factors that influence the at-risk status of this pop-

ulation: biological, psychological, sociocultural, and environmental factors (Fig. 35–1).

Biologic Factors

Certain biologic factors can place people at increased risk for mental illness. Neurobiologic and genetic mechanisms play a significant role, usually in combination with other factors. An example is autism, which has a familial pattern and is often associated with mental retardation (American Psychiatric Association, 2000). Although no single gene has been found to cause a specific mental disorder, variations in multiple genes can disrupt healthy brain function and, under certain environmental conditions, lead to mental illness. Age is another factor. Many mental illnesses appear to have their origins in early childhood, or even in the way the brain develops prenatally, but lie dormant until adulthood.

Biologic risk factors in children for development of a mental disorder include the following (SAMHSA, 1999):

- Prenatal damage from exposure to alcohol, illegal drugs, or tobacco
- Low birth weight
- Inherited predisposition to mental disorder
- Physical problems (such as abnormalities of the central nervous system [CNS] that affect behavior, thinking, or feeling and are caused by infection, injury, poor nutrition, or environmental toxins)
- Intellectual disabilities such as retardation

Some individuals may acquire mental impairment as a result of traumatic brain injuries or illnesses that cause tissue damage or anoxia. Birth defects and injuries sustained at birth also contribute to risk.

Psychological Factors

Psychological factors also influence the vulnerability of this population. Stress connected with employment, financial worries, family problems, death of a loved one, and other life events can contribute to mental illness if the in-

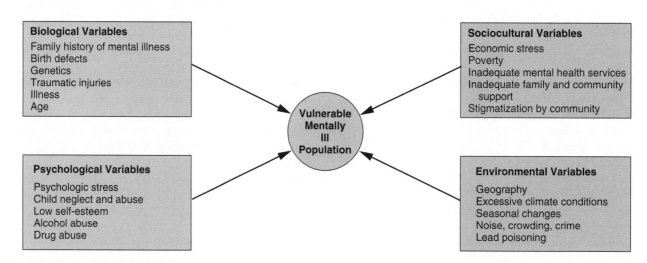

FIGURE 35-1. Factors that influence the vulnerability of the mentally ill population.

dividuals affected have not developed healthy coping patterns. Neglect and abuse during childhood place individuals at greater risk for various mental disorders, and dysfunctional family life can predispose to conduct disorders and antisocial personality disorders. Low self-esteem also seems to accompany poor mental functioning. Alcohol and drug abuse can lead to chemical dependence, physiologic damage, and mental impairment; also, a family history of mental and addictive disorders is a risk factor for children (SAMHSA, 1999).

Sociocultural Factors

Economic hardship affects the mental health of many individuals. Anxiety over such things as inadequate income and housing, increasing debt, or unemployment can create emotional stress with which some people cannot cope. Multigenerational poverty continues to place individuals at greater risk for mental disorders.

Data on racial and ethnic distribution among the mentally ill are limited and inconclusive. A higher proportion of minorities appear among the impoverished mentally ill in the community. However, mental health problems and mental disorders exist in families of all social classes and cultural backgrounds; no one is immune. What is clear is that minority group members who need mental health care are "less likely to receive needed care" and "when they receive care, it is more likely to be poor in quality" (SAMHSA, 2001, p. 3)

Inadequate mental health services in the community, lack of adequate community support systems, and little emphasis on prevention are major sociocultural factors increasing vulnerability to mental illness. Overall, research is demonstrating that most mental disorders are caused by some combination of genetic, biologic, and psychosocial influences (SAMHSA, 1999) (see Research: Bridge to Practice).

Environmental Factors

Geographic environmental factors play a lesser role in affecting vulnerability to mental illness. Nonetheless, climate and geography can cause severe stresses if there are threats of frequent hurricanes, tornadoes, floods, or earthquakes. Some individuals are affected by absence of natural sunlight during long, grey winters. They experience a type of depression called *seasonal affective disorder* (SAD), which is far more common in northern regions. Additionally, many conditions in urban areas are anxiety-producing, including transportation problems, excessive noise, crowded streets, inadequate sanitation, high crime rates, and impersonal services.

Lead poisoning continues to be a serious public health problem contributing to mental impairment. Children are especially vulnerable to lead poisoning, whose sources include peeling paint in older homes and workplaces, exhaust fumes, drinking water channeled through lead pipes, the glaze on ceramic mugs or bowls that have not been properly fired, various home remedies, foreign-made candy, and crystal glassware whose lead has leached after repeated dishwasher use or extended contact with acidic beverages. The risk of lead poisoning is not confined to children living in poverty. With the growing popularity of home improvement and renovation, individuals who are unaware of the risks or choose not to have professional guidance in lead paint abatement may inadvertently place their children at risk for lead poisoning. Although poverty is strongly associated with lead poisoning in children, other risk factors must also be considered.

RESEARCH: BRIDGE TO PRACTICE

Hines-Martin, V., Malone, M., Kim, S., & Brown-Piper, A. (2003). Barriers to mental healthcare access in an African American population. *Issues in Mental Health Nursing, 24,* 237–256.

Disparities in access to mental health services affect all racial and ethnic groups but are of particular concern within minority, low-income populations. This study used a qualitative, grounded theory approach to explore barriers in accessing mental health care services. Participants included 24 African-American, low-income adults who had sought mental health treatment at selected public health inpatient or outpatient settings during the past 12 months. An 11-question, semistructured interview guide was used to explore the issues related to access and help-seeking behaviors. The participants identified three levels of barriers (individual, environmental, and institutional) and 14 subcategories corresponding to those levels. Most frequently reported were barriers related to thoughts/knowledge deficit, and beliefs/attitudes/values (both at the Individual level), and family/significant others/community (environmental level). The institutional barriers included time/limitations/capacity; gatekeepers; and rules but appeared less critical to perceived access limitations. Many of the participants had experienced mental health problems beginning in childhood or adolescence. Barriers to obtaining care, whether real or perceived, resulted in delays in treatment, often for many years. The findings of the study provide a basis for exploration of access issues in mental health care in order to decrease barriers experienced by those most in need of care and reduce or eliminate the disparities that currently exist for many minority populations.

INTERVENTIONS FOR COMMUNITY MENTAL HEALTH

Epidemiologic data and information about risk factors help to guide the community mental health nurse in planning for community mental health services. Such services, to be truly comprehensive, should encompass the entire range of prevention levels—primary, secondary, and tertiary. The majority of community mental health services in the past have focused their efforts on addressing the needs of the mentally ill. Although this population must continue to be a priority, it is now becoming clear that community mental health efforts must also focus to a much greater degree on preventing mental illness and promoting mental health. These latter two emphases hold the key to a healthier future for the nation and the world.

Healthy People 2010 Objectives for Mental Health and Substance Abuse

For the focus area of mental health and mental disorders, *Healthy People 2010* states the following goal: "Improve mental health and ensure access to appropriate, quality mental health services" (USDHHS, 2000a). Fourteen objectives were developed to accomplish this goal, to be completed by the year 2010. These objectives, listed in Table 35–1, emphasize the reduction and prevention of suicide, better access to and utilization of services, early detection of mental illness, and improved functioning for persons with mental disorders in the community. All levels of prevention—primary, secondary and tertiary—are included.

Healthy People 2010 also addresses the issues of tobacco and substance use, with an emphasis on both primary and secondary prevention efforts (see Table 35–1). Use of tobacco products and use of substances (alcohol and illicit drugs) are included in the list of leading health indicators within the document. The combined impact of cigarette smoking and the use of alcohol and illicit drugs exacts a high price in terms of both individual health and the resultant economic costs. Preventable illnesses and deaths can be both directly and indirectly linked to substance use and abuse and, as such, are a high priority. The five specific objectives address smoking, illicit drug use, and alcohol consumption by adults and adolescents.

Three of the 10 leading health indicators within *Healthy People 2010* are devoted specifically to issues of mental health and substance use. This fact serves to emphasize the need within our communities for the vital resources of time, money, and personnel to affect a real and lasting change; the cost of inaction will be far higher.

Serving the Mentally Ill Population

In order to design appropriate services for the mentally ill population, it is important for the community health nurse to build on knowledge of epidemiologic data, risk factors, and

other information, then work in concert with other health team members for planning and implementing services. To begin with, it is important to know the needs of people with mental disorders.

TABLE 35–1

Healthy People 2010: Objectives for Mental Health and Substance Abuse

Mental Health: Health Status Improvment	• Reduce the suicide rate. • Reduce the rate of suicide attempts by adolescents. • Reduce the proportion of homeless adults who have serious mental illness. • Increase the proportion of persons with serious mental illnesses who are employed. • Reduce the relapse rates for persons with eating disorders, including anorexia nervosa and bulimia nervosa. • Increase the number of persons seen in primary health care who receive mental health screening and assessment. • Increase the proportion of children with mental health problems who receive treatment. • Increase the proportion of juvenile justice facilities that screen new admissions for mental health problems. • Increase the proportion of adults with mental disorders who receive treatment. • Increase the proportion of persons with co-occurring substance abuse and mental disorders who receive treatment for both disorders. • Increase the proportion of local governments with community-based jail diversion programs for adults with serious mental illnesses.
Mental Health: State Activities	• Increase the number of States and the District of Columbia that track consumers' satisfaction with the mental health services they receive. • Increase the number of states, territories, and the District of Columbia with an operational mental health plan that addresses cultural competence. • Increase the number of states, territories, and the District of Columbia with an operational mental health plan that addresses mental health crisis interventions, ongoing screening, and treatment services for elderly persons.
Tobacco Product and Substance Use: Health Status Improvement	• Reduce cigarette smoking by adolescents. • Reduce cigarette smoking by adults. • Increase the proportion of adolescents not using alcohol or any illicit drugs during the past 30 days. • Reduce the proportion of adults using any illicit drug during the last 30 days. • Reduce the proportion of adults engaging in binge drinking of alcoholic beverages during the past month.

Needs of the Mentally Ill

As the needs of this population are assessed, various health-related problems will be found. The nature of these problems, and the degree to which they are preventable, vary with the type and severity of the mental disorder, whether the affected individuals are receiving and complying with needed treatment, and the degree of independence with which they can function in the community. Although the mentally ill population is disparate in terms of its wide range of diagnoses and conditions, there are nonetheless many problems shared by members of this group. Furthermore, interventions designed to address specific needs for an individual or a group can often provide wide-reaching benefits to the whole population. The problems of this group, like those of other vulnerable populations, can be divided into three categories: physical, psychological, and social.

Physical Problems

The physical problems of the mentally ill are numerous. Because many people in this population take medications for a prolonged period, a major problem for them is dealing with serious medication side effects. Prolonged tranquilizer use, for example, can cause tardive dyskinesia, an irreversible condition in which damage to the cerebral cortex caused by the drug leads to tremors and loss of motor control. Clients taking psychotropic drugs tend to have increased problems with constipation and regular elimination. They frequently have sleep disturbances that lead to sleep deprivation and make them vulnerable to other physical health problems. Poor compliance in taking prescribed medications is an additional problem for this population. Many forget to take their medications or do not value their importance; others lose track in moving from one group home or living situation to the next. Psychotropic medications can affect clients' vision, making it difficult to read or even to decipher medication label instructions. The medications usually are needed to enable mentally ill individuals to function and live independently; if treatment protocols are not followed consistently, many will be at risk for exacerbation of symptoms.

Poor nutrition is another serious concern within the mentally ill population, particularly for those living on their own. Eating disorders and poor eating habits are prevalent in this group and include undernutrition due to lack of access to consistent food sources. Because of their impaired function or limited finances or both, many mentally ill clients are unable to shop, prepare food for themselves, or make appropriate food choices. A high-fat, high-carbohydrate, "junk food" diet leads to obesity for many in this population, as well as promoting greater risk for coronary artery disease, diabetes, and dental problems. The mentally ill population, particularly the men, are also vulnerable to liver disease, heart disease, and cancer because of their high rate of dependency on alcohol, drugs, and cigarette smoking.

As a population, the mentally ill are vulnerable to a number of communicable diseases, including sexually transmitted diseases, HIV/AIDS, and tuberculosis. Depending on their extent of mental dysfunction, these clients, particularly those with SMIs, also face problems associated with limited motor coordination and self-care ability, including personal hygiene.

Psychological Problems

The psychological problems of the mentally ill vary depending on the type and severity of the disorder. The stresses of coping with daily living, compounded by the complexities of city life or the isolation resulting from rural living, may create responses such as confusion, depression, frustration, and anger. Psychological isolation, loneliness, and poor self-esteem are interrelated problems for most people with mental disorders. People with these conditions are often unable to establish supportive relationships and feel the stigma that society places on mental illness. In addition, few have adequate, if any, family or friendship supports.

Chemical dependency and other forms of addiction are a serious concern for many of the mentally ill. Lacking adequate coping skills to deal with daily life and seeking relief or escape from the stresses they feel, people with mental disorders frequently turn to alcohol, drugs, cigarette smoking, and gambling, singly or in combination. Dependence on these habits leads to additional physical, emotional, social, and financial problems.

Social Problems

Stigma, discussed earlier, poses a major problem for the mentally ill. Fear and misunderstanding of mental disorders by the larger society lead to disrespect, mistreatment, lack of acceptance, and social isolation, which in turn reduce this population's already limited resources. Without needed support from family, friends, and community, the mentally ill are further handicapped and even more vulnerable.

System inadequacies cause another set of problems for the mentally ill. Income for these individuals is limited, and finding and sustaining employment is difficult given their disabilities. If they have worked, they are eligible in the United States for Social Security Disability income; if they have never worked, they can receive supplemental income under the Social Security Act. However, in both cases only a subsistence level of living is provided. Many clients have unstable housing, which creates mobility with additional problems. A further problem is limited finances for treatment or health care benefits. The Mental Health Parity Act of 1996 limits mental health coverage compared with non–mental health conditions. It has resulted in increased numbers of the poor going without their prescribed psychotropic medications and psychotherapy because they do not have the means to pay for them. It has also resulted in several high-visibility crimes committed by individuals with SPMIs who were without treatment at the time of the crime. Services for the mentally ill are often fragmented and inadequate; improved services and collaboration among providers who serve this population are needed. A summary of these problems is listed in Table 35–2.

T A B L E   3 5 – 2

Health-Related Problems of the Mentally Ill

Physical Problems	Psychological Problems	Social Problems
Medication side effects	Depression	Low income
Loss of motor control	Confusion	Unemployment
Constipation	Anger/frustration	Physical isolation
Sleep disturbances	Lack of motivation for compliance	Unstable housing
Poor nutrition	with treatment	System does not foster independence
Dental problems	Anxiety	Disjointed and inconsistent mental
Obesity	Low self-esteem	health services
Chronic diseases (coronary artery disease,	Unable to establish relationships	Stigma
diabetes, heart disease, liver disease, cancer)	Feelings of stigmatization	Parity problems
Limited self-care ability	Psychological isolation	
Communicable diseases (sexually transmitted diseases,	Neuroses	
acquired immunodeficiency syndrome, tuberculosis)	Psychoses	
	Addictive behaviors	

Service Interventions for the Mentally Ill Population

The needs of the mentally ill are addressed primarily through either biomedical or psychotherapeutic approaches. Often a combination of both is found to be effective.

Biomedical Approaches

Biomedical therapy for persons with mental disorders involves the use of medications or electroshock therapy.

Pharmacotherapy

Historically, the treatment of the mentally ill consisted of isolation, restraint, ice packs, insulin shock therapy, electroconvulsive therapy, brain surgery, and minimal drug use. The most common drugs in use were paraldehyde, chloral hydrate, and barbiturates. In the early 1950s, the first tranquilizer, thorazine, was prescribed, ushering in a new wave of pharmacologic treatment for mental illness. Psychotropic medications not only have resulted in relief of symptoms but also have significantly improved the quality of life for millions of clients worldwide. Many clients previously held in long-term psychiatric facilities are now treated in community mental health centers or group homes or access outpatient facilities from their homes. The successful addition of medications to the treatment regimen of mental illness has promoted the position that mental illness is often biologically based or responsive to biologic treatment.

Electroconvulsive Therapy

Electroconvulsive therapy (ECT), also called *shock therapy,* uses electrically induced seizures primarily to treat severe depression. It has proved to be a safe and effective therapy and is often used for clients whose disease has not responded to drug therapies, for the elderly, and for highly suicidal clients, when there is no time to wait for the onset of the effects of antidepressants (Kalb, Ellinger, & Reulbach, 2003; Skye, 2001).

Psychotherapy

Psychotherapy is the treatment of mental or emotional disorders through psychologically based interventions. These interventions may be used alone, in combination with pharmacotherapies, or with complementary therapies such as yoga, relaxation exercises, or visualization. It is not uncommon for many of the therapy groups or modalities used in conjuction with professional psychotherapy to be facilitated by allied health personnel or lay individuals. The community mental health nurse, as case manager, may often participate in these activities or provide overall supervision of the activities and personnel, ensuring that the overall therapeutic needs of the clients are being met and that the activities are both safe and effective.

Common Psychotherapeutic Strategies

Additional psychotherapeutic strategies that may be provided based on individual needs, include the following:

- *Art therapy*—used as a means for expression through drawings, sculpture, or music. It is particularly effective with children and with clients whose verbal skills are limited.
- *Behavior therapy*—aims to reduce or eliminate certain behaviors through concentrated, specific guidelines. Smoking cessation and weight-loss groups are examples of behavior-modification approaches.
- *Client-centered therapy*—focuses on enabling clients to identify and actualize their own internal resources to work through their concerns.
- *Cognitive behavioral therapy*—focuses on clients' beliefs and actions and on reducing these beliefs and actions into more positive moods.
- *Insight-oriented therapy*—assists clients to improve their functioning through insight into themselves and their situation.
- *Interpersonal therapy*—focuses on clients' ability to gain

insight into their psychological distress in relation to disturbed interpersonal relationships.

- *Group therapy*—makes use of the interactions among several clients who share an interest in a common issue, such as anxiety, panic, depression, or eating disorders. Therapy groups may also be used for survivors of sexual assault, sexual abuse, or domestic violence, as well as many other topics.

Psychotherapy, sometimes called "talk therapy," uses one or more of these strategies. It is offered in a variety of settings and is available either individually or on a group basis. Private psychotherapy services can be accessed through referral or word-of-mouth for clients who are financially able to pay. Managed care organizations often restrict the number of therapy visits, posing a challenge to both clients and therapists. Clients with limited funds may access individual and group therapies through mental health clinics or community agencies. In addition to these therapies, there are community resources that enhance primary treatment.

Community Mental Health Resources

A variety of resources exist in the community to promote mental health, prevent mental illness, and serve the needs of the mentally ill. They include sources for education, advocacy, treatment, support, referral, rehabilitation, financial assistance, case management, and more. Community mental health centers, halfway houses, support programs, mobile crisis teams, self-help groups, and private mental health services provide the support mentally ill clients need.

Community Mental Health Centers

Community mental health centers (CMHCs) provide comprehensive, publicly funded services to the mentally ill population. In order for a CMHC to receive reimbursement through either Medicare or Medicaid, the following services must be provided (USDHHS, 2002):

- Outpatient services, including specialized services for children, the elderly, individuals who are chronically ill, and residents of the CMHC's mental health services area who have been discharged from inpatient treatment at a mental health facility
- Emergency services available 24 hours a day
- Day treatment, other partial hospitalization services, or psychosocial rehabilitation services
- Screening for patients being considered for admission to state mental health facilities to determine the appropriateness of such admission
- Consultation and education services

In addition to the required services, each client must have a physician-established **Individualized Treatment Plan** (ITP) indicating the type, amount, frequency, and duration of furnished services along with the clinical diagnosis and anticipated goals. The CMHCs are staffed by a multidisciplinary team who provide these on-site services. The community mental health nurse is an important member of this team.

Halfway Houses

A **halfway house** is a residential program for individuals with SPMIs. In addition to housing, the halfway house offers supervision, treatment, safety, socialization, recreation, and support. One of the difficulties experienced by many clients with mental illness is an inability to form attachments or have meaningful interactions with others. Halfway houses offer an opportunity to work within a framework of social support. The benefits include

- Learning from the experiences of others
- Observing social interventions
- Feeling a sense of belonging
- Drawing on the strengths of others
- Learning new strategies for problem-solving

Halfway houses provide the seriously mentally ill with the opportunity to function in a setting with their peers. Although they often cause some initial concern in neighborhoods in which they are located, problems anticipated by neighboring residents are rarely seen. They may be part of a CMHC or located elsewhere in the community.

Community Support Programs

Community support programs are a publicly funded set of services designed to assist persons with SPMIs. At the federal level, the Center for Mental Health Services (CMHS) is designed to work with states, local communities, mental health consumers, and their families to help mentally ill individuals access the treatment and services they need. These services include assistance in meeting basic needs such as housing, jobs, education, social services, transportation, and medical and nursing care. The overriding purpose of CMHS is to bridge the gap between research knowledge of best-practice models for community mental health services and the application of those models within the local community (SAMHSA, 1998).

Mobile Crisis Teams

A mobile crisis team is a multidisciplinary group of clinicians who travel to the scene of a crisis or critical event. They provide on-site evaluation of both the individuals involved in the crisis and the circumstances surrounding the incident. Although the immediate goal of this method of intervention is crisis management, education and facilitation of community support are also important objectives.

Self-Help Groups

A self-help group is a group of individuals who meet regularly with or without a professional leader or consultant to work on personal problems and issues. Leadership is frequently facilitated by the members, who rotate responsibilities. The goals of self-help groups usually include the following:

- Instillation of hope—that solutions to the problem are possible
- Imparting of information—that resources for help are available
- Increasing feelings of universality—that the individual is not alone with the problem

- Increasing feelings of altruism—that others can be trusted to care

Alcoholics Anonymous (AA) is a classic example of a self-help group with a long history of success. Based on a program of 12 Steps and 12 Traditions, it has been used as a model for other groups dealing with mental health and addictions, such as Narcotics Anonymous and Gamblers Anonymous (discussed later). Codependents Anonymous (CODA) is a self-help group for individuals struggling with issues of self-esteem and dysfunctional families. It assists individuals who grew up in homes where violence, substance abuse, neglect, or child abuse occurred and compromised the individuals' abilities to relate to others.

Private Mental Health Services

Many independent mental health treatment options are available in the community. Examples include individual, group, or family therapy with a psychiatrist, a psychologist, a nurse with advanced training in mental health, or a psychiatric social worker. Payment for these services may come from clients themselves, from managed care or other insurance agencies, or through community assistance funds.

Preventing Mental Disorders

With the burden of disease imposed by mental disorders, both nationally and worldwide, there is a growing urgency felt in the field of public health to put more effort into prevention. There is currently much more scientific information available on the treatment of mental illness than on how to prevent it. To enhance preventive intervention efforts, more clarity on the causes of mental illness, better information on whom to target, and more accurate measures for evaluating program effectiveness are needed. Yet there is still much that can be done.

Models for Preventing Mental Disorders

Some models have proved useful in approaching prevention of mental disorders. Two are examined here: the Public Health Model and the Mental Health Intervention Spectrum Model.

The Public Health Model

Early efforts to prevent illness used the Public Health Model of prevention, which was originally designed to control infectious diseases. This model includes three levels of prevention: primary prevention keeps a health problem from occurring, secondary prevention seeks to detect a health problem at its earliest stage and keep it from getting worse, and tertiary prevention aims to reduce the disability associated with the health problem. Applying the Public Health Model to the mentally ill population, Gerald Caplan (1964), in his classic work using this model, proposed population interventions at three prevention levels:

- *Primary prevention* activities with a population would decrease the number of new cases (incidence) of a mental disorder or reduce the rate of their development.
- *Secondary prevention* activities would lower the number

of existing cases of a mental disorder, thereby reducing its rate (prevalence). Examples of these activities are screening, early case finding, and early treatment.

- *Tertiary prevention* activities would decrease the severity of a mental disorder and its associated disabilities through rehabilitation. An example is a program of intensive case management and social skills training for schiziphrenics.

Mental health prevention efforts in the United States have used this model for many years in addressing the range of prevention levels. However, its application in terms of funding and support has been strongest in the area of secondary prevention.

The Mental Health Intervention Spectrum Model

In recent years, research has enhanced the understanding of risk factors and their association with health outcomes in relation to mental disorders. As a result, in 1994 the Institute of Medicine's Committee on Prevention of Mental Disorders developed a comprehensive model called the Mental Health Intervention Spectrum Model (MHISM) (Institute of Medicine, 1994).

The MHISM model presents a range of interventions for mental illness that includes prevention, treatment, and maintenance. The prevention aspects of the model are most relevant to the discussion here.

The prevention section of the MHISM model lists three types of interventions: universal, selective, and indicated. *Universal* preventive interventions target a whole population group or the general public who are not identified as being at risk for a specific mental disorder. This approach is useful for planning large-scale preventive interventions, such as a comprehensive program of prenatal services that could promote healthy brain development with a subsequent reduction in the incidence of schizophrenia.

The second type, *selective* preventive interventions, targets selected at-risk groups or individuals within a population. These are individuals or groups who have been identified as having a much higher risk of developing a mental disorder. An example of a selective preventive intervention is a support group and bereavement counseling for elderly persons who have lost a spouse, to prevent the onset of or lessen the degree of depression.

The third type, *indicated* preventive intervention, targets high-risk individuals who show signs of a beginning mental disorder or who have other evidence of a predisposition for a mental disorder. An example is parenting training and support for young mothers who were abused as children, especially if they show early signs of repeating that abuse with their own children.

Both the Public Health Model and the MHISM provide useful perspectives for designing preventive interventions and continue to be used today.

Preventive Interventions

Prevention is a fundamental role of the community health nurse working with mentally ill clients or with communities attempting to respond to the problems of mental disorders.

Primary, secondary, and tertiary prevention activities are discussed here.

Primary Prevention

With primary prevention, the goal is to both anticipate potential threats and prevent the actual development of a mental disorder. Combining the Public Health Model with "universal" preventive intervention from the MHISM, an intervention for a population or group can be designed by following these steps:

- *Select a mental disorder,* one that epidemiologic data have shown to be a significant problem for intervention (eg, adolescent alcoholism).
- *Identify the target population for intervention* (eg, all adolescents in a given community).
- *Determine causes and risk factors that contribute to the disorder* from research data in the literature. For example, identify factors that appear to contribute to teenagers' wanting to use and abuse alcohol (eg, peer pressure, risk-taking behaviors, escape).
- *Design, implement, and evaluate an intervention.* Conduct an educational program in the schools that addresses the contribution of risk factors to the development of adolescent alcoholism.

Other examples of primary prevention include support groups for children of divorced parents or spouses considering divorce, safe-housing projects, programs to prevent substance abuse, suicide prevention programs, and parenting classes. Informing parents of developmental milestones, age-related behaviors, and stress-reducing strategies can significantly reduce the risk of abuse. Other opportunities for primary prevention include supportive care for teenage mothers, well-baby classes, and stress-management classes.

Secondary Prevention

Secondary prevention efforts attempt to reduce the prevalence of mental disorders in the community or the severity of disorders in affected individuals. Health screening for mental illness is an important secondary prevention strategy to detect illness in its earliest stages. National Anxiety Screening Day, National Depression Screening Day, and similar programs are community-based examples and should be promoted in local media, clinics, libraries, schools, churches, welfare offices, and even on bulletin boards in supermarkets. Also, the community health nurse provides secondary prevention through monitoring of medication use. It is essential that the nurse be familiar with medications that clients are taking, particularly drug interactions and contraindications. This is particularly true for elderly clients, who may be taking medications for physical conditions as well. The nurse may be the primary person to identify breakthrough symptoms, noncompliance, or failure of clients or family members to fill prescriptions. As discussed later, the nurse's advocacy role can enable the client or family to negotiate systems that may be interfering with medication compliance.

Secondary prevention efforts also include case-finding and referral for primary or follow-up care. This means alertness and vigilance to find people in the community who show early signs of developing problems. Examples are a support program for family caregivers of patients with Alzheimer disease and an educational and support program for parents of autistic children. Facilitation of a self-help group, depending on its precise nature and goals, can also be an effective secondary prevention measure.

Tertiary Prevention

The goal with tertiary preventive intervention is to decrease the amount of disability associated with mental disorders. A tertiary preventive program can be designed for a population or group, combining techniques from the Public Health Model and the MHISM.

1. Select a significant mental disorder (eg, ADHD).
2. Identify the target population for intervention (eg, schoolchildren with diagnosed ADHD or with symptoms that suggest the onset of this disorder).
3. Identify the causes and risk factors that contribute to the problem. For example, it is known that boys are four times more likely to have ADHD than girls, that it is found in all cultures, that it runs in families (ie, genetics may play a part), and that multimodal therapies combining psychosocial and pharmacologic approaches are most effective for treatment of ADHD (SAMHSA, 1999).
4. Design, implement, and evaluate an intervention (eg, a combined individual and group therapy program for the targeted children).

Psychiatric rehabilitation, in which the intervention goal is to promote clients' functioning and independence, is another means of accomplishing tertiary prevention. An example is a rehabilitation program for depressed clients who have attempted suicide. Tertiary preventive activities seek not only to reduce symptoms and the overall disabling effects of the disorder but also to improve clients' quality of life. These interventions may include activities such as focusing on clients' strengths, increasing coping skills, helping clients develop better support systems, providing skill coaching for new settings, and encouraging self-determination.

Resocialization programs for people with SMIs are another form of tertiary prevention. These include sheltered workshops, development of life skills, and recreational programs with social events that enable clients to improve the quality of their lives and have more meaningful contact with society.

Finally, a tertiary preventive intervention of great significance is stigma eradication. Stigmatization of the mentally ill has resulted in lost opportunities for individuals to seek treatment, to improve, or to recover. Discrimination and social isolation only exacerbate the problems of the mentally ill; reversing this process could reduce their disabilities and enhance the quality of their lives. Widespread public education and information programs about mental disorders help to erase the obstacle of stigma. The community mental health nurse may promote stigma eradication through involvement in educational programs for the public, by serving on committees and boards in the community, and by influencing community leaders, lawmakers, and health policy development.

MENTAL HEALTH PROMOTION

As the field of mental health has matured through advances in epidemiologic methods, research, and treatment, there has been increasing interest in illness prevention and health promotion (SAMHSA, 1999). Treatment and prevention of mental illness are important and ongoing priorities in community mental health, but promoting mental health, which is essential to healthier people for the future, needs greater emphasis.

What Is Mental Health Promotion?

WHO (2001) has defined **mental health promotion** as an "umbrella term that covers a variety of strategies, all aimed at having a positive effect on mental health. The encouragement of individual resources and skills and improvements in the socioeconomic environment are among them." Another way to think about mental health promotion is to review the definition of mental health in *Healthy People 2010*. It is a successful performance of mental function that results in (1) productive activities, (2) fulfilling relationships, (3) the ability to adapt to change, and (4) the ability to cope with adversity (USDHHS, 2000a, p.37). Targeting of these areas becomes a way of prioritizing in planning for health-promoting interventions. In other words, it would be useful to design programs in community mental health that encourage productive activities (eg, sports, hobbies), fulfilling relationships (eg, foster grandparenting), adapting to change (eg, volunteering), and coping with adversity (eg, preparing for developmental crises).

Interventions for Mental Health Promotion

Several different approaches can be used in designing interventions for mental health promotion. Two of them are discussed here: development of interventions to protect people who are potentially at risk for mental disorders, and promotion of healthy activities and lifestyles to the general public.

Risk-Protective Activities

Epidemiologic data, along with the results of a growing body of other kinds of research, provide the community mental health nurse with increasing information about the factors that place people at risk for mental disorders. Targeting at-risk individuals with health promotion interventions gives them the resources needed to raise their own levels of health and protects them from mental disorders. It is known, for example, that consumption of alcohol, illegal drugs, and tobacco during pregnancy can damage the fetus. Consequently, extensive prenatal education and support programs can promote parental health and reduce this risk for the next generation. It also is known that abuse and neglect during child-

hood are risk factors for certain mental disorders. Promoting healthy parenting and stress-reducing activities through classes, group work, and other means can promote the health of parents and protect the health of their children.

Lifestyle and Behavior Activities

To promote the well-being of the public, health promotion interventions that are both life-sustaining and life-enhancing can be planned. Life-sustaining activities include proper nutrition and exercise, healthy sleep patterns and adequate rest, healthy coping with stress, and the ability to use family and community supports and resources. Health promotion programs in the community may address any or all of these. An example is educating schoolchildren about the food guide pyramid and encouraging the provision of healthy snacks and well-balanced meals in the home. Other examples include fitness programs for all ages, promotion of community playgrounds and walking or biking trails, and establishing networks of support in the community such as Meals on Wheels and other volunteer programs.

Life-enhancing activities include meaningful work, whether through or outside employment, creative outlets, interpersonal relationships, recreational activities, and opportunities for spiritual and intellectual growth. Again, mental health promotion interventions can address any or all of these areas. For example, arts and crafts classes and fairs encourage creative expression, community sports events promote social outlets, participation in Elderhostel (see Chapter 30) and other kinds of learning experiences promotes spiritual and intellectual stimulation, volunteer programs encourage community participation, and classes to develop new skills promote meaningful vocation (see Clinical Corner).

ROLE OF THE COMMUNITY MENTAL HEALTH NURSE

The nurse's role in community mental health is multifaceted; this has been evident throughout the chapter. First of all, the nurse must be able to *access and use epidemiologic data* in order to understand and serve the mentally ill population. This means identifying the incidence and prevalence of mental disorders, examining the causes and risk factors associated with mental illness, and identifying the needs of people with mental disorders. Nurses sometimes serve as part of the epidemiologic investigative team to conduct surveys and assist with data collection.

Next, an important part of the nurse's role with the mentally ill is *advocacy*. In this role, the nurse seeks to increase client access to mental health services, to reduce stigma and promote improved public understanding of this population, and to improve services in community mental health (Christoffel, 2000). The advocacy role requires being politically involved by serving on decision-making boards and committees, lobbying for legislative changes, and helping to influence mental health policy development that will better

CLINICAL CORNER

SCENARIO 1

You are a community health nurse in Smithville. Today you will begin working with a new client, Emmit. Emmit is a 50-year-old man who lives with his 83-year-old mother, Alice, in rural Smithville. Emmit is a veteran of the Vietnam War. His diagnoses include

- Paranoid schizophrenia with delusions
- Hypertension
- Coronary artery disease
- Peripheral neuropathy
- Hypertension

Emmit receives home health nursing services in order to monitor compliance with medications and for assessment of complications related to his multiple diagnoses. Because the nearest Veteran's Administration (VA) Hospital is located in Capitol City, Emmit's physician determined that home health services would provide the most cost-effective means of ongoing care. Emmit's case is currently under review for possible benefits related to Agent Orange exposure leading to peripheral neuropathy.

Emmit's daily medication regimen includes seven drugs prescribed qd or bid and nitroglycerin prn. He receives home health nursing visits three to four times each week for the purposes of

- Assessment and education about compliance with medications
- Physical assessment, including cardiovascular and pulmonary systems
- Assessment of mental health status and adequacy of caregiver support
- Follow-up on complaints of fatigability with activities of daily living
- Assessment and referrals about caregiver support
- Foot care

Before your initial visit with Emmit, you discuss the case with his previous nurse, James. James informs you that he has provided home health nursing services to Emmit for more than 2 years. He states that Emmit is pleasant, but that he frequently exhibits inappropriate behavior and adds, "You'd better be ready to deal with it." Primarily, Emmit's behavior focuses on expressing his anger about issues in the news. James reports that Emmit keeps abreast of political and other news events and that he has a propensity to become loud and angry when expressing his views. Emmit is also very insistent that he is capable of living independently. Despite numerous complications due to inappropriate self-medicating, Emmit has stated repeatedly, "I don't want any help from anyone, I don't mind you all visiting us, but I can take care of myself and my mother just fine."

James informs you that Alice seemed very resistant to his intervention during the first year of the home visitation but that she "came around" eventually. Due to Emmit's inconsistency in self-medicating, Alice has assumed responsibility for administering all medications. She has made formal requests to Emmit's physician and the VA Hospital to receive daily home health visits as well as a live-in support person. In reviewing previous notations in the chart, you see that Alice relates an inability to pay "with my pension"; besides, she added, "they messed up his mind . . . they should pay to take care of him." She informed James that "if something happens to me they'll just let him die . . . we have no other family to take care of him." She has frequently stated that the responsibility of caring for Emmit "is taking its toll on me."

Given the information available to you, you identify the goals of the involved parties:

Agency goals: assessment, monitoring, and education of existing medical conditions and caregiver support

VA Hospital and physician goals: maintenance of ongoing care needs in a cost-effective manner

Caregiver goals: emotional and financial support, increased level of supportive services

Client goals: increased independence

QUESTIONS

1. Based on this information, what are *your goals* for the initial visit with this family?
2. If you were to approach this situation with the goal of accomplishing all of the agency's goals each visit, what do you anticipate would occur during your initial visit? Why?
3. Conversely, what do you predict the outcome of the visit would be if you attempted to address only the issues that Emmit and Alice felt were important?
4. How will you "sell" yourself and your services in this situation?
5. Prioritize your goals and objectives:
   #1:
   #2:
   #3:
   #4:

After working with Emmit for 6 months, you attend a case conference held at the V.A. In attendance are Emmit's VA physician, a medical social worker, and the VA benefits specialist. During the course of your discussion with the other health care professional after the case conference, you realize that there are many families in your community who are in situations similar to that of Emmit and his mother.

(continued)

CLINICAL CORNER (CONTINUED)

The group decides that, given your success in working with Emmit and Alice, they would like you to begin a support group in Smithville for veterans and family members or support persons who are dealing with mental illness.

6. What more do you need to know about your aggregate?
7. How will you go about getting this information?

8. How will you define your aggregate (eg, criteria)?
9. Brainstorm about a program that would offer a holistic approach to medical and psychosocial support for your aggregate, the veterans, and their families.
10. How will you outreach to your aggregate?
11. Where might you begin to obtain assistance in your endeavors? How will you solicit funding, volunteers, donations of meeting space and foot, and so on?

---

serve this population. Membership in state and national nursing organizations can be helpful in establishing collaborative partnerships to benefit the mentally ill. Membership in the National Alliance for the Mentally Ill or other advocacy groups can also effect positive change. In any of these venues, the vision and expertise of the community mental health nurse can be used to advocate for the enhancement of existing services, the development of new services, and increased access for the mentally ill to all services.

Another aspect of the nurse's role is *education*. The community mental health nurse teaches clients individually and in groups about their mental health conditions, their treatment protocols, ways to function more independently in the community, prevention and health-promoting strategies, and much more. The nurse also teaches the public through community education programs and has an educational role with caregivers, family and community members, and health care decision makers by providing information for service planning.

Case management for persons with SMIs is also part of the community mental health nurse's role. This includes screening, assessment, care planning, arranging for service delivery, monitoring, reassessment, evaluation, and discharge. It is often offered within the context of a CMHC. Case management helps the person with an SMI to access services and live as independently as possible.

The nurse's role also involves *case-finding and referral*. This means early identification of persons with mental disorders who are in need of treatment and referral of those persons to the appropriate resources for treatment. The purpose of this role is secondary prevention, because early identification and treatment help to ameliorate the severity of the mental disorder and promote a speedier recovery.

Finally, the nurse's role includes *collaboration*. Whether serving individual clients, groups, or populations, the nurse is part of the larger community mental health team and works in collaboration with many people to accomplish the goals of community mental health. The composition of the team—made up of clients, psychiatric nurses, physicians, social workers, nutritionists, epidemiologists, psychologists, health planners, and many more—is diverse and varies depending on the community health nurse's work set-

ting. Collaboration allows for a pooling of professional expertise that enhances the quality and effectiveness of services for the mentally ill.

When working with the mentally ill, the nurse must be aware of issues of personal safety. Although most mentally ill clients are no more prone to violence than the population at large, conditions involving paranoia, hallucinations, or mania can increase clients' tendency toward physical violence. There are many cases in which social workers, physicians, or nurses have been harmed by psychotic clients. Clients who are under the influence of drugs or alcohol pose a potentially serious threat to the nurse's safety. The nurse should be prepared for this eventuality with those clients suffering from addictions. Nurses working with this population must use caution in any situation that suggests danger and must take action immediately to protect themselves and their clients. This may require the nurse to take self-defense classes or assertiveness training or to carry protective gear. It may help to use an escort from a security service, collaborate with the police, or establish a "buddy system" in which two nurses work together in isolated or dangerous homes or areas. Additionally, the public health agency may consider hiring risk-management consultants to examine dangerous situations and recommend actions to preserve safety.

The nurse serving in community mental health plays many roles that are practiced in a variety of settings in collaboration with other members of the community mental health team. It is the challenge of this role and the opportunity to assist in raising the level of mental health for individuals and communities that make this field of practice so rewarding.

ADDICTION

This chapter has included some discussion of substance abuse as it relates to the broader issue of mental health. Viewing each individual holistically, it is difficult not to appreciate the mental health issues that may precipiate substance use or abuse, as well as the aftermath of that use, be it psychological, biologic, sociocultural, or environmental. What differentiates substance use and abuse from the broader issue of mental health is the significant cost incurred by society in terms of poor health, decreased quality of life, shortened life-span, and the inherent economic implications. WHO reported that 4.9 million deaths worldwide were attributable to tobacco use in 2000, 1 million more than in 1990. Most striking in these figures is the marked increase in deaths in developing countries. This same report also noted that the gobal disease burden from alcohol has reached 4% (representing 1.8 million alcohol-related deaths), with the highest proportion occuring in the Americas and Europe (WHO, 2002). In the United States alone, alcohol abuse is estimated to result in annual economic costs of $167 billion, with drug abuse closely following at $110 billion (1995 estimates); these disorders claim resources that are desperately needed in other areas of health services. Costs aside, cigarrette smoking accounts for more deaths in this country than the combined

deaths attributed to AIDS, alcohol, cocaine, heroin, homicide, suicide, motor vehicle crashes, and fires (USDHHS, 2000a). The preventable nature of tobacco and substance use clearly set them apart in terms of national and international priorities (see The Global Community). For the community health nurse, the opportunity to influence the community through education, referral, and support is vital to meeting the *Healthy People 2010* goals.

AN OVERVIEW OF ADDICTION

Community health nurses have encountered populations with addiction problems for decades. Consider, for example, the rural nurse who serves a Native American population with a

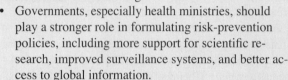

THE GLOBAL COMMUNITY

The recent WHO report, *Reducing Risks, Promoting Healthy Life* (2002), raises the attention of the international community regarding what are believed to be the greatest challenges facing world health in the 21st century. Worldwide efforts to reduce morbidity and mortality resulting from poor sanitation, communicable diseases, and under-nutrition have improved the lives of many, especially in the underdeveloped areas of the world. Although these problems remain a high priority for the world community, the greatest threats to individual and global health may be more related to life style and behavioral choices—threats no longer confined to the wealthier societies. The list of leading risks includes underweight, unsafe sex, high blood pressure, tobacco consumption, alcohol consumption, unsafe water, sanitation and hygiene, iron deficiency, indoor smoke from solid fuels, high cholesterol, and obesity. The burden of these risks is especially felt by the developing world, which must battle both extremes of risk—having too little and having too much.

Alcohol consumption has grown most dramatically in developing countries, fostered in part by a rapid increase in the marketing of alcoholic products to low- and middle-income countries. Almost 2 million deaths have been caused by alcohol consumption, representing 4% of the global disease burden. Although the proportion of deaths is highest in the Americas and Europe (as might be expected), the increase in alcohol-related deaths continues to climb across the globe. Roughly 20% to 30% of diseases such as esophageal cancer, liver disease, and epilepsy, as well as motor vehicle accidents, homicide, and other intentional injuries are attributed to alcohol.

WHO has recommended a number of actions that governments can take in order to reduce the health risks to their citizens. Those most applicable to the issue of al-

cohol include the following:

- Governments, especially health ministries, should play a stronger role in formulating risk-prevention policies, including more support for scientific research, improved surveillance systems, and better access to global information.
- Cost-effectiveness analysis should be used to identify high-, medium-, and low-priority interventions to prevent or reduce risks, with highest priority given to those interventions that are cost-effective and affordable.
- International and intersectional collaboration should be strengthened to improve risk management and increase public awareness and understanding of risks to health.
- A balance between government, community, and individual action is necessary. For example, community action should be supported by nongovernmental organizations, local groups, the media, and others. At the same time, individuals should be empowered and encouraged to make positive, life-enhancing health decisions for themselves on matters such as tobacco use, alcohol consumption, unhealthy diet, and unsafe sex.

The full report offers a road map for governments and the world community to address health risks, such as alcohol consumption, including strategies to reduce risk and the development and strengthening of risk-prevention policies. What is unique about this approach is that it shifts the focus from disease treatment for the minority to health promotion for the entire population. The challenge has been made—it will now be up to the world community to embrace prevention as a necessary and vital part of national and international programs. If the U.S. experience in funding prevention programs is any indication, this will be a hard road.

high rate of fetal alcohol syndrome, or the school nurse who sees an increasing number of adolescents reporting experimentation with methamphetamine and "Ecstasy." Sometimes the nurse has no idea what to do or where to turn to help clients begin to maintain healthful lifestyles. Before assessment, interventions, and resources for addiction are discussed, the terms commonly used when characterizing the problem need to be clarified and the history and demographics of addiction reviewed. Also, because the community health nurse may have personal issues to overcome before she or he is able to intervene in a therapeutic manner, this discussion will assist the nurse with values clarification as it relates to addiction.

Terminology of Addiction

Addiction is defined as a compulsive use and impaired control over use of a substance, preoccupation with obtaining and using the drug, and continued use despite adverse consequences. It also describes a compulsion to participate in and a preoccupaton with a certain activity, such as gambling or binge eating. The word "compulsive" indicates that the addictive behavior is beyond the individual's self-control; for this reason, addictions are very difficult to treat.

Several terms relate specifically to the abuse of chemical substances. **Chemical dependence** is a strong, overwhelming preoccupation with and desire to have a drug. It is often described as a *craving*. Chemical dependence usually accompanies addiction but does not necessarily signify the presence of addiction. **Detoxification** is a term used to describe the process of ridding the body of harmful substances. **Relapse** refers to use of a chemical or participation in an activity after a period of abstinence. **Substance abuse** refers to excessive and prolonged use of some chemical (alcohol, tobacco, drugs) that leads to serious physical, emotional, and social problems. Under these definitions, an individual may face a problem of substance abuse without actually being chemically dependent or addicted. **Polysubstance use and abuse** occurs when a person is using or abusing more than one chemical. Typical combinations of drugs are alcohol and marijuana, alcohol and tobacco, alcohol and cocaine, cocaine and marijuana, alcohol and antianxiety medications, and even tobacco and caffeine. Addiction to chemicals is characterized by **tolerance**, which is a need for increasing amounts of a substance to achieve the desired effects or a significantly diminished effect with continued use of the same amount of the same substance (American Psychiatric Association, 2000). **Triggers** are events and activities that may cause a person to continue addictive activities. If an addicted individual does not use the addictive substance for a certain period of time, he or she may experience **withdrawal symptoms**, physical and psychological symptoms such as tremors, lethargy, anxiety, or depression that are typically opposite to the effects of the addictive substance.

This discussion focuses primarily on chemical addictions to alcohol, tobacco, and other drugs, which together are commonly referred to as "ATOD." The other drugs usually include caffeine, marijuana, cocaine, CNS depressants and stimulants, hallucinogens, opiates, over-the-counter (OTC) drugs, pre-scription drugs, and inhalants. Non-substance addictions, such as addiction to gambling, are also briefly discussed.

History of Addictive Behavior in the United States

A look at the U. S. history of taxation and legislation regarding alcohol, tobacco, and other drugs reveals that most of these substances were not regulated until fairly recently but have been sources of national revenue for centuries. As early as 1600, tobacco, introduced to European settlers by Native Americans, had become a cash crop in North Carolina. A federal tax was imposed on tobacco in 1862 to help finance the Civil War. In 1864, the first federal cigarette excise tax was imposed. This began a long history of taxation of cigarettes.

Cocaine is derived from the coca plant. Cocaine was first extracted from coca leaves in the 1800s. Coca is grown in South America and was chewed as early as 3000 BC. In 1862, the pharmaceutical company Merck produced one-fourth pound of cocaine. In the 1870s, Parke, Davis manufactured a fluid extract of coca. Freud published *On Coca* in 1884, in which he recommended the use of cocaine to treat various conditions. That same year, cocaine was being used as a local anesthetic in eye surgery (Gootenberg, 1999; Spillane, 2000).

Opium has been imported, albeit illegally, for many years. Opium was used by the Sumerians as early as 3000 BC. In the 1700s, opium-tobacco mixtures began to be used in the East Indies, and their use spread to Formosa and the South China coast. The Chinese emperor prohibited the sale of opium and the operation of smoking houses. In the mid-1700s, Hong Kong merchants served as intermediaries between foreigners and the Chinese authorities. Patent medicines were readily available in the United States without restrictions. Many people used opium instead of alcohol because it was cheaper. This caused many people to become addicted. In 1800 it was legal to smoke opium and cocaine, and in 1900 patent medicines, tonics, and elixirs commonly included significant amounts of opium, cocaine, and alcohol. Not surprisingly, by 1914 many U. S. citizens were addicted to one or more of these substances. In that year, the Harrison Act was passed, requiring that narcotics dealers register with the Internal Revenue Service; however, no attempt was made at that time to criminalize the trade in or use of narcotics. It was not until the 1930s that the federal government established the first treatment programs for narcotics addiction, in Lexington, Kentucky, and Fort Worth, Texas (Allen, 1996).

The Women's Christian Temperance Union was established in 1874 to decrease the consumption of alcohol and cigarettes. Federal legislation prohibiting the manufacture and sale of alcohol did not take effect until 1919. Prohibition has been seen as a failed experiment for many reasons. It spawned illegal trafficking in liquor, which in turn resulted in increasing rates of violent crime, and it did not significantly decrease the consumption of alcohol, in part because it did not stop people from making their own spirits.

Until the early 20th century, no treatment was available for addiction to alcohol. In 1935, a stockbroker named Bill Wilson and a physician, Robert Smith, both alcoholics, founded AA to help themselves and others struggling with alcohol addiction. AA is still an important treatment option for those struggling with alcohol abuse. This 12-step self-help model is the basis for many other groups that help people deal with addictions.

More recently, Presidents Richard Nixon and George Bush declared a "war on drugs," First Lady Nancy Reagan tirelessly promoted an antidrug campaign called "Just Say No," and President Bill Clinton signed the "three strikes" crime bill, calling for life imprisonment after three convictions for drug offenses. Despite these efforts, substance abuse and chemical addiction remain serious national problems. Indeed, the incidence and prevalence of addiction to certain drugs actually increased in the final decades of the 20th century.

Population Statistics

Drug abuse is found among all socioeconomic classes, age groups, races, and genders. Data from the 2001 National Household Survey on Drug Abuse show that almost 11 million Americans aged 12 years and older had abused or were dependent on alcohol during the past year, with more than 2 million abusing or dependent on both alcohol and another illicit drug (SAMHSA, 2002).

Incidence and Prevalence

The prevalence of alcohol and drug use varies according to gender, age, and race/ethnicity. According to the 2001 National Household Survey on Drug Abuse, young adults are more likely to binge drink (consuming five or more drinks on one occasion during the past 30-day period) and to drink heavily (consuming at least five drinks on the same occasion on at least five different days in the past month). In the 18- to 25-year-old age group, almost half of current drinkers were binge drinkers and appoximately 14% to 18% were heavy drinkers (SAMHSA, 2002). Binge drinking was more common among underaged whites (22%) and least likely among Asians and Blacks (11% each). Men were more likely than women to binge drink (22% versus 16%) and to drink heavily (SAMHSA, 2002).

Trends in adolescent drug abuse and use have been measured for the past two decades in grades 8, 10, and 12. The three most prevalent drugs of abuse by adolescents are alcohol, cigarettes, and marijuana. The overall rate of drug use among adolescents has declined since 1975, although marijuana and cigarette use among students at all three grade levels actually increased during the period between 1990 and early 2000. Between 1991 and 2001, marijuana use rose from 14% to 24% among those age groups, and the percentage of students who admitted smoking cigarettes on 20 or more of the past 30 days rose from 12.7% to 13.8%. The percentage of youths admitting to having at least one alcoholic drink in the past 30 days dropped slightly between 1991 (51%) and 2001 (47%), but the numbers remain staggering. There was also a change in the attitudes of adolescents during the 1990s, with a decline in the percentage of students who believed that marijuana was harmful and disapproved of its use (Youth Risk Behavior Surveillance System, 2001).

Almost one third of heavy drinkers were also current illicit drug users. By comparison, only 1.7% of nondrinkers were illicit drug users.

Demographics

Drug abusers are individuals, primarily adolescents and young adults, who try drugs on an experimental and impulsive basis, often because of peer pressure. Repeated use in many cases leads to addiction. Some individuals are well adjusted but become addicted as a result of overprescription of medications for treatment of insomnia, pain, obesity, or some other medical condition. Others are having trouble coping with the stresses of life or have personal problems. There are individuals who become addicted as they repeatedly seek escape or release through illicit drug use. Individuals in certain professions tend to have higher rates of alcohol and drug abuse than in others. Nurses have been plagued by addiction problems, probably because of the easy access to drugs and the stresses related to the profession.

Community health nurses need to be particularly alert to aggregates that appear to be at greater risk than others. One of the populations at higher risk for abuse of chemicals is adolescents, who are particularly vulnerable to peer pressure and have a tendency to be impulsive. Recently there has been an increase in the number of senior citizens with addictions. Senior citizens often suffer from medical problems, loneliness, loss, and grief, from which they seek relief through alcohol and drugs. They also may be taking medications that can cause them to forget when they have taken them, or they may not be receiving the relief they expected from their medication; either situation may lead to overmedication, which can cause addiction problems. Another, more common practice is the concurrent use of medications and alcohol. Many individuals are unaware of the potentiation of side effects of many medications if taken with alcohol—the result could be fatigue, dizziness, falls, or medical complications.

Etiology of Addiction

There is no consensus about the causes of alcohol and drug addiction. Research approaches to studying the population of substance abusers have pointed to a variety of possible causal factors, some physiologic, some social, and some psychological. There is evidence, for example, that certain individuals using alcohol seem to "need" more, even at the onset of their drinking, suggesting a chemical predisposition leading to addiction. Other evidence points to psychological factors such as low self-esteem, or behavioral patterns such as drug experimentation, that promote use and abuse. Social factors such as overprescription and drug advertising also influence use and abuse. The environmental milieu surrounding certain individuals, which may include peer pressures, dysfunctional families, and societal attitudes about drugs (both "good" and "bad" drugs can promote use and eventual dependence). There seem to be few, if any, single causes but rather an interaction of multiple factors operating to influence substance abuse.

Biologic causative factors include a family history of alcoholism or drug abuse. Although there is little conclusive evidence that genetic predisposition is an actual cause, there is reason to believe that in some cases individuals who begin using alcohol or certain drugs are more readily susceptible to addiction. Neurobiologic theory research is beginning to identify the affects that alcohol has on the neurotransmitters in the brain. Drugs inhibit, stimulate, or change the release or action of these neurotransmitters. The disease theory was first described by Jellinek (1946) and later by Vaillant (1983). The rationale behind the disease theory is that alcoholism has a biologic cause and that there is a predictable natural history to the disease (the disease is progressive and ultimately fatal). In any case, the belief that alcohol or drug dependence and addiction are diseases has a basis in fact when one considers the effects on the health of substance abusers.

The behavioral/psychological causative factors are varied. For children and adolescents, trying new and risky things is part of normal developmental behavior and often includes experimentation with drugs, alcohol, and tobacco. Peer pressure for adolescents is a major influence and, when combined with drug experimentation, can lead to dependence. Even people who are relatively well adjusted emotionally turn to alcohol or drugs as a way to relieve stress from such things as divorce, death of a loved one, chronic pain, job loss, work pressures, family conflict, or simply a life that is too fast paced. Drug choices may range from excessive coffee consumption and smoking, to self-medication with OTC medications such as tranquilizers, to the use of illicit drugs. Social activities incorporating alcohol consumption are commonplace, and even illicit drugs such as marijuana or cocaine are encouraged in some social groups. When these patterns persist, tolerance and dependence can result. People with low self-esteem are at greater risk for substance abuse, as are those with personality disorders or other psychological disturbances who may be seeking thrills or defying authority through drug use. Their mental impairment contributes to maladaptive coping patterns, prompting some in society to unfairly label substance abuse as a "moral failing."

Sociocultural factors form another set of variables influ-

encing substance abuse. Substance abusers include all ages, sexes, races, and economic levels, but the poor and minorities are often more vulnerable because they lack the education and resources to cope with life stresses and find needed assistance. Many individuals do not realize the dangers inherent in certain drugs or do not know how to use drugs safely. They may drink alcohol while taking tranquilizers, a combination that can be lethal. Misleading information is another factor. OTC drugs are often not considered drugs, and their ready access and heavy promotion through advertising lead to abuse. Examples are the excessive use of diet pills, cold remedies, and nonprescription painkillers. Overprescription of medications, such as morphine for pain or valium for anxiety, can also lead to addiction. The quality of illegal drugs cannot be controlled, so that many drugs, such as heroin and cocaine, may be poorly mixed and have unpredictable dosages. Marijuana is now 20 times more potent than it was in the 1960s and 1970s. Social values that promote competition, productivity, and involvement in too many activities further contribute to stress that can lead to alcohol and drug abuse. Drug laws labeling users as criminals often prevent these individuals from seeking appropriate help that might prevent addiction or treat dependence. Some cultural groups promote moderate use of substances or even abstention, but in the United States these influencing variables usually are not present.

Environmental factors related to the physical and social milieu can influence substance abuse. Dysfunctional families and abusive relationships contribute to both alcohol and drug use leading to dependence. Peer pressure, with a desire for social acceptance among adolescents and young adults especially, is a strong contributing factor. The ready availability of legal and illegal drugs, particularly in highly populated urban settings, further promotes use. Widespread public misconceptions about which drugs are dangerous to health can influence abuse; many people believe that alcohol, tobacco, and OTC and prescription drugs are acceptable because they are legal. A summary of these influencing factors is shown in Figure 35–2.

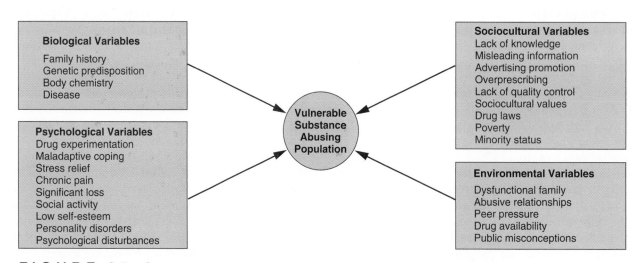

FIGURE 35–2. Factors that influence the vulnerability of the substance-abusing population.

Epidemiologic Model Applied to Addiction

Because the goal of public health is to attain the highest level of wellness for the greatest number of people, addictions are a grave public health concern. The nurse can apply the host-agent-environment epidemiologic model, shown in Figure 35–3 and further described in Chapter 8, to ATOD addiction as follows. The *host* is the individual or population affected. One must consider ethnicity, race, gender, age, and occupation, as well as the biochemical, physiologic, and psychological aspects of the disease. The disease-causing *agent* is the substance of use. The *environment,* which may foster the substance abuse, includes the values, beliefs, and norms of the culture, community, and society, as represented through governmental and nongovernmental organizations, faith communities, volunteer groups, peer groups, schools, and local, state, and federal governments. Even other nations must be considered part of the environment of addiction; because many substances that are illegal in the United States are smuggled in from other countries, it is essential that policy-making with foreign governments support activities to eliminate international trafficking in drugs.

Common Assumptions About Clients Living With Addiction

Our society holds conflicting views about addictions. The moralistic view proposes that individuals should simply "stop the behavior"; if they would only exercise their willpower, they could cease the abuse and overcome the addiction. This view is grounded in the belief that substance abuse, even when accompanied by chemical dependence and addiction, is a choice. On the other hand, as discussed earlier in this chapter, the overwhelming evidence of scientific research in the 20th century indicates that addiction, especially chemical addiction, is a disease. Proponents of this scientific view advocate the same level of compassionate assessment and intervention that would be appropriate for clients with physical

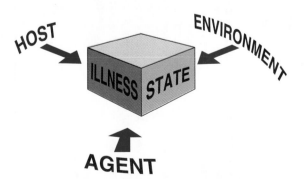

FIGURE 35–3.   Epidemiologic triad. Epidemiologists study the causal agent, the susceptible host, and environmental factors that contribute to an illness state (or a wellness state). Intervention may focus on any of these three to prevent the spread of illness or to improve health in a population.

disorders. Community health nurses must look at the reasons behind their own beliefs and values so that they can establish a therapeutic relationship with the clients involved. Some questions you might ask yourself are listed in Display 35–1.

PROBLEMS RELATED TO ADDICTION

Addiction is typically accompanied by a variety of other problems, many of which affect the addict's family and community. Each substance or addictive activity has its own particular side effects and possible consequences; these are listed more specifically in Table 35–3. The overall health needs of this at-risk population can be grouped into four categories: physical problems, psychosocial problems, economic problems, and problems experienced by the fetus, newborn, and children of addicted parents.

DISPLAY 35–1

Values Clarification

Some questions you might ask yourself include:
- What do I believe about chemical dependency?
- Is it a disease, or is it a choice people make?
- Did I have close contact with someone (mother, father, sibling, husband) who had an addiction?
- How did I feel about this person and their behavior?
- Do my religious beliefs influence my attitudes toward addictions?
- How do I ask questions about the individual and his or her use?
- Am I uncomfortable asking assessment questions?
- If I am uncomfortable, what are the reasons for this?
- Is it that I might have to intervene?
- What are my feelings when I'm making a home visit to a mother who is using chemicals?
- Do I relate to her with empathy or disdain?
- Do I distrust this mother when she states she will quit using chemicals, or do I find support systems for her and encourage her to seek help?
- How do I feel about the mother who is living with a man who is chemically dependent and abusive to her?
- Do I get annoyed that she won't leave?
- Do I understand why she stays with him?
- Do I suspect emotional and/or physical abuse?
- How do I feel about women and men who are in abusive relationships?
- How do I ask the questions to assess whether she is being abused without offending her?
- How do I assess whether he is being abused?
- What is my role if I suspect both parents are addicted?
- Are the children safe? How can I protect the children from harm?
- Am I looking at the clients' strengths?

T A B L E   3 5 – 3

Drugs Involved in Substance Abuse

Drug Type	Facts	Possible Signs of Use/Abuse	Possible Health Risks of Use/Abuse
Cannabis			
Hashish (hash, herb, kif) Hashish oil (hash oil, honey) Marijuana (grass, weed, dope, ganja, reefer, pot, Acapulco gold, Thai sticks)	Cannabis is made from the hemp plant, *Cannabis sativa*. When smoked or ingested produces mild euphoria, relaxation, and intense sensory perception. Users may develop tolerance and physical dependence. Sinsemilla is a highly potent form of marijuana.	Relaxation and euphoria Altered perceptions of time and space Hallucinations or anxiety attacks with sinsemilla use	Damage to heart and lungs Damage to brain nerve cells Memory disorders Temporary loss of fertility Psychological dependence
Depressants			
Alcohol (brew, juice, liquor) Barbiturates (downers, barbs) Benzodiazepines (Valium, Librium, tranquilizers) Chloral hydrate (knockout, Mickey Finn) Glutethimide (Doriden) Methaqualone (Quaalude, Ludes) Other Depressants (Equanil, Miltown, Noludar, Placidylm, Valmid)	Depressants depress or slow down the central nervous system by relaxing muscles, calming nerves and producing sleep. Alcohol is a depressant. Depressants are composed of sedative-hypnotic and tranquilizer drugs. Depressants are addictive. Users of depressants develop a tolerance to the drugs, meaning larger doses must be taken each time to produce the same effect.	Relaxation and drowsiness; lack of concentration; disorientation; loss of inhibitions; lack of coordination; dilated pupils; slurred speech; weak and rapid pulse; distorted vision; low blood pressure; shallow breathing; staggering; clammy skin; fever, sweating; stomach cramps; hallucinations, tremors; and delirium	Liver damage; convulsions; addiction with severe withdrawal symptoms; coma; death due to overdose. For pregnant women: the newborn may be dependent and experience withdrawal or suffer from birth defects and behavioral problems
Hallucinogens			
Lysergic acid diethylamide (LSD) Phencyclidine (PCP, angel dust) Mescaline and peyote (Mesc, buttons, cactus) Psilocybin (mushrooms) Amphetamine variants (MDMA/Ecstasy, MDA/Love Drug, TMA, DOM, DOB, PMA, STP, 2.5-DMA) Phencyclidine analogues (PCE, PCPy, TCP) Other hallucinogens (Bufotenine, Ibogaine, DMT, DET)	Hallucinogens are psychedelic, mind-altering drugs that affect a person's perception, feelings, thinking, self-awareness, and emotions. A "bad trip" may result in the user's experiencing panic, confusion, paranoia, anxiety, unpleasant sensory images, feelings of helplessness, and loss of control. A "flash back" is a reoccurrence of the original drug experience without taking the drug again.	Dilated pupils, increased body temperature, heart rate, and blood pressure; sweating; loss of appetite; sleeplessness; dry mouth; tremors; hallucinations; disorientation; confusion; paranoia; violence; euphoria; anxiety; and panic	Agitation; extreme hyperactivity; psychosis; convulsions; mental or emotional problems; death

(continued)

TABLE 35-3 (continued)

Drugs Involved in Substance Abuse

Drug Type	Facts	Possible Signs of Use/Abuse	Possible Health Risks of Use/Abuse
Inhalants			
Amyl nitrate (poppers, snappers) Butyl nitrate (rush, bolt, bullet) Chlorohydrocarbons (aerosol sprays, cleaning fluids) Hydrocarbons (solvents, airplane glue, gasoline, paint thinner) Nitrous oxide (laughing gas, whippets)	Inhalants are substances that are breathed or inhaled through the nose. Inhalants are depressants and depress or slow down the body's functions. Inhalants are normally not thought of as drugs because they are often common household or industrial products. However, inhalants are often the most dangerous drugs per dose.	Euphoria and lightheadedness; excitability; loss of appetite; forgetfulness; weight loss; sneezing; coughing; nausea and vomiting; lack of coordination; bad breath; red eyes; sores on nose and mouth; delayed reflexes; decreased blood pressure; flushing (skin appears to be reddish); headache; dizziness; and violence	Depression; damage to the nervous system and body tissues; damage to liver and brain; heart failure; respiratory arrest; suffocation; unconsciousness; seizures; heart failure; sudden death from sniffing
Narcotics			
Codeine (school boy) Heroin (H, harry, junk, brown sugar, smack) Meperidine (doctors) Methadone (dollies, methadose) Morphine (morpho, Miss Emma) Opium (Dover's powder) Other narcotics (Percodan, Talwin, Lomotil, Darvon, Numorphan, Percocet, Tylox, Tussionex, fentanyl)	Narcotics are composed of opiates and synthetic drugs. Opiates are derived from the seed pod of the Asian poppy. Synthetic drugs called opioids are chemically developed to produce the effects of opiates. Initially, narcotics stimulate the higher centers of the brain, but then slow down the activity of the central nervous system. Narcotics relieve pain and induce sleep. Narcotics, such as heroin, are often diluted with other substances (i.e., water, sugar) and injected. Other narcotics are taken orally or inhaled. Narcotics are extremely addictive. Users of narcotics develop a tolerance to the drugs, meaning larger doses must be taken each time to produce the same effect.	Euphoria; restlessness and lack of motivation; drowsiness; lethargy; decreased pulse rate; constricted pupils; flushing (skin appears to be reddish); constipation; nausea and vomiting; needle marks on extremities; skin abscess at injection sites; shallow breathing; watery eyes; and itching	Pulmonary edema; respiratory arrest; convulsions; addiction; coma; death due to overdose. For users who share or use unsterile needles to inject narcotics: tetanus, hepatitis, HIV/AIDS. For pregnant women: premature births; stillbirth, and acute infections among newborns

(continued)

T A B L E   35-3   (continued)

Drugs Involved in Substance Abuse

Drug Type	Facts	Possible Signs of Use/Abuse	Possible Health Risks of Use/Abuse
Steroids			
Anabolic-Androgenic (roids, juice, d-ball)	Steroids may contribute to increases in body weight and muscular strength. The acceleration of physical development is what makes steroids appealing to athletes and young adults. Anabolic-androgenic steroids are chemically related to the male sex hormone testosterone. Anabolic means to build up the muscles and other tissues of the body. Steroids are injected directly into the muscle or taken orally.	Sudden increase in muscle and weight; increase in aggression and combativeness; violence ("roid rage"); hallucinations; jaundice; purple or red spots on body, inside mouth, or nose; swelling of feet or lower legs (edema); tremors; and bad breath. For women: breast reduction, enlarged clitoris, facial hair and baldness, deepened voice. For men: enlarged nipples and breasts, testicle reduction, enlarged prostate, baldness.	Acne; high blood pressure; liver and kidney damage; heart disease; increased risk of injury to ligaments and tendons; bowel and urinary problems; gallstones and kidney stones; liver cancer. For men: impotence and sterility. For women: menstrual problems. For users who share or use unsterile needles to inject steroids: hepatitis, tetanus, AIDS
Stimulants			
Amphetamines (uppers, pep pills) Cocaine (coke, flake, snow) Crack (rock) Methamphetamines (ice, crank, crystal) Methylphenidate (Ritalin) Phenmetrazine (Preludin, Preludes) Other stimulants (Adipex, Cylert, Didrex, Ionamin, Melfiat, Plegine, Sanorex, Tenuate, Tepanil, Prelu-2)	Stimulants stimulate the central nervous system, increasing alertness and activity. Users of stimulants develop a tolerance, meaning larger doses must be taken to get the same effect. Stimulants are psychologically addictive.	Increased alertness; excessive activity; agitation; euphoria; excitability; increased pulse rate, blood pressure, and body temperature; insomnia; loss of appetite; sweating; dry mouth and lips; bad breath; disorientation; apathy; hallucinations; irritability; and nervousness	Headaches; depression; malnutrition; hypertension; psychosis; cardiac arrest; damage to the brain and lungs; convulsions; coma; death

(From Spradley, B.W., & Allender, J.A. [1996]. *Community health nursing* [4th ed.]. Philadelphia; Lippincott-Raven.)

T A B L E   3 5 – 4

Health-Related Problems of the Substance-Abusing Population

Physical Problems	Psychological Problems	Social Problems
Physical damage (liver, brain, heart, central nervous system, kidneys, skin, ligaments and tendons, bowel, lungs)	Psychological dependence	Poverty
Disease (heart, lung cancer, AIDS, cirrhosis of liver, hepatitis)	Anxiety	Unemployment
Exposed newborns (low birth weight, birth defects, addiction, stillbirth, premature birth, infections)	Depression	Stigma
	Agitation	Punishment for crimes committed to support habits
	Hyperactivity	Family disruption
Polysubstance interactions	Hallucinations	Family neglect/abuse
Sterility	Neuroses	Depleted family resources
Headaches	Psychoses	Increased violence in community
Malnutrition	Violence	Homicide
Addiction and withdrawal	Suicide	Crime
Memory disorders		High cost of drug treatment and rehabilitation
Pulmonary edems		
Convulsions		
Respiratory arrest		
Cardiac arrest		
Suffocation		
Unconsciousness		
Coma and death		

(From Spradley, B.W., & Allender, J.A. [1996]. *Community health nursing* [4th ed.]. Philadelphia; Lippincott-Raven.)

Physical Problems

Serious physical health problems can arise from substance abuse. Damage to organs and other body parts is common with most drugs and includes damage to the liver, brain, CNS, heart, kidneys, skin, ligaments and tendons, bowel, and lungs. Disease resulting from substance abuse includes cirrhosis of the liver with alcohol abuse, heart disease and liver cancer with abuse of steroids, AIDS and hepatitis from needle sharing with narcotics, and lung cancer with tobacco and marijuana abuse. Abuse of steroids can cause impotence and sterility in men and menstrual problems in women, and marijuana abuse can lead to infertility in both women and men. Other physical problems include headaches, malnutrition, severe withdrawal symptoms from addiction, memory disorders with marijuana, pulmonary edema with narcotics, convulsions, respiratory arrest, heart failure, suffocation, unconsciousness, and, with overdose, coma and death. Polysubstance use and abuse can also lead to serious results from multiple drug interactions (American Psychiatric Association, 2000; USDHHS, 2001).

Psychosocial Problems

Social problems resulting from substance abuse cover a broad area affecting individual abusers, their families, and the community. Monetary and social costs to the individual of maintaining a drug habit can lead to poverty, unemployment, social stigma, and punishment for crime. Abuse of alcohol and drugs creates family disruption, neglect, and abuse and depletes financial and emotional resources. For the community, problems include an increased incidence of violence, traffic accidents and deaths, homicides, and crimes related to obtaining money or possessing illicit drugs. Further problems for the community come from the added costs of law enforcement, welfare programs, drug abuse surveillance, and drug treatment and rehabilitation services (Table 35–4).

Psychological Dependence

Psychological dependence occurs when the user perceives the need for a substance to maintain his or her optimal state of well-being, interpersonal relationships, or skill performance. Often the user does not recognize that he or she has an addiction to the drug. This is common with people who abuse antianxiety drugs; the drugs may have been prescribed, but the user increases the dose as increased problems with coping are experienced. Other problems observed in substance abusers include anxiety and depression (with use of inhalants); agitation, hyperactivity, and hallucinations (with hallucinogens); and neuroses, psychoses, violence, and suicide.

Depression and Suicide

Depression is a common disorder that is associated with chemical use and abuse. Many of the drugs involved are CNS depressants. People who experience clinical depression and other psychological disorders use drugs to self-medicate or to help diminish their symptoms. Some people are suicidal when they use drugs or alcohol. It is important for nurses to assess the level of depression, previous suicide attempts, and suicidal ideation. It is not uncommon for people who are intoxicated to talk about suicide and later, when they are sober, deny any suicidal ideation. These symptoms cannot be ignored. It is a myth that people who are intoxicated will not or cannot commit suicide. People who are intoxicated often commit suicide.

Codependence

Codependence is a term used to describe dysfunctional behaviors that are evident among family members. It describes individuals who are able to achieve a sense of control through fulfilling the needs of others. An example of a codependent person is a wife who controls the family finances and gives her alcoholic husband an allowance to prevent him from spending all his money on alcohol. People who are codependent are unable to meet their needs for autonomy and self-esteem and feel a sense of powerlessness.

There is no criterion available to describe this behavior as a psychiatric condition. Some of the behaviors seen in people who are codependent are controlling or attempting to control others; assuming responsibility for meeting others' needs; exhibiting anxiety and boundary distortions; and being enmeshed in relationships, especially with people who have personality disorders, are chemically dependent, or are also codependent. It is not uncommon for people who are chemically dependent to seek help for their own issues of codependency. Several resources are available to help people overcome some of the problems related to codependency; the most available and widely used is Al-Anon, which is designed on the principles of AA. Providing a safe environment for the individual to explore feelings and share experiences with others in a nonjudgemental atmosphere is a hallmark of self-help groups such as Al-Anon. A similar group designed exclusively for teenagers living with alcoholism (often of a parent) is Alateen. Both groups are available in most communities. The 12 Steps and 12 Traditions of Al-Anon are shown in Table 35–5. It should be noted that the term "God" is used throughout these tenents, although the alternative "Higher Power" is also used by members of Al-Anon who do not feel comfortable with use of the term "God."

Family Disruption, Neglect, and Abuse

Families are almost always adversely affected when someone in the family is using or abusing drugs or alcohol, and it is not uncommon for marriages to fall apart as the result of addictions. There are often family secrets and abuse, both physical and emotional. It is not uncommon to see bruises on family members that are hard to explain. Children do not bring friends home for fear of being embarrassed by the behavior of the person in the household who is chemically dependent. There is often poverty, related to the amount of money that goes for drugs or alcohol. Children may have to go without food because there is no money for groceries. The toll that gambling takes on a family is especially difficult. Family members are usually the last to know that there is a gambling problem; by that time, the gambling addict has often mortgaged the house and spent all the savings (see Chapter 25).

Community Problems

There is a high cost to communities related to addiction problems. Children miss school because no one is available to get them there. States must increase jail and prison space to house more and more people who are convicted of drug-related crimes. Communities are often spending more tax dollars on jails than on schools. In many communities, parents are afraid to let their children play outside because of fears that they may be caught in the crossfire of rival drug-dealing gangs or approached by drug dealers. Children often are living in deplorable situations in "crack houses" because their caregivers are addicts. These conditions are often very unsafe because children may have access to drugs, needles, and weapons. Because many people leave inner-city communities to avoid the problems of poverty, drug and alcohol abuse and related crimes, and poor school systems, the remaining tax base for prevention programs is reduced (see Chapters 32 and 36).

Economic Problems

Many economic problems are associated with addiction. Clients often are poor as a result of their inability to keep a job; they may end up working for temporary agencies or at low-paying jobs. It is not uncommon for people to move frequently because they are unable to pay rent or are evicted because of their destructive behavior. Legal problems often are encountered by the addict. These problems may be a result of stealing money to support their habit. There are endless costs in disability, treatment programs, unemployment, and low productivity on the job, as well as welfare costs when a family loses a breadwinner.

Problems of the Fetus, Newborn, and Children of Addicted Parents

The problem of alcohol use during pregnancy has led to a significant amount of research covering the range of child bearing in women. One of the leading preventable causes of birth defects, mental retardation, and neurodevelopmental disorders is prenatal exposure to alcohol (Jacobs et al., 2000). During 1999, approximately one-half million pregnant women nationwide reported having had one or more drinks during the preceding month, and more than 130,000 reported seven or more drinks per week (Centers for Disease Control and Prevention, 2003). This has warranted several goals in *Healthy People 2010*. One goal that relates to pregnant women who may use or abuse drugs during pregnancy is to increase abstinence from alcohol, cigarettes, and illicit drugs among pregnant women. Another goal is to decrease the incidence of fetal alcohol syndrome. Prenatal use of alcohol causes many birth defects, and there is a wide window of opportunity during pregnancy for alcohol to affect the CNS of the fetus. It is not known what affect alcohol has on the sperm or on the woman before she is pregnant. Adolescents are becoming sexually active and consequently pregnant at a young age. Teenage sexual promiscuity and teen pregnancy have been linked to adolescent substance abuse (Winters,

TABLE 35-5

12 Steps and 12 Traditions of Al-Anon

12 Steps	12 Traditions
• We admitted we were powerless over alcohol—that our lives had become unmanageable.	• Our common welfare should come first; personal progress for the greatest number depends upon unity.
• Came to believe that a Power greater than ourselves could restore us to sanity.	• For our group purpose there is but one authority—a loving God as He may express Himself in our group conscience. Our leaders are but trusted servants; they do not govern.
• Made a decision to turn our will and our lives over the care of God *as we understood Him.*	• The relatives of alcoholics, when gathered together for mutual aid, may call themselves an Al-Anon Family Group, providing that, as a group they have no other affiliation. The only requirement for membership is that there be a problem of alcoholism in a relative or friend.
• Made a searching and fearless moral inventory of ourselves.	
• Admitted to God, to ourselves and to another human being the exact nature of our wrongs.	• Each group should be autonomous, except in matters affecting another group of Al-Anon or AA as a whole.
• Were entirely ready to have God remove all these defects of character.	• Each Al-Anon Family Group has but one purpose: to help families of alcoholics. We do this by practicing the Twelve Steps of AA *ourselves,* by encouraging and understanding our alcoholic relatives, and by welcoming and giving comfort to families of alcoholics.
• Humbly asked Him to remove our shortcomings.	
• Made a list of all persons we had harmed, and became willing to make amends to them all.	• Our Al-Anon Family Groups ought never endorse, finance, or lend our name to any outside enterprise, lest problems of money, property and prestige divert us from our primary spiritual aim. Although a separate entity, we should always cooperate with Alcoholics Anonymous.
• Made direct amends to such people wherever possible, except when to do so would injure them or others.	
• Continued to take personal inventory and when we were wrong promptly admitted it.	• Every group ought to be fully self-supporting, declining outside contributions.
• Sought through prayer and meditation to improve our conscience contact with God *as we understood Him,* praying only for knowledge of His will for us and the power to carry that out.	• Al-Anon Twelfth Step work should remain forever nonprofessional, but our service centers may employ special workers.
• Having had a spiritual awakening as the result of these Steps, we tried to carry this message to others, and to practice these principles in all our affairs.	• Our groups, as such, ought never be organized; but we may create service boards or committees directly responsible to those they serve.
	• The Al-Anon Family Groups have no opinion on outside issues; hence our name ought never be drawn into public controversy.
	• Our public relations policy is based on attraction rather than promotion; we need always maintain personal anonymity at the level of press, radio, TV and films. We need guard with special care the anonymity of all AA members.
	• Anonymity is the spiritual foundation of all our Traditions, ever reminding us to place principles above personalities.

(From Al-Anon Family Group Headquarters. [2003a]. *The twelve steps.* Virginia Beach, VA: Author. Available at: *http://www.al-anon.org/12steps.html*; Al-Anon Family Group Headquarters. [2003b]. *The twelve traditions.* Virginia Beach, VA: Author. Available at: *http://www.al-anon.org/12traditions.html*)

1999). Many women are drinking alcohol before they know they are pregnant, which can cause problems during fetal development. Primary prevention information can be disseminated throughout a community through the schools, public service announcements, doctors' offices, fliers, and newspaper articles.

ALCOHOL ADDICTION

One of the most widely available and deadly chemicals is alcohol. It has been used for thousands of years for "recreational purposes," to induce relaxation, disinhibition, or euphoria. Alcohol has also been used as a beverage when water supplies were contaminated, as a medicine, for pain relief and sedation, and in religious ceremonies to promote visions or feelings of community or ecstasy. Even today a community's social, cultural, and religious values influence the level of alcohol use observed in that community.

Community health nurses have an opportunity to implement appropriate prevention strategies once they have become informed about the uniqueness of the community they serve. Community assessment is the first activity that should be accomplished: What does the population look like, in terms of age, level of education, ratio of families to singles, employment, and so on? What local statutes or programs focus on preventing alcohol abuse? What resources are currently available? The community health nurse is in a unique position to facilitate community-wide coalitions to address alcohol abuse, dependence, and addiction.

Preventive Measures

Because experimentation with alcohol commonly begins in the early teen years, prevention strategies work best if they are begun with young children. Also, a multidimensional approach that includes family, social groups, school, church, local community, and local media is also important at all stages of prevention.

Primary Prevention

Primary prevention is extremely important to help decrease the multitude of problems associated with alcohol use and abuse. Primary prevention methods in regard to alcohol addiction need to take into consideration the current theories of addiction (eg, the probability of a genetic predisposition). It is important that the community health nurse include this aspect in presentations to the community. Because many people begin using alcohol by the junior high school years or earlier, primary prevention must begin before junior high school.

Secondary Prevention

Secondary prevention strategies begin with individuals who have been assessed and found to be at risk for development of an addiction. The nurse assesses the amount of use; the impact the use is having on the family, job, and other relationships; and the safety of the family if the alcoholic is violent when drinking. Binge drinking must also be assessed, because it is a very common phenomenon among young adults (USDHHS, 2000a). Many people do not think they have a problem with alcohol if they "just drink on weekends." Binge use was defined in the 2001 National Household Survey on Drug Abuse as "five or more drinks on the same occasion at least once in the 30 days prior to survey." The survey results showed that young adults aged 18 to 25 years had the highest rate of binge drinking, peaking at 21 years of age (SAMHSA, 2002).

Many tools have been developed to assist with screening people for alcohol addiction problems. Use of the DSM-IV cri-

teria and the screening tool known as CAGE (acronym for **c**ut down, **a**nnoyed by criticism, **g**uilty about drinking, and **e**ye-opener drinks) helps the community health nurse assess the severity of the drinking problem (Display 35–2). The CAGE screening tool, developed in 1984, is simple, easy to use, and has been widely applied (Ewing, 1984). Studies have suggested, however, that with the elderly additional queries beyond the standard CAGE survey may improve identification of at-risk individuals (Bradley et al., 2001; Moore, et al., 2002).

Once a problem is identified, the nurse must assess the readiness of the individual for treatment and the kind of intervention that is most appropriate. The progression from substance abuse or dependence to recovery was researched extensively by Prochaska and DeClemente (1992). Five stages of change in addictive behaviors were identified:

- *Precontemplation,* in which there is no intention to change behavior in the foreseeable future. At this stage, the individual may be denying that there is a problem; family and friends either are not aware of the problem or are also denying it.
- *Contemplation,* in which the individual is seriously thinking about overcoming the problem but has not yet made a commitment to take action.
- *Preparation,* in which the individual makes a commitment to change and prepares for action.
- *Action,* in which the individual modifies his or her behavior to overcome alcohol use.
- *Maintenance,* in which the individual works to prevent relapse.

Once the problem has been identified, the nurse explores the most appropriate kind of intervention. AA is an excellent referral resource that is available in most communities. The meetings are anonymous, because many people are afraid they will be looked down on, lose their jobs, or be isolated from family or friends if their addiction is found out. Since the mid-20th century there has been a proliferation of treatment programs for people with alcohol problems. Employers began to recognize that alcoholism was costing them money from accidents on the job, lost time from work due to alcohol use on weekends, and other problems. Many corporations began to set up or contract with agencies to provide counseling to employees and their families. These programs are generally called Employee Assistance Programs (EAPs). Counseling often includes issues related to substance abuse, family relationships, anger management, and financial management.

The nursing assessment must include a determination of whether the individual is experiencing withdrawal symptoms. Withdrawal symptoms can include increased anxiety, diaphoresis, tremors, increased vital signs, nausea and vomiting leading to dehydration, seizures (if not given immediate medical attention), delirium tremens, and ultimately death. Individuals often self-medicate with alcohol when the withdrawal symptoms appear, thus continuing the vicious circle of alcoholism. The nurse must be supportive and assist the client to access detoxification services. These services are available in most communities and provide medical inter-

DISPLAY 35–2

CAGE Screening Tool

C Have you felt you ought to **cut down** on your drinking?

A Have people **annoyed** you by criticizing your drinking?

G Have you felt bad or **guilty** about your drinking?

E Have you ever had a drink first thing in the morning—an **eye opener**—to steady your nerves or get rid of a hangover?

Note: More than one positive response indicates a probable drinking problem.

(Ewing, J.A. [1984]. Detecting alcoholism: The CAGE questionnaire. *Journal of the American Medical Association, 252*(14), 1905–1907.)

LEVELS OF PREVENTION MATRIX

SITUATION: A neighboring community in a Midwestern state recently suffered the los of several high school students in alcohol-related traffic accidents. This has prompted a rural high school to look at ways to prevent similar tragedies with their own population.

GOAL: Using the three levels of prevention, negative health conditions are avoided, or promptly diagnosed and treated, and the fullest possible potential is restored.

PRIMARY PREVENTION		SECONDARY PREVENTION		TERTIARY PREVENTION		
Health Promotion and Education	*Health Protection*	*Early Diagnosis*	*Prompt Treatment*	*Rehabilitation*	*Primary Prevention*	
					Health Promotion and Education	*Health Protection*
• Health education: a school nurse arranges for a school-wide presentation by a local teenager who was involved in an alcohol-related traffic fatality and now shares his experiences with other teenagers.	• A school nurse works with the Parent Teacher Association to plan senior graduation activities that are safe, entertaining, reasonably priced, and alcohol/drug free.	• Screening and case-finding: a nurse works with a local addictions counseling center to administer a simple screening tool to self-identify alcohol abuse and misuse in teenagers during a class on substance abuse.	• Treatment: teenagers who take the screening test and would like additional information regarding available counseling services are provided with a local phone number to call. They are assured that the services are free and confidential.	• Restore function: the school nurse works with school administrators to make space available for meetings of Alcoholics Anonymous and AlaTeen on school premises, both after school and on weekends.	• Health teaching: a nurse provides ongoing classroom education on the risks of alcohol use by teenagers and resources available within the community.	• Maintenance: a nurse works with local law enforcement to provide a visible police presence during and especially after major school events, to help identify teenagers who may be under the influence of alcohol or drugs.

vention, which includes giving the client medications that will decrease the withdrawal symptoms.

The next step after detoxification is to get the client into a treatment program or AA. Many treatment programs are conducted on an outpatient basis. For most people who are addicted to alcohol, abstinence is the only option for sobriety. Sobriety is difficult for many people because they must change their old lifestyle, habits, ways of thinking, and ways of dealing with life's problems in addition to dealing with the problems of physiologic withdrawal (eg, cravings).

Tertiary Prevention

The most important aspect of tertiary prevention is to help the individual remain drug free. There should be rapid inter-

vention if the client relapses. Interventions implemented before the relapse help the client build self-esteem and positive feelings about the ability to stay sober. Growing evidence shows that memories of places and events experienced while using alcohol can cause cravings and can trigger a relapse in people who have some sobriety. Helping the client identify the triggers that precipitate alcohol use, so that those situations can be avoided, is very helpful. It is especially important that the client be able to talk about and work through these feelings with nonjudgmental, sober people.

Another aspect is helping the client with residual health problems as a result of former alcohol abuse to maintain as active and healthy a lifestyle as possible. Health problems can cause depression, which can lead to using alcohol again.

Role of the Community Health Nurse

The community health nurse plays a vital role in working with clients, their families, and communities. The nurse provides the community with prevention information and works with other agencies to provide prevention programs to pregnant women, adolescents, and other high-risk populations. Because the community health nurse has access to individuals and families, he or she can provide information, assess the level of the alcohol addiction, and assist in the referral process. One of the most important aspects of intervention is the support the nurse can provide to the client and family during very difficult times. The nurse should work with the family to ensure that a safety plan is in place if there is a possibility of violence. The nurse knows the referral resources in the community for the family as well as the client and can facilitate appropriate referrals.

TOBACCO ADDICTION

The first report on the detrimental effects of tobacco on the health of individuals was the Surgeon General's Report to Congress in 1964. Since that time, there has been an increasing awareness of the impact of tobacco on the health of the nation. Specifically, smoking or using other forms of nicotine, such as snuff and chewing tobacco, increases the risk of coronary artery disease, chronic obstructive pulmonary disease, and cancers of the mouth, throat, and lungs.

Nicotine is also highly addictive, providing both relaxation and an increase in energy. When smoked, it reaches the brain in just 7 seconds, and one pinch of chewing tobacco produces the effects of three to four cigarettes. Finally, because it is legal, widely available, relatively inexpensive, and socially acceptable in many peer groups, tobacco is often the first substance to which adolescents form an addiction.

Preventive Measures

All health care workers see the effects of tobacco use daily. For the elderly client facing surgery for lung cancer, even tertiary measures may be of little consequence. Prevention measures are most effective before tobacco use begins and are also moderately successful in achieving long-term cessation before the onset of addiction.

Primary Prevention

There appears to be a set of stages that adolescents go through when beginning to use tobacco. In the *preparatory stage,* the adolescent develops attitudes about smoking. In the *trying stage,* he or she tries a few cigarettes. The *experimental stage* is marked by repeated but irregular use of tobacco. This stage often advances to the *regular use* stage and then to *addiction,* with physiologic dependence on tobacco (USDHHS, 2000b).

Given this information, it is important for the community health nurse to use aggressive primary prevention strategies.

As usual, a multidimensional approach is most effective, with families, schools, neighborhood groups, and governmental agencies working together. The earlier that information is disseminated to parents and children, the more likely it is that tobacco use will never start. Teaching should include the problems nicotine can cause to the health of the individual, the effects of secondhand smoke, and the highly addictive nature of nicotine, including chewing tobacco and snuff. Teaching strategies for children could employ colorful pictures, simple language, role-playing, and other interactive games.

In many communities, law-enforcement officials and citizens monitor cigarette machines to prevent underage smoking. Cigarette machines are being discouraged, and merchants are being encouraged to keep cigarettes and smokeless tobacco behind the counter and to require some identification before purchase of these products.

Secondary Prevention

Secondary prevention includes identifying people who are using tobacco or who are addicted. There are four stages that people go through when trying to quit using tobacco:
- Stage I: The client is not thinking seriously about quitting.
- State II: The client is seriously thinking about quitting.
- Stage III: The client is actively trying to quit.
- Stage IV: The client has quit and is trying to maintain abstinence from nicotine.

Understanding which stage the client is in can help the nurse identify appropriate interventions. Some of the resources available for clients who are addicted are health insurance plans that offer education materials and support groups. The American Cancer Society and the American Lung Association have excellent materials; state and local health departments often have developed materials to help people quit using tobacco. The community health nurse can help the client identify triggers that cause the desire to use tobacco.

Pregnant women who use tobacco are at high risk of causing harm to the fetus. Prenatal exposure has been linked to risk of miscarriage, premature delivery, and sudden infant death syndrome (USDHHS, 2000a), The community health nurse can be very helpful and supportive to this population. Useful materials are available, and in some cases nurses have established support groups in the community. Parents who smoke are exposing their children to problems such as asthma and bronchitis, not to mention the higher risk of injury and death resulting from smoking-related household fires (USDHHS, 2000a).

Tertiary Prevention

Many people who have smoked are suffering from the long-term effects of their addiction. The health problems can be life-threatening and include emphysema, lung cancer, other forms of cancer, and heart disease. Many people who develop diseases related to tobacco often continue to use tobacco products long after the initial diagnosis, despite the obvious decline in their overall health. It is important for the community health nurse to continue to provide encouragement to those who have quit and to support the efforts of those who have been less successful. Because you as a community health nurse may provide care to individuals who are suffering from life-threatening diseases caused by tobacco use, it may be helpful for you to again evaluate your own attitudes about addictions (see Display 35–1).

Role of the Community Health Nurse

Community health nurses play a significant role in working with communities to prevent tobacco addiction. The community may need to be educated about the addictive qualities of tobacco, and the nurse may work with educators to help prevent students from beginning to use tobacco. The nurse plays an important role in helping pregnant women to quit using tobacco, to prevent the problems related to low-birth-rate infants and other medical problems associated with tobacco use. The nurse can provide the support and resources necessary to help people who are addicted to tobacco to quit. In the community, the nurse can work with law enforcement agencies and community members to ensure that laws regarding sales to minors are enforced.

OTHER CENTRAL NERVOUS SYSTEM DEPRESSANTS

Marijuana is the most widely used illicit drug. It is widely available, easy to grow, relatively inexpensive, and used by all age groups. There is considerable disagreement about the medicinal effects of marijuana use in decreasing the nausea associated with chemotherapy, AIDS, and other disorders. There is also disagreement about the addictive qualities of marijuana. Marijuana affects the CNS, cardiovascular system, and respiratory system. It causes intoxication, euphoria, relaxation, impaired judgment, memory failure, increased heart rate, reddened eyes, and dry mouth.

Other depressants used by people are the benzodiazepines, opiates, and sedatives/hypnotics. The benzodiazepines that are the most widely used and abused are diazepam (Valium), chlordiazepoxide (Librium), lorazepam (Ativan), clonazepam (Klonopin), and alprazolam (Xanax). They are addictive, and withdrawal is similar to the withdrawal from alcohol. Almost all CNS depressants cross the blood–brain and placental barriers, so women who are pregnant should not be prescribed these medications. Withdrawal symptoms include drowsiness, slurred speech, unsteady gait, mood lability, lack of coordination, impaired judgment, memory failure, and seizures. It is important to assess the client for suicidal tendencies, anxiety, depression, and alcoholism.

Sedatives/hypnotics are the drugs of choice for people who have other addictions. These drugs include the barbiturates secobarbital (Seconal), phenobarbital, pentobarbital (Nembutal), amobarbital (Amytal), Tuinal, and other barbiturate-like drugs. The toxic effects of these drugs cause symptoms similar to those caused by the benzodiazepines. They produce drowsiness, euphoria, emotional lability, poor judgment, and decreased blood pressure, respirations, temperature, pulse, and urinary output. Respiratory and cardiac failure can occur with an overdose. Accidental overdoses are fairly common, becase the individual cannot remember how much or when the drug was last taken.

Opiates are common analgesics that are often abused and cause addiction. The most frequently abused opiates are morphine, heroin, hydromorphone (Dilaudid), methadone, and, more recently, designer drugs. They affect the CNS receptors, respiratory system, and peripheral nervous system.

Preventive Measures

People who use and abuse depressants are usually obtaining the drugs through illegal methods. Preventive measures can be effective when the drugs are prescribed and education is provided to the client about the effects and side effects. Working with law enforcement agencies can help curb some of the illegal drug activity.

Primary Prevention

Primary prevention methods used in preventing abuse of and addiction to depressants are similar to those used with other chemicals. It is important that the community health nurse assess the amount of use and the availability of the drugs in the community. Sources of information include emergency departments, police departments, drug and alcohol counselors, and drug treatment programs.

Benzodiazepines are prescribed for people suffering from anxiety, panic attacks, and other mental health problems. Educating the client regarding the importance of taking the medication as prescribed and the potentially addictive quality of the medication is useful. The client should feel free to contact the prescribing physician if the medication is not working, rather than increase the dose or begin self-medicating. Pregnant women should be educated about the problems that can be caused by ingesting CNS depressants, including the fact that the fetus will experience the same effects that the woman experiences. It is especially important for the community health nurse to be vigilant with older people, who often forget when they have taken their medication. They may also have adverse effects from the medication, which can include confusion.

Secondary Prevention

Nurses often are confronted with problems of clients who are, or whom they suspect are, addicted to CNS depressants. If the nurse believes that a client is abusing any of the depressants, it is important that the client be medically withdrawn and detoxified from the chemical. Benzodiazepine withdrawal is similar to alcohol withdrawal. The withdrawal symptoms are anxiety, tremors, diaphoresis, increased vital signs, and possible seizures. Withdrawal from opiates causes "flulike" symptoms, including nausea, vomiting, muscle aching and cramping, rhinorrhea, diaphoresis, dilated pupils, pilorection, diarrhea, fever, insomnia, yawning, irritability, increased sensitivity to pain, and "craving." Gradual tapering of the chemical may be indicated, but this is more safely done in a medical facility than on a self-monitored outpatient basis, which can be risky for the client and the family. It is relatively easy to access chemicals illegally, so it is important that treatment be started immediately after the withdrawal is completed.

Tertiary Prevention

Tertiary prevention includes ongoing support groups and staying away from places and people who might cause the client to remember past use and cause cravings. The family will need ongoing support. Clients must be encouraged to share with their physicians and care providers the fact that they once had a substance abuse problem, so that they will not inadvertently be prescribed their drug of choice, thus starting the cycle over again. There may be long-term health problems related to the addiction, including hepatitis, AIDS, lung problems, heart problems, and other systemic disorders. Community health nurses will provide nursing care to clients with these long-term problems.

Role of the Community Health Nurse

Many people do not know what can be done for someone who is addicted to depressants. The community health nurse is in a unique position to provide education and information about the effects and side effect of these drugs and can help assess the level of use or abuse. Helping the family or client access appropriate referral sources and giving the client and family support are important activities of the nurse.

STIMULANTS

People use stimulants for a variety of reasons: for recreational purposes to "get high," for weight loss to decrease the appetite, and to increase energy levels. Chemicals used include methylphenidate (Ritalin), cocaine, and crack (the solid form of cocaine). Crack and cocaine are used and abused by all age and income groups. Because cocaine costs more than crack, cocaine is most likely to be used by people with higher income levels. Cocaine and crack stimulate the CNS, peripheral nervous system, and cardiovascular system. Cardiac arrest and heart failure are not uncommon side effects of cocaine and crack use. Cocaine blocks reabsorption of the neurotransmitter dopamine by nerve cells, or neurons, in one of the brain's key pleasure centers. There is buildup of dopamine in the space between the nerve cells, which causes stimulation of the receiving neurons ("New Report Provides," 1999).

Most people who use cocaine or crack also use either marijuana or alcohol to counteract the effects of cocaine. Crack and cocaine are particularly life-threatening when they are first administered and the "rush" occurs. Nurses need to identify what depressant the client is using to counteract the impact of the cocaine. If the client uses alcohol, there is a chance that alcohol withdrawal symptoms will appear. The addicting feature of crack and cocaine is the need of the addict to increase the dose to intensify and prolong the euphoric effects.

Cocaine appears to affect the fetus, but the exact nature of the impact is as yet unclear. A review of studies conducted between 1984 and 2000 that examined prenatal cocaine exposure and possible links to (1) physical growth, (2) cognition, (3) language skills, (4) motor skills, and (5) behavior, attention, affect, and neurophysiology was less than conclusive (Myles, 2001). The independent effect of prenatal cocaine exposure on physical growth, cognition, or language skills was not supported in any of the studies examined. In another study exploring the possible impact on Bayley Scales of Infant Development scores, heavier cocaine use did not independently result in depressed scores when compared with lighter use. Low birth weight and caregiver factors appeared to have more impact on poor developmental outcomes (Frank et al., 2002). Multiple drug use, low birth weight, lack of prenatal care, and a variety of other related issues make it extremely difficult to determine the exact contribution of cocaine to developmental and physical problems experienced by drug-exposed newborns.

More individuals are using amphetamines and methamphetamines. They are readily available, fairly inexpensive, and easy to manufacture in unsophisticated laboratories. These stimulants produce euphoria, grandiosity, increased energy, suppressed appetite, aggressive feelings, and paranoia. They increase the blood pressure and heart and respiration rates, cause pupils to dilate, and cause depression after the initial rush. Amphetamines and methamphetamines are used at "rave parties" by college students and others. Methamphetamine is referred to by various street names, including "ice," "crystal," "glass," and "crank." It is stronger in its effects than amphetamines. Methamphetamines are being used more and more by youths and young women as a weight-loss agent. Ecstasy (methylenedioxymethamphetamine) shares many of the same properties as methamphetamine, but also has hallucinogic properties. It is known by the additional names "Adam" or "XTC." There has been a significant increase in the number of young people referred for treatment for use of these and many other illegal drugs.

It is very difficult to keep track of all the drugs that are used by various people or groups of people. Immigration not only brings new people into the country but also brings drugs that are not familiar in this country. One such drug that has entered the scene is "Khat" (pronounced "cot"), which is grown in East Africa, southern Arabia, and the Middle East. It is used socially and medicinally for its stimulant properties. Cathinone, the active ingredient, is found only in the fresh Khat leaves (Mela & McBride, 2000).

It is often very difficult for the nurse to get accurate information from an individual when he or she is using these drugs. The only thing a nurse might be able to assess is the level of consciousness, the affect, and the mood the individual is displaying.

Preventive Measures

Stimulants are usually received by the addict from illegal sources. Some of these drugs are manufactured in unsophisticated laboratories. Prevention includes working with law enforcement agencies and communities to force drug dealers out of neighborhoods by exposing their activities and by arresting the dealers. Education of the community about the dangers of various stimulants can decrease the sale of these drugs by preventing youth from engaging in drug use and sales.

Primary Prevention

Community health nurses working with other community agencies can identify high-risk populations and provide information about stimulants. Parents and community members should be informed about the availability of stimulants in their communities. They should be educated to identify the effects of stimulants. Young people in the community are especially vulnerable as they experiment with stimulants. Another aspect that the community must face is the illegal dealing of drugs. Drug dealers often recruit young people to sell drugs on the streets. The lure for young people is easy money, which is not available through jobs in poor neighborhoods.

The community health nurse can be alert to possible drug dealing and crack houses in the neighborhoods where he or she is visiting clients. Working closely with the police can help to eliminate some of the dangers of drugs in communities. Community health nurses can work with other community agencies to help provide job opportunities to youth. These efforts are working in many neighborhoods where youth are providing much-needed services, such as doing work for the elderly. These activities help to maintain the elderly longer in their homes while providing youths with meaningful activities and preventing them from getting involved in illegal activities.

Another primary prevention activity focuses on providing a "sense of belonging," which many youths feel is lacking in their lives. This lack makes gang membership very attractive, because the gang provides the sense of belonging. Faith communities and community centers provide activities that help youths feel a sense of belonging and are excellent referral sources for the community health nurse. Parenting courses are available in many communities to help parents and adolescents communicate more effectively, and they help prevent feelings of alienation between young people and their parents. In many communities, the community health nurse provides parenting classes.

Secondary Prevention

Stimulants are extremely addicting. People who are addicted to stimulants, especially crack and cocaine, have a difficult time staying drug free. The addict spends more and more money on the drug of choice. The effects of crack and cocaine are so short-lived that the addict rapidly increases his or her daily dosage. The addict's days are filled with activities that are directed at getting the next "fix." The addict is often malnourished because all his or her money goes for drugs. People are often driven into prostitution and other illegal activities to support their habit.

The nursing assessment must be comprehensive, including questions about sexual practices, sexually transmitted diseases, and safe sex practices. It is also important to assess how the children are being cared for when the mother is away from home. Are the children left alone? Are they left with someone the mother knows and trusts? Assessing the situation for safety and the nutritional status of the mother and children is a high priority. The nurse assesses for bruising or any other signs of abuse or neglect. If there are concerns about child abuse or neglect, the nurse is required to report these findings to the local child protection agency.

One of the problems with individuals who are addicted to crack or cocaine is that there are often children living in very unsafe situations. Community health nurses often receive referrals to these residences to assess the health of children. The safety of the children and the nurse must be assessed. It may be necessary to do joint visits with other nurses, child protection workers, or police officers. There is always a dilemma: should the nurse attempt to establish a trusting relationship with the mother who is living in the crack house, or is it so unsafe that it is better to involve the police immediately and have the children removed from the home? These are hard decisions for the community health nurse, because often the mother views the nurse as safe and a helper. It may be possible to negotiate with the mother to meet her someplace other than her residence, allowing for better communication and safety. It is especially important to try to get pregnant mothers into prenatal care as early as possible and into treatment. Many more treatment programs are now available for pregnant women who have children. These may be outpatient programs that provide day care or inpatient programs with facilities for day care and some kind of communal living situation for mothers and their children.

Tertiary Prevention

Relapse, or returning to drug use, is very common among individuals who are addicted to crack or cocaine. To stay drug free, the individual must change his or her lifestyle, which includes developing friendships with people who are sober. The recovering addict may have to move away from the neighborhood because there are too many triggers or reminders that cause cravings. Much is still not understood about the causes of relapse, but it is known that abstinence is the only way to ensure recovery.

Many people suffer from the residual effects of their drug use. These individuals may be referred to the community health nurse for care related to a medical problem. Some clients have had seizures, heart attacks, or gunshot wounds as a result of their drug activity. Some of these individuals have adjusted to their disability, whereas others are angry and have made poor adjustments. Often these are young adults who are not able to lead a normal life due to their disability. Medication compliance, rehabilitation, sober social support systems, relapse programs, and aftercare groups are all important factors in helping the addict remain sober and lead as normal a life as possible.

The Role of the Community Health Nurse

There are various activities the community health nurse can perform related to persons addicted to stimulants. The nurse

USING THE NURSING PROCESS

ASSESSMENT

Ann Maxwell is a 23-year-old single mother of a 1-year-old son. She abused cocaine for 2 years before the birth of her son. Early in her pregnancy she sought help for her drug abuse, and she has remained drug free since. She currently lives with a middle-aged aunt in the aunt's house in a low-income but well maintained neighborhood in the city. Ann attended Narcotic Anonymous (NA) on a regular basis until 6 months ago, when she began working part-time at a local convenience store to help with expenses for her son and herself. With her aunt's encouragement, she has also enrolled in a night program to complete her GED, because she dropped out of high school in her senior year. She has regular visits from the community health nurse to follow the progress of her son, who was born prematurely and has shown signs of some minor developmental delays. At the last visit by the nurse, Ann voiced concern over feeling stressed by all the new responsibilities of work and school and her ability to be a "good mother" to her son. She appears tired and has lost some weight since the last visit. Ann holds the child in her lap during the visit, and he appears to be very happy, clean, and well nourished.

NURSING DIAGNOSIS

1. The client is at risk for resumption of drug abuse due to lack of ongoing support from the self-help group NA and increased stress levels.
2. The child is at risk for abuse and neglect due to the mother's stress and potential resumption of drug use.

PLAN/IMPLEMENTATION

Diagnosis 1: Because the client has attended NA in the past, the community health nurse discusses how she can fit regular meetings into her current schedule. It is possible that there are meetings held at sites closer to her workplace or school that will be easier to attend. The nurse also discusses ways that the client can reduce her stress levels by eating regular healthy meals and getting physical activity.

Diagnosis 2: The nurse discusses the issue of child abuse and neglect with the client, stressing the need for her to keep herself healthy and drug free.

EVALUATION

The client finds that there are meetings of NA at the same site that she has her GED courses, and can attend right after the classes. After attending on a regular basis for 2 months, she expresses feeling "more in control" of her life and feeling less stressed. Her classes are going well, and she has regained the weight that she had lost. With the increased focus on her sobriety, she states that she is enjoying caring for her son more and has even discussed attending the community college with her aunt once she completes her GED. Although she has not found a way to include some physical activity in her daily routine, she plans to look at some exercise classes held at the local community center. At the NA meetings, she has made a couple of friends who also have young children, and they have begun meeting once a week at a local park with their children.

---

can provide the community with information about the availability of stimulants and the signs and symptoms of stimulant intoxication and work to provide youth with activities that help them feel they belong to the family and community. Nurses can work with women to help them obtain access to drug treatment and prenatal services. Children are often in need of safe housing; by working with other community agencies, the nurse can help provide safety for children. The nurse is often called on to provide nursing care to people who have health problems related to their drug use.

GAMBLING

Over the last 2 decades gambling has become a large-scale issue, and it is now recognized as being potentially addictive. The etiology of gambling appears to be somewhat more evasive to researchers than that of substance abuse. Some theo-

ries suggest that there are sociologic, biologic, and psychologic processes interacting with respect to problem gambling (Lesieur, 1994). Researchers are studying the effect that gambling has on the brain and the neurotransmitters. It appears that many people experience a rush, which seems to be associated with the "process" rather than the "win." Often people "chase," which means that they return the next day in an attempt to win back losses. Until recently, most studies of gambling behavior were conducted on the male population. One study of 40 problem gamblers in an outpatient treatment program suggested that the reasons for gambling were a desire for excitement or to win; risk-taking; an attempt to change mood states, especially boredom or depression; escape; and to relieve physical pain (Specker et al., 1996). Female gamblers have a higher percentage of psychiatric hospitalizations and suicide attempts, compared with male gamblers. It appears that men seek treatment more frequently than women do. In one outpatient program, 80% of the clients were men.

There has been an increase in problem gambling with the increased availability of gambling opportunities. The elderly and poor populations are often targeted by gambling establishments through advertisements and free bus transportation to casinos. Gambling provides older adults with an opportunity to fill their idle time, socialize with other people, and possibly win some money to supplement their incomes; however, they may lose money needed to live on, or social gambling may become "problem gambling." A cross-sectional study involving 80 elderly African-Americans identified 64% as nongamblers or occasional gamblers, 19% as light to moderate gamblers, and 17% as heavy to pathologic gamblers. There were also statistically significant relationships between gambling behaviors and measures of (1) psychological well-being, (2) anxiety, (3) obsessive-compulsive symptoms, (4) perceived health status, (5) health locus of control, (6) religiousness, and (7) stressful life-event (Bazargan, Bazargan, & Akanda, 2001).

Preventive Measures

There has been increasing concern about problem gambling and the effect it has on individuals, families, and communities. Some state lottery organizations have begun placing advertisements warning people to be cautious when buying lottery tickets. Many people buy numerous tickets in the hope that they will have a better chance at winning the lottery. Public education is helpful to warn people of the potential dangers of gambling. Education should start with youth, who are gambling at greater rates than ever before.

Primary Prevention

When performing the community assessment, the community health nurse needs to identify the opportunities for people to gamble. Are there many opportunities to play the lottery? Are there casinos near the community with easy access (eg, free transportation)? Are there pull-tabs in the bars and restaurants? Then the at-risk populations must be identified. Are there large numbers of idle elderly and poor people in the population? Are there buses of people bound for casinos? What other activities are being provided for high-risk populations?

Gambling is not just a problem of the elderly and the poor populations. Data may be available from state gambling organizations, treatment programs, or court systems to help with the community assessment. This information helps the community health nurse focus primary prevention strategies on at-risk populations. Excellent educational materials are available, and in some communities speakers are available to discuss their own experiences with a gambling problem.

Secondary Prevention

When the nurse assesses a family or individual, it is important to assess for all addictions, including gambling. In one study of 30 people recruited through advertising, 67% reported a gambling problem, 60% had a lifetime mood disorder, and 64% had a lifetime substance-use disorder (Black & Moyer, 1998).

Skills for the nurse include observation, assessment, and careful attention to the client's history. Duncan (1996)

identified 10 key points to help in assessing whether gambling has become a problem (Display 35–3). Depending on the individual, the community health nurse may want to leave an assessment tool with the client; this provides for more privacy, and the client may feel less shame and fill out the tool more honestly. It is very important for the nurse to maintain a nonjudgmental attitude, allowing the client to be more open and honest. The assessment must include a suicide and chemical dependency assessment. As Lesieur stated, "Gambling did not replace alcohol abuse, it joined it" (Lesieur & Blume, 1987).

There is a high rate of suicide among problem gamblers, particularly women who are also using substances. The client may need help both with the gambling addiction and with other mental health issues. It is important for the community health nurse to work with the client to obtain the appropriate help. Gamblers Anonymous, a self-help group based on the principles of AA, is available in most communities. More programs, both inpatient and outpatient, are now available for problem gamblers.

Withdrawal from gambling poses some of the same symptoms as withdrawal from chemicals. Some of the symptoms that have been reported are restlessness, irritability, and "cravings." It is important for the family to be aware of these symptoms, because they are common during withdrawal.

DISPLAY 35–3

Nine Key Indicators of Pathologic Gambling

Skills in identifying compulsive gambling revolve around observation, assessment, and careful attention to detail in a client's history. The following nine key points help in establishing whether the person's gambling behavior is pathologic:

- Preoccupation with gambling and dreaming of the "big win"
- Concealment of gambling behavior; loss of money and defaults
- Increasing the frequency and quantity of bets to get a buzz
- A history of failed attempts at controlling or curtailing gambling
- "Withdrawal-like" symptoms such as headache, irritability, restlessness, agitation, and feeling on edge when reducing or curtailing gambling
- Relief gambling to ease feelings of anxiety, tension, depression, and guilt
- Criminal activities sponsor gambling
- "Chasing," that is, betting in an attempt to recoup past and future losses and come good again
- A history of loss of friends', relatives', colleagues' support, employment and career opportunities, and social contact

(Duncan, S. [1996]. Just a flutter. *Nursing Standard, 10*[48], 22–23.)

Unlike with chemical dependency, the family of the gambler may be the last to know there is a problem. It is common for the gambler to keep his or her activities hidden from other family members for a long time. When the family discovers the gambling problem, they are often very angry and not supportive of the individual. The family may find that bills have not been paid; there may be legal problems or huge debts that the family is ill prepared to handle. It is important that the nurse understand and work with the family to help them cope with their anger in appropriate ways. It may be necessary for the family to seek financial counseling. There may be irreparable damage to relationships, so additional family counseling may be necessary.

Tertiary Prevention

Considerations in providing tertiary care are the emotional and financial drain on the problem gambler and his or her family. The community health nurse needs to provide ongoing support to the client and family. This is especially important if the gambler also has had a chemical dependency problem, because alcoholics are more likely to relapse when they have a gambling problem. After the client has been through treatment, it is important to provide support so that he or she can maintain abstinence from gambling. There are as many opportunities to gamble as there are to use substances, so it is necessary for the client to establish relationships with people who do not gamble and who are in recovery. The client is likely to be faced with large debts, possible legal problems, and fragile relationships with family and old friends. Attending Gamblers Anonymous is critical to maintaining abstinence.

OTHER ADDICTIONS

Community health nurses need to be aware of other types of addictions that can inhibit an individual's ability to lead a healthy lifestyle. There are many addictions that can affect a person's quality of life, including work, exercise, shopping, sex, food (often classified in the literature as eating disorders), and, in recent years television, video games, the Internet, and—last but not least—day trading on the stock market via the Internet. The community health nurse needs to include in a comprehensive assessment information about numerous types of addictions.

GLOBALIZATION OF ADDICTION PROBLEMS

Addiction problems are not unique to the United States. There has been concern about gambling in other countries, including England and Canada, where research is being conducted on the reasons people become addicted to gambling. Much of the research currently being conducted looks at the physiologic aspects, including a possible genetic link or a predisposition to addictions. Many countries are struggling with chemical addiction problems and laws governing the use, sale, and availability of chemicals. History has shown that many countries have outlawed certain drugs, but they are still being imported illegally. WHO (2002) has challenged the global community to address the issues of alcohol and tobacco abuse, noting that more than one third of deaths worldwide can be attributed to 10 leading health risks:

1. Underweight
2. Unsafe sex
3. High blood pressure
4. Tobacco consumption
5. Alcohol consumption
6. Unsafe water, sanitation, and hygiene
7. Iron deficiency
8. Indoor smoke from solid fuels
9. High cholesterol
10. Obesity

Clearly, the significant threat to health that substance abuse poses extends well beyond U. S. borders and involves needed interventions at all levels of prevention.

There are many issues involved in the use and abuse of drugs. Few incentives are available for the people of Colombia who raise coca to replace their cash crop with something else; any other crop would not produce the same income. The farmers are often very poor but are enticed by drug lords to continue growing coca. There is so much corruption related to drugs, especially cocaine, that many people working in governments are also involved in the illegal activities of selling and distributing drugs. Curbing drug traffic from country to country is very difficult, and it is costly to enforce drug laws. Countries have varying laws regarding legal and illegal drugs, and this inconsistency makes drug enforcement almost impossible. The United States spends much money on trying to curb drug trafficking across borders and at airports, but this expenditure has still not made a dent in the illegal drugs coming into the country. Poor countries do not have the sophistication or the resources to fight drug trafficking.

SUMMARY

Although there have been significant improvements with some diseases, mental illness and addictions remain serious, persistent, and even increasing problems, both in the United States and globally. Mental health has become a growing priority nationally for research and services, yet there is still much more to be done. The significant role that addictions and substance abuse play in quality-of-life issues and premature death continue to strain available services. The need for effective and efficient efforts at all levels of prevention—primary, secondary, and tertiary—has never been greater.

Most community mental health efforts have focused on treatment, and only lately has there been a growing emphasis on prevention and health promotion. The national *Healthy People 2010* objectives particularly target suicide and seri-

ACTIVITIES TO PROMOTE CRITICAL THINKING

1. As a community health nurse, you have been asked to design and present a 2-hour program on suicide to the entire student body of the local high school. This activity is representative of which level of prevention? What are some of the considerations involved in planning this program to promote optimal success? How might you measure the effectiveness of this intervention?

2. John is a 26-year-old Asian man who has been diagnosed with schizophrenia for 5 years. He lives with his parents, who moved to the United States from China 10 years ago. He participates in a resocialization program at the local YMCA. He told the nurse that his parents do not want him to take medication and believe that he is not sick at all. What cultural influences should be considered in this situation? How can the community health nurse assist this client and his family to prevent further exacerbation of the client's symptoms? What other services might be helpful in this situation?

3. You are part of a multidisciplinary team whose goal is to identify families in your city who are at risk for crisis (eg, single parent, divorce, teen pregnancy, loss of job) and develop a set of interventions. How would you determine who these families are? What interventions would be appropriate to meet their needs? What level of prevention would you be targeting?

4. Susan, is a 38-year-old high school teacher who, along with three of her students, was just attacked by a student with a gun, who was threatening to kill all of them. The teacher and students are hysterical, sobbing and screaming about the fear and terror they experienced. The school nurse has been called to the scene and has contacted the mobile crisis unit to report to the school. What priorities would the school nurse establish? What plan would be the most realistic? What interventions would be most applicable under these circumstances?

5. You have met a few elderly men in your area who live alone and are widowed, and you have heard that there are others. Assuming your advocacy role in community mental health, you decide to take some action to ensure that their needs are being met. How would you determine the risks and needs for this group? What interventions would be appropriate to meet their needs?

6. Select a problem that places people at risk for mental disorders (eg, child abuse and neglect, drug abuse) and do a search on the Internet to learn all you can about it. What is the incidence and prevalence of this problem? What interventions are most effective in addressing it? What can be done to prevent it?

ous mental illnesses but include some prevention objectives as well. Knowing the needs of the mentally ill population assists in planning services. Many resources exist in the community to serve the mentally ill population and those affected by addiction. Among them are CMHCs, halfway houses, and community support programs. Two models for preventing mental illness are the Public Health Model and the MHISM. Separately or combined, they provide a focus for designing preventive interventions at the primary, secondary, and tertiary levels.

The issues surrounding mental illness are clearly very complex. If mental illness is complicated by the presence of addiction, the problems for the client, the family, and the community escalate. For the community health nurse, the ability to approach these issues with all the professionalism, dedication, and concern as would be applied to any other illness is crucial. Through ongoing community education, the mystery and stigma of mental illness and addictions can be eliminated in our communities, improving the potential health and well-being of those suffering from these maladies and their families.

REFERENCES

Allen, K.M. (1996). *Nursing care of the addicted client.* Philadelphia: Lippincott-Raven.

Al-Anon Family Group Headquarters. (2003a). *The twelve steps.* Virginia Beach, VA: Author. Retrieved February 16, 2004, from *http://www.al-anon.org/12steps.html*

Al-Anon Family Group Headquarters. (2003b). *The twelve traditions.* Virginia Beach, VA: Author. Retrieved February 16, 2004, from *http://www.al-anon.org/12traditions.html*

American Psychiatric Association (2000). *Diagnostic and statistical manual of mental disorders* (4th ed., Text Revision) (DSM-IV-TR). Washington DC: Author.

American Psychiatric Association (1994). *Diagnostic and statistical manual of mental disorders* (4th ed.) (DSM-IV). Washington DC: Author.

Bazargan, M., Bazargan, S., & Akanda, M. (2001). Gambling habits among aged African Americans. *Clinical Gerontologist, 22*(3/4), 51–62.

Black, D.W., & Moyer, T. (1998). Clinical features and psychiatric comorbidity of subjects with pathological gambling behavior. *Psychiatric Services, 49*(11), 143–149.

Bradley, K.A., Kivlahan, D.R., Bush, K.R., McDonell, M.B., &

Fihn, S.D. (2001). Variations on the CAGE alcohol screening questionnaire: Strengths and limitations in VA general medical patients. *Alcoholism: Clinical and Experimental Research*, 25, 1472–1478.

Caplan, G. (1964). *Principles of preventive psychiatry*. New York: Basic Books.

Centers for Disease Control and Prevention. (2003). Multinational intervention to reduce alcohol-exposed pregnancies—Florida, Texas, and Virginia, 1997–2001. *MMWR, 52*, 441–444.

Christoffel, K.K. (2000). Public health advocacy: Process and product. *American Journal of Public Health, 90*(5), 722–726.

Duncan, S. (1996). Just a flutter. *Nursing Standard, 10*(48), 22–23.

Ewing, J. (1984). Detecting alcoholism: The CAGE questionnaire. *Journal of the American Medical Association, 252*(14), 1905–1907.

Frank, D.A., Jacobs, R.R., Beeghly, M., Augustyn, M., Bellinger, D., Cabral, H., et al. (2002). Level of prenatal cocaine exposure and scores on the Bayley Scales of Infant Development: Modifying effects of caregiver, early intervention, and birth weight. *Pediatrics, 110*, 1143–1152.

Gamwell, L., & Tomes, N. (1973). *Madness in America: Cultural and medical perceptions of mental illness before 1914*. New York: Cornell University Press.

Gootenberg, P. (1999). *Cocaine*. New York: Routledge

Grob, G.N. (1991). *From asylum to community: Mental health policy in modern America*. Princeton, NJ: Princeton University Press.

Grob, G.N. (1994). *The mad among us: A history of the care of America's mentally ill*. New York: Free Press.

Hines-Martin, V., Malone, M., Kim, S., & Brown-Piper, A. (2003). Barriers to mental healthcare access in an African American population. *Issues in Mental Health Nursing, 24*, 237–256.

Hurry, J.B. (1978). *Imhotep, the vizier and physician of King Zoser, and afterwards the Egyptian god of medicine*. New York: AMS Press.

Institute of Medicine (1994). *Reducing risks for mental disorders*. Washington, DC: National Academy Press.

Jacobs, E.A., Copperman, S.M., Jeffe, A., & Kulig, J. (2000). Fetal alcohol syndrome and alcohol-related neurodevelopmental disorders. *Pediatrics, 106*, 358–361.

Jellinek, E.M. (1946). Phases in the drinking history of alcoholics: An analysis of a survey conducted by the official organization of Alcoholics Anoymous. *Quarterly Journal of Studies in Alcohol, 7*, 188.

Kalb, R., Ellinger, K., & Reulbach, U. (2003). Improvement in response times for simple and complex tasks after electroconvulsive therapy. *Progress in Neuropsychopharmacology and Biological Psychiatry, 27*, 459–465.

Kiple, K.F. (1995). *The Cambridge world history of human disease*. Cambridge, UK: Cambridge University Press.

Lee, S., & Kleinman, A. (1997). Mental illness and social change in China. *Harvard Review of Psychiatry, 5*(1), 43–46.

Lesieur, H.R. (1994). Epidemiological surveys of pathological gambling: Critique and suggestions for modification. *Journal of Gambling Studies, 10*, 385–398.

Lesieur, H., & Blume, S. (1987). The South Oaks Gambling Screen (SOGS): A new instrument for identification of pathological gamblers. *American Jourrnal of Psychiatry, 144*, 1184–1188.

Luoma, J.B., & Pearson, J.L. (2002). Suicide and marital status in the United States, 1991–1996: Is widowhood a risk factor? *American Journal of Public Health*, 92, 1518–1522.

Mela, M., & McBride, A. J. (2000). Khat and khat misuse: An overview. *Journal of Substance Use, 5,* 218–226.

Minino, A.M., Arias, E., Kochanek, K.D., Murphy, S.L., & Smith, B.L. (2002). Deaths: Final data for 2000. *National Vital Statistics Reports, 50*(15), 1–119.

Moore, A.A., Seeman, T., Morgenstern, H., Beck, J.C., & Reuben D.B. (2002). Are there differences between older persons who screen positive on the CAGE questionnaire and the Short Michigan Alcoholism Screening Test–geriatric version? *Journal of the American Geriatrics Society, 50*, 858–862.

Myles, J. (2001). Review: Prenatal exposure to cocaine does not independently affect physical growth, cognition, or language skills. *Evidenced Based Mental Health, 4*(4), 121.

National Institute of Mental Health. (2001). The numbers count: Mental disorders in America. Retrieved February 16, 2004, from *www.nimh.nih.gov/publicat/numbers.cfm*

New report provides information on cocaine abuse and treatment. (1999). *NIDA Notes, 14*(3). Retrieved February 16, 2004, from *http://www.drugabuse.gov/NIDA_Notes/NNVol14N3/Tearoff.html*

Ng, V. (1990). Madness in late imperial China: From illness to deviance. Norman, OK: University of Oklahoma Press.

Prochaska, J.P., & DiClemente, C.C. (1992). Stages of change in the modification of problem behaviors. In M. Hersen, R.M. Eisler, & P.M. Miller (Eds.). *Progress in behavior modification* (pp. 184–214). Sycamore, IL: Sycamore Press.

Rosen, G. (1968). *Madness in society*. Chicago: University of Chicago Press.

Simon, B. (1978). *Mind and madness in ancient Greece: The classical roots of modern psychiatry*. New York: Cornell University Press.

Skye, (2001). Electroconvulsive therapy: An acceptable and therapeutic intervention? *Assignment, 7*(4), 16–19.

Specker, S.M., Carlson, G.A., Edmonson, K.M., Johnson, P.E., & Marcotte, M. (1996). Psychopathology in pathological gamblers seeking treatment. *Journal of Gambling Studies, 10*, 67–81.

Spillane, J.F. (2000). *Cocaine: From medical marvel to modern menace in the United States, 1884–1920*. Baltimore: Johns Hopkins University Press.

Spradley, B.W., & Allender, J.A. (1996). *Community health nursing* (4th ed.) Philadelphia: Lippincott-Raven.

Substance Abuse and Mental Health Services Administration. (1998). *Community support: About the program*. Rockville, MD: U. S. Department of Health and Human Services, National Institutes of Health. Retrieved February 16, 2004, from *http://www.mentalhealth.org/cmhs/CommunitySupport/about.asp*

Substance Abuse and Mental Health Services Administration. (1999). *Mental health: A report of the Surgeon General*. Rockville, MD: U. S. Department of Health and Human Services, National Institutes of Health. Retrieved February 16, 2004, from *http://www.surgeongeneral.gov/library/mentalhealth/home.html*

Substance Abuse and Mental Health Services Administration. (2001). *Mental health: Culture, race, ethnicity—Supplement*. Rockville, MD: U. S. Department of Health and Human Services, National Institutes of Health. Retrieved February 16, 2004, from *http://www.mentalhealth.org/cre/default.asp*

Substance Abuse and Mental Health Services Administration. (2002). *Results from the 2001 National Household Survey on Drug Abuse, vol. 1. Summary of national findings*. (Office of Applied Studies, NHSDA Series H-17, DHHS Publication No. SMA 02-3758). Rockville, MD: U. S. Department of Health and Human Services, National Institutes of Health. Retrieved

February 16, 2004, from *http://www.samhsa.gov/oas/nhsda/2k1nhsda.vol1/toc.htm*

U. S. Department of Health and Human Services. (2000a). *Healthy People 2010: Understanding and improving health.* Washington, DC: U. S. Government Printing Office. Retrieved February 16, 2004, from *http://www.health.gov/healthypeople/Document/*

U. S. Department of Health and Human Services. (2000b). *Reducing tobacco use: A report of the Surgeon General.* Washington, DC: U. S. Government Printing Office. Retrieved February 16, 2004, from *http://www.cdc.gov/tobacco/sgr_2000/FullReport.pdf*

U. S. Department of Health and Human Services. (2001). *Healthy People 2000: Final review.* Washington, DC: U. S. Government Printing Office. Retrieved February 16, 2004, from *http://www.cdc.gov/nchs/products/pubs/pubd/hp2k/review/highlightshp2000.htm*

U. S. Department of Health and Human Services (2002). *Centers for Medicare and Medicaid Services intermediary manual, part 3. Chapter II—Coverage (continued).* Washington, DC: U. S. Government Printing Office. Retrieved February 16, 2004, from *http://www.cms.hhs.gov/manuals/13_int/a3im3190.asp*

Vaillant, G. (1983). *The natural history of alcoholism.* Cambridge, MA: Harvard University Press.

Winters, K.C., Latimer, W.W., & Stinchfield, R.D. (1999). *Screening and assessing adolescent substance involvement.* Minneapolis, MN: Department of Psychiatry, University of Minnesota.

World Health Organization. (1999). *The world health report 1999* (Chapter 2). Geneva, Switzerland: Author. Retrieved February 16, 2004, from *http://www.who.int/whr2001/2001/archives/1999/en/index.htm*

World Health Organization. (2001). *Fact sheet: Strengthening mental health promotion.* Geneva, Switzerland: Author. Retrieved February 16, 2004, from *http://www.who.int/inf-fs/en/fact220.html*

World Health Organization. (2002). *The world health report 2002: Reducing risks, promoting healthy life.* Geneva, Switzerland: Author. Retrieved February 16, 2004, from *http://www.who.int/whr/2002/en/*

Youth Risk Behavior Surveillance System. (2001). *YRSSS: 2001 information and results.* Washington, DC: U. S. Department of Health and Human Services. Retrieved February 16, 2004, from *http://www.cdc.gov/nccdphp/dash/yrbs/2001/youth01online.htm*

SELECTED READINGS

Chaudry, R.V., Polivka, B.J., & Kennedy, C.W. (2000). Public health nursing directors' perceptions regarding interagency collaboration with community mental health agencies. *Public Health Nursing, 17*(2), 75–84.

Collier, M., Harrison, G.W., & McInnes, M.M. (2002), Evaluating the tobacco settlement damage awards: Too much or not enough? *American Journal of Public Health, 92,* 984–989.

Falkowski, C. (1998). *Drug abuse trends: Minneapolis/St. Paul.* Center City, MN: Hazelden Institute, Butler Center for Research and Learning.

Hampton, M.D., & Chafetz, L. (2002). Factors associated with residential placement in an assertive community treatment program. *Issues in Mental Health Nursing, 23,* 677–689.

Happell, B., Carta, B., & Pinikahana, J. (2002). Nurses' knowledge, attitudes and beliefs regarding substance use: A questionnaire survey. *Nursing and Health Sciences, 4,* 193–200.

Lambers, D., & Clark, K. (1996). The maternal and fetal physiological effects of nicotine. *Seminars in Perinatology, 20*(2), 115–126.

Magyary, D., & Brandt, P. (2002). A decision tree and clinical paths for the assessment and management of children with ADHD. *Issues in Mental Health Nursing, 23,* 553–566.

Meisenhelder, J.B. (2002). Terrorism, posttraumatic stress, and religious coping. *Issues in Mental Health Nursing, 23,* 771–782.

Paul, J.P., Catania, J., Pollack, L., Moskowitz, J., Canchola, J., Mills, T., et al. (2002). Suicide attempts among gay and bisexual men: Lifetime prevalence and antecedents. *American Journal of Public Health, 92,* 1338–1345.

Smoyak, S.A. (2000). The history, economics, and financing of mental health care, part 2: The 20th century. *Journal of Psychosocial Nursing and Mental Health Services, 38*(10), 26–37, 44–45.

Snowden, L.R. (2003). Bias in mental health assessment and intervention: Theory and evidence. *American Journal of Public Health, 93,* 239–243.

Swartz, M.S., Swanson, J.W., & Burns, B.J. (1998). Mental disorder, substance abuse, and community violence: An epidemiological approach. In J. Monahan & H.J. Steadman (Eds.). *Violence and mental disorder: Developments in risk assessment.* Chicago: University of Chicago Press.

Weist, M.D. (2001). Toward a public mental health promotion and intervention system for youth. *Journal of School Health,* 73, 101–104.

West, M.M. (2002). Early risk indicators of substance abuse among nurses. *Journal of Nursing Scholarship, 34,* 187–193.

Zickler, P. (2000). NIDA studies clarify effects of prenatal cocaine exposure. *NIDA Notes, 14*(3), 1–4. Retrieved February 16, 2004, from *http://165.112.78.61/NIDANotes/NNVol14N3/Prenatal.html*

Internet Resources

Al-Anon Family Group Headquarters, Inc.: *http://www.al-anon.org/index.html*

American Medical Association: *http://www.ama-assn.org/ama/pub/category/3558.html*

American Psychological Association: *http://www.apa.org/*

Bazelon Center for Mental Health Law: *http://www.bazelon.org/*

Mother's Against Drunk Driving (MADD): *http://www.madd.org/home*

National Alcohol Screening Day: *http://www.mentalhealthscreening.org/alcohol.htm*

National Center on Addiction and Substance Abuse at Columbia University: *http://www.casacolumbia.org*

National Institute on Alcohol Abuse and Alcoholism (NIAAA): *http://www.niaaa.nih.gov/*

National Institute of Mental Health: *http://www.nimh.nih.gov*

National Mental Health Association: *http://www.nmha.org/*

Practitioners Research Reports and Current Information on the Diagnosis and Treatment for Mental Disorders: *http://www.nimh.nih.gov/practitioners/index.cfm*

Robert Wood Johnson Foundation: *http://www.rwjf.org/index.jsp*

Substance Abuse and Mental Health Administration (SAMHSA): *http://www.samhsa.gov/*

36

Clients in Correctional Facilities

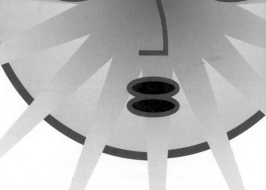

Key Terms

- Correctional facility
- Felony
- Forensics
- Jail
- Inmates
- Literacy
- Maximum security
- Minimum security
- Penitentiary
- Prison
- Recidivism

Learning Objectives

Upon mastery of this chapter, you should be able to:

- Define terms associated with correctional health care and correctional institutions.
- Describe the correctional culture and environment.
- Describe the history of correctional health care.
- Identify the key issues and challenges of correctional health care.
- Describe at least four organizations associated with inmates of correctional facilities.
- Identify the communicable diseases and physical and mental health disorders commonly seen in correctional populations.
- Discuss the special areas of concern for nurses who work with incarcerated women.
- Describe the role of the community health nurse who works with populations in correctional facilities.

Have you ever been inside a jail, prison, or other correctional facility? Do you know anyone who is or was incarcerated? Do you know where your city or county correctional facility is located? Have you ever considered a career in correctional nursing? If you answered "No" to all of these questions, you are not alone. To most people, correctional facilities, incarcerated populations, and the nurses who serve them are invisible. With our Western ideals of independence, we tend to dislike even thinking about those who have had their freedom taken away. Nurses who work with incarcerated clients face multiple challenges; they work in a physically and emotionally stressful environment, with a client population that most people would rather ignore and the nurses themselves face the challenge of being the least visible members of their profession.

Nevertheless, correctional nursing can be an exciting opportunity to practice compassionate community health nursing. Most prisoners have a history of poverty, substance abuse, physical and emotional abuse, and mental illness with episodic health care. Indeed, incarceration may represent the first time an inmate has received comprehensive, continuous health care or has had the opportunity to develop a therapeutic relationship with a nurse (Price, 2001). Correctional nursing also gives nurses an opportunity to practice skills, including the therapeutic use of self (Miller, 1999), and to apply the principles of public health and **forensics**—the science of health care jurisprudence wherein legal argument is used to advocate for offenders.

This chapter introduces basic concepts and terminology in correctional health care, and describes the facility environment and the inmates. The history of correctional health care is then reviewed, and the issues and challenges of correctional nursing are explored. The health care concerns that are most common among inmate populations are described, as are the unique health care issues of women prisoners. Finally, the roles of educator, client advocate, and discharge "bridge" that are so vital to community health nursing with the incarcerated population are examined.

BASIC CONCEPTS IN CORRECTIONAL HEALTH CARE

Because most people have had little if any exposure to correctional issues, environments, or populations, a review of basic terminology and concepts is in order.

Terminology of Corrections

A **correctional facility** is one whose primary objective is to provide safety to the public by incarcerating those who have committed crimes and who are deemed to be threats to the community. People detained in correctional facilities are called **inmates** or offenders; more progressive institutions are moving toward the latter term. As indicated by the term *correction,* a correctional facility also ideally serves to improve inmates—to provide them with new perspectives and options so that, on release, they can live as productive citizens. For some people, the ideal of improvement seems frivolous; they see correctional facilities as warehouses for "undesirable elements" and programs to improve inmates' physical and mental health, literacy, and employability as a waste of public funds.

People accused of committing a crime may be held for arraignment (the summons to appear in court to answer charges) in a *detention center* or *holding cell* within a local jail. **Jails** also confine individuals both before and after sentencing for minor offenses (*misdemeanors*) and parole violations. In addition, intoxicated individuals may be held in jails overnight to "dry out." Incarceration for detainees usually ranges from 1 month to 1 year, although some individuals stay for less than 3 weeks; therefore, jails often have a high turnover rate.

State departments of corrections (DOC) detain individuals who are convicted of crimes against the state. State DOC facilities are usually referred to as **prisons** and are assigned a security level ranging from **minimum security** to **maximum security**, depending on the type of prisoners housed there. For example, prisoners who have committed **felonies** (serious crimes such as murder, rape, or burglary) are typically housed in maximum-security prisons.

The Federal Department of Corrections detains individuals who have committed crimes against the United States government, as well as those who have committed interstate crimes. Most federal correctional facilities are called **penitentiaries**; they are commonly referred to among prisoners as "the big house." Like state prisons, federal penitentiaries have security levels ranging from minimum to maximum. Most states and counties also have prison camps that are available for minimum-security criminals. Such camps usually have a rehabilitative or work-related focus.

The Correctional Environment

The environment within which correctional nurses perform their duties differs greatly from that of the hospital, clinic, or home setting. In addition to a variety of unfamiliar rules and restrictions, the nurse in a correctional setting must adapt to constant security monitoring that may be unnerving for the novice. The nurse must also work to inspire hope in an atmosphere often filled with despair.

Overcrowding is another aspect of the typical correctional environment that the nurse must cope with. Indeed, 1998 became the year in which the United States incarcerated 1 million nonviolent prisoners (Irwin, 2000). This statistic represented a threefold increase in prison and jail populations over the previous two decades and was a direct result of more stringent sentencing laws (described later). In any environment where large numbers of people live together in small, confined quarters, the rapid spread of infectious diseases emerges as a public health concern. In addition, the increased rates of incarceration lead to increased staffing needs, health care costs, and fragmentation of families and communities.

The "chain of command" within correctional institutions also differs greatly from that of traditional health care settings. Nurses usually report directly to the administrator of the correctional institution. As employees, they are bound by the rules of the institution, which often are made by personnel unfamiliar with health care. A statement commonly heard from prisoners and staff within correctional facilities is, "This is the warden's house." The warden, or chief administrator, sets the rules that are to be followed. Ethical dilemmas may arise if an inmate's health care needs require actions that challenge the institution's standard policies and procedures. In some situations, advance practice nurses report to a managed care agency that specializes in correctional health care. This situation can allow nurses greater freedom to provide nursing care according to professional nursing standards. In any case, the nurse is employed by the correctional facility, strict adherence to state nursing practice guidelines and to the American Nurses Association's *Scope and Standards of Nursing Practice in Correctional Facilities* (2003) provide the foundation on which to base the most therapeutic outcomes (Display 36–1).

Profile of the Inmate

Although it is difficult to give exact numbers because of the high turnover rate, the Bureau of Justice Statistics reported

DISPLAY 36-1

Guidelines for Correctional Nursing Practice

In the correctional health setting, the nurse:
1. Adapts to an environment of strict rules, regulations, and monitoring where client custody is of primary importance.
2. Expands the scope of nursing practice to meet the unique needs and demands of a prison population with a variety of physical and mental health conditions.
3. Utilizes the nursing process to assess, plan for, implement, and evaluate treatment, prevention, and health promotion services to individuals and groups of inmates.
4. Seeks to establish a trusting professional relationship and carry out needed teaching and counseling activities as inmates' length of incarceration permits.
5. Recognizes that health services are the nurse's sole responsibility and refrains from involvement in security or correctional procedures.
6. Seeks to ensure inmates' human rights and the provision of equitable health care, both in prison and upon release, through advocacy and collaborative efforts.
7. Exercises care to maintain professional conduct and personal safety.

that the number of prisoners incarcerated in the United States in 2002 was 2,019,234 (0.7% of the population), exceeding 2 million for the first time (Butterfield, 2003). If individuals on probation or parole are added to this number, more than 3% of the U. S. population (6.6 million persons) are under the jurisdiction of corrections systems at any given time (Conklin, Lincoln, & Tuthill, 2000; Freudenberg, 2001). Approximately 10% of these are federal prisoners (Federal Bureau of Prisons, 2000). Of these,

- 93% are male
- 37 years is the average age
- 36% are in medium- or high-security institutions
- 38% have a sentence of 10 or more years
- 55% were imprisoned because of a conviction for drug trafficking or possession

Although whites make up the majority of federal prisoners (56%), blacks are represented in numbers disproportionate to their presence in the population as a whole—41% according to the Federal Bureau of Prisons (2000). Asian-American and Native American inmates make up roughly 3% of the remaining federal prisoners. However, 32% of the white and black racial groups in federal prisons identify their ethnicity as Hispanic. People of color, especially blacks and Latinos, are disporportionately represented in the entire criminal justice system (Cole, 1999). In 2003, the U. S. Justice Department reported that an estimated 12% of African-American men aged 20 to 34 years were in jail or prison, the highest rate ever measured. By comparison, 1.6% of white men in the same age group were incarcerated on a given day. Over the course of a lifetime, the rates are much higher. The Bureau of Justice has calculated that 28% of African-American men will be sent to jail or prison during their lifetimes (Butterfield, 2003).

Since 1980, the number of women in prison has increased at almost double the rate for men. Between 1990 and 1998, the number of incarcerated women increased by 71%. In 1998, women constituted 16% of the correctional population in the United States. African-American women are especially over-represented; although they make up a small percentage of the total U. S. population, they represent 52% of women incarcerated in jails, prisons, and penitentiaries (Freudenberg, 2001).

Many incarcerated individuals have a history of abuse, neglect, or other troubling circumstances in childhood. For example, children arrested for a violent crime had a history of abuse four times greater than that of the general population. One study demonstrated that exposure to childhood sexual abuse "conveys a greater risk for experiencing other violence, psychological and physical morbidity, and high-risk behaviors" (Cohen et al., 2000, p. 564). Approximately 50% of incarcerated juveniles had a parent who was also incarcerated; one-third were living in families without fathers when arrested.

Approximately 75% of prisoners incarcerated today are nonviolent offenders. Their offenses include drug trafficking and possession, robbery, arson, extortion, fraud, bribery, immigration offenses, and other nonviolent crimes. They are usually incarcerated in different institutions from violent felons who have committed crimes such as murder, rape, kidnapping, armed robbery, aggravated child molestation, aggravated sodomy, and aggravated sexual battery.

In many prison populations, there is a hierarchy of "prestige" related to the type of offense committed. In particular, sex offenders represent a broad and diverse segment of the correctional population that is often stigmatized by other inmates. Child molesters are even more discriminated against. Because crimes against children are considered by most inmates as the most despicable, child molesters are not only excluded from recreational activities and friendships but also are often harmed by fellow prisoners. The correctional nurse may need to take on an additional role as protector when caring for a child molester—for example, by scheduling appointments to avoid confrontations with other inmates. For sex offenders and child molesters, outcome-based interventions designed with a clear understanding of the characteristics of the offender can play an important role in rehabilitation and secondary prevention.

EVOLUTION OF CORRECTIONAL HEALTH CARE

The manner in which health care is delivered within a correctional institution reflects the social and political milieu of the time. Understanding the history of prison health care as well as the development of legislation and professional organizations related to prisoners provides insight into the current challenges of correctional nursing.

Historical Overview

Until recently, prisons were designed to be punitive and prisoners were considered to have forfeited all rights. Consequently, incarcerated individuals were often mistreated, tortured, and malnourished, were denied exercise, sanitation, and the means for basic hygiene, and had no rehabilitative care or health care. Because of these deplorable conditions, prisoners historically have been at high risk for plagues, sexually transmitted diseases (STDs), tuberculosis (TB), typhus, gangrene, and scurvy.

The history of corrections in the United States is tied to that of England and Europe. In 1775, an epidemic of typhus hit the United States and Europe, prompting reforms in hygienic practices in institutions, including poor houses, hospitals, and prisons. Delousing prisoners on arrival, issuing them clean clothing, and providing examinations by a physician were practices that originated during this time. There were also crusades to improve prisoners' diets.

In the 1800s, mortality attributable to the social and health conditions of prisons was again examined. For the first time, epidemiologic studies of prisoners were conducted. In particular, the work of Louis René Villerme led to prison re-

forms that included reduced crowding, exercise, increased lighting and ventilation, provision of fresh food, opportunities for productive work, and fair treatment of prisoners. It was believed that these reforms would improve prisoners' mental outlook and that this would contribute to their rehabilitation.

It was also at this time that physicians began to treat prisoners with more regularity and to re-examine them just before release, a practice that has continued to this day. Additionally, reform-minded physicians noted that medical understaffing was contributing to a severe lack of health education among prisoners.

In 1929, the 15 reports were published that eventually gave rise to correctional care as it is practiced today: the report of the National Society on Penal Information and the 14 reports of the Wickersham Commission, appointed by President Herbert Hoover (Harvard Law School, 2003). These were the first national and comprehensive surveys of the American criminal justice system, and changes recommended by the reports in parole, probation, and incarceration treatments laid the foundation for significant correctional care reform.

In 1955, the First United Nations Congress on the Prevention of Crime and the Treatment of Offenders adopted a set of international standards for the treatment of incarcerated persons. These standards, which were updated in 1977, provide guidelines on food, clothing, exercise, health care, discipline, books, religion, contact with the outside world, and many other aspects of prison life. The fundamental thread throughout this document is respect for the humanity and dignity of all prisoners and detainees regardless of race, religion, color, creed, political affiliation, gender, or economic status.

In 1975, the National Institute of Law Enforcement and Criminal Justice published another report that directly addressed the issues of health care within correctional institutions (Brecher & Della Penna, 1975). *The Prescriptive Package: Health Care in Correctional Institutions* was a landmark document calling for significant social and medical reforms and providing guidance on organizing medical services within prisons and jails. In particular, it advocated the following actions:

- Use of outside health care agencies in an effort to increase the variety of services offered, decrease costs, and reduce the isolation of health care personnel within correctional facilities
- Collaboration with community liaisons in all aspects of correctional care, including ties to medical and nursing schools and to professional organizations
- Development of a high-quality, consistent, and reliable system of health care as the antidote for numerous class-action lawsuits that were plaguing prison administrations
- Improvements in medical record-keeping systems

The *Prescriptive Package* has resulted in more humane and expert health care of prisoners. It has also increased the use of health care agencies, which in turn has increased health care workers' autonomy to provide quality care. On the other hand, *The Prescriptive Package* has been criticized for its lack of emphasis on rehabilitative and mental health care, issues that were addressed in the 1929 reports.

Correctional health care today continues to improve, but many problems remain. The relationship between health care provider agencies and correctional institutions is still undefined. Overcrowding has increased since the late 1980s, as has the number of prisoners infected with the human immunodeficiency virus (HIV). Perhaps the greatest problem is correctional care workers' lack of a united professional voice, which leads to a lack of comprehensive standards of care for incarcerated persons. The bureaucratic nature of federal, state, and local policies and procedures in the various correctional facilities further compounds this fragmentation.

Legislation Affecting Correctional Health Care

The Eighth Amendment to the U. S. Constitution guarantees the right of prisoners to a safe and humane environment. The 1976 U. S. Supreme Court decision in *Estelle v Gamble* further clarified that correctional facilities could not deliberately show indifference to serious medical needs of prisoners (Levine, 2002). This decision opened the door to questions about what constitutes a minimum standard of health care for prisoners, and community standards for health care began to be applied within correctional institutions. As a result, inmates are the only people in America who today are guaranteed medical treatment (see What Do You Think?)

In 1987, as part of the "War on Drugs," Congress passed legislation enacting stiffer prison sentences for trafficking in or possession of drugs. A further refinement of this law was the 1994 Violent Crime Control and Law Enforcement Act, commonly called the Crime Bill. It calls for mandatory sentencing for certain drug offenses, including a mandatory prison sentence for first-time possession of crack cocaine. These laws have contributed to the escalation in the prison population since that time and the resulting overcrowding of correctional facilities across the country.

The 1994 Crime Bill also empowered the Federal Department of Justice to enforce the constitutional rights of incarcerated individuals through civil suits. This provision enabled the Department to investigate and bring legal action against state institutions when there is a question of civil rights violations. This provision was weakened by the 1996 Prison Litigation Reform Act, which significantly decreased the ability of the federal courts, nongovernmental organizations, and individuals to intervene in class-action suits pertaining to prison conditions. The newer law did, however, require correctional institutions to be responsible for the quality of health care delivered to individuals while incarcerated.

In 1996, the American Correctional Association's Task Force on Health Care in Corrections stated, "Correctional jurisdictions must utilize a comprehensive, holistic approach to providing health and mental health care services which are sensitive to the cultural, subcultural, age, and gender-specific needs of a growing and diverse population. All services provided must be consistent with contemporary health standards".

Professional Organizations Affecting Inmates

Integral to correctional health care are many professional organizations and agencies. The official federal law enforcement agency is the National Institute of Law Enforcement and Criminal Justice, currently referred to as the National Institute of Justice (NIJ). Professional organizations contributing to correctional health care standards include the International Association of Forensic Nurses, the American Nurses Association, the American Public Health Association's Jail and Prison Health Council, the American Correctional Health Care Services Association, and the National Commission on Correctional Health Care. In addition, organizations such as the World Health Organization, United Nations, Amnesty International, and the Human Rights Watch Women's Rights Project monitor human rights of incarcerated persons internationally.

ETHICAL ISSUES IN CORRECTIONAL HEALTH CARE

The priorities of the correctional system are confinement and security. The priority of the nurse is caring. Correctional nurses often get caught in ethical dilemmas when security policies of the institution require actions that threaten the therapeutic nurse–client relationship. These actions include body searches (called "pat downs"), body-cavity searches, collection of forensic evidence, use of restraints and force, and writing up inmates' behavior or complaints. Many professional organizations suggest that, whenever possible, the primary caregiver who has developed a relationship of trust and respect with an inmate shoud not be required to perform any of those actions or to discipline that inmate. Alternatively, performing such procedures with respect, sensitivity, and compassion can make them less traumatic for the inmate.

WHAT DO YOU THINK?

Should a killer in a Minnesota prison have received a life-saving, $900,000 bone marrow transplant? Should a California robber have received a new heart? Both states said yes, because "no" would violate the Constitution's ban on cruel and unusual punishment.

(From Levine, S. [2002]. Criminal care at a high price. *U.S. News & World Report, 133*[5], 44–45).

Any procedure having to do with the "chain of evidence" is done by outside health agencies; for example, blood is drawn for the determination of blood alcohol levels by an unaffiliated contractor.

An ethical dilemma may also surface regarding the conflict between the imposition of a death penalty or life sentence versus the nursing goal of rehabilitation. In 2003, 38 states had death penalties, and more than 400 executions have occurred between 1980 and 2003. Most professional health care organizations prohibit their members from participating in executions (Display 36–2). The American Nurses Association states that it is "inappropriate for nurses practicing in corrections to participate in disciplinary decisions or committees or to participate directly or indirectly in executions by lethal injection" (American Nurses Association, 1995, p. 3). This situation prompts a variety of ethical questions for correctional nurses: Who will ensure compassionate care at the time of execution? Who will ensure that appropriate doses of medications are administered? Who will certify the death?

Confidentiality is another difficult issue, because little privacy exists within correctional institutions. For example, in many prisons, care of inmates with HIV is provided in special HIV clinics; everyone knows who attends these clinics, yet the nurse must be careful not to reveal the name of anyone attending the clinic to any nonauthorized person. However, the person in charge of the facility, the commander or warden, must be notified of all HIV-positive inmates in the facility. Regardless of setting, it is the responsibility of the nurse to be careful where and when she or he speaks about confidential issues.

It may also be difficult for some nurses to remain objective and provide compassionate care while knowing the prisoner's criminal history. This may be especially true when the nurse cares for inmates who have committed murder, rape, or crimes against children. In most cases, it is best and easiest to not know the charges. As was emphasized earlier, strict adherence to state practice guidelines and nursing standards, coupled with outcome-oriented interventions, will help the nurse in these situations to provide appropriate, compassionate care.

Correctional nurses may also be required to provide care to inmates who exhibit a personal or sexual interest in them. It may help the nurse to remember that incarcerated adults have the same sexual needs and desires as the population at large; at the same time, the nurse must recognize that the prisoner's behavior is inappropriate. The importance of maintaining strict and specific boundaries without compromising the nurse–client relationship cannot be stressed enough. Inmates who have poorly developed coping skills often seek methods to hold staff hostage emotionally, and such persons may have difficulty acknowledging the nurse's boundaries or limits. The best approach is to treat the inmate with respect and to avoid showing partiality or accepting gifts and favors from offenders.

These are just a few of the ethical issues that arise in cor-

---

D I S P L A Y   3 6 – 2

The American Correctional Health Services Association Code of Ethics

The correctional health professional should

- Evaluate the inmate as a patient or client in each and every health care encounter.
- Render medical treatment only when it is justified by an accepted medical diagnosis. Treatment and invasive procedures after informed consent.
- Afford inmates the right to refuse care and treatment. Involuntary treatment shall be reserved for emergency situations in which there is grave disability and an immediate threat of danger to the inmate or others.
- Provide sound privacy during health services in all cases and sight privacy whenever possible.
- Provide health care to all inmates regardless of custody status.
- Identify themselves to their patients and not represent themselves as other than their professional license or certificaton permits.
- Collect and analyze specimens only for diagnostic testing based on sound medical principles.
- Perform body cavity searches only after training in proper techniques and when not in a patient-provider relationship with the inmate.
- Not be involved in any aspect of execution of the death penalty.
- Ensure that all medical information is confidential and health care records are maintained and transported in a confidential manner.
- Honor custody functions but do not participate in such activities as escorting inmates, forced transfers, security supervision, strip searches, or witnessing use of force.
- Undertake biomedical research on prisoners only if the research methods meet all requirements for experimentation on human subjects and individual prisoners or prison populations are expected to derive benefits from the results of the research.

(American Correctional Health Services Association. *ACHSA code of ethics.* Retrieved February 12, 2004, from *http://www.corrections.com/achsa*)

---

rectional nursing. Resolving these issues and continuing to practice within corrections can be very difficult; however, active involvement in professional nursing associations and development of a support system of colleagues within correctional nursing can be extraordinarily beneficial in helping the nurse face these complex concerns.

In addition, correctional nurses should maintain accurate information regarding laws that influence their practice. Among the resources available are state bar association publications, state codes, publications of the state's Office of the Attorney General, federal and state registers, and case law.

The computerized search tool called "Lexis" and a service from the Library of Congress called "Scorpio" are also helpful legal resources for nurses.

HEALTH CARE CONSIDERATIONS

The health care needs of incarcerated individuals pose a myriad of concerns. Prisoners may have had poor access to health care before incarceration and therefore may have entered with unmet or unrecognized health care needs, such as chronic systemic illnesses, traumatic injuries, substance abuse, mental illness, STDs, or a history of physical or sexual abuse. In addition, because the prison population is aging, correctional nurses must address increased incidences of acute and chronic illnesses common to aging populations, as well as exacerbations of those illnesses that may be related to long-term incarceration. On occasion, nurses are required to provide end-of-life care for terminally ill inmates.

Communicable Diseases in Correctional Facilities

It is difficult to ascertain the exact rates of communicable disease within correctional facilities because most institutions do not require mandatory testing. This may be in part because mandatory testing can be considered an infringement of human rights; however, another factor is that if the facility has not identified a health problem, there is no obligation to treat it. For these reasons, diligent assessment, surveillance, and reporting are key tasks of the correctional nurse. These activities can assist not only in the detecting and preventing the spread of communicable disease but also in developing educational programs and other initiatives for inmates and staff.

Tuberculosis

TB was in the past one of the leading causes of death in the United States. After nationwide reporting began in 1953, the number of TB cases declined each year until the 1980s, at which time the disease was no longer considered a public health hazard. Thereafter, TB rates began to climb, peaking in 1992. After a subsequent 5-year decline, the incidence appears to be on the rise again, as a result of the HIV epidemic, immigration from other countries, ongoing transmission, and deterioration of the TB control infrastructure (California Department of Corrections, 1999).

Within correctional facilities in the United States, TB remains the single most important communicable disease (Hammett, Harmon, & Maruschak, 1999). TB cases may occur three times more often in the correctional system than in the general adult population. In some large systems, TB case rates have been reported at 6 to 11 times the rate in the general community (California Department of Corrections, 1999). Several factors contribute to such high incidence rates. The prison population has a higher percentage of med-

ically underserved people (eg, the poor, HIV-positive people, illegal drug users) than is seen in the general public. In addition, inmates are confined to relatively small areas, which augments spread of the bacteria by aerosol droplets. Multidrug-resistant TB (mTB) is an even more serious concern; currently, mTB is the causal organism in 7% of TB infections reported in state and federal prisons and 10% of those reported in jails.

Testing for TB is mandatory in 73% of all correctional facilities; it is conducted in more than 90% of state and federal prisons and half of jails on admission (Hammett, Harmon, & Maruschak, 1999). However, many inmates are released before skin tests can be read, particularly in jails. Most prisons and jails report that inmates with suspected or confirmed TB disease are isolated in negative-pressure rooms. Testing of the rooms to ensure that the air exchange is working properly may be lax, and such rooms may remain in use even when the air exchange is known to be out of order.

Health education for inmates and staff with respect to testing, identification, management, and policies regarding TB within correctional institutions is an important role for the correctional nurse. Investigation and follow-up on release are essential. Many non–English-speaking inmates have additional dilemmas with continuing treatment; correctional nurses are their links to ongoing treatment and community health resources.

Sexually Transmitted Diseases

Rates of STDs among prisoners are almost double those in the population in general. Screening for syphilis, gonorrhea, and chlamydia may be conducted on admission to the correctional facility. The majority of prisons are in a difficult position with respect to sexual behavior and STDs; sex between inmates or between inmates and staff is a punishable crime in many jurisdictions, and the possession of condoms is prohibited as well. Most prison officials consider condoms contraband that can be used to hide drugs or other illegal substances or objects. They also fear that condoms promote the message that sex among prisoners is acceptable. However, the prohibition of condoms is under review in many prison systems because of high rates of STDs and the rising rate of HIV infection in the prison population (see Research: Bridge to Practice).

Human Immunodeficiency Virus/Acquired Immunodeficiency Syndrome

Only 16 states require mandatory testing for HIV infection on admission to correctional facilities. Many more states provide voluntary testing, testing after an incident, or testing after medically related problems are identified.

Prevalence rates vary widely around the country, but approximately 2.3% of state and federal inmates are known to be HIV positive. Data from a national survey of jails and prisons showed that acquired immunodeficiency syndrome (AIDS) is almost six times more prevalent among inmates

RESEARCH: BRIDGE TO PRACTICE

Chen, J., Callahan, D.B., & Kerndt, P.R. (2002). Syphilis control among incarcerated men who have sex with men: Public health response to an outbreak. *American Journal of Public Health, 92*(9), 1473–1475.

Syphilis has retreated from its epidemic years of 1986–1990, with the rates steadily declining in the United States to an all-time low of 2.5 cases per 100,000 population in 1999. Such a dramatic decline led the Centers for Disease Control and Prevention (CDC) to create a national plan for syphilis elimination. However, multiple areas in the United States continue to experience outbreaks. Rapid outbreak response should include enhanced surveillance of groups at high risk, such as incarcerated men who have sex with men (MSM).

The Los Angeles County Men's Central Jail has an inmate unit that houses about 300 self-identified MSM who are voluntarily segregated from the general inmate population. A syphilis control program was initiated with this population that included screening, mass prophylactic treatment, high-risk behavior detection, and education.

The voluntary screening for syphilis and human immunodeficiency virus (HIV) included all segregated inmates, with screening for chlamydia and gonorrhea added 1 month later. Prophylaxis using azithromycin was begun 2 months later. After 6 months, 811 inmates (94% received azithromycin threapy) had been screened for syphilis; 38 (5%) had tested positive, with 29 previously treated for syphilis and 9 newly identified. In addition, there was a 9% HIV rate. On surveillance, high-risk behaviors were identified among newly incarcerated MSM. Failure to use condoms and anonymous sex with different partners appeared to be common practice for this population, warranting public health interventions.

Screening in the correctional setting aided in disease control by enabling identification and treatment of nine new cases of syphilis. The high acceptance of azithromycin prophylaxis indicates the feasibility of mass therapy as a disease containment measure among incarcerated MSM, who are especially vulnerable because of coinfection with HIV and participation in high-risk sex.

---

than in the total population, which has a rate of 0.09%. It was estimated that 25% of all people with HIV infection have been released from prison or jail within the past year (Freudenberg, 2001). AIDS was responsible for 29% of inmate deaths in state prisons in 1995, and it is currently the leading cause of death for female inmates (Centers for Disease Control and Prevention, 1999; Hammett, Harmon, & Maruschak, 1999).

HIV-infected inmates have the same health care needs as HIV-infected individuals in the general population, but incarceration may increase the complexity of such needs. Many inmates did not have continuous health care before they entered prison, so their viral loads are often higher and they are generally sicker. Prisoners who have elevated viral loads and who do not receive highly active antiretroviral therapy (HAART) are more susceptible to opportunistic infections, including TB. They have reduced treatment outcomes; they are potentially more contagious to others during sexual intercourse, needle exchanges, and violent altercations (including biting); and they are at higher risk for end-of-life complications. Finally, they may be more likely to miss doses, to take medications improperly, or to be unable to meet the complex dietary regimens that many HIV medications require. Educating prison staff and inmates about the importance of strict compliance with all aspects of HIV medication administration is an essential responsibility of the correctional nurse. In addition, the nurse must address such issues as how to

- Get offenders to volunteer for testing

- Ensure that prisoners have HAART available during lockdowns and transfers
- Ensure that prisoners have prerelease plans that include housing, employment, HIV clinic appointments, and medications for at least 1 month

Confidentiality is difficult to maintain within a prison. Many prisons contract out for HIV care. Leaving the institution to attend an outside HIV clinic instantly identifies a prisoner as HIV-positive. Such a label carries tremendous stigmatization from other inmates. Additionally, prisoners are often taken in shackles to outside HIV clinics, where they feel that both their HIV-positive status and their status as prisoners are "on display." Finally, prisoners may fear the loss of their partners or children outside the prison if their HIV status becomes known. Rather than endure such stigmatization, humiliation, and loss, many inmates do not disclose their HIV status or do not complain of symptoms that they fear will lead to a diagnosis of AIDS.

Other ethical issues related to the care of HIV-infected prisoners include the following:
- Notification of sexual partners and those who share needles
- Disclosure of status
- Methods for halting transmission via sexual intercourse or injection drug use
- Post-exposure care
- Pregnancy and vertical transmission
- Access to medicines from clinical trials
- Discharge planning to provide for the optimal health of the client and the safety of the community

Hepatitis

Hepatitis C virus (HCV), which often accompanies HIV infection, has a 9 to 10 times higher prevalence in correctional facilities than in the general population (Freundenberg, 2001). Epidemiologic data suggest that 30% to 40% of the nation's inmates are infected with HCV, primarily as a result of drug use. HCV seroconversion while in prison is relatively low; however, inmates may arrive with HCV and few correctional facilites have adequate HCV control programs (Freudenberg, 2001). The Occupational Safety and Health Administration recommends that correctional staff receive hepatitis A, B, and C vaccines. Hepatitis C threatens to become a significant problem because of treatment costs and poor compliance with control programs designed to reduce incidence in the incarcerated population.

Mental Illness in Correctional Facilities

Correctional care nursing includes caring for the mentally ill. The entire range of mental illnesses, including depression, bipolar disorder, post-traumatic stress disorder (PTSD), behavioral disorders, and schizophrenia, may be seen in the prison population. Rates of mental illness are two to three times higher in offenders than in the general population, data supported by studies conducted in Chicago and by the Bureau of Justice Statistics in 1998 (Freudenberg, 2001).

The risk of suicide attempts and completions is also of significant concern. Clients withdrawing from alcohol or drugs have significant treatment needs. Suicide is the leading cause of death in jails and prisons. Inmates have a suicide rate 11 to 14 times higher than that of the general population. Researchers suggest that these high rates are associated with high rates of untreated depression. Intervention programs can play an important role in lowering suicide rates (Freudenberg, 2001). The nurse can oversee the development of written policies and guidelines for risk assessment and management of at-risk inmates and can assist with proper referral and transportation to medical facilities when needed. Nurses in correctional care must be prepared to perform the same assessments and interventions as would nurses in psychiatric facilities. Corrrectional care nurses also assist with design and implementation of intervention programs in collaboration with other health professionals in the setting.

Correctional facilities have large populations of mentally ill persons whose mental health needs are often poorly addressed. Such people are incarcerated for behavior that generally results from their mental illnesses; if they are released without adequate treatment or community follow-up, the cycle tends to be repeated. It is a dangerous situation for the mentally ill as well as for the community. Diversion programs for mentally ill offenders are slowly being developed in many states and in other countries to address this problem (Draine & Solomon, 1999). These programs team mental health nurses and other mental health workers with police personnel to monitor and assist mentally ill offenders who live in the community (see Clinical Corner).

Family Considerations

The importance of providing support to the parents, partners, and children of inmates cannot be emphasized strongly enough. Assisting a family with the grief, embarrassment, and humiliation of losing a loved one to incarceration and providing for the inmate's needs for love and belonging are essential components of compassionate and effective nursing care. Inmates who receive no visitors or communication from "outside the walls" are at risk for suicidal behavior, depression, and violence. If transportation or financial issues interfere with visitation, the correctional nurse can suggest community resources to assist the family.

In 1999, an estimated 767,200 black children, 384,500 white children, and 301,600 Hispanic children had one parent in prison (National Practitioners Network for Fathers and Families [NPNFF], 2000). The impact on children of a parent's incarceration is immeasurable. First, the loss of the parent's physical presence can create anxiety, fear, sadness, and anger. Of all parents in state and federal prisons, 46% said they were living with their children just before admission to prison (NPNFF, 2000). Explaining the parent's absence to friends and schoolmates can cause the child deep humiliation. The child's attitude toward people in authority, including teachers and law enforcement officials, may become fearful or resentful. These factors may influence the child to run away from home; engage in self-destructive behaviors such as drinking, drug use, sexual promiscuity, or suicide attempts; or commit petty crimes. As noted earlier, many of the children of incarcerated parents go on to become criminals themselves. In consideration of these effects, the correctional nurse may wish to develop support groups for the partners and children of inmates; such groups can provide participants with a safe forum for dealing with their feelings, thoughts, and experiences after the incarceration. On a broader scale, nurses can advocate for the elimination of poverty conditions that spawn violence and crime.

WOMEN IN PRISON

There are approximately 67,500 women incarcerated on any given day in the United States. This number represents 11.3% of the nation's adult jail population, an increase from 8.0% in 1985 (Beck, 2000). In actual numbers, it is a 300% increase. About 85% of these women are mothers, the overwhelming majority of whom have children younger than 18 years of age. An average of 6% to 10% of women enter prison pregnant, and there are 1300 live births and 900 miscarriages or abortions annually (Richardson, 1998).

Some Gender Differences in Corrections

More women than men live in poverty, and women earn just 75 cents to every dollar that men earn (U. S. Bureau of the Census, 2000). Economic power buys better legal advice,

CLINICAL CORNER

IMPROVING THE HEALTH OF AN INCARCERATED POPULATION

SCENARIO

You have been working as a nurse in a large prison outside Metropolis for 4 years. Recently you were promoted to the role of supervisor. You are now responsible for analysis of health care services for the prison. You look forward to the opportunity to address some of the suboptimal health practices that you have observed in your time as a staff nurse working in the system. You feel strongly that previous supervisors have been remiss in failing to address serious health issues facing the prison population. You plan to implement policies and programs that will address these issues and lead to a healthier environment for the inmates and staff.

The health issues that you plan to address include:
- substance use among inmates
- noncompliance with medications
- unsafe sex among inmates

Demographics of Prison Population
- Gender: all male inmates and guards
- Number: 700–900 inmates on average

Staff
- Guards are employees of the state correctional department.
- Health care providers are employees of the local health department.

- Health care staff consists of one male physician, one male and one female nurse practitioner, and four female and two male registered nurses.

Substance Abuse Among Inmates

The problem of substance abuse among inmates in Metropolis Prison has been identified and discussed by previous administrators. Attempts have been made to address the issue. Interventions have included group education, counseling by local drug diversion program staff, and weekly AA/NA meetings. Although some inmates have expressed interest in these approaches, the problem of substance abuse remains rampant.

You have gathered anecdotal information from health service staff, correctional officers, and inmates regarding the extent of the problem and believe that the drug-using population in this facility comprises a demographically mixed subculture of about 30% of the total population. It is generally believed that the most common drugs being utilized by prisoners include "crack" cocaine or heroin. Needles and syringes are valuable commodities and are used in the underground bartering system. It is highly likely that these IV drug "works" are being shared by inmates without cleaning between users.

QUESTION

1. Discuss your application of the nursing process to address the issue presented above. Use information available to you given the scenario and extrapolate when information is unknown.

---

which translates into reduced sentences for crimes. Furthermore, women tend to lack comprehensive knowledge about crimes in which they have participated and therefore have little information to trade for reduced sentences. This lack of power extends into the prison system, especially with male prison guards. Studies have shown that anxiety and depression are escalated during incarceration because of perceived powerlessness and fear of retribution such as sexual assault for speaking out.

Violence Against Women in Prison

Most women enter prison with a history of domestic violence or sexual assault or both. Studies estimate that more than 75% have experienced sexual abuse as children or adults (Browne, Miller, & Maguin, 1999). Another study suggests that 44% have been beaten by one or both parents, and it is estimated that 90% come from homes where hitting, slapping, and striking are commonplace (Browne, Miller, & Maguin, 1999; Fogel & Belyea, 1999).

Physical and sexual abuse continue to be problematic for women within prison. Although the Fourth Amendment to the U. S. Constitution provides protection against sexual abuse of prisoners, several states currently have no laws prohibiting sexual abuse and misconduct in correctional facilities. In 1999, Amnesty International released a report called *Not Part of My Sentence,* which detailed numerous instances of sexual assault and inappropriate conduct of male guards toward female prisoners (Amnesty International USA, 1999). The findings of this report were so appalling that two television networks, ABC and CNN, followed up with investigations of sexual assault and misconduct against women in U. S. prisons. Some women "consent" to sexual relations with guards, a practice known as "trading favors." However, consent between a prisoner and a guard is legally impossible (as it is between a minor and an adult); such behavior may reflect the woman's overwhelming sense of powerlessness and her fear that she will not be able to survive within the system unless she consents. Indeed, retribution by guards against women for withholding sex has been documented to include putting feces in prisoners' food, urinating on prisoners, refusing prisoners medical care, and even forced hanging.

Reproductive and Family Issues

Women in prison have the same reproductive and family issues as women in the population at large. Those who are mothers are as concerned about their children's welfare and safety as any mother who is separated from her child anywhere. Some children are left with abusive fathers, uncaring relatives, or in foster care. Some imprisoned women lose their children to adoption. Even those children who remain at home with loving fathers or grandparents may, because of financial constraints or their geographic distance from the prison, be unable to visit more than once every few months. For these reasons, many imprisoned women suffer from "empty nest syndrome" and are almost unbearably lonely.

The correctional nurse can do much in this area. Support groups that allow women to express their feelings for their families and provide techniques for healing these wounds can be tremendously beneficial. For instance, the nurse can offer suggestions about how to heal the pain of loss and how to reach out to the children that may have been harmed. Alleviation of shame and guilt can spur incarcerated mothers to connect more meaningfully with their loved ones (see Voices From the Community).

As noted earlier, approximately 6% to 10% of women entering prison are pregnant. Some miscarry, others choose abortion, and others carry their babies to term, only to lose them immediately after birth to foster care. New York State's Bedford Hills is one of only a few programs that allow women prisoners to keep their babies. Comprehensive prenatal care, parenting classes, and counseling are provided to mothers in an attempt to break the cycle of crime, violence, and substance abuse that typically contributes to incarceration.

Gynecologic examinations to screen for STDs, pregnancy, and concealed contraband or weapons can be part of the admission process. This can be a difficult experience for a woman with a history of sexual abuse because it may trigger memories of the incident and cause extreme anxiety or tears. A gentle, stepped process of providing gynecologic care to traumatized inmates was described by Dole (1999). Taking the additional time with traumatized inmates is imperative if the painful wounds of sexual abuse are ever to heal. The prison environment affords the correctional nurse this opportunity, because many inmates are incarcerated for several years.

ROLE OF THE COMMUNITY HEALTH NURSE

According to the Federal Bureau of Prisons (2000), nurses constitute 19% of the federal prison health services population. In some settings, nurses work with health care–trained custody staff as partners in delivering care. The nurse who works with the prison population assumes a variety of roles similar to those in the outside world. The correctional nurse's role in education, advocacy, and provision of a bridge for inmates into the community are discussed in the following paragraphs.

Educational and Literacy Issues

Literacy is defined as the ability to read and write to an extent that allows the individual to function in daily life. Low literacy levels have been associated with increased rates of incarceration, in part because literacy is usually a requirement for employment.

Screening for illiteracy among prisoners is important in combating recidivism and ensuring that written health education materials are understood. In addition, poor readers are typically ill informed and hold many misconceptions about their bodies, illness, and health care. Screening can be difficult because many illiterate individuals have learned to compensate for this shortcoming and hide it very well. When asked directly, most deny their inability to read. Suggested questions for ascertaining literacy might include the following: "Some people find it hard to understand what they read. Is this true for you?" "Do you like to read?" "What have you read recently?"

Correctional nurses can be helpful not only in identifying illiteracy, but also in encouraging improvement in literacy and health knowledge among prisoners. Almost all correctional facilities have educators and existing educational programs, including health education programs and materials (see Chapter 12). The nurse works with educational staff to ensure that

VOICES FROM THE COMMUNITY

I worked in a psychiatric hospital on the campus of a large women's prison. It was perhaps the most challenging job I will ever have! Among other assignments, I facilitated a group for 1 hour each afternoon. The issues we discussed were similar to those most women struggle with in the "real world": self-esteem, family concerns, interpersonal relationships, loneliness, and many more. However, here when a woman spoke of concern for her child, it was that she might never see the child again—"Will my child ever remember me?" or even, "Where is my child and who has her?" Loneliness was profound. One inmate told me with tears in her eyes, "Ms. Lind, I know I can do one life term but I don't think I can do two." Her sentences ran back to back.

The group remained relatively stable the year I was there. Some women would improve and leave the acute unit, returning to the general population. Many cycled through on a regular basis, and a few remained acute the whole time.

The reward for the nurse working in this type of setting is great. These women have so few resources or coping skills that you can have tremendous impact on their ability to find some inner strength or peace to cope with their dismal future.

Barbara Lind, RN

health education materials are comprehensible to all inmates. For example, videos and cartoon-like instructional materials with vivid pictures and few words can be used effectively. The nurse also uses informal opportunities to provide health education to inmates such as during "sick call" contacts.

In addition, correctional nurses have an opportunity to provide inmates with an increased understanding of their bodies, their diseases, or their medications. The nurse may be the first person to ever offer this information. Health education in these areas empowers inmates and improves their outcomes, ultimately benefiting the institution as well. Educating prisoners about the medication system and sick-call procedures is mandated. Additionally, education of correctional staff about use of universal precautions, transmission of communicable diseases, the need to report changes in health of inmates, the importance of monitoring for depression and suicide risk, and the unacceptability of withholding medications as punishment is an important responsibility of the correctional nurse.

Advocacy

An important role of the correctional nurse is that of advocate and activist. Inmates have essentially no power and often experience abusive and health-damaging treatment from fellow prisoners, as well as custody personnel. Nurses can and must advocate for prisoners if they suspect improprieties. However, they need to understand that they may be labeled "a snitch" by inmates or "a troublemaker" by staff or administrators. Advocacy and empowerment are not highly valued by most prison authorities, who fear that prisoners will become agitated and cause riots or other problems. Nonetheless, although advocacy for prisoners' health care may be met with resistance, the nurse must remain undaunted. Custody staff and administration personnel understand chain of command and authority. The nurse must earn respect of custody personnel and act with authority, using the chain of command with impunity.

The nurse's advocacy role can be enhanced significantly by consulting with or using the services of a forensic nurse if one is available. Forensics allows for legal arguments to be used to advocate for the health and well-being of clients.

Bridge Programs With the Community

As prisoners are released into the community, the correctional nurse again plays a vital role. Unless prisoners are prepared and their release plans coordinated, **recidivism** (eg, a relapse into criminal behavior with subsequent incarceration) is likely to occur. Recidivism is highest in the first 24 hours and the earliest days of release; rates vary but are generally about 35%. Comprehensive prerelease programs can decrease recidivism by half (Freudenberg, 2001). Corrections systems can assist in successful release by providing discharge planning, community aftercare, and other postrelease supportive services. Attention must be paid to issues of housing, employment, and

continuity of medical care. Providing these necessities actually decreases public costs because of the corresponding decrease in recidivism. Some correctional facilities use peer education programs to provide inmates with information and beginning skills for application outside (Boudin et al., 1999).

Some prerelease programs bring health care providers into the prison for a first appointment before the inmate's release. Most prisoners have difficulty maneuvering within the health care system outside the prison, and this allows them to make a meaningful advance contact with their health care providers. It is helpful to arrange a "drop-in" policy for inmates initially and to schedule an appointment for the second week after release. This gives prisoners a sense that someone cares about them and is invested in their successful transitions to life outside prison. Giving inmates a business card and encouraging them to call for any problem also increases their confidence and provides a safety net for social and health care support. Prisoners are typically anxious on release and must deal with many life stressors concurrently. Having a safe place to drop in may mean the difference between success and a return to a life of crime.

Preparing inmates for release is an expanded role for the correctional nurse. Reentry into a community that may be hostile poses significant challenges, in terms of both successful reintegration and the avoidance of a return to criminal behaviors. Substance abuse, self-destructive behavior, and recidivism commonly occur when released inmates are shunned by their communities or denied employment or housing. The correctional nurse must work with community liaisons to design discharge plans that will result in positive outcomes for the client. Nursing practice at its most comprehensive level benefits clients, society, and the system within which it occurs (see Using the Nursing Process).

In discharge planning, the nurse must remember to consider the needs of the inmate's family. While the inmate is incarcerated, the family has adjusted to his or her absence and has reorganized the family system to fill the roles and responsibilities of the missing member. The return home of an ex-convict can create upheaval and conflict. Family therapy and support throughout the reintegration process can result in smoother readjustment. Long-term support rather than brief intervention is more effective in enabling family members to begin communicating and interacting in a positive manner, allowing them to resolve their anger, disappointment, humiliation, and grief.

Personal Safety, Stress Reduction, and Self-Care

Working within the confines of the prison system poses significant stress for the nurse. Stressors include the following:

- An environment fraught with rules, restrictions, and constant monitoring
- A philosophically conflicting culture that poses ethical dilemmas
- An unknown, often unstable, and potentially dangerous client population
- A setting wherein nursing decisions often must be made

USING THE NURSING PROCESS

When Working With Incarcerated Women

You have been working at Central Women's Prison for 2 years. This is a minimum-security prison for 200 women. Most of the women are serving 2- to 5-year sentences and have school-age children they can see only on Sundays for one unfocused hour. Some of the women have families who live close enough for regular visitation. From the comments shared in a weekly support group you initiated along with mental health services, you are aware that the women are desperately lonely and miss being meaningfully involved in their children's lives.

ASSESSMENT

About 25% of the women have less than 1 year remaining in their sentences. Most have family nearby who bring their children to visit each Sunday. The women are interested in working with the administration and the community to enhance the parent-child relationship, prepare them for an improved parenting role, and promote reentry into the community. It is also believed that focusing on working with their children for an extended period of time will decrease the women's stress and feelings of isolation and loneliness.

NURSING DIAGNOSES

- Disruption of the interactive processes between parent and child due to long-term separation
- Altered parenting related to knowledge deficit of parenting skills and long-term separation

PLAN—PHASE I

- A pilot group of 12 women who expressed an interest and were selected by the administration will meet with you twice a week for 2 weeks to plan a "community reentry program" focused on developing their parenting skills and reattaching with children they have been separated from for 2 years or longer.
- You will meet with the warden, mental health services personnel, and a representative from the community school district during week 3 to explore potential program directions.
- You will set up a meeting with the pilot group of women and the above-mentioned administration and community members in week 4 to outline a program of parent/child enhanced bonding.
- In weeks 3 and 4 the women will make a list of things they hope to achieve by enhancing the Sunday visiting hours with their children. The list will address their needs, the perceived needs of their children, and the goals they want to achieve.

PLAN—PHASE II

- In week 5 you meet with the pilot group of women and discuss the role the administration, community, and women will take in the "community reentry program." It has been decided to have a three-pronged approach to the program: educational, social, and family oriented.
- The administration will allow the visiting hours to be increased from 1 hour to 3 hours each Sunday. They will provide a counselor each Sunday for 2 hours to guide discussion groups during the social and family segments of the program. The school district will provide a teacher for 2 hours each Sunday to assist with the educational and family-oriented segments of the program. The pilot group of women have contacted family members regarding the new program, and they have agreed to participate regularly during the length of the program which is tentatively scheduled to be 12 weeks long and to be reevaluated for continuation after 10 weeks.

IMPLEMENTATION

- The first hour of the 12-week "community reentry program" focuses on parent/child bonding through homework assistance. Each parent works with her children at their school levels and learns how to be supportive and noncritical and enjoy the time engaged in their children's learning.
- The second hour has a social focus with some guided group exercises initiated by the counselor and guided by you and the counselor. Various simulation games and parent/child interactive activities are scheduled.
- During the third hour, the focus is on family. Grandparents and other caretakers, along with the children and the incarcerated parent, enjoy each other's company and refreshments. The teacher shares with the caretakers and mothers areas in which the children are working and how both set of "stakeholders" can enhance learning during the week until their next Sunday together.

EVALUATION

During the educational hour, it was discovered after the first 10 weeks that many of the women are intimidated by the levels of school work of their children and feel inadequate to help them. After two formative evaluation meetings with the women, it was decided to begin a tutoring program for women in the afternoons to enhance their educational skills; this program eventually included all interested women in the facility.

(continued)

USING THE NURSING PROCESS   (CONTINUED)

When Working With Incarcerated Women

It was also decided to increase the educational hour to 90 minutes and shorten the family hour to 30 minutes, allowing time for you to teach some specific parenting skills through gaming (see Chapter 12) and time for practice. The women found greater satisfaction working one-on-one with their children, and much "socializing" occurred during that time.

Finally, it was decided to continue the program until the 12 women in the pilot group were released, while begin-

ning with another group of women after the first 12 weeks.

It was decided to follow-up with the first 12 women for 3 months after release and compare their reentry into the community with that of other women released at the same time who did not go through the program. Even though the women, children, and family members initially involved evaluated the program very positively, the administration and school district wanted to see data that would support continuation.

in isolation, without immediate access to other health team members or resources

Self-care, stress reduction, relaxation, and planned "time out" are essential for the success of community health nursing practice within the correctional system. Personal safety issues must be addressed and incorporated into daily practice. This includes avoiding health risks though immunization, using safety precautions around inmates with infectious diseases, and having correctional officers in close proximity when working with potentially dangerous clients. Avoidance of "vicarious traumatization" is essential to prevent burnout and the development of significant emotional distress. Correctional nurses face additional concerns in terms of personal relationships and their ability to separate from the multifaceted stressors associated with professional responsibilities so that they can maintain a positive and healthy personal life. Establishing a peer support group with the correctional care team and with other correctional nurses can reduce the sense of professional isolation that often accompanies this particular area of specialization.

SUMMARY

Serving clients in correctional facilities poses unique challenges and opportunities for community health nurses. To understand prisoners and the issues affecting their health, the nurse must be familiar with the correctional environment, know its rules, restrictions, and strict chain of command, adapt to security monitoring, and recognize problems associated with an atmosphere of overcrowding, despair, and numerous negative health conditions.

The number of inmates in the United States is growing; the majority are white men, many of whom have a history of abuse or neglect in childhood. About three fourths of the inmates are nonviolent offenders. They tend to be poor, undereducated, and at risk for many chronic and infectious diseases.

Historically, prisoners were mistreated and the conditions in correctional facilities were deplorable. Reforms in the 1700s and 1800s gradually improved conditions; international standards were adopted in 1955 that promoted respect for inmates' humanity and rights. Correctional health care today has greatly improved, but many problems remain.

Various laws enacted in recent decades have improved prison conditions, standards, and inmates' rights. Some laws, intended to curb drug trafficking and other offenses, have contributed to an escalation in the number of prisoners, with resultant overcrowding of correctional facilities.

A variety of professional organizations and agencies influence the incarcerated population's living conditions, rights, and policies that govern their treatment.

Ethical dilemmas arise in correctional health care including the death penalty, which conflicts with nursing goals of rehabilitation. The need to preserve client confidentiality and privacy poses additional problems. Furthermore, it is difficult for the nurse to practice objectively with offenders who have committed heinous crimes or with inmates who make sexual advances.

Incarcerated offenders have many health problems and needs. Communicable diseases are a major problem; they include TB, STDs, and HIV/AIDs, along with hepatitis and other associated illnesses. Caring for an incarcerated population with these health problems is complex because treatment compliance, confidentiality, and follow-up after discharge are difficult to ensure. Mental illness affects a large portion of the prison population and leads to a vicious circle of recidivism if not treated adequately. Inmates' families, particularly children, suffer in many ways as a result of the inmate's incarceration; affected family members need support.

Women are a minority of the prison population but have many special health care needs because of their vulnerability and powerlessness. Many were abused as children and as adults; they may suffer from depression, loneliness, and the misconduct of guards. Inmates who are mothers suffer loss and the grief of separation from their children.

The correctional community health nurse can make a significant difference with the incarcerated population and can play various roles. In particular, the nurse serves as health educator to combat illiteracy and ignorance, as advocate to correct improprieties and promote inmates' health, and as a "bridge" to assist with predischarge planning and preparation for release into the community.

Finally, correctional health nurses must protect their own personal safety, take measures to cope with a stressful work environment, and find needed outlets and support.

ACTIVITIES TO PROMOTE CRITICAL THINKING

1. You are treating several women who are incarcerated in a medium-security prison for PTSD. All of these inmates have been sexually abused or assaulted. They express significant distress at the constant monitoring of all their activities day and night by male guards. How would you handle this situation? What are the issues inherent in this case?

2. John S., age 58 years, was recently incarcerated for the second time for armed robbery. He has been monitored for suicidal risk and is being treated for hypertension. He reports to the nurse that he is not being given his medications at night because the guards "don't like him." This inmate has been labeled a troublemaker. How would you handle this situation? What are some of the issues inherent in this case?

3. You are responsible for examining the health issues affecting the incarcerated population at your all-male facility. In particular, you learn that unsafe sexual practices among inmates are a major problem that is emotionally charged and that no one has been willing to address. You learn that
   • Sexual acts are used in the underground bartering system.
   • STDs often go untreated during the period of incarceration.

   • Nonconsensual sexual violence occurs frequently, yet is rarely reported to staff.
   • By the estimate of one inmate, more than 30% of inmates are practicing unsafe sex.
   • Condoms are not available to inmates.
   • Previous attempts to make condoms available to inmates were unsuccessful because the Department of Corrections believed that supplying condoms would encourage illegal activities such as sodomy and drug smuggling.

   With a group of your classmates, discuss how you would apply the nursing process to these issues, using the information given and extrapolating for information that is unknown. Identify the host, agent, and environment factors in the epidemiologic triad that are present in this situation. Develop a plan for primary, secondary, and tertiary prevention for unsafe sex, sexual abuse, and STDs with this population.

4. Assume that you are a correctional nurse researching information about a health problem that affects your inmates. Search at least two Web sites for information on this problem. Summarize what you learn about the problem and describe its application to your practice.

REFERENCES

American Correctional Association. (1996). *Public policy on correctional health care.* Retrieved February 14, 2004, from *http://www.corrections.com*

American Correctional Health Services Association. *ACHSA code of ethics.* Retrieved February 12, 2004, from *http://www.corrections.com/achsa/*

American Nurses Association. (2003). *Scope and standards of nursing practice in correctional facilities.* ANA Publ. NP-104. Washington, DC: Author.

Amnesty International USA. (1999). *"Not part of my sentence": Violations of the human rights of women in custody.* New York: Author.. Retrieved February 14, 2004, from *http://www.amnestyusa.org/countries/usa/document.do?id=D 1F037D8618F4F6D8025690000692F87*

Beck, A.J. (2000). *Prison and jail inmates at midyear 1999.* Washington, DC: Bureau of Justice Statistics.

Boudin, K., Carrero, I., Clark, J., Flournoy, V., Loftin, K., Martindale, S., et al. (1999). ACE: A peer education and counseling program meets the needs of incarcerated women with HIV/AIDS issues. *Journal of the Association of Nurses in AIDS Care, 10*(6), 90–98.

Brecher, E.M., & Della Penna, R.D. (1975). *The prescriptive package: Health care in correctional institutions.* Washington, DC: National Institute of Law Enforcement and Criminal Justice, U. S. Department of Justice.

Browne, A., Miller, B., & Maguin, E. (1999). Prevalence and severity of lifetime physical and sexual victimization among incarcerated women. *International Journal of Law and Psychiatry, 22*(3–4), 301–322.

Butterfield, F. (2003, April 7). Rates of incarceration for young blacks hits record. *The Fresno Bee,* p. A3.

California Department of Corrections, Office of Continuing Education and Training and Public Health Section. (1999). *Tuberculosis training for correctional employees.* Sacramento, CA: Author.

Centers for Disease Control and Prevention. (1999). Decrease in AIDS-related mortality in a state correctional system—New York, 1995–1998. *Mortality and Morbidity Weekly Report, 47*(51), 1115–1117. Retrieved April 16, 2004 from *http://www.cdc.gov/nchstp/od/mmwr/47/(51);1115-1117.htm*

Chen, J.L., Callahan, D.B., & Kerndt, P.R. (2002). Syphilis control among incarcerated men who have sex with men: Public health response to an outbreak. *American Journal of Public Health, 92*(9), 1473–1475.

Cohen, M., Deamant, C., Barkan, S., Richardson, J., Yound, M.,

Holman, S., et al. (2000). Domestic violence and childhood sexual abuse in HIV-infected women and women at risk for HIV. *American Journal of Public Health, 90*(4), 560–565.

Cole, D. (1999). *No equal justice: Race and class in the American criminal justice system.* New York: New Press.

Conklin, T.J., Lincoln, T., & Tuthill, R.W. (2000). Self-reported health and prior health behaviors of newly admitted correctional inmates. *American Journal of Public Health, 90*(12), 1939–1941.

Dole, P. (1999). Examining sexually traumatized incarcerated women. *HEPP News, 2*(6), 5 [HIV Education Prison Project, Brown University]. Retrieved April 16, 2004 from *http://www.aegis.com/files/hepp/hepp1999-06.pdf*

Draine, J., & Solomon, P. (1999). Describing and evaluating jail diversion services for persons with serious mental illness. *Psychiatric Services, 50,* 56–61.

Federal Bureau of Prisons. (2000, April 27). *Public information: Quick facts and statistics.* Washington, DC: Office of Public Affairs. Retrieved February 14, 2004, from *http:// www.bop.gov*

Fogel, C.I., & Belyea, M. (1999). The lives of incarcerated women: Violence, substance abuse, and at risk for HIV. *Journal of the Association of Nurses in AIDS Care, 10*(6), 66–73.

Freudenberg, N. (2001). Jails, prisons, and the health of urban populations: A review of the impact of the correctional system on community health. *Journal of Urban Health: Bulletin of the New York Academy of Medicine, 78*(2), 214–235.

Hammett, T.M., Harmon, P., & Maruschak, L.M. (1999). *1996–1997 update: HIV/AIDS, STDs, and TB in correctional facilities.* Washington, DC: U. S. Department of Justice.

Harvard Law School. (2003). United States Wickershem Commission Records 1928–1931. Retrieved April 16, 2004, from *http://oasis.harvard.edu/html/law00114.html*

Irwin, J. (2000). *America's one million nonviolent prisoners.* Washington, DC: Justice Policy Institute. Retrieved February 14, 2004, from *http://cjcj.org/pubs/one_million/onemillion.html*

Levine, S. (2002). Criminal care at a high price. *U.S. News & World Report, 133*(5), 44–45.

Miller, S.K. (1999). New directions for nurse practitioners: Correctional health care. *Patient Care for the Nurse Practitioner, 2*(11), 53.

National Pratitioners Network for Fathers and Families. (2000). 1.5 million children have an incarcerated parent. *The Practitioner, 1*(3), 1.

Price, M. (2001). When your patient is an inmate. *Nursing Spectrum: Career Management. New England Edition.* [online]. Retrieved February 14, 2004, from *http://nsweb.nursingspectrum.com/MagazinArticles/article.cfm?AID=5650*

Richardson, S.Z. (1998). Preferred care of the pregnant inmate. In M. Puisis, *Clinical practice in correctional medicine* (pp. 181–187). St. Louis: Mosby.

United States Bureau of the Census. (2000). *Men still make more.* Washington, DC: Author.

SELECTED READINGS

Butterfield, F. (2000, November 29). Often, parole is one stop on the way back to prison. *New York Times,* pp. A1, A32.

Byock, I.R. (Ed.). (2001). *A handbook for end-of-life care in correctional facilities.* Alexandria, VA: Volunteers of America.

Charuvastra, A., Stein, J., Schwartzapfel, B., Spaulding, A., Horowitz, E., Macalino, G., et al. (2001). Hepatitis B vaccination practices in state and federal prisons. *Public Health Reports, 116*(3), 203–209.

DeLone, M. (2003). *Standards for health services in correctional institutions* (3rd ed.). Waldorf, MD: American Public Health Association.

Dubler, N., & Post, L.F. (2001). *Improving palliative care practice in jails and prisons.* Rockville, MD: Health Resources and Services Administration.

Fickenscher, A., Lapidus, J., Silk-Warner, P., & Becker, T. (2001). Women behind bars: Health needs of inmates in a county jail. *Public Health Reports, 116*(3), 191–196.

Hammett, T.M., Harmon, M.P., & Rhodes, W. (2002). The burden of infectious disease among inmates of and releasees from U.S. correctional facilities, 1997. *American Journal of Public Health, 92*(11), 1789–1794.

May, J.P. (2000). *Building violence.* Thousand Oaks, CA: Sage.

Prison Health Policy Unit. (2000). *Nursing in prisons: Report by the working group considering the development of prison nursing, with particular reference to health care officers.* London: Department of Health.

Saunders, D.L., Olive, D.M., Wallace, S.B., Lacy, D., Leyba, R., & Kendig, N.E. (2001). Tuberculosis screening in the federal prison system: An opportunity to treat and prevent tuberculosis in foreign-born populations. *Public Health Reports, 116*(3), 210–218.

Spaulding, A., Lubelczyk, R.B., & Flanigan, T. (2001). Can unsafe sex behind bars be barred? *American Journal of Public Health, 91*(8), 1176–1177.

Stringer, H. (2001, March 12). Prison break: Correctional nurses enjoy greater degree of professional freedom behind bars. *NurseWeek.* Retrieved February 14, 2004, from *http://www.nurseweek.com/news/features/01-03/correctional.asp*

Tsenin, K. (2000). One judicial perspective on the sex trade. In *Research on women and girls in the justice system* (Vol. 3, pp. 15–26). Washington, DC: National Institute of Justice.

United States Department of Health and Human Services. (2000). *Health issues specific to incarcerated women: Information for state maternal and child health programs.* Washington, DC: Health Resources and Services Administration.

Varghese, B., & Peterman, T.A. (2001). Cost-effectiveness of HIV counseling and testing in U. S. prisons. *Journal of Urban Health, 78,* 304–312.

Vicini, J. (2000, January 18). Supreme Court upholds segregation of HIV-infected inmates. *Reuters Medical News on Medscape.* Retrieved February 14, 2004, from *http://www.hiv.medscape.com*

Resources

A sister's story (free comic book for female offenders about HIV; available in Spanish and English). Bristol-Meyers Squibb.

Cell wars (comic book on HIV in prison populations). Bristol-Meyers Squibb.

Get tested (video on HIV in correctional facilities). Glaxo Wellcome.

HIV Inside: A Quarterly Newsletter for Correctional Professionals. New York: World Health CME, telephone 212-481-8534. Free subscription supported by a grant from Glaxo-Wellcome.

Peternelj-Taylor, C.A., & Johnson, R. *Custody and caring: A challenge for nursing* (video documentary).

Reeder-Bey, V., & Wilburn, A.M. *My grandma has AIDS: Annisha's story*. Agouron Pharmaceuticals, Inc., telephone 1-888-847-2237.

A strategy to increase HIV/AIDs medication adherence in correctional settings (Inmate Adherence Videotape Series). Albany Medical Center, telephone 518-262-6864 or santosm@mail.amc.edu.

Internet Resources

American Civil Liberties Union. Stop Prisoner Rape Affidavit. In ACLU et al v. Reno. Available at *http://www.aclu.org/privacy/privacy.cfm?ID=13959%c=252*

Amnesty International: *http://www.amnestyusa.org*

Association of Nurses in AIDS Care: *http://www.anacnet.org*

Clinician's Educational Resource: *http://www.hivline.com*

HEPP News, Brown University HIV Education Prison Project: *http://www.hivcorrections.org*

Human Rights Watch: *http://www.hrw.org*

Justice Policy Institute: *http://www.cjcj.org*

Justice Works: *http://www.justiceworks.org*

Medscape, HIV/AIDS Home Page (operated by UCLA; has a range of HIV articles updated regularly): *http://medscape.com/hiv-aidshome*

National Commission on Correctional Health Care: *http://www.ncchc.org*

The Bureau of Justice Statistics: *http://www.ojp.usdoj.gov/bjs*

The Corrections Connection Network: *http://www.corrections.com*

37

Clients Receiving Home Health and Hospice Care

Key Terms

- Durable medical equipment
- Formal caregivers
- Home health care
- Home health nursing
- Homebound
- Homemaker agency
- Hospice
- Hospital-based agency
- Informal caregivers
- Ombudsman
- Palliative care
- Respite
- Terminally ill

Learning Objectives

Upon mastery of this chapter, you should be able to:

- Describe the home care and hospice populations.
- Discuss standards and credentialing for home care and hospice nursing.
- Provide an overview of the evolution of home care and hospice nursing.
- Identify the variety of agencies providing home care and hospice services.
- Explain the roles and responsibilities of the various members of the home health care and hospice teams.
- Describe the reimbursement systems common to home health and hospice care.
- Describe the role of the community health nurse in meeting the health care needs of the homebound population.
- Describe the role of the community health nurse in meeting the health care needs of the hospice family.

Have you ever sat with a frail, elderly gentleman with chronic obstructive pulmonary disease receiving oxygen at home and listened to his stories of the "good old days" when he was young, full of vigor, and taking on the world? Have you ever tried to comfort a middle-aged woman dying of cancer and fearful for the welfare of her teenage daughter after she is gone? Have you ever listened to the fears and concerns expressed by family members of chronically ill or terminally ill clients? These are just three of the myriad of experiences that make up the daily lives of nurses who work with home care and hospice clients. Indeed, these programs allow nurses to practice what some see as the very heart of compassionate nursing care.

This chapter discusses home care and hospice nursing as domains of practice. The reader is also referred to the discussions in Chapters 24 and 30 on how to plan for, implement, and evaluate the family visit at home; issues of personal safety; and the older adult. Home care and hospice programs have become a growing part of the existing health care system and are work setting choices being made by more and more nurses.

AN OVERVIEW OF HOME CARE

The need for health care at home has been growing steadily in the last two decades. Drastic changes in financing, changing provider roles, and increasing client acuity have contributed to this trend. For example, early hospital discharges resulting from third-party payers' efforts toward cost containment have forced clients back into their homes to recuperate from surgeries and severe illnesses far more quickly than 20 years ago. Moreover, third-party payers are now requiring that certain procedures be performed only on an outpatient basis. As a result, such complex procedures as intravenous (IV) chemotherapy, parenteral nutrition, and mechanical ventilation, all of which were once provided only in hospitals or in skilled nursing care facilities, are today routinely provided and maintained in the client's home. Hospital stays for mothers and newborns have been shortened to an average of 24 to 48 hours, necessitating postpartum and infant home care. Advances in technology have led to the development of machines that can provide dialysis, pain control, and ventilatory care in the client's home. In addition, **terminally ill** clients—those with less than 6 months to live—find that the supportive services of hospice care allow them to live as fully as possible and die at home rather than in a hospital. Finally, there are now simply more elderly people in the United States than there were two decades ago; this means a corresponding increase in clients with chronic illnesses, many of whom prefer to be cared for at home.

As a result, many community health nurses are spending more of their time caring for clients in their homes. Therefore, it is important to take a look at the terminology of home care, the demographics of the home care population, and the standards and credentials associated with home care nursing.

Terminology of Home Health Care

Home health care, broadly defined, refers to all of the services and products provided to clients in their homes to maintain, restore, or promote their physical, mental, and emotional health. Its purpose is to maximize the client's level of independence and to minimize the effects of existing disabilities through noninstitutional services. Its primary goal is to use these supportive services to decrease rehospitalization and prevent or delay institutionalization (Martinson, Widmer, & Portillo, 2002; Rice, 2001).

There is a distinct difference between professional and technical home care services provided to clients. Professional home care services are practice driven; that is, the boundaries of practice are determined by standards based on scientific theory and research. Professional home care is provided by professionals with licenses, certification, or specific qualifications. These professionals typically work for home care agencies with internal and external standards that guide the provision of their services. Nurses, social workers, physical therapists, occupational therapists, and home health aides are examples of professional home care practitioners.

Technical home care services are product driven and therefore do not always consider what is best for the client. Providers of technical home care do not necessarily have standards or regulations that govern how they serve clients. **Durable medical equipment** (DME) includes equipment that is used for a long period of time and can be used again by others, such as wheelchairs, walkers, hospital beds, ventilators, IV therapy poles, and so on. DME suppliers, oxygen providers, and other equipment home delivery providers make up the majority of providers in this category.

Home health nursing is a specialized area of nursing practice with its roots firmly placed in community health nursing (American Nurses Association [ANA], 1999). The nurse provides home health nursing care to acute, chronic, and terminally ill clients of all ages in their homes while integrating community health nursing principles that focus on the environmental, psychosocial, economic, cultural, and personal health factors affecting a client's and family's health status and well-being. It is a unique field of nursing practice that requires a synthesis of community health nursing principles with the theory and practice of medical/surgical, maternal–child, geriatric, and mental health nursing. Home care nurses care for clients who have procedures and treatments conducted in their homes and for those who wish to live out the final days of their lives in their homes rather than in an institution.

The focus of home care nursing is the treatment of human responses. Home health nursing demands that the varied human responses seen in home care clients be addressed in a holistic framework so that the client and family can be assisted to reach their goals.

The Home Care Population

The client cared for in home care nursing is not only the individual patient but also the family and any significant others. Therefore, the nurse must consider numerous factors related to the client's family, community, culture, society, and religion (Navaie-Waliser, et al., 2001). The nurse must consider how the environmental, psychosocial, economic, cultural, and personal health–related factors affect the client's illness and ability to meet the goals outlined in the plan of care.

In 2000, more than 7.8 million people received home care services for acute illnesses, long-term health conditions, permanent disabilities, or terminal illnesses (National Association for Home Care [NAHC], 2001). The demographics of home care clients in the United States reveal a predominantly female (66.8%) and white (61.6%) population. The majority of home care clients (68.6%) are 65 years of age or older, although home care is provided to clients of all ages, from birth to death.

The most common diagnoses for home care clients are shown in Display 37–1. Notably absent are cancer diagnoses. A primary diagnosis of malignant neoplasm is present in only 4.7% of home care clients, whereas it accounts for the majority of hospice clients.

Most clients receiving home care are registered with urban home care agencies. As reimbursements for home care nursing continue to decrease, the costs of visiting clients in geographically remote areas have forced many rural home care agencies to close, limiting home care access for populations in rural regions.

Although home care nursing is provided to a large number of people in the United States, it still represents a small percentage of the national health care expenditures, which topped $1057 billion in 1999. Whereas hospital care consumed 36% of health care dollars in 2000, physician services consumed 25%, and prescription drugs consumed 10%, home care represented only 3% of health care spending (NAHC, 2001). This statistic supports many researchers' observations of the cost-effectiveness of home care practice.

Standards and Credentials in Home Care Nursing

The ANA (1999) has developed the *Scope and Standards of Home Health Nursing Practice* (Display 37–2). These 14

DISPLAY 37–1

Most Common Diagnoses for Home Care Clients

- Heart disease
- Musculoskeletal and connective tissue disease
- Diabetes mellitus
- Diseases of the respiratory system
- Injury
- Poisoning

DISPLAY 37–2

Scope and Standards of Home Health Nursing Practice

Standards of Care

Standard I Assessment
The home health nurse collects client health data.

Standard II Diagnosis
The home health nurse analyzes the assessment data in determining diagnoses.

Standard III Outcome Identification
The home health nurse identifies expected outcomes to the client and client's environment.

Standard IV Planning
The home health nurse develops a plan of care that prescribes intervention to attain expected outcomes.

Standard V Implementation
The home health nurse implements the interventions identified in the plan of care.

Standard VI Evaluation
The home health nurse evaluates the client's progress toward attainment of outcomes.

Standards of Professional Performance

Standard I Quality of Care
The home health nurse systematically evaluates the quality and effectiveness of nursing practice.

Standard II Performance Appraisal
The home health nurse evaluates his or her own nursing practice in relation to professional practice standards, scientific evidence, and relevant statutes and regulations.

Standard III Education
The home health nurse acquires and maintains current knowledge and competency in nursing practice.

Standard IV Collegiality
The home health nurse interacts with and contributes to the professional development of peers and other health care practitioners as colleagues.

Standard V Ethics
The home health nurse's decisions and actions on behalf of clients are determined in an ethical manner.

Standard VI Collaboration
The home health nurse collaborates with the client, family, and other health care practitioners in providing client care.

Standard VII Research
The home health nurse uses research findings in practice.

Standard VIII Resource Utilization
The home health nurse assists the client or family in becoming informed consumers about the risks, benefits, and cost of planning and delivering client care.

(Reprinted with permission from American Nurses Association [1999]. *Scope and standards of home health nursing practice.* Washington, DC: American Nurses Publishing, American Nurses Foundation/American Nurses Association.)

standards guide professional nursing practice in home care settings and are based on the association's work in 1986 and 1992. Because there are several types of home care agencies (discussed later), these standards are designed to assist nurses in providing a level of service that meets a minimal expectation while being appropriate for clients, regardless of the home care agency from which they receive services.

In addition to standards of practice, home care nurses can hold advanced credentials and belong to professional organizations in order to enhance skills in this practice area.

The American Nurses' Credentialing Center (ANCC) credentials nurses in many specialty areas, including home care nursing. This credential can be granted after the required years of home care practice and passing a nationally administered test. Information about accreditation can be found on their Website (*http://www.nursingworld.org/ancc*).

The NAHC provides a bevy of direct services to members, including the publication *Caring* and monthly newsletters. Such focused organizations give their members the most recent information in their specialty area. Hospice nursing and community health nursing organizations also are useful resources for the home care nurse.

AGENCIES, PERSONNEL, AND REIMBURSEMENT

The types of agencies engaged in providing home care services have changed drastically as reimbursement policies have changed and as specializations in various domains of health care have evolved. The following paragraphs describe these agencies, their personnel, and their reimbursement structures.

Types of Home Care Agencies

Currently, many types of agencies provide home care to clients. In the early days of home care most providers worked in visiting nurses associations (VNAs). In some parts of the United States this continues to be true, but in most parts of the country the mix of home care agencies includes voluntary agencies, proprietary agencies, hospital-based agencies, official agencies, homemaker agencies, and hospices. Official, voluntary, and proprietary agencies are discussed more fully in Chapter 6 but are reviewed here for clarity. Table 37–1 lists the number of Medicare-certified home care agencies by type in the United States for selected years.

Voluntary Agencies

A *voluntary agency* is a home health agency that does not depend on state and local tax revenues but instead is financed with nontax funds such as donations, endowments, United Way contributions, and third-party provider payments. Voluntary agencies are usually governed by a voluntary board of directors; they are considered community-based because they provide services within a well-defined geographic location.

An example of a voluntary agency system is the VNAs. They are nonprofit agencies with a charitable mission. Like all non-profits, VNAs are exempt from paying taxes. Whereas in the past VNAs were assured of receiving almost

T A B L E 37–1

Number of Medicare-Certified Home Care Agencies by Type, for Selected Years, 1967–2000

Year	Freestanding Agencies				Facility-Based Agencies	
	VNA	PUB	PROP	PNP	HOSP	REHAB/SNF
1967	549	939	0	0	133	0
1975	525	1228	47	0	273	14
1985	514	1205	1943	832	1277	149
1995	575	1182	3951	667	2470	170
2000	436	909	2863	560	2151	151

VNA: Visiting Nurse Associations are freestanding, voluntary, nonprofit organizations governed by a board of directors and usually financed by tax-deductible contributions as well as by earnings.

PUB: Public agencies are government agencies operated by a state, county, city, or other unit of local government that have a major responsibility for presenting disease and for community health education.

PROP: Proprietary agencies are freestanding for-profit home care agencies.

PNP: Private not-for-profit agencies are freestanding and privately developed, governed, and owned nonprofit homecare agencies. These agencies were not counted separately before 1980.

HOSP: Hospital-based agencies are operating units or departments of a hospital. Agencies that have working arrangements with a hospital, or perhaps are even owned by a hospital but operated as separate entities, are classified as freestanding agencies under one of the categories listed.

REHAB/SNF: Refers to agencies based in rehabilitation and skilled nursing facilites.

(From National Association for Home Care [2001]. *Basic statistics about home care.* Washington, DC. Retrieved February 12, 2004, from *http://www.nahc.org*)

all of the home care referrals in their community, the proliferation of other agencies has eroded their traditional base and put them in a competitive mode; VNAs are therefore expanding their services to appeal to a broader market.

Proprietary Agencies

A private, for-profit home health agency is known as a *proprietary agency*. Although proprietary agencies can be governed by individual owners, many are part of large, national chains that are administered through corporate headquarters. Proprietary agencies are expected to turn a profit on the services they provide, either for the individual owners or for their stockholders. Although some participate in the Medicare program, others rely solely on "private-pay" clients.

Hospital-Based Agencies

A hospital may operate a separate department as a home health agency. This agency is governed by the sponsoring hospital's board of directors or trustees. The referrals to such **hospital-based agencies** usually come from the hospital staff itself, and the missions of the agency and the sponsoring hospital are similar. The same is true for rehabilitation and skilled-nursing facilities where home health departments exist.

Official Agencies

Governmental home health agencies are called *official agencies*. They are created and empowered through statutes enacted by legislation. Services are frequently provided by the nursing divisions of state or local health departments and may or may not combine care of the sick with traditional public-health nursing services, including health promotion, illness prevention, communicable disease investigation, environmental health services, and maternal–child care. Administrative support for these agencies is the responsibility of the city, county, or state government. Funding comes from taxes and is usually distributed on the basis of a per capita allocation.

Homemaker Agencies

Homemaker agencies provide homemaker aides, who perform services such as cooking, cleaning, and shopping, or home health aides, who perform personal client care such as bathing, dressing, feeding, assistance in ambulating, and companionship; they may provide both. These agencies are usually private and derive their funding from direct payment by the client or from private insurers. They may be governed by individual owners or by corporations.

Hospices

Hospice philosophy promotes a care perspective that recognizes that death is inevitable and near and that cure is not at present a possibility. Hospice services are comprehensive and are delivered by an interprofessional team, including volunteers, that focuses on "care" rather than "cure." The caregiving team has physician leadership, and care can be provided on an inpatient basis or through home health care where the client lives.

Hospices have received certification from the federal government to provide end-of-life care to the terminally ill in the community. Some hospices are freestanding and serve only hospice clients, whereas others are programs of larger organizations such as a VNA or a hospital-based agency. Alternative housing centers, such as assisted living and long-term care settings, can apply for a "hospice waiver" and be reimbursed for end-of-life caregiving for people in the last months of life. This enables residents to achieve a more peaceful death by dying "at home" rather than being transferred to different surroundings with a medical and curative focus.

Types of Home Care Personnel

Most people receiving home care receive care from two or more caregivers, either formal or informal.

Informal Caregivers

Informal caregivers are family members and friends who provide care in the home and are unpaid. It is estimated that almost three fourths of elderly individuals with multiple comorbidities and severe disabilities who receive home care rely on family members or other sources of unpaid assistance. Most of the estimated 18 million family caregivers in the United States are women, and 10% to 17% of the working public also care for an elderly relative (Sultz & Young, 1999). The type of care they provide ranges from routine custodial care such as bathing and feeding to sophisticated skilled care, including tracheostomy care and IV medication administration.

Informal caregivers assume a considerable physical, psychological, and economic burden in the care of their significant other in the home. When layered on top of existing responsibilities, caregiver tasks compete for time, energy, and attention. As a result, caregivers often describe themselves as emotionally and physically drained and may very much need information about resources to assist them (D'Amico-Panomeritakis & Sommer, 1999). Home care nurses can teach caregivers how to manage clients successfully at home following these guidelines:

Approach
- Keep a positive attitude that is focused on abilities, not limitations, of the caregivers.
- Keep safety at the forefront of all interventions.
- Include all family members and caregivers in the plan.
- To help keep caregiver frustration low, choose to teach first an area that the client is motivated to learn.

Things to Include
- Provide tips on energy conservation for the caregiver and client.
- Include how to manage and maintain equipment.
- Provide resources for support, information, equipment, and assistance.
- Help the family develop a home emergency escape plan.

The economic cost of providing home care places a significant burden on informal caregivers. Out-of-pocket expenditures include medications, transportation, home medical equipment, supplies, and respite services. These costs may be nonreimbursable and are often invisible, but they are very real to families struggling to provide care on a fixed income. In addition, often the primary informal caregiver is an elderly spouse who is physically and emotionally involved (D'Angelo, 1999).

Formal Caregivers

Formal caregivers are professionals and paraprofessionals who are compensated for the in-home care they provide. In 2000, it was estimated that there were almost 600,000 persons employed in home health agencies. Registered nurses represent 44.7% of formal caregiver full time equivalent (FTE) positions in Medicare-certified agencies, whereas licensed practical (vocational) nurses represent 11%. Home health aides account for 34% of the FTE positions (Bureau of Labor Statistics, 2001). Table 37–2 lists the range of formal home care providers in Medicare-certified home health agencies and their roles and responsibilities.

In addition to the personnel described in the table, the business and office personnel of a home health agency are critical to the agency's ability to deliver services to clients. Home health nurses must acquire an understanding of the financial aspects of their clients' care and provide this information to the agency staff so that appropriate and full reimbursement can be obtained for the services provided.

Reimbursement Systems in Home Care

Home health services are reimbursed by both corporate and governmental third-party payers as well as by individual clients and their families. Corporate payers include insurance companies, health maintenance organizations (HMOs), preferred provider organizations, and case-management programs. Government payers include Medicare, Medicaid, the Civilian health and Medical Program of Uniformed Services (CHAMPUS), and the Veterans Administration system. These governmental programs have specific conditions for coverage of services, which are often less flexible than those of corporate payers. For a general description of these reimbursement systems, see Chapter 7.

MEDICARE CRITERIA FOR HOME CARE SERVICES

Medicare is the largest single payer for home care services in the United States and has set the standard in establishing reimbursement criteria for other payers (Nathanson & Cuervo, 2002). Therefore, it is essential that home care nurses understand Medicare and its criteria for determining eligibility for

TABLE 37–2

Types of Providers in Home Care	
Type of Provider	**Role and Responsibilities**
Nurses	
Registered nurse	Deliver skilled care to clients in the home under the direction of the physician. Considered the coordinator of care.
Licensed practical nurse	Deliver routine care to clients under the direction of a registered nurse.
Advanced practice nurse	Provide total client care to complex clients, supervise other nurses in difficult cases related to their speciality, and direct a special program.
Therapists	
Physical therapist	Deliver skilled care that includes assessment for assistive devices in the home. Perform therapy procedures with the client and teach the client and family to assist in treatment. Assist client to improve mobility.
Occupational therapist	Focus on improving physical, mental and social functioning. Rehabilitation of the upper body and improvement of fine motor ability.
Speech therapist	Rehabilitation of clients with speech and swallowing problems.
Respiratory therapist	Provide support to clients using respiratory home medical equipment such as ventilators. Perform professional respiratory therapy treatments.
Other Clinical Staff	
Social workers	Help clients and families identify needs and refer to community agencies. Assist with applications for community-based services and provide financial assistance information.
Dieticians	Provide diet counseling to clients with special nutritional needs. *Direct service of a dietician is not a reimbursable service in home care.*
Paraprofessionals	
Home health aide	Perform personal care, basic nursing tasks (as opposed to skilled), and incidental homemaking.
Homemaker	Perform housekeeping and chores to ensure a safe and healthy home care environment.

home care services. As of 2004, a client must meet all five criteria to be eligible for reimbursement by Medicare (Display 37–3).

MEDICARE'S PROSPECTIVE PAYMENT SYSTEM

The number of home health agencies grew by approximately 10% each year during the 1990s. This pattern of increased utilization was a source of increasing concern for government agency officials, policy analysts, and some members of Congress ("Home Health Payments," 1999). As part of the Balanced Budget Act of 1997, Congress adopted changes in payment for home health services. These included implementation of a prospective payment system (PPS). During the transition period in the year 2000, an interim payment system (IPS) was used. The PPS bases reimbursement on an episode of illness. Clients are assigned to one of approximately 80 reimbursement schemes depending on their clinical and functional characteristics. Theoretically, the more clinically and functionally complex the case, the greater the potential reimbursement.

Once admitted to the agency, the client receives the necessary care to assist in achieving clinical outcomes. If the agency is efficient and the client achieves the identified goals in a few visits, the overall expenses for the client might be less than the Medicare reimbursement and the agency might realize a profit. However, if the client has problems in the course of treatment and requires unanticipated visits, the agency must assume the financial burden of this care. Because of the PPS system, agencies have become very careful about the amount and type of services they provide to Medicare clients. Each home health care encounter must be carefully designed to assist clients to achieve their clinical goals.

Because of the PPS approach to reimbursement, many home health agencies went out of business in the late 1990s. The law affected Medicare's 39 million recipients as well as insurers, providers, suppliers, physicians, and home health agency staff, including nurses, as projected federal government spending on the program was reduced by $116 billion between 1998 and 2002 (Harris, 1998).

AN OVERVIEW OF HOSPICE CARE

The concept of hospice care is relatively new to the United States, with most programs less than 25 years old. Hospice is a philosophy of care and not a place. Hospice is a service most Americans would choose, if they understood it. With these thoughts in mind, the more a community health nurse knows about hospice the better she or he is prepared to introduce the concept to terminally ill clients.

In 1983, Medicare recognized hospice services and began to assume a major portion of the costs. Today, hospice services are recognized by Medicare, Medicaid, and insurance companies as legitimate services for which the third-party payers assume the costs. It was not unusual for hospice programs in the early 1980s to be supported by sponsoring institutions or private-pay clients or to fail due to a lack of steady reimbursement sources. In 1995, Medicare paid for 74% of hospice care in the United States, and private health plans paid for about 12% (Health Care Financing Administration, 1999).

Hospices have a unique philosophy and serve a population who are not best served in acute care settings, which focus on cure and have technology, services, and personnel geared toward diagnosis, treatment, and recovery (Display 37–4). The dying client needs a focus on care rather than cure. Community health nurses often work in hospice programs or with hospice personnel in the community, because much of the hospice care is delivered in the community.

D I S P L A Y   3 7 – 3

Medicare Criteria for Reimbursement

1. Services provided must be reasonable and necessary. This refers to the type of services provided and the frequency. The decision as to whether this criterion has been met is based on a review of the client's medical record and plan of care and the client's current health status. For example, daily visits may not be deemed reasonable for a client who requires weekly blood-glucose monitoring. Also, if a care plan has been ineffective with a client over a long period of time, continuation of that care plan would not be considered reasonable. Therefore, comprehensive documentation is essential to validate that the provided care was both reasonable and necessary.
2. The client must be **homebound**. This means that the client leaves the home with difficulty in mobility and only for medical appointments or adult day care related to the client's medical care.
3. The plan of care must be entered onto specific Medicare forms. The forms require very specific information regarding the client's diagnosis, prognosis, functional limitations, medications, and types of services needed. The home health nurse often has the primary responsibility for ensuring that the forms are completed appropriately.
4. The client must be in need of a skilled service. In the home, skilled services are provided only by a nurse, physical therapist, or speech therapist. *Skilled nursing services* include skilled observation and assessment, teaching, and performing procedures that require nursing judgment.
5. Services must be intermittent and part-time. It is anticipated that clients requiring more than intermittent, part-time care could be cared for more cost-effectively in a setting other than the home, such as a skilled nursing facility.

D I S P L A Y   3 7 – 4

Myths and Facts about Hospice Care

Myth	Fact
Medicare provides only 6 months of hospice care.	Medicare law does not time-limit the hospice benefit. Clients may enroll when their physicians judge that the illness is terminal, with an estimated life expectancy of 6 months or less.
All hospice care is the same.	Hospices vary markedly, especially in the kinds of treatment clients can receive, even within the same community.
Clients cannot receive curative treatments while in hospice.	Although the Medicare Hospice Benefit (MHB) requires that beneficiaries forego curative treatments, some hospices accept clients into their special palliative care programs who prefer to continue receiving therapies directed toward reversal of disease and prolongation of life.
Hospice means giving up hope.	Hospice workers help people revise what they may hope for and help them achieve comfort when death is inevitable. They do nothing to hasten or prevent death.
Hospice is useful only for heavy-duty pain medicines.	Hospice care is designed to provide not only medical care but social, psychological, and spiritual support given by an interdisciplinary team that includes a nurse, social worker, chaplain, and other professionals.
You cannot keep your own doctor at hospice.	Most hospices establish working relationships with a wide base of referring physicians so that clients can keep their own doctors on admission to hospice care.
Hospice is only for cancer patients.	Hospice care is available to an increasing number of clients with noncancer diagnoses; however, people who die of cancer are more likely to choose hospice care than are those who die of other conditions.
Hospice is only for the sick family member.	Hospice is designed to support all family members during the illness and to offer at least 1 year of bereavement support after a death.
Hospice is a place, so you must leave home to receive hospice.	In America, most hospice care is delivered in the home. Inpatient care is generally available (in a variety of settings) to serve those with special needs, such as pain control.
Hospice is expensive.	In general, hospice costs less than hospital or nursing home care and saves significant Medicare money.

(Adapted from Labyak, M. [August, 2001]. Ten myths and facts about hospice care. Focus: Hospice Care, Part I. *State Initiatives in End-of-Life Care, 11,* 3.)

The Philosophy of Hospice Care

Hospices focus on providing holistic, family-centered care to the terminally ill person, with death being accepted as a human experience. Holistic care is delivered to terminally ill people who are in the final phase of their illness, are expected to die, and are not receiving curative treatment. Any activities or services that will enhance the comfort and well-being of the hospice client are employed. Hospice care goals can be achieved in the client's home or, if needed or desired, in an inpatient hospice program (see Voices From the Community I).

The hospice philosophy is a caregiving philosophy that does not depend on the setting but on the holistic nature of caring, delivered through an interprofessional team, that encompasses the family and client values. Hospices rely heavily on family members and volunteers, who work in collaboration with a broad range of professional caregivers. The nurse works as a key member of the caregiving team, working with the primary care provider, pharmacy, clergy, social services, family, volunteers, and other support personnel to orchestrate well-coordinated caregiving services.

Precepts underlying hospice care are essential principles for all end-of-life care (Display 37–5). These precepts are in accord with the International Council of Nurses' mandate that nurses have a unique and primary responsibility for ensuring that individuals at the end of life experience a peaceful death (International Council of Nurses, 1997).

The Hospice Population

The hospice population can include any person diagnosed with an illness that cannot be cured, who chooses not to con-

"Those who use the Medicare Hospice Benefit see it as setting the standard for compassionate, holistic end-of-life care. It provides the kind of care most of us would want when we face the end of our lives. The need to educate the public at large, as well as health care providers who advise us on our options, is very urgent."

Senator Chuck Grassley (R-Iowa), Chair of the Senate's Special Committee on Aging's September 2000 Hearings on the Medicare Hospice Benefit

THE EVOLUTION OF HOSPICE CARE

The concept of hospice is derived from medieval Europe, when hospice was a place where travelers on long and arduous journeys could stop to rest and replenish themselves before they moved onward. As early as the 19th century, hospices in England evolved to provide palliative care in hospitals and in homes. **Palliative care** is comfort care directed at the alleviation of pain and other symptoms. Dying, like birthing, has always been known as a natural process that was most effectively managed in the home with the assistance of family and friends. As health care became more complex, these natural events were shifted from the home to the hospital.

England has been a leader in the modern hospice movement, with nurse Dame Cicely Saunders being the visionary guide at St. Christopher's Hospice (Schroeder & Towle, 1999). She is a former nurse, medical social worker, and doctor. With a small stipend from a dying patient in 1948, she started the hospice movement by opening St. Christopher's Hospice in 1967. The first American hospice, in Connecticut, was created as a freestanding inpatient hospice in 1974 (NAHC, 2001). After this initial endeavor, hospices began to emerge throughout the United States. Once reimbursement systems were actualized for this care in the mid-1980s, the hospice movement expanded to more than 2000 separate programs sharing the same philosophy of care. Most major cities in the country have an inpatient hospice program for short-term admissions and respite care. In addition, all communities with home care services have the potential to receive in-home hospice services through the home care agency.

tinue active treatment and has a life expectancy of 6 months or less. Because the time of death cannot be precisely determined, it is the decision of the health care provider responsible for the client to determine hospice status.

Traditionally, the largest number of hospice-eligible clients have been diagnosed with cancer and have been older than 65 years of age. Increasingly, clients have been diagnosed with AIDS, heart disease, end-stage renal or respiratory disease, or a variety of other diseases with terminal diagnoses. Some hospice programs focus caregiving programs on clients with AIDS. Such hospices are often affiliated with community outreach services for gay communities and are located where there is the greatest need and close to the client's support systems.

HOSPICE SETTINGS, TEAM MEMBERS, AND REIMBURSEMENT

As mentioned earlier, hospice is not a place but a philosophy. As part of that philosophy, skilled and volunteer team members deliver care. In addition, there is a well-developed reimbursement system for hospice clients who are eligible for Medicare.

Inpatient Hospices

The prototype for an inpatient hospice is a freestanding hospice. This is a small inpatient setting not associated with an acute care facility. In some communities, an inpatient hospice is created in a large house or a renovated existing building or is built to meet community preferences. These facilities are usually small, accommodating 6 to 30 clients. They have a large volunteer staff and a professional staff of registered nurses who demonstrate the primary caregiving model of nursing care. Each nurse has a small group of clients (ideally three to four clients) for whom she or he is responsible

DISPLAY 37–5

Precepts of Hospice Care

- Individuals live fully until the moment of death.
- Care offered until death may be offered by a variety of professionals, family members, and volunteers.
- Care is coordinated, sensitive to diversity, and offered around the clock, and respects client's dignity and worth.
- Care gives attention to the physical, psychological, social, and spiritual concerns of the client and the client's family.

(From American Association of Colleges of Nursing [1998]. *Peaceful death: Recommended competencies and curricular guidelines for end-of-life nursing care.* Washington, DC: Author; and Schulkin, V. [1999]. Providing palliative care for the dying elderly client. In S.M. Zang & J.A. Allender, *Home care of the elderly* [pp. 486–505]. Philadelphia: Lippincott Williams & Wilkins.)

as the primary nurse. Volunteers are used extensively to assist with personal care. Alternative or complementary care methods are integrated with traditional Western medical practices to alleviate pain and provide comfort. Imagery, biofeedback, massage, and music are just a few of the care methods used in addition to medications, positioning, and bathing (see Voices from the Community II).

The inpatient hospice, like hospice care in the home, is free of most high-tech equipment seen in the acute care setting. All clients have a "no-code" status, and technology is present for comfort alone. Oxygen is available to ease difficult breathing. IV lines are used to deliver pain medication or alleviate symptoms of nausea or diarrhea, not to hydrate the client. Suction equipment is used to clear the airway of a client with throat or neck cancer who is unable to swallow. There are no crash carts or diagnostic equipment. The environment is as homelike as possible.

The typical routines of acute care facilities are forfeited to meet the client's wishes. The type of arrangement that is more typical of an inpatient hospice may be that of a client who chooses to have his wife help to bathe him in the evening, eats eight small meals a day of home-cooked foods plus a beer or glass of wine, sleeps with all the lights on and with music playing, and has his wife and pet dog snuggle in bed with him.

Clients come into inpatient hospices for a variety of medical and social reasons. Hospice clients are usually cared for through in-home hospice services but may come into the inpatient hospice for pain management, symptom control, family respite, or to die. Family members who give care 24 hours a day, 7 days a week, may need **respite**, or a break from the intensity of caregiving. They may plan a weekend trip or just want to rest and care for themselves for a few days. Such respite is not a luxury; it is a necessity.

In some situations, the family has been able to manage the dying family member's care well, but during the final days of life they are unable to see the person die at home. They may have culturally based feelings that would make the home difficult to live in if a family member had died in it, or they may feel uncomfortable or inadequate in dealing with the actual death experience at home. Home health hospice nurses work closely with the family, the primary care provider, and the inpatient hospice staff to accommodate client and family wishes in such situations.

In-Home Hospices

Most hospice care is provided to clients and families in their homes. People typically want to remain in familiar surroundings, in the comfort of their own bed, and prefer to die at home. This decision should be assessed early in the hospice care services and planned for throughout the care. At times the decision to die in an acute care setting or inpatient hospice may be made near the end of the client's life, and the nurse should be prepared for this change in plans. It may be a serious decision or a fleeting fear of what to expect; the nurse needs to provide the support needed to help the family and client make either decision.

Home health hospice nurses provide the support the family needs throughout the hospice care, but especially at the time of death. The nurse encourages a relationship with the family in which the nurse is notified if the client's condition changes, regardless of the time of day or night. The hospice nurse talks to the family or comes to be with the client and family if desired. She or he assists with providing comfort measures, terminal caregiving needs, and immediate bereavement care to family members when death occurs.

There are legal aspects of care at the time of death. In many states, hospice nurses can pronounce a person deceased and call to arrange for the body to be removed from the home by the selected funeral parlor or cremation society. In other states, the community ambulance service is called for the body to be transported to an emergency department to be pronounced by a physician. This does not end the hospice services to the family. The nurse often attends the funeral or traditional ceremony or memorial service selected by the family. The nurse keeps in contact with the family, providing support and bereavement care and counseling long after the client's death. Many hospice programs have annual memorial services to which they invite family members of deceased clients in the year after the death, continuing a holistic approach as they deliver hospice care to an entire family.

Skilled Team Members

The skilled hospice team includes a broad array of professionals, each providing a unique service that the hospice client and family needs. The primary care provider, nurse, and social worker are core team members. For hospice clients, the team is broader and includes the pharmacist, clergy member, and psychologist (see Research: Bridge to Practice).

Medically ordered combinations of medications, or "cocktails," can be provided in liquid form by the pharmacist to alleviate pain, nausea, syncope, constipation or diarrhea, edema, anxiety, and shortness of breath. Giving these med-

VOICES FROM THE COMMUNITY II

Hospice nursing, even more than home health nursing, gives me such a full feeling of satisfaction. I know I make a difference in these families' lives when they allow me into the most personal aspect of their lives during the dying of a loved one. They accept me as a family member, and I cry with them as I feel their pain and laugh with them as they recall happier days. This kind of nursing is everything I always thought nursing would be.

Ann, RN, BSN, hospice nurse

RESEARCH: BRIDGE TO PRACTICE

Tolle, S.W., Tilden, V.P., Rosenfeld, A.G., & Hickman, S.E. (2000). Family reports of barriers to optimal care of the dying. *Nursing Research, 49*(6), 310–317.

There is intense national pressure to improve end-of-life care. There are problems or barriers to optimal care that must be determined in order to eliminate them.

In this study the researchers contacted 475 informants via telephone interviews over a 14-month period. Those contacted were family members (spouse or adult child) who had experienced the death of a close family member within the previous 2 to 5 months. Researchers used a 58-item questionnaire developed from other investigations or from experience with patients and families at the end of life. The questionnaire was designed to assess family perceptions of end-of-life care in three areas: (1) health care practitioners' respect for family preferences for location of death and for amount of life-sustaining treatments given in the last month of life; (2) satisfaction with support from health care providers in the week before death; (3) and barriers to successful management of pain experienced by the terminally ill client in the week before death.

Data showed that most families (68%) experienced a high frequency of advance planning (deceased had a living will or family members were aware of the deceased's preferences for life-supportive measures) and a high level of respect by health care practitioners for patient-family preferences about end-of-life location and

treatment decisions. Family satisfaction with care (emotional support and attention to pain and comfort) was generally high; however, 20% of the sample indicated that they were dissatisfied with physician availability, and 8% were dissatisfied with the availability of nurses and had considered making a complaint. Thirty-four percent of the family decendants stated that health care practitioner's attention to comfort and pain control was unsatisfactory and did not relieve suffering in the last week of life, because the client was in moderate to severe pain at that time.

Barriers to optimal end-of-life care remain, despite a generally positive overall profile. Barriers include the level of pain, management of pain, and some dissatisfaction with physician availability.

An important note about this study is that it took place in Oregon. This state has a capitated health care plan that covers health care for otherwise uninsured persons up to 100% of the poverty level, which makes end-of-life care more accessible for all citizens. This state has one of the highest rates of hospice use and one of the highest rates of morphine prescriptions per capita in the country. This suggests that health care providers aggressively manage pain in Oregon. In addition, there has been intense media coverage regarding debates on physician-assisted suicide and public education about rights to good palliative care. Therefore, the findings in this study may assist in initiating changes in end-of-life care in other states in the United States.

ications orally, in combination, eliminates use of injections and IV tubes and the need to swallow multiple pills. In addition, large doses of narcotics may be delivered in smaller amounts of IV fluids. At times a pharmacist may need to provide 2000 mg of morphine in 500 mL of fluid. With pain and discomfort from other symptoms a major concern for the terminally ill client, the pharmacist becomes a valuable team member.

A clergy member is frequently available in hospice programs to provide support for the clients, family, and staff. Professional and volunteer staff members become emotionally involved with hospice clients, and regular support or debriefing sessions help the staff cope with their own feelings when providing such intimate and emotional care. In addition, the team members may work with the client's own clergyperson. For clients not involved in an organized religion, the clergyperson on staff is an important resource; he or she works with all clients as desired and can work collegially with the religious leader the client prefers.

Some hospice programs have the services of a psychologist. This team member provides one-on-one or group

meeting support to staff and to clients and families. The psychologist works with clients who are having difficulty with their disease progression and with family members who are having a hard time coping with the impending loss of a family member or the stress of caregiving. Clerical and psychological services are often part-time appointments and can be shared by inpatient and in-home hospice programs on a part-time basis. Sometimes these professionals volunteer their time to hospice programs.

Volunteer Team Members

Volunteerism is the backbone of a succesful hospice program. Volunteers fill an important need in both inpatient and in-home hospice programs. They act as companions to the client when the family must be somewhere else or is away for short respite. They run errands for family members, organize hot meals prepared by friends and neighbors, babysit children in the family—the list can go on and on. Inpatient volunteers may act like nursing assistants and assist the nurse with personal care by helping to hold or position clients during treatments, bathing, or dressing. They cook foods the client feels like eating. Most inpatient hospices have a kitchen available for the staff and family to use. Client appetites often tend to be small and selective, so nurses, volunteers, and family members become short- order cooks. One inpatient hospice volunteer recalls caring for a 23-year-old man with an inoperable brain tumor who rarely had an appetite. One day he asked for an egg, fried in the middle of a piece of bread with a hole in it for the egg to sit, covered in catsup and served with a warm bottle of beer. The volunteer was so excited that he had an appetite that she worked very hard to make his choice to perfection—and even warmed the refrigerated beer in a pan of hot water (see Using the Nursing Process).

Reimbursement Systems in Hospice Care

As mentioned earlier, hospice care is a covered service in Medicare. In fact, services are covered more fully for inpatient and in-home hospice care than for home health clients in general. Display 37–6 compares criteria and ben-

---

USING THE NURSING PROCESS

Caring for the Terminally Ill at Home

OVERVIEW/ASSESSMENT

Jeffrey Johnson, age 52, struggled with pancreatic cancer for a year. His wife and teenage daughters, aged 15 and 17, were very involved in his treatment, progress, and, eventually, the end-of-life care that was provided by your hospice agency. Mrs. Johnson called your agency regarding her daughters' behavior since her husband died 1 month ago. Mrs. Johnson works full-time but has liberal family leave benefits, which she used during her husband's illness, and has a strong support system from coworkers. She is concerned about her daughters, who have been quiet, not going out with friends or having them over, and who have had a dip in their grades in school. She is concerned about them and would like you to visit the family to assist them to function at a higher level of wellness.

NURSING DIAGNOSES

- Alterations in functioning related to grieving the death of their father.
- Family process disruption due to the loss of their husband/father.

PLANNING/IMPLEMENTATION

Planning and implementation specifically for the teenage daughters include the following:
- Meeting with the daughters to discuss what support systems they use and their feelings about their father's illness, entry into hospice, and death.
- Exploring coping methods the girls use and how effective they have been.
- Assessing their interest in your agency's hospice programs for family members: a grief support group for older teens and adults and a support group for children ages 6 to 18 who have experienced a loss.

- Asking Mrs. Johnson to speak to a school counselor regarding support services, teacher expectations, and the girls' general attitudes and behavior while in school.

EVALUATION

- After you meet with the daughters on three occasions, they revealed that they were very involved in caring for their father while their mother continued to work and are sad about losing him. They just "don't feel like having friends over or going out." They are confused that their mother is back to work and "adjusting" so well.
- The girls say they don't seem to have a "family" any more. They feel like "outsiders" when friends talk about their lives.
- The girls expressed an interest in the support groups, especially the one for teens. You encouraged them to also attend the one for teens and adults with their mother. They attended both groups regularly. After 6 weeks, they noticed that their relationship with their mother is stronger and they were seeing their friends again.
- Mrs. Johnson found out that the girls were receiving support from both teachers and friends, and the teachers indicated that their grades were improving and the "dip" was temporary.

(As you were evaluating the initial plans and interventions for the daughters, you met with Mrs. Johnson to discuss her own level of coping and perceptions of the "new family structure." You encouraged her to participate in the grief support group and to reevaluate her new role as parent. After 2 months, the family have improved their adjustment to their new family structure and are continuing to attend the support groups.)

efits of home care and hospice according to Medicare reimbursement.

Most private insurers cover costs for clients who are not eligible for Medicare. For clients with no health insurance and no Medicare, there are voluntary agencies that assist with covering the costs of caregiving. For instance, the American Cancer Society provides dressings and assists with the costs of medications for up to 3 months. Local churches and disease-specific agencies have funds available to support people during the terminal phase of an illness. In addition, hospices reserve a certain number of beds for the medically indigent so that no one needing hospice care is refused care.

ROLE OF THE COMMUNITY HEALTH NURSE IN HOME HEALTH AND HOSPICE CARE

Community health nurses working in home health and hospice care settings have aspects to their caregiving that are similar. Caregiving includes direct care; detailed Medicare- and Medicaid-specific documentation; supervision of other professional, family, and volunteer caregivers; and client advocacy.

Direct Care

Direct care always involves assessment of the client's physical and psychosocial status and client and family education. However, in these roles direct care includes the performance of a skilled procedure. Family assessment is discussed in Chapter 23 and assessment of clients at various developmental stages in Chapters 26 to 30. In addition, we discussed the community health nurse's role in client education in

DISPLAY 37–6

Home Care and Hospice—Medicare Benefits

Criteria	Home Care	Hospice
Client must be homebound	Yes	No
Skilled need required	Yes	No
Prognosis of 6 months to live	No	Yes
Short in-patient stay and respite available	No	Yes
Supplies and equipment covered	With limitations	No limitations
Chaplain, volunteers, bereavement support	No	Yes
Medications covered	No	Yes (pain and symptom management only)

Chapter 12. Some of the other skilled and technologic procedures more commonly performed by home care and hospice nurses are shown in Display 37–7.

Infection Control

As hospital stays have shortened, clients with communicable diseases and multiple invasive devices are now being cared for in the home. There are two major concerns for the nurse in caring for these clients:

- How to prevent infection in clients who are debilitated and may be immunocompromised
- How to protect the nurse, family, and community from a client who has an infectious or communicable disease

The home setting poses special challenges for the nurse in preventing the spread of infection or protecting the immunocompromised client from pathogens. For example, the primary caregivers, usually family members, are often untrained in procedures and know little about aseptic technique. The home may also lack facilities to care for the client under optimal conditions. In some homes, there is no access to run-

DISPLAY 37–7

Procedures Performed by Home Care and Hospice Nurses

1. Intravenous services—initiating, monitoring, and teaching family members to monitor and maintain.
2. Wound care—can be simple or complex and includes old and new pressure ulcers, burns and surgical wounds, clean or sterile wet or dry dressings, irrigations, and treatments.
3. Oxygen therapy—assessing the need for, use of, and safe use of oxygen delivery systems.
4. Phlebotomy—skillful drawing, storage, and transportation of blood from client veins or arteries as needed to perform ordered blood tests.
5. Ventilators—operating and monitoring stationary and portable units based on client need.
6. Pumps—setting up, monitoring, and in-home care; teaching clients to deliver client-controlled pain medication, insulin, and antibiotics.
7. Nutritional supplementation—setting up, monitoring, and teaching clients and families about TPN or nasal and gastric feeding tubes.
8. Elimination technology—teaching, initiating, and/or monitoring; dialysis methods, biofeedback for incontinence, indwelling catheters, suprapubic catheters, obtaining sterile urine specimens from catheters or clean-catch urine specimens, enemas to treat elimination problems and for medication instillation as a treatment.
9. New or experimental therapies—inpatient and in-home care for clients with specific diagnoses, such as AIDS, and cancer clients receiving state-of-the-art treatments; portable in-home phototherapy for infants with hyperbilirubinemia.

ning water, a heating unit to boil equipment, or adequate facilities to dispose of contaminated equipment. These conditions may necessitate the development of unique solutions to control infection. To guide the nurse, agencies have developed policies and procedures that deal with infection control; these typically are based on national policies, such as the Centers for Disease Control and Prevention's universal blood and body fluid precautions.

Infection control in inpatient hospice settings is similar to that in the acute care setting, with some exceptions. This facility is home for weeks or months for many of the clients. When a group of clients with compromised immune systems related to old age and debilitating illnesses live together, communicable diseases can become epidemic. Good handwashing technique for the staff, volunteers, and clients offers a first line of defense to avoid the spread of communicable diseases.

Nuisance diseases such as scabies and pediculosis may infect clients and caregivers alike. Good hygiene, proper bedding change and cleaning techniques, and client assessment help to keep such annoying diseases to a minimum.

Client Education

Most care provided in the home is the responsibility of someone other than the nurse. Teaching, then, becomes the most common intervention performed by home care nurses. Nurses are responsible for providing the client and family with the necessary information and skills to provide safe and effective care between home visits and after discharge from the home care agency.

In inpatient hospice settings, the nurse's role focuses on family instruction and in-service teaching of paraprofessional staff and volunteers. Topics to be taught vary depending on the client mix, the experience of the family members in caregiving, and volunteer experience.

In home care, the nurse may need to conduct one-on-one teaching if a client is diagnosed with a new disease (eg, diabetes) or is to receive a new medication or treatment for an existing condition (eg, asthma, arthritis). Family members are an integral part of home care and hospice care services. Depending on the client's condition and cognitive ability, family members may become the primary contacts with whom the nurse teaches and interacts.

Documentation

Accurate and thorough documentation is a critical component of home health and hospice care. In addition to conveying the clinical course of care for the client, documentation must address reimbursement and regulatory requirements. The record will be inspected by the payer, not only for the number of home care visits made or the health status of a client in a hospice program, but also for the types of services provided, to determine whether they were appropriate to meet the determined goal. As an indication of the magnitude of the task of documenting in home care, the NAHC has developed a task force of administrative and clinical experts to examine methods for reducing the paperwork burden for home care providers. Many agencies already have developed strategies to reduce the amount of time a nurse spends on documentation: these include the use of dictaphones, computerized care plans, and flow sheets or standardized care plans.

Supervision and Case Management

The home health and hospice care nurse is responsible for coordination of the other professionals and paraprofessionals involved in the client's care. Additionally, the nurse is the primary contact with the client's physician, both reporting changes in the client's condition and securing changes in the plan of care.

As the home health or hospice care case manager, the nurse conducts case conferences among team members to share information, discuss problems, and plan actions to effect the best possible outcomes for the client. Medicare mandates such case conferences every 60 days in home care. Additionally, the nurse must have the knowledge to refer clients to community resources for services not provided by the agency. Finally, the nurse manager supervises the paraprofessionals, such as home health aides, who also serve the homebound client. This may entail visiting the client at a time when the home health aide is present to observe the care provided.

Supervisory responsibilities are key roles for community health nurses in home health care and inpatient hospices. The registered nurse is the case manager for each client and follows through with all the functions identified as part of the case manager's role. In hospices, the staff consists primarily of professionals and volunteers, and nurses function as case managers for the clients they have as their primary clients.

Two additional responsibilities of the nurse as case manager in home health care include determining financial coverage and determining the frequency and duration of home care services.

Determining Financial Coverage

A unique aspect of the role of the home health nurse as case manager is involvement in securing and maintaining reimbursement for the client's care. The home care nurse must know who is going to pay for services from the first visit to the time of discharge from the agency. If the client does not have a source of payment for the care that is needed, the agency must determine whether the client will receive the care free of charge or at a reduced rate. Many agencies have a sliding fee scale, which means that the charge for the services is based on the client's ability to pay. Nurses who deliver in-home hospice care have similar responsibilities. In skilled nursing facilities, the nurse tracks caregiving days to inform the primary care provider of Medicare coverage dates and works closely with billing departments, social workers, and ombudsmen so that arrangements can be made for clients who continue to need care after insurance coverage comes to an end (see Bridging Financial Gaps).

BRIDGING FINANCIAL GAPS

IMPROVING ACCESS AND FINANCIAL VIABILITY TO HOSPICE

Proposed policy changes to improve access and financial viability. (2002, November). Focus: Hospice care, Part II. *State Initiatives in End-of-Life Care, 17,* 6.

Improved access to and financial viability for end-of-life care is needed. Several proposed policy changes from hospice advocates and independent researchers have been made through either regulatory or legislative changes and are shared here.

RETHINK HOSPICE REIMBUSEMENT

- Make Medicare Hospice Benefits (MHB) per diem reflect true costs—which will take an act of Congress.
- Pay a higher rate for first and last days, when hospice costs are highest.
- Adopt an outlier policy for high-cost patients—those patients whose costs of care lie outside the average.
- Re-examine the MHB and ensure that all states' Medicaid programs include hospice (six states in 2002 did not cover hospice in their Medicaid programs).

RE-EVALUATE ELIGIBILITY REQUIREMENTS

- The appropriateness of the 6-month certification rule needs to be examined. Clients with a minimal chance of survival do not choose hospice because, if they do, they will have to forgo active treatment. Even with a 10% chance of survival, people will elect treatment over hospice.

EDUCATE PHYSICIANS AND BENEFICIARIES

- Initiate Medicare-funded seminars and continuing education courses to clarify hospice benefit regulations and to publicize existing policies of which few physicians are aware.

CONSIDER DEMONSTRATION PROJECTS

- Conduct demonstration projects that could temporarily and in a limited fashion lift current reimbursement and eligibility polices in order to test potential adjustments in those areas. Trial changes to hospice reimbursement, to account for patients with short stays, or for those who need unusually costly palliative treatments, could reveal useful solutions to the difficulties with the current per diem that hospices report.

Determining Frequency and Duration of Services

The home care nurse is also responsible for determining the frequency and duration of the client's care. Will home visits be made twice weekly, once weekly, or once a month? For how long will visits continue? As the care is provided and the client's condition improves, the home care nurse, in collaboration with the physician, determines whether the frequency of visits should be reduced or whether the client can be discharged.

Advocacy

Although the role of advocate is not unique to home health and hospice care, the way in which the nurse advocates for the client requires unique knowledge and skills. One of the most common advocacy issues is helping the older client or older spouse to negotiate the complex medical care reimbursement system. This may involve assisting clients to interpret bills from previous hospitalizations, organizing their receipts for submission to their insurance company, or informing them of the services of hospice programs. Although these advocacy actions may not seem significant, nurses must be aware that the stress of financial worries can interfere with the client's recovery or peaceful death.

Advocacy in home health or hospice programs is important to the quality of care the clients receive. There needs to be a system in place to ensure client advocacy. Some home care agencies and inpatient hospices have an **ombudsman** available—someone who speaks for the client and acts as an advocate in all matters concerning the client's participation in the agency. The nurse can ensure that these systems are in place and are not just symbols but active and integral components of the services and functioning of the agency.

SUMMARY

Community health nurses have an important role in working with elders who receive home care or hospice services. As the population continues to age, the need for nurses to work with older adults where they live, as they are discharged from acute care settings earlier and earlier and, if they are terminally ill, during their final months and days, will only increase.

Home care services comprise the entire array of health care and nursing care services brought to a person's home. Rapid discharge from acute care settings does not allow the client to completely recover in that setting, which puts demands on family members when the client goes home.

Most home care clients are older than 65 years of age, female, and white. Health monitoring, medication instruction, client advocacy, and teaching about disease or treatment processes to the client and family members are the focus of the home health nurse's role. Whatever the caregiving needs are, they must be conducted so that goals are achieved within a few home visits if Medicare is reimbursing for the care given. This has become even more important since the

Balanced Budget Act of 1997 brought about legislative changes restricting the numbers of home visits. If the client pays for the visits or has a private insurance policy, more visits may be available to achieve the goals.

There are many types of home care agencies: voluntary, proprietary, hospital-based, official, homemaker, and hospice. Care is provided by formal and informal caregivers. Professional staff members, such as nurses, social workers, therapists, and certified nursing assistants, work in collaboration with family members, and in some situations with friends and neighbors.

Hospice is a fairly new concept in the United States but has a longer history in England. Medicare covers hospice care without the restrictions experienced by non-hospice home care clients. Hospice programs provide holistic care to clients during the last months of life. Many programs are home-based, and they often are a service of a home health agency. In addition to in-home hospices, there are inpatient hospices. These can be located in a freestanding building, in part of a skilled nursing facility, or in a section of an acute care facility. What is different is the focus of care—it is not aimed at cure, and it employs holistic caregiving practices that involve family members, professionals, and volunteers.

The nurse provides direct physical nursing care in home health care and with hospice clients. In additon, the nurse teaches clients, family members, and volunteers; supervises; and case manages. Assessing clients to determine health status and eligibility for additional services and acting as a client advocate occurs with both groups of clients. Determining the frequency and duration of services occurs in home care. With both home care and hospice clients the nurse must become familiar with the requirements of documentation to promote continuity of care and ensure reimbursement.

REFERENCES

American Association of Colleges of Nursing. (1998). *Peaceful death: Recommended competencies and curricular guidelines for end-of-life nursing care.* Washington, DC: Author.

American Nurses Association. (1999). *Scope and standards of home health nursing practice.* Washington, DC: American Nurses Foundation/American Nurses Association.

D'Angelo, A.M. (1999). Effectively managing the elderly client in the community. In S.M. Zang & J.A. Allender. *Home care of the elderly* (pp. 3–16). Philadelphia: Lippincott Williams & Wilkins.

D'Amico-Panomeritakis, D., & Sommer, J.K. (1999). Promoting and maintaining mobility in the homebound elderly client. In S.M. Zang & J.A. Allender, *Home care of the elderly* (pp. 78–97). Philadelphia: Lippincott Williams & Wilkins.

Harris, M.D. (1998). The impact of the Balanced Budget Act of 1997 on home health care agencies and nurses. *Home Healthcare Nurse, 16*(7), 435–437.

Health Care Financing Administration. (1999). *Medicare and you, 2000* (Publication No. HCFA-10050). Baltimore: U. S. Department of Health and Human Services, HCFA.

Home health payments: Turbulent times. (1999). *Nursing Trends and Issues, 4*(2). Retrieved February 16, 2004, from *http://www.nursing world.org/readroom/nti/9909nti.htm*

International Council of Nurses. (1997). *Basic principles of nursing care.* Washington, DC: American Nurses Publishing.

Labyak, M. (2001, August). Ten myths and facts about hospice care. Focus: Hospice Care, Part I. *State Initiatives in End-of-Life Care, 11,* 3. Retrieved February 12, 2004, from *http://www.lastacts.org/files/publications/hospiceone-final.pdf*

Martinson, I.M., Widmer, A.G., & Portillo, C.J. (2002). *Home health care nursing* (2nd ed.). Philadelphia: W.B. Saunders.

Nathanson, M., & Cuervo, A.M. (Eds). (2002). *Home care compliance manual* (2nd ed.) (AHLCC Compliance Series). Gaithersburg, MD: Aspen.

National Association for Home Care (2001). *Basic statistics about home care.* Washington, DC: Author. Retrieved February 12, 2004, from *http://www.nahc.org/Consumer/hcstats.html*

Navaie-Waliser, M., Feldman, P.H., Gould, D.A., Levine, C., Kuerbis, A.N., & Donelan, K. (2001). The experiences and challenges of informal caregivers: Common themes and differences among whites, blacks, and Hispanics. *The Gerontologist, 41(6),* 733–741.

Proposed policy changes to improve access and financial viability. (2002, November). Focus: Hospice Care, Part II. *State Initiatives in End-of-Life Care, 17,* 6. Retrieved February 12, 2004, from *http://www.lastacts.org/files/publications/hospice2.pdf*

Rice, R., (2001). *Home care nursing practice: Concepts and applications* (3rd ed.). St. Louis: Mosby.

Schroeder, B. & Towle, S.M. (1999). Care of the terminally ill patient at home. *NurseWeek, 12*(7), 32–34.

Schulkin, V. (1999). Providing palliative care for the dying elderly client. In S.M. Zang & J.A. Allender, *Home care of the elderly* (pp. 486–505). Philadelphia: Lippincott Williams & Wilkins.

Sultz, H.A., & Young, K.M. (1999). *Health care USA: Understanding its organization and delivery* (2nd ed.). Gaithersburg, MD: Aspen.

Tolle, S.W., Tilden, V.P., Rosenfeld, A.G., & Hickman, S.E. (2000). Family reports of barriers to optimal care of the dying. *Nursing Research, 49*(6), 310–317.

U. S. Bureau of Labor Statistics. (2001). *Employment statistics: Home health care agencies.* Washington, DC: Author.

SELECTED READINGS

Alexander, C., & McKenna, S. (2001). A sound partnership for end-of-life care. *American Journal of Nursing, 101*(12), 75–77.

Balaban, R. (2000). A physician's guide to talking about end-of-life care. *Journal of General Internal Medicine, 15,* 195–200.

Barnum, B.S. (2001). Interview with Karen Soto, RN, BSN and Rosalee Whyte, RN, BSN: The challenge of providing nursing care for the dying. In Feldman, H.R. (Ed.). *Nursing leaders speak out: Issues and opinions* (pp.159–169). New York: Springer.

Brogden, M. (2001). *Geronticide: Killing the elderly.* Philadelphia: Jessica Kingsley.

Childress, S.B. (2001). Enhance end-of-life care. *Nursing Management, 32*(10), 32–35.

DePalma, J.A. (2002). Proposing an evidence-based policy process. *Nursing Administration Quarterly, 26*(4), 55–61.

DiCicco-Bloom, B., & Cohen, D. (2003). Home care nurses: A study of the occurrence of culturally competent care. *Journal of Transcultural Nursing 14*(1), 25–31.

Hougton, P. (2001). *On death, dying and not dying.* Philadelphia: Jessica Kingsley.

Lipman, A.G., Jackson, K.C. II, & Tyler, L.S. (Eds.). (2000). *Evidence based symptom control in palliative care.* Binghamton, NY: The Haworth Press.

McNamara, B. (2001). *Fragile lives: Death, dying and care.* Philadelphia: Open University Press.

Murashima, S., Nagata, S., Magilvy, J.K., Fukui, S., & Kayama, N. (2002). Home care nursing in Japan: A challenge for providing good care at home. *Public Health Nursing, 19*(2), 94–103.

Norlander, L. (2001). *To comfort always: A nurse's guide to end of life care.* Washington, DC: American Nurses Association.

Pool, R. (2000). *Negotiating a good death: Euthanasia in the Netherlands.* Binghamton, NY: The Haworth Press.

Rutledge, D.N., & Grant, M. (2002). Introduction to evidence-based practice in cancer nursing. *Seminars in Oncology Nursing, 18*(2), 1–2.

Sankar, A. (2000). *Dying at home: A family guide for caregiving.* Baltimore, MD: The John Hopkins University Press.

Weiner, D.K., Herr, K., & Rudy, T.E. (Eds.). (2002). *Persistent pain in older adults: An interdisciplinary guide for treatment.* New York: Springer.

Worden, J.W. (2002). *Grief counseling and grief therapy: A handbook for the mental health practitioner* (3rd ed.). New York: Springer.

Resources and Internet Sites

AARP Grief & Loss Programs: *http://www.aarp.org/griefandloss*

American Cancer Society: *http://www.acs.org*

Complementary Therapies: *http://www.wholenurse.com/*

Family Caregiver Alliance: *http://www.caregiver.org*

Last Acts Family Committee Consumer/Family Resources for End-of-Life Care: *http://www.lastacts.org/files/publications/familyresources.pdf*

Medicare: telephone 1-800-633-4227, *http://www.medicare.gov*

National Association of Home Care: *http://www.nahc.org*

National Eldercare Locator: telephone 1-800-677-1116

Partnership for Caring: *http://www.lastacts.org*

The Agency for Health Care Policy and Research (AHCPR): *http://www.AHCPR.gov/clinic*

The Heart Failure Society of America (HFSA): *http://www.hfsa.org*

GLOSSARY

Accommodation—being sufficiently mature so that previously unsolved problems can now be solved.

Acquired immunodeficiency syndrome (AIDS)—a severe, life-threatening condition representing the late clinical stage of infection with the human immunodeficiency virus (HIV), in which there is progressive damage to the immune and other organ systems.

Active immunity—a long-term resistance to a specific disease-causing organism, acquired naturally or artificially.

Active listening—the skill of assuming responsibility for and understanding the feelings and thoughts in a sender's message.

Adaptation—the ability to cope with the demands of the environment.

Addiction—compulsive use of or impaired control over use of a substance; preoccupation with obtaining and using a drug, substance, or activity; and continued use despite adverse consequences.

Adult—anyone between 18 and 64 years of age.

Advocate—someone who pleads clients' causes or acts on their behalf.

Affective domain—learning that involves changes in emotion, feeling, or affect.

Ageism—stereotyping of older adults, perpetuating false information and negative images and characteristics about them.

Agent—a factor that causes or contributes to a health problem or condition.

Aggregate—a mass or grouping of distinct individuals who are considered as a whole and who are loosely associated with one another.

Alcoholics Anonymous (AA)—a self-help program designed to keep alcoholics sober one day at a time and based on the "12-step" model that includes a belief in a higher power.

Al-Anon—a self-help organization designed around the principles of Alcoholics Anonymous and intended for family members and close friends of alcoholics.

Alateens—a self-help organization modeled after Al-Anon, designed around the principles of Alcoholics Anonymous, and intended for older children and teenagers affected by an alcoholic in the family.

Alzheimer's disease (AD)—a progressive dementia affecting older adults in increasing numbers as people age; judgment and reasoning are lost, eventually affecting the person physically with increased weakness, wasting, and immobility.

Analytic epidemiology—seeks to identify associations between a particular human disease or health problem and its possible causes.

Anorexia nervosa—an eating disorder of emotional etiology that is characterized by body image disturbance, an intense fear of becoming fat or gaining weight, and refusal to maintain an adequate body weight.

Anticipatory guidance—a process of assisting the client in preparing for a future role or developmental stage.

Arson—the deliberate burning of buildings.

Assault and battery—the threat to use force against another person, and the accomplishment of that threat.

Assessment—gathering and analyzing information that will affect the health of the people to be served.

Assets assessment—an assessment that focuses on the strengths and capacities of the community rather than on the problems alone.

Assimilation—reacting to new situations by using skills already possessed.

Assisted living—a special combination of housing, supportive services, personalized assistance, and health care designed to respond to the individual needs of those who need help with activities of daily living and instrumental activities of daily living.

Assurance—those activities that make certain that services are actually provided.

Attention-deficit disorder (without hyperactivity) (ADD)—a cluster of problems related mainly to inattention, poor motivation, and disorganization.

Attention-deficit/hyperactivity disorder (ADHD)—a cluster of problems related to hyperactivity, impulsivity, and inattention.

Audit—an organized effort whereby practicing professionals monitor, assess, and make judgments about the quality and appropriateness of nursing care provided by peers as measured against professional standards of practice.

Autocratic leadership style—an authoritarian style in which leaders use their power to influence their followers.

Autonomous leadership style—a facilitative style of leadership that encourages group members to select and carry out their own activities and function independently.

Autonomy—freedom of choice and the exercise of people's rights.

Baby boomers—those people born after World War II, specifically between 1946 and 1964.

Battered child syndrome—the collection of injuries sustained by a child as a result of repeated mistreatment or beatings.

Benchmarking—studying another's processes in order to improve one's own processes.

Beneficence—doing good or benefiting others.

Bilateral agencies—agencies that usually deal directly with other individual governments, such as the U. S. Agency for International Development, the Peace Corps, and the U. S. Centers for Disease Control and Prevention.

Biostatistics—the science of statistically measuring population health conditions.

Bioterrorism—the use of living organisms, such as bacteria, viruses, and other organic materials, to harm or intimidate others in order to achieve political ends.

Blended family—a family in which single parents marry and raise the children from each of their previous relationships together.

Brainstorming—an idea-generating process that encourages group members to freely offer suggestions.

Bulimia—an eating disorder characterized by recurrent episodes of binge eating with repeated compensatory mechanisms to prevent weight gain, such as causing vomiting or taking laxatives.

Burden of disease—the impact of premature death and disability on a population's health status; assessed by measuring the gap between the population's health status and some reference status.

Camp health aides—bilingual and bicultural individuals, usually women, who help reinforce positive health values and create a sense of self-esteem and empowerment among migrant farmworkers.

Capitation rate—a fixed amount of money paid per person by the health plan to the provider for covered services.

Case management—a systematic process by which a nurse assesses clients' needs, plans for and coordinates services, refers to other appropriate providers, and monitors and evaluates progress to ensure that clients' multiple service needs are met in a cost-effective manner.

Casualty—a human being who is injured or killed during or as a direct result of a traumatic event.

Causal thinking—relating disease or illness to its cause.

Causality—the relationship between a cause and its effect.

Change—any planned or unplanned alteration of the status quo in an organization, situation, or process.

Channel—the medium through which the sender conveys the message.

Chemical dependence—a strong, overwhelming preoccupation with and desire to have a drug.

Child abuse—the maltreatment of children, including any or all of the following: physical, emotional, medical, or educational neglect; physical punishment or battering; or emotional or sexual maltreatment and exploitation.

Chronic disease—a set of diseases occurring mainly among adults and including degenerative diseases, diseases of the circulatory system, cancer, and diabetes.

Client myth—the belief that the primary clients in community health nursing are individuals and families.

Clinician—a nursing role in the community that ensures that health services are provided to individuals, families, groups, and populations.

Coalition—an alliance of individuals or groups working together to influence outcomes of a specific problem.

Codependence—dysfunctional behaviors that are evident among family members.

Cohabiting couples—the forming of a family alliance outside marriage or through a private ceremony not legally recognized as marriage.

Cohort—a group of people who share a common experience in a specific time period.

Cognitive domain—the area of leaning that involves the mind and thinking processes.

Collaboration—working together in cooperation with other team members, coordinating services and addressing the needs of population groups.

Collaborator—a role in which the nurse works jointly with others in a common endeavor.

Common-interest community—a collection of people who, although they are widely scattered geographically, have an interest or goal that binds them together.

Commune family—a group of unrelated, monogamous couples living together and collectively rearing their children; considered a nontraditional family.

Communicable disease—a disease that can be transmitted from one person to another.

Communication—transferring meaning and enhancing understanding.

Community—a collection of people who interact with one another and whose common interests or characteristics form the basis for a sense of unity or belonging.

Community as client—the concept of a community-wide group of people as the focus of nursing service.

Community-based—a term used to describe the setting for nursing care delivery.

Community collaboration—the ability of the community to work together as a team of citizens, professional and lay people alike, to meet an identified need in the community.

Community development—the process of collaborating with community members to assess their collective needs and desires for a positive change and to address those needs through problem-solving, use of community experts, and resource development.

Community diagnoses—nursing diagnoses about the community's ineffective coping ability and potential for enhanced coping.

Community health—the identification of needs and the protection and improvement of collective health within a geographically defined area.

Community health advocacy—efforts aimed at creating awareness of and generating support for meeting the community's health needs.

Community health nursing—a field of nursing combining nursing science with public health science to formulate a practice that is community based and population focused.

Community mental health—a field of practice that seeks

to address the needs of the mentally ill, prevent mental illness, and promote the mental health of the community.

Community mental health centers (CMHC)—sites that provide comprehensive, publicly funded services to the mentally ill population.

Community needs assessment—the process of determining the real or perceived needs of a defined community of people.

Community of solution—a group of people who come together to solve a problem that affects all of them.

Community-oriented, population-focused care—care that is shaped by the characteristics and needs of a given community and employs population-based skills.

Community subsystem assessment—an assessment that focuses on a single dimension of community life, such as churches or schools.

Community support programs—a publicly funded set of services designed to assist persons with serious and persistent mental illness (SPMI).

Commuter family—a family in which both partners work but have jobs in different cities; one parent raises the children in the "home" city while the second partner lives in the other city and commutes home for weekends or less frequently, depending on the distance.

Competition—a contest between rival health care organizations for resources and clients.

Comprehensive assessment—an assessment that seeks to discover all relevant community health information.

Conceptual model—a framework made up of ideas for explaining and studying a phenomenon of interest, conveying a particular perception of the world.

Conceptual skills—the mental ability to analyze and interpret abstract ideas for the purpose of understanding and diagnosing situations and formulating solutions.

Concurrent review—an assessment of care while in the process of being given; often combined with a retrospective review.

Confidant—a close friend; someone in whom an older adult can confide, reflect on the past, and trust.

Contaminant—organic or inorganic matter that enters a medium, such as water or food, and renders it impure.

Contemporary families—emerging family patterns that did not exist a few years earlier, such as "loose shirt" families, in which parents work from home via the computer and Internet.

Continuing care center—a type of housing facility for older adults that provides a homelike setting for people at all levels of functioning, from total independence to dependence on skilled nursing care, offering older adults a home for life; often referred to as a total life center.

Continuous needs—the birth-to-death developmental health care needs of populations in all age groups.

Contracting—negotiating a working agreement in which two or more parties come to a shared understanding and mutually consent to the purposes and terms of the transaction.

Control group—randomly assigned subjects in a research study who are not receiving the intervention.

Control of communicable disease—the point at which a specific disease has ceased to be a public health threat.

Controller—a management function of the community health nurse in which the nurse monitors the plan and ensures that it stays on course.

Coping—those actions and ways of thinking that assist people in dealing with and surviving difficult situations.

Core public health functions—three basic areas of public health services (assessment, policy development, and assurance) that encompass a wide variety of activities.

Corporal punishment—violence against a child as a form of discipline.

Correctional facility—one whose primary objective is to provide safety to the public by incarcerating those who have committed crimes and who are deemed a threat to the community.

Cost sharing—a cost-containment strategy in which consumers pay a portion of health care costs.

Crew leader—a person who acts as a mediator between a group of migrant laborers, called crews, and a farmer; often the farmer pays the crew leader, who then pays the laborers.

Crisis theory—a body of knowledge that helps to explain why people respond in certain ways; it is useful to predict the phases that people will go through in a crisis of any kind.

Critical incident stress debriefing (CISD)—a mechanism for providing victims emotional reconciliation after a disaster, ideally between 24 and 72 hours after the event.

Critical pathway—written plans and outcomes for patient care with a timetable; a term used synonymously with clinical pathway.

Cross-sectional study—exploring the relationship of a health condition to other variables in a specific population at a particular point in time.

Culture—the beliefs, values, and behaviors that are shared by members of a society and that provide a design or "map" for living.

Cultural assessment—obtaining health-related information about a designated cultural group concerning their values, beliefs, and practices.

Cultural brokering—facilitating health care for migrant workers who are unable to overcome the barriers of existing health care.

Cultural diversity—a variety of cultural patterns that co-exist within a designated geographic area.

Cultural relativism—recognizing and respecting alternative viewpoints and understanding values, beliefs, and practices within their cultural context.

Cultural self-awareness—recognition of one's own values, beliefs, and practices that make up one's culture.

Cultural sensitivity—recognizing that culturally based values, beliefs, and practices influence people's health and lifestyles.

Culture shock—a state of anxiety that results from cross-cultural misunderstanding and an inability to interact appropriately in the new context.

Curanderas—Mexican folk healers.

Custodial care—personal care that is considered non-skilled, such as bathing, dressing, feeding, and assisting with mobility and recreation.

Cycle of violence—the repetitive cyclic pattern of abuse seen in domestic violence situations.

Dating violence—physical, sexual, emotional, or verbal abuse between persons who are or have been in a casual or serious dating relationship.

Decoding—translating a message into understandable form.

Deforestation—the clearing of tropical and temperate forests for cropland, cattle grazing, or urbanization.

Deinstitutionalization—the process of transferring the mentally ill from public institutions to community-based care settings.

Delphi technique—a method of arriving at group consensus through a systematic pooling of separate individuals' judgments by written questionnaire and suggestions.

Demographic entrapment—the effect on a population of exceeding the ability of its ecosystem to support it or to acquire the support needed, or exceeding its ability to migrate to other ecosystems in a manner that preserves its standard of living.

Department of Health and Human Services (DHHS)—the federal level of five primary agencies concerned with health and organized under the umbrella of the DHHS: the Public Health Service, the Office of Human Development Services, the Health Care Financing Administration, the Family Support Administration, and the Social Security Administration.

Descriptive epidemiologic study—a study that examines the amount and distribution of a disease or health condition in a population by person, place, and time.

Descriptive epidemiology—investigations that seek to observe and describe patterns of health-related conditions that naturally occur in a population.

Descriptive statistics—those that describe in quantitative or mathematical terms the data collected.

Desertification—the conversion of fertile land into desert that is unable to support crop growth or wildlife.

Detoxification—the process of ridding the body of harmful substances.

Developmental crisis—periods of disruption that occur at transition points during normal growth and development.

Developmental disability—any of a broad scope of limitations, including intellectual limitations and the inability to perform certain activities of daily living, that is identified before age 22 years.

Developmental framework—studies families from a life-cycle perspective by examining members' changing roles and tasks in each progressive life-cycle stage.

Diagnostic-related groups—a billing classification system based on 23 major diagnostic categories and 467 diagnosis-related groups that provides fixed Medicare reimbursement to hospitals.

Direct transmission—immediate transfer of infectious agents from a reservoir to a new host.

Direct victim—a person who experiences an event such as a fire, volcanic eruption, war, or bomb.

Disabling injury—an injury that results in restriction of normal activities of daily living beyond the day on which the injury occurred.

Disability-Adjusted Life Year (DALY)—the combination of years of life lost due to premature mortality and years of life lived with disability, adjusted for the severity of disability; developed to compare across conditions and risk factors.

Disaster—any event that causes a level of destruction that exceeds the abilities of the affected community to respond without assistance.

Disenfranchised—someone who does not have full privileges and rights as a citizen.

Displaced persons—those who are forced to leave their homes to escape the effects of a disaster.

Distributive health policy—promotes nongovernmental activities thought to be beneficial to society as a whole.

Distributive justice—a belief that benefits should be given first to the disadvantaged or those who need them the most.

District nursing—the formal organization of visiting nursing, known as district nursing in England; the period in the history of community health/public health nursing from the mid-1800s to 1900.

Domestic violence—morbidity and mortality attributed to violence within the home setting.

Dominant values—the beliefs and sanctions of the dominant or majority culture.

Drug-dependent—a person who physically and psychologically requires use of drugs to function and, if pregnant, gives birth to an infant exhibiting withdrawal symptoms.

Drug-exposed—a person who uses drugs intermittently and, if pregnant, gives birth to a drug-exposed infant.

Durable medical equipment (DME)—the equipment used for a long period of time in a person's home that can be used again by others, such as wheelchairs, walkers, hospital beds, ventilators, and IV poles.

Ecologic perspective—a viewpoint about the community of living organisms and their interrelated physical and chemical environments.

Eco-map—a diagram of the connections between a family and the other systems in its ecologic environment; originally devised to depict the complexity of the client's story.

Ecosystem—a community of living organisms and their interrelated physical and chemical environments.

Educator—the role of health teacher; a major function of the community health nurse.

Egalitarian justice—a system that promotes decisions based on equal distribution of benefits to everyone, regardless of need.

Elder abuse—the mistreatment or exploitation of older adults.

Electronic meetings—a method of meeting that applies nominal group technique combined with computer technology.

Elimination—reduction of prevalence to a level of less than 1 case per million population in a given area.

Elite-old—those older than 100 years of age, or centenarians.

Emotional abuse—psychological mistreatment and/or neglect, such as when caregivers or family members do not provide the normal experiences producing feelings of being loved, wanted, secure, and worthy.

Empathy—the ability to communicate understanding and vicariously experience the feelings and thoughts of others.

Empiric-rational change strategies—strategies used to effect change based on the assumption that people are rational and when presented with empiric information will adopt new practices that appear to be in their best interest.

Employee assistance programs—programs cooperatively sponsored by employers and bargaining agencies with the intent to promote the mental health of the employee by providing an outlet for employee concerns.

Empowerment—a process of developing knowledge and skills that increase one's mastery over the decisions that affect one's life.

Encoding—the sender's conversion of a message into symbolic form.

Enculturation—learning one's own culture through socialization with the family or significant group.

Endemic—the continuing presence of a disease or infectious agent in a given geographic area.

Energy exchange—materials or information that families exchange with their environment.

Environment—all the external factors surrounding the host that might influence vulnerability or resistance.

Environmental health—assessing, controlling, and improving the impact people make on their environment and the impact of the environment on them.

Environmental impact—the effect of positive or negative changes on the environment and on the people, animals, and plants living in it.

Environmental justice—a movement that has sought to ensure that no particular part of the population is disproportionately burdened by the negative effects of pollution.

Epidemic—a disease occurrence that clearly exceeds the normal or expected frequency in a community or region.

Epidemiology—the study of health, disease, and injury determinants and distribution in populations.

Episodic needs—one-time, specific negative health events, such as illness or injury, that are not an expected part of life.

Equity—being treated equally or fairly.

Eradication—the interruption of person-to-person transmission and a limitation of the reservoir of infection such that no further preventive efforts are required.

Ergonomics—a field of study in occupational health concerned with the design of workplaces, tools, and tasks to match the physiologic, anatomic, and psychological characteristics and capabilities of the worker; sometimes called human engineering.

Ethical decision-making—making a choice that is consistent with a moral code or that can be justified from an ethical perspective.

Ethical dilemma—a decision involving a potential conflict between moral values.

Ethics—a set of moral principles or values; a theory or system of moral values.

Ethnic group—a collection of people with common origins and with a shared culture and identity.

Ethnicity—that group of qualities that mark a person's association with a particular ethnic group.

Ethnocentrism—the belief and feeling that one's own culture is best.

Evaluation—the process by which a practice is analyzed, judged, and improved according to established goals and standards.

Evaluator—a management function in which the nurse compares and judges performance and outcomes against previously set goals and standards.

Evolutionary change—change that is gradual and requires adjustment on an incremental basis.

Experimental design—a research method in which the investigators institute an intervention and then measure its consequences.

Experimental epidemiology—follows and builds on information gathered from descriptive and analytic approaches; used to study epidemics, the etiology of human disease, the value of preventive and therapeutic measures, and the evaluation of health services.

Experimental group—randomly assigned subjects who are receiving the intervention in a research study.

Experimental study—a study in which the investigator controls or changes factors suspected of causing a condition and observes the results.

Extinction—the loss of a species from the earth forever.

Familialism—taking responsibility for one's own family and protecting them from harm.

Familiarization assessment—studying data already available on a community, and gathering a certain amount of firsthand data, in order to gain a working knowledge of the community; sometimes called a "windshield" survey.

Family—two or more individuals who share a residence or live near one another; possess some common emotional bond; engage in interrelated social positions, roles, and tasks; and share a sense of affection and belonging.

Family crisis—a stressful and disruptive event, or series of events, that comes with or without warning and disturbs the equilibrium of the family.

Family culture—the acquired knowledge that family members use to interpret their experiences and to generate behaviors that influence family structure and function.

Family functioning—those behaviors or activities by family members that maintain the family and meet family needs, individual member needs, and society's views of family.

Family health—how well the family functions together as a unit.

Family map—a diagram that illustrates the pattern of interactions and interdependence among family members.

Family nursing—a kind of nursing practice in which the family is the unit of service.

Family structure—comprises the characteristics of individuals who make up a family unit: age, gender, and number.

Family system boundary—the greater concentration of energy that exists within the family than between the family and its external environment.

Family violence—action by a family member with the intent to cause harm to or control another family member.

Feedback loop—Indication by the receiver that the message has been understood (decoded) in the way that the sender intended (encoded).

Felony—a serious crime such as murder, rape, or burglary, for which the criminal is typically housed in a maximum-security prison.

Feminization of poverty—the growing numbers of women who have fallen into poverty, caused by weakening of the nuclear family as more women head households alone, by low-wage jobs for unskilled work, and by the dismantling of social programs for women.

Fetal alcohol effects (FAE)—a combination of birth anomalies characterized by some, but not all, of the symptoms of fetal alcohol syndrome.

Fetal alcohol syndrome (FAS)—a combination of birth anomalies characterized by structural abnormalities of the head and face including microcephaly and flattening of the maxillary area, intrauterine growth retardation, decreased birth weight and length, developmental delays, intellectual impairment, hyperactivity, altered sleep pattern, feeding problems, perceptual problems, mood problems, and language dysfunction; caused by maternal alcohol consumption during pregnancy.

Fidelity—keeping one's promises.

Force field analysis—a technique for examining all the positive and negative forces influencing a change situation.

Forensics—the science of medical or health care jurisprudence in which legal argument is used to advocate for offenders.

Formal caregivers—professionals and paraprofessionals who are compensated for in-home care they provide.

Formal contracting—a process in which all parties negotiate a written contract by mutual agreement, sign the agreement, and sometimes have it witnessed or notarized.

Foster families—families who have had formal training and are licensed to accept nonrelated children into their homes to raise temporarily while the families of origin resolve their problems.

Frail elderly—those older than 85 years of age who need assistance in attending to activities of daily living.

Frontier area—sparsely populated place with six or fewer persons per square mile.

Gang—a loose-knit organization of individuals between the ages of 14 and 24 years that has a name, is usually territorial or claims a certain territory as under its exclusive influence, and is involved in criminal acts.

Generalizability—the ability to apply research results to other similar populations.

Genetic engineering—gene manipulation in a laboratory setting.

Genocide—the killing of a group of people because of their race, politics, or culture.

Genogram—a display of family information in a graphic form that provides a quick view of complex family patterns.

Geographic community—a community defined by its geographic boundaries.

Geriatrics—the medical specialty that deals with the physiology of aging and with the diagnosis and treatment of diseases affecting the aged.

Gerontology—a broad, interdisciplinary practice that includes all aspects of the aging process (economic, social, clinical, and psychological) and their effects on the older adult and society.

Gestalt-field—a family of cognitive theories that assumes that people are neither good nor bad; they simply interact with their environment, and their learning is related to perception.

Gestational diabetes—glucose intolerance of variable degree with onset or first recognition during pregnancy.

Global burden of disease (GBD)—disparities, verified with quantifiable data, in the burden of disease worldwide among the developing countries, especially among children.

Global economy—international trade, investment, travel, and ownership of information and ideas.

Global health patterns - the route, form, and virulence with which diseases appear in countries around the world, based on environmental, ecologic, human, technologic, and political factors.

Global nursing—paid employment or volunteer nursing in foreign/developing countries in a variety of nursing positions based on interest, experience, skills, and credentials.

Global warming—the trapping of heat radiation from the earth's surface that increases the overall temperature of the world, causing a "greenhouse" effect.

Goals—broad statements of desired end results.

Gross national product—the total value of all goods and services produced in the national economy in 1 year.

Group homes—homes designed to meet the needs of specific populations, such as the mentally ill, the developmentally disabled, the elderly, or people with Alzheimer's disease.

Group-marriage family—several adults who share a common household, consider that all are married to one another, and share everything, including sex and child rearing.

Group-network family—nuclear families not related by birth or marriage but bound by a common set of values, such as a religious system, who share goods, services, and child-rearing responsibilities.

Halfway house—a residential program for individuals with serious and persistent mental illness (SPMI) that, in addition to housing, offers supervision, treatment, safety, socialization, recreation, and support.

Head Start—federally funded preschool programs for 3- to 5-year-old children from low-income families in disadvantaged communities.

Health—a holistic state of well-being that includes soundness of mind, body, and spirit.

Health care economics—a branch of the science that describes and analyzes the production, distribution, and consumption of health care goods and services.

Health continuum—a range of degrees from optimal health at one end of a spectrum to total disability or death at the other end.

Health for all—a major social goal of governments and the World Health Organization (WHO), initially declared at Alma-Ata in 1978; the attainment by all people by the year 2000 of a level of health that would allow them to lead a socially and economically productive life.

Health maintenance organizations (HMOs)—systems in which participants pay a fixed monthly premium to receive comprehensive health services delivered by a defined network of providers to plan participants.

Health policy—any policy that constitutes the governing framework for providing health services on a local, state, national, or international level.

Health promotion—efforts that seek to move people closer to optimal well-being or higher levels of wellness.

Hearty elderly—people older than 65 years of age who maintain a level of wellness and activity well above current expectations for that age.

Hebrew hygienic code—possibly the first written code in the world, which serves as a prototype for personal and community sanitation.

Herd immunity—the immunity level present in a particular population of people.

High-risk families—families exhibiting the symptoms of potentially abusive or neglectful behavior or who are under the types of stress associated with abuse or neglect.

High-risk infant—an infant whose mother has not received adequate nutrition or care during pregnancy due to a lack of proper prenatal care, economic disadvantage, or disease exposure.

Home care nurse—a community health nurse who provides skilled nursing services focusing on physical nursing care needed by family members who are ill, injured, or in the acute or terminal phase of a disease process.

Home health care—all of the services and products provided to clients in their homes to maintain, restore, or promote their physical, mental, and emotional health.

Home health nursing—the provision of nursing to acute, chronic, and terminally ill clients of all ages in their homes, while integrating community health nursing principles that focus on the environmental, psychosocial, economic, cultural, and personal health factors affecting the client's and family's health status and well-being.

Home visit—visiting a family where they live in order to assist them to achieve as high a level of wellness as possible.

Homebase—a migrant farmworker's permanent address.

Homebound—as defined by Medicare, a person who can leave the home only with difficulty in mobility and only for medical appointments or adult day care related to the client's medical care; as a general definition, a person who can leave the home only with great difficulty, for short periods of time, and with assistance.

Homemaker agency—provides homemaker aides, who perform services such as cooking, cleaning, and shopping, or home health aides, who perform personal client care such as bathing and dressing, or both.

Homeless family—a family who finds itself without permanent shelter due to a lack of marketable skills, negative economic changes, or chronic mental health problems.

Homicide—any action taken to cause non–war-related death to another person.

Hospice—a philosophy of care that recognizes that death is inevitable and near and that a cure is not within current human reach.

Hospice care—a philosophy of holistic caregiving to families with a dying family member; the purpose is to make the dying process as dignified, free from discomfort, and emotionally, spiritually, and socially supportive as possible.

Hospital-based agencies—outreach services, including home health care, provided by an acute-care facility with missions similar to those of the sponsoring hospital.

Host—a susceptible human or animal who harbors and nourishes a disease-causing agent.

Human immunodeficiency virus (HIV)—a retrovirus that attacks the body's immune system; transmitted through sexual contact, through sharing of HIV-contaminated needles or syringes, through transfusion of blood or blood byproducts, and from infected mother to child during the perinatal period.

Human skills—the ability to understand, communicate, motivate, delegate, and work well with people.

Illness—a state of being relatively unhealthy.

Immunity—the host's ability to resist a particular infectious disease-causing agent.

Immunization—the process of introducing some form of a disease-causing organism into a person's system in order to cause the development of antibodies that will resist that disease.

Implementation—putting a plan into action and carrying out the activities delineated in the plan.

Incest—sexual abuse among family members who are related by blood.

Incidence—all of the new cases of a disease or health condition that appear during a given time.

Incubation period—the time interval between exposure and onset of symptoms.

Indigent—people who are impoverished and deprived of basic comforts.

Indirect transmission—occurs when the infectious agent is transported within contaminated inanimate materials such as air, water, or food.

Indirect victims—the relatives and friends of direct victims.

Individualism—a belief that the interests of the individual are or ought to be paramount.

Infant—child from birth to 1 year old.

Infectious—capable of producing infection.

Inferential statistics—making inferences about features of a population based on observations of a sample.

Informal caregivers—family members and friends who provide care in the home and are unpaid.

Inmates—people detained in correctional facilities.

Insanity—a legal term reserved for mental impairment that may relieve a person from the legal consequences of his or her actions.

Instrument—the specific tool, often a questionnaire or interview guide, used to measure the variables in a study.

Instrumental values—codes of conduct, such as confidentiality, keeping promises, or being honest.

Integrated management of childhood Illness (IMCI)—an intervention that promotes wider immunization coverage, rapid referral of serious cases, prompt recognition of secondary conditions, and improved nutrition.

Intensity—the physical or emotional level of something; in a disaster, the level of destruction and devastation.

Interaction—reciprocal exchange and influence between people.

Interactional framework—describes the family as a unit of interacting personalities and emphasizes communication, roles, conflict, coping patterns, and decision-making processes.

Intermediate care—a level of caregiving at which the amount and type of skilled care given is decreased.

Intrafamilial sexual abuse—sexual activity between family members not related by blood.

Intrarole functioning—playing several roles at the same time, such as when one woman is a wife, mother, grandmother, aunt, teacher, volunteer, author, neighbor, and friend.

Isolation—separation of infected persons or animals for the period of communicability in order to limit transmission of the infectious agent to susceptible others.

Jail—a facility where people accused of committing a crime await arraignment, the summons to appear in court to answer charges; also called a detention center or holding cell.

Justice—treating people fairly.

Key informants—persons who know much about their community and are willing to share their information with the community health nurse.

Kin-network—several nuclear families who live in the same household, or near one another, and share goods and services.

Lay workers—migrant camp members who are trained and supervised by community health nurses and who form formal and informal links with the community to promote health and provide continuity of care.

Leader—a function of the community health nursing role in which the nurse directs, influences, or persuades others to effect change that will positively affect people's health and move them toward a goal.

Leadership—an interpersonal process in which one person influences the activities of another person or group of persons toward accomplishment of a goal.

Learning—the process of assimilating new information that promotes a permanent change in behavior.

Learning disability—a genetic, environmental, or cultural influence that affects a child's ability to learn; it is estimated that 2% to 10% of school-age children have some type of learning disability.

Life expectancy—the average number of years that an individual member of a specific cohort (usually a single birth year) is projected to live.

Literacy—the ability to read and write to an extent that allows the individual to function in daily life.

Lobbying—the process by which an individual or group acts on behalf of others to influence specific decisions of policy makers, such as legislators.

Location myth—a belief that community health nursing can be described in terms of where it is practiced (ie, in a specific setting or location such as outside of the hospital).

Location variables—a profile of the community that includes community boundaries, location of health services, geographic features, climate, flora and fauna, and the human-made environment.

Long-term care—an assortment of settings that are residences for people who are unable to physically care for themselves independently due to physical or cognitive alterations.

Looting—stealing goods.

Low birth weight—weight less than 2500 g at birth.

Lynching—executing without due process of law.

Machismo—male qualities of dominance that include pride, honor, and dignity.

Macroeconomic theory—concerned with the broad variables that affect the status of the total economy.

Mandated reporters—people who have responsibility for the welfare of children, such as nurses, doctors, teachers, counselors, and certain other professionals.

Managed care—a broad system, under which case management exists, that is designed to be a cost-containing system of health care administration.

Managed competition—combining market competition to achieve cost savings with government regulation to achieve expanded coverage.

Manager—a nursing role in which the nurse exercises administrative direction toward the accomplishment of specified goals by assessing clients' needs, planning and organizing to meet those needs, directing and leading to achieve results, and controlling and evaluating the progress to ensure that goals are met.

Marginalized—people who live on the margins, or edges, of society, rather than in the mainstream.

Maximum security—a correctional facility with the highest security level, generally housing prisoners who have committed violent crimes.

Medicaid—known as Title XIX of the Social Security Act Amendments of 1965; provides medical assistance for certain individuals and families with low incomes and resources.

Medically indigent—those who are unable to pay for and totally lacking in medical services.

Medicare—known as Title XVIII of the Social Security Act Amendments of 1965; provides mandatory federal health insurance for adults age 65 years and older and certain disabled persons.

Mental health—a state of successful mental functioning, resulting in productive activities, fulfilling relationships, and the ability to change and cope with adversity.

Mental health promotion—interventions that enhance well-being and strengthen life-sustaining and life-enhancing activities.

Mental illness—collectively, all mental disorders; health conditions that are characterized by alterations in thinking, mood, or behavior (or some combination thereof) associated with distress or impaired functioning.

Message—an expression of the purpose of communication.

Meta-analysis—a research method that allows researchers to evaluate the results of many similar quantitative research studies in an attempt to integrate the findings.

Metropolitan—counties that include one or more cities of 50,000 or more residents and a total population of 100,000 or greater.

Microcultures—systems of cultural knowledge characteristic of subgroups within larger societies.

Microeconomic theory—concerned with the supply and demand of goods and services as these relate to consumer income allocation and distribution.

Migrant farmworkers—farmworkers who travel to find agricultural work throughout the year, usually from state to state with the seasons.

Migrant health programs—health programs for migrant workers that depend on referrals and vouchers to address gaps in health care services.

Migration—the act of moving from one region or country to another, often temporarily or seasonally.

Minimum security—a correctional facility with a minimum level of security, generally housing prisoners who have committed nonviolent crimes.

Minority group—a part of the population that differs from the majority and often receives differential and unequal treatment.

Model—a description or analogy used as a pattern to enhance understanding of some reality.

Moral—conforming to a standard that is right and good.

Moral evaluations—judgments concerning adherence to standards of what is right and good.

Morbidity rate—the relative incidence of disease in a population.

Mortality rate—the relative death rate or the sum of deaths in a given population over a given time.

Multigenerational family—several generations within one family, such as the aged mother of the husband, wife, teenage children, and one teen's infant.

Multilateral agencies—multinational agencies that support development efforts of governments and organizations in less developed nations of the world, such as the United Nations, the World Health Organization (WHO), and the World Bank.

Munchausen syndrome by proxy—a psychological disorder in which clients bring medical attention to themselves by injuring or inducing illness in their children; they fabricate the symptoms of a disease so that the child will undergo medical tests, hospitalization, or even medical or surgical treatment.

Mutual goals—goals that the family and the nurse plan and take action on together.

National health insurance (NHI)—a solution to the high cost and inaccessibility of health services whereby health insurance coverage would be provided for all citizens through a single-payer system.

Natural history—events that occur preceding a disease's development, during its course, and during its conclusion.

Neglect—a state in which the physical, emotional, or educational resources necessary for healthy growth and development are withheld or unavailable.

Neurosis—a general term denoting any of a variety of mental or emotional disorders involving anxiety, phobia, or other abnormal behavioral symptoms.

New and emerging diseases—diseases not known previously and diseases that were previously thought to be under control.

Nominal group technique—a group decision-making method that pools face-to-face group ideas after members initially think and write down their ideas independently.

Nonexperimental design—a research design used to describe and explain phenomena or examine relationships among phenomena; also called a descriptive design.

Nongovernmental organizations (NGO)—organizations not under government sponsorship or control; also called private voluntary organizations (PVO).

Nonmetropolitan—counties that do not have a city of 50,000 residents within their borders.

Nonmaleficence—avoiding or preventing harm to others as a consequence of one's own choices and actions.

Nontraditional family—a family pattern that has not traditionally been socially acceptable, such as a single-parent household headed by a woman.

Nonverbal messages—messages that are conveyed without words; constitute almost two thirds of the messages transmitted in normal communication.

Normative-reductive change strategies—strategies used to influence change that not only present new information but also directly influence people's attitudes and behaviors through persuasion.

Nuclear family—a mother, father, and one or more biologic or adopted children living together, separate from others.

Nuclear-dyad family—husband and wife.

Nursing bag—a carry-all nurses take on home visits that contains supplies needed on the visits.

Nursing informatics—a term for the collective technologic sciences available to nurses in the health care delivery system today for the delivery of nursing care.

Objectives—specific statements of desired outcomes stated in behavioral terms that can be measured and that include target dates.

Occupational disease—any condition or disorder caused by an exposure that resulted from employment.

Occupational health—a specialty health practice that focuses on the health and well-being of the working population, including both paid and unpaid laborers, thus covering most of the country's well adults.

Occupational health nurse—a nurse employed to ensure that the work force is, and remains, healthy and productive.

Official health agencies—health care agencies that are publicly funded and operated by federal, state, or local governments and supported by taxes.

Ombudsman—a person hired through the Area Agency on Aging (AAA) or agency, who serves the residents of assisted living or skilled nursing facilities by speaking for them and acting as an advocate in all matters concerning the residents' stay in the facility.

Operationalizing—putting ideas or concepts into words that can be used.

Opposition defiant disorder (ODD)—a set of "externalizing" behavior problems, including noncompliance, temper tantrums, and other socially provocative behaviors, first diagnosed in the preschool years.

Organizer—a function of the community health nurse's manager role that involves designing a structure within which people and tasks can function to reach desired objectives.

Osteoporosis—a systemic skeletal disease characterized by low bone mass and microarchitectural deterioration of bone tissue, leading to increased bone fragility and a consequent increase in fracture risk.

Outcome criteria—measurable criteria toward which the community will work and by which they will measure their success as they attempt to improve the health of their community.

Outcome evaluation—the assessment of change in the family's (client's) health status based on mutually agreed upon activities.

Outmigration—the phenomenon of young and middle-age adults leaving their rural homes for a more urban environment.

Palliative care—comfort care directed at the alleviation of pain and other symptoms.

Pan American Health Organization (PAHO)—an arm of the World Health Organization (WHO) that serves as the central coordinating organization for public health in the Western hemisphere.

Pandemic—an epidemic that is worldwide in distribution.

Paraphrasing—stating back to the sender what you thought you heard.

Participative leadership style—a democratic style in which leaders involve followers in the decision-making process.

Partnerships—agreements between people and agencies to benefit a joint purpose.

Passive immunity—short-term resistance to a specific disease-causing organism that may be acquired naturally or artificially through inoculation with a vaccine that gives temporary resistance.

Passive smoking—exposure to tobacco smoke from other people smoking in one's environment.

Peer review—an organized system by which peer professionals assess the quality of care being delivered.

Penitentiary—a federal correctional facility, commonly referred to among prisoners as "the big house," which may have a minimum or maximum security level.

Personal-care homes—homes that offer basic personal care, such as bathing, grooming, and social support, but provide no skilled nursing services.

Pediculosis (pediculus humanus capitis; head lice)—parasites that live and feed on the human scalp; considered a nuisance disease and affecting one in four elementary schoolchildren.

Pedophile—an adult whose main sexual interest is a child.

Personalismo—the quality of pleasant conversation appreciated by Hispanics.

Physical abuse—the intentional harm to someone by another person that results in pain, physical injury, or death.

Planned change—a purposeful, designed effort to effect improvement in a system with the assistance of a change agent.

Planner—a function in the management process that requires the nurse to set goals and directions for the organization or project and determine the means for achieving them.

Planning—a logical, decision-making process of designing an orderly, detailed program of action to accomplish specific goals and objectives.

Pluralistic medical systems—consist of traditional healing systems, lay practices, household remedies, transitional health workers, and Western medicine.

Polarization—the process by which a group is split into two or more factions over a political issue.

Policy—an authoritatively stated course of action that guides decision making.

Policy analysis—the systematic identification of causes or consequences of policy and the factors that influence it.

Policy development—formulating local and state health policies and directing resources toward those policies with information gathered during assessment.

Policy system—an entity that receives input from external sources and has legal authority to generate or revise policies governing or managing the constituents it represents.

Political action—action taken by an individual or group to influence the political decisions of others toward issues or policies beneficial to the welfare of the individual or group.

Political action committee (PAC)—a group or organization that endorses and financially backs candidates and supports the group's position on issues.

Political empowerment—a conscious state in which an individual, group, or organization becomes recognized as influential in determining policy.

Politics—an interactive process of influencing others to make decisions that favor a person's or group's chosen position and the allocation of scarce resources to support that position.

Pollution—the contamination of natural resources such as air, water, and soil, making them foul and unfit for human use.

Polysubstance use and abuse—when a person uses or abuses more than one chemical, such as alcohol with marijuana or cocaine with antianxiety medications.

Population—all of the people occupying an area or all of those sharing one or more characteristics.

Population-focused—the concern for the health status of population groups and their environment.

Population variables—the size, density, composition, rate of growth or decline, cultural characteristics, social class, and mobility of people within a designated community.

Poverty threshold—an income line below which people are defined as poor.

Power—the ability to influence or control other people's behavior to accomplish a specific purpose.

Power bases—knowledge or skills the powerholder possesses that enable him or her to exert influence over others.

Power sources—the qualities or situations from which the power holder gains a power base.

Power-coercive change strategies—use of coercion based on fear to effect change.

Preferred provider organizations (PPOs)—a model of managed or coordinated care that consists of a network of physicians, hospitals, and other health-related services that contract with a third-party payer organization to provide comprehensive health services to subscribers on a fixed fee-for-service basis.

Preschooler—a child 3 or 4 years of age.

Prevalence—all of the people with a health condition existing in a given population at a given point in time.

Prevalence studies—those that describe patterns of occurrence, always looking at factors from the same point in time and in the same population.

Primary health care—in developed countries, the partnership between health professionals and communities; in most developing countries, a voluntary health service created at the village level.

Primary prevention—measures taken to keep illness or injury from occurring.

Primary relationship—two or more people interacting in a continuing manner within the greater environment.

Prison—a state department of corrections facility that may be assigned a security level ranging from minimum to maximum.

Private voluntary organizations (PVO)—organizations not under government sponsorship or control: also known as nongovernmental organizations (NGO).

Problem-oriented assessment—an assessment that begins with a single problem and then assesses the community in terms of that problem.

Proprietary health services—privately owned and managed health care services.

Prospective payment—a payment method based on rates derived from predictions of annual service costs that are set in advance of service delivery.

Prospective study—looking forward in time to find a causal relationship.

Psychomotor domain—visible, demonstrable performance skills that require some kind of neuromuscular coordination.

Psychosis—a mental disorder characterized by partial or complete withdrawal from reality.

Public health—the science and art of preventing disease, prolonging life, and promoting health and efficiency through organized community efforts for the sanitation of the environment, the control of communicable infections, the education of the individual in personal hygiene, the organization of medical and nursing services for early diagnosis and preventive treatment of disease, and the development of the social machinery to ensure everyone a standard of living that is adequate for the maintenance of health, so organizing these benefits as to enable every citizen to realize his or her birthright of health and longevity.

Public health nursing—the term describing community health nursing from 1900 to 1950; replaced by the term community health nursing to better describe where the nurse practices. In this text, the terms are used interchangeably.

Public Health Service (PHS)—a federal umbrella organization concerned with the broad health interests of the country.

Public policy—decisions made by government at the local, state, or federal level that affect the public.

Qualitative research—emphasizes subjectivity and the meaning of experiences to individuals.

Quality assurance—initial setting of standards, formal auditing, and peer review in the health care delivery system to ensure quality.

Quality care—the state in which services provided match the needs of the population, are technically correct, and achieve beneficial results.

Quality circles—a participative management approach in which employees and managers share the responsibility for decision making and problem-solving in client care.

Quality improvement—studying the impact of intervention and instituting tighter controls on the delivery of specific community health nursing services.

Quality indicators—quality-focused objectives used as markers to determine whether a goal has been achieved and to measure client outcomes or process outcomes.

Quality measurement—the ability to identify services and programs that best serve the needs of the community.

Quantitative research—concerns data that can be quantified or measured objectively.

Quarantine—a period of enforced isolations of persons exposed to a communicable disease during the incubation period to prevent spread of the disease should infection occur.

Quasi-experiment—a research method that lacks one of the elements found in a true experiment, such as randomization of the subjects.

Race—a biologically designated group of people whose distinguishing features are inherited.

Randomization—the systematic selection of research subjects so that each one has an equal probability of selection.

Rape—an act of sexual aggression in which the perpetrator is motivated by a desire to dominate, control, and degrade the victim.

Rate—a statistical measure expressing the proportion of persons with a given health problem among a population at risk.

Rationing—limiting the provision of adequate health services in order to save costs, but in so doing jeopardizing the well-being of some groups of people.

Receiver—person to whom the message is directed and who is its actual recipient.

Recidivism—an inmate's relapse into criminal behavior after release, with subsequent reincarceration.

Referral—a request for service from another agency or person.

Refugee—a person who is forced to leave his or her homeland because of war or persecution.

Regulation—mandated procedure and practice affecting health services delivery that is enforced by law.

Regulatory health policy—policy that attempts to control the allocation of resources by directing those agencies or persons who offer resources or provide public services.

Rehabilitation—efforts that seek to reduce disability and, as much as possible, restore function.

Relapse—continuing to use a chemical after a period of nonuse.

Relationship-based care—care that incorporates the values of establishing and maintaining a reciprocal, caring relationship with the community.

Reliability—how consistently an instrument measures a given research variable within a particular population.

Research—the systematic collection and analysis of data related to a particular problem or phenomenon affecting community health and community health practice.

Researcher—a role of the community health nurse in which the nurse engages in systematic investigation, collection, and analysis of data for the purpose of solving problems and enhancing community health practice.

Reservoir—any person, animal, or substance in which an infectious agent normally lives and multiplies and then is transmitted from its source to a susceptible host.

Resource directory—a published source of community services developed for professionals and the broader community.

Respect—treating people as unique, equal, and responsible moral agents.

Respite care—a break for caregivers from the intensity of caregiving, in which they can care for themselves for a few days; not a luxury but a necessity for successful caregiving.

Restorative justice—a belief that benefits should go primarily to those who have been wronged by prior injustice, such as victims of crime or racial discrimination.

Retrospective payment—reimbursement for a service after it has been rendered.

Retrospective review—a quality assessment process that examines patterns of care over a specified period in health records of care given in the past.

Retrospective study—looking backward in time to find a causal relationship.

Revolutionary change—change that is rapid, drastic, and threatening and that may completely upset the balance of a system.

Riot—a violent disturbance created by a large number of people assembled for a common purpose.

Risk—the probability that a disease or other unfavorable health condition will develop.

Risk assessment—the process of identifying factors that lead to negative events.

Roles—the assigned or assumed parts that members play during day-to-day family living; they are bestowed and defined by the family.

Rural—communities with fewer than 10,000 residents and a county population density of fewer than 1000 persons per square mile.

Sanitation—the promotion of hygiene and prevention of disease through maintenance of health-enhancing (sanitary) conditions.

School-based health centers (SBHC)—clinics on school sites that provide ready access to health care for large numbers of children and adolescents during school hours, making absences from school due to health care appointments unnecessary.

School nurse—a specialty branch of professional nursing that serves the school-age population.

School nurse practitioner—a registered nurse with advanced academic and clinical preparation and experience in physical assessment, diagnosis, and treatment, who provides primary care to schoolage children.

Scope—the range of effects.

Screening—delivering a testing mechanism to detect disease in groups of asymptomatic, apparently healthy individuals.

Seasonal farm worker—a farm worker who lives in one geographic location and labors in the fields of that particular area.

Secondary prevention—efforts that seek to detect and treat existing health problems at the earliest possible stage when disease or impairment already exists.

Self-care—the process of taking responsibility for developing one's own health potential.

Self-care deficit—when people's ability to continue self-care activities drops below their need.

Self-determination—a person's exercise of the capacity to shape and pursue personal plans for his or her life.

Self-help group—peers who come together for mutual assistance to satisfy a common need, such as overcoming a handicap or life-disrupting problem.

Self-interest—the fulfillment of one's own desires without regard for the greater good.

Sender—person conveying a message.

Senility—a term widely used by health professionals and lay people alike to denote deteriorating mental faculties associated with old age.

Serious and persistent mental illness (SPMI)—the preferred term for serious mental illness of a chronic nature.

Serious mental illness (SMI)—any mental illness that has compromised both the client's level of function and the quality of life.

Setting priorities—assigning rank or importance to clients' needs to determine the order in which goals should be addressed.

Sexual abuse—acts of sexual assault or sexual exploitation of a person; may consist of a single incident or many acts over a long period of time.

Sexual exploitation—conduct or activities related to pornography depicting people in sexually explicit situations.

Shaken baby syndrome—the effect of the intentional abusive action of violently shaking an infant or toddler, usually younger than 18 months of age.

Shattuck Report—a landmark document, written in 1850 and called the "Report of the Sanitary Commission of Massachusetts," that described public health concepts and methods on which much of today's public health practice is based.

Simpatica—the quality of positive interpersonal relationships appreciated by Hispanics.

Single-adult family—one adult living alone either by choice to remain single or because of separation from spouse and/or children because of divorce, death, or distance from children.

Single-parent family—a mother or father (but not both) and their children.

Single-payer system—an approach to health care that emphasizes universal health insurance coverage through a stronger role played by government.

Situational crisis—a stressful disruption arising from an external event that occurs suddenly, often without warning, to a person, group, aggregate, or community.

Skilled nursing facilities (SNF)—residences designed to meet the caregiving needs of the frailest of society's citizens who need long-term rehabilitative, recuperative, or custodial care, including the skilled procedures and equipment.

Skilled nursing services—includes skilled observation and assessment, teaching, and performing procedures that require nursing judgment.

Skills myth—a belief that community health nurses employ only the skills of basic clinical nursing when working with community clients.

Smokeless tobacco products—products such as snuff or chewing tobacco, which provide tobacco exposure without exposure to smoke.

Social class—the ranking of groups within society by income, education, occupation, prestige, or a combination of these factors.

Social status—a person's ranking or standing in society, which can be affected by gender, age, and race.

Social support—the quality of interpersonal ties between individuals and the strength and extent of these personal ties.

Social support network map—a detailed display regarding the quality and quantity of social connections.

Social system variables—the various parts of a community's social system that interact and influence the system.

Special interest group—any group of people sharing a common goal who are politically active in attempting to influence policy makers to support their goal.

Spousal abuse—acts of violence against an intimate partner.

Stages of change—the three sequential steps leading to change (unfreezing, changing, and refreezing), which have become a cornerstone for understanding the change process; first described by Lewin.

Standards of care—desired goals that can help in planning and evaluation of nursing practices.

Stigma—an unjustified mark of shame and discredit attached to mental illness.

Strengthening—a communication technique in which, either verbally or in writing, the nurse lists positive points about an otherwise negative situation.

Structural-functional framework—describes the family as a social system relating to other social systems in the external environment, such as church, school, work, and the health care system.

Subcultures—relatively large aggregates of people within a society who share separate distinguishing characteristics.

Substance abuse—excessive and prolonged use of some chemical (alcohol, tobacco, drugs) that leads to serious physical, emotional, and social problems.

Suicide—taking action that causes one's death.

Surveillance—the continuous scrutiny of all aspects of occurrence and spread of a disease that are pertinent to effective control.

Survey—an assessment method in which a series of questions is used to collect data for analysis of a specific group or area.

Tacit—describes a guide for human interaction that is mostly unexpressed and at the unconscious level.

Teaching—a specialized communication process in which desired behavior changes are achieved.

Technical skills—the ability to apply special management-related knowledge and expertise to a particular situation or problem.

Technology—the application of science for changing processes of production or industry.

Telehealth—electronically transmitted clinician consultation between the client and the health care provider.

Temporary Aid to Needy Families (TANF)—the restructuring of Aid to Families with Dependent Children in 1996, which created federal funding to be channeled to individual states; each state has great latitude in setting up programs, with support limited to 5 years in a person's lifetime.

Tenet—any principle or doctrine held as true.

Terminal values—end-states of existence, such as spiritual salvation, peace of mind, or world peace.

Terminally ill—people with less than 6 months to live.

Terrorism—the unlawful use of force or violence against persons or property to intimidate or coerce a government or civilian population in the furtherance of political or social objectives.

Tertiary prevention—attempts to reduce the extent and severity of a health problem to its lowest possible level so as to minimize disability and restore or preserve function.

Theory—a set of systematically interrelated concepts or hypotheses that seek to explain or predict phenomena.

Third-party payments—monetary reimbursements made to providers of health care by someone other than the consumer who received the care.

Toddler—a child just out of infancy, from age 1 to 2 years.

Tolerance—the need for increasing amounts of a substance to achieve the desired effects, or a significantly diminished effect with continued use of the same amount of the same substance.

Total quality management (TQM)—a comprehensive term referring to the systems and activities used to achieve all aspects of quality care within a given agency.

Toxic agent—a poisonous substance in the environment that produces harmful effects on human, animal, or plant health.

Traditional family—the family structures that are most familiar and that are most readily accepted by society.

Traditional health care systems—ancient, ethno-cultural-religious health beliefs and practices that have been handed down through generations.

Transactional leadership—a process in which leader and followers engage in a reciprocal transaction whereby the roles and tasks of the followers are clarified and assigned as the group works to accomplish its goals.

Transcultural nursing—culturally sensitive nursing service to people of an ethnic or racial background different from that of the nurse.

Transformational leadership—leadership that inspires followers to high levels of commitment and effort in order to achieve group goals.

Triage—the process of sorting multiple casualties in the event of a war or major disaster.

Triggers—events and activities that may cause a person to continue addictive activities.

True experiment—characterized by instituting an intervention or change, assigning subjects to groups in a specific manner, and comparing the group of subjects who experience the manipulation to the control group.

Unintentional injuries—injuries resulting from unintended exposure to physical agents, including heat, mechanical energy, chemicals, or electricity; usually referred to as accidents.

United Nations International Children's Emergency Fund (UNICEF)—organized in 1946 as a temporary emergency program to assist children of war-torn countries after World War II; now promotes child and maternal health and welfare globally through programs and services.

United States Agency for International Development (USAID)—an agency that provides economic and humanitarian assistance overseas.

Universal coverage—provision of health care coverage to all citizens through one system, replacing the 1500 health insurance companies currently involved in reimbursement for health care coverage.

Unsafe condition—any environmental factor, either social or physical, that increases the likelihood of an unintentional injury.

Vaccine—a preparation made from killed, living attenuated, or living fully virulent organisms and administered to produce or artificially increase immunity to a particular disease.

Validity—the assurance that an instrument measures the variables it is supposed to measure.

Value—a notion or idea designating relative worth or desirability.

Value systems—organizations of beliefs that are of relative importance in guiding individual behavior.

Values clarification—a process that helps one identify the personal and professional values that guide actions by prompting examination of what one believes about the worth, truth, or beauty of any object, thought, or behavior, and where this belief ranks compared with one's other values.

Vector—a nonhuman carrier of disease, such as an animal or insect.

Veracity—telling the truth.

Verbal messages—communicated ideas, attitudes, and feelings transmitted by speaking or writing.

Violent crimes—those involving physical or psychological injury or death, or the threat of injury or death.

Very low birth weight—weight less than 1500 g at birth.

Voluntary health agencies—privately funded and operated health care agencies not supported by taxes.

Wellness—includes the definition of health but incorporates the capacity to develop one's potential to lead a fulfilling and productive life; can be measured in terms of quality of life.

Well-being—a state of positive health or a person's perception concerning positive health.

Wetlands—natural inland bodies of shallow water, such as marshes, ponds, river bottoms, and flood plains, that filter contaminated surface waters and support wildlife reproduction and growth.

Wider family—a family that emerges from lifestyle, is voluntary, and is independent of necessary biologic or kin connections.

Withdrawal symptoms—physical and psychological symptoms (eg, tremors, lethargy, anxiety, depression) that typically are opposite to the effects of the addictive substance and that occur when an addicted individual does not use the substance for a certain period of time.

World Bank (WB)—a major international health-related agency founded in 1944 with a goal of "a world free of poverty."

World Health Organization (WHO)—the body that promotes health on a global basis, with 191 member countries; its mandates include acting as the directing and coordinating authority on international health work.

INDEX

Note: Page numbers followed by *d* indicate display material, *f* indicates figures, and *t* indicates tables.